9TH Edition

BURNS & GROVE'S

THE PRACTICE OF
Nursing Research

Appraisal, Synthesis, and Generation of Evidence

Jennifer R. Gray, PhD, RN, FAAN
Dean
College of Professional Studies
Oklahoma Christian University
Edmond, Oklahoma
Professor Emeritus
College of Nursing and Health Innovation
The University of Texas at Arlington
Arlington, Texas

Susan K. Grove, PhD, RN, ANP-BC, GNP-BC
Professor Emeritus
College of Nursing and Health Innovation
The University of Texas at Arlington
Arlington, Texas
Adult Nurse Practitioner

ELSEVIER

Elsevier
3251 Riverport Lane
St. Louis, Missouri 63043

BURNS AND GROVE'S THE PRACTICE OF NURSING RESEARCH: ISBN: 978-0-323-67317-4
APPRAISAL, SYNTHESIS, AND GENERATION OF EVIDENCE, NINTH EDITION

Notice

Previous editions copyrighted 2017, 2013, 2009, 2005, 2001, 1997, 1993, and 1987.

Library of Congress Control Number: 2020938477

Executive Content Strategist: Lee Henderson
Senior Content Development Manager: Luke Held
Senior Content Development Specialist: Maria Broeker
Publishing Services Manager: Shereen Jameel
Senior Project Manager: Karthikeyan Murthy
Design Direction: Margaret Reid

Printed in China

Last digit is the print number: 9 8 7 6 5 4 3 2 1

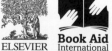

Dedication

*To nurses who are on the frontlines of caring for patients with COVID-19
and other emerging infections. These nurses demonstrate the best of our profession,
by providing competent and compassionate care, advocating for effective infection
control measures to protect all healthcare workers, and participating in ground-
breaking studies to guide safe, quality practice.*

Jennifer and Susan

CONTRIBUTORS

Christy Bomer-Norton, BSN, MSN, PhD
Consultant
Concord, Massachusetts

Daisha J. Cipher, PhD
Associate Professor
College of Nursing and Health Innovation
University of Texas at Arlington
Arlington, Texas

Polly A. Hulme, PhD, MA, MSN, MS
Professor
College of Nursing
South Dakota State University
Brookings, South Dakota

Suzanne Sutherland, PhD, RN
Professor Emeritus and Part-Time Lecturer
School of Nursing
California State University–Sacramento
Staff Nurse II (Retired)
Burn Unit
University of California Davis Medical Center
Sacramento, California

PREFACE

Evidence-based practice is critically important to nursing. Nurses need additional evidence to guide their practice in clinical, educational, and policy settings. To generate this evidence, nurses must be able to design and implement rigorous studies and critically appraise published studies. Our aim in developing the ninth edition of *The Practice of Nursing Research: Appraisal, Synthesis, and Generation of Evidence* is to increase your knowledge of research and evidence-based practice. It is critically important that all nurses, especially those in roles as advanced practice registered nurses (APRNs) (i.e., nurse practitioners, clinical nurse specialists, nurse anesthetists, nurse midwives) and in advanced roles as administrators and educators, have a strong understanding of the research methods conducted to generate evidence-based knowledge for nursing practice. Graduate and undergraduate nursing students and practicing nurses must be actively involved in critically appraising and synthesizing research evidence for the delivery of quality, safe, cost-effective care.

The world is currently experiencing a pandemic due to a novel coronavirus (COVID-19). Research is critical for determining how this virus is spread, individuals' responses to the virus, effectiveness of diagnostic tools, and methods for managing the disease. Nurses are on the frontline in the diagnosis and management of this virus and the collection of data related to it. More than ever before we see the importance of research in promoting health, preventing illness, and managing acute and chronic diseases.

This text provides detailed content and guidelines for implementing critical appraisal and synthesis processes. The text also contains extensive coverage of the research methodologies—quantitative, qualitative, mixed methods, and outcomes—commonly used in nursing. Doctoral students and practicing nurses might use this text to facilitate their conduct of quality studies essential for generating nursing knowledge.

The depth and breadth of content presented in this edition reflect the increase in research activities and the growth in research knowledge since the previous edition. Nursing research is introduced at the baccalaureate level and becomes an integral part of graduate education (master's and doctoral) and clinical practice. We hope that this new edition might increase the number of nurses at all levels involved in research activities to improve outcomes for nursing practice.

This ninth edition is written and organized to facilitate ease in reading, understanding, and implementing the research process. Two major strengths of this text are comprehensive, relevant content and an accessible style.

Comprehensive Relevant Content

- State-of-the-art description and discussion of evidence-based practice (EBP)—a topic of vital and growing importance in a healthcare arena focused on quality, safe, cost-effective patient care.
- Broad coverage of quantitative, qualitative, mixed methods, and outcomes research strategies.
- Rich and frequent illustration of major points and concepts from the most current nursing research literature, emphasizing a variety of clinical practice areas.
- A strong conceptual framework that links nursing research with EBP, theory, knowledge, and philosophy.
- An introduction to ethical issues related to the conduct of genomics research, especially future use of DNA samples.
- Expansion of the chapter on mixed methods research, a methodology that is used today with increasing frequency, reflecting the modern proliferation of multifaceted problems.
- A balanced coverage of qualitative and quantitative research methodologies.

Accessible Style

- A clear, concise writing style for facilitation of student learning that is consistent throughout all chapters.
- New figures that display the critical elements of quantitative research designs.
- Websites and electronic references with digital object identifiers (DOIs) that direct the student to an extensive array of information that is important for conducting studies and using research findings in practice.

Our text provides a comprehensive introduction to nursing research for graduate and practicing nurses. Of particular usefulness at the master's and doctoral levels, the text provides not only substantive content related to research but also practical applications based on the authors' experiences in conducting various types of nursing research, familiarity with the research literature, and experience in teaching nursing research at various educational levels.

The ninth edition of this text is organized into five units and 29 chapters. Unit One provides an introduction to the general concepts of nursing research. The content and presentation of this unit have been designed to introduce evidence-based practice (EBP), quantitative research, and qualitative research.

Unit Two provides an in-depth presentation of the research process for quantitative, qualitative, mixed methods, and outcomes research, including two detailed chapters on measurement. As with previous editions, this text provides extensive coverage of study designs and statistical analyses.

Unit Three addresses the implications of research for the discipline and profession of nursing. Content is provided to direct the student in conducting critical appraisals of both quantitative and qualitative research. A detailed discussion of types of research synthesis and strategies for promoting EBP is provided.

Unit Four provides students and practicing nurses the content they need to implement their own research studies. This unit includes chapters focused on data collection and management, statistical analysis, interpretation of research outcomes, and dissemination of research findings.

Unit Five addresses proposal development and seeking support for research. Readers are given direction for developing successful research proposals and seeking funding for their proposed research.

The changes in the ninth edition of this text reflect advances in nursing research and incorporate comments from outside reviewers, colleagues, and students. Our desire to promote the continuing development of the profession of nursing was the incentive for investing the time and energy required to develop this new edition.

NEW CONTENT

The ninth edition provides current comprehensive coverage of nursing research and is focused on the learning needs and styles of today's nursing students and practicing nurses. Several exciting new areas of content based on the changes and expansion in the field of nursing research are included in this edition. Some of the major changes from the previous edition are as follows:

- Chapter 1, "Discovering the World of Nursing," provides an updated introduction to EBP and an example applying the most current evidence-based guidelines for the management of dehydration in older adult patients.
- Chapter 2, "Evolution of Research in Building Evidence-Based Nursing Practice," describes the history of research within the nursing profession with an emphasis on more recent initiatives at the federal level to link evidence-based interventions to patient outcomes. The processes for synthesizing research knowledge (systematic reviews, meta-analyses, meta-syntheses, and mixed methods research syntheses) are defined and applied to nursing practice.
- Chapter 3, "Introduction to Quantitative Research," was rewritten by Dr. Polly Hulme, a noted nurse researcher, to provide a clearer overview of the quantitative research process and the different types of quantitative research (descriptive, correlational, quasi-experimental, and experimental). Detailed examples from published studies are provided to assist students in identifying and understanding the steps of the quantitative research process.
- Chapter 4, "Introduction to Qualitative Research," describes the philosophical foundations of qualitative research and four designs frequently used by nurse researchers: phenomenological, grounded theory, ethnographical, and exploratory-descriptive qualitative research. Two additional designs, case studies and narrative inquiry, are introduced.
- Chapter 5, "Research Problem and Purpose," was revised to include clear, concise figures and content to direct students in identifying the problems and purposes in different types of nursing studies and developing the problem and purpose for a study.
- Chapter 6, "Objectives, Questions, Hypotheses, and Study Variables" has been rewritten to guide students in the wording of research questions and objectives and constructing various types of hypotheses for different types of quantitative and qualitative designs. In addition, different types of variables are described with directions for writing conceptual and operational definitions for major study variables.

- Chapter 7, "Review of Relevant Literature," provides practical steps for searching electronic databases for relevant sources and for synthesizing the information into a cohesive, written review.
- Chapter 8, "Frameworks," describes selected grand nursing theories and middle range theories that have been used as frameworks for guiding nursing research studies. The chapter also describes developing a study framework from an integration of theoretical perspectives and research findings.
- Chapter 9, "Ethics in Research," features new coverage of genomics research, historical and recent ethical violations, and changes in the legal requirements to protect human subjects.
- Chapters 10 and 11 were redesigned to present designs for noninterventional quantitative studies (Chapter 10) and interventional quantitative studies (Chapter 11). Each chapter begins with the definition of key terms and the threats to validity for the study designs that are included. New tables define each threat to design validity and provide an example of the threat in a study. The algorithms to determine which design has been used or should be used and the figures representing the different designs have been updated for clarity.
- Chapter 12, "Qualitative Research Methods," guides researchers through the steps of the research process as applied to qualitative research. The usual data collection methods of observation and interviewing individuals or groups are covered as well as collecting data through Web-based social media platforms and online surveys. The chapter includes new information on collecting visual data, such as photovoice.
- Chapter 13, "Outcomes Research," a unique feature of our text, was revised by our colleague, Dr. Suzanne Sutherland. Outcomes research will continue to expand because of the exponential growth of electronic data in administrative and clinical databases.
- Chapter 14, "Mixed Methods Research," was rewritten with new examples for three broad categories of mixed methods research: exploratory sequential design, explanatory sequential design, and convergent concurrent designs. Continued emphasis is given to the critical step of integrating the two types of data into a coherent set of findings.
- Chapter 15, "Sampling," was revised to reflect the most current coverage of sampling methods and the

processes for determining sample size for quantitative and qualitative studies in nursing. Discussion of sampling methods and settings are supported with examples from current, relevant studies. Current, creative strategies are provided for recruiting and retaining research participant in nursing studies.
- Chapter 16, "Quantitative Measurement Concepts," features detailed, current information for examining the reliability and validity of measurement methods and the precision and accuracy of physiological measures used in nursing studies. The discussions of sensitivity, specificity, and likelihood ratios are expanded and supported with examples from current studies.
- Chapter 17, "Measurement Methods Used in Developing Evidence-Based Practice," provides updated detail on the use of physiological measurement methods in research with current examples from published nursing studies.
- Chapter 18, "Critical Appraisal of Nursing Studies," continues to include three steps of critical appraisal that are consistent to all types of research studies: (1) identifying the steps or elements of the research process, (2) determining study strengths and limitations, and (3) evaluating the credibility, trustworthiness, and meaning of study findings. Specific questions to consider when appraising quantitative, qualitative, and mixed method studies are provided in the chapter.
- Chapter 19, "Evidence Synthesis and Strategies for Implementing Evidence-Based Practice," has undergone revision to promote the conduct of research syntheses and the use of best research evidence in nursing practice. The chapter contains current, extensive details for conducting systematic reviews, meta-analyses, meta-syntheses, and mixed methods research syntheses. The increased use of EBP models are evident in the nursing literature and expanded in this chapter.
- Chapter 20, "Collecting and Managing Data," was revised by Dr. Daisha Cipher, a noted statistician and healthcare researcher. She included new figures and content to assist nurses in collecting quality data for their studies.
- Revisions have been made in the chapters focused on statistical concepts and analysis techniques (Chapters 21 through 25). The content is presented in a clear, concise manner and supported with current examples of analyses conducted on actual

clinical data. Dr. Cipher continues to provide the quality revisions of these chapters.

- Chapter 26, "Interpreting Research Outcomes," has been revised, expanding on the design validity-based model as an underpinning for identification of limitations, generalizations, and recommendations for further research.
- Chapter 27, "Disseminating Research Findings," provides descriptions and helpful hints for disseminating research findings to different audiences through abstracts, poster and podium presentations, and manuscripts for peer-reviewed journals. Strategies to effectively use tables and figures are described and examples provided. The chapter also includes selecting an appropriate journal for dissemination of your study findings.
- Chapter 28, "Writing Research Proposals," identifies different types of proposals and what should be included in each chapter or section of a proposal. The process of submitting and defending a proposal before an institutional review board is also described. An example proposal concludes the chapter.
- Chapter 29, "Seeking Funding for Research," describes how a program of research can be built through the integration of capital, contribution, and

capacity. A program of research begins with funding by local agencies, regional research societies, and professional organizations and eventually can lead to receiving funding from federal sources for multi-site and multi-year studies.

Evolve Student Resources

An **Evolve Resources website,** which is available at http://evolve.elsevier.com/Gray/practice/, includes the following:

- Interactive Review Questions, which have been revised. A considerable amount of questions are at the application, analysis, or synthesis level.
- Research Article Library includes 10 full-text Elsevier articles.

Evolve Instructor Resources

The **Instructor Resources** are available on Evolve at http://evolve.elsevier.com/Gray/practice/. Instructors also have access to the online student resources. The Instructor Resources feature a revised Test Bank (now available in ExamView) of more than 600 items reflecting ninth-edition changes and revisions, PowerPoint presentations totaling more than 700 slides, updated to ninth-edition changes and revisions, and an Image Collection consisting of the images from the text.

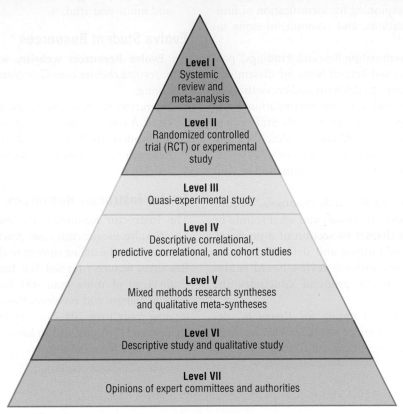

Levels of evidence.

Processes Used to Synthesize Research Evidence

Synthesis Process	Purpose of Synthesis	Types of Research Included in the Synthesis (Sampling Frame)	Analysis for Achieving Synthesis
Systematic review	Systematically identify, select, critically appraise, and synthesize research evidence to address a particular problem in practice (Cullen et al., 2018; Higgins & Thomas, 2019; Johnson & Hennessey, 2019; Liberti et al., 2009; Melnyk & Fineout-Overholt, 2019).	Quantitative studies with similar methodology, such as randomized controlled trials (RCTs) and meta-analyses focused on a practice problem	Narrative and statistical
Meta-analysis	Pooling of the results from several previous studies using statistical analysis to determine the effect of an intervention or the strength of relationships (Cullen et al., 2018; Higgins & Thomas, 2019; Johnson & Hennessey, 2019; Liberti et al., 2009; Melnyk & Fineout-Overholt, 2019).	Quantitative studies with similar methodology, such as quasi-experimental and experimental studies focused on the effect of an intervention or correlational studies focused on selected relationships	Statistical
Meta-synthesis	Systematic compilation and integration of qualitative studies to expand understanding and develop a unique interpretation of the studies' findings in a selected area (Cullen et al., 2018; Johnson & Hennessey, 2019; Melnyk & Fineout-Overholt, 2019; Sandelowski & Barroso, 2007).	Original qualitative studies and summaries of qualitative studies	Narrative
Mixed methods research synthesis	Synthesis of the findings from independent studies conducted with a variety of methods (quantitative, qualitative, and mixed methods) to determine the current knowledge in an area (Heyvaert, Mases, & Onghena, 2013; Higgins & Thomas, 2019; Pluye & Hong, 2014; Sandelowski, Voils, Leeman, & Crandell, 2012).	Variety of quantitative, qualitative, and mixed methods studies	Narrative and sometime statistical

ACKNOWLEDGMENTS

Writing the ninth edition of this textbook has allowed us the opportunity to examine and revise the content of the previous edition based on input from our colleagues and students. We spend many hours searching the literature for trends in research methods, examples of rigorous studies, and perspectives of accomplished researchers. We are truly grateful for the scholars who have published their work, sharing their knowledge with the rest of us in nursing. By doing this, they have made their work accessible to us for inclusion in this textbook. We owe a special debt to a group of researchers who review our textbook and researchers who share their expertise with students in public and private universities across North America. A textbook such as this requires synthesizing the ideas of many people and resources.

We also want to thank the people who contributed to this new edition. Dr. Daisha J. Cipher provided an excellent revision of Chapters 21 through 25 with her strong statistical expertise and ability to explain data analysis in an understandable way. New in this edition, Dr. Cipher used her knowledge of data collection to revise Chapter 20 on collecting and managing data. Dr. Christy Bomer-Norton graciously worked with us again and revised Chapters 7, 8, and 18 on a wide range of topics: reviewing the literature, selecting a theoretical framework, and critically appraising published studies. We want to thank Dr. Polly A. Hulme for her expert revision of Chapter 3 on the introduction to quantitative research. We also extend a special thank you to Dr. Suzanne Sutherland for the quality revision of Chapters 12, 27, 28, 29, and the textbook glossary.

We are fortunate to have had a network of support during the long and time-consuming experience of revising a book of this magnitude. The administrators and fellow faculty at our respective universities have offered their encouragement and tangible assistance for our writing. Our families and friends have been patient and understanding, even when they occasionally needed to remind us to take care of ourselves and our relationships.

Finally, we thank the people at Elsevier, who have been extremely helpful to us in producing a scholarly, attractive, appealing text. We extend a special thank you to the people most instrumental in the development and production of this book: Lee Henderson, Executive Content Strategist; and Maria Broeker, Associate Content Development Specialist. We also want to thank others involved with the production and marketing of this book: Karthikeyan Murthy, Project Manager; Maggie Reid, Designer; and Bergen Farthing, Marketing Manager.

Jennifer R. Gray, PhD, RN, FAAN

Susan K. Grove, PhD, RN, ANP-BC, GNP-BC

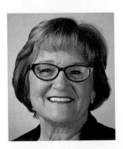

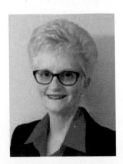

CONTENTS

APPENDICES

1

Discovering the World of Nursing

Jennifer R. Gray

http://evolve.elsevier.com/Gray/practice/

Welcome to the world of nursing research. Entering a new world requires learning a unique language, identifying and applying new rules, and having new experiences. As you learn about the world of research, you will gain the knowledge and skills to critically appraise and appropriately use study findings in clinical practice. This knowledge includes how to locate, read, and comprehend research reports—and much more. Right now, you may view research as a barrier between you and completing a degree to expand your nursing practice. You probably did not choose nursing because you wanted to learn research, but to be better prepared to take care of patients. Nurses prepared as advanced practice nurses (APNs), administrators, educators, and researchers have increased responsibility to use the best evidence in their own practice and lead efforts to implement clinical practice guidelines (Grinspun & Bajnok, 2018; Hall & Roussel, 2017). Evidence-based practice (EBP) in nursing requires the ability to critically appraise available studies and synthesize credible findings. Once synthesized, nurses can use their knowledge to promote quality care for their patients, families, and communities, thereby facilitating better patient outcomes. We developed this text to facilitate your understanding of nursing research and its contribution to the implementation of evidenced-based nursing practice.

This chapter broadly explains the world of research, including a definition of nursing research. The majority of the chapter is structured around the framework for this textbook that connects the practice of nursing in the empirical world to the body of nursing knowledge. The body of nursing knowledge is based on science, which includes theory and research. The chapter concludes with an overview of types of research and the roles of nurses in research and EBP.

DEFINITION OF NURSING RESEARCH

The root meaning of the word *research* is "search again" or "examine carefully." More specifically, **research** is the diligent, systematic inquiry or investigation to generate new knowledge, validate existing knowledge, and refine knowledge by incorporating new research findings. The concepts *diligent* and *systematic* are critical to the meaning of research because they imply planning, organization, rigor, and persistence. Because most disciplines conduct research, you may ask, "What distinguishes nursing research from research in other disciplines?" In some ways, there are no differences, because the knowledge and skills required to conduct ethical and valid research are similar from one discipline to another. Also, nursing knowledge frequently overlaps with knowledge produced by researchers in biology, economics, genetics, psychology, sociology, and physiology (American Nurses Association [ANA], 2015; Smith, 2019).

Nursing research, however, uniquely addresses questions relevant to the "largest healthcare profession," as we seek to improve the quality of life of individuals, families, and communities (National Institute of Nursing Research, 2016, p. 3). Nurse researchers need to implement the most effective research methodologies to develop nursing's unique body of knowledge (Smith, 2019).

The ANA has defined nursing as "the protection, promotion, and optimization of health and abilities, prevention of illness and injury, facilitation of healing, alleviation of suffering through the diagnosis and treatment of human response, and advocacy in the care of individuals, families, groups, communities, and populations" (ANA, 2015, p. 1). On the basis of this definition, nursing research is needed to generate knowledge about human responses and determine the best interventions to improve health outcomes for "diverse and complex populations" (Battaglia & Glasgow, 2018, p. 431). The idea of nurses improving the health of the public is not a new idea. For over 10 years, the American Association of Colleges of Nursing (AACN, 2006) has been advocating for the role of nurse researchers in improving the health of populations.

Many nurses hold the view that nursing research should focus on generating knowledge that can be directly implemented in clinical practice. This type of research is often referred to as **applied** (or practical) **research** (Leedy, Ormrod, & Johnson, 2019). Some nurses may not see the value of **basic** (or bench) **research** that is not immediately applicable to practice. Basic research findings are needed to build and strengthen the scientific foundation of practice (Leedy et al., 2019). Some nurses also may not see the value of studies of nursing education and nursing administration. However, research to determine effective teaching-learning strategies (Morton, 2017), the resources needed for effective nursing teams (Rashkovits & Drach-Zahavy, 2017), and the strategies to prevent burnout (Hunsaker, Chen, Maughan, & Heston, 2015; Szczygiel & Mikolajczak, 2018) are critical to having an adequate number of well-prepared nurses to provide high-quality care. Thus some nurse researchers focus on advancing the science of nursing education, with the desire to have evidence-based strategies to prepare future nurses (National League for Nursing, 2019). Nurse administrators

are involved in research to enhance nursing leadership and the delivery of quality, cost-effective patient care (Hall & Rousell, 2017; Statler & Mota, 2018). In addition, studies of interdisciplinary health services are important to quality outcomes in the nursing profession and the healthcare system (Wu, Rubenstein, & Yoon, 2018). Consistent with research being applicable to all aspects of nursing, you will notice that throughout this text we provide examples of studies from practice, education, administration, and health services.

To summarize, the body of knowledge generated through nursing research provides the scientific foundation essential for all areas of nursing and encompasses the vision and social mandate for the profession. In this text, **nursing research** is defined as a scientific process that validates and refines existing knowledge and generates new knowledge that directly and indirectly influences the delivery of evidence-based nursing.

FRAMEWORK LINKING NURSING RESEARCH TO THE WORLD OF NURSING

To best explore nursing research, we have developed a framework to help establish connections between research and the various aspects of nursing. The framework presented in the following pages links nursing research to the world of nursing and is used as an organizing model for this textbook (Fig. 1.1). Instead of viewing nursing research as an entity disconnected from the rest of nursing, nursing research is influenced by and influences all other aspects of nursing. The use of two-way arrows in the model indicates the dynamic interaction among the aspects of nursing. The following discussion introduces a continuum of concrete to abstract and progresses from the concrete concept of the empirical world of nursing practice to the most abstract concept of nursing philosophy.

Concrete-Abstract Continuum

On the right side of Fig. 1.1, you will notice a vertical line labeled "Concrete" at the bottom and "Abstract" at the top, representing the concrete-abstract continuum. **Concrete** is a descriptor of thinking that is oriented toward and limited by tangible things or by events that we experience objectively through our senses. The focus of concrete thinking is immediate events limited by time and space. Nurses frequently are more comfortable with concrete thinking because they use it frequently as they

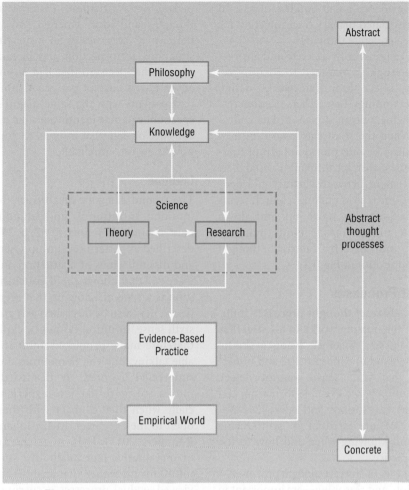

Fig. 1.1 Framework linking nursing research to the world of nursing.

evaluate patients' vital signs, urinary output, and other physiological and psychological factors to implement specific, objective actions in their practice.

Abstract is a concept oriented toward the development of an idea without application to or association with a particular instance (Chinn & Kramer, 2018). Abstract thinkers consider the broader situation or system and look for meaning, patterns, and relationships rather than at a specific behavior or incident. Concepts such as competence, quality, social support, and hope emerge from abstract thinking. This type of thinking is independent of time and space. Graduate nursing educators foster abstract thinking because it is an essential skill for developing theory and generating ideas for study.

Nurses assuming advanced roles need both abstract and concrete thinking. For example, when APNs assess a patient, they use abstract thinking to consider applicable research evidence, the possible impact of the patient's age and family situation, and a wide range of differential diagnoses (Reinoso, Bartlett, & Bennett, 2018). They use their clinical expertise to diagnose and develop a plan of action for the patient's care (i.e., concrete thinking) (Chen, Hsu, Chang, & Lin, 2016). Hospitals are implementing care bundles, a group of interventions that, when implemented together, promote improved patient outcomes (Gilhooly, Green, McCann, Black, & Moonesinghe, 2019). Registered nurses (RNs) review agency-based bundles of care to ensure they are evidence based (i.e., abstract thinking) and implement the evidence-based bundles of care to prevent a catheter-associated urinary tract infection for a specific patient (i.e., concrete thinking).

Nursing research requires both concrete and abstract thinking. Abstract thought is required to identify researchable problems, select study frameworks, design studies, and interpret findings. Researchers use concrete thinking when following a detailed plan of data collection and analysis. When the researcher considers how the statistical results can be interpreted in light of findings from other studies, abstract thinking is used. The back-and-forth movement between abstract and concrete thought may be one reason nursing research seems complex and challenging. To move up and down between the concrete and abstract requires a range of thinking processes, indicated by "abstract thought processes" on the continuum in Fig. 1.1.

Abstract Thought Processes

As described earlier, **abstract thought processes** influence every aspect of the nursing world. In a sense, they link all aspects of nursing together. Being a skillful abstract thinker allows you to conceptualize and understand phenomena that your senses cannot detect. Through abstract thinking, we are able to reason, test our reality, and draw conclusions and inferences. Abstract thought processes are essential for synthesizing research evidence and knowing when and how to use this knowledge in practice.

Three major categories of abstract thought processes—introspection, intuition, and reasoning—are important in nursing (Silva, 1977). These thought processes are used in critically appraising and applying best research evidence in practice and in planning and implementing research (Melnyk & Fineout-Overholt, 2019).

Introspection

Introspection is the process of turning your attention inward toward your own thoughts. It occurs at two levels. At the more superficial level, you are aware of the thoughts you are experiencing. You have a greater awareness of the flow and interplay of feelings and ideas that occur in constantly changing patterns. These thoughts or ideas can rapidly fade from view and disappear if you do not quickly write them down. When you allow introspection to occur in more depth, you examine your thoughts more critically and in detail. You reflect on how your behaviors may have influenced a person or a situation. Patterns and links between thoughts and ideas emerge, and you may recognize fallacies or weaknesses in your thinking. In clinical situations, introspection may include thinking about a patient care decision that had an unexpected result or about how a current patient is similar or dissimilar to past patients with the same diagnosis. Through introspection, you may identify specific data that you did not consider or data that influenced your decision but you now know was unreliable.

Intuition

The second category of abstract thought processes is intuition. **Intuition** is "understanding without a rationale" (Benner & Tanner, 1987, p. 23). Intuition is often described as pattern recognition, seeing the similarities and dissimilarities of a situation and seeing the whole in a way that allows rapid conclusions. Because intuition is a type of knowing that seems to come unbidden, it may also be described as a gut feeling, hunch, or sixth sense. Intuition cannot be explained scientifically, therefore many people discount it or are uncomfortable talking about it. Sometimes the feeling or sense is suppressed, ignored, or dismissed as inane. Expert nurses are more likely to experience intuition, especially when they connect with their patients and are open to their feelings (Melin-Johansson, Palmqvist, & Ronnberg, 2017). These researchers conducted a review of quantitative and qualitative studies about clinical intuition and argued that analysis and intuition may be viewed as dual processes occurring almost simultaneously. An expert nurse may recognize a subtle change in a patient's condition (intuition), gather additional data, and draw a conclusion through analysis (Smyth & McCabe, 2017). Through clinical experience and the use of intuition, nurses are able to recognize a pattern of deviations from the normal clinical course and know how and when to act.

Intuition has a place in research, but does not apply to all aspects of research. Having a hunch about significant differences between one set of scores and another set of scores is not particularly useful (Grove & Cipher, 2020). However, a burst of intuition may identify a problem for study, indicate important concepts to be described, or link two ideas together in interpreting the findings. Some researchers keep a journal to capture elusive thoughts or hunches as they think about their phenomenon (singular) or phenomena (plural) of interest. Research **phenomena** are nurses' topics of interest that may be the focus of current or future studies.

Reasoning

Within abstract thought processes, reasoning is the third category. When you are processing ideas, organizing insights, and drawing inferences from evidence (Hayes, Stephens, Ngo, & Dunn, 2018), you are using **reasoning** to reach conclusions. Through reasoning, you are able to make sense of your thoughts and experiences. Several types of reasoning will be described, including logical, problematic, operational, dialectical, and collaborative reasoning.

Logical reasoning. **Logic** is a science that involves valid ways of relating ideas to promote understanding. The aim of logic is to determine truth or to explain and predict phenomena. **Logical reasoning** is used to dissect components of a situation or conclusion, examine each carefully, and analyze relationships among the parts. Nurses use logical reasoning in clinical practice by recognizing that the whole is the sum of the parts and that the parts organize the whole. For example, a patient states that she is hot. You logically examine the following parts of the situation and their relationships: (1) room temperature, (2) patient's blankets, and (3) sunlight in the room. You take the patient's temperature and it is 98.8° F. The room temperature is 75° F due to direct sunlight entering the windows through open blinds. The patient is covered by three blankets. Based on your conclusion that the patient's perception of being hot is due to room temperature, extra blankets, and sunlight, you will lower the blinds, remove the blankets, and offer to refill the patient's pitcher with water and ice. Dissecting individual parts and examining their contribution to the whole also occurs in research as you select a study design and develop a plan for recruitment and data collection. Logical reasoning is also used when researchers examine the results of their data analysis and formulate their studies' findings in the context of existing knowledge.

The science of logic includes inductive and deductive reasoning. People use these modes of reasoning constantly, frequently switching back and forth between the modes. Cognitive scientists do not agree on whether a single process or dual processes can best explain how humans use inductive and deductive reasoning (Hayes et al., 2018). **Inductive reasoning** moves from the specific to the general, whereby a fairly small number of instances are observed and then combined into a general statement that may be applicable to a larger set of observations (Gravetter & Forzano, 2018; Leedy et al., 2019). An example of inductive reasoning follows:

An episode of hypoglycemia is an altered level of health that is stressful.

A fractured bone is an altered level of health that is stressful.

A terminal illness is an altered level of health that is stressful.

Therefore all altered levels of health are stressful.

In this example, inductive reasoning is used to move from the specific instances of altered levels of health that are stressful to the general belief that all altered levels of health are stressful. By examining the findings of many studies of stress in subjects with altered levels of health, you could determine the strength of the evidence supporting the general statement that all types of altered health are stressful.

Inductive reasoning is used when analyzing qualitative data. For example, a research team might conduct five focus groups about medication adherence. As the researchers analyze the transcribed narratives of the focus groups, they identify the following significant statements made by different participants:

"I have a schedule and do things at specific times so I can take my medications as prescribed."

"I set a timer on my phone to remind me when to take my medications."

"I know which medicines I take at 8 a.m., then at noon, and at 6 p.m."

"My husband is better at keeping track of the time, so he reminds me when it is time to take my pills."

Therefore medication adherence involves awareness of time.

In this example, inductive reasoning is used to move from the specific instances of schedules and timing to the general belief that medication adherence involves awareness of time.

Deductive reasoning moves from the general to the specific or from a general premise to a particular situation or conclusion (Leedy et al., 2019). A **premise** is a statement predicting characteristics of specific instances (Gravetter & Forzano, 2018). An example of deductive reasoning follows:

PREMISES:

All human beings experience loss.

All adolescents are human beings.

CONCLUSION:

All adolescents experience loss.

In this example, deductive reasoning is used to move from the two general premises about human beings experiencing loss and adolescents being human beings to the specific conclusion, "All adolescents experience loss." However, the conclusions generated through deductive reasoning are valid only if they are based on valid premises. Consider another example:

PREMISES:

All health professionals are caring.

All nurses are health professionals.

CONCLUSION:

All nurses are caring.

The premise that all health professionals are caring is not an accurate reflection of reality. Research is a means to test and demonstrate support for or refute a premise so that valid premises can be used as a basis for reasoning in nursing practice and research.

Problematic reasoning. **Problematic reasoning** involves (1) identifying a problem and the factors influencing it, (2) selecting solutions to the problem, and (3) resolving the problem. For example, nurses use problematic reasoning in the nursing process to identify diagnoses and to implement nursing interventions to resolve these problems. Problematic reasoning is also evident in research. During the planning of a study, the researcher identifies a gap in what is known (the research problem) and selects a method to examine it (Bourgault, 2018; Creswell & Creswell, 2018). Problematic reasoning is used when a researcher selects the setting for a study, assesses the environmental and attitudinal challenges to collecting data in the setting, and develops a solution that will hopefully resolve the problem.

Operational reasoning. **Operational reasoning** is the identification of and discrimination among many alternatives and viewpoints. If you are thinking this definition overlaps with the description of problematic reasoning, you are correct. We use different types of reasoning simultaneously and are seldom aware of the processes we are using. Operational reasoning focuses on the process (debating alternatives) rather than on the resolution. Nurses use operational reasoning to develop realistic, measurable health goals with patients and families. Nurse practitioners (NPs) and clinical nurse specialists (CNSs) use operational reasoning to debate which pharmacological and nonpharmacological treatments to use in managing patient illnesses. In research,

operationalizing a treatment or intervention to implement, comparing measurement methods, and debating the appropriate data analysis techniques to use in a study require operational thought (Grove & Cipher, 2020).

Dialectical reasoning. **Dialectical reasoning** involves looking at situations in a holistic way. A dialectical thinker believes that the whole is greater than the sum of the parts and that the whole organizes the parts. For example, instead of viewing a patient as "the stroke in room 219," a nurse using dialectical reasoning would view the patient as a retired army colonel who was widowed 8 years ago, takes care of his grandchildren 3 days a week, and is experiencing an illness. Dialectical reasoning also involves examining factors that are opposites and making sense of them by merging them into a single idea or by finding a middle ground (de Oliveira & Nisbett, 2017). For example, dialectical reasoning is required to analyze studies with conflicting findings and summarize these findings to determine the current knowledge base for a research problem. Conflicting findings may also occur in a mixed methods study when the findings from the qualitative and quantitative phases of the study are dissimilar. Dialectical reasoning is used to synthesize the findings and present the implications of the study for practice and future research.

Collaborative reasoning. **Collaborative reasoning** occurs when individuals with different perspectives "reason together" to develop a coordinated plan of action (Laursen, 2018). Collaborative reasoning frequently overlaps with dialectical reasoning; however, collaborative reasoning involves multiple people. For example, you have a male patient who has had 4 years of chemotherapy and radiation for hepatic tumors. The cancer has metastasized to the spine, and pain has become a constant problem. You convene a meeting of the physician, the social worker, the pharmacist, and the patient's daughter, who is her father's power of attorney. The physician wants to try a new chemotherapy medication; in contrast, the social worker asserts that the patient is appropriate for hospice care. The pharmacist wants the patient to remain hospitalized so that his team can continue to try different medications and delivery methods to manage the patient's pain. The patient's daughter is overwhelmed with the contradictory plans for her father. You identify that the common goal is to improve and maintain the patient's quality of life. Then you begin to ask questions about each approach, such as risks, benefits, and costs. The social worker explains the benefits of palliative care, such as pain management. The physician acknowledges the low likelihood that the chemotherapy would improve the patient's symptoms and could cause unpleasant side effects. The pharmacist recognizes the cost of continued hospitalization and agrees to share with the hospice's pain management team the medications that have been most effective for the patient. As you reason together, gradually a plan emerges that improves the patient's quality of life.

Collaborative reasoning is needed within research teams, especially interdisciplinary research teams that may have conflicting views on various aspects of the research process. They may disagree on the level of significance required for a specific statistical analysis, the value of qualitative research, the need to train data collectors, or the meaning of the findings (Laursen, 2018). Respect for each other and open dialogue can be critical factors in the collaborative reasoning needed to effectively function as a research team.

Empirical World

In Fig. 1.1, you notice that the empirical world is located at the bottom of the diagram to represent the concrete portion of our experiences. The **empirical world** is what you experience through your senses (i.e., what makes up your reality). Reality involves kinetic activities, or what we call "doing." The empirical or real world seems more certain, understandable, predictable, and even controllable. You may be a concrete thinker who want facts and focuses on the empirical world. You may want to be able to apply whatever you learn to the current situation.

The practice of nursing takes place in the empirical world. Within the empirical world of nursing, the goal is to provide evidence-based interventions, which are more likely to improve patient outcomes (Melnyk & Fineout-Overholt, 2019). The scope of nursing practice varies for the RN and the APN, including in the area of EBP. RNs provide care to and coordinate care for patients, families, and communities in a variety of settings. They initiate evidence-based nursing interventions and carry out treatments authorized by other healthcare providers (ANA, 2015). APNs, such as NPs, CNSs, nurse anesthetists (NAs), and nurse midwives, have an advanced nursing degree and, as a result, have an expanded clinical practice. Their knowledge, skills, and expertise promote role autonomy as providers of care to patients and families. In addition, APNs are expected to lead the implementation of EBP.

APNs are not the only nurses with graduate degrees and defined roles that include EBP. Nursing faculty have the responsibilities of serving as role models to students, teaching nursing knowledge that is evidence based, and using evidence-based teaching strategies (Morton, 2017). Nursing administrators and leaders are expected to create work environments that are supporting of implementing EBP (Statler & Mota, 2018).

Evidence-Based Practice for Nursing

Evidence-based practice is shown in Fig. 1.1 as being connected by two-way arrows to the empirical world. The ultimate goal of nursing is to provide evidence-based care that promotes quality outcomes for patients, families, healthcare providers, and the healthcare system (Straus, Glasziou, Richardson, Rosenberg, & Haynes, 2019). EBP evolves from the integration of the best research evidence with clinical expertise and patient needs and values (Straus, Glasziou, Richardson, Rosenberg, & Haynes, 2019). This definition of EBP has been widely accepted since 2012, when the AACN initiated the Quality and Safety Education for Nurses (QSEN) Education Consortium. The consortium developed undergraduate- and graduate-level competencies to guide the preparation of future nurses and provide them with the advanced knowledge, skills, and attitudes needed to deliver quality, safe health care. The QSEN competencies include a focus on EBP defined as "the integration of best current evidence with clinical expertise and patient/family preferences and values for the delivery of optimal health care" (QSEN, 2019).

Fig. 1.2 was developed to demonstrate the interrelationships between the three major concepts—best

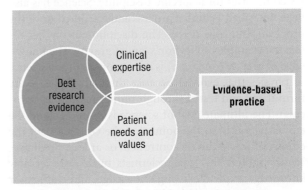

Fig. 1.2 Model of evidence-based practice.

research evidence, clinical expertise, and patient needs and values—that are merged to produce EBP. **Best research evidence** is the empirical knowledge generated from the synthesis of quality study findings to address a practice problem. **Clinical expertise** is the knowledge and skills of the healthcare professional providing care. A nurse's clinical expertise is determined by years of practice, institutional policy, current knowledge of the research and clinical literature, and educational preparation. The stronger the clinical expertise, the better the nurse's clinical judgment is in the delivery of quality care (Reinoso et al., 2018). The **patient's need(s)** may include perceived and actual deficits in the resources needed to promote health, prevent illness, manage acute and chronic illness, or rehabilitate following an injury or medical event. In addition, the **patient's values** or unique preferences, expectations, concerns, and cultural beliefs will shape the clinical encounter but may be the most difficult to determine when patients are acutely ill (Bourgault, 2018). With EBP, patients and their families are encouraged to take an active role in managing their health care. In summary, expert clinicians use the best research evidence available to deliver quality, safe, cost-effective care to patients and families with specific health needs and values to achieve EBP (Hall & Roussel, 2017; Melynk & Fineout-Overholt, 2019). Evidence-based practice will be covered in greater depth in Chapters 2 and 19.

Science

In the middle of Fig. 1.1 is a blue box that represents science. **Science** is a coherent, comprehensive body of knowledge, "the knowledge of a discipline that has been developed rigorously and systematically" (Rodgers, 2018, p. 21) and is composed of research findings and tested theories for a specific discipline. Science has also been described as both a process and the outcome of the process (Polifroni, 2018). The discipline of physics offers the example of Newton's law of gravity. The knowledge of gravity (outcome) is a component of the science of physics that evolved because theoretical ideas were formulated and tested through numerous studies (process). The ultimate goal of science is to understand the empirical world to the point that the conditions of the empirical world can be controlled, or at least predicted. To accomplish this goal, scientists must discover new knowledge, expand existing knowledge, and reaffirm or disconfirm previously held knowledge.

One method for expanding the science of a discipline is the traditional research process, or quantitative research (Sakamoto, 2018). The information gained from one quantitative study, however, is not sufficient for its inclusion in the body of science. A study must be replicated several times and yield similar results each time before that information can be considered to be scientific (Chinn & Kramer, 2018).

Consider the scientific knowledge related to smoking, lung damage, and cancer. Numerous studies conducted on animals and humans for at least seven decades indicate causative relationships between smoking and lung damage and between smoking and lung cancer. Science clearly supports that everyone who smokes experiences lung damage, and although not everyone who smokes develops lung cancer, smokers are at a much higher risk for cancer. Extensive, replicated quantitative and outcome studies have been conducted to generate empirical evidence about the health hazards of smoking, and this evidence has resulted in smoke-free environments and medications to support a person's efforts to stop smoking.

Although some sciences rigidly limit the types of research that can be conducted to obtain knowledge, nursing science has recognized the importance of multiple types of research and knowledge (Sakamoto, 2018). Nurses recognize and value the knowledge gained through quantitative research about the risks of smoking. However, nurses are also interested in adolescents' perceptions of media campaigns to prevent smoking and in the strategies that motivate female patients to consider smoking cessation. Knowledge of this type might be generated by qualitative studies and studies that combine quantitative and qualitative studies (mixed methods studies). Nursing science is being developed using a variety of research methodologies, including quantitative, qualitative, mixed methods, and outcomes research (Creswell & Clark, 2018; Creswell & Creswell, 2018; Creswell & Poth, 2018; Doran, 2011; Thorne, 2018). The focus of this textbook is to increase your understanding of these different types of research and how they are used to develop and test nursing theory for EBP.

Theory and Research

In Fig. 1.1, theory and research are included within science. Research was defined earlier in this chapter as a systematic investigation that creates new knowledge, validates or refines existing knowledge, and raises additional questions for study. A **theory** is a scientific representation of reality that includes concepts and relationships among concepts (Reed, 2019). A theory consists of a set of concepts that are defined and interrelated to present a unified view of a selected phenomenon (Roy, 2019). An example from nursing science is Roy's adaptation model that classifies types of stimuli and identifies four adaptive modes that persons use to cope with stimuli (Flanagan, 2018; Roy, 2011). Nurses can use this model to structure assessment of their patients, select interventions to support adaptive modes, and evaluate the impact on coping. More directly, theoretical concepts of the model are linked to research. Statements of relationships among the theoretical concepts (propositions) of Roy's model have been tested in 360 studies (Roy, 2011). Therefore a theory can be understood to provide a framework for studying a phenomenon, and the study findings support or fail to support the theory. This knowledge then influences the revision or refinement of the theory. Roy used the findings of these studies to reconceptualize coping as being transactional and multidimensional.

Theory and research are closely connected. The theorist may use findings from research as a starting point and then organize the findings to best explain the empirical world and advanced nursing practice (Rega, Telaretti, Alvaro, & Kangasniemi, 2017). Alternatively, the theorist may use abstract thinking, personal knowledge, and intuition to develop a theory of a phenomenon. This theory then requires testing through research to determine whether it is an accurate reflection of reality (Durepos, Orr, Ploeg, & Kaasalainen, 2018). Thus research has a major role in theory development, testing, and refinement. Some forms of qualitative research focus on developing new theories or extending existing theories (Marshall & Rossman, 2016). Various types of quantitative research are often implemented to test the accuracy of theory. The study findings either support or fail to support the theory, providing a basis for renovation of the theory (Hickman, 2019).

Knowledge

Knowledge is a complex, multifaceted concept that is expected to be an accurate reflection of reality (Durepos et al., 2018). Nursing theory, research findings, and clinical experience increase the knowledge of nursing as a discipline (Rega et al., 2017). There are different types

of knowing, such as knowing another person, knowing how to perform a clinical skill, or knowing the best course of action based on ethical values. There is a need for certainty in the world, and individuals seek it by trying to decrease uncertainty through knowledge. In the same way, there is a need for certainty in nursing that imposes or recognizes order on thoughts and ideas. Think of the questions you ask another nurse who presents you with a bit of knowledge, such as a patient's fasting blood sugar: "How long has the patient fasted?" "Was the glucometer calibrated?" "Did you use standard technique to obtain a blood sample?" We expect knowledge to be an accurate reflection of reality.

Ways of Acquiring Nursing Knowledge

Knowledge for the discipline of nursing is increased by theory and research, as shown by the two-way arrows among the three terms in Fig. 1.1. A critical aspect of preparing for expanded roles is to increase your knowledge of nursing. It is important to evaluate how you acquired your current knowledge and select reliable methods of acquiring new knowledge. The ways of acquiring nursing knowledge can be categorized as being informal and formal (Box 1.1). Ways of informally acquiring knowledge include tradition, authorities, borrowing, personal experiences, and trial and error. These are briefly described in this section.

Informal ways of acquiring knowledge. When a patient or new graduate questions why vital signs are taken before 6 a.m., you may respond, "That is the way we have always done it." Traditions consist of truths or beliefs that are based on customs and past trends. Nursing traditions from the past have been transferred to the present by written and verbal communication. Traditions create structure and useful processes in the delivery of care, but too often limit the knowledge sought for nursing practice. Traditions are difficult to change

BOX 1.1 **Informal and Formal Ways of Acquiring Knowledge**	
Informal	**Formal**
Traditions	Role modeling
Authority	Mentoring
Borrowing	Education
Personal experience	Research
Trial and error	Theory development

because they have been accepted and embedded in the culture of a group.

You may have also gained your current knowledge by observing and listening to authorities. An **authority** is a person, who because of his or her expertise and power, can influence opinion and behavior. Authorities are people who have more knowledge in a specific area than others do. Persons viewed as authorities in one field are not necessarily authorities in other fields. An expert is an authority only when addressing his or her area of expertise.

New employees may unconsciously learn the traditions of a specific work group by observing actions of leaders or consciously as an authority orients them to the group. You may acknowledge an authority when you credit another person as the source of the information. Frequently, nurses who publish articles and books or develop theories are considered authorities. Students usually view their instructors as authorities, and clinical nursing experts are considered authorities within their clinical settings. When you were a new graduate, you may have unconsciously learned how to administer an enema or approach patients and families from the more experienced nurse who oriented you to the setting. Observation, however, is limited because you may learn a skill, but not know the supporting rationale of when to use the skill or how to assess for potential adverse effects.

Nurses frequently use knowledge from other disciplines (Roy, 2019), such as using psychological knowledge to communicate with a patient therapeutically. Using knowledge developed in other disciplines is called **borrowing**. Borrowing knowledge is using the theories, laws, and information belonging to other disciplines as the rationale for nursing actions. Nurses have borrowed knowledge from authorities in other disciplines for years and applied it directly to nursing practice. This information was not integrated within the unique focus of nursing. For example, some nurses have used the medical model to guide their nursing practice, thus focusing on the diagnosis and treatment of physiological diseases with limited attention to the patient's holistic nature. This type of borrowing continues today as nurses use technological advances to focus on the detection and treatment of disease, to the exclusion of health promotion and illness prevention. A more appropriate way of borrowing is to integrate information from other disciplines into nursing knowledge.

Personal experience can be defined as the knowledge that comes from being personally involved in an event, situation, or circumstance. Early in nursing's history, the profession evolved through the nurses' personal experiences. Personal experience is a key element of developing clinical expertise (Benner, 1984). With no other sources of knowledge available, nurses used **trial and error**, selecting an action based on guesses or prior experiences. As knowledge of effective practices was codified in textbooks and manuals, the need to rely on personal experience was decreased. The trial-and-error way of acquiring knowledge was time consuming because nurses tried multiple interventions before one was found to be effective. When an effective intervention is identified through personal experience, the nurse may choose to use it again in the future, only to discover that the unique characteristics of the patient resulted in a different outcome. The trial-and-error approach to developing knowledge would be more efficient if nurses documented the patient and situational characteristics that provided the context for the patient's unique response.

Formal ways of acquiring knowledge. Informal ways of acquiring knowledge may result in learning that is inconsistent and knowledge that is not reliable. In contrast, formal ways of acquiring knowledge are deliberate, purposeful actions (see Box 1.1). **Role-modeling** is learning by imitating the behaviors of an exemplar, such as a clinical faculty (Baldwin, Mills, Birks, & Budden, 2017). You may have learned about how to be a nurse in specific situations by "imitating and identifying with role models who represent what is achievable and desirable" (Garcia, Restubog, Ocampo, Wang, & Tang, 2019, p. 40).

The behaviors and attitudes of role models provide a template or framework within which less experienced nurses develop their own professional identity. In nursing, role-modeling enables the novice nurse to learn from interacting with expert nurses or following their examples. Examples of role models are admired teachers, expert practitioners, researchers, and illustrious individuals who inspire students, practicing nurses, educators, and researchers through their examples.

An accentuated form of role-modeling is **mentorship**. In a mentorship, the expert nurse, or **mentor**, serves as a teacher, sponsor, facilitator, clinical guide, and preceptor for the novice nurse (or **mentee**) (Tuomikoski, Ruotsalainen, Mikkonen, Miettunen, & Kääriäinen, 2018). The mentee imitates and internalizes the values, attitudes, and behaviors of the mentor while gaining intuitive knowledge and personal experience. Mentorship is important for building research competence in nursing. A graduate student may become part of a research team conducting a funded study to assist with the work of the study but also to be mentored in how to conduct research.

Another formal way of knowing is to increase one's education by enrolling in graduate school or completing a professional development activity. **Education** is purposeful with the teacher selecting teaching-learning activities and evaluation methods, guided by learning objectives. The curricula of graduate nursing programs are developed according to standards established by professional organizations, such as the AACN. Members of the organization serve as a panel of authorities to discuss and come to a consensus about what different types of nursing education programs should include. Universities establish the policies by which it is determined that a student has completed the educational program.

Research and **theory development** are also formal ways of knowing. Studies are conducted to address a gap in what is known (research problem) and are implemented according to standards of rigor, such as reliability and validity. In Chapter 18, you will find guidelines for determining the credibility of a study's findings. A theory is a creative and rigorous structuring of ideas that includes defined concepts, existence statements, and relational statements that are interrelated to present a systematic view of a phenomenon. Theories are tested by research and can also be generated by qualitative research (see Chapter 8 for more on theories).

To summarize, in nursing, a body of knowledge must be acquired (learned), incorporated, and assimilated by each member of the profession and collectively by the profession as a whole (Smith, 2019). This body of knowledge guides the thinking and behavior of the profession and of individual practitioners. It also directs further development and influences how science and theory are interpreted within the discipline (see Fig. 1.1). This knowledge base is necessary for health professionals, consumers, and society to recognize nursing as a science and a unique discipline (Smith, 2019).

Philosophy

Philosophy provides a broad, global explanation of the world. It is the most abstract and most all-encompassing concept in the model (see Fig. 1.1). Philosophy gives unity and meaning to the world of nursing and provides a framework for examining the complexity of nursing and health (Thorne & Sawatzky, 2014). Nursing's philosophical position influences its knowledge base, because how nurses conduct research to gain new knowledge and apply knowledge to practice in the form of theories and research findings depends on their philosophy related to science (Durepos et al., 2018). Ideas about truth and reality, as well as beliefs, values, and attitudes, are part of philosophy. Philosophers ask questions such as, "Is there an absolute truth, or is truth relative?" and "Is there one reality, or is reality different for each individual?"

Everyone's world is modified by her or his philosophy, as a pair of eyeglasses modifies vision. Your philosophy creates a perspective or lens through which you make sense of the world (Kwon, Thorne, & Sawatzky, 2019). If what you see is not within your ideas of truth or reality, if it does not fit your belief system, you may not see it. Your mind may reject it altogether or may modify it to fit your philosophy. For example, you might notice that a husband who has been visiting his wife in the hospital leaves without kissing his wife. Within a philosophy (perspective) that evaluates one's level of concern by behaviors, you may conclude that the couple has a distant or strained relationship. Over time, through conversation with the wife, you learn, however, that the wife and husband believe public displays of affection are inappropriate. Your perspective caused you to evaluate a behavior incorrectly instead of being open to what the behavior meant within the perspective of the patient. Learning to remain open to different philosophies and perspectives is an important skill as you advance your education. As you start to discover the world of nursing research, it is important to keep an open mind about the value of research and your future role in the development or use of research evidence in practice.

Philosophical positions commonly held within the nursing profession include the view that human beings are holistic, rational, and responsible. Nursing's focus on holistic human beings can be traced back to Florence Nightingale's assertion that the mind, body, and spirit (the whole person) were affected by environmental factors (Smith, 2019). Because nurses believe that people desire health and that health is better than illness, they intervene to promote health and quality of life. Nurses care for patients within their physical, emotional, and social contexts or environments and value knowing the uniqueness of each person (Bender, 2018). Nurses focus on people as humans, which includes facilitating finding meaning in events, providing choice, promoting quality of life, and fostering healing in living and dying (Roy, 2019). Although nurses' philosophies for practice and research vary, they are influenced by nursing's metaparadigm, the interactions among the constructs of person, health, environment, and nursing that are foundational to the profession (Bender, 2018).

In nursing, truth is often perceived as being relative, and reality tends to vary with perception and bias (Wieringa, Engebretsen, Heggen, & Greenhalgh, 2018). For example, because nurses believe that reality varies with perception and that truth is relative, they would not try to impose their views of truth and reality on patients. Rather, they would accept patients' views of the world and help them seek health from within those worldviews, an approach that is a critical component of EBP.

Research can seem abstract and irrelevant. That is why we have described the framework of the interactions between the empirical world, EBP, science, research, theory, and philosophy (see Fig. 1.1). The framework may serve to remind you of the importance of research as you continue to develop your knowledge and ability to use evidence in your practice.

FOCUS OF RESEARCH EVIDENCE IN NURSING

The empirical evidence in nursing focuses on description, explanation, prediction, and control of phenomena important to professional nursing. The following sections address the types of knowledge that are needed as nursing moves toward EBP.

Description

Description involves observing and documenting a phenomenon, in essence providing a snapshot of reality (Adams & Lawrence, 2019; Melnyk & Fineout-Overholt, 2019). This type of research may be used to explore a new concept or to gain understanding of the variable in its natural setting (Gravetter & Forzano, 2018). Descriptive designs can be qualitative, quantitative, mixed methods, and outcomes studies. Through descriptive research, nurses are able to (1) explore and describe what exists in nursing practice, (2) discover new information and

meaning, (3) promote understanding of situations, and (4) classify information for use in the discipline. Some examples of research evidence from descriptive research include the following:

- Identification of individuals' experiences related to a variety of health conditions and situations
- Exploration of the health promotion and illness prevention strategies used by various populations
- Determination of the incidence of a disease locally, nationally, and internationally
- Identification of the cluster of symptoms and responses for a particular disease

Elbilgahy, Hashem, and Alemam (2019) conducted a descriptive study in a children's hospital in Egypt to determine the extent to which mothers of children in the pediatric intensive care unit (PICU) were satisfied with the care provided for their children. The mothers ($N = 108$) completed a survey and provided clinical and demographic information about themselves and their children. The researchers found that respiratory problems were the most frequent reason for children being admitted to the PICU. The mothers were most satisfied with the "care and cure" aspects of the hospitalization followed by the professional attitudes of the staff.

> . . . the mothers' satisfaction with care provided for their children was influenced by many factors such as maternal education level, length of hospital stay, communication and parental participation in care. Moreover, the clinical conditions and the diagnosis of the child also affected mothers' satisfaction. (Elbilgahy et al., 2019, p. 26)

The researchers determined that training programs were needed to improve communication between the health team and the mothers. The descriptive study fulfilled its purpose of providing information about existing conditions in the PICU and recommendations for improvement.

Explanation

Explanation clarifies the relationships among concepts or variables with the goal of understanding how they work with each other. Explanation can be accomplished through qualitative, quantitative, mixed methods, and outcomes research (Adams & Lawrence, 2019; Creswell & Clark, 2018; Creswell & Creswell, 2018; Hall & Roussel, 2017; Marshall & Rossman, 2016). Research focused on explanation provides the following types of evidence essential for practice:

- Link of concepts to develop an explanation, model, or theory of a phenomenon in nursing
- Determination of the assessment data (both subjective data from the health history and objective data from physical examination) needed to address a patient's health need
- Link of assessment data to determine a diagnosis (both nursing and medical)
- Link of causative risk factors or etiologies to illness, morbidity, and mortality
- Determination of the relationships among health risks, health status, and healthcare costs

The concepts of burnout and resilience, as responses to workplace adversity, were examined in a grounded theory (qualitative) study of nurses in critical care units (Jackson, Vandall-Walker, Vanderspank-Wright, Wishart, & Moore, 2018). Through open-ended interviews, the researchers explained conditions that fostered workplace adversity and identified four techniques the nurses used to manage their exposure to workplace adversity: protecting, processing, decontaminating, and distancing. Awareness was a prerequisite of managing exposure. Nurses who were unaware of workplace adversity were more likely to burn out. In contrast, nurses who were aware of workplace adversity learned to use techniques that promoted resilience. The grounded theory of managing exposure was displayed as a diagram of the process with indicators of the results being thriving, resilience, surviving, and burnout. Through the study, Jackson et al. (2018) provided an explanation of a relevant nursing issue, along with techniques that other nurses may find helpful.

Prediction

Through **prediction**, one can estimate the probability of a specific outcome in a given situation (Chinn & Kramer, 2018). However, predicting an outcome does not necessarily enable one to modify or control the outcome (Dane, 2018). Through prediction, the risk of illness is identified and linked to possible screening methods that will identify the illness. Knowledge generated from research focused on prediction is critical for EBP and includes the following:

- Prediction of the risk for a disease in different populations
- Prediction of the accuracy and precision of a screening instrument, such as mammogram, to detect a disease

- Determination of the likelihood of surviving 10 years following a cancer diagnosis based on the stage of the cancer
- Prediction of the impact of nursing actions on selected outcomes
- Prediction of behaviors that promote health, prevent illness, and increase longevity
- Determination of the likelihood of specific nursing actions being acceptable to the patient based on the patient's personality

Numerous researchers have determined that serum albumin at admission is a strong predictor of morbidity and mortality in surgical patients and those who are admitted to intensive care units (ICUs). Kendall, Abreu, and Cheng (2019) reviewed these studies and identified a gap in knowledge as to whether trends in serum albumin after admission predicted mortality in patients admitted to an ICU with sepsis. Using retrospective analysis of medical records, the researchers identified a sample of 577 ICU patients admitted with sepsis and extracted five different albumin values for each: admission albumin, minimum albumin, maximum albumin, serum albumin trend, and average albumin. Each of the albumin variables was predictive of mortality with high sensitivity and specificity, with serum albumin trend and minimum albumin level being the most sensitive and specific predictors. Age was the only demographic variable that contributed to the prediction of mortality (Kendall et al., 2019).

Control

If one can predict the outcome of a situation, the next step is to control or manipulate the situation to produce the desired outcome. Using the best research evidence, nurses can prescribe specific interventions to meet the needs of patients. Nurses need this type of research evidence to provide EBP (see Fig. 1.2). Research in the following areas is important for generating EBP in nursing:

- Testing interventions to improve the health status of individuals, families, and communities
- Testing leadership strategies to improve healthcare delivery
- Determination of the quality and cost effectiveness of interventions
- Implementation of an evidence-based intervention to determine whether it is effective in managing a patient's health need (health promotion, illness

prevention, acute and chronic illness management, and rehabilitation) and producing quality outcomes
- Synthesis of research evidence for use in practice.

Example of Applying an EBP Guideline

Dehydration in older adults, especially those with cognitive changes, is a challenging nursing problem that was addressed by the Hartford Institute for Geriatric Nursing (Mentes, 2008, 2012). Older adults who are required to be nil per os (nothing by mouth) prior to a procedure, who experience febrile episodes and vomiting/diarrhea, or who have an increased risk for dehydration based on a standardized assessment tool are the target population for the clinical practice guideline "Managing oral hydration." The guideline was developed from the findings of over 20 studies, which were evaluated for quality and level of evidence. For the older adult who has ongoing threats to hydration such as dementia and incontinence, the recommended nursing actions are to (1) calculate a daily fluid goal, (2) compare current intake to fluid goal, (3) offer a variety of fluids routinely during rounds at designated times, (4) schedule "happy hours" or "tea times" to increase fluid intake, and (5) monitor urine color and amount (Mentes, 2012). By implementing the specific nursing actions for an older adult, the nurse can correct a fluid deficit or prevent dehydration.

YOUR ROLE IN RESEARCH

Many more studies and research syntheses are needed to generate evidence for practice (Bourgault, 2018; Clanton, 2017; Melnyk & Fineout-Overholt, 2019). Your level of education in nursing prepares you for different roles related to nursing. As a baccalaureate-educated nurse, you were prepared to critically appraise existing studies and participate in studies as data collectors (Table 1.1). Through masters-level education, your ability to critically appraise studies will grow and you may share your clinical expertise as part of a research team. The nurse with a Doctorate of Nursing Practice degree will be able to conduct a systematic review of existing studies with application to a clinical problem or patient concern. The nurse who seeks a doctoral degree focused on research, Doctor of Philosophy in (PhD) Nursing, will be equipped to plan and implement studies with a team of nurse researchers (see Table 1.1). Following graduation, some PhD-prepared nurses may realize that they need additional education or mentoring to reach their career goals. These nurses may apply to postdoctoral education programs, which provide individualized plans of courses and research experiences guided by a high-skilled, funded researcher. The critical need for additional nursing studies and for critical appraisal of existing studies provide you with many opportunities to be involved in the world of nursing research.

TABLE 1.1	Nurses' Participation in Research at Various Levels of Education
Educational Preparation	**Research Expectations and Competencies**
BSN	Read and critically appraise studies. Use best research evidence in practice with guidance. Assist with problem identification and data collection.
MSN	Critically appraise and synthesize studies to develop and revise protocols, algorithms, and policies for practice. Implement best research evidence in practice. Collaborate in research projects and provide clinical expertise for research.
DNP	Participate in evidence-based guideline development. Develop, implement, evaluate, and revise as needed protocols, policies, and evidence-based guidelines in practice. Conduct clinical studies, usually in collaboration with other nurse researchers.
PhD	Assume a major role, such as primary investigator, in conducting research and contributing to the empirical knowledge generated in a selected area of study. Obtain initial funding for research. Coordinate research teams of BSN, MSN, and DNP nurses.
Postdoctoral	Implement a funded program of research. Lead and/or participate in nursing and interdisciplinary research teams. Identified as experts in their areas of research. Mentor PhD-prepared researchers.

BSN, Bachelor of Science in Nursing; *DNP,* Doctorate of Nursing Practice; *MSN,* Master of Science in Nursing; *PhD,* Doctor of Philosophy.

This chapter introduced you to the world of nursing research and the connections among EBP, research, theory, and science (see Fig. 1.1). As you study the following chapters, you will expand your understanding of different research methodologies so you can critically appraise studies, synthesize research findings, and use the best research evidence available in clinical practice. This text also gives you a background for conducting research in collaboration with expert nurse researchers. We think you will find that nursing research is an exciting adventure that holds much promise for the future practice of nursing.

KEY POINTS

- Nursing research is defined as a scientific process that validates and refines existing knowledge and generates new knowledge that directly and indirectly influences the delivery of EBP.
- The empirical world interacts with EBP, research, theory, science, knowledge, and philosophy. The framework moves from the concrete empirical world of practice to the abstract philosophical views affecting the profession of nursing (see Fig. 1.1).
- Research is a way to test reality, and nurses use a variety of research methodologies (quantitative, qualitative, mixed methods, and outcomes) to test their reality and generate knowledge.
- A theory is a creative and rigorous structuring of ideas that includes defined concepts, existence statements, and relational statements that are interrelated to present a systematic view of a phenomenon.
- Science is a coherent, comprehensive body of knowledge that is composed of research findings and tested theories for a specific discipline. Science evolves as scientists discover new knowledge, expand existing knowledge, and reaffirm or disconfirm previously held knowledge.
- EBP evolves from the integration of best research evidence with clinical expertise and patient needs and values (see Fig. 1.2).
- The best research evidence is the empirical knowledge generated from the synthesis of quality studies to address a practice problem.
- The clinical expertise of a nurse is determined by years of clinical experience, current knowledge of the research and clinical literature, and educational preparation.
- The patient brings values—such as unique preferences, expectations, concerns, cultural beliefs, and health needs—to the clinical encounter, which are important to consider in providing evidence-based care.
- Nurses are consumers of research and use research evidence to improve their nursing practice.
- Three major abstract thought processes—introspection, intuition, and reasoning—are important in nursing. Abstract thinking processes and sources of knowledge were described along with their application to research and advanced practice.
- The informal ways of knowing, tradition, authority, borrowing, personal experience, and trial and error are no longer an adequate basis for sound nursing practice.
- The formal ways of knowing include role modeling, mentoring, research, theory development, and structured education.
- The goal of nurses and other healthcare professionals is to deliver evidence-based health care to patients and their families.
- The knowledge generated through research is essential for describing, explaining, predicting, and controlling nursing phenomena.
- All nurses have a role in research that is delineated by their levels of education and influenced by their practice environments. Some nurses will develop and conduct studies to generate and refine the knowledge needed for nursing practice, and other nurses will critically appraise completed studies to identify evidence to be used in practice.

REFERENCES

Adams, K., & Lawrence, E. (2019). *Research methods, statistics, and applications* (2nd ed.). Thousand Oaks, CA: Sage.
American Association of Colleges of Nursing (AACN). (2006). *AACN position statement on nursing research.* Washington, DC: AACN. Retrieved from http://www.aacn.nche.edu/Publications/positions/NsgRes.htm
American Association of Colleges of Nursing (AACN) QSEN Education Consortium. (2012). *QSEN learning module series.* Retrieved from https://www.aacnnursing.org/Faculty/Teaching-Resources/QSEN/QSEN-Learning-Module-Series

American Nurses Association. (2015). *Nursing: Scope and standards of practice* (3rd ed.). Silver Spring, MD: Author.

Baldwin, A., Mills, J., Birks, M., & Budden, L. (2017). Reconciling professional identity: A grounded theory of nurse academics' role modelling for undergraduate students. *Nurse Education Today, 59*, 1−5. doi:10.1016/j.nedt.2017.08.010

Battaglia, C., & Glasgow, R. (2018). Pragmatic dissemination and implementation research models, methods and measures and their relevance for nursing research. *Nursing Outlook, 66*(5), 430−445. doi:10.1016/j.outlook.2018.06.00

Bender, M. (2018). Re-conceptualizing the nursing metaparadigm: Articulating the philosophical ontology of the nursing discipline that orients inquiry and practice. *Nursing Inquiry, 25*, e12243. doi:10.1111/nin.12243

Benner, P. (1984). *From novice to expert: Excellence and power in clinical nursing practice.* Menlo Park, CA: Addison-Wesley.

Benner, P., & Tanner, C. (1987). How expert nurses use intuition. *American Journal of Nursing, 87*(1), 23−31.

Bourgault, A. (2018). Guest editorial: Bridging evidence-based practice and research. *Critical Care Nurse 38*(6), 10−12. doi:10.4037/ccn2018278

Chen, S. L., Hsu, H. Y., Chang, C., & Lin, E. C. (2016). An exploration of the correlates of nurse practitioners' clinical decision-making abilities. *Journal of Clinical Nursing, 25*(7-8), 1016−1024. doi:10.1111/jocn.13136

Chinn, P. L., & Kramer, M. K. (2018). *Knowledge development in nursing: Theory and process* (10th ed.). St. Louis, MO: Mosby.

Clanton, C. (2017). Introduction to evidence-based research. In H. Hall & L. Roussel (Eds.), *Evidence-based practice: An integrative approach to research, administration, and practice* (2nd ed., pp. 283−300). Burlington, MA: Jones & Bartlett Learning.

Creswell, J. W., & Clark, V. (2018). *Designing and conducting mixed methods research* (3rd ed.). Thousand Oaks, CA: Sage.

Creswell, J. W., & Creswell, J. D. (2018). *Research design: Qualitative, quantitative, and mixed methods approaches* (5th ed.). Thousand Oaks, CA: Sage.

Creswell, J. W., & Poth, C. (2018). *Qualitative inquiry and research design: Choosing among five approaches* (4th ed.). Thousand Oaks, CA: Sage.

Dane, F. (2018). *Evaluating research: Methodology for people who need to read research* (2nd ed.). Thousand Oaks, CA: Sage.

de Oliveira, S., & Nisbett, R. (2017). Culture changes how we think about thinking: From "human inference" to "geography of thought." *Perspectives on Psychological Science, 12*(5), 782−790. doi:10.1177/1745691617702718.

Doran, D. M. (2011). *Nursing-sensitive outcomes: State of the science* (2nd ed) Sudbury, MA: Jones & Bartlett Learning.

Durepos, P., Orr, E., Ploeg, J., & Kaasalainen, S. (2018). The value of measurement for development of nursing knowledge: Underlying philosophy, contributions and critiques. *Journal of Advanced Nursing, 74*(10), 2290−2300. doi:10.1111/jan.13778

Elbilgahy, A., Hashem, S., & Alemam, D. (2019). Mothers' satisfaction with care provided for their children in pediatric intensive care unit. *Middle East Journal of Nursing, 13*(2), 17−28. doi:10.5742MEJN.2019.93636

Flanagan, N. (2018). Persistent pain in older adults: Roy's adaptation model. *Nursing Science Quarterly, 31*(1), 25−28. doi: 10.1177/089431841774109

Garcia, P., Restubog, S., Ocampo, A., Wang, L., & Tang, R. (2019). Role modeling as a socialization mechanism in the transmission of career adaptability across generations. *Journal of Vocational Behavior, 111*(1), 39−48. doi:10.1016/j.jvb.2018.12.002

Gilhooly, D., Green, S., McCann, C., Black, N., & Moonesinghe, S. (2019). Barriers and facilitators to the successful development, implementation and evaluation of care bundles in acute care in hospital: A scoping review. *Implementation Science, 14,* Document 47. doi:10.1186/s13012-019-0894-2

Gravetter, F., & Forzano, L. A. (2018). *Research methods for the behavioral sciences.* Boston, MA: Cengage.

Grinspun, D. (2018). Transforming nursing through knowledge: The conceptual and programmatic underpinnings of RNAO's BPG program. In D. Grinspun, & I. Bajnok (Eds.), *Transforming nursing through knowledge: Best practices for guideline development, implementation science, and evaluation* (pp. 3−27). Indianapolis, IN: Sigma Theta Tau International.

Grinspun, D., & Bajnok, I. (2018). *Transforming nursing through knowledge: Best practices for guideline development, implementation science, and evaluation.* Indianapolis, IN: Sigma Theta Tau International.

Grove, S., & Cipher, D. (2020). *Statistics for nursing research: A workbook for evidence-based practice* (3rd ed.). St. Louis, MO: Elsevier.

Hall, H., & Roussel, L. (2017). *Evidence-based practice: An integrative approach to research, administration, and practice* (2nd ed.). Burlington, MA: Jones & Bartlett Learning.

Hayes, B., Stephens, R., Ngo, J., & Dunn, J. (2018). The dimensionality of reasoning: Inductive and deductive inference can be explained by a single process. *Journal of Experimental Psychology, Learning, Memory, and Cognition, 44*(9), 1333−1351. doi:10.1037/xlm0000527

Hickman, R. (2019). Nursing theory and research: The path forward. *Advances in Nursing Science, 42*(1), 85−86. doi:10.1097/ANS.0000000000000255

Hunsaker, S., Chen, H.-C., Maughan, D., & Heston, S. (2015). Factors that influence the development of compassion fatigue, burnout, and compassion satisfaction in emergency department nurses. *Journal of Nursing Scholarship, 47*(2), 186–194. doi:10.1111/jnu.12122.

Jackson, J., Vandall-Walker, V., Vanderspank-Wright, B., Wishart, P., & Moore, S. (2018). Burnout and resilience in critical care nurses: A grounded theory of managing exposure. *Intensive & Critical Care Nursing, 48,* 28–35. doi:10.1016/j.iccn.2018.07.002

Kendall, H., Abreu, E., & Cheng, A. L. (2019). Serum albumin trend is a predictor of mortality in ICU patients with sepsis. *Biological Research for Nursing, 21*(3), 237–244. doi:10.1177/1099800419827600

Kwon, J., Thorne, S., & Sawatzky, R. (2019). Interpretation and use of patient-reported outcome measures through a philosophical lens. *Quality of Life Research, 28*(3), 629–636. doi:10.1007/s11136-018-2051-9

Laursen, B. (2018). What is collaborative, interdisciplinary reasoning? The heart of interdisciplinary team research. *Informing Science: The International Journal of Emerging Transdiscipline, 21,* 75–106. doi:10.28945/4010

Leedy, P., Ormrod, J., & Johnson, L. (2019). *Practical research: Planning and design* (12th ed.). New York City, NY: Pearson.

Marshall, C., & Rossman, G. B. (2016). *Designing qualitative research* (6th ed.). Los Angeles, CA: Sage.

Melin-Johansson, C., Palmqvist, R., & Ronnberg, L. (2017). Clinical intuition in the nursing process and decision-making—A mixed-studies review. *Journal of Clinical Nursing, 26*(23-24), 3936–3949. doi:10.1111/jocn.13814

Melnyk, B. M., & Fineout-Overholt, E. (2019). *Evidence-based practice in nursing & healthcare: A guide to best practice* (4th ed.). Philadelphia, PA: Wolters Kluwer.

Mentes, J. (2008, 2012). *Nursing standard of practice: Managing oral hydration.* Retrieved from https://consultgeri.org/geriatric-topics/hydration-management

Morton, P. G. (2017). Nursing education research: An editor's view. *Journal of Professional Nursing, 33*(5), 311–312. doi:10.1016/j.profnurs.2017.08.002

National Institute of Nursing Research (NINR). (2016). *The NINR strategic plan: Advancing science, improving lives: A vision for nursing science.* Retrieved from https://www.ninr.nih.gov/sites/files/docs/NINR_StratPlan2016_reduced.pdf

National League for Nursing (NLN). (2019). *About the NLN: Mission and goals.* Retrieved from http://www.nln.org/about/mission-goals

Polifroni. E. (2018). Philosophy of science: An introduction and a grounding for your practice. In J. Butts & K. Rich (Eds.), *Philosophies and theories for advanced nursing practice* (3rd ed., pp. 3–18). Burlington, MA: Jones & Bartlett Learning.

Quality and Safety Education for Nurses (QSEN) Institute. (2019). *Graduate QSEN competencies.* Retrieved from http://qsen.org/competencies/graduate-ksas/

Rashkovits, S., & Drach-Zahavy, A. (2017). The moderating role of team resources in translating nursing teams' accountability into learning and performance: A cross sectional study. *Journal of Advance Nursing, 73*(5), 1124–1136. doi:10.1111/jan.13200

Reed, P. G. (2019). Intermodernism: A philosophical perspective for development of scientific nursing theory. *Advances in Nursing Science, 42*(1), 17–27. doi:10.1097/ANS.0000000000000249

Rega, M., Telaretti, F., Alvaro, R., & Kangasniemi, M. (2017). Philosophical and theoretical content of the nursing discipline in academic education: A critical interpretative synthesis. *Nursing Education Today, 57*(1), 74–81. doi:10.1016/j.nedt.2017.07.001

Reinoso, H., Bartlett, J., & Bennett, S. (2018). Teaching differential diagnosis to nurse practitioner students. *The Journal of Nurse Practitioners, 14*(10), e207–e212. doi:10.3928/01484834-20140724-02

Rodgers, B. (2018). The evolution of nursing science. In J. Butts & K. Rich (Eds.), *Philosophies and theories for advanced nursing practice* (3rd ed., pp. 19–50). Burlington, MA: Jones & Bartlett Learning.

Roy, C. (2011). Research based on the Roy adaptation model: Last 25 years. *Nursing Science Quarterly, 24*(4), 314–320. doi:10.1177/0894318411419218

Roy, C. (2019). Nursing knowledge in the 21st century: Domain-derived and basic science practice shaped. *Advances in Nursing Science, 42*(1), 28–42. doi:10.1097/ANS.0000000000000240

Sakamoto, M. (2018). Nursing knowledge: A middle ground exploration. *Nursing Philosophy, 19*(3), e12209. doi:10.1111/nup.12209

Silva, M. C. (1977). Philosophy, science, theory: Interrelationships and implications for nursing research. *Image-Journal of Nursing Scholarship, 9*(3), 59–63.

Smith, M. (2019). Regenerating nursing's disciplinary perspective. *Advances in Nursing Science, 42*(1), 3–16. doi:10.1097/ANS.0000000000000241

Smyth, O., & McCabe, C. (2017). Think and think again! Clinical decision making by advanced nurse practitioners in the emergency department. *International Emergency Nursing, 31*(1), 72–74. doi:10.1016/j.ienj.2016.08.001

Statler, A., & Mota, A. (2018). Using systems thinking to envision quality and safety in healthcare. *Nursing Management, 42*(9), 32–39. doi:10.1097/01.NUMA.0000529925.66375.d0

Straus, S. E., Glasziou, P., Richardson, W. S., Rosenberg, W., & Haynes, R. B. (2019). *Evidence-based medicine: How to practice and teach EBM* (5th ed.). Edinburgh: Churchill Livingstone Elsevier.

Szczygiel, D., & Mikolajczak, M. (2018). Emotional intelligence buffers the effects of negative emotions on job burnout of female nurses. *Frontiers in Psychology, 9,* 2649. doi:10.3389/fpsyg.2018.02649

Thorne, S. (2018). What can qualitative studies offer in a world where evidence drives decisions? *Asia-Pacific Journal of Oncology Nursing, 5*(1), 43–45. doi:10.4103/apjon.apjon_51_17.

Thorne, S., & Sawatzky, R. (2014). Particularizing the general: Sustaining theoretical integrity in the context of an evidence-based practice agenda. *Advances in Nursing Science, 37*(1), 5–18. doi:10.1097/ANS.0000000000000011

Tuomikoski, A.-M., Ruotsalainen, H., Mikkonen, K., Miettunen, J., & Kääriäinen, M. (2018). The competence of nurse mentors in mentoring students in clinical practice—A cross-sectional study. *Nurse Education Today, 71,* 78–83. doi:10.1016/j.nedt.2018.09.008

Wieringa, S., Engebretsen, E., Heggen, K., & Greenhalgh, T. (2018). Rethinking bias and truth in evidence-based health care. *Journal of Evaluation in Clinical Practice, 24*(5), 930–938. doi:10.1111/jep.13010

Wu, F., Rubenstein, L., & Yoon, J, (2018). Team functioning as a predictor of patient outcomes in early medical home implementation. *Health Care Management Review, 43*(3), 238–248. doi:10.1097/HMR.0000000000000196

Evolution of Research in Building Evidence-Based Nursing Practice

Jennifer R. Gray

http://evolve.elsevier.com/Gray/practice/

Research in nursing began when Florence Nightingale investigated patient morbidity and mortality during the Crimean War. She applied her findings in hospitals in England and disseminated her experiences through the books she wrote such as *Notes on Hospitals* (1859/ 2015). Nursing research, however, did not become a focus for the profession until nurses began conducting studies of nursing education in the 1930s and 1940s. Nurses and nursing roles were the focus of research in the 1950s and 1960s. However, in the late 1970s and 1980s, the focus of many nurse researchers shifted to studies to improve nursing practice. This emphasis continued in the 1990s with research focused on describing nursing phenomena, testing the effectiveness of nursing interventions, and examining patient outcomes. The goal in this millennium is the development of evidence-based nursing practice.

Evidence-based practice (EBP) is the conscientious integration of the best research evidence with clinical expertise and patient values and needs in the delivery of quality, cost-effective health care (Straus, Glasziou, Richardson, & Haynes, 2011). Chapter 1 presents a model depicting the elements of EBP (see Fig. 1.2) and an example of applying a clinical practice guideline for the assessment, prevention, and treatment of dehydration of older adults. Chapter 2 was developed to increase your understanding of how nursing research evolved over the past 160 years and of the current movement of the profession toward EBP. The chapter includes the historical events relevant to nursing research, identifies the methodologies used in nursing to develop research evidence, and concludes with a discussion of the best research evidence needed to build an EBP (Melnyk & Fineout-Overholt, 2019).

HISTORICAL DEVELOPMENT OF RESEARCH IN NURSING

Following Nightingale's work (1840–1910), nursing research received minimal attention until the mid-1900s. Today, nurses obtain federal, corporate, and foundational funding for their research; conduct complex studies in multiple settings; and generate sound research evidence for practice. The transformation of nursing research did not occur easily or quickly; it required increased education and sustained effort to arrive where we are today. Tables 2.1 and 2.2 identify key historical events that have influenced the development of nursing research and the movement toward EBP. Table 2.3 provides a linear record of the growth in the number and type of nursing research journals, the means for disseminating the findings of nurse-conducted studies. These historical events are discussed in the following sections.

Florence Nightingale

Nightingale has been described as a researcher and reformer who influenced nursing specifically and health care in general. Nightingale, in her book *Notes on Nursing* (1859), described her initial research activities, which focused on the importance of a healthy environment in promoting the patient's physical and mental

TABLE 2.1	Historical Events Influencing Research in Nursing (1850-1980)
Years	**Era and Events**
1850–1900	**Birth of a Profession** • Florence Nightingale is recognized as first nurse researcher. • The National League for Nursing (NLN) is founded. • *American Journal of Nursing,* a journal for nurses, is published for the first time.
1901–1930	**Graduate Education in Nursing** • Teachers College, Columbia University, offers first doctorate of education specifically for nurses. • Yale University offers first master's in nursing degree.
1931–1960	**Nursing Organizations and Research** • The Association of Collegiate Schools of Nursing (AACN) is formed to promote conduct of research. • The American Nurses Association (ANA) conducted a study of nursing functions and activities. • The ANA established the American Nurses Foundation (ANF) to fund nursing research. • Teachers College, Columbia University, established the Institute of Research and Service in Nursing Education. • Regional nursing organizations are developed to support and disseminate nursing research: Southern Regional Education Board (SREB), Western Interstate Commission for Higher Education (WICHE), and New England Board of Higher Education (NEBHE).
1961–1970	**ANA Focus on Research** • ANA sponsors the first nursing research conferences. • ANA establishes the Commission on Nursing Research.
1971–1980	**Foundations of Evidence-Based Practice (EBP)** • Dr. Cochrane publishes the book, *Effectiveness and Efficiency,* introducing concepts relevant to EBP. • ANA establishes the Council of Nurse Researchers. • Nursing diagnoses are being developed and the first Nursing Diagnosis Conference is held. The group later becomes the North American Nursing Diagnosis Association (NANDA). • The Stetler/Marram Model for Application of Research Findings to Practice is published, with focus on using research to improve nursing practice. • The Midwest Nursing Research Society (MNRS), a regional nursing research organization, is established with members in 13 states. • WICHE Regional Nursing Research Development Project is conducted.

well-being. To determine the extent of the environments' influence, she gathered data on the environment, such as ventilation, cleanliness, temperature, purity of water, and diet (Herbert, 1981).

Nightingale's data collection and statistical analyses during the Crimean War were sophisticated for that period (Palmer, 1977). After she collected data on soldier morbidity and mortality rates, she presented her results in tables and pie charts that communicated the causes of death, factors influencing the deaths, and outcomes of changes that she and her nurses made. Nightingale was the first woman elected to the Royal Statistical Society (Oakley, 2010), and her research was highlighted in the periodical *Scientific American* in 1984 (Cohen, 1984).

Through her research and her effective communication, Nightingale was able to instigate attitudinal, organizational, and social changes. She changed the attitudes of the military and society toward the care of the sick. The military began to view the sick and injured as having the right to adequate food, suitable quarters, and appropriate medical treatment, a change that greatly reduced the mortality rate (Cook, 1913). Nightingale improved the hospital construction, hospital management, and army administration. Because of Nightingale's research evidence and influence, society began to accept responsibility for testing public water, improving sanitation, preventing starvation, and decreasing morbidity and mortality rates (Palmer, 1977).

TABLE 2.2	Historical Events Influencing Research in Nursing (1981–2020)
1981–1990	**Nursing Research and National Efforts** • Sackett and his collaborators develop methodologies to determine the best evidence for practice. • The findings of the Conduct and Utilization of Research in Nursing (CURN) Project are published. • The National Center for Nursing Research (NCNR) is established as part of the National Institutes of Health (NIH). • The federal government also establishes the Agency for Health Care Policy and Research (AHCPR). • The American Nurses Credentialing Center (ANCC) implements the Magnet Recognition Program® for Excellence in Nursing Services, which includes criteria related to nurse-led research.
1991–2000	**Evidence-Based Practice (EBP), Prevention, and Health Promotion** • The Centers for Disease Control and Prevention (CDC) provides research priorities in the form of health promotion and disease prevention objectives, published as *Healthy People 2000*. • The NCNR is renamed the National Institute of Nursing Research (NINR), increasing the recognition of the importance of nursing research. • The Cochrane Collaboration begins its efforts to produce and disseminate systematic reviews and EBP guidelines. • The AHCPR is renamed Agency for Healthcare Research and Quality (AHRQ). • The CDC continues its efforts to improve the health of the nation by publishing *Healthy People 2010*.
2001–2010	**Linking Quality Care and EBP** • Stetler publishes model Steps of Research Utilization to Facilitate EBP. • The Institute of Medicine (IOM) shines the spotlight on the need for improved health care by publishing *Crossing the Quality Chasm: A New Health System for the 21st Century*. • The Joint Commission (JC) revises accreditation policies for hospitals to include the use of EBP. • North American Nursing Diagnosis Association (NANDA) becomes an international organization—NANDA-I. • The Robert Wood Johnson Foundation funds Quality and Safety Education for Nurses (QSEN) initiative involving 15 schools. • The American Association of Colleges of Nursing (AACN) releases Position Statement on Nursing Research. • QSEN website (http://qsen.org/) is launched that features teaching strategies and resources.
2011–2020	**Quality Care and Patient-Oriented Care Outcomes** • The QSEN collaboration publishes Graduate QSEN Competencies online. • The NINR refines its mission statement. • The CDC makes *Healthy People 2020* available online. • The Patient-Centered Outcomes Research Institute is launched to refocus research on the topics and outcomes most important to patients. • The AHRQ conducts studies to identify innovative ways to produce and disseminate EBP guidelines. • The CDC begins the development of *Healthy People 2030*. • NINR leads NIH efforts to establish Symptom Science Center.

Early 1900s

From 1900 to 1950, research activities in nursing were limited. Most nursing education programs were situated in hospitals, lasted 3 years, and culminated in a diploma. Diploma programs were the norm until the

Goldmark Report was published in 1923. The report described the results of a national study related to nursing education (Abdellah, 1972; Johnson, 1977). The researchers and consultants who prepared the Goldmark Report recommended that schools of nursing needed to

TABLE 2.3	Growth in the Number and Types of Nursing Research Journals
Year Publication Began	**Name of Journal**
1952	*Nursing Research*
1960	*International Nursing Review (International Council of Nurses Journal)*
1963	*International Journal of Nursing Studies*
1967	*Image,* now titled *Journal of Nursing Scholarship*
1969	*Canadian Journal of Nursing Research*
1978	*Research in Nursing & Health*
1978	*Advances in Nursing Science*
1979	*Western Journal of Nursing Research*
1983	*Annual Review of Nursing Research*
1983	*Nursing Economics*
1987	*Scholarly Inquiry for Nursing Practice*
1988	*Applied Nursing Research*
1988	*Nursing Science Quarterly*
1990	*Nursing Diagnosis,* now titled *International Journal of Nursing Terminologies and Classifications*
1992	*Clinical Nursing Research*
1993	*Journal of Nursing Measurement*
1994	*Qualitative Health Research*
1996	*Journal of Research in Nursing*
1998	*Evidence-Based Nursing*
1999	*Journal of Hospice and Palliative Nursing*
2000	*Pain Management Nursing*
2000	*Biological Research for Nursing*
2001	*Journal of Nursing Research* (previously available only in Taiwanese)
2001	*Newborn and Infant Nursing Reviews*
2002	*BioMed Central (BMC) Nursing*
2004	*Worldviews on Evidence-Based Nursing*
2007	*Asian Nursing Research (Korean Society of Nursing Society)*

be established in university settings and culminate in a baccalaureate degree. The baccalaureate degree in nursing was needed for many reasons, one of which was the degree provided a foundation for graduate nursing education. The first master's of nursing degree program was offered by Yale University in 1929. Teachers College at Columbia University offered the first Doctor in Education for nurses in 1923 to prepare teachers for the profession (see Table 2.1). The Association of Collegiate Schools of Nursing was organized in 1932 to represent the interests of faculty and administrators of baccalaureate and graduate nursing programs. In 1969, the association was renamed the American Association of Colleges of Nursing (AACN). The AACN continues today with its mission being to serve as a "catalyst for excellence and innovation in nursing education" (AACN, 2019b). This organization

also sponsored the publication of the first research journal in nursing, *Nursing Research,* in 1952 (Fitzpatrick, 1978) (see Table 2.3). AACN continues to influence nursing research by promoting research-intensive environments to support nursing science and delineating the research-related roles for nurses educated at different levels (AACN, 2006).

In 1922, six nursing students at Indiana University Training School for Nurses started a school-based honor society, which became Sigma Theta Tau International. Sigma now has over 134,000 members in more than 90 countries (Sigma, 2019a). In addition to promoting leadership development and international collaboration, Sigma has funded studies and sponsored national and international research conferences. The university-based chapters of Sigma provide research funds to members and frequently sponsor research conferences to promote the dissemination of research findings. *Image* was a peer-reviewed journal initially published in 1967 by Sigma. This journal, now titled *Journal of Nursing Scholarship,* includes many international nursing studies and global health articles. A major goal of Sigma is to advance scholarship in nursing by promoting the conduct of research, communication of study findings, and use of research evidence in nursing (Sigma, 2019a).

Beginning in the 1940s, the focus of nursing shifted from nursing education to the organization and delivery of nursing services. Studies were conducted on the numbers and kinds of nursing personnel, staffing patterns, patient classification systems, patient and nurse satisfaction, and unit arrangement. Types of care, such as comprehensive care, home care, and progressive patient care, were evaluated to determine the best approach to patient care. These evaluations of care laid the foundation for standards of care and the development of self-study manuals. The self-study manuals later evolved into the quality improvement processes that we use today (Gortner & Nahm, 1977).

Nursing Research in the 1950s and 1960s

In 1950, the American Nurses Association (ANA) initiated a 5-year study on nursing functions and activities. The findings were reported in the book, *Twenty Thousand Nurses Tell Their Story* (Hughes, Hughes, & Deutscher, 1958). This study enabled the ANA to develop statements on functions, standards, and qualifications for professional nurses. During the same time, clinical research expanded as groups of nurses developed standards of care for specialty areas, such as community health, psychiatric, medical-surgical, pediatric, and obstetrics nursing. The research conducted by ANA and the specialty groups provided the basis for the nursing practice standards that currently guide professional nursing practice (Fitzpatrick, 1978).

Educational studies were conducted in the 1950s and 1960s to determine the most effective educational preparation for the registered nurse (RN). During World War II, the need for nurses was acute and the Cadet Nursing Corps was started. The Corps program demonstrated that nursing education programs could be less than 3 years long and produce clinically skilled and knowledgeable nurses (Appalachian State University [ASU], 2019). After the war, nurse educator Mildred Montag completed her doctoral degree and in her dissertation she advocated for a 2-year nursing program.

Dr. Montag was the first to develop and evaluate an associate degree nursing program (Harker, 2017; McBride, 1996). The Kellogg Foundation funded a demonstration project for associate degree nursing programs, with seven schools in four states (ASU, 2019). The characteristics of each school and nursing students were different so the researchers could determine which characteristics were important to student persistence and quality. The debate as to the appropriate length of nursing education programs continued. Nurse researchers studied student characteristics, such as admission and retention patterns and the elements that promoted success in nursing education and practice, for both associate degree–prepared and baccalaureate degree–prepared nurses (Downs & Fleming, 1979). These early studies did not end the debate.

Research initiatives were instigated by universities and the ANA during the 1950s. In 1953, an Institute for Research and Service in Nursing Education was established at Teachers College, Columbia University, which provided research-learning experiences for doctoral students (Werley, 1977). The American Nurses Foundation (ANF) was chartered in 1955 to work alongside ANA in the promotion of research. From 1955 to 2012, the ANF used donor funding to provide early career small grants to over 1000 nurse researchers. Messmer, Zalon, and Phillips (2014) studied the careers of these nurses and learned that approximately one-third of the researchers were later recipients of federal research funding. In 1956, the Committee on Research and Studies was established to guide ANA research (See, 1977).

The Department of Nursing Research was established in the Walter Reed Army Institute of Research in 1957 (see Table 2.1). This was the first nursing unit in a research institution that emphasized clinical nursing research (Werley, 1977). The same year, the Southern Regional Education Board, the Western Interstate Commission for Higher Education (WICHE), and the New England Board of Higher Education were created. These organizations remain actively involved today in promoting research and disseminating the findings. ANA sponsored the first of a series of research conferences in 1965. Only studies relevant to nursing and conducted by a nurse researcher were presented (See, 1977). During the 1960s, nurse leaders advocated for research resources, such as laboratories and funding, and for nurses to receive research preparation through PhD programs. A growing number of clinical studies focused on quality care and the development of criteria to measure patient outcomes. Intensive care units were being developed, promoting the investigation of nursing interventions, staffing patterns, and cost effectiveness of care (Gortner & Nahm, 1977).

During the 1960s, nursing research was also being disseminated through international venues. The International Council of Nurses began publishing the *International Nursing Review* in 1960, and British nursing leaders started the *International Journal of Nursing Studies*. Near the end of the decade, the *Canadian Journal of Nursing Research* was launched (see Table 2.3).

Nursing Research in the 1970s

In the 1970s, the nursing process became the focus of many studies, with investigations of assessment techniques, nursing diagnosis classification, goal-setting methods, and specific nursing interventions. The first Nursing Diagnosis Conference, held in 1973, evolved into the North American Nursing Diagnosis Association (NANDA). In 2002, NANDA became international and is now known as NANDA International, Inc. (NANDA-I). The organization supports research activities focused on identifying appropriate diagnoses for nursing and generating an effective diagnostic process. NANDA's journal, *Nursing Diagnosis,* was published in 1990 and was later renamed *International Journal of Nursing Knowledge* (NANDA-I, 2018).

The educational studies of the 1970s evaluated teaching methods and student learning experiences. The first nursing organization, known today as the National League for Nursing (NLN), has been a consistent supporter of research related to nursing education (Duffy, Fren, & Patterson, 2011). In the early days, the NLN established standards for nursing programs and advocated for nursing education to be controlled by nurses. In more recent years, the NLN "is committed to the promotion of evidence-based nursing education through research, scholarship, publication, pedagogical excellence, and collaboration" (NLN, 2019). In addition to providing small grants, the NLN has identified and disseminated research priorities and serves as a resource for tools and instruments for nursing education research (NLN, 2019).

During the 1970s, the Midwest Nursing Research Society (MNRS) began from a group of nurses collaborating on a research project. They recognized the need to support each other's research efforts and formed a society with members in 13 states (Lach & Gaspar, 2018; MNRS, 2019). In 1976, the *Journal of Advanced Nursing* was published for the first time. Its aim was to publish high-quality research and scholarship that would influence practice, policy, and management strategies (Zeleznik, Vosner, & Kokol, 2017).

Different approaches to structuring nursing care were tried during the 1970s. One was primary nursing care, which involved assigning an RN to a patient at admission. The primary nurse was accountable for the patient's care 24 hours a day (Hambleton, 1998). Primary nurses provided daily care for their assigned patients, served as a liaison between the family and the physician, planned the patient's nursing care, and prepared the family and patient for discharge. Studies were conducted to examine the outcomes of primary nursing care delivery models, compared to team nursing. Hospitals began to have challenges filling all their RN positions and moved away from the primary nursing care delivery model, except in critical care areas. Today, on medical surgical units, hospitals use some modification of team nursing with teams comprised of RNs, licensed practical nurses, and nursing assistants.

The number of nurse practitioners (NPs) and clinical nurse specialists (CNSs) with master's degrees increased rapidly during the 1970s. The NP, CNS, nurse midwifery, and nurse anesthetist roles have been researched extensively to measure their impact on productivity, quality, and cost of health care. In addition, those clinicians with master's degrees acquired the background to conduct research and to use research evidence in practice.

In the 1970s, nursing scholars began developing models, conceptual frameworks, and theories to guide nursing practice (Chinn & Kramer, 2018). The profession's body of knowledge included the writings of nursing theorists (Parse, 2017), whose works also provided frameworks for nursing studies. In 1978, a new journal, *Advances in Nursing Science*, began publishing the works of nursing theorists and the research related to their theories. In the early 1970s, an increased number of nurses were earning doctor of philosophy (PhD) degrees in other disciplines (Hawkins & Nezat, 2009). By the end of the decade, the number of PhD programs in nursing increased as well as the number of nurses prepared at the doctoral level (Chinn & Kramer, 2018). Some of the nurses with doctoral degrees were active researchers, increasing the number and complexity of nursing studies; however, other nurses prepared at the doctoral level did not become actively involved in research. In 1970, the ANA Commission on Nursing Research was established; in turn, this commission established the Council of Nurse Researchers in 1972 to advance research activities, provide an exchange of ideas, and recognize excellence in research. The commission also prepared position papers on subjects' rights in research and on federal guidelines concerning research and human subjects (see Chapter 9), and it sponsored research programs nationally and internationally (See, 1977). The Council of Nurse Researchers was dissolved in the late 1990s when ANA changed its organizational structure. Board members from the American Academy of Nursing formed a national organization to promote "Better Health through Nursing Science." The organization, the Council for the Advancement of Nursing Science (CANS), was and continues today as a partner with regional nursing research societies and other research-focused organizations (CANS, 2016).

Prior to 1955, nurses rarely received federal research funding. From 1955 to 1976, federal funds for nursing research increased significantly, up to a total slightly more than $39 million. Although the increase was significant, it could not compare to the funding for medical research. The federal government paid $493 million to medical researchers in 1974 alone (de Tornyay, 1977).

Two new research journals begun in the 1970s, *Research in Nursing & Health* in 1978 and *Western Journal of Nursing Research* in 1979, increased the communication of nursing research findings. However, the findings of many studies conducted and published in the 1970s were not being used in practice, so Stetler and Marram (1976) developed a model to promote the communication and use of research findings in practice (see Table 2.1). Over time, Stetler (1994, 2001) refined the model to reflect a conceptual framework of knowledge utilization and to be more useful to nurses in practice (see Chapter 19 for a description of this model). By following the Stetler model, nurses were able to identify a study with potential application to their clinical area and critique the study. If the study was rigorous, the nurses were guided by the model to state the findings, substantiate the study's findings, and determine if the findings fit the setting and whether they could be feasibly used in practice. Then the nurses would decide whether to apply the findings and exactly

how. Research utilization was a precursor to EBP (Melnyk & Fineout-Overholt, 2019).

Professor Archie Cochrane originated the concept of EBP with a book published in 1972 titled *Effectiveness and Efficiency: Random Reflections on Health Services*. In the book, Cochrane argued that most healthcare interventions being implemented were not supported by evidence (Shah & Chung, 2009). Because he had a disorder called porphyria, he knew first hand that interventions were not based on evidence (Brucker, 2016). He advocated valid and reliable evidence was required to improve the quality of care and other patient outcomes. To facilitate the use of research evidence in practice, the Cochrane Center was established in 1992, and the Cochrane Collaboration in 1993 (Shah & Chung, 2009), the name being given in recognition of Cochrane's advocacy. The staff of the Cochrane Collaboration and Library curate and store numerous EBP resources, such as systematic reviews of research on specific topics and evidence-based guidelines for practice (discussed later in this chapter) (see the Cochrane Collaboration at http://www.cochrane.org/).

Nursing Research in the 1980s and 1990s

The conduct of clinical nursing research was the focus in the 1980s and 1990s. Research reports began to appear in a variety of clinical journals, such as *Archives of Psychiatric Nursing, Cancer Nursing, Heart & Lung,* and *Rehabilitation Nursing.* One new research journal was started in 1987, *Scholarly Inquiry for Nursing Practice,* and two in 1988, *Applied Nursing Research* and *Nursing Science Quarterly.* Sigma introduced a new journal in 1994, called *WORLDviews on Evidence-Based Nursing,* primarily to disseminate knowledge synthesis articles and reports of large-scale studies that have implications for EBP. The journal's focus is to link evidence to action in clinical settings and other settings where nurses practice (Sigma, 2019b).

The need for additional nursing research was the impetus for the formation of regional nursing organizations focusing on research. The Western Institute of Nursing (WIN) began in 1985, Southern Nursing Research Society (SNRS) in 1986, and Eastern Nursing Research Society (ENRS) in 1988 (ENRS, n.d.; SNRS, n.d.; WIN, 2016). The annual conferences of the regional nursing research organizations have provided an environment for new nurse researchers to present their work and be mentored by more experienced researchers.

The body of empirical knowledge generated through nurses conducting clinical research continued to increase. Unfortunately, little of this knowledge was used in practice. Two major projects were launched to promote the use of research-based nursing interventions in practice: The WICHE Regional Nursing Research Development Project and the Conduct and Utilization of Research in Nursing (CURN) Project (see Table 2.1). In these projects, nurse researchers, with the support of federal funding, designed and implemented strategies for using research findings in practice. The WICHE Project participants selected research-based interventions for use in practice and then functioned as change agents to implement the selected intervention in a clinical agency. Because of the limited amount of research that had been conducted, the project staff and participants had difficulty identifying adequate clinical studies with findings ready for use in practice (Krueger, Nelson, & Wolanin, 1978).

The CURN Project was a 5-year venture (1975–1980) directed by Horsley, Crane, Crabtree, and Wood (1983) to increase the utilization of research findings. To accomplish this goal, CURN participants disseminated study findings, identified modifications to be made at the organizational level to facilitate research utilization, and encouraged researchers to collaborate to design and implement research with direct transferability to clinical practice. Research utilization was seen as a process to be implemented by an organization rather than by an individual nurse. The project team defined the activities of research utilization as identifying and synthesizing the findings of multiple studies on a specific topic or conceptual area, describing these findings of similar studies in a meaningful way, and transforming the findings into a solution or clinical protocol. The clinical protocol was then transformed into specific nursing actions (innovations) that were administered to patients. The implementation of the innovation was to be followed by clinical evaluation of the new practice to ascertain whether it produced the predicted result (Horsley et al., 1983). The clinical protocols developed during the project were published to encourage nurses in other healthcare agencies to use these research-based intervention protocols in their practice (CURN, 1981–1982).

To ensure that the studies were incorporated into nursing practice, the findings needed to be synthesized for different topics. In 1983, the first volume of the *Annual Review of Nursing Research* was published (Werley

& Fitzpatrick, 1983). Following synthesis of research findings, authors frequently describe priorities for this area of research. The *Annual Review of Nursing Research* continues to be published once a year to (1) expand the synthesis and dissemination of research findings, (2) promote the use of research findings in practice, and (3) identify directions for future research.

Many nurses obtained master's and doctoral degrees during the 1980s and 1990s, and postdoctoral education was encouraged for nurse researchers. The ANA (1989) stated that nurses at all levels of education have roles in research, which extend from reading and critically appraising studies to designing and conducting complex funded programs of research (see Chapter 1).

Nurse visionaries had a goal that nursing research would be recognized as essential to health research (Grady, 2018). Most of the federal funds in the 1980s were designated for studies involving the diagnosis and cure of diseases. Therefore nursing received a small percentage of the federal research and development funds (approximately 2% to 3%) as compared with medicine (approximately 90%), even though nursing personnel greatly outnumbered medical personnel (Larson, 1984). However, in 1986, the ANA achieved a major political victory when the National Center for Nursing Research (NCNR) was created within the National Institutes of Health (NIH) (Grady, 2018). This center was created after years of work and two presidential vetoes (Bauknecht, 1986; National Institute of Nursing Research [NINR], 2010; Williams, 1984). The purpose of the NCNR was to support the conduct of basic and clinical nursing research and the dissemination of findings. With its creation, nursing research had visibility at the federal level for the first time. Since the beginning, the focus has been on the advancement of nursing science (NINR, 2010).

In the early years, the leaders of NCNR developed the mission, established programs of research, and decided how to best organize the activities of the center to have the greatest impact on improving health (Grady, 2018). During the tenure of its first director, Dr. Ada Sue Hinshaw, the NCNR became the NINR (see Table 2.2). This change in title in 1993 reflected a change in status and enhanced the recognition of nursing as a research discipline with expanded funding.

Outcomes research emerged as an important methodology for documenting the effectiveness of healthcare services in the 1980s and 1990s. This type of research evolved from the quality assessment and quality assurance functions that originated with the professional standards review organizations in 1972. During the 1980s, William Roper, the director of the Health Care Finance Administration, promoted outcomes research for determining the quality and cost effectiveness of patient care (Johnson, 1993). Nurse researchers in the 1990s addressed the need for nurses to join teams who were studying the effectiveness of different treatments (Cummings, 1992) and the challenges of measuring patient satisfaction as an outcome of nursing care (Lin, 1996).

In 1989, the Agency for Health Care Policy and Research (AHCPR) was established to facilitate the conduct of outcomes research (Rettig, 1991). The agency also had an active role in communicating research findings to healthcare practitioners and was responsible for publishing the first national evidence-based clinical practice guidelines in 1989. Several of these guidelines, including the latest research findings with directives for practice, were published in the 1990s. The Healthcare Research and Quality Act of 1999 reauthorized the AHCPR, changing its name to the Agency for Healthcare Research and Quality (AHRQ). This significant change positioned the AHRQ as a scientific partner with a mission to "produce evidence to make health care safer, higher quality, more accessible, equitable, and affordable" (AHRQ, 2019a). AHRQ works with other federal health-related departments and agencies to ensure that "evidence is understood and used" (AHRQ, 2019a).

Building on the process of research utilization, physicians, nurses, and other healthcare professionals focused on the development of EBP during the 1990s. A research group led by Dr. David Sackett at McMaster University in Canada developed explicit research methodologies to determine the *best evidence* for practice. The term *evidence-based* was first used by David Eddy in 1990 (Eddy, 2011), with the focus on providing evidence to support medicine decision making (Straus et al., 2011).

In 1990, the leaders of ANA established the American Nurses Credentialing Center (ANCC) and approved a program for hospitals called the Magnet Recognition Program® for Excellence in Nursing Services. The establishment of the Magnet designation evolved from a 1983 study by the American Academy of Nursing. In this study, characteristics of hospitals that attracted and retained nurses were identified (ANCC, n.d.). These hospital characteristics became the foundation for Magnet designation. The Magnet program has evolved over the last 30 years but has remained true to its commitment to improve patient outcomes by supporting nurses and promoting the conduct of research by nurses at the bedside (Hatfield et al., 2016).

Nursing Research in the 21st Century

The focus on EBP has become stronger over the last decade. The Joint Commission's (JC) accreditation standards promote the use of evidence-based clinical practice guidelines and screening tools to ensure patient safety and quality care (JC, 2019). In nursing, CANS was initiated in 2000 to expand the development of research evidence. The council has as its goal to foster better health through nursing science (CANS, 2016). The focus on EBP in nursing has resulted in the conduct of more biological studies and randomized controlled trials (RCTs) and the publication of *Biological Research for Nursing* in 2000 and *WORLDviews on Evidence-Based Nursing* in 2004.

The vision for nursing research in the 21st century includes conducting quality studies through the use of a variety of methodologies, synthesizing the study findings into the best research evidence, using this research evidence to guide practice, and examining the outcomes of EBP (Melnyk & Fineout-Overholt, 2019; Moorhead, Swanson, Johnson, & Maas, 2018). Leaders for healthcare systems are pushing for implementation of EBP, and examples are being published. For example, Cullen et al. (2018) published how the University of Iowa Hospitals and Clinics have implemented EBP. Grinspun and Bajnok (2018) published a book of best practices to develop, implement, and evaluate EBP guidelines. These publications as well as others provide a strong foundation for national research initiatives.

CURRENT NATIONAL RESEARCH INITIATIVES

Different agencies and institutes within the US government play key roles in current research initiatives, from developing goals for health promotion to identifying priorities for funding. Nurse educators and researchers also play key roles in promoting quality and safety. They teach students about research and EBP and conduct studies to improve health outcomes. These and other topics are covered in this section.

Research Focused on Health Promotion and Illness Prevention

The focus of healthcare research and funding has expanded from the treatment of illness to include health promotion and illness prevention. *Healthy People 2000, Healthy People 2010,* and *Healthy People 2020* have identified the national goals related to improving the health of the country's citizens (see Table 2.2). The Office of Disease Prevention and Health Promotion (ODPHP) within the US Department of Health and Human Services (ODPHP, 2019b) is the lead organization for these efforts. Work has begun on the objectives for *Healthy People 2030* (ODPHP, 2019a). One of the differences that will be reflected in the new objectives is the focus on leading health indicators (LHIs). The LHIs will be selected based on their public health burden, the magnitude of the health disparity, the degree to which changes in the LHI could indicate a potential threat to the health of the nation, and the actionability of the objective (ODPHP, 2018). One nurse is serving on the Secretary's Advisory Committee for *Healthy People 2030,* and nurses and other citizens will have opportunities to provide input during the development process. These objectives will indicate the federal priorities for research, including nursing research.

Outcomes Research With Patient Engagement

In 2010, the Patient-Centered Outcomes Research Institute (PCORI) was established by the Affordable Care Act to engage patients in research—not just as subjects, but as partners in determining the topics that should be studied and the methods that should be used (Bernstein, Getchell, & Harwood, 2019; PCORI, 2018). PCORI brings stakeholders together from healthcare facilities, insurance companies, scientists, and communities to identify funding priorities. PCORI began funding studies in 2012 and continues to do so, with the most studied health conditions being mental/behavioral health followed by cancer (PCORI, n.d.). The institute seeks studies that address the priorities and concerns of patients and that compare the clinical outcomes of two different courses of treatment.

Linking Nurse Characteristics and Staffing to Quality Outcomes

The Institute of Medicine published a report in 2001, *Crossing the Quality Chasm: A New Health System for the 21st Century,* that emphasized the importance of quality and safety in the delivery of health care. When the report was published, nurse researchers were already studying patient outcomes related to nursing resources. For patients with acquired immunodeficiency syndrome (AIDS), mortality had been found to be lower in hospitals with Magnet designation and those with dedicated-AIDS units than in hospitals without Magnet designation and dedicated-AIDS units (Aiken, Sloane, Lake, Sochalski, & Weber, 1999). Using data from hospitals in four countries, Aiken, Clarke, and Sloane (2002) found high levels of job dissatisfaction and burnout among nurses, which were increased in hospitals with weak organizational support.

The education of nurses was also studied as a factor in patient outcomes. In 2003, Aiken, Clark, Cheung, Sloane, and Silber published the findings of their study with data from 168 hospitals in Pennsylvania that provided evidence of the importance of nurses being educated at the baccalaureate level. When the proportion of direct-care RNs with baccalaureate degrees increased, more surgical patients survived. The findings of the Aiken et al. (2003) study linked lower patient-nurse ratio with improved patient survival. Aiken and colleagues conducted several studies of the effects of nurse staffing, education, patient-nurse ratios, and organizational characteristics on patient outcomes of mortality and morbidity (Aiken, Clarke, Sloane, Sochalski, & Silber, 2002; Finlayson, Aiken, & Nakarada-Kordic, 2007; Lake et al., 2018). The impact of nurse staffing, nursing education, and work environments continued to be studied as the healthcare system evolved over the next 10 years. These are still priority areas for future research to improve the healthcare system.

Linking QSEN Competencies and Nursing Research

The Quality and Safety Education for Nurses (QSEN, 2019a) was an initiative in response to concerns about poor patient outcomes and errors by healthcare professionals. QSEN's ultimate goal is to improve the quality and safety of healthcare systems (QSEN, 2019a), beginning with nursing education (see Table 2.2). Improving the knowledge, skills, and attitudes (KSAs) of nursing graduates was the first step toward improving practice. Table 2.4 includes the six essential competencies for graduate nursing education identified by QSEN (2019b). In addition, KSA statements were developed for prelicensure and graduate education related to each

TABLE 2.4   Graduate QSEN Competencies and Knowledge, Skills, or Attitudes Statements (2019b)

Competency	Examples of Knowledge, Skills, or Attitude Statements
Evidence-Based Practice	Evaluate organizational cultures and structures that promote evidence-based practice (Knowledge).
Quality Improvement	Propose appropriate aims for quality improvement efforts (Skill).
Safety	Describe human factors and other basic safety design principles as well as commonly used unsafe practices (such as workarounds and dangerous abbreviations) (Knowledge).
Teamwork and Collaboration	Respect the unique attributes that members bring to a team, including variation in professional orientations, competencies, and accountabilities (Attitude).
Patient-Centered Care	Assess and treat pain and suffering in light of patient values, preferences, and expressed needs (Skill).
Informatics	Appreciate the need for consensus and collaboration in developing systems to manage information for patient care (Attitude).

Quality and Safety Education for Nurses (QSEN) Institute. (2019b). *Graduate-level competencies: Knowledge, skills, and attitudes (KSAs)*. Retrieved from http://qsen.org/competencies/graduate-ksas

competency. Since 2007, the QSEN Institute website (http://qsen.org) has provided teaching strategies and resources to facilitate the accomplishments of the QSEN competencies in nursing education programs. Nursing faculty have revised the curricula of their programs to incorporate QSEN competencies and have conducted studies to evaluate the impact of QSEN competencies on students' practice (Altmiller, 2019; Lewis, Stephens, & Ciak, 2016; Pauly-O'Neil, Cooper, & Prion, 2016). Sherwood (2019) and other nurse leaders are advocating for international adoption of the QSEN competencies for nursing education and practice.

The most current QSEN KSAs for graduate nursing education programs are presented in Table 2.4 and can be found online (QSEN, 2019b). The EBP competency is defined as "integrating the best current evidence with clinical expertise and patient/family preferences and values for delivery of optimal health care." Graduate-level nursing students must have KSAs to conduct critical appraisals of studies; summarize current research evidence; develop protocols, algorithms, and policies for use in practice based on research; and participate in the conduct of research activities. An expanded knowledge of research is necessary to accomplish the QSEN competencies.

Current Mission of the Agency for Healthcare Research and Quality

As mentioned previously in this chapter, the AHRQ has been designated the lead federal agency supporting research designed to improve the quality and safety of health care in the United States. "The AHRQ sponsors and conducts research that provides evidence-based information on healthcare outcomes, quality, cost, use, and access" (AHRQ, 2019c). AHRQ (2019d) maintains over 20 other websites to help fulfill its mission. The websites include one for clinical decision support with tools to apply clinical guidelines to specific situations in practice, another website with resources to connect primary care clinicians with research they can use in practice, and yet another is a repository for systematic reviews (AHRQ, 2019d).

This research information promotes effective healthcare decision making by patients, clinicians, health system executives, and policymakers. AHRQ identifies funding opportunities, training opportunities, and research findings on their website (AHRQ, 2019c, d). Currently, the AHRQ and NINR work collaboratively to promote funding for nursing studies. These agencies often issue joint calls for proposals for studies of high priority to both agencies.

National Institute of Nursing Research Mission and Strategic Plan

NINR has the mission to "promote and improve the health and quality of life of individuals, families, and communities" (NINR, n.d.). When it came time to develop a new strategic plan, the NINR sought input to "encourage new thinking and creativity in nursing science, explore unanswered questions, promote results-oriented research, and guide the science over the next five to ten years" (NINR, 2016, p. 8). The most recent strategic plan for NINR (2016) identified four areas of scientific focus: Symptom science, wellness, self-management for persons living with chronic illness, and end-of-life and palliative care. As part of the focus on symptom science, the NINR recently led the other institutes at the NIH to create a Symptom Science Center within the NIH's Division of Intramural Research (NINR, 2019).

The NINR has also supported the development of nurse scientists in genetics and genomics by sponsoring the Summer Genetics Institute (SGI) since 2000 (Cimino, 2014). The SGI is a month-long intensive laboratory and classroom opportunity at the NIH that provides the participants the knowledge and skills to make significant contributions to genetic research. The funding priorities, funding process, and current research findings are available on the NINR website (http://www.ninr.nih.gov/). With the support of the NINR, nurses can conduct studies using a variety of research methodologies to generate the essential knowledge needed to promote EBP and quality health outcomes.

Doctoral Degrees in Nursing

In 2004, the AACN released a position statement encouraging the development of a practice doctorate within nursing, stating that there was a need for both research-focused doctorates and practice-focused doctorates. The research-focused degree would continue to be the PhD in Nursing, whereas the graduates of the new practice-focused doctoral programs would earn the Doctor of Nursing Practice (DNP) (AACN, n.d.). By virtue of their education, PhD graduates are prepared to develop and implement research studies to generate new knowledge. DNP graduates are prepared through their education to critically appraise and synthesize research findings, integrate these findings into practice, and conduct translational research. Trautman, Idzik, Hammersla, and Rosseter (2018, para. 3) described the career of a PhD nurse as one "devoted to intellectual inquiry and conducting original research studies," in contrast to the career of a DNP nurse, which would "concentrate on developing practice expertise and implementing evidence-based practice innovations at the macro or microsystems level." Some DNP programs have focused on advancing the education of advanced practice registered nurses. Others

have focused on preparing graduates to be leaders in complex healthcare systems (Trautman et al., 2018).

The number of DNP programs has grown quickly. Loomis, Willard, and Cohen (2006) reported 10 DNP programs in operation and 190 programs in development. In 2019, the number of programs with currently enrolled students is 348 and the number of programs in development is 98 (AACN, 2019a). The number of PhD students is only a quarter of the number of DNP students (Groer & Clochesy, 2019). The concern has been raised whether nursing will have an adequate number of nurse scientists if these trends continue.

The roles of DNP-prepared nurses continue to evolve (Beeber, Palmer, Waldrop, Lynn, & Jones, 2019). Morton (2018) identified a lack of evidence for the characteristics of the roles and the outcomes of the contributions made by DNP-prepared nurses. Nursing science would benefit from collaboration among PhD-prepared and DNP-prepared nurses to generate new nursing knowledge and to ensure its translation into practice.

METHODOLOGIES FOR DEVELOPING RESEARCH EVIDENCE IN NURSING

Nursing science generates the evidence to support nursing interventions and cannot be separated from nursing practice. All types of research are needed "to enhance the practice of nursing and stimulate further scientific work" (Pickler, 2018, p. 1). Pickler goes on to say, "limiting our research to certain methods, phenomena, or level of discovery would only constrain our future" (p. 1). Since the 1930s, many researchers have narrowly defined **scientific method** to include only objective, numerical research known as quantitative research. The view has prevailed in the health sciences and may be consistent with what you previously learned in school. Kaplan (1964), however, defined the scientific method as incorporating all procedures that scientists have used, currently use, or may use in the future to pursue knowledge. Another definition of the scientific method is asking and answering questions in a systematic way to ensure the answers are as accurate as possible (Gravetter & Forzano, 2018). These broad definitions embrace the use of both quantitative and qualitative research methodologies in developing research evidence for practice.

Historically, quantitative research methods were based on logical positivism or empiricism, philosophies consistent with the belief that absolute truth existed and only needed to be discovered. Over time, the philosophy of postpositivism emerged as scientists grew to believe that truth was not absolute and science could reveal knowledge with a probability of being accurate (Creswell & Creswell, 2018; Gravetter & Forzano, 2018). Scientific knowledge is generated through the testing of deductive theories, an application of logical principles, and reasoning whereby the researcher adopts a distant and noninteractive posture with the research subject to prevent bias (Borglin & Richards, 2010). Thus **quantitative research** is best defined as a formal, objective, systematic study process implemented to obtain numerical data to answer a research question. This research method is used to describe variables, examine relationships among variables, and determine cause-and-effect interactions between variables (Kerlinger & Lee, 2000; Shadish, Cook, & Campbell, 2002).

Qualitative research is a systematic, interactive, subjective, holistic, scholarly approach used to describe life experiences, cultures, and social processes from the perspectives of the persons involved in their natural settings (Creswell & Creswell, 2018; Creswell & Poth, 2018; Marshall & Rossman, 2016). Qualitative research is not a new idea in the social and behavioral sciences (Glaser & Strauss, 1967), including nursing. Nurses may find an affinity for qualitative research because of our focus on relationships with patients and our concern for the needs of the individual. This type of research is conducted to explore, describe, and promote understanding of human experiences, situations, events, and cultures over time.

Comparison of Quantitative and Qualitative Research

Quantitative and qualitative research complement each other because they generate different kinds of knowledge that are useful in nursing practice. The problem to be studied and purpose to be achieved determine the type of research to be conducted, and the researcher's knowledge of both types of research promotes accurate selection of the methodology for the problem identified (Creswell & Creswell, 2018; Kazdin, 2017). Quantitative and qualitative research methodologies have some similarities because both require researcher expertise, follow steps of the research process, involve rigor in implementation, and result in the generation of scientific knowledge for nursing practice. Some of the differences between the two methodologies are presented in Table 2.5. Some researchers include both quantitative and qualitative research methodologies in their studies, an approach referred to as **mixed methods research** (see Chapter 14) (Creswell & Clark, 2018).

Philosophical Origins of Quantitative and Qualitative Research Methods

The quantitative approach to scientific inquiry emerged from a branch of philosophy called **logical positivism**, which operates on strict rules of logic, truth, laws, axioms, and predictions. Quantitative researchers hold the position that truth is absolute and that there is a single reality that one could define by careful measurement. To find truth as a quantitative researcher, you need to be

TABLE 2.5 **Characteristics of Quantitative and Qualitative Research Methods**		
Characteristic	**Quantitative Research**	**Qualitative Research**
Philosophical origin	Logical positivism, postpositivism	Naturalistic, interpretive, humanistic
Focus	Concise, objective, reductionistic	Broad, subjective, holistic
Reasoning	Logical, deductive	Dialectic, inductive
Basis of knowing	Cause-and-effect relationships	Meaning, discovery, understanding
Theoretical focus	Tests theory	Develops theory and frameworks
Researcher involvement	Control	Shared interpretation
Data collection methods	Structured interviews, questionnaires, observations, scales, physiological measures	Unstructured interviews, observations, focus groups
Data	Numbers	Words
Analysis	Statistical analysis	Text-based analysis
Findings	Acceptance or rejection of theoretical propositions, generalization	Uniqueness, dynamic, understanding of phenomena, new theory, models, and/or frameworks

completely objective, meaning that your values, feelings, and personal perceptions cannot influence the measurement of reality. Quantitative researchers believe that all human behavior is objective, purposeful, and measurable. The researcher needs only to find or develop the *right* instrument or tool to measure the behavior.

Today, however, many nurse researchers base their quantitative studies on more of a postpositivist philosophy (Clark, 1998; Creswell & Creswell, 2018). This philosophy evolved from positivism but focuses on the discovery of reality that is characterized by patterns and trends that can be used to describe, explain, and predict phenomena. With postpositivism, "truth can be discovered only imperfectly and in a probabilistic sense, in contrast to the positivist ideal of establishing cause-and-effect explanations of immutable facts" (Ford-Gilboe, Campbell, & Berman, 1995, p. 16). For example, you may implement a preoperative educational intervention about deep breathing and ambulation with the goal of decreasing the *probability* of postoperative complications after abdominal surgery, but the intervention does not prevent all complications in these patients. The postpositivist approach also rejects the idea that the researcher is completely objective about what is to be discovered but continues to emphasize the need to control environmental influences (Creswell & Creswell, 2018; Newman, 1992; Shadish et al., 2002).

Qualitative researchers value an interpretive methodological approach consistent with subjective science more than quantitative researchers may value this approach. Qualitative research evolved from the behavioral and social sciences as a method of understanding the unique, dynamic, holistic nature of human beings. The philosophic basis of qualitative research is interpretive, humanistic, and naturalistic and is concerned with helping those involved understand the meaning of their social interactions. Qualitative researchers believe that truth is both complex and dynamic and can be found only by studying persons as they interact with and within their sociohistorical settings (Creswell & Poth, 2018; Creswell & Creswell, 2018; Denzin & Lincoln, 2018; Munhall, 2012; Padgett, 2017).

Focuses of Quantitative and Qualitative Research Methods

The focus or perspective for quantitative research is usually concise and reductionistic. **Reductionism** involves breaking the whole into parts so that the parts can be examined. Quantitative researchers remain detached from the study and try not to influence it with their values (objectivity). Researcher involvement in the study is thought to bias or sway the study toward the perceptions and values of the researcher, and biasing a study is considered poor scientific technique (Borglin & Richards, 2010; Shadish et al., 2002).

The focus of qualitative research is usually broad, and the intent is to reveal meaning about a phenomenon from the naturalistic perspective. The qualitative researcher has an active part in the study and acknowledges that personal values and perceptions may influence the findings. Thus this research approach is subjective, because it assumes that subjectivity is essential for understanding human experiences (Creswell & Creswell, 2018; Denzin & Lincoln, 2018).

Uniqueness of Conducting Quantitative Research and Qualitative Research

Quantitative research is conducted to describe variables or concepts, examine relationships among variables, and determine the effect of an intervention on an outcome. Thus this method is useful for testing a theory by testing the validity of the relationships that compose the theory (Chinn & Kramer, 2018). Quantitative research incorporates logical, deductive reasoning, as the researcher examines particulars to generalize about the universe.

Qualitative research generates knowledge about meaning through discovery. Inductive reasoning and dialectic reasoning are predominant in these studies. For example, the qualitative researcher studies the whole person's response to pain by examining his views about human pain and determining the meaning that pain has for a particular person. Because qualitative research is concerned with meaning and understanding, researchers using qualitative approaches may identify possible relationships among the study concepts, and these relational statements may be used to develop and extend theories (Creswell & Poth, 2018).

Quantitative research requires control (see Table 2.5). The investigator uses control to identify and limit the problem to be researched and attempts to limit the effects of extraneous or other variables that are not the focus of the study. For example, as a quantitative researcher, you might study the effects of nutritional education on serum lipid levels (total serum cholesterol, low-density lipoprotein cholesterol, high-density lipoprotein [HDL] cholesterol, and triglycerides). You would control the educational program (the intervention) by manipulating the content and teaching methods, the length and setting for the program, and the selection and training of the instructor. The nutritional program might be consistently implemented with the use of a video shown to subjects in a structured setting. You could also control other extraneous variables, such as a participant's age, exercise level, history of cardiovascular disease, and exposure to prior cholesterol education, because these extraneous variables might affect the serum lipid levels. The intent of these measures of control is to examine more precisely the effects of a nutritional education program (intervention) on the outcomes of serum lipid levels.

Quantitative research requires the use of (1) structured interviews, questionnaires, or observations; (2) scales; and (3) physiological measures that generate numerical data. Statistical analyses are conducted to reduce and organize data, describe variables, examine relationships, predict outcomes, and determine differences among groups (Grove & Cipher, 2020). Control, precise measurement methods, and statistical analyses are used to increase the validity of the research findings. In other words, the findings accurately reflect reality so that the study findings can be generalized. **Generalization** involves the application of trends or general tendencies (which are identified by studying a sample) to the population from which the sample was drawn. Researchers must be cautious in generalizing, because a sound generalization requires the support of many studies with a variety of samples (Kazdin, 2017; Shadish et al., 2002).

Qualitative researchers use observations, interviews, and focus groups to gather data. Qualitative data are words recorded on paper or electronically. For example, the researcher may ask study participants to share their experiences of engagement with a healthcare professional and record their narrative responses. The interactions between the researcher and participants are guided by standards of rigor but are not controlled in the way that quantitative data collection is controlled. In some qualitative designs, researchers begin analyzing data during data collection (Creswell & Poth, 2018; Kazdin, 2017; Rieger, 2019; Squires & Dorsen, 2018).

Qualitative data are analyzed according to the qualitative approach that is being used. The intent of the analysis is to organize the data into a meaningful, individualized interpretation, framework, or theory that describes the phenomenon studied. Qualitative researchers recognize that their analysis and interpretations are influenced by their own perceptions and beliefs. The findings from a qualitative study are unique to that study, and it is not the researcher's intent to generalize the findings to a larger population (see Table 2.5). Qualitative researchers are encouraged to question generalizations and to interpret meaning based on individual participants' perceptions and realities (Kazdin, 2017; Marshall & Rossman, 2016; Rieger, 2019).

CLASSIFICATION OF RESEARCH METHODOLOGIES PRESENTED IN THIS TEXT

Research methods used frequently in nursing can be classified in different ways, so a classification system was developed for this textbook and is presented in Box 2.1. This textbook includes quantitative, qualitative, mixed methods, and outcomes research for generating nursing knowledge.

In this text, the quantitative research methods are classified into four categories: (1) descriptive, (2) correlational, (3) quasi-experimental, and (4) experimental (Gravetter & Forzano, 2018). Different types of quantitative research are used to test theories and generate and refine knowledge for nursing practice. Over the years, quantitative research has been the most frequently conducted methodology in nursing. Quantitative research

---

BOX 2.1 Classification of Research Methodologies for This Textbook

Types of Quantitative Research
Descriptive research
Correlational research
Quasi-experimental research
Experimental research

Types of Qualitative Research
Phenomenological research
Grounded theory research
Ethnographical research
Exploratory-descriptive qualitative research

Mixed Methods Research
Outcomes Research

methods are introduced in this section and described in more detail in Chapter 3.

The qualitative research methods included in this textbook are (1) phenomenological research, (2) grounded theory research, (3) ethnographical research, and (4) exploratory-descriptive qualitative research (see Box 2.1) (Creswell & Poth, 2018; Marshall & Rossman, 2016; Rieger, 2019). These approaches, all methodologies for discovering knowledge, are introduced in this section and described in depth in Chapters 4 and 12. Unit Two of this textbook focuses on understanding the research process and includes discussions of quantitative, qualitative, mixed methods, and outcomes research methodologies.

Quantitative Research Methods

In this section, you will find descriptions of the four categories of quantitative research as introduced earlier. Research designs for the descriptive and correlational categories will be covered in Chapter 10. For the quasi-experimental and experimental categories, appropriate research designs are covered in Chapter 11.

Descriptive Research

Descriptive research provides an accurate portrayal or account of characteristics of a specific individual, situation, or group (Gravetter & Forzano, 2018). Descriptive studies offer researchers a way to (1) discover new meaning, (2) describe what exists, (3) determine the frequency with which something occurs, and (4) categorize information. Descriptive studies are usually conducted when little is known about a phenomenon and provide the basis for the conduct of correlational studies.

Correlational Research

Correlational research involves the systematic investigation of relationships between or among two or more variables that have been identified in theories, observed in practice, or both (Gravetter & Forzano, 2018; Kazdin, 2017). If the relationships exist, the researcher determines the type (positive or negative) and the degree or strength of the relationships. In positive relationships, variables change in the same direction, either increasing or decreasing together. For example, the number of hours of sleep per day is positively related to a perception of being rested, which means as the hours of sleep increase, the perception of being rested increases. In a negative relationship, variables change inversely or in

opposite directions. For example, hours of exercise per week is negatively related to a person's weight, which means as the hours of exercise per week increase, the lower the person's weight is. The primary intent of correlational studies is to explain the nature of relationships, *not to determine cause and effect*. However, correlational studies are the means for generating hypotheses to guide quasi-experimental and experimental studies that focus on examining cause-and-effect interactions (Gravetter & Forzano, 2018; Kazdin, 2017).

Quasi-Experimental Research

The purposes of **quasi-experimental studies** are (1) to identify causal relationships, (2) to examine the significance of causal relationships, (3) to clarify why certain events happened, or (4) a combination of these objectives (Kazdin, 2017; Shadish et al., 2002). These studies test the effectiveness of nursing interventions for possible implementation to improve patient and family outcomes in nursing practice.

Quasi-experimental studies are less powerful than experimental studies because they involve a lower level of control in at least one of three areas: (1) manipulation of the treatment or independent variable, (2) manipulation of the setting, and (3) assignment of subjects to groups. When studying human behavior, especially in clinical areas, researchers are commonly unable to manipulate or control certain variables (Gravetter & Forzano, 2018). Subjects cannot be required to participate in research and are usually not selected randomly but on the basis of convenience. Thus, as a nurse researcher, you will probably conduct more quasi-experimental than experimental studies.

Experimental Research

Experimental research is an objective, systematic, controlled investigation conducted for the purpose of predicting and controlling phenomena. This type of research examines causality (Gravetter & Forzano, 2018). Experimental research is considered the most powerful quantitative method because of the rigorous control of variables. Experimental studies have three main characteristics: (1) a controlled manipulation of at least one treatment variable (independent variable), (2) administration of the treatment to some of the subjects in the study (experimental group) and not to others (control group), and (3) random selection of subjects or random assignment of subjects to groups, or both (Shadish et al.,

2002). Experimental studies usually are conducted in highly controlled settings, such as laboratories or research units in clinical agencies. An RCT is a type of experimental research that produces the strongest research evidence for practice from a single source or study (Melnyk & Fineout-Overholt, 2019).

Qualitative Research Methods

Qualitative research methods and methodologies are distinct in that the focus is on the perspective of the participants or group in the study (Bazeley, 2013). This section will provide descriptions of phenomenological, grounded theory, ethnographical, and exploratory-descriptive qualitative research (see Box 2.1).

Phenomenological Research

Phenomenological research is a humanistic study of phenomena. The aim of phenomenology is to explore an experience as it is lived by the study participants and interpreted by the researcher. During the study, the researcher's experiences, reflections, and interpretations influence the data collected from the study participants (Creswell & Poth, 2018; Munhall, 2012). Thus the participants' lived experiences are expressed through the researcher's interpretations that are obtained from immersion in the study data and the underlying philosophy of the phenomenological study. For example, phenomenological research might be conducted to describe the experience of living with heart failure or the lived experience of losing a family member in a flood.

Grounded Theory Research

Grounded theory research is an inductive research method initially described by Glaser and Strauss (1967). This research approach is useful for discovering what problems exist in a social setting and the processes people use to handle them. Grounded theory is particularly useful when little is known about the area to be studied or when what is known does not provide a satisfactory explanation (Rieger, 2019). Grounded theory methodology emphasizes interaction, observation, and development of relationships among concepts. Throughout the study, the researcher explores, proposes, formulates, and validates relationships among the concepts until a theory evolves. The basis of the social process within the theoretical explanation is described. The theory developed is *grounded in,* or has its

roots in, the data from which it was derived (Charmaz, 2014; Rieger, 2019).

Ethnographical Research

Ethnographical research was developed by anthropologists to investigate cultures through in-depth study of the members of the cultures. This type of research attempts to tell the story of people's daily lives while describing the culture in which they live. The ethnographical research process is the systematic collection, description, and analysis of data to develop a description of cultural behavior. The researcher (ethnographer) may live in or become a part of the cultural setting to gather the data. Ethnographical researchers describe, compare, and contrast different cultures to add to our understanding of the impact of culture on human behavior and health (Creswell & Poth, 2018; Rasmussen & McLiesh, 2019).

Exploratory-Descriptive Qualitative Research

Exploratory-descriptive qualitative research is conducted to address an issue or problem in need of a solution and/or understanding. Qualitative nurse researchers explore an issue or problem area using varied qualitative techniques with the intent of describing the topic of interest and promoting understanding. Although the studies result in descriptions and could be labeled as descriptive qualitative studies, most of the researchers are in the exploratory stage of studying the area of interest. This type of qualitative research usually lacks a clearly identified qualitative methodology, such as phenomenology, grounded theory, or ethnography (Denzin & Lincoln, 2018). In this text, studies that the researchers identified as being qualitative without indicating a specific approach will be labeled as being exploratory-descriptive qualitative studies.

Mixed Methods Research

Mixed methods research is conducted when the study problem and purpose are best addressed using both quantitative and qualitative research methodologies. Researchers might have a stronger focus on either a quantitative or a qualitative research method based on the purpose of their study. Quantitative and qualitative research methods are implemented concurrently or consecutively based on the knowledge to be generated (Creswell & Clark, 2018; Currie & Nunez-Smith, 2015). Integration of the qualitative and quantitative results is the strength of the method (Morse & Cheek, 2015). For example, a researcher may use a standardized tool to collect quantitative data from nurses with human immunodeficiency virus (HIV) infection about their work experiences. The researcher also interviews some of the nurses who participated in the quantitative part of the study to collect qualitative data on their work experiences since becoming HIV positive. Then the quantitative and qualitative data are analyzed for areas of agreement and disagreement, and a more holistic description of the nurses' experiences can be reported. The different strategies for combining qualitative and quantitative research methods in mixed methods studies are described in Chapter 14.

Outcomes Research

The spiraling cost of health care has generated many questions about the quality and effectiveness of healthcare services and the patient outcomes. Consumers want to know what services they are buying and whether these services will improve their health. Healthcare policymakers want to know whether the care is cost effective and of high quality. These concerns have promoted the proliferation during the past decade of **outcomes research**, which examines the results of care and measures the changes in health status of patients (Doran, 2011; Moorhead et al., 2018). As noted earlier, the work of PCORI has placed an increased emphasis on patient-centered outcomes and patient engagement. Key ideas related to outcomes research are addressed throughout the text, and Chapter 13 contains a detailed discussion of this methodology. In summary, nurse researchers conduct a variety of research methodologies (quantitative, qualitative, mixed methods, and outcomes research) to develop the best research evidence for practice (see Box 2.1).

INTRODUCTION TO BEST RESEARCH EVIDENCE FOR PRACTICE

EBP involves the use of best research evidence to guide clinical decision making in practice. As a nurse, you make numerous clinical decisions each day that affect the health outcomes of your patients and their families. By using the best research evidence available, you can make informed clinical decisions that will improve health outcomes for patients, families, and communities. This section introduces you to the concept of best

research evidence for practice by providing (1) a definition of the term *best research evidence,* (2) a model of the levels of research evidence available, and (3) a link of the best research evidence to evidence-based guidelines for practice.

Definition of Best Research Evidence

Best research evidence is a summary of the highest quality, current empirical knowledge in a specific area of health care that is developed from a synthesis of quality studies in that area (Cullen et al., 2018; Melnyk & Fineout-Overholt, 2019; Straus et al., 2011). The synthesis of study findings is a complex, highly structured process that is conducted most effectively by at least two researchers or even a team of expert researchers and healthcare providers. There are various types of research syntheses, and the type of synthesis conducted varies according to the quality and types of research evidence available. The quality of the research evidence available in an area depends on the number and strength of the studies. Replicating or repeating of studies with similar methodology adds to the quality of the research evidence. The strengths and weaknesses of the studies are determined by critically appraising the credibility or trustworthiness of the study findings (see Chapter 18).

The types of research commonly conducted in nursing were identified earlier in this chapter as quantitative, qualitative, mixed methods, and outcomes (see Box 2.1). The research synthesis process used to summarize knowledge varies for quantitative, qualitative, and mixed methods research methods. In building the best research evidence for practice, the quantitative experimental study, such as an RCT, has been identified as producing the strongest research evidence for practice (Cullen et al., 2018; Melnyk & Fineout-Overholt, 2019).

The following processes are usually conducted to synthesize research in nursing and health care: (1) systematic review, (2) meta-analysis, (3) meta-synthesis, and (4) mixed methods research synthesis. Depending on the quantity and strength of the research findings available, nurses and other healthcare professionals use one or more of these four synthesis processes to determine the current best research evidence in an area. Table 2.6 identifies the common processes used in research synthesis, the purpose of each synthesis process, the types of research included in the synthesis (sampling frame), and the analysis techniques used to achieve the synthesis of research evidence (Higgins, &

TABLE 2.6 Processes Used to Synthesize Research Evidence

Synthesis Process	Purpose of Synthesis	Types of Research Included in the Synthesis (Sampling Frame)	Analysis for Achieving Synthesis
Systematic review	Systematically identify, select, critically appraise, and synthesize research evidence to address a particular problem in practice (Cullen et al., 2018; Higgins & Thomas, 2019; Johnson & Hennessey, 2019; Liberti et al., 2009; Melnyk & Fineout-Overholt, 2019).	Quantitative studies with similar methodology, such as randomized controlled trials (RCTs), and meta-analyses focused on a practice problem	Narrative and statistical
Meta-analysis	Pooling of the results from several previous studies using statistical analysis to determine the effect of an intervention or the strength of relationships (Cullen et al., 2018; Higgins & Thomas, 2019; Johnson & Hennessey, 2019; Liberti et al., 2009; Melnyk & Fineout-Overholt, 2019).	Quantitative studies with similar methodology, such as quasi-experimental and experimental studies focused on the effect of an intervention, or correlational studies focused on selected relationships	Statistical
Meta-synthesis	Systematic compilation and integration of qualitative studies to expand understanding and develop a unique interpretation of the studies' findings in a selected area (Cullen et al., 2018; Johnson & Hennessey, 2019; Melnyk & Fineout-Overholt, 2019; Sandelowski & Barroso, 2007).	Original qualitative studies and summaries of qualitative studies	Narrative
Mixed methods research synthesis	Synthesis of the findings from independent studies conducted with a variety of methods (quantitative, qualitative, and mixed methods) to determine the current knowledge in an area (Heyvaert, Mases, & Onghena, 2013; Higgins & Thomas, 2019; Pluye & Hong, 2014; Sandelowski, Voils, Leeman, & Crandell, 2012).	Variety of quantitative, qualitative, and mixed methods studies	Narrative and sometime statistical

Thomas, 2019; Melnyk & Fineout-Overholt, 2019; Sandelowski & Barroso, 2007).

A **systematic review** is a structured, comprehensive synthesis of the research literature conducted to determine the best research evidence available to address a healthcare question. A systematic review involves identifying, locating, appraising, and synthesizing quality research evidence for expert clinicians to use to promote an EBP (Higgins & Thomas, 2019; Johnson & Hennessey, 2019; Liberti et al., 2009). Teams of expert researchers, clinicians, and sometimes students conduct these reviews to determine the current best knowledge for use in practice. Systematic reviews are also used in the development of national and international standardized

guidelines for managing health problems such as depression, hypertension, and type 2 diabetes. The processes for critically appraising and conducting systematic reviews are detailed in Chapter 19.

A **meta-analysis** is conducted to statistically pool the results from previous studies into a single quantitative analysis that provides one of the highest levels of evidence about an intervention's effectiveness (Higgins & Thomas, 2019; Johnson & Hennessey, 2019; Liberti et al., 2009). The studies synthesized are usually quasi-experimental or experimental types of studies that are measuring the same outcome variable in similar ways. In addition, a meta-analysis can be performed using correlational studies to determine the type (positive or negative) and strength of relationships among selected variables (see Table 2.6). Because meta-analyses involve statistical analysis to combine study results, the synthesis of research evidence is more objective. Some of the strongest evidence for using an intervention in practice is generated from a meta-analysis of multiple, controlled quasi-experimental and experimental studies. Thus many systematic reviews conducted to generate evidence-based guidelines include meta-analyses. The process for conducting a meta-analysis is presented in Chapter 19.

Qualitative research synthesis is the process and product of systematically reviewing and formally integrating the findings from qualitative studies (Melnyk & Fineout-Overholt, 2019). Sandelowski and Barroso (2007) were funded by NINR to develop a process for synthesis of qualitative studies. Several other methods of integrating the findings from qualitative studies have also been described in the literature (Kelly et al., 2018; Korhonen, Hakulinen-Viitanen, Jylhä, & Holopainen, 2013; Melnyk & Fineout-Overholt, 2019). In this text, the concept of meta-synthesis is used to describe the process for synthesizing qualitative research. **Meta-synthesis** is defined as the systematic compiling and integration of qualitative study results to expand understanding and develop a unique interpretation of study findings in a selected area (Johnson & Hennessey, 2019). The focus is on interpretation rather than the combining of study results as with quantitative research synthesis (see Table 2.6). The process for conducting a meta-synthesis is presented in Chapter 19.

Over the past 10 to 15 years, nurse researchers have conducted an increasing number of mixed methods studies (previously referred to as triangulation studies) that include both quantitative and qualitative research methods (Creswell & Creswell, 2018; Korhonen et al., 2013). In addition, determining the current research evidence in an area might require synthesizing both quantitative and qualitative studies. In the nursing research literature, this synthesis of quantitative, qualitative, and mixed methods studies is commonly referred to as a **mixed methods research synthesis** (see Table 2.6; Heyvaret et al., 2013; Sandelowski et al., 2012). Mixed methods research syntheses, sometimes referred to as mixed methods systematic reviews (Higgins & Thomas, 2019), might include a variety of study designs, such as quasi-experimental, correlational, and/or descriptive quantitative studies and different types of

qualitative studies (Creswell & Clark, 2018; Heyvaert et al., 2013; Sandelowski et al., 2012). In this text, the synthesis of a variety of quantitative and qualitative study findings is referred to as a mixed methods research synthesis. The value of these reviews depends on the application of rigorous standards during the synthesis process. The process for conducting a mixed methods research synthesis is discussed in Chapter 19.

Levels of Research Evidence

The strength or validity of the best research evidence in an area depends on the quality and quantity of the studies conducted in the area. Consistent findings among the studies, such as the effectiveness of a specific intervention, also strengthen the evidence. Quantitative studies, especially experimental studies like RCTs, are thought to provide the strongest research evidence from a single source. In addition, the conduct of studies with similar frameworks, research variables, designs, and measurement methods increase the strength of the research evidence generated in an area (Cohen, Thompson, Yates, Zimmerman, & Pullen, 2015). The levels of the research evidence can be visualized as a pyramid with the highest quality of research evidence at the top and the weakest research evidence at the base (Melnyk & Fineout-Overholt, 2019). Many pyramids have been developed to illustrate the levels of research evidence in nursing; Fig. 2.1 was developed to identify the seven levels of evidence relevant to this text. Systematic reviews and meta-analyses of high-quality experimental studies (RCTs) provide the strongest or best research evidence for use by expert clinicians, administrators, and educators in nursing. Systematic reviews and meta-analyses of quasi-experimental and experimental studies also provide strong research evidence for managing practice problems (see Level I). Level II includes evidence from an RCT or experimental study, and Level III includes evidence from a quasi-experimental study. Nonexperimental correlational and cohort studies provide evidence for Level IV. Mixed methods research synthesis of quantitative and qualitative studies and meta-syntheses of qualitative studies comprise the evidence for Level V (see Table 2.6 for a summary of these synthesis methods). Level VI includes a descriptive study or qualitative study, often conducted on a new area of research, and these types of studies provide limited evidence for making

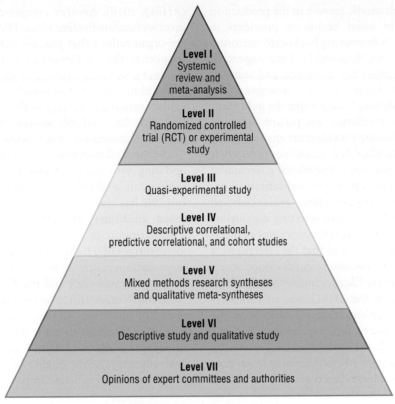

Level I
Systemic review and meta-analysis

Level II
Randomized controlled trial (RCT) or experimental study

Level III
Quasi-experimental study

Level IV
Descriptive correlational, predictive correlational, and cohort studies

Level V
Mixed methods research syntheses and qualitative meta-syntheses

Level VI
Descriptive study and qualitative study

Level VII
Opinions of expert committees and authorities

Fig. 2.1 Levels of evidence.

changes in practice (see Fig. 2.1). The base of the pyramid includes the weakest evidence, which is generated from opinions of expert committees and authorities that are not based on research.

The levels of research evidence identified in Fig. 2.1 help nurses determine the quality, trustworthiness, and validity of the evidence that is available for them to use in practice. Advanced practice nurses must seek out the best research evidence available in an area to ensure that they promote health, prevent illness, and manage patients' acute and chronic illnesses with quality care (Butts & Rich, 2018; Melnyk & Fineout-Overholt, 2019). Nursing faculty must seek out the best research evidence for teaching, learning, and creating environments that support students and faculty development. Nursing administrators need the best research evidence to ensure safety of providers and patients, systems of care that promote quality outcomes, and staffing models that maximize the use of limited resources. The best research evidence generated from

research syntheses and meta-analyses is used most often to develop standardized or evidence-based guidelines for practice.

INTRODUCTION TO EVIDENCE-BASED PRACTICE GUIDELINES

EBP guidelines are rigorous, explicit clinical guidelines that are based on the best research evidence available in an area. These guidelines are usually developed by a team or panel of expert researchers; expert clinicians (physicians, nurses, pharmacists, and other health professionals); and sometimes consumers, policymakers, and economists. The expert panel seeks consensus on the content of the guideline to provide clinicians with the best information for making clinical decisions in practice. However, expert clinicians must implement these generalized guidelines to meet the unique needs and values of the patient and family (Melnyk & Fineout-Overholt, 2019).

There has been a dramatic growth in the production of EBP guidelines to assist healthcare providers in building an EBP and in improving healthcare outcomes for patients, families, providers, and healthcare agencies. Every year, new guidelines are developed, and some of the existing guidelines are revised when new research is published. These guidelines have become the **gold standard** (or standard of excellence) for patient care, and nurses and other healthcare providers are encouraged to incorporate these standardized guidelines into their practice. Expert national and international government agencies, professional organizations, and centers of excellence have made many of these evidence-based guidelines available online. When selecting a guideline for practice, be sure that a credible agency or organization developed the guideline and that the reference list reflects the synthesis of extensive research evidence.

The National Guideline Clearinghouse (NGC), which was initiated in 1998 by the AHRQ, was an extremely important source of evidence-based guidelines in the United States. By the time its funding ended in 2018, the NGC contained more than 1500 EBP guidelines. AHRQ is conducting a year-long study to determine innovative methods for making evidence-based guidelines available

(AHRQ, 2018). Another component of AHRQ's work involves funding Evidence-based Practice Centers, which are organizations that provide technology assessments, support to the US Preventive Services Task Force, and conduct systematic reviews (AHRQ, 2019b).

Building on Dr. Cochrane's legacy, the Cochrane Collaboration and Library in the United Kingdom continues to be a reliable source of systematic reviews and EBP guidelines (http://www.cochrane.org/). The Cochrane Collaboration is known for producing and updating systematic reviews to ensure that the best evidence is available to clinicians. The Joanna Briggs Institute has also been a leader in developing evidence-based guidelines for nursing practice but requires a subscription to access the guidelines (http://www.joannabriggs.org/). In addition, professional nursing organizations, such as the Oncology Nursing Society (http://www.ons.org/) and the National Association of Neonatal Nurses (http://www.nann.org/), have developed EBP guidelines for their specialties. These websites will introduce you to some guidelines that exist nationally and internationally. Chapter 19 will help you critically appraise the quality of an EBP guideline and implement that guideline in your practice.

▊ KEY POINTS

- Florence Nightingale initiated nursing research more than 160 years ago. Her work was followed by several decades when very little research was done by nurses about nursing.
- During the 1950s and 1960s, research became a higher priority with the development of graduate programs in nursing that increased the number of nurses with doctoral and master's degrees.
- Since the 1980s, the major focus of nursing research has been on the conduct of clinical research to improve nursing practice.
- Outcomes research emerged as an important methodology for documenting the effectiveness of healthcare service in the 1980s and 1990s.
- In 1989, the AHCPR (later renamed the AHRQ was established to facilitate the conduct of outcomes research.
- The vision for nursing in the 21st century is the development of a scientific knowledge base that enables nurses to implement an EBP.

- Nursing research incorporates quantitative, qualitative, mixed methods, and outcomes research methodologies.
- Quantitative research is classified into four types for this textbook: Descriptive, correlational, quasi-experimental, and experimental.
- Qualitative research is classified into four types for this textbook: Phenomenological research, grounded theory research, ethnographical research, and exploratory-descriptive qualitative research.
- Mixed methods research is conducted when the study problem and purpose are best addressed by using both quantitative and qualitative research methodologies.
- Outcomes research focuses on determining the results of care or a measure of the change in health status of the patient and family, as well as determining what variables are related to changes in selected outcomes.
- Best research evidence is a summary of the highest quality, current empirical knowledge in a specific area of health care that is developed from a synthesis

of high-quality studies (quantitative, qualitative, mixed methods, and outcomes) in that area.
- Research evidence in nursing and health care is synthesized using the following processes: (1) systematic review, (2) meta-analysis, (3) meta-synthesis, and (4) mixed methods research synthesis.
- The levels of the research evidence can be visualized as a pyramid with the highest quality of research

evidence at the top and the weakest research evidence at the base.
- A team or panel of experts synthesizes the best research evidence to develop EBP guidelines.
- EBP guidelines have become the gold standard (or standard of excellence) for patient care, and nurses and other healthcare providers are encouraged to incorporate them into their practice.

REFERENCES

Abdellah, F. G. (1972). Evolution of nursing as a profession. *International Nursing Review, 19*(3), 219–235.

Agency for Healthcare Research and Quality (AHRQ). (2018). *Guidelines and measures updates.* Retrieved from https://www.ahrq.gov/gam/updates/index.html

Agency for Healthcare Research and Quality (AHRQ). (2019a). *About AHRQ: Mission & budget.* Retrieved from https://www.ahrq.gov/cpi/about/mission/index.html

Agency for Healthcare Research and Quality (AHRQ). (2019b). *Evidence-based Practice Centers (EPC) program overview.* Retrieved from https://www.ahrq.gov/research/findings/evidence-based-reports/overview/index.html.

Agency for Healthcare Research and Quality (AHRQ). (2019c). *Funding & grants.* Retrieved from https://www.ahrq.gov/funding/index.html

Agency for Healthcare Research and Quality (AHRQ). (2019d). *Other AHRQ web sites.* Retrieved from https://www.ahrq.gov/cpi/about/otherwebsites/Index.html

Aiken, L., Clark, S., Cheung, R., Sloane, D., & Silber, J. (2003). Educational levels of hospital nurses and surgical patient mortality. *Journal of the American Medical Association, 290*(12), 1617–1623. doi:10.1001/jama.290.12.1617

Aiken, L., Clarke, S., Sloane, D., for the International Hospitals Outcomes Research Consortium. (2002). Hospital staffing, organization, and quality of care: Cross-national findings. *International Journal for Quality in Health Care, 14*(1), 5–13.

Aiken, L., Clarke, S., Sloane, D., Sochalski, J., & Silber, H. (2002). Hospital nurse staffing and patient mortality, nurse burnout, and job dissatisfaction. *Journal of the American Medical Association, 288*(16), 1987–1993. doi:10.1001/jama.288.16.1987

Aiken, L., Sloane, D., Lake, E., Sochalski, J., & Weber, A. (1999). Organization and outcomes of inpatient AIDS care. *Medical Care, 37*(8),760–772.

Altmiller, G. (2019). Care bundles, QSEN, and student learning. *Nurse Educator, 44*(1), 7–8. doi:10.1097/NNE.0000000000000617

American Association of Colleges of Nursing (AACN). (n.d). *DNP education.* Retrieved from https://www.aacnnursing.org/Nursing-Education-Programs/DNP-Education

American Association of Colleges of Nursing (AACN). (2004). *AACN position statement on the practice doctorate in nursing.* Retrieved from https://www.aacnnursing.org/DNP/Position-Statement

American Association of Colleges of Nursing (AACN). (2006). *AACN position statement on nursing research.* Retrieved from https://www.aacnnursing.org/Portals/42/News/Position-Statements/Nursing-Research.pdf

American Association of Colleges of Nursing (AACN). (2019a). *DNP fact sheet.* Retrieved from https://www.aacnnursing.org/DNP/Fact-Sheet

American Association of Colleges of Nursing (AACN). (2019b). *Missions and values.* Retrieved from https://www.aacnnursing.org/About-AACN/AACN-Governance/Vision-and-Mission

American Nursing Association (ANA). (1989). *Education for participation in in nursing research.* Kansas City, MO: Author.

American Nurses Credentialing Center (ANCC) (n.d.). *History of the Magnet program.* Retrieved from https://www.nursingworld.org/organizational-programs/magnet/history/.

Appalachian State University (ASU). (2019). *The beginnings of associate degree nursing education in North Carolina.* Retrieved from https://nursinghistory.appstate.edu/beginnings-associate-degree-nursing-education-nc

Bauknecht, V. L. (1986). Congress overrides veto, nursing gets center for research. *American Nurse, 18*(1), 24.

Bazeley, P. (2013). *Qualitative data analysis: Practical strategies.* Thousand Oaks, CA: Sage.

Beeber, A., Palmer, C., Waldrop, J., Lynn, M., & Jones, C. (2019). The role of doctor of nursing practice-prepared nurses in practice settings. *Nursing Outlook, 67*(4), 354–364. doi:10.1016/j.outlook.2019.02.006

Bernstein, E., Getchell, L., & Harwood, L. (2019). Partnering with patients, families, and caregivers in nephrology nursing research. *Nephrology Nursing Journal, 46*(3), 340–343.

Borglin, G., & Richards, D. A. (2010). Bias in experimental nursing research: Strategies to improve the quality and explanatory power of nursing science. *International Journal of Nursing Studies, 47*(1), 123–128. doi:10.1016/j.ijnurstu.2009.06.016

Brucker, M. (2016). Applying evidence to health care with Archie Cochrane's legacy. *Nursing for Women's Health, 20*(5), 441–442. doi:10.1016/j.nwh.2016.08.011

Butts, J. B., & Rich, K. L. (2018). *Philosophies and theories for advanced nursing practice* (3rd ed.). Burlington, MA: Jones & Bartlett Learning.

Charmaz, K. (2014). *Constructing grounded theory* (2nd ed.). Thousand Oaks, CA: Sage.

Chinn, P. L., & Kramer, M. K. (2018). *Knowledge development in nursing: Theory and process* (10th ed.). St. Louis, MO: Elsevier.

Cimino, A. (2014). From Hela cells to nanotechnology: NINR celebrates 15th anniversary of its Summer Genetics Institute. *The NIH Catalyst, 22*(6). Retrieved from https://irp.nih.gov/catalyst/v22i6/from-hela-cells-to-nanotechnology

Clark, A. M. (1998). The qualitative-quantitative debate: Moving from positivism and confrontation to post-positivism and reconciliation. *Journal of Advanced Nursing, 271*(6), 1242–1249.

Cohen, B. (1984). Florence Nightingale. *Scientific American, 250*(3), 128–137. Retrieved from https://www.jstor.org/stable/24969329

Cohen, M. Z., Thompson, C. B., Yates, B., Zimmerman, L., & Pullen, C. H. (2015). Implementing common data elements across studies to advance research. *Nursing Outlook, 63*(2), 181–188. doi:10.1016/j.outlook.2014.11.006

Conduct and Utilization of Research in Nursing (CURN) Project. (1981–1982). *Using research to improve nursing practice.* New York, NY: Grune & Stratton.

Cook, E. (1913). *The life of Florence Nightingale* (Vol. 1). London, England: Macmillan.

Council for the Advancement of Nursing Science (CANS). (2016). *Council history.* Retrieved from http://www.nursingscience.org/about/council-history

Creswell, J. W., & Clark, V. L. P. (2018). *Designing and conducting mixed methods research* (3rd. ed.). Thousand Oaks, CA: Sage.

Creswell, J. W., & Creswell, J. D. (2018). *Research design: Qualitative, quantitative, and mixed methods approaches* (5th ed.). Thousand Oaks, CA: Sage.

Creswell, J. W., & Poth, C. N. (2018). *Qualitative inquiry & research design: Choosing among five approaches.* Thousand Oaks, CA: Sage.

Cullen, L., Hanrahan, K., Farrington, M., DeBerg, J., Tucker, S., & Kleiber, C. (2018). *Evidence-based practice in action: Comprehensive strategies, tools, and tips from the University of Iowa Hospitals and Clinics.* Indianapolis, IN: Sigma Theta Tau International.

Cummings, M. (1992). Patient outcomes research—Nursing, an important component. *Journal of Professional Nursing, 8*(6), 318.

Curry, L., & Nunez-Smith, M. (2015). *Mixed methods in health sciences research: A practical primer.* Thousand Oaks, CA: Sage.

de Tornyay, R. (1977). Nursing research—the road ahead. *Nursing Research, 26*(6), 404–407.

Denzin, N., & Lincoln, Y. (2018). *The Sage handbook of qualitative research.* Thousand Oaks, CA: Sage.

Doran, D. M. (2011). *Nursing-sensitive outcomes: State of the science.* Sudbury, MA: Jones & Bartlett.

Downs, F. S., & Fleming, W. J. (1979). *Issues in nursing research.* New York, NY: Appleton-Century-Crofts.

Duffy, J., Fren, M., & Patterson, B. (2011). Advancing nursing education science: An analysis of the NLN's grants program 2008-2010. *Nursing Education Perspectives, 32*(1), 10–13.

Eastern Nursing Research Society (ENRS). (n.d.). *About us.* Retrieved from http://communities.enrs-go.org/about/mission-vision

Eddy, D. (2011). The origins of evidence-based medicine: A personal perspective. *Virtual Mentor, 13*(1), 55–60. doi:10.1001/virtualmentor.2011.13.1.mhst1-1101

Finlayson, M., Aiken, L., & Nakarada-Kordic, I. (2007). New Zealand nurses' reports on hospital care: An international comparison. *Nursing Praxis in New Zealand, 23*(1), 17–28.

Fitzpatrick, M. L. (1978). *Historical studies in nursing.* New York, NY: Teachers College Press.

Ford-Gilboe, M., Campbell, J., & Berman, H. (1995). Stories and numbers: Coexistence without compromise. *Advances in Nursing Science, 18*(1), 14–26.

Glaser, B. G., & Strauss, A. L. (1967). *The discovery of grounded theory: Strategies for qualitative research.* Chicago, IL: Aldine.

Gortner, S. R., & Nahm, H. (1977). An overview of nursing research in the United States: The development of research in nursing practice (Part 3). *Nursing Research, 26*(1), 18–21.

Grady, P. (2018). The National Institute of Nursing Research: A glance back, and a vision for the future. *Journal of Nursing Scholarship, 50*(6), 579–581. doi:10.1111/jnu.12432

Gravetter, F., & Forzano, L. (2018). *Research methods for the behavioral sciences.* Boston, MA: Cengage.

Grinspun, D., & Bajnok, I. (2018). *Transforming nursing through knowledge: Best practices for guideline development, implementation science, and evaluation.* Indianapolis, IN: Sigma Theta Tau International.

Groer, M., & Clochesy, J. (2019). Conflicts within the discipline of nursing: Is there a looming paradigm war? *Journal of Professional Nursing,* in press. doi:10.1016/j.profnurs.2019.06.014.

Grove, S. K., & Cipher, D. (2020). *Statistics for nursing research: A workbook for evidence-based practice* (3rd ed.). St. Louis, MO: Saunders.

Hambleton, J. (1998). A patient resource program: Strengthening primary nursing. *Nursing Management, 29*(3), 33–34.

Harker, M. (2017). History of nursing education evolution Mildred Montag. *Teaching and Learning in Nursing, 12*(4), 295–297. doi:10.1016/j.teln.2017.05.006

Hatfield, L., Kutney-Lee, A., Hallowell, S., Guidice, M., Ellis, L., Verica., L., & Aiken, L. (2016). Fostering clinical nurse research in a hospital context. *Journal of Nursing Administration, 46*(5), 245–249. doi:10.1097/NNA.0000000000000338

Hawkins, R., & Nezat, G. (2009). Education news. Doctoral education: Which degree to pursue? *American Association of Nurse Anesthetists, 72*(2), 92–96.

Herbert, R. G. (1981). *Florence Nightingale: Saint, reformer or rebel?* Malabar, FL: Robert E. Krieger.

Heyvaert, M., Maes, B., & Onghena, P. (2013). Mixed methods research synthesis: Definition, framework, and potential. *Quality & Quantity, 47*(2), 659–676. doi:10.1007/s11135-011-9538-6.

Higgins, J. P. T., & Thomas, J. (2019). *Cochrane handbook for systematic reviews of interventions* (2nd ed.). West Sussex, UK: Wiley Cochrane Series.

Horsley, J. A., Crane, J., Crabtree, M. K., & Wood, D. J. (1983). *Using research to improve nursing practice: A guide; CURN Project.* New York, NY: Grune & Stratton.

Hughes, E., Hughes, H., & Deutscher, I. (1958). *Twenty thousand nurses tell their story.* Philadelphia, PA: J. B. Lippincott.

Institute of Medicine (IOM). (2001). *Crossing the quality chasm: A new health system for the 21st century.* Washington, DC: National Academy Press.

Johnson, B., & Hennessey, E. (2019). Systematic reviews and meta-analysis in the health sciences: Best practices for research synthesis. *Social Science & Medicine, 233*(1), 237–251. doi:10.1016/j.socscimed.2019.05.035

Johnson, J. E. (1993). Outcomes research and health care reform: Opportunities for nurses. *Nursing Connections, 6*(4), 1–3.

Johnson, W. L. (1977). Research programs of the National League for Nursing. *Nursing Research, 26*(3), 172–176.

Kaplan, A. (1964). *The conduct of inquiry: Methodology for behavioral science.* New York, NY: Chandler.

Kazdin, A. (2017). *Research design in clinical psychology* (5th ed.). Boston, MA: Pearson.

Kelly, M., Ellaway, R., Reid, H., Ganshorn, H., Yardley, S., Bennett, D., & Dornan, T. (2018). Considering axiological integrity: A methodological analysis of qualitative evidence syntheses, and its implications for health professions education. *Advances in Health Sciences Education, 23*(4), 833–851. doi:10.1007/s10459-018-9829-y

Kerlinger, F. N., & Lee, H. B. (2000). *Foundations of behavioral research* (4th ed.). Fort Worth, TX: Harcourt.

Korhonen, A., Hakulinen-Viitanen, T., Jylhä, V., & Holopainen, A. (2013). Meta-synthesis and evidence-based health care—a method for systematic review. *Scandinavian Journal of Caring Science, 27*(4), 1027–1034. doi:10.1111/scs.12003

Krueger, J. C., Nelson, A. H., & Wolanin, M. A. (1978). *Nursing research: Development, collaboration, and utilization.* Germantown, MD: Aspen.

Lach, H., & Gaspar, P. (2018). Progress and changes in gerontological nursing research in the Midwest: A review. *Research in Gerontological Nursing, 11*(5), 231–237. doi:10.3928/19404921-20180809-01

Lake, E., Roberts, K., Agosto, P., Ely, E., Bettencourt, A., Schierholz, E., … Aiken, L. (2018). The association of the nurse work environment and patient safety in pediatric acute care. *Journal of Patient Safety.* Epub ahead of print. doi:10.1097/PTS.0000000000000559

Larson, E. (1984). Health policy and NIH: Implications for nursing research. *Nursing Research, 33*(6), 352–356.

Lewis, D., Stephens, K., & Ciak, A. (2016). QSEN: Curriculum integration and bridging the gap to practice. *Nursing Education Perspective, 37*(2), 97–100. doi:10.5480/14-1323

Liberati, A., Altman, D., Tetzlaff, J., Mulrow, C., Gøtzsche, P., … Moher, D. (2009). The PRISMA statement for reporting systematic reviews and meta-analyses of studies that evaluate health care interventions: Explanation and elaboration. *Journal of Clinical Epidemiology, 62*(10), e1–e34. doi:10.1016/j.jclinepi.2009.06.006

Lin, C. C. (1996). Patient satisfaction with nursing care as an outcome variable: Dilemmas for nursing evaluation researchers. *Journal of Professional Nursing, 12*(4), 207–216.

Loomis, J., Willard, B., & Cohen, J. (2006). Difficult professional choices: Deciding between the PhD and the DNP in nursing. *OJIN: The Online Journal of Issues in Nursing, 12*(1). doi:10.3912/OJIN.Vol12No1PPT02

Marshall, C., & Rossman, G. B. (2016). *Designing qualitative research* (6th ed.). Los Angeles, CA: Sage.

McBride, A. (1996). Professional nursing education—today and tomorrow. In G. Wunderlich, F. Sloan, & C. Davis (Eds.), *Nursing staff in hospitals and nursing homes: Is it adequate?* (pp. 333–360). Washington, DC: National Academy Press.

Melnyk, B. M., & Fineout-Overholt, E. (2019). *Evidence-based practice in nursing and healthcare: A guide to best practice* (4th ed.). Philadelphia, PA: Lippincott Williams & Wilkins.

Messmer, P., Zalon, M., & Phillips, C. (2014). ANF scholars: Stepping stones to a nursing research career. *Applied Nursing Research, 27*(1), 2–24. doi:http://dx.doi.org/10.1016/j.apnr.2013.10.009

Midwest Nursing Research Society (MNRS). (2019). *Everyone has a story: We love to share ours.* Retrieved from https://mnrs.org/about/history/

Moorhead, S., Swanson, E., Johnson, M., & Maas, M. L. (2018). *Nursing outcomes classification (NOC): Measurement of health outcomes* (6th ed.). St. Louis, MO: Elsevier.

Morse, J., & Cheek, J. (2015). Introducing qualitatively-driven mixed-method designs. *Qualitative Health Researcher, 25*(6), 731–733. doi:10.1177/1049732315583299

Morton, P. (2018). The doctor of nursing practice: A recap of resources. *Journal of Professional Nursing, 34*(3), 147–148. doi:10.1016/j.profnurs.2018.04.003

Munhall, P. L. (2012). *Nursing research: A qualitative perspective* (5th ed.). Sudbury, MA: Jones & Bartlett Learning.

NANDA International. (2018). *About us.* Retrieved from http://www.nanda.org/about-us/

National Institute of Nursing Research (NINR). (n.d.). *NINR mission statement.* Retrieved from https://www.ninr.nih.gov/aboutninr/ninr-mission-and-strategic-plan

National Institute of Nursing Research (NINR). (2016). *The NINR strategic plan: Advancing science, improving lives.* Retrieved from https://www.ninr.nih.gov/sites/files/docs/NINR_StratPlan2016_reduced.pdf

National Institute of Nursing Research (NINR). (2019). *Symptom Science Center: A resource for precision health.* Retrieved from https://www.ninr.nih.gov/newsandinformation/events/sscevent

National Institute of Nursing Research (NINR), with Cantelon, P. (2010). *NINR: Bringing science to life* (NIH Publication No. 10-7502). Washington, DC: National Institutes of Health.

National League for Nursing (NLN). (2019). *Research.* Retrieved from http://www.nln.org/professional-development-programs/research

Newman, M. A. (1992). Prevailing paradigms in nursing. *Nursing Outlook, 40*(1), 10–13, 32.

Nightingale, F. (1859). *Notes on nursing: What it is, and what it is not.* Philadelphia, PA: Lippincott.

Nightingale, F. (2015). *Notes on hospitals.* Mineola, NY: Dover Publications (Original published in 1859).

Oakley, K. (2010). Nursing by the numbers. *Occupational Health, 62*(4), 28–29.

Office of Disease Prevention and Health Promotion (ODPHP), U.S. Department of Health and Human Services (DHHS). (2018). *Secretary's Advisory Committee on National Disease Health Promotion and Disease Prevention Objectives for 2030: Recommendations for the Healthy People 2030 Leading Health Indicators.* Retrieved from https://www.healthypeople.gov/sites/default/files/Committee-LHI-Report-to-Secretary_1.pdf

Office of Disease Prevention and Health Promotion (ODPHP), U.S. Department of Health and Human Services (DHHS). (2019a). *Development of the National Health Promotion and Disease Prevention Objectives for 2030.* Retrieved from https://www.healthypeople.gov/2020/About-Healthy-People/Development-Healthy-People-2030

Office of Disease Prevention and Health Promotion (ODPHP), U.S. Department of Health and Human Services (DHHS). (2019b). *History and development of Healthy People.* Retrieved from https://www.healthypeople.gov/2020/About-Healthy-People/History-Development-Healthy-People-2020

Padgett, D. K. (2017). *Qualitative methods in social work research* (3rd ed.). Thousand Oaks, CA: Sage.

Palmer, I. S. (1977). Florence Nightingale: Reformer, reactionary, researcher. *Nursing Research, 26*(2), 84–89.

Parse, R. (2017). Where have all the *nursing* theories gone? *Nursing Science Quarterly, 29*(2), 101–102. doi:10.1177/0894318416636392

Patient-Centered Outcomes Research Institute (PCORI). (n.d.). *Research funding.* Retrieved from https://www.pcori.org/sites/default/files/PCORI-Research-Funding.pdf

Patient-Centered Outcomes Research Institute (PCORI). (2018). *Research done differently.* Retrieved from https://www.pcori.org/sites/default/files/PCORI-Research-Done-Differently.pdf

Pauly-O'Neil, S., Cooper, E., & Prion, S. (2016). Student QSEN participation during an adult medical-surgical rotation. *Nursing Education Perspectives, 37*(3), 165–167. doi:10.5480/14-1410

Pickler, R. (2018). Honoring the past; Pursuing the future. *Nursing Research,67*(1), 1–2. doi:10.1097/NNR.0000000000000255

Pluye, P., & Hong, Q. (2014). Combining the power of stories and the power of numbers: Mixed methods studies and mixed studies review. *Annual Review of Public Health, 35*(1), 29–45. doi:10.1146/annurev-publhealth-032013-182440

Quality and Safety Education for Nurses (QSEN) Institute. (2019a). *About QSEN.* Retrieved from http://qsen.org/about-qsen/

Quality and Safety Education for Nurses (QSEN) Institute. (2019b). *Graduate-level competencies: Knowledge, skills, and attitudes (KSAs).* Retrieved from http://qsen.org/competencies/graduate-ksas

Rasmussen, P., & McLiesh, P. (2019). Understanding research: Qualitative research in orthopaedic and trauma nursing. *International Journal of Orthopaedic and Trauma Nursing, 32*(2), 41–47. doi:10.1016/j.ijotn.2018.10.003

Rettig, R. (1991). History, development, and importance to nursing of outcomes research. *Journal of Nursing Quality Assurance, 5*(2), 13–17.

Rieger, K. (2019). Discriminating among grounded theory approaches. *Nursing Inquiry, 26*(1), e12261. doi:10.1111/nin.12261

Sandelowski, M., & Barroso, J. (2007). *Handbook for synthesizing qualitative research*. New York, NY: Springer.

Sandelowski, M., Voils, C. I., Leeman, J., & Crandell, J. L. (2012). Mapping the mixed methods-mixed research synthesis terrain. *Journal of Mixed Methods Research, 6*(4), 317–331. doi:10.1177/1558689811427913

See, E. M. (1977). The ANA and research in nursing. *Nursing Research, 26*(3), 165–171.

Shadish, S. R., Cook, T. D., & Campbell, D. T. (2002). *Experimental and quasi-experimental designs for generalized causal inference*. Boston, MA: Houghton Mifflin Company.

Shah, H., & Chung, K. (2009). Archie Cochrane and his vision for evidence-based medicine. *Plastic and Reconstructive Surgery, 124*(3), 982–988. doi:10.1097/PRS.0b013e3181b03928

Sherwood, G. (2019). A global call to action: Cultivating a safety mindset. *International Nursing Review, 66*(1), 1–3. doi:10.1111/inr.12543

Sigma (2019a). *Sigma organizational fact sheet*. Retrieved from https://www.sigmanursing.org/why-sigma/about-sigma/sigma-organizational-fact-sheet

Sigma (2019b). *WORLDviews on Evidence-Based Nursing guidelines for authors*. Retrieved from https://sigmapubs.onlinelibrary.wiley.com/hub/journal/17416787/about/forauthors.

Southern Nursing Research Society (SNRS). (n.d.). *History*. Retrieved from https://www.snrs.org/history

Squires, A., & Dorsen, C. (2018). Qualitative research in nursing and health professions regulation. *Journal of Nursing Regulation, 9*(3), 15–24. doi:10.1016/S2155-8256(18)30150-9

Stetler, C. B. (1994). Refinement of the Stetler/Marram model for application of research findings to practice.

Nursing Outlook, 42(1), 15–25. doi:10.1016/0029-6554(94)90067-1

Stetler, C. B. (2001). Updating the Stetler Model of research utilization to facilitate evidence-based practice. *Nursing Outlook, 49*(6), 272–279. doi:10.1067/mno.2001.120517

Stetler, C. B., & Marram, G. (1976). Evaluating research findings for applicability in practice. *Nursing Outlook, 24*(9), 559–563. doi:10.1016/0029-6554(94)90067-1

Straus, S. E., Glasziou, P., Richardson, W. S., & Haynes, R. B. (2011). *Evidence-based medicine: How to practice and teach it* (4th ed.). London, England: Churchill Livingstone Elsevier.

The Joint Commission (JC). (2019). *About us*. Retrieved from https://www.jointcommission.org/mobile/about_us.aspx

Trautman, D. E., Idzik, S., Hammersla, M., & Rosseter, R. (2018). Advancing scholarship through translational research: The role of PhD and DNP prepared nurses. *OJIN: The Online Journal of Issues in Nursing, 23*(2). doi:10.3912/OJIN.Vol23No02Man02

Werley, H. H. (1977). Nursing research in perspective. *International Nursing Review, 24*(3), 75–83.

Werley, H. H., & Fitzpatrick, J. J. (Eds.). (1983). *Annual review of nursing research* (Vol. 1). New York, NY: Springer.

Western Institute of Nursing (WIN). (2016). *History of WIN*. Retrieved from https://www.winursing.org/about-win/the-history-of-win/

Williams, M. K. (1984). Nursing, a new institute for NIH. *Nursing Economic$, 2* (March-April), 113–114.

Zeleznik, D., Vosner, H., & Kokol, P. (2017). A bibliometric analysis of the *Journal of Advanced Nursing*, 1976–2015. *Journal of Advanced Nursing, 73*(10), 2407–2419. doi:10.1111/jan.13296

3

Introduction to Quantitative Research

Polly A. Hulme

http://evolve.elsevier.com/Gray/practice/

What comes to mind when you think of the word *research*? Frequently, the word *experiment* pops up. One might equate experiments with randomizing subjects into groups, collecting data, and conducting statistical analyses. Many people believe that an experiment is conducted to answer a clinical question, such as: Is this pain intervention more effective than another? These ideas are associated with the classic experimental design originated by Sir Ronald Fisher (1935). Fisher is noted for adding the terms *structure* and *control* to the steps of the quantitative research process to decrease the potential for error and improve the accuracy of study findings.

From previous research and statistical classes, you have probably learned that the classic experimental design is not the only way to conduct quantitative research. Indeed, not all research questions posed by nurses can be answered by using the experimental approach. For example, some research questions focus on exploring and describing nursing phenomena. For these questions, the descriptive approach is best. Other research questions address relationships among nursing phenomena for the purpose of explaining or predicting. The correlational approach is best for these questions. Additional research questions involve testing a nursing intervention, and the quasi-experimental and experimental approaches are best for these questions. The quasi-experimental approach is used when the amount of control that the experimental approach requires is unattainable. These four approaches— descriptive, correlational, quasi-experimental, and experimental—are synonymous with the four research

methodologies used most frequently by quantitative nurse researchers.

The steps of the quantitative research process are the same for all four approaches. However, the philosophy and strategies for implementing these steps vary with the approach. As a brief background, the fields of sociology, education, and psychology are noted for their development and expansion of strategies for conducting descriptive research (Kerlinger & Lee, 2000). Karl Pearson developed statistical methods for examining relationships among variables, which helped lay the foundation for correlational research (Porter, 2004). Likewise, Campbell and Stanley (1963) are well known for developing quasi-experimental designs, and, as already noted, Fisher's experimentation provided the groundwork for what is now known as experimental research.

Let's pause and go back to the original question: What comes to mind when you think of the word *research*? Many people also use the word to mean educating oneself on a topic of interest. An example from conversation is, "I researched the side effects of vaccines." Such activities usually center on informal searches for information from professional sources and the internet. Although this use of the word *research* is common, you will want to distinguish it from the meaning and methods of research as taught in this text. To avoid miscommunication in professional and academic settings, such verbs as *looked up*, *read about*, and *studied up on* are good alternatives when describing informal activities to increase personal knowledge by examining existing sources.

This chapter walks you through the steps of the quantitative research process and provides examples from a descriptive correlational study for each of the steps. Prior to the description of these steps, relevant terms are defined, including the scientific method, basic research, applied research, rigor, and control. The chapter concludes with a discussion of the steps of the research process from a quasi-experimental study.

METHODS FOR QUANTITATIVE RESEARCH

The research methods for quantitative research included in this text are presented in Fig. 3.1. The method—or type—chosen by the researcher is influenced by current knowledge about a research problem. When little knowledge is available, descriptive studies are conducted that provide a basis for correlational research. Descriptive and correlational studies are conducted frequently to provide a basis for quasi-experimental and experimental studies, which are more highly controlled.

It is important to appreciate that some healthcare disciplines use different terms than nursing uses for quantitative research methods. For example, medicine and epidemiology tend to label both descriptive and correlational studies as observational studies and quasi-experimental and experimental studies as intervention studies. However, whether the study is descriptive, correlational, quasi-experimental, or experimental is usually

discernable with further reading of the research report. This text uses similar logic in dividing its in-depth discussion of quantitative research design into two categories: nonintervention research (Chapter 10) and intervention research (Chapter 11).

Descriptive Research

Descriptive research is the exploration and description of phenomena in real-life situations. Its purpose is to provide an accurate account of characteristics of particular individuals, situations, or groups using numbers (Leedy, Ormrod, & Johnson, 2019). Quantitative descriptive studies are usually conducted with large numbers of subjects or study participants, in natural settings, with no manipulation of the situation. Through descriptive studies, researchers describe what exists to increase knowledge on a phenomenon. They determine the frequency with which a phenomenon occurs, categorize the attributes of a phenomenon and measure the relative amount of each category, and determine quantity when a phenomenon can be characterized by amount. In descriptive studies, researchers also often compare the results across different groups and/or time. The underlying research questions in descriptive research are: To what extent does this variable exist? What are the principal types of this variable? What are the relative amounts of this variable? Are there differences between groups on this variable? Do individuals change over time regarding this variable?

An example of descriptive research is a study conducted by Schoenfisch et al. (2019). The authors sought to better understand the use of assistive devices by nursing staff with hospitalized patients. Using a self-report questionnaire, 108 participants from three different hospitals answered questions on (a) their training in available assistive devices; (b) the frequency of assistive device use in the past 4 weeks; and (c) the presence of known barriers to assistive device use at the time of lifting, transferring, or repositioning a patient. The results showed that all participants had training in assistive devices, but only 40% used assistive devices for half or more of their lifts or transfers. Comparisons were made between participants who did and did not use assistive devices for half or more of their lifts and transfers on age, gender, race, hospital type, unit type, job title, and patient care experience with no significant differences overall. However, there was a significant increase of

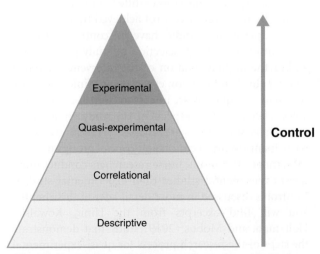

Fig. 3.1 Types of quantitative research conducted in nursing.

reported assistive device use over the first 5 years of patient care experience. Barriers to assistive device use were multiple and consisted of a combination of patient, nurse, equipment, and situational categories. A correlational study on the relative strength of relationships among barriers and assistive device use would be a logical next step for expanding knowledge on this important nursing topic.

Correlational Research

Correlational research involves the systematic investigation of relationships between or among variables. The numerical strength of relationships is determined to discover whether a change in the value of one variable is likely to occur when another variable increases or decreases. The intent of correlational studies is either to explain the nature of relationships or to allow prediction, all in the context of the real world. Importantly, the relationships revealed in correlation studies are not cause-and-effect relationships, but associations (Kazdin, 2017; Leedy et al., 2019). The associations identified by correlational studies are the means for generating hypotheses to guide quasi-experimental and experimental studies that do focus on cause-and-effect relationships (see Fig. 3.1). Examples of underlying research questions in correlational research are: What is the nature of the relationship between these two variables? To what extent do each of these variables contribute to this outcome? How well does this theory explain this phenomenon? What are the risk factors for this health condition?

Correlational analysis allows the researcher to determine the degree or strength of the relationship and the type (positive or negative) of relationship. The strength of a relationship varies, ranging from -1 (perfect negative correlation) to $+1$ (perfect positive correlation), with 0 indicating no relationship (Grove & Cipher, 2020). A **positive relationship** indicates that the variables vary together; that is, both variables increase or decrease together. For example, research has shown that the more minutes people exercise each week the greater their bone density. A **negative relationship** indicates that the variables vary in opposite directions; thus as one variable increases, the other will decrease. As an example, research has shown as the number of smoking pack-years (number of years smoked multiplied by the number of packs smoked per day) increases, people's life spans decrease. You will find a synopsis of a correlational study by Adynski, Zimmer, Thorp, and Santos (2019) later in this chapter. Table 3.1 contains a list of the studies provided as examples in this chapter.

Quasi-Experimental Research

The purpose of **quasi-experimental research** is the objective and systematic study of cause-and-effect relationships. Cause-and-effect relationships are examined by using numerical means to determine whether manipulating one variable affects other variables. These studies involve implementing an intervention (the manipulated variable) and examining the effects of this intervention using selected methods of measurement (Kazdin, 2017; Shadish, Cook, & Campbell, 2002). For example, an intervention of a swimming exercise program might be implemented to improve balance and muscle strength of older women with osteoarthritis. The underlying research question for a study of the effectiveness of this intervention is: Does this particular swimming exercise program improve balance and muscle strength of older women with osteoarthritis? Secondary research questions could be addressed as well, such as: What dose of the swimming exercise program yields the most improvements? Does the swimming exercise program also reduce osteoarthritic pain in these women? In quasi-experimental and experimental research, once the underlying primary research question has been clearly identified, a hypothesis is formulated to predict the study outcome and guide subsequent research planning (Friedman, Furberg, DeMets, Reboussin, & Granger, 2015).

Quasi-experimental studies differ from experimental studies by the level of control achieved by researchers. Quasi-experimental studies have less control over management of the setting, selection of study participants, and/or the implementation of the intervention. When studying human behavior, especially in clinical settings, researchers frequently are unable to control certain variables related to these aspects of the study. In addition, researchers sometimes are unable to randomly assign participants to intervention and control groups in clinical settings. As a result, nurse researchers conduct more quasi-experimental studies than experimental studies. Control is discussed in more detail later in this chapter. You will find excerpts from the Hinic, Kowalski, Holtzman, and Mobus (2019) study that demonstrate the steps of the research process for quasi-experimental research toward the end of this chapter. The study by

TABLE 3.1 **List of Quantitative Research Examples in Chapter 3 with Control and Setting Characteristics for Each Type of Research**

Authors	Title	Type	Control	Typical Setting
Schoenfisch et al. (2019)	Use of assistive devices to lift, transfer, and reposition hospital patients	Descriptive	No intervention; limited or no control of extraneous variables	Natural or partially controlled setting
Adynski, Zimmer, Thorp, & Santos (2019)	Predictors of psychological distress in low-income mothers over the first postpartum year	Correlational	No intervention; limited or no control of extraneous variables	Natural or partially controlled setting
Theeke, Carpenter, Mallow, & Theeke (2019)	Gender differences in loneliness, anger, depression, self-management ability, and biomarkers of chronic illness in chronically ill mid-life adults in Appalachia	Descriptive Correlational	No intervention; limited or no control of extraneous variables	Natural or partially controlled setting
Hinic, Kowalski, Holtzman, & Mobus (2019)	The effect of a pet therapy and comparison intervention on anxiety in hospitalized children	Quasi-experimental	Controlled intervention; rigorous control of extraneous variables	Partially controlled setting
Ma et al. (2019)	Role of exercise activity in alleviating neuropathic pain in diabetes via inhibition of the proinflammatory signal pathway	Experimental	Highly controlled intervention and extraneous variables	Research unit or laboratory setting

Hinic and colleagues examined the effect of pet therapy on anxiety in hospitalized children (see Table 3.1).

Experimental Research

Experimental research is the objective, systematic, and highly controlled investigation of cause-and-effect relationships (Shadish et al., 2002). Experimental research is the most powerful quantitative method because of the rigorous control of variables. At least two separate groups must be present, one of which is a distinct control group that does not receive the intervention. In addition, subjects must be randomly assigned to either the intervention group or the control group in experimental research. Random assignment is the process of assigning subjects so that each has an equal opportunity (or probability) of being in either group. Conducting the study in a laboratory or a research facility further strengthens control in a study. An example

of experimental research by Ma et al. (2019) is described later in this chapter (see Table 3.1).

The special terminology for the variables in quasi-experimental and experimental research is important for you to understand. The manipulated variable (the intervention) is called the **independent variable**. The delivery of the independent variable is highly controlled in experimental research and is less controlled in quasi-experimental research due to constraints in the environment. The variables subjected to controlled manipulation of the independent variable are the **dependent variables** or outcomes. Returning to the example of a swimming exercise program designed to improve the balance and muscle strength of older women with osteoarthritis, the independent variable is the swimming exercise program. The dependent variables are balance and muscle strength. Correlational research that proposes to explain or predict also uses the independent and dependent variable terminology. However, in correlational research the independent variable is not manipulated as it is in quasi-experimental and experimental research.

DEFINING TERMS RELEVANT TO QUANTITATIVE RESEARCH

The Scientific Method

When people think of science, the natural sciences such as biology, chemistry, and physics often come to mind. Nurses who conduct quantitative research use the same methods for their research as natural scientists do (Kazdin, 2017). They use these methods to help build nursing's distinct domain of knowledge. The methods of the natural sciences have resulted in remarkable advances in knowledge about the natural world with valued applications to medicine, nursing, technology, and other fields ("What has science done," 2013). Therefore it is not surprising that the scientific methods used by natural scientists are often referred to as *the* scientific method. However, as noted in Chapter 2, the scientific method for nursing is broader than that used by the natural sciences because it encompasses other scientific traditions as well, including those used for conducting qualitative and mixed methods research (Creswell & Creswell, 2018).

The scientific method for quantitative studies is grounded in the philosophy of logical positivism (see Chapter 2 for a summary). It rests on the process of stating hypotheses, testing them, and then either disproving them or testing them more fully. Hence its purpose is to develop knowledge by testing hypotheses. When not enough about a phenomenon is known to develop a hypothesis (as is often the case with descriptive research), the aim shifts to gaining enough knowledge to formulate testable hypotheses for future studies. A principle of quantitative research includes the notion that measurement is never 100% accurate. In other words, error intrudes in all measurement to some extent. Because of this, one test of a hypothesis is never sufficient. Before research results are considered dependable, the same hypothesis should be retested in a subsequent study, called a **replication study** (Kazdin, 2017) (see Chapter 5). Even if a study's findings are supported by a replication study, the setting, location, and population

to which the findings are applicable must be similar to those of the original and replication studies.

Basic Research

Quantitative research can be divided into two types: basic and applied. **Basic research** aims to increase knowledge or understanding of the "fundamental aspects of phenomena and of observable facts *without specific application . . . in mind* [emphasis added]" (Basic Research, n.d.). In the health sciences, basic research contributes to (a) a broad understanding of human biology and behavior and (b) a fundamental knowledge regarding specific health needs (Lauer, 2016). Normal physiology and pathophysiology are studied at the molecular, cellular, tissue, and organism levels (Grady, 2010). A common assumption is that knowledge gained from basic research in the health sciences will have a clear application to solving real-life health problems. However, a guiding principle for basic research is that there is no "obligation to apply [the knowledge gained through basic research] to practical ends" (Rubio et al., 2010, p. 470).

Basic research is conducted in a research laboratory or other artificial setting with animals, paid human volunteers, or animal or human tissue. Because basic research is often conducted in research laboratories on long tables or benches, it is sometimes referred to as bench research. Nurses who conduct basic research are by necessity trained in the biological or behavioral sciences through their doctoral studies or postdoctoral programs. An alternate strategy for nurses interested in conducting basic research or in conducting applied research with biological or behavioral variables is to seek a scientist mentor in the appropriate field. The scientist mentor would enter into the arrangement with the expectation of facilitating the nurse researcher's knowledge development in key aspects of bench science (Dorsey & Pickler, 2019). The advantage for the scientist mentor—especially those who work mainly with animals—is future collaboration with the nurse researcher on studies of humans.

An example of basic research conducted by nurses is found in an experimental study by Ma et al. (2019). The researchers chose a rat model of diabetes to study the effect of exercise on (a) neuropathic pain and (b) proinflammatory cytokines in peripheral nerve tissue. The rats were randomly assigned to healthy and diabetic groups, and in turn these groups were randomly assigned to exercise and no exercise groups, making four groups all together. Diabetes was induced in the rats assigned to the diabetic group with streptozotocin, a drug that kills pancreatic beta cells. A rodent treadmill was used to exercise the rats assigned to exercise. Pain was measured by an established rodent protocol called the mechanical paw withdrawal threshold in which a series of filaments of varying sizes and force is applied to the hind paw. Proinflammatory cytokines were assayed from nerve tissue, specifically the dorsal root ganglion. The results revealed that over time the rats with diabetes who exercised had less pain and lower levels of proinflammatory cytokines in their nerve tissue than controls. These findings suggested that exercise reduces the pain of diabetic neuropathy and that reduced levels of proinflammatory cytokines in peripheral nerve tissue help explain why.

Applied Research

The purpose of **applied research** in the health sciences is to create knowledge that will improve health, lengthen life, and decrease illness and disability (Lauer, 2016). Applied research in nursing focuses specifically on generating knowledge that will directly influence or improve nursing practice. Therefore this type of research is conducted to solve real-life problems, to make decisions, or to predict or control outcomes in real-life practice situations. Applied research also pertains when theory is tested and validated for its usefulness in nursing practice. Because the questions that applied researchers seek to answer arise from practice situations, applied research is conducted in practice settings quite similar to the settings in which the results will be applied. Most nursing research is applied, not basic. Nonetheless, both basic and applied studies are needed to develop knowledge for evidence-based practice (EBP) in nursing (Melnyk & Fineout-Overholt, 2019; Tappen, 2016). Nurses who conduct applied research often incorporate findings from basic research to determine their usefulness for nursing practice. For example, a nurse researcher interested in reducing the pain of diabetic peripheral neuropathy would find the Ma et al. (2019) article supportive for developing an exercise intervention to reduce neuropathic pain in humans due to diabetes.

Applied research is often called clinical research in the health sciences. Correspondingly, basic research is often designated preclinical research. However, the scope of applied nursing research is broader than clinical research in its strictest sense because nurses practice their expertise in a variety of roles, settings, and populations (see Chapter 1). Nursing practice includes direct care of patients and families in clinical and community settings as well as indirect care that focuses on populations. In addition, a substantial number of nurses with advanced education are nurse administrators or nurse educators, and their research reflects these pursuits. Health services delivery and nursing informatics are also topics of interest for nurse researchers. Therefore direct patient care is not the only form of nursing practice that can be influenced or improved through nursing research. Nonetheless, the development and testing of nursing interventions in clinical settings to improve patient outcomes remains nursing's quintessential contribution to clinical research in the health sciences (Kearney, 2019).

A unique and defining feature of nursing research is the discipline's holistic view of health. Nursing upholds a view of health that is inclusive of biological, psychological, social, and spiritual dimensions. Applied nurse researchers may study just one of these dimensions in a given study or more than one. Nursing's holistic view of health is also well suited for interdisciplinary research on complex health problems that are difficult to solve with purely medical approaches. For example, cutting-edge research conducted by nurses and their teams is using omics—examples being genetics, epigenetics, and the microbiome—to help build knowledge for precision health science (Dorsey & Pickler, 2019) and symptom science (Dorsey et al., 2019). Knowledge development in both of these fields is being revolutionized by advancements in data science (big data), another cutting-edge topic in which nurse informaticists are substantially contributing to building the knowledge base (AL-Rawajfah, Aloush, & Hewitt, 2015; Bakken, 2019).

An example of applied research conducted by nurses that incorporates a holistic view of health is the study conducted by Adynski et al. (2019) that was introduced earlier (see Table 3.1). These researchers examined potential biological and social predictors of psychological distress in mothers during the first postpartum year. The sample consisted of approximately 850 low-income women recruited from five locations across the United States. The data for these women had already been collected for another study and were made available to the researchers in a deidentified data set (see Chapter 9).

Biological predictors were a composite of laboratory values and body measurements labeled the allostatic load score. Social predictors were measures of the social determinants of health and a measure of interpersonal violence. Psychological distress was measured in three ways: stress symptoms, depressive symptoms, and anxiety symptoms. Interestingly, interpersonal violence reported prior to delivery was a predictor for all three of the psychological distress measures over the first postpartum year, but the allostatic load score was a predictor for none. A few of the social determinants of health, such as food insecurity, were predictors of psychological distress, but most were not. The results, which need to be replicated, suggested that interpersonal violence is a risk factor for psychological distress in low-income women over the first postpartum year.

Rigor in Quantitative Research

Rigor is the striving for excellence in research, which requires discipline, adherence to detail, consistency, and precision. A rigorously conducted quantitative study has a tightly controlled study design, a representative sample, and precise measuring tools. In rigorous quantitative research, deductions are flawlessly reasoned, and decisions are based on the scientific method. The logical reasoning conducted to link the phenomena to be studied at an abstract level to the actual variables and their measurement needs to be meticulous. Consistency in applying this logical reasoning to all aspects of a study—including its theory, design, and data analysis—is a necessity (Hinshaw, 1979). A strategy called substruction is an excellent method for threading logical consistency throughout a study. Briefly, substruction consists of visually mapping out (1) the constructs and concepts of the phenomenon to be studied, (2) their relationships among each other, (3) their corresponding variables, and (4) the measurement method for each variable (Ryan, Weiss, & Papanek, 2019). Box 3.1 provides definitions for constructs, concepts, and variables to which you can refer throughout this chapter (for more details see Chapters 6 and 8).

Another aspect of rigor is **precision**, which encompasses accuracy, detail, and order. Precision is evident in the concise statement of the research purpose and detailed development of the study design. However, the most explicit example of precision is the measurement or quantification of the study variables (Kazdin, 2017; Waltz, Strickland, & Lenz, 2017). For example, a researcher

---

BOX 3.1   Definitions of Constructs, Concepts, and Variables

Constructs
Concepts at very high levels of abstraction that have general meanings.

Concepts
Terms that abstractly describe and name objects or phenomena, thus providing them with a separate identity or meaning.

Variables
Qualities, properties, or characteristics of persons, things, or situations that change or vary and are manipulated, measured, or controlled in research.

---

might use a cardiac monitor to measure and record the heart rate of subjects during an exercise program, rather than palpating a radial pulse for 30 seconds and recording it on a data collection sheet. Precision is essential for **transparency** in research so that other investigators know as explicitly as possible the exact steps and elements that make up a study. Precision allows for replication and for variation, which is necessary for other scientists to validate or extend the findings. The ways in which these methods were put into practice need to be stated in the research report for transparency.

Control in Quantitative Research

Control involves the imposing of rules by researchers to decrease the possibility of error, thereby increasing the probability that the study's findings are an accurate reflection of reality. Error can be introduced into a study due to the presence of extraneous variables. These variables can influence or confound findings for the study variables, thus altering study results. Error can also be introduced when an intervention is not enacted in a precise and consistent manner. The rules used to achieve control in research are referred to as **design**. Quantitative studies include various degrees of control, ranging from uncontrolled to highly controlled, depending on the type of study (see Fig. 3.1). Descriptive and correlational studies are rigorously conducted but are often designed with minimal researcher control because no intervention is implemented, and study participants are examined as they exist in their natural setting, such as work, school, or healthcare clinic. Quasi-experimental studies focus on determining the effectiveness of an intervention in producing a desired outcome in partially controlled settings. Experimental studies are the most highly controlled type of quantitative study with controlled settings and interventions, as well as random assignment to intervention and control groups.

Extraneous Variables

Through control, the researcher can reduce the influence of extraneous variables. An **extraneous variable** is something that is not the focus of a study but can make the independent variable appear more powerful or less powerful than it really is. Extraneous variables exist in all studies and can interfere with obtaining a clear understanding of the relationships among the study variables. For example, if a study focused on the effect of relaxation therapy on the perception of incisional pain, the researchers would have to control the extraneous variables, such as type of surgical incision and time, amount, and type of pain medication administered after surgery, to prevent their influence on the patient's perception of pain. Selecting only patients with abdominal incisions who are hospitalized and receiving only one type of pain medication intravenously after surgery would control the extraneous variables identified in this example.

The extent to which a researcher controls for the effects of extraneous variables in the study's design is referred to as **internal validity**. While a study is in its early planning stages, the researcher identifies pertinent extraneous variables that can potentially affect the results of the study. Adjustments are then made in the research design and methods to control for the effects of these variables on the study results. One effective method for the control of extraneous variables is to carefully designate who will be eligible to participate in the study, as in the earlier example of the study that focused on the effect of relaxation therapy on the perception of incisional pain. Another key method is to randomly assign participants of experimental studies into intervention and control groups. Random assignment to groups reduces the effects of extraneous variables by increasing the likelihood of their even distribution across groups. A third method is to measure potential extraneous variables and then control for their effects on the dependent variables by means of statistical procedures (Kazdin, 2017; Kerlinger & Lee, 2000; Leedy et al., 2019). Control can also be exerted on (1) research settings, (2) sampling and attrition, and (3) study interventions, as discussed next.

Research Settings

The **setting** is the location in which a study is conducted. There are three common settings for conducting research—natural, partially controlled, and highly controlled (see Table 3.1). A natural (or field) setting is an uncontrolled real-life situation or environment. Conducting a study in a natural setting means that the researcher does not manipulate or change the environment for the study. Descriptive and correlational studies often are conducted in natural settings. A partially controlled setting is a natural setting that the researcher has manipulated or modified in some way to limit the effects of extraneous variables on the findings. For example, a researcher is designing an intervention study that tests a new method for a nursing procedure conducted in the hospital setting. The researcher plans for the control group to receive the nursing procedure as usually provided. One method to increase control in this natural setting is for the researcher to reduce variability in the way the current nursing procedure is performed. A review session with the nurses could be held to discuss hospital policy for provision of the procedure and the importance of consistently following the hospital policy. Finally, a highly controlled setting is an artificially constructed environment developed for the sole purpose of conducting research. Laboratories, research centers, and test units in universities or healthcare agencies are highly controlled settings in which bench and experimental studies often are conducted. Chapter 15 discusses the process for selecting a setting for the conduct of quantitative research.

Sampling and Attrition

Sampling is a process of selecting participants who are representative of the population being studied. In performing quantitative research, you will use a variety of random and nonrandom sampling methods to obtain study samples. Random sampling methods usually provide a sample that is representative of a population, because each member of the population has a probability greater than zero of being selected for a study. In addition, random sampling helps prevent **bias** (slanting of findings away from what is true or accurate) in who is selected for the study or who is assigned to an intervention or control group. Thus random or probability sampling methods require greater researcher control and rigor than nonrandom or nonprobability sampling methods. Sample sizes in quantitative studies are usually determined with a power analysis to ensure adequate numbers of study participants throughout the study (Aberson, 2019). Researchers are rigorous in reducing **attrition**, or loss of study subjects. Attrition can introduce bias and reduce confidence that the results of data analysis reveal true findings (Babic et al., 2019). Chapter 15 provides a detailed discussion of the sampling process and determining sample size for quantitative studies.

Study Interventions

Quasi-experimental and experimental studies examine the effect of an intervention (the independent variable) on an outcome(s) (the dependent variable[s]). Rigorous nursing intervention studies are vital for establishing an EBP for nursing. Controlling the development and implementation of a study intervention increases the validity of the study design and credibility of the findings. A study intervention needs to be (1) clearly and precisely developed, (2) consistently implemented, and (3) examined for effectiveness through quality measurement of the dependent variables (Melnyk & Fineout-Overholt, 2019; Morrison-Beady & Melnyk, 2018). The detailed development of a quality intervention and the consistent implementation of this intervention are known as **intervention fidelity** (Bova et al., 2017). Chapter 11 provides detailed directions for the development and implementation of a study intervention.

There are several ways to strengthen a study by decreasing threats to design validity. Chapters 10 and 11 address the various types of design validity and the process for selecting an appropriate study design. Your understanding of rigor and control provides the basis for the implementation of the steps of the quantitative research process, which are precisely executed in descriptive, correlational, quasi-experimental, and experimental research.

STEPS OF THE QUANTITATIVE RESEARCH PROCESS

The **quantitative research process** consists of conceptualizing a research project, planning and implementing that project, and communicating the findings. Fig. 3.2 identifies the steps of the quantitative research process and shows the logical flow of this process as each step progressively builds on the previous steps. The process is depicted in a circle with two-way arrows because

there is a back-and-forth flow while the different steps of the study are developed, clarified, strengthened, and implemented. Fig. 3.2 also contains a feedback arrow to "Generating Further Research," indicating that the research process is cyclical, for each study provides a basis for generating further research in the development of knowledge for EBP.

In this chapter, you are briefly introduced to the steps of the quantitative research process that are presented in detail in Units Two and Four. The descriptive correlational study conducted by Theeke, Carpenter, Mallow, and Theeke (2019) on loneliness in chronically ill midlife adults in Appalachia is used as an example to introduce the steps of the quantitative research process. The study is classified as descriptive correlational research because the authors used both descriptive and correlational methods.

Formulating a Research Problem and Purpose

In nursing, a **research problem** is an area in which there is a gap in nursing's knowledge base. This gap may relate only to general understanding (basic research) or it may have practice implications (applied research). Perhaps it represents an area in which theoretical knowledge is incomplete. It is, by implication, an area about which you have some curiosity.

In a research proposal or research report, a **problem statement** is often included that clearly identifies the problem as based on a review of relevant literature. The problem statement includes a brief summary (only a few sentences) of the current state of knowledge about a phenomenon for a given population and then a sentence that identifies the knowledge gap, such as "However, little is known about . . .," "Other examples are . . .," "... is a new concept and must be investigated," and "... is not well described in the literature." In clear language, the problem statement identifies the principal concepts upon which the study will focus. Frequently included with the problem statement is the reason the problem is significant to nursing.

The **research purpose** is generated from the problem (see Fig. 3.2) and identifies the specific focus or goal of the study. It is a short, usually one-sentence, statement that identifies itself in a research proposal or report by such wording as *purpose, objective,* or *intent* (Creswell & Creswell, 2018). In a research proposal, the present tense is used: "The purpose of this research is to investigate . . .,"

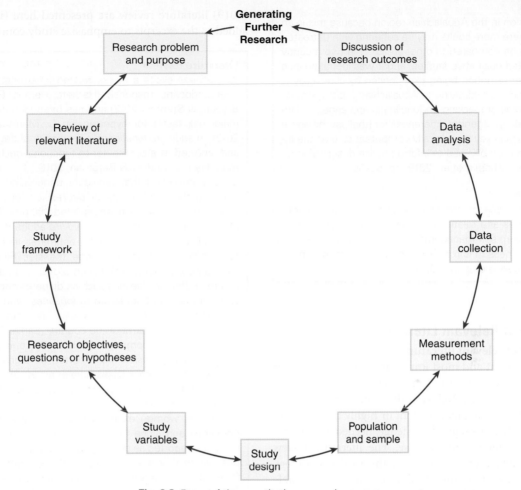

Fig. 3.2 Steps of the quantitative research process.

and in a research report the past tense is used: "The purpose of this research was to demonstrate . . .." The purpose often indicates the type of study to be conducted (descriptive, correlational, quasi-experimental, or experimental) and usually includes the major variables, population, and setting for the study. Chapter 5 provides a background for formulating a research problem and purpose for study.

Theeke and colleagues (2019) were interested in loneliness and its impact on physical health, psychosocial functioning, and quality of life, particularly in midlife adults with chronic illnesses in Appalachia. The researchers sought to better understand the ways in which loneliness, anger, depression, self-management ability, and biomarkers of chronic illness (a) differ by gender and (b) are related to each other. No one problem

statement was included in the research report; instead, gaps in the knowledge were woven into the literature review (see the following study excerpt). The study purpose excerpt comes from the abstract, where it was most clearly stated.

Research Problem

"Loneliness, a significant biopsychosocial stressor with a prevalence of 17% in U.S. adults, is linked to poor outcomes for multiple chronic health conditions and poor health behaviors.... Understanding loneliness as a major predictor of depression is paramount because depression is estimated to become the number one cause of disability in the United States within the next 2 decades.... It is critical to understand loneliness and depression in the Appalachian region because this is an area where more adults may be suffering with untreated depression compared to other areas.... In two recently completed qualitative studies, anger was identified as a significant emotion being experienced by chronically ill lonely older adults living in Appalachia..., but quantitative studies are lacking on loneliness and anger.... Understanding... gender differences for [the] psychological constructs is key to culturally competent care as the information can be used to inform precise design of interventions." (Theeke et al., 2019, pp. 55–56)

Purpose

"[The purpose of this study was to describe] gender differences and relationships among loneliness, anger, depression, self-management ability and biomarkers of chronic illness in chronically ill mid-life adults in Appalachia." (Theeke et al., 2019, p. 55)

Review of Relevant Literature

A **review of relevant literature** is conducted to discover the most recent and most important information about a particular phenomenon and to identify any knowledge gaps that exist. **Relevant literature** refers to those sources that are highly pertinent or highly important in providing the in-depth knowledge needed to study a selected problem and purpose. The literature review enables researchers to build on the works of others. By reviewing relevant studies, researchers are able to clarify (1) which problems have been investigated, (2) which require further investigation or replication, and (3) which have not been investigated. In addition, the literature review can direct researchers in designing the study and interpreting outcomes. Although a review of the literature includes research reports, it may contain other nonresearch information, such as theories, clinical practice articles, and other professional sources. Often one or two theories are included in the research report to help explain connections between and among study variables. Chapter 7 provides greater depth regarding the review of relevant literature.

Theeke et al.'s (2019) literature review focused on health effects and costs of loneliness and loneliness's links to anger, depression, chronic illness, and gender. Loneliness's links to self-management ability and biomarkers of chronic illness were not included in the literature review. Key excerpts from the Theeke et al.

(2019) literature review are presented here (italics are added to the excerpts to emphasize study concepts):

Literature Review

"*Loneliness* elicits a stress related inflammatory and neuroendocrine response (Hackett, Hamer, Endrighi, Brydon, & Steptoe, 2012) and has been identified as a major risk factor for hypertension (...Momtaz et al., 2012). In addition, *loneliness* is predictive of depression and reported as a contributor to functional decline, and mortality (. . . Bodner & Bergman, 2016...).... It is particularly important that providers understand *depression* and the antecedents of *depression* for adults in *mid-life* because it has been reported that prevalence of *depression* is highest among *mid-life* adults (Cacioppo et al., 2010) who have a 29.9% estimated lifetime risk for a major depressive episode (Kessler, Petukhova, Sampson, Zaslavsky, & Wittchen, 2012).... In addition, common *chronic illnesses* such as diabetes and cardiovascular disease, both linked to *loneliness* and *depression*, are most prevalent in Appalachia, compared to other more urban parts of the country (Barker, Kirtland, Gregg, Geiss, & Thompson, 2011).... Since *loneliness, anger*, and *depression* are reported as significant to cardiovascular disease (Nakamura et al., 2013)..., *anger* [is] an important related concept to consider when studying *loneliness*.

Men and women experience psychological distress differently and since the early 1980's [sic], *loneliness* has been reported as differing by *gender* with incongruous results. It was recently reported that lower levels of family and social support can contribute more so to *loneliness* in women (Lee & Goldstein, 2016) yet social network characteristics are predictive of *loneliness* more so in men.... In one qualitative study of older adults, it was determined that women experience *loneliness* differently than man with higher scores on personal growth and discovery scales..." (Theeke et al., 2019, pp. 55–56)

Frameworks

In research, a **concept** is a term to which abstract meaning is attached (see Box 3.1), and a **framework** is a combination of concepts and the connections between them. A **relational statement** explains the connection between two concepts. In the statement, "Fatigue can impair performance," *fatigue* and *performance* are concepts; *can impair* is the relational term that explains the connection between those concepts. A framework is an abstract version of the relationships between the study's variables. The relational statements or **propositions** in a study's framework are tested through research (Smith & Liehr, 2018).

A **theory** is similar to a framework: Both are abstract, both guide the development of research, and both are tested through quantitative research. A theory can exist by itself and be used to explain the concepts of various studies. A framework is usually linked to one given study—related to the major concepts being researched and the relationships among them. Because a framework provides an idea of how the concepts in a given study are related, it should both guide the research and help the reader of the research report understand the connections among study variables. Sometimes a framework is represented graphically as a diagram in a published research report. It may be called a map, a research framework, or a model. Chapter 8 provides an explanation of frameworks, theories, and related terms. An excerpt from Theeke et al.'s (2019) study of their framework statements follows:

Framework

"This study design and variable choice was framed using the Psychoneuroimmunology (PNI) paradigm (McCain, Gray, Walter, & Robins, 2005). This paradigm emphasizes that psychosocial stressors elicit both neurological and immunological stress responses that impact physical health, psychosocial functioning, and quality of life. For this study, the focus was on understanding relationships among the person factors (identified as sociodemographic variables and chronic illness diagnoses), the psychosocial variables (loneliness, anger, and depression), and measures of physical health which included blood pressure, BMI, [waist-hip ratio], blood glucose, and self-management ability." (Theeke et al., 2019, p. 56)

Making Assumptions Explicit

An **assumption** is a belief that is accepted as true, without proof and provides the basis for the phenomenon described by a theory (Meleis, 2018). Assumptions can also relate directly to the research process, the population, the sample, the intervention, the data obtained in the course of conducting the research, or some other aspect of the study. It is important that researchers make explicit their assumptions related to the conduct of the research. This involves a considerable amount of reflection on the researcher's part, in the nature of: What is

---

BOX 3.2 Making Assumptions Explicit: Hypothetical Example

A student designs a study to measure the relationship between a happy childhood and the number of marriages in American adults who are now themselves parents. Study subjects are to be recruited online through a parent support chat room and data collected anonymously using an online survey tool. In the study, each subject will self-rate childhood happiness on a 0-point to 10-point scale and report number of marriages. The student correctly recognizes assumptions that relate to how well the study variables will be measured. The assumptions are (1) subjects will honestly report number of marriages, and (2) subjects can remember their childhoods enough to make an accurate assessment of childhood happiness. Each of these assumptions would affect the study's credibility, were it not true.

Encouraged to reflect further, the student identifies additional assumptions. For example, a theoretical assumption underlying the student's proposed research is that divorce has some relationship to childhood happiness, and perhaps the relationship is predictive. The findings of the research may contradict the student's assumption. Another assumption, related to generalization of the results, is that the inhabitants of an online parent support chat room are fairly representative of the population of American adults who are parents. If this is not true, generalizability of the study results will be limited.

---

assumed in this study? What is taken for granted as true? What are the beliefs that guide this study? If the assumptions a researcher holds are not true, the findings will not be credible. Research reports often do not identify assumptions. When assumptions are addressed, researchers tend to report only those that affect the framework or accurate measurement of variables. In their research report, Theeke et al. (2019) did not mention any assumptions. To provide you with an idea of the importance of identifying assumptions, Box 3.2 presents a hypothetical research scenario with identified and unidentified assumptions.

Formulating Research Objectives, Questions, or Hypotheses

Investigators formulate research objectives (often labeled specific aims), questions, or hypotheses to bridge the gap between the more abstractly stated research problem and purpose and the study design and plan for data collection and analysis (see Fig. 3.2). Objectives, questions, and hypotheses are narrower in focus than the purpose and often specify only one or two research variables. They also identify the relationship between the variables and indicate the population to be studied. Some descriptive studies include only a research purpose, whereas others include a purpose and objectives or questions to direct the study. Correlational studies often include a purpose and objectives or questions. Hypotheses may or may not be included in descriptive and correlational studies. However, quasi-experimental and experimental studies need to include hypotheses to direct the conduct of the studies and the interpretation of findings (see Chapter 6). Theeke et al.'s (2019) research objectives and hypotheses are presented as follows:

Objectives

"[The study] had two specific aims: 1) to describe the gender differences for prevalence and characteristics of loneliness, anger, depression, self-management ability and biomarkers of chronic illness in a sample of chronically ill middle-aged adults living in Appalachia and 2) to describe the relationships among loneliness, anger, depression, self-management ability, biomarkers of chronic illness in chronically ill middle-aged adults living in Appalachia." (Theeke et al., 2019, p. 56)

Hypotheses

"Based on our extensive literature review on psychological constructs in persons living in Appalachia, the study team hypothesized that...

1. Women would have higher self-reports of loneliness and depression.
2. Men would have higher self-reports of anger.
3. Men would have higher mean scores for blood pressure when compared to women.
4. In both men and women, higher loneliness scores would be inversely related to self-management ability.
5. Loneliness would be predictive of poor self-management ability even while controlling for the possible effect of age, depression, and anger.
6. In both men and women, loneliness scores would be positively related to depressive symptoms, anger, and [biomarkers of chronic illness].
7. Mean loneliness scores would differ based on diagnosis of depression.
8. Mean anger would differ based on diagnosis of hypertension."
(Theeke et al., 2019, p. 56)

Defining Study Variables

The research objectives, questions, or hypotheses identify the variables to be examined in a study. **Variables** are concepts at various levels of abstraction that are measured, manipulated, or controlled in a study (see Box 3.1). Variables and concepts often share the same label or name. For example, in the Theeke et al. (2019) study, loneliness is both a concept and a variable. Sometimes more than one variable is needed to measure a concept, so the labels by necessity will differ. An example comes from a study by Lan et al. (2018) of an intervention to improve the sleep of hospitalized premature infants. The concept of sleep was measured by four variables—sleep efficiency, total sleep time, sleep latency, and frequency of wake bouts.

In quantitative research, variables are operationalized by developing conceptual and operational definitions. A **conceptual definition** provides a variable with theoretical meaning (Fawcett & Garity, 2009; Smith & Liehr, 2018) and is derived from a theorist's definition of the concept, a concept analysis, or a definition from the expert literature. Variables that measure abstract concepts such as creativity, empathy, and social support are best operationally defined by using a theorist's definition or a concept analysis. Variables that measure more concrete concepts such as temperature, weight, and blood pressure are best operationally defined by using the expert literature. An **operational definition** indicates how a variable will be measured, manipulated, or controlled in a study. The knowledge you gain from studying the variable will increase your understanding of the concept that the variable represents (see Chapter 6). In their study of loneliness in chronically ill midlife adults in Appalachia, Theeke et al. (2019) did not conceptually define their variables in the research report. Table 3.2 provides the operational definition for each variable as identified by the authors in the narrative.

Selecting a Research Design

The **research design** provides a blueprint for maximizing control over factors that could interfere with a study's desired outcome. The choice of research design depends on what is known and not known about the research problem, the researcher's expertise, the purpose for the study, and the desire to generalize findings. A variety of descriptive, correlational, quasi-experimental, and experimental designs have been generated over time to meet the evolving needs of researchers

TABLE 3.2	Operational Definitions of Study Variables in Theeke et al. (2019)
Variable	**Operational Definition**
Gender	Self-report of sociodemographic characteristic
Loneliness	Revised University of California, Los Angeles (UCLA) Loneliness Scale (Russell, 1996)
Anger	Clinical Anger Scale (CAS) (Snell, Gum, Shuck, Mosley, & Hite, 1995)
Depression	Patient Health Questionnaire-9 (PHQ-9) (Arroll et al., 2010)
Self-Management Ability	Self-Management Ability Scale–Short form (SMAS-S) (Cramm, Strating, deVreede, Steverink, & Nieboer, 2012)
Biomarkers of Chronic Illness	Blood pressure, body mass index, waist-hip ratio, and fasting finger stick glucose
Chronic Illness	Clinical diagnosis of hypertension, diabetes, depression, arthritis, obesity, hyperlipidemia, anxiety, emotional problems, heart disease, stroke, and/or lung disease
Mid-life Adults	Persons between the ages of 45 and 64 years old

(Kazdin, 2017; Leedy et al., 2019). In descriptive and correlational studies, no intervention is administered, so the purposes of these study designs include improving the precision of measurement, describing what exists, and clarifying relationships that provide a basis of quasi-experimental and experimental studies. Quasi-experimental and experimental study designs usually involve intervention and control groups and focus on achieving high levels of control, as well as precision in measurement (see Table 3.1). Chapters 10 and 11 present a variety of designs that are frequently implemented in quantitative studies.

Choice of a design commits the researcher to various details of the research process. These details may include number of subject groups, methods of sample selection and assignment to group, sample size, type of research setting, whether the researcher performs an intervention, timing of the research intervention, duration of the research process, method of data collection, method of data analysis, statistical tests chosen, conclusions able to be drawn from the study results, and scope of recommendations made. Because alterations in design may be necessary between the researcher's first general plan and the study's actual implementation, there ensues a ripple effect for the various components of the study. These components must be altered, as well, to maintain overall congruence among the components of the research plan. For example, the research purpose and questions or hypotheses must be edited to reflect any changes that are later made to the methodology and design of the study.

Some studies are designed as pilot studies. A **pilot study** can be defined as a "small-scale investigation conducted preparatory to a subsequent adequately powered trial" (Conn, 2010, p. 991) or other method of research. A typical reason to conduct a pilot study is to determine whether the proposed methods are effective in locating and obtaining consenting subjects, and in collecting useful data. This type of pilot study is often referred to as a feasibility study. Feasibility studies can determine whether subjects will actually consent to study participation, how many subjects really are available, how much time is required to gather data on one subject, and how well the instruments work. Some pilot studies strive to determine whether an intervention produces a measurable difference in the dependent variable and how large that difference is. For these studies, sample size needs to be carefully considered for meaningful results (Hertzog, 2008). Another reason for a pilot study is to pretest some aspect of the study. For example, a pilot study may be conducted to develop or refine an intervention or a measurement method. Other pilot studies may trial a data collection tool or even the entire data collection process. Conducting pilot studies usually results in stronger and more rigorous full-scale studies (Kazdin, 2017).

Theeke et al. (2019) describe their study design as "descriptive, cross-sectional" (p. 56). Their research objectives presented earlier suggest instead a descriptive correlational study design. The first specific aim focuses on describing gender differences in the study variables. As a comparison without manipulation of any variables, this aim indicates a descriptive design. The second aim focuses on describing relationships among the study variables, again without any manipulation of variables, which signifies a correlational study design. It is a common practice to combine the components of both descriptive and correlational designs in one study. The term *cross-sectional* means the data were collected during one slice in time without variable manipulation (Leedy et al., 2019).

Defining the Population and Sample

In research, the **population** is the set of all members of a defined group that serves as the focus of a study (Grove & Cipher, 2020). The defined group's members are known as elements. Elements of a population can be people, animals, plants, events, venues, or substances. The elements share at least one characteristic in common, such as an income level or a health condition. A population contains a finite number of elements (Thompson, 2012). There are many ways a researcher might choose to define the population of a study. For example, a researcher wants to conduct a study to describe patients' responses to nurse practitioners (NPs) as their primary care providers (PCPs). Some of the ways that the population might be defined are (1) all patients seen for their primary health care in clinics that employ NPs, (2) all patients who have already been under the care of NPs as their PCPs for at least a year, and (3) all adult patients covered by a health plan. The definition of the population depends on anticipated sampling criteria, type of research design, amount of time in which the study must be completed, method of data collection, costs, and researcher access. The part of the population to which the researcher has reasonable access is called the **accessible population**.

A **sample** is a subset of the accessible population that the researcher selects for participation in a study. Sampling defines the process for selecting a group of people or other elements with which to conduct a study. As mentioned earlier in this chapter, nursing studies use both random (probability) and nonrandom (nonprobability) sampling methods, and sample size is usually determined by conducting a power analysis (Aberson, 2019) (see Chapter 15). Excerpts from the Theeke et al. (2019) article that describe their study population and sample are presented next. The authors used a nonrandom sample recruited from a community-based primary care center located in West Virginia. The headers were provided to clarify the focus of the excerpts.

Population

"The target population included all adult patients between the ages of 45 and 64 who were experiencing chronic illness and who were being seen for a primary care visit at the clinical site." (Theeke et al., 2019, p. 56)

Sample

"Scheduled patients were made aware of the study using approved posters and flyers in the clinical site. Interested participants were screened using the inclusion and exclusion criteria prior to being invited to participate. Inclusion criteria were: diagnosis of least one chronic illness, living in Appalachia, and living in a community setting. Exclusion criteria were: current diagnosis of dementia, Folstein Minimental Status Examination (MMSE) (Folstein, Folstein, & McHugh, 1975) less than or equal to 23, significant psychiatric illness requiring antipsychotic medicine, or inability to understand and respond to survey questions. Each interview took approximately 20 min. With a 5% margin of error and 95% confidence interval, an estimated minimum sample of 70 was needed [as calculated by power analysis]. Oversampling of 90 participants was accomplished to allow for additional subgroup comparisons." (Theeke et al., 2019, p. 56)

Selecting Methods of Measurement

Measurement is the process of assigning "numbers to objects (or events or situations) in accord with some rule" (Kaplan, 1964, p. 177). A component of measurement is instrumentation, which is the application of specific rules to the development of a measurement method or instrument (Waltz et al., 2017). An instrument is a device selected by the researcher to measure a specific variable. Examples of common measurement devices used in nursing research are (1) rating scales for behavioral observations such as whether or not a patient is capable of self-feeding, (2) biomedical devices such as a pulse oximeter, (3) calculated laboratory tests such as sodium value, and (4) patient self-rating scales such as the Patient Health Questionnaire-9 (PHQ-9) (Arroll et al., 2010).

Data collected with measurement devices range from the nominal level through the ratio level of measurement. At the nominal level of measurement, only named or category values are present, such as male/female or nurse specialties. The values are names, from the Latin term *nomina*. Before or during data entry, these category names are coded as numbers for the process of descriptive statistical analysis. At the ratio level of measurement, using real numbers, there is an infinite array of possible values, such as −4.821, 82.5, and 373. The level of measurement, with nominal being the lowest form of measurement and ratio being the highest, is a determinant of the type of statistical analysis that can be performed on the data (Grove & Cipher, 2020).

Proper use of an instrument in a study includes examination of its reliability and validity. **Reliability** assesses how consistently the measurement technique measures a concept. The **validity** of an instrument is the extent to which it actually reflects the abstract concept being examined (Waltz et al., 2017). Chapter 16 introduces concepts of measurement and explains the different types of reliability and validity for instruments, and precision and accuracy for physiological measures (Ryan-Wenger, 2017). Chapter 17 provides a background for selecting measurement methods for a study. Excerpts from the Theeke et al. (2019) study on each of the self-rated scales that they used (see Table 3.2), including reliability and validity data, are presented as follows. An excerpt is also included in which Theeke et al. (2019) touched on the precision and accuracy of their measures of the biomarkers of chronic illness. Italics are added to the excerpts to emphasize study variables.

Methods of Measurement

"*Anger* was assessed using the Clinical Anger Scale (CAS). The CAS is a 21-item inventory that was chosen because it was developed to assess clinical anger which is conceptualized as a comprehensive assessment of anger and how it may be interfering with health and thinking (Snell [et al.], 1995). Each CAS score ranges from 0 to 63 with scores 0–13 indicating minimal anger, 14–19 indicating mild anger, 20–28 indicating moderate anger, and 29–63 indicating severe anger. Initial psychometrics support reliability (Cronbach's alpha = 0.94) and factor analysis supported a single factor analysis for men and women combined with an eigenvalue > 1. The SMOG [Simple Measure of Gobbledygook] score for readability is educational grade 3.4.

Loneliness was assessed using the 20-item scale Revised UCLA [University of California, Los Angeles] Loneliness Scale (Russell, 1996). This scale has been widely used in research for over 20 years with confirmed reliability and validity for assessing loneliness in multiple populations, including mid-life adults.... Participants rank answers on a Likert scale that ranges from *Never* (1) to *Always* (4) and then 9 questions are reverse-coded for total scoring. Scores range from 20 to 80 with 40 considered to be moderate loneliness... and 80 being very high loneliness....

Self-Management Ability... was operationalized using the self-management ability scale (SMAS-S). This 18-item version (total scores ranging from 0 to 84) was designed to operationalize the six core abilities of self-management as subscales with varying score ranges. They are identified as Taking Initiatives (range 0–15), Investment Behavior (range 0–15), Variety (range 0–15), Multifunctionality (range 0–12), Self-Efficacy (range 0–12), and positive Frame of Mind (range 0–15) (Cramm, Starting, deVreede, Steverink, & Nieboer, 2012). Internal consistency measures of the six subscales are reported to range from Cronbach's alpha 0.69–0.77. The SMOG readability score for the SMAS-S is educational grade 8.

Depressive symptoms were assessed using the Patient Health Questionnaire-9 (PHQ-9) (Arroll et al., 2010), which consists of nine items, each of which corresponds to a symptom of major depressive disorder. Patients report how often they experience these symptoms over two weeks on a 4-point Likert scale ranging from 0 (not at all) to 3 (nearly every day). The summed scores can range from 0 to 27, with scores of ≥ 5, ≥ 10, ≥ 15, and ≥ 20, representing mild, moderate, moderately severe, and severe levels of depressive symptoms, respectively. The reliability and validity of the PHQ-9 has been demonstrated extensively (Arroll et al., 2010). The SMOG score for readability is educational grade 6.

Biomarkers of chronic illness included blood pressure, body mass index, [waist-hip ratio], and fasting finger stick glucose. Blood pressure was measured by a registered nurse using a sphygmomanometer, BMI was calculated after obtaining . . . height and weight measures, and finger stick glucose was assessed using a calibrated plasma referenced glucometer and test strip." (Theeke et al., 2019, p. 57)

Developing a Plan for Data Collection and Analysis

A **data collection plan** in quantitative research is your plan for obtaining the output of the study instruments (see Fig. 3.2). Planning data collection will enable you to anticipate problems that are likely to occur and to explore possible solutions. Usually, detailed procedures for implementing an intervention and collecting data are developed, with a schedule that identifies the initiation and termination of the process (see Chapter 20). The expected location for the data collection plan in a research proposal is under the Methods section, often with the subheading Procedures. The same is true for reports of completed research, except that the Procedures section is worded in the past tense and includes any modifications of the original data collection plan that occurred.

A **data analysis plan** in quantitative research is your plan for how the data will be managed and which statistical tests will be conducted. Planning for data analysis occurs prior to implementation of the study to avoid the study findings influencing which statistics are conducted, the latter being an action that would reduce study rigor. Plans for data analysis are based on (1) objectives, questions, or hypotheses (or research purpose, if these are lacking); (2) type and volume of data; and (3) the level of measurement achieved by the research instruments (Grove & Cipher, 2020). Most researchers consult a statistician for assistance in developing analysis plans. Planning data analysis is the final step before the study commences.

Implementing the Research Plan

Implementing the research plan involves preparation of data collection materials, sample selection, collection of data (descriptive and correlational research) or intervention implementation and collection of data (quasi-experimental and experimental research), data analysis, and interpretation of research outcomes (see Fig. 3.2).

Data Collection

Data collection is the precise, systematic gathering of information relevant to the research purpose of a study. The data collected in quantitative studies are usually numerical, or in the case of nominal data, converted to numbers before data analysis. The process of data collection extends from before the first subject's data are obtained and ends as the last subject's data are obtained. Study variables are measured through a variety of techniques, depending on the measurement device(s) used. Common techniques include (1) observing with the use of checklists or similar devices to record observations, (2) collecting self-reported data through interviews and self-administered questionnaires and scales, (3) extracting existing data from such repositories as patient

records, and (4) assessing biomarkers such as anthropomorphic and physiological measures. The data are collected and recorded systematically for each subject in a computer file(s), which facilitates retrieval and analysis.

Prior to data collection, you must obtain permission for access to the research setting for the duration of the study. When this has been established, you will then obtain permission to collect data from human subjects, including approval of the consent form. That permission is obtained from the facility itself, if it has a committee for the protection of human subjects, usually called the institutional review board (IRB). You most likely will be required to complete training or certification related to data collection and ethical responsibilities to subjects. Students and faculty members conducting research in healthcare facilities usually need approval of both the university IRB and the facility IRB or the facility head (see Chapter 9). Two excerpts from the Theeke et al. (2019) study on the topic of data collection are presented as examples next. The first excerpt is a description of the permission process used for collecting the data. The second excerpt includes the techniques they used for data collection: face-to-face interviews, surveys (another term for self-administered questionnaires and scales), and physical measure testing (biomarker assessment).

Data Collection

"A letter of approval for the ethical conduct of research was obtained from the West Virginia University Institutional Review Board. Informed consent was obtained from each participant and the consent form was reviewed with the potential participants prior to signing. Participants were interviewed in a secure and private interview room within the Family Medicine Clinic. All members of the research team were trained to meet confidentiality requirements." (Theeke et al., 2019, p. 56)

"Data collection was conducted using three techniques. Face to face interviews to collect sociodemographic information and surveys of loneliness (UCLA), anger (CAS), depression (PHQ-9),... and [self-management ability] (SMAS-S).... The study team then performed physical measure testing to establish BMI, blood pressure, waist-hip ratio, and blood glucose levels. Chronic illness diagnoses were obtained by self-report in the interviews and verified with the electronic health records." (Theeke et al., 2019, p. 57)

Data Analysis

Data analysis is the reduction, organization, and statistical testing of information obtained in the data collection phase. Study subjects are first analyzed in terms of preexistent demographics. Then statistical tests are applied to the data collected on the study variables. The analysis of data from quantitative research involves the conduct of the following analyses: (1) descriptive analysis techniques (see Chapter 22) to describe demographic variables and study variables, (2) correlational statistical techniques to test proposed relationships among the variables (see Chapter 23), (3) regression analysis techniques to make predictions (see Chapter 24), and (4) analysis techniques to examine group differences, such as differences between genders or differences between intervention and control groups (see Chapter 25). As mentioned, decisions about data analysis are usually made a priori—before implementation of the research—to maintain the integrity of the research.

Procedures for data analysis used and the results of data analysis in Theeke et al.'s (2019) study are found in the following excerpts. Headings that identify the variables and hypotheses being tested were added to the results for learning purposes. Based on the results, the authors noted that their hypotheses 1, 2, 3, and 8 were not supported; hypotheses 4, 5, and 7 were supported; and hypothesis 6 was partially supported (see the hypothesis list presented earlier).

Data Analysis

"Data was [sic] entered into an SPSS [Statistical Package for the Social Sciences] data file and analyzed using SPSS Version 21. Prior to analysis, data was [sic] cleaned to look for outliers or impossible or missing values. Missing data patterns did identify < 5 cases of missing data on individual scale items and for these missing cells, mean substitutions based on gender were used. Analysis included repeating analyses with and without missing data to assess for any differences and none were present. To achieve the study aims, analysis included exploration of variables for descriptive information and bivariate analysis as appropriate based on variable type to determine gender differences and significant relationships among study variables. Once significant relationships were determined, hierarchical multiple regressions were performed if it was logical to do so based on the bivariate analyses. Regression was seeking the [predictive] value of loneliness, while controlling for age, anger and depression on self-management ability." (Theeke et al., 2019, p. 57)

Results

Sociodemographic Data Compared by Gender

"The sample of 90 adults [mean age 55.86, *SD* [standard deviation] 5.5, range 45–64 years] was majority female (68%), white (89%), married (50%) or divorced (20%), high school educated or higher (91%), and living at or near poverty level (mean number of people in the home > 2 and 65% with household incomes less than $40,000 per annum), working full-time (53%), and living in Appalachia > 10 years (79%). Eighty percent were born in Appalachia.… there were no significant differences in sociodemographics by gender." (Theeke et al., 2019, p. 58)

Chronic Illness Diagnoses Compared by Gender

"Overall, the study participants had a mean of 3.4 chronic illness diagnoses (*SD* 1.95). Men and women did not differ on diagnoses of hypertension, diabetes, anxiety[/emotional problems], arthritis, obesity, hyperlipidemia, or heart disease. However, men and women did differ on depression ($p < .01$). Women had a higher incidence of depression (47.4%) compared to men (15.6%)." (Theeke et al., 2019, p. 58)

Loneliness, Anger, Depression, and Self-Management Ability Compared by Gender (Hypotheses 1 and 2)

"In the overall sample, moderate loneliness was prevalent (mean UCLA score 41.29, *SD* 12.06, range 20–79) with only 1 participant having no loneliness. Depressive symptoms were low (mean PHQ-9 = 5.89, *SD* 5.54, range 0–22), and anger was low (mean [CAS] 5.67, *SD* 7.12, range 0–37).… Men were lonelier than women ($p < .01$). Men and women did not differ on anger, depressive symptoms, or self-management ability." (Theeke et al., 2019, p. 58)

Biomarkers of Chronic Illness Compared by Gender (Hypothesis 3)

"For the entire sample, all means for [biomarkers of] chronic illness… were elevated above the clinically accepted values.… Men had a higher mean waist-hip ratio when compared to women ($p = .001$).…men and women did not differ on blood pressure." (Theeke et al., 2019, p. 58)

Correlations Among Study Variables (Hypotheses 4 and 6)

"High loneliness correlated with anger ($r = 0.415$, $p < .01$) and depressive symptoms ($r = 0.558$, $p < .01$), and anger was correlated with depressive symptom[s] ($r = 0.621$, $p < .01$). Loneliness was inversely correlated with overall [self-management ability] ($r = -0.698$).... Anger inversely correlated to overall [self-management ability] ($r = -0.229$, $p < .01$).... and depression inversely correlated with overall SMA [self-management ability] ($r = -0.442$, $p < .01$)...." (Theeke et al., 2019, p. 58)

"Loneliness did correlate with depressive and anger symptoms but not with [the biomarkers of] chronic illness. . . ." (Theeke et al., 2019, p. 59)

Loneliness as a Predictor of Self-Management Ability (Hypothesis 5)

"Hierarchical multiple regression was used to assess the ability of loneliness to predict levels of self-management ability after controlling for the influence of age, anger, and depression. Age, anger, and depression were entered at step 1, explaining 23% of the variance in self-management ability. After entering loneliness at step 2, the total variance explained by the model was 54.8%, $F (4, 67) = 20.34$, $p < .001$. After controlling for age, anger, and depression, loneliness explained an additional 32% of the variance in SMA [self-management ability], R squared change $= 0.32$, F change $(1, 67) = 47.67$, $p < .01$." (Theeke et al., 2019, pp. 58–59)

Loneliness and Anger Compared by Chronic Illness Diagnosis (Hypotheses 7 and 8)

"Comparisons were conducted for differences in loneliness and anger based on chronic illness diagnoses.... mean loneliness scores did differ for chronic illness diagnoses of depression ($p = .05$) and emotional problems ($p < .01$).... Mean scores for anger... did differ based on chronic illness diagnoses of depression ($p < .01$) and emotional problems ($p < .01$) but not on the diagnosis of hypertension...." (Theeke et al., 2019, p. 59)

Interpreting Research Outcomes

The results obtained from data analysis require interpretation to be meaningful. **Interpretation of research outcomes** involves (1) examining the results of data analysis, (2) explaining what the results mean in light of current practice and previous research, (3) identifying study limitations, (4) forming conclusions, (5) deciding on the appropriate recommendation for generalization of the findings, (6) considering the implications for nursing's body of knowledge, and (7) suggesting the direction of further research. The study results from data analyses are translated and interpreted to become **findings**, and these findings are synthesized to form conclusions. Study conclusions are influenced by the limitations of the study. Implications for nursing's body of knowledge include ways to incorporate the conclusions into nursing theory and practice (Melnyk & Fineout-Overholt, 2019). Suggesting the direction of further research helps close the feedback loop of the steps of the quantitative research process with wise guidance for generating further research (see Fig. 3.2).

Limitations are aspects of the study that decrease the generalizability of the findings. These may or may not be due to problems or weaknesses of the study. There are four types of limitations, and they are related to the four types of validity discussed in Chapters 10 and 11. Construct limitations, sometimes called theoretical limitations, are failures of logic related to the researcher's definitions or reasoning, which limit the ability to interpret study findings on the theoretical level, the application level, or both. Internal validity limitations amount to incomplete or poor control of important extraneous variables and weaken the logical argument for the study's findings. External validity limitations refer to the actual population to which the study results can legitimately be generalized. Statistical limitations refer to inadequate or inappropriate statistical conclusions, often based on poor choices by the researcher. Limitations can diminish the credibility of study findings and conclusions or restrict the population to which findings can be generalized. It is important to remember that quantitative research is generalized to populations similar with respect to the study variables and to other attributes or conditions that might have impacted the results. Study conclusions provide a basis for identifying nursing implications and suggesting further studies in most research reports (see Chapter 26).

Theeke et al. (2019) interpreted all aspects of their research outcomes in the Discussion section of their research report, which is the typical location. Excerpts from the article that demonstrate interpretation of the research outcomes are presented next. The results were examined and explained in light of previous research and public health data. Both expected and surprising results were identified with an exploration of the meaning of these results. Subsections on Limitations, Implications for Clinical Practice, Implications for Future Research, and Conclusions completed the Discussion section.

Interpretation of the Research Outcomes

"Discussion

This study is the first to explore loneliness, anger, depression, self-management ability, and chronic illness control in this population. Although loneliness had been reported in some studies of mid-life adults who face traumatic life events..., empty nest...and retirement..., little was known about loneliness as it relates to other health variables. The sociodemographic and health-related descriptive findings were not surprising and are consistent with knowledge about determinants of health in Appalachia (Marshall et al., 2017). The overall prevalence of multiple chronic conditions is consistent with prevalence rates reported in [West Virginia].... The finding that women were more often diagnosed with depression is congruent with findings from other studies in samples of adults in this region of Appalachia (Theeke et al., 2012). While the descriptive findings of this study are not surprising for this population, they do highlight the experience of social determinants of health in Appalachia as the findings differed from national statistics of mid-life adults on education and income. Nationally, over 30% of adults have a college degree or higher and the median household income is greater than $51,000 per year (...Ryan & Baumen, 2016). It is known that social determinants of health, such as lower income and less educational attainment, have significant impact on physical and mental health.

The prevalence of loneliness reported by the mid-life adults in this study is similar to other studies that report loneliness as prevalent and moderately high in older Appalachian adults (Theeke et al., 2012). This is contrary to reports from other countries that adults in mid-life have generally less loneliness when compared to young or older adults (Victor & Yang, 2012). This finding makes it logical to consider that loneliness may be prevalent across the lifespan for Appalachian adults. This would be problematic as recent studies have reported that loneliness in mid-life adults is associated with systemic inflammation and contributes to poor physical health outcomes.... Little is known about the link between elevated inflammatory markers at mid-life and the seemingly reciprocal relationships among functional decline, illness burden, and feelings of loneliness, anger, and depression...." (Theeke et al., 2019, p. 59)

"The findings on anger were surprising and challenged existing qualitative findings that anger is very prevalent in lonely people.... Social relationships are needed for good mental and physical health. People who experience difficulties in establishing and maintaining mutual relationships with others are likely to experience loneliness, anger, depression, and anxiety.... However, it is difficult to establish the causal direction of the relationship between loneliness and anger because it is most likely that a reciprocal relationship exists.... We speculate, based on qualitative work, that anger in lonely persons is related to functional decline, frustration with healthcare system issues, disappointment in family or social relationships, and emotional dyscontrol from mental and physiological stress.... Hence, the fact that high loneliness was positively correlated with anger, even with anger being less prevalent, indicates that more work is needed to better measure anger in lonely persons...." (Theeke et al., 2019, p. 60)

"Limitations

The sample consisted of a convenience sample of mid-life adults from the north central region in Appalachia and potential participants were aware that the study included loneliness. Therefore, these findings represent loneliness in the mid-life Appalachian population, not the broader national population. It is also possible that sample bias exists and that men who were lonely volunteered to participate in the study since convenience sampling was used. Sociodemographic and survey responses were self-reported. Hence, these variables carry with them the limitations inherent in self-reported data. Given the characteristics of the anger described in this study, it is possible that the clinical anger scale did not capture the unique experience of anger specific to loneliness in this group. It is also possible that participants who value social desirability did not wish to disclose anger as an emotional response to loneliness. Lastly, it is possible that participants were experiencing other prevalent life circumstances that are not reflected in the survey questions." (Theeke et al., 2019, p. 60)

"Implications for clinical practice

Advanced understanding of how loneliness relates to anger and depression could lead to assessment programs, improved behavioral health services, new interventions, or refinement of existing interventions. Knowing that depression is on the rise and a major contributor to national disability, makes understanding the antecedents to diagnosis important. Developing treatment plans for patients in mid-life who are at high risk for depression should include the assessment of loneliness. Intervening when people are moderately lonely, not severely lonely, may be the key to prevention of depression, improving self-management ability, and preventing poor chronic illness outcomes later in life, especially for those living in Appalachia and experiencing health disparities." (Theeke et al., 2019, p. 61)

"*Implications for future research*
Future studies are needed to fill gaps in understanding the links between the determinants of health and loneliness as a predictor of depression and poor health outcomes, especially in mid-life. The prevalence of loneliness across the life-span and the known disparity of diabetes, stroke, and cardiovascular disease in Appalachia, makes it imperative to understand the reciprocal relationships among loneliness, functional decline, illness burden, chronic illness, and self-management ability. Identifying moderating and mediating variables using the PNI paradigm as a framework is potential future research. Further exploration of gender differences in the experience of loneliness, chronic illness burden and illness could lead to more precise interventions that are precise to gender. Findings related to anger in this study and those voiced in previous qualitative research warrants future investigation aimed at understanding anger in relation to functional decline, frustration, social relationships, and emotional dyscontrol within the experience of loneliness. Future studies of mid-life women are also needed to understand the high depression scores that were concurrent with reports of adequate support and positive SMA [self-management ability]." (Theeke et al., 2019, p. 61)

"*Conclusions*
Enhanced understanding of the relationships among loneliness, anger, depressive symptoms, and SMA in mid-life adults provides foundational information for future studies. This paper presents new information that loneliness is prevalent in mid-life adults in Appalachia and that loneliness is predictive of diminished self-management ability, even while controlling for the possible effects of age, anger, and depression. Including loneliness in behavioral health assessments in clinical practice and developing and studying the impact of interventions designed to target loneliness as a health problem will be imperative to continued understanding of loneliness and its impact on health." (Theeke et al., 2019, p. 61)

Communicating Research Findings

Research is not considered complete until the findings have been communicated. **Communicating research findings** involves developing and disseminating a research report to appropriate audiences. The research report is disseminated through presentations and publication (see Chapter 27). Theeke et al.'s (2019) study was published in *Applied Nursing Research*, a long-standing and prestigious nursing research journal.

STEPS OF THE QUANTITATIVE RESEARCH PROCESS FOR A QUASI-EXPERIMENTAL STUDY

The final example of quantitative research presented in this chapter is a quasi-experimental study (see Table 3.1). The Hinic and colleagues (2019) study, introduced earlier, sought to determine the effect of pet therapy on anxiety in hospitalized children. The researchers also measured coping in the hospitalized children and parent satisfaction as secondary aims, but only excerpts related to the primary aim are shown in the following example. Excerpts from the research report that capture the research problem, research purpose, and review of literature are found in the example.

A framework was not provided in the research report. In addition, a hypothesis was not formulated, which is atypical for quasi-experimental research. However, conceptual and operational definitions of both the independent and dependent variables were clearly stated. This study is an excellent example of the reasons it can be difficult to randomize study participants into intervention and control groups. The researchers could not seclude the control group from pet therapy because pet therapy was provided several times a week on the hospital unit where the study took place. The control group received a puzzle activity on the days that pet therapy was not scheduled. The limitations that this approach placed on the study are described by the researchers in their discussion section. The researchers used a pretest-posttest design with comparison group (see Chapter 11) in which the dependent variable was measured both before and after the pet therapy or puzzle activity. Data analysis demonstrated that the intervention and control groups did not differ by anxiety before the activities, but anxiety was significantly lower after these activities in the intervention group. The researchers interpreted their research outcomes in the context of prior research findings, which helped define the state of the science for pet therapy in this population.

Steps of the Research Process in a Quasi-Experimental Study

Research Problem

"Hospitalization of a child is a stressful life event for a child and family, causing a sudden disruption in the daily routines of home and school that are fundamental to well-being....Specific stressors can include physical pain, fear associated with both procedures and un-known healthcare workers, separation from familiar people, foods, environment, belongings, and pets. Specialists in pediatric care including pediatric nurses and childlife specialists are dedicated to promoting healing by normalizing the acute care hospital for the child and family. Animal assisted activities (AAA), also referred to as pet therapy, are a practice widely used in a variety of healthcare settings (Goddard & Gilmer, 2015, ...).... Pet therapy provides a non-pharmacological, complementary intervention to help alleviate anxiety and fear related to hospitalization in children. *While there has been an increase in research related to pet therapy and children in recent years, this is still a developing body of knowledge. Empirical support for the use of complementary therapies to reduce anxiety among children in the acute care setting is needed* [emphasis added to indicate the problem statement]." (Hinic et al., 2019, p. 55)

Research Purpose

"The purpose of this study was to evaluate the effect of a brief pet therapy visit and a comparison intervention on anxiety in hospitalized children" (Hinic et al., 2019, p. 55)

"The main research question that guided the study was: What is the effectiveness of a brief pet therapy intervention in comparison to a puzzle activity on state anxiety among children receiving care in a US hospital?" (Hinic et al., 2019, p. 56)

Review of Relevant Literature

"Pet Therapy and Children

Among children, pet therapy has long been used as a complementary therapy for those with or at risk for mental health problems. A recent systematic review identified equine therapy for autism and canine therapy for trauma as those areas with the strongest evidence base for children with or at risk for mental health problems (Hoagwood, Acri, Morrissey, & Peth-Pierce, 2017). Three out of three studies reviewed showed beneficial effects of AAA for children who experienced trauma. Another systematic review specifically focused on trauma, but not limited to children, found reduced depression, anxiety

and posttraumatic stress disorder (PTSD) symptoms across studies among people participating in pet therapy activities (O'Haire, Guérin, & Kirkham, 2015)...." (Hinic et al., 2019, pp. 55–56)

"Pet therapy and anxiety in hospitalized children

In a recent randomized study, Barker, Schubert, Green, & [sic] Ameringer (2015) explored the impact of a 10-minute pet therapy visit on pain and anxiety in hospitalized children between the ages of 8 and 18 years of age (m = 11.3 years of age). Children were hospitalized for 31 different unspecified conditions, with the most commonly reoccurring being appendicitis and abdominal pain. The study also evaluated whether the child's attachment level to family had a mediating effect on the response to the animal visit. Participants (N = 40) were randomly assigned to either the intervention group, which consisted of a 10-minute pet therapy visit (n = 20), or the control group (n = 20), which involved the child completing an age-appropriate jigsaw puzzle. There were no significant differences between or within the intervention or control groups in terms of self-reported pain or anxiety, suggesting that the pet therapy treatment did not significantly impact pain or anxiety in this sample. However, baseline anxiety levels were low, with 60% of participants reporting no anxiety. This low baseline could provide some explanation for the lack of significant changes in the outcome variables." (Hinic et al., 2019, p. 56)

Independent Variable (Pet Therapy Intervention)

Conceptual Definition

"The International Association of Human-Animal Interaction Organizations (IAHAIO, 2014) defines AAA as an informal interaction between a patient and a therapy animal for motivational, educational, or recreational purposes. These activities can include visits with a therapy animal and its handler, who is typically a non-medically trained volunteer, and are spontaneous in nature." (Hinic et al., 2019, p. 55)

Operational Definition

"[P]articipants in the pet therapy group received an eight to 10-minute visit from a therapy dog and handler team along with the research assistant.... The coordinator of our pet therapy program worked with the certifying agencies to ensure consistent visits with these particular dog-handler teams throughout the period of data collection." (Hinic et al., 2019, p. 57-58)

Dependent Variable (State Anxiety)

Conceptual Definition

"The S[tate]-anxiety scale is designed to measure temporary anxiety states, defined as 'subjective, consciously perceived feelings of apprehension, tension, and worry that vary in intensity and fluctuate over time' (Spielberger, 1973, p. 1)." (Hinic et al., 2019, p. 57)

Operational Definition

"Study data were collected using the STAIC [State-Trait Anxiety Inventory for Children] S-Anxiety Scale (Spielberger, 1973). . . ." (Hinic et al., 2019, p. 57)

Sample

"A convenience sample of children and adolescents who were hospitalized at the study site were invited to participate in the study. Participants were limited to English speaking children between the ages of six and 17 without cognitive impairment who were hospitalized in the general pediatric inpatient unit. Therefore, those receiving care in the outpatient areas, pediatric day hospital, or pediatric intensive care unit were excluded from participation. Additional exclusion criteria were consistent with the institution's pet therapy policy and included allergy to or fear of dogs, need for any type of isolation precautions, open sores or burns, neutropenia, splenectomy, bone marrow transplants, and certain types of infection. Children who had received a prior pet therapy visit during the current hospitalization were also excluded.... An *a priori* power analysis, based on moderate effect size ($d = 0.5$) and $p \leq .05$, indicated that a sample of 84 participants, with 42 in the intervention group and 42 in the control group, was required for the study." (Hinic et al., 2019, p. 57)

Procedures

"Families for both the control and intervention group were approached by a member of the research team and invited to participate in a study related to anxiety in children. If the parent and child expressed interest, the child was then screened for study eligibility. The study, along with its voluntary nature, was explained to eligible families and written consent was obtained from a parent and assent obtained and documented from the child. Participants were assigned to either the pet therapy or comparison group based upon the day on which data collection was occurring. Randomization was not feasible due to the open nature of the pediatric unit and the general excitement among the children when the therapy dog and handler teams enter the unit. Instead, data collection was scheduled for 2 days of each week—1 day when pet therapy visits were scheduled and the other where no pet therapy visits were scheduled and participants were grouped accordingly. The parent was present for all study related activities, including the consent process, the duration of the pet therapy visit and puzzle completion [(the control group)], and completion of questionnaires.

Following explanation of the study and the consent and assent process, participants in both groups were invited by the research staff to complete the State-Trait Anxiety [Inventory] for Children (STAIC) S-Anxiety Scale (Spielberger, 1973), also referred to as the 'How I feel Questionnaire.' ... Following the visit, the child again completed the STAIC S-Anxiety Scale ...." (Hinic et al., 2019, p. 57)

Data Analysis

"Data were cleaned and entered on an ongoing basis throughout the study. The sample was compared descriptively between control and intervention groups using *t*-test and chi square analysis. Descriptive analysis provided an overview of factors related to state anxiety levels.

Because STAIC S-Anxiety scores did not follow a normal distribution, non-parametric analyses were employed to evaluate changes in the construct of state anxiety. Wilcoxon matched-pair signed rank test was used to evaluate change in anxiety before and after each intervention within group. Mann–Whitney *U* test was employed to evaluate differences in anxiety between groups pre and post and to evaluate the difference in anxiety change scores between groups. Data were analyzed with IBM [International Business Machines] SPSS Statistics, Version 23, (Armonk, NY), and $p < .05$ was considered significant." (Hinic et al., 2019, p. 58)

Results

"Wilcoxon matched-pair signed rank tests were conducted to measure whether there was a change in state anxiety level in the control and intervention groups, as illustrated in the table below. Within the pet therapy group, there was a significant difference in state anxiety scores before the intervention (med = 31, min–max = 20–46) and after the intervention (med = 25, min–max = 20–40); $p < .001$. Similarly, in the comparison group, there was a significant difference in state anxiety score before completing the puzzle (med = 30, min–max = 20–48) and after completing the puzzle (*m* = 28, min–max = 20–40); $p < .001$. These findings suggest that both the puzzle and the pet therapy visits decreased children's experiences of state anxiety. However, while there was no significant difference in baseline state anxiety scores between the intervention and control groups ($p = .537$), postintervention state anxiety scores were significantly lower in the pet therapy intervention group than in the puzzle comparison group ($p = .002$). Additionally, change in anxiety scores was calculated based upon decrease from baseline to post-intervention. Median change score for the

Anxiety comparison across groups.

	Pre-anxiety	Post-anxiety	p-Value
	med (min-max)	*med* (min-max)	
Puzzle comparison group	30 (20–48)	28 (20–40)	<0.001*
Pet therapy intervention group	31 (20–46)	25 (20–40)	<0.001*
p value difference	0.537**	0.002**	

* Wilcoxon matched-pair signed rank test used to calculate p-values.
** Mann-Whitney *U* test used to calculate p-values.

From Hinic, K., Kowalski, M. O., Holtzman, K., & Mobus, K. (2019). The effect of a pet therapy and comparison intervention on anxiety in hospitalized children. *Journal of Pediatric Nursing, 46,* 55–61.

puzzle group was a decrease by two points and for the pet therapy group was a decrease of six points. A Mann–Whitney *U* test confirmed that this represented a statistically significant difference ($p = .004$) in anxiety change score between the two groups. These findings suggest that while both the pet therapy and comparison interventions positively affected participants' state anxiety level, the pet therapy intervention more effectively reduced anxiety levels." (Hinic et al., 2019, p. 58)

Interpretation of Research Outcomes
"Discussion

Families of children who are hospitalized identify stress, anxiety, and pain as key factors that contribute to an overall negative hospital experience (Muscara et al., 2015). Findings from this study add to the body of knowledge related to non-pharmacologic strategies to increase wellbeing in both children receiving care in the hospital and their families. Strengths of this study include an adequate sample size, standardized intervention, and the presence of an active comparative intervention.

Anxiety

Study findings suggest that a brief pet therapy visit more effectively reduces state anxiety than a comparative activity of completing a jigsaw puzzle. These findings are congruent with results of a recent meta-analysis (Waite, Hamilton, & O'Brien, 2018) that supported the positive effect of pet therapy on anxiety, distress, and pain in 22 studies, including 13 that involved children in medical settings. Other studies, however, including those by Barker et al. (2015) and by Tsai et al. (2010) contrast with our study findings and have found no significant decrease in state anxiety following pet therapy. The effect of pet therapy on state anxiety may be mediated by other factors such

as trait anxiety level, presence of a chronic condition, new diagnosis of a serious illness, and other medical, psychological and social factors...." (Hinic et al., 2019, p. 59)

"Limitations

The findings from this study need to be interpreted in the context of several limitations. This was a convenience sample and it is not known how families who chose to participate in the study may have differed from children and families who did not participate. Also, ... because we did not use randomization, it is possible that other biases could have been introduced since participants knew which group they were assigned upon enrollment. In addition, we did not collect information related to circumstances that may have affected baseline anxiety levels in participants such as exposure to an invasive procedure, a visit from family, or length of stay. We also did not collect data related to medications the child may have received prior to study participation that could have affected anxiety levels....

The majority of research, including this study, related to pet therapy in children focuses on baseline and immediate post-intervention data. This type of study design does not provide information about whether the immediate benefits of pet therapy are sustained after the early post-intervention period. Also, much of the data in pet therapy studies are collected by self-report. Many of the conditions pet therapy aims to address, such as pain and anxiety, are intrinsically subjective constructs.

Finally, while the study sample was diverse in relation to reasons for hospitalization, age, presence of chronic condition, it was conducted at a single site so this may limit generalizability of findings." (Hinic et al., 2019, p. 60)

"Clinical implications [and implications for future studies]

Incorporating a brief pet therapy visit into routine pediatric care can be a relatively low cost, non-pharmacologic intervention to decrease anxiety and promote patient satisfaction in children and families receiving care in the hospital setting. Nurses and childlife specialists routinely assess children and families for stress, anxiety, and effectiveness of coping strategies. Study findings provide empirical support for a brief pet therapy visit as a tool to decrease anxiety in hospitalized children and promote family satisfaction. When resources for providing pet therapy visits are limited, clinicians may consider prioritizing children who are most affected by anxiety or are having difficulty coping with the stress of hospitalization.

There is a great need for future studies that explore longer term effects of pet therapy on patient outcomes that continue after the novelty of the visit wears off as well as rigorous evaluation of pet therapy interaction beyond a brief visit (Waite et al., 2018). Future study of anxiety could additionally include further investigation into biomarkers, salivary cortisol measurement, or other physiologic parameters such as heart rate and blood pressure." (Hinic et al., 2019, p. 60)

"Conclusions

Pet therapy can be an effective complementary therapy to decrease anxiety in children receiving care in the hospital. Additional development and implementation of evidence-based pet therapy programs can have a positive effect on children and families. Rigorous study of psychological and physiological outcomes associated with these programs both in the immediate and long-term periods is needed to continue to expand the evidence-base for this potentially powerful tool." (Hinic et al., 2019, p. 60)

KEY POINTS

- Nurses use a broad range of quantitative approaches—including descriptive, correlational, quasi-experimental, and experimental—to develop nursing knowledge (see Fig. 3.1).
- In this chapter, examples from published studies are used to illustrate the steps of the quantitative research process for these different types of quantitative research.
- Some of the terms relevant to quantitative research are (1) the scientific method, (2) basic research, (3) applied research, (4) rigor, and (5) control.
- The scientific method is the basis for decision making related to testing hypotheses.
- Basic research, often called preclinical research in the health sciences, is a scientific investigation that involves the pursuit of knowledge for knowledge's sake, without a specific application in mind.
- Applied or clinical research is a scientific investigation conducted to generate knowledge that will directly influence or improve clinical practice.
- Rigor involves discipline, scrupulous adherence to detail, and strict accuracy.
- Control involves the imposing of rules by the researcher to decrease the possibility of error and thus increase the probability that the study's findings are an accurate reflection of reality.

- The steps of the quantitative research process are as follows (see Fig. 3.2):
  1. Formulating a research problem and purpose identifies an area of concern and the specific focus or aim of the study.
  2. Reviewing relevant literature allows the researcher to build a picture of what is known about a particular situation or phenomenon and identify the knowledge gaps that exist.
  3. Developing a framework guides the development of the study and enables the researcher to link the findings to the body of knowledge in nursing.
  4. Formulating research objectives, questions, or hypotheses allows the researcher to bridge the gap between the more abstractly stated research problem and purpose and the study design and plan for data collection and analysis.
  5. Defining study variables involves developing a conceptual definition and operational definition for each variable.
  6. Selecting a research design directs the selection of a population, sampling procedure, implementation of the intervention, methods of measurement, and a plan for data collection and analysis.
  7. Defining the population and sample determines who will participate in the study.

8. Developing a detailed intervention plan involves the detailed steps or elements of the intervention and the consistent implementation of the intervention during the study (for quasi-experimental and experimental research).

9. Selecting methods of measurement involves determining the best method(s) to measure each study variable.

10. Developing a plan for data collection and analysis directs the precise, systematic gathering of information relevant to the research purpose or the specific objectives, questions, or hypotheses of a study and involves the selection of appropriate statistical techniques to analyze the study data.

11. Implementing the research plan involves intervention implementation for quasi-experimental and experimental research, data collection, data analysis, and interpretation of research outcomes.

12. Interpreting the research outcomes involves examining the results from data analysis, exploring the significance of the findings, identifying study limitations, forming conclusions, generalizing findings as appropriate, considering implications for nursing practice, and suggesting further studies.

13. Communicating findings includes the development and dissemination of a research report to appropriate audiences through presentations and publication.

REFERENCES

Aberson, C. L. (2019). *Applied power analysis for the behavioral sciences* (2nd ed.). New York, NY: Routledge Taylor & Francis Group.

Adynski, H., Zimmer, C., Thorp, J., & Santos, H. P. (2019). Predictors of psychological distress in low-income mothers over the first postpartum year. *Research in Nursing & Health, 42*(3), 205–216. doi:10.1002/nur.21943

AL-Rawajfah, O. M., Aloush, S., & Hewitt, J. B. (2015). Use of electronic health-related datasets in nursing and health-related research. *Western Journal of Nursing Research, 37*(7), 952–983. doi:10.1177/0193945914558426

Arroll, B., Goodyear-Smith, F., Crengle, S., Gunn, J., Kerse, N., Fishman, T., ... Hatcher, S. (2010). Validation of PHQ-2 and PHQ-9 to screen for major depression in the primary care population. *Annals of Family Medicine, 8*(4), 348–353. doi:10.1370/afm.1139

Babic, A., Tokalic, R., Silva Cunha, J. A., Novak, I., Suto, J., Vidak, M., ... Puljak, L. (2019). Assessments of attrition bias in Cochrane systematic reviews are highly inconsistent and thus hindering trial comparability. *BMC Medical Research Methodology, 19*, 76. doi:10.1186/s12874-019-0717-9

Bakken, S. (2019). Not the medical informatics of our founding mothers and fathers, or is it? *Journal of the American Medical Informatics Association, 26*(5), 381–382. doi:10.1093/jamia/ocz027

Barker, L. E., Kirtland, K. A., Gregg, E. W., Geiss, L. S., & Thompson, T. J. (2011). Geographic distribution of diagnosed diabetes in the U.S.: A diabetes belt. *American Journal of Preventive Medicine, 40*(4), 434–439. doi:10.1016/j.amepre.2010.12.019

Barker, S. B., Schubert, C. M., Green, J. D., & Ameringer, S. (2015). The effect of an animal assisted intervention on anxiety and pain in hospitalized children. *Antrozoös, 28*(1), 101–112. doi:10.2752/089279315X14129350722091

Basic Research. (n.d.) In *Glossary of NIH terms*. Retrieved from https://grants.nih.gov/grants/glossary.htm

Bodner, E., & Bergman, Y. S. (2016). Loneliness and depressive symptoms among older adults: The moderating role of subjective life expectancy. *Psychiatry Research, 237*, 78–82. doi:10.1016/j.psychres.2016.01.074

Bova, C., Jaffarian, C., Crawford, S., Quintos, J. B., Lee, M., & Sullivan-Bolyai, S. (2017). Intervention fidelity: Monitoring drift, providing feedback, and assessing the control condition. *Nursing Research, 66*(1), 54–59. doi:10.1097/NNR.0000000000000194

Cacioppo, J. T., Hawkley, L. C., & Thisted, R. A. (2010). Perceived social isolation makes me sad: 5-year cross-lagged analyses of loneliness and depressive symptomatology in the Chicago Health, Aging, and Social Relations Study. *Psychology and Aging, 25*(2), 453–463. doi:10.1037/a0017216

Campbell, D. T., & Stanley, J. C. (1963). Experimental and quasi-experimental designs for research on teaching. In N. L. Gage (Ed.), *Handbook of research on teaching* (pp. 171–246). Chicago, IL: Rand McNally.

Conn V. S. (2010). Rehearsing for the show: The role of pilot study reports for developing nursing science. *Western Journal of Nursing Research, 32*(8), 991–993. doi:10.1177/0193945910377161

Cramm, J. M., Strating, M. M., deVreede, P. L., Steverink, N., & Nieboer, A. P. (2012). Validation of the self-management ability scale (SMAS) and development and validation of a shorter scale (SMAS-S) among older adult patients shortly after hospitalisation. *Health and*

Quality of Life Outcomes, 10(9), 1–7. doi:10.1186/1477-7525-10-9

Creswell, J. W., & Creswell, J. D. (2018). *Research design: Qualitative, quantitative, and mixed methods approaches* (5th ed.). Los Angeles, CA: Sage.

Dorsey, S. G., Griffioen, M. A., Renn, C. L., Cashion, A. K., Colloca, L., Jackson-Cook, C. K., … Lyon, D. (2019). Working together to advance symptom science in the precision era. *Nursing Research, 68*(2), 86–90. doi:10.1097/NNR.0000000000000339

Dorsey, S. G., & Pickler, R. H. (2019). Precision science in nursing research. *Nursing Research, 68*(2), 85. doi:10.1097/NNR.0000000000000333

Fawcett, J., & Garity, J. (2009). *Evaluating research for evidence-based nursing practice.* Philadelphia, PA: F. A. Davis.

Fisher, Sir, R. A. (1935). *The designs of experiments.* New York, NY: Hafner.

Folstein, M. F., Folstein, S. E., & McHugh, P. R. (1975). "Mini-mental state": A practical method for grading the cognitive state of patients for the clinician. *Journal of Psychiatric Research, 12*(3), 189–198. doi:10.1016/0022-3956(75)90026-6

Friedman, L. M., Furberg, C. D., DeMets, D. L., Reboussin, D. M. & Granger, C. B. (2015). *Fundamentals of clinical trials* (5th ed.). Switzerland: Springer International.

Goddard, A. T., & Gilmer, M. J. (2015). The role and impact of animals with pediatric patients. *Pediatric Nursing, 41*(2), 65–71.

Grady P. A. (2010). Translational research and nursing science. *Nursing Outlook, 58*(3), 164–166. doi:10.1016/j.outlook.2010.01.001

Grove, S. K., & Cipher, D. J. (2020). *Statistics for nursing research: A workbook for evidence-based practice* (3rd ed.). St. Louis, MO: Elsevier.

Hackett, R. A., Hamer, M., Endrighi, R., Brydon, L., & Steptoe, A. (2012). Loneliness and stress-related inflammatory and neuroendocrine responses in older men and women. *Psychoneuroendocrinology, 37*(11), 1801–1809. doi:10.1016/j.psyneuen.2012.03.016

Hertzog, M. (2008). Considerations in determining sample size for pilot studies. *Research in Nursing & Health, 31*(2), 180–191. doi:10.1002/nur.20247

Hinic, K., Kowalski, M. O., Holtzman, K., & Mobus, K. (2019). The effect of a pet therapy and comparison intervention on anxiety in hospitalized children. *Journal of Pediatric Nursing, 46*, 55–61. doi:10.1016/j.pedn.2019.03.003

Hinshaw, A. S. (1979). Theoretical substruction: An assessment process. *Western Journal of Nursing Research, 1*(4), 319–324. doi:10.1177/019394597900100410

Hoagwood, K. E., Acri, M., Morrissey, M., & Peth-Pierce, R. (2017). Animal-assisted therapies for youth with or at risk for mental health problems: A systematic review. *Applied Developmental Science, 21*(1), 1–13. doi:10.1080/10888691.2015.1134267

International Association of Human-Animal Interaction Organizations. (2014). *The IAHIO definitions for animal assisted intervention and guidelines for wellness of animals involved.* Retrieved from http://iahaio.org/wp/wp-content/uploads/2017/05/iahaiowhite-paper-final-nov-24-2014.pdf

Kaplan, A. (1964). *The conduct of inquiry: Methodology for behavioral science.* New York, NY: Chandler.

Kazdin, A. E. (2017). *Research design in clinical psychology* (5th ed.). Boston, MA: Pearson.

Kearney, M. H. (2019). Intervention research is hard to find: Reflections on RINAH's history and future. *Research in Nursing & Health, 42*(1), 2–4. doi:10.1002/nur.21932

Kerlinger, F. N., & Lee, H. B. (2000). *Foundations of behavioral research* (4th ed.). Fort Worth, TX: Harcourt College Publishers.

Kessler, R. C., Petukhova, M., Sampson, N. A., Zaslavsky, A. M., & Wittchen, H. (2012). Twelve-month and lifetime prevalence and lifetime morbid risk of anxiety and mood disorders in the United States. *International Journal of Methods in Psychiatric Research, 21*(3), 169–184. doi:10.1002/mpr.1359

Lan, H., Yang, L., Hsieh, K., Yin, T., Chang, Y., & Liaw, J. (2018). Effects of a supportive care bundle on sleep variables of preterm infants during hospitalization. *Research in Nursing & Health, 41*(3), 281–291. doi:10.1002/nur.21865

Lauer, M. (2016). *NIH's commitment to basic science.* Retrieved from https://nexus.od.nih.gov/all/2016/03/25/nihs-commitment-to-basic-science/

Lee, C. Y., & Goldstein, S. (2016). Loneliness, stress, and social support in young adulthood: Does the source of support matter? *Journal of Youth & Adolescence, 45*(3), 568–580. doi:10.1007/s10964-015-0395-9

Leedy, P., Ormrod, J., & Johnson, L. (2019). *Practical research: Planning and design* (12th ed.). New York City, NY: Pearson.

Ma, X. Q., Qin, J., Li, H. Y., Yan, X. L., Zhao, Y., & Zhang, L. J. (2019). Role of exercise activity in alleviating neuropathic pain in diabetes via inhibition of the pro-inflammatory signal pathway. *Biological Research for Nursing, 21*(1), 14–21. doi:10.1177/1099800418803175

Marshall, J., Thomas, L., Lane, N., Holmes, G., Arcury, T. A., Randolph, R., … Ivey, K. (2017). *Health disparities in Appalachia.* Washington, DC: Appalachian Regional Commission. Retrieved from https://www.arc.gov/research/researchreportdetails.asp?REPORT_ID=138

McCain, N. L., Gray, D. P., Walter, J. M., & Robins, J. (2005). Implementing a comprehensive approach to the study of health dynamics using the psychoneuroimmunology paradigm. *Advances in Nursing Science, 28*(4), 320–332. doi:10.1097/00012272-200510000-00004

Meleis, A. I. (2018). *Theoretical nursing.* Philadelphia, PA: Wolters Kluwer.

Melnyk, B. M., & Fineout-Overholt, E. (2019). *Evidence-based practice in nursing and healthcare: A guide to best practice* (4th ed.). Philadelphia, PA: Wolters Kluwer.

Momtaz, Y. A., Hamid, T. A., Yusoff, S., Ibrahim, R., Chai, S. T., Yahaya, N., & Abdullah, S. S. (2012). Loneliness as a risk factor for hypertension in later life. *Journal of Aging & Health, 24*(4), 696–710. doi:10.1177/0898264311431305

Morrison-Beady, D., & Melnyk, B. (2018). *Intervention research and evidence-based quality improvement: Designing, conducting, analyzing, and funding* (2nd ed.). New York: Springer.

Muscara, F., McCarthy, M. C., Woolf, C., Hearps, S. J. C., Burke, K., & Anderson, V. A. (2015). Early psychological reactions in parents of children with a life threatening illness within a pediatric hospital setting. *European Psychiatry, 30*(5), 555–561. doi:10.1016/j.eurpsy.2014.12.008

Nakamura, S., Kato, K., Yoshida, A., Fukuma, N., Okumura, Y., Ito, H., & Mizuno, K. (2013). Prognostic value of depression, anxiety, and anger in hospitalized cardiovascular disease patients for predicting adverse cardiac outcomes. *American Journal of Cardiology, 111*(10), 1432–1436. doi:10.1016/j.amjcard.2013.01.293

O'Haire, M. E., Guérin, N. A., & Kirkham, A. C. (2015). Animal-assisted intervention for trauma: A systematic literature review. *Frontiers in Psychology, 6*, 1–13. doi:10.3389/fpsyg.2015.01121

Porter, T. M. (2004). *Karl Pearson: The scientific life in a statistical age.* Oxfordshire, United Kingdom: Princeton University Press.

Rubio, D. M., Schoenbaum, E. E., Lee, L. S., Schteingart, D. E., Marantz, P. R., Anderson, K. E., … Esposito, K. (2010) Defining translational research: Implications for training. *Academic Medicine: Journal of the Association of American Medical Colleges, 85*(3), 470–475. doi:10.1097/ACM.0b013e3181ccd618

Russell, D. W. (1996). UCLA Loneliness Scale (Version 3): Reliability, validity, and factor structure. *Journal of Personality Assessment, 66*(1), 20-40. doi:10.1207/s15327752jpa6601_2

Ryan, C. L., & Bauman, K. (2016, March). *Educational attainment in the United States: 2015* (P20-578). Washington, DC: U.S. Census Bureau. Retrieved from https://www.census.gov/library/publications/2016/demo/p20-578.html

Ryan, P., Weiss, M., & Papanek, P. (2019). A substruction approach to assessing the theoretical validity of measures. *Journal of Nursing Measurement, 27*(1), 126–145. doi:10.1891/1061-3749.27.1.126

Ryan-Wenger, N. A. (2017). Precision, accuracy, and uncertainty of biophysical measurements for research and practice. In C. F. Waltz, O. L. Strickland, & E. R. Lenz (Eds.), *Measurement in nursing and health research* (5th ed.) (pp. 427–445). New York, NY: Springer.

Schoenfisch, A. L., Kucera, K. L., Lipscomb, H. J., McIlvaine, J., Becherer, L., James, T., & Avent, S. (2019). Use of assistive devices to lift, transfer, and reposition hospital patients. *Nursing Research, 68*(1), 3–12. doi:10.1097/NNR.0000000000000325

Shadish, W. R., Cook, T. D., & Campbell, D. T. (2002). *Experimental and quasi-experimental designs for generalized causal inference.* Chicago: IL: Rand McNally.

Smith, M. J., & Liehr, P. R. (2018). *Middle range theory for nursing* (4th ed.). New York, NY: Springer Publishing Company.

Snell Jr., W. E., Gum, S., Shuck, R. L., Mosley, J. A., & Hite, T. L. (1995). The clinical anger scale: Preliminary reliability and validity. *Journal of Clinical Psychology, 51*(2), 215–226. doi:10.1002/1097-4679(199503)51:2%3C215::AID-JCLP2270510211%3E3.0.CO;2-Z

Spielberger, C. D. (1973). *Preliminary test manual for the State-Trait Anxiety Inventory for Children.* Palo Alto, CA: Consulting Psychologists Press, Inc.

Tappen, R. (2016). *Advanced nursing research: From theory to practice* (2nd ed.). Burlington, MA: Jones & Bartlett Learning.

Theeke, L., Carpenter, R. D., Mallow, J., & Theeke, E. (2019). Gender differences in loneliness, anger, depression, self-management ability and biomarkers of chronic illness in chronically ill mid-life adults in Appalachia. *Applied Nursing Research, 45*, 55–62. doi:10.1016/j.apnr.2018.12.001

Theeke, L., Goins, R. T., Moore, J., & Campbell, H. (2012). Loneliness, depression, social support, and quality of life in older chronically ill Appalachians. *Journal of Psychology, 146*(1/2), 155–171. doi:10.1080/00223980.2011.609571

Thompson, S. K. (2012). *Sampling* (3rd ed.). Hoboken, NJ: Wiley.

Tsai, C. C., Friedmann, E., & Thomas, S. A. (2010). The effects of animal-assisted therapy on stress responses in hospitalized children. *Anthrozoös, 23*(3), 245–258. doi:10.2752/175303710X12750451258977

Victor, C. R., & Yang, K. (2012). The prevalence of loneliness among adults: A case study of the United Kingdom. *The Journal of Psychology: Interdisciplinary and Applied, 146*(1–2), 85–104. doi:10.1080/00223980.2011.613875

Waite, T. C., Hamilton, L., & O'Brien, W. (2018). A meta-analysis of animal assisted interventions targeting pain, anxiety, and distress in medical settings. *Complementary*

Therapies in Clinical Practice, 33, 49–55. doi:10.1016/
j.ctcp.2018.07.006

Waltz, C. F., Strickland, O. L., & Lenz, E. R. (2017). *Measurement in nursing and health research* (5th ed.). New York,
NY: Springer.

"What has science done for you lately?" (2013). *Understanding
science.* University of California Museum of Paleontology.
Retrieved from https://undsci.berkeley.edu/article/
whathassciencedone_01

Introduction to Qualitative Research

Jennifer R. Gray

http://evolve.elsevier.com/Gray/practice/

Qualitative research is a scholarly approach used to describe life experiences, cultures, and social processes from the perspectives of the persons involved. Qualitative researchers gain insights without measuring concepts or analyzing statistical relationships. Rather, they improve our comprehension of a phenomenon from the viewpoint of the people experiencing it. Qualitative researchers focus on hearing "the voices of the individuals themselves," rather than turning the experience into a number on an inventory or scale (Kazdin, 2017, p. 227). Qualitative research allows us to explore the depth, richness, and complexity inherent in the lives of human beings (Creswell & Creswell, 2018). Insights from this process build nursing knowledge by fostering understanding of patient needs and problems, guiding emerging theories, and describing cultural and social forces affecting health (Marshall & Rossman, 2016).

Comprehending qualitative research methodologies will allow you to critically appraise published studies, use findings in practice, and develop skills needed to conduct qualitative research. Nurse researchers conducting qualitative studies contribute important information to our body of knowledge, information often unobtainable by quantitative means. For example, an instrument to measure the person's assessment of coping after a loss, a quantitative method, will provide valuable information but not have the individual richness of interviewing the person about coping after a loss, a qualitative method.

This chapter presents the philosophical foundations of qualitative research followed by a general overview of the following qualitative methodologies: phenomenological research, grounded theory research, ethnographical research, and exploratory-descriptive qualitative research. These are the methodologies that seem to be used most frequently by qualitative nurse researchers. Two other approaches, narrative analysis and case study methods, will be described briefly. Although each qualitative approach is unique, they share common ground, and that is where we will begin.

PHILOSOPHICAL PERSPECTIVES FOR QUALITATIVE RESEARCH

All researchers have philosophical perspectives that guide the topics they study and their choices about methodology (Creswell & Creswell, 2018). The **philosophical perspectives** of researchers are the worldviews that guide their research decisions. Three interrelated and essential components of philosophical perspectives are axiology, ontology, and epistemology. The meaning of these components and their implications for qualitative research will be described.

Foundational Concepts
Axiology

Axiology is the value structure of a person—in this case, a researcher (Creswell & Poth, 2018). A researcher's axiology is based on answers to questions such as "What is right?" and "What is the value of a person?" The ethical foundation of nursing goes back to the Nightingale Oath written in 1893 (Fowler, 2017). The *Code of Ethics for Nurses with Interpretive Statements* (American Nurses Association, 2015) has been updated over the intervening years as society and health care changed, although basic ethical standards have not changed. For example, privacy and confidentiality are ethical values explicitly addressed in the *Code* that have not changed and are applicable to all areas of nursing, including research. The ethical values of nursing as applied to research will be described in Chapter 9. Although all nurses would agree on ethical values of the profession, such as privacy and confidentiality, other values may vary from nurse to nurse and from researcher to researcher.

Axiology related to research encompasses subtle values that influence the types of research that a nurse prefers to read or to conduct. Qualitative researchers value the experiences of research participants and the meaning they have constructed for those experiences (subjective data) more than the numerical values describing variables related to a phenomenon (objective data). For example, qualitative researchers value participants' description of how they provide self-care more than participants' scores on a self-care instrument. Among qualitative researchers, there may be even subtler differences, such as whether a proposed study should focus on social processes, cultural practices, or pressing problems that need to be solved. Qualitative researchers are explicit about their values by positioning themselves in relation to a study (Creswell & Poth, 2018; Patton, 2015).

Positioning is the communication of a researcher's characteristics related to the study topic, such as the researcher's social status, gender, age, personal experiences, and political party. This positioning may be discussed with other members of a research team or a student's faculty advisor but may also be included in the report of the study. Positioning helps the reader understand the researchers' axiology and the characteristics that influenced their axiology. Estefan, Moules, and Laing (2019) conducted a narrative inquiry study about sexuality and the development of sexual identity among adolescents who had been treated for cancer. To position themselves, they included a description of their backgrounds in a section entitled "Narrative Beginnings."

> "We are nurses with diverse backgrounds and experiences, which inform our approach to practice and to this inquiry. Andrew has long been interested in experiences that interrupt a person's sense of fit in the world and, consequently, their well-being. He remembers awakening over time to his own sexuality, amid other self-stories of childhood and adolescent illness. Andrew remembers these stories of himself as an awkward child, an outsider on the periphery, always looking in but unable to play.
>
> Over 30 years ago, Nancy's background in child and adolescent psychiatry and family therapy led to a position as a support nurse in pediatric oncology in the United States. On returning to Calgary, Nancy met Catherine (Author 3) who stimulated her clinical imagination, quickly earned her friendship, and reminded her that she had once been 'captured' by the young oncology patients and their families. Nancy returned to pediatric oncology as a researcher, focusing on psychosocial oncology.
>
> Throughout her career Catherine has noticed that despite gaining a tremendous amount of practical and theoretical knowledge there remains a privacy to the experience of cancer that even after 20 years in this field she cannot access. Catherine reflects on how, as much as she would like to think she knows about this experience, it can never really be known unless it has been lived. . . .
>
> Narrative beginnings do more than provide stories that situate researchers. Narrative beginnings also offer insights into the personal, practical, and social justification (Clandinin, 2013) for a given narrative inquiry." (Estefan et al., 2019, p. 192)

Closely linked to positioning is **reflexivity**, defined as researchers' self-awareness, understanding, and acknowledgment of their personal biases and their influence on the topic and the participants (Probst, 2015). One way to practice reflexivity is to write in a journal how your characteristics and experiences interact with the study. Positioning is an acknowledgment of these characteristics, and reflexivity is the ongoing process of considering how one's position and life experience may be influencing the study. Reflexivity also includes the researcher's self-awareness (recognition) of the influence of the study and participants on oneself. One of the challenges of identifying biases is that they may be unconscious. Members of a research team can facilitate reflexivity by discussing their perceptions of each other's biases and values in a safe environment (Buetow, 2019). Reflexivity is the process of using your insights from positioning and continuing to reflect at each stage of the study on how your values and biases may be affecting your thinking.

Ontology

Ontology is defined as the study of the nature of being and existence. It addresses questions such as "What does it mean to exist?" and "What is real?" (Brancati, 2018; Creswell & Poth, 2018). When selecting qualitative methodologies, researchers indicate they believe in multiple realities. A qualitative researcher demonstrates this belief by reporting these multiple realities, providing evidence of these multiple realities, and including "multiple forms of evidence in themes using the actual words of different individuals and presenting different perspectives" (Creswell & Poth, 2018, p. 20). Our realities as human beings influence our language and are influenced by our language (Jackson & Mazzei, 2018). An example is, in the lower 48 US states, the English language includes one word for snow. Yes, we use such words as *fluffy, wet, drifting,* or *icy* as adjectives but these adjectives are describing the same noun, *snow*. In the Eskimo languages, there are at least 50 different words for snow (Boas, 1911; Robson, 2013). The reality of snow has resulted in multiple words for description. Language can be a window into the experiences of an individual or group.

Qualitative researchers believe that reality is constructed and interpreted by individuals within their historical, social, family, geographical, economical, and spiritual contexts. In contrast to assessing the pieces to understand the whole, the qualitative researcher's ontology includes the reality of humans and existence being holistic and embedded in an environment that cannot be divided into pieces (van Wijngaarden, van der Meide, & Dahlberg, 2017).

Epistemology

Distinct but related, **epistemology** is the study of knowledge: "What is knowledge?" or "How is knowledge produced?" or "How can I know what is real?" The ontology and epistemology of the researcher are inseparable. Writing specifically about phenomenological research, van Wijngaarden et al. (2017, p. 1740) argue that qualitative methods have the "potential to describe the fundamental meaning structure of phenomena" and thus, provide "insight into the ontological nature of reality…." Stated a different way, Walsh and Evans (2014, p. e1) wrote that "unless the right questions are asked about the reality we are attempting to describe, explore or explain, then our knowledge of that reality will remain superficial and impoverished."

Consistent with qualitative perspectives of ontology is the epistemology that knowledge is subjective and varies from person to person (Corry, Porter, & McKenna, 2019). For that reason, when you study nonfatal suicidal behavior, you recruit a sample of persons who have made attempts on their own lives. You do not ask their significant others to participate in the study, unless your topic is their reactions to their loved ones' nonfatal suicidal behavior. As an example, Sommer, Kelley, Norr, Patil, and Vonderheid (2019) conducted a qualitative study with Mexican American mothers who were adolescents.

"In this study, we focused on Mexican American adolescent mothers, whose voices are largely absent in the literature, albeit their particularly relevant eminence. Among Mexican American adolescent mothers, common challenges inherent to early parenting as described in previous literature are complicated further by sociocultural stressors such as multiple ethnic identities grounded in their Mexican heritage and mainstream dominant Anglo-American influences…we concentrated on adolescent mothers who were second-generation Mexican Americans, defined as either born in the United States or born in Mexico, but having lived in the United States 5 or more years (Portes & Rumbaut, 2001). Nineteen young mothers who self-identified as Mexican American were recruited from the pool of mothers…The first author conducted first-person interviews with the 18 young mothers. Conversations took place situated in their own homes. Having their babies present was conducive for thinking about their mothering experiences. Observing the young mothers interact with their babies allowed the interviewer to enter their lifeworld and 'stay close to the experience as lived' (van Manen, 2016, p. 316). One young mother was not able to meet in her own home due to privacy issues, so we spoke with her in a private room at the university." (Sommer et al., 2019, pp. 3–4)

Notice that because they believed in the inseparable nature of human beings and their environment, Sommer et al. (2019) interviewed the women in their homes when possible. The interviewer was also able to observe a mother's interaction with her baby. As the researcher interviews the participant, the interaction and language co-construct his or her knowledge of the participant's reality.

Social Constructivism

In learning theories, **constructivism** is the premise that knowledge is individually constructed (Ward, Hoare, & Gott, 2015). Based on this philosophical perspective, lived experiences would be considered to be individually constructed. The philosophical perspective consistent with different, multiple, subjective views of reality is known as **constructionism**, the reality that is co-constructed with others (White, 2004). However, the differences between the two become less clear when writers use the terms interchangeably (Ward et al., 2015) or insert *social* before constructionism or constructivism to account for the social aspect of learning or the social co-construction of lived experience. We have chosen to use the term *social constructivism*.

Social constructivism is a philosophy that supports different, multiple, subjective views of experiences that are co-constructed with others (Creswell & Poth, 2018). The philosophy has been used to understand social institutions, such as family, religion, and profession, within the context of time: "socially constructed realities are understood to vary with the historical societies that construct them" (Lynch, 2016, p. 105). In addition to the macro-level view as applied to institutions, social constructivism is also useful for understanding the complexities of the meanings of lived experiences across different individuals (Creswell & Poth, 2018). For example, Molzahn et al. (2019) conducted a narrative inquiry of death and dying among 11 persons with chronic kidney disease (CKD) and 9 family members. The study was designed to "explore people's experiences of living with the uncertainties of illness and the likelihood of dying. A social constructionist perspective framed the approach to the study" (Molzahn et al., 2019, p. 131). The participants realized that "life has a boundary" and talked about "living close to the edge between life and death" (Monzahn et al., 2019, pp. 132–133). In their social world of dialysis, these themes were constructed through interactions with fellow patients who had CKD. The participants and families had also observed deaths during dialysis and known patients who stopped dialysis. Two other themes that emerged were "I'm not afraid to die; but…" and "remembering loss and death experiences" (Molzahn et al., 2019, pp. 133–134). The importance of social constructivism was summed up in one sentence: "Living and dying with a life-limiting illness such as CKD is clearly a family experience and not only the experience of the individual" (Molzahn et al., 2019, p. 134).

In addition to the methodology of narrative inquiry, the methodology of phenomenology is founded on social constructivism and has an individual level of focus (Creswell & Poth, 2018). Social constructivism, the co-construction of meaning, is not limited to the individual focus, however. It can focus on the social processes that are embedded and influence the participants' movement through an experience. This application of social constructivism supports the grounded theory methodology. Ethnography is also consistent with social constructivism, but the focus is on the macro level. Ethnographical methods are used to describe the meanings, processes, and structures that are co-constructed by groups, such as an indigenous people living in a remote location or employees in a clinic within a healthcare system. Table 4.1 displays social constructivism as the broad philosophical foundation for phenomenology, grounded theory, and ethnography.

Pragmatism

Pragmatism is another perspective that has philosophical implications for researchers. Pragmatism is a worldview for the researcher who is seeking to find a solution for a problem (Creswell & Poth, 2018). The pragmatist researcher is not concerned about how the issue or problem was created, unless that understanding

---

TABLE 4.1 Qualitative Methodologies in Nursing Research and Their Foundations

Qualitative Methodology	Discipline	Broad Philosophical Perspective	Philosophical and Theoretical Orientations
Phenomenological research	Psychology	Social constructivism	Phenomenology
Grounded theory research	Sociology	Social constructivism	Symbolic interaction theory
Ethnographical research	Anthropology	Social constructivism	Cultural relativism
Exploratory-descriptive qualitative research	Health disciplines, social sciences	Pragmatism	Varies depending on the discipline and purpose of the study

is necessary to finding the solution. The focus is on the solution or the consequences (Kankam, 2019). What do participants suggest as solutions to the identified problem?

Several early philosophers in the United States wrote about pragmatism (Creswell & Creswell, 2018). Charles Peirce (1839–1914) was a scientist, philosopher, and innovative thinker who found value in many philosophies and laid a foundation for pragmatism. Although his work was never published in his lifetime, Peirce shaped the views of his colleagues (Peirce, 1955), one of whom was William James. James (1840–1910) was educated as a physician, but decided not to practice, becoming a lecturer instead on the subjects of physiology, psychology, and philosophy at Harvard University (Goodman, 2017). He wrote a seminal book on psychology (James, 1890) and, in later life, a book on pragmatism (James, 1907/2007). James viewed pragmatism as the middle ground between the extremes in philosophy, because pragmatism used ideas from several philosophies (Goodman, 2017). John Dewey (1859–1952), better known for his contributions to education, was another philosopher who discussed pragmatism. Building on James's writing, one of Dewey's (1916/2012) goals in writing about pragmatism was to "…affirm that the term 'pragmatic' means only the rule of referring all thinking, all reflective considerations, to consequences for final meaning and test" (p. 330).

Pragmatism does not bind the researcher to a specific philosophy or methodology (Kankam, 2019). Therefore researchers choose the methodology that allows them to honor the perspectives of those affected, understand the problem, and identify ways to appropriately address the problem (Creswell & Poth, 2018). Researchers who value pragmatism may collect several forms of data, including quantitative and qualitative data. For that reason, pragmatism is an appropriate basis of mixed methods studies (Corry et al., 2019; Kankam, 2019). Pragmatism, however, has also been used as the foundation for grounded theory methodology in the study of the mental health issues of Iraqi immigrants in the United States (Davenport, 2017). Lith (2014) informed her case study of recovery from mental illness with pragmatism and phenomenology. Because of its focus on problem solving, pragmatism may also support the exploratory-descriptive qualitative methodology. We are including pragmatism here for this latter purpose but will also address it in Chapter 14 in describing mixed methods research.

In our effort to make the content of the chapter accessible to beginning graduate students, we have limited our description of philosophical perspectives to those supporting the methodologies that we have chosen to include. We have notably omitted the philosophies supporting social justice, feminism, and critical theory, philosophies that may become increasingly relevant (Denzin & Lincoln, 2018). As you progress in your scholarly journey, we encourage you to read the original authors of the qualitative philosophies and methodologies to broaden and deepen your understanding of this complex field.

UNIQUE CHARACTERISTICS OF QUALITATIVE RESEARCH

Scientific rigor is valued because it is associated with the trustworthiness and significance of research findings. **Rigor** means the extent to which a study was implemented consistently with the standards accepted by scientists. The credibility of the findings of qualitative studies is appraised differently from the rigor of quantitative studies because of differences in the underlying philosophical perspectives. Based on positivistic or postpositivism philosophies, quantitative studies are considered rigorous when planned procedures are followed precisely, the sample represents the population, and objectivity is maintained. Deviating from those procedures is a threat to the rigor of the study.

Rigorous qualitative researchers are characterized by flexibility and openness while ensuring the methods used are congruent with the underlying philosophical perspective. The qualitative researcher collects data with sensitivity and thoroughness, listening carefully to participants (Morse, 2018). The researcher may adjust the interview or focus group questions in response to emergent patterns and themes found during simultaneous data collection and analysis. The ability to be responsive during a study is consistent with qualitative standards for rigor (Miles, Huberman, & Saldaña, 2020).

Qualitative findings contribute to new understanding of an experience by elaborating with richness and depth on thoughts and emotions (Kazdin, 2017; Miles et al., 2020). Because the perspective of each qualitative researcher is unique, the meanings drawn from the data vary from researcher to researcher, especially in the naming of the key ideas and describing these concepts and the relationships among them (Morse, 2018). The researcher keeps records of his or her thinking processes, analysis, findings, and conclusions so that others can audit or retrace the analysis and thinking processes that resulted in the researcher's conclusions. Betriana and Kongsuwan (2019) described the steps they took to establish the quality of their phenomenological study of Muslim nurses' lived experiences of caring for a patient who died. The researchers met with the nurses individually, gave them a blank paper and colored pens, and asked the nurses to draw a picture of their grief (Betriana & Kongsuwan, 2019). Then each nurse was interviewed and asked to talk about his or her drawing.

"The triangulation methods used in this study involved the use of two data sources, including graphic representations and interview transcriptions. After each interview, the researcher restated the answer for the participants in order to clarify whether the information gained matched each participants' meaning. These data were clarified in the daily journal written up by the researcher during data collection. The daily journal was used to achieve confirmability by recording the time and date of data collection, features of the context, the physical setting where the data collection took place, the researcher's own reflections and questions and interpretations that came up during interviews. Transferability was established by providing 'thick' or detailed descriptions of the phenomenon. Dependability was established by external audit with expert review." (Betriana & Kongsuwan, 2019, p. 11)

The themes found in the data fit within the "five lived worlds used in van Manen's approach (2014)" (Betriana & Kongsuwan, 2019, p. 11). The study's findings are shown in Box 4.1. (See Chapter 12 for

BOX 4.1 Betriana and Kongsuwan's (2019) Study of Muslim Nurses Caring for Dying Patients: Themes Within van Manen's Life Worlds

Lived other: Empathetic understanding
Lived body: Balancing self
Lived space: Avoidance
Lived time: Anticipating the future of own death
Lived things: Relating technologies in bargaining

From Betriana, F., & Kongsuwan, W. (2019). Lived experiences of grief of Muslim nurses caring for patients who died in an intensive care unit. *Intensive & Critical Care, 52*(1), 9–16. doi:10.1016/j.iccn.2018.09.003

additional information on qualitative data analysis and other qualitative methods.)

Critical appraisal is necessary before you can incorporate qualitative research findings into the development of evidence-based practice (Melnyk & Fineout-Overholt, 2019). Critical appraisal of the rigor of qualitative studies is discussed in more detail in Chapter 18.

METHODOLOGIES FOR QUALITATIVE RESEARCH

Studies using a wide variety of qualitative methodologies have been reported in the literature. We have chosen to focus on four methodologies, with the expectation that you will seek additional references for other methodologies that you encounter in the literature. Each of the qualitative methodologies have unique characteristics primarily because they originated in different disciplines (see Table 4.1). Phenomenological research emerged from psychology and the philosophy of phenomenology (Creswell & Creswell, 2018; Morley, 2019). Grounded theory was developed as a methodology by sociologists Glaser and Strauss, following their collaborative study of death and dying in hospitals (Charmaz, 2014). Anthropologists developed ethnography with its focus on culture (de Chesnay, 2014; Ladner, 2014). Exploratory-descriptive qualitative research has emerged from the disciplines of nursing and medicine and is focused on using the knowledge gained to benefit patients and families and improve health outcomes. Although no philosophy is formally linked to exploratory-descriptive qualitative research in the literature, its problem-solving approach is consistent with pragmatism (Creswell & Creswell, 2018; Creswell & Poth, 2018). Table 4.1 provides an overview of the disciplinary roots and philosophical and theoretical foundations of each of the methodologies described in this chapter.

Phenomenological Research

Phenomenology is both a philosophy and a research method. The purpose of **phenomenological research** is to describe the essence of experiences (or phenomena) from the participant's perspective or, as frequently stated, capture the lived experience (Creswell & Poth, 2018; Patton, 2015). A **phenomenon** is an experience of an individual, or multiple individuals who have a similar experience. A phenomenon (singular term) might be applying for graduate school, mothering a child with a congenital cardiac defect, or experiencing joy. **Phenomena,** as the plural term, would be used to refer to all of these experiences plus more. The philosophy of phenomenology undergirds the research methods of listening to participants and analyzing verbal and nonverbal communication to gain a more comprehensive and deep understanding of their experiences—their lived experiences.

Philosophical and Theoretical Orientations

Phenomenologists perceive the person as being in constant interaction with the environment and making meaning of experiences in that context. The environment, or world around each of us, influences us, and we, in turn, influence the world through our actions and relationships. Beyond this, however, phenomenologists diverge in their beliefs about the person and the experience. The key philosophers who developed phenomenology are Husserl and Heidegger (Creswell & Poth, 2018).

A mathematician, Edmund Husserl (1859–1938) is considered the father of phenomenology (van Wijngaarden et al., 2017). Departing from the positivist tradition of knowing, Husserl posited that phenomena make up the world of experience. Hussserl argued that these experiences cannot be explained by examining causal relations but must be studied as the very things they are. Husserl wrote *Logical Investigations* (1901/1970) in which he developed his ideas about phenomena, contrasting human sciences (primarily psychology) and the basic or natural sciences (such as physics). Husserl articulated the importance of **subjectivity**, the awareness of one's own being, feelings, and thoughts that can lead to self-understanding. Being aware of an experience's meaning while it is being experienced, as well as through

later reflection, is an indication of attentiveness, which can be passively or actively engaged (Jansen, 2016). During an interview, the researcher may elicit the active attention of a study participant to the selected experience or to the memory of that experience. The person experiencing his or her life must be the one to share the meaning of the experience.

Four concepts are critical to understanding Husserl's philosophy and related research methods: epoche, bracketing, essence, and reduction. These concepts with descriptions are provided in Table 4.2. **Epoche** can be defined as the blank tablet that a researcher attempts to create by suspending "our automatic and deep-seated belief in the mind-independent existence of reality" (Zahavi & Martiny, 2019, p. 154). The idea of suspending our beliefs about reality allows the researcher to be surprised by or intuitively drawn to the meanings shared across participants, the meanings embedded in the data. The idea of suspending judgment is somewhat counterintuitive to constructivism (Rockenbach, Walker, & Luzader, 2012) but is linked frequently to positioning (see earlier definition) and to bracketing. To describe the experience, the researcher must be open to the participant's worldview, set aside personal perspectives, and allow meanings to emerge. Setting aside one's beliefs during qualitative research is **bracketing**. Researchers who use bracketing describe journaling and discussing with members of the team their assumptions and presuppositions about the phenomenon, so the researcher's viewpoint does not affect data collection and analysis.

To make the definitions of essence and reduction more understandable, let's begin with an example. Imagine you are conducting a phenomenological study of the experience of seeing red. You begin the interviews by asking participants to describe something that is red. One participant describes an exquisite red rose, another

TABLE 4.2	Descriptive Phenomenology: Key Ideas
Key Ideas	**Role in Interpretive Phenomenology**
Positioning	Understanding past experiences related to the phenomenon, for the purpose of setting one's own assumptions and values
Bracketing	Setting aside the assumptions and experiences identified during positioning
Epoche	The blank slate created by positioning and bracketing; purpose is to focus only on the phenomenon
Reduction	Removing the details of the participants' descriptions of the lived experience so that the essence can be seen
Essence	Articulating what is the phenomenon and what is not the phenomenon

describes a house with a red door, and a third describes a woman wearing a red dress. You then ask each participant, "What feelings does red evoke when you see [object he or she described]?" or "What message does red communicate to you?" As you analyze the data generated by the interviews, you set aside your presuppositions about what red is, your experiences of hearing or stating the phrase "seeing red," and your feelings related to red (bracketing). Your goal is to experience and describe the essence of red. The **essence** of a phenomenon is its abstract meaning and central structures (Bynum & Varpio, 2018). **Reduction** is removing the influence of your preunderstanding of the experience and focusing on the lived experience of the participant. The goal is to remove any accidental or nonessential details or elements described by the participants and your own assumptions until only the essence of the phenomenon remains (Hopkins, Regehr, & Pratt, 2017), until you can see what is truly red.

The four concepts and a fifth, positioning, interact with each other. For example, you plan to conduct a phenomenological study of the lived experience of surviving tragedy. Before the study, you realized the importance of positioning yourself by journaling about your own experience of surviving the 2011 earthquake in Japan, the subsequent tsunami waves, and the aftermath of the disaster. By positioning yourself, you have made explicit your feelings of terror, persistent sadness, and overwhelming loss. You also relived and documented the physical exhaustion of disaster relief and the sense of comradery among the survivors. You begin interviewing participants who have experienced tragedies, such as the loss of multiple family members in a car crash and a skiing accident that resulted in a spinal cord injury on the eve of one's wedding. While interviewing the participants and analyzing the data, you bracket your experience, attitudes, and assumptions about surviving tragedies. The goal of positioning and bracketing is to move to the epoche, which in turn facilitates the process of reduction with the goal of describing the essence of surviving a disaster. Because of Husserl's insistence on bracketing and analyzing data without interpretation, his phenomenological methods became known as **descriptive phenomenology** (Derico, 2017).

An example of a descriptive phenomenological study was conducted by Shardonofsky et al. (2019), who interviewed 20 fathers caring for children with cystic fibrosis (CF). The researchers were explicit about their selection of Husserl's descriptive phenomenology and the use of bracketing.

"Husserl's (1970) descriptive phenomenology was used in this study. Foundational to Husserl's methodology is the belief that a one-on-one interaction with study participants creates a reflection of reality more explicit than what was earlier understood... The basic tenets of phenomenology corresponded with the goal of this study, which was to explore and better understand the lived experiences of fathers who have children living with CF.... An important aspect of Husserl's (1970) descriptive phenomenology is the use of bracketing.... Bracketing was used to meet the rigor criterion of clarification of researcher bias.... Several themes emerged from the interviews with fathers about their experiences of caring for their child with CF. These included being overwhelmed, feeling isolated, experiencing altered family dynamics, actively seeking resources, experiencing financial strain, and feeling hopeful." (Shardonofsky et al., 2019, pp. 87–88)

Shardonofsky et al. (2019) described the process used for data analysis and being aware of the insights gained from the data. To be consistent with Husserl's phenomenology, their report of the findings did not include interpreting the results or framing the results through their own experiences. Bracketing was clearly used, but they did not report positioning or reduction as other characteristics of Husserl's approach. They noted two study limitations, one of which was potential differences between fathers who agreed to participate and those who did not. The second limitation was not screening the fathers for anxiety and depression, either of which may have affected the descriptions of their experiences. The fathers were interviewed in person, by video calling, and by voice calling, but the researchers did not note as a limitation the differences in their ability to see and interact with the fathers during data collection.

Martin Heidegger (1889–1976) was a student of Husserl but expanded the goal of phenomenology from description of lived experience to the interpretation of lived experiences (Derico, 2017). The focus is on the meaning of the experience to the person experiencing it. Heidegger's seminal work was *Being and Time*

(1927/2010). Heideggerian phenomenologists believe that the self exists within a body, or is **embodied** (Munhall, 2012). This was a major shift in ontology from Husserl who viewed the person as comprised of a duality, the person as body (objective) and the person as spirit (subjective). In contrast, Heidegger believed, experiences cannot occur except through the body and its senses. The objective and subjective aspects of the situation are merged in the participant's mind, known as **embodiment**.

All knowledge is an interpretation (Amos, 2016). Because human beings are situated in the world and "cannot be separated from their culture, relationships, or history" (Burns & Peacock, 2019, p. 3), the researcher interprets the data within its context to understand the lived experience. The person interprets experiences while they are occurring. Because of this, researchers who follow the philosophy proposed by Heidegger do not agree with Husserl's ideas on bracketing. Rather, they take the position that bracketing is not possible. One always remembers and is influenced by what one knows.

Table 4.3 explains characteristic processes of Heidegger's view of phenomenology, known as interpretive phenomenology. To distinguish Husserl's emphasis on bracketing from Heidegger's purposeful inclusion of the researcher's perspective into data collection and analysis, the latter has been called **interpretive phenomenological research** (Burns & Peacock, 2019).

Heidegger also described **situated freedom**. To explain, you as a person are situated in specific context and time that shapes your experiences, paradoxically freeing and constraining your ability to establish meanings through language, culture, history, purposes, and values (Munhall, 2012). Part of your uniqueness is that you live in a historical, cultural, geographical, and temporal context. Consider the adolescent female athlete diagnosed with sarcoma who lives in 2020 in a US urban area with a nationally acclaimed cancer treatment center less than 5 miles away. Contrast the adolescent's experience of cancer with that of an 82-year-old man who lived on a farm in Europe in 1932 and was diagnosed with prostate cancer. Gender roles, availability of treatment, financial resources, geographical location, and historical era are only a few of the factors that would shape the cancer experience for these individuals. Each of them has only situated freedom, not total freedom. The adolescent has the freedom to choose physicians from among those who will accept her insurance. The older man may have the freedom only to choose whether he will use traditional herbs or not seek treatment at all. Until a disruption such as an unexpected diagnosis of cancer occurs, the person may not consider the limits on meaning and choices imposed by context and time.

A team of Canadian nurse researchers conducted an interpretive phenomenological study of the lived experience of making a conscientious objection as a nurse. Because of the extensive data collected and the relevance of the topic, the findings of the study were reported in two articles (Lamb, Babenko-Mould, Evans, Wong, & Kirkwood, 2018; Lamb, Evans, Babenko-Mould, Wong, & Kirkwood, 2019). The first author indicated she had made a conscientious objection, and her experiences with the research topic were incorporated as she interviewed participants and analyzed data. Excerpts from both articles will be used to describe the study. In Lamb et al. (2019), the researchers focused on the meaning of conscience and provided the context of the study in the introduction.

TABLE 4.3	Interpretive Phenomenology: Key Ideas	
Key Ideas	**Role in Descriptive Phenomenology**
Positioning	Understanding past experiences related to the phenomenon, for the purpose of considering own experiences along with the collected data
Embodiment	Subjective perceptions are experienced within the objective physical world, including one's own body
Situated freedom	The possibilities and limitations created by one's position in history, social and geographical locations, and personal characteristics such as income and education
Interpretation	Researcher's and participants' combined view of their lived experiences related to the phenomenon; higher level of abstraction than themes produced by descriptive phenomenology

"... it is relevant to note that recent legislation in Canada (where this study was conducted), decriminalizing euthanasia has also led to contentious discussion, legal precedent, and confusion over how to specifically support nurses who are ethically opposed to assisting their patients to die.... While regulatory guidelines on euthanasia vary across the provincial and territorial landscape in Canada, this recent provincial ruling leaves Canadian nurses in need of further professional support on how to maintain a moral balance between personal belief, professional obligations, and provincial legislation.... Since human experiences vary from one person to another, Heidegger's (1927/2010) method was also selected since he calls for lived experiences to be interpreted in a subjective context to lend insight into how particular humans (such as nurses) contextually live through encountering a specific phenomenon (making meaning of conscience)." (Lamb et al., 2019, pp. 595–596)

Lamb et al. (2018) described the interpretive phenomenology methodology of Heidegger in greater detail. Heidegger's (1927/2010) term *daesin* was defined as human existence. **Intersubjectivity** was defined as the interaction between persons subjectively encountering the objective world around them. van Manen (2017) built on Heidegger's work in phenomenology. Lamb et al. (2018) identified van Manen's life worlds, the basic ways of being in the world. Remember that Betriana and Kongsuwan (2019) connected their study results to van Manen's life worlds in their phenomenological study of Muslim nurses' experiences with dying (see Box 4.1). Lamb et al. (2018) also considered van Manen's ideas in their explanation of interpretive phenomenology.

"... In these different modes of being-in-the-world, one can grasp their experiences as being in a certain space, in time, as beings that relate inter-subjectively to one another and in the material things that one encounters in the world. A life world is the way in which a day-to-day experience presents itself to *dasein*, such as the daily moments of being a nurse. On a given day, if a nurse makes a conscientious objection, the meaning that can be derived from that lived experience is what an interpretive phenomenological researcher would aim to capture, to understand the meaning embedded in that experience (Mackey, 2005). For example, being (existing) in the now (time), as nurses (life world) shape how an experience (making a conscientious objection) with a phenomenon (conscientious objection) can be understood through relating to patients or colleagues (inter-relationality, corporeality) and through the things (material objects, that is, codes of ethics), that tell nurses something about who they are (van Manen, 2014)." (Lamb et al., 2018, p. 3)

Lamb et al. (2018, 2019) used quotations from the nurses in the study to support each of six themes for making a conscientious objection as a nurse. The themes began with encountering a situation in which the nurse faced a decision followed by the themes of knowing oneself, taking a stand, feeling alone and uncertain, caring for others, and perceiving support. Through two interviews with each of the eight participants and detailed data analysis, the researchers went beyond describing the data to provide an interpretation of the meaning.

"Across participants' narratives, making a conscientious objection in clinical practice was meaningfully experienced by participants as an opportunity to transcend the status quo, to acknowledge that they each had a conscience, and to take a stand to live by a moral code. Conscientious objection meant doing what was right. These nurses wanted to be clear that they did not personally want to do harm, from a professional standpoint, toward themselves, their patients, or their nursing profession.... Prior to making their conscientious objections, the nurse informants shared that they each encountered an ethical problem in their professional practice.... Nancy recalled this encounter as a time of deep, personal struggle because she did not ethically agree with assisting patients to die, and seeing this person [woman planning to die by euthanasia] on a day-to-day basis as a nurse brought her close to an issue in her nursing experience that she did not agree with.... Kate shared that as a Catholic, her ethics are informed by her faith, but she noted that her faith is based on reason and working through ethical scenarios with deliberation, which is something that takes moral discernment and education.... For these nurse participants, conscience and conscientious objection were not mutually exclusive—conscience is about discerning what is right for one to do, and making a conscientious objection is based on one's conscience-based perceptions of morality and then expressed as that right action (ethics)." (Lamb et al., 2018, pp. 4–7)

Lamb et al. (2019) noted the need for future research to understand the thinking processes of nurses between encountering a situation with which they do not agree and conscientiously objecting to participating.

Multiple adjectives, in addition to descriptive and interpretive, have been used to describe types of phenomenological studies. One of the more prominent is **hermeneutic phenomenological research**. Hermeneutical phenomenology emphasizes the importance of language and written texts. Some would argue that Heidegger's interpretive phenomenology is hermeneutical in nature (Bynum & Varpio, 2018; Vagle, 2018). In fact, some studies are labeled interpretive hermeneutical phenomenology (Kelly & Kelly, 2019). Gadamer (1992, 2011) and van Manen (1990, 2007, 2017) were proponents of hermeneutical phenomenology (Annells, 1996; Bynum & Varpio, 2018).

Another type of phenomenological research in the nursing literature is empirical phenomenology. Horne and Paul (2019) studied the lived experience of chronic pain among persons with diabetes and a lower limb amputation and used the empirical phenomenological methodology. Instead of hermeneutical phenomenology that uses rich, thick descriptions, the researchers used empirical phenomenology that emphasizes "structure and commonality of experiences" (Horne & Paul, 2019, p. 271). Horne and Paul purposively recruited patients being seen in an orthotic and prosthetic practice, interviewing 11 participants whose amputation had occurred at least 6 months prior to the study. When asked about their pain, the participants indicated they had none, but when asked specifically about phantom pain, they described it in detail, including how it interfered with their daily lives. Surgical pain was understood, but phantom pain was not considered part of their overall pain experience. Because the participants did not believe there were any treatments for phantom pain, they did not discuss it with their healthcare providers (HCPs).

These two subthemes, pain nonexistent and helplessness, became the theme "Phantom pain is untreatable pain" (Horne & Paul, p. 271). The second theme was "Non-empathetic support systems" (Horne & Paul, p. 272). The family and friends were supportive of the participants in many ways, but the participants perceived that their support system did not want to hear about the pain (subtheme: lack of understanding). If and when they mentioned their phantom pain to their HCPs, the response was to prescribe pain medications (subtheme: analgesics are the only option). The final theme was "Identification of a new normal" (Horne & Paul, 2019, pp. 271–272). One of the subthemes was that amputation was a choice. Most of the participants felt positive about the decision to amputate their legs, because it was a decision that they made willingly. The participants were surprisingly hopeful and considered themselves blessed, indicating that their faith and spirituality had made the difference in learning to live a "new normal" life. The study provided a glimpse into the lived experiences of the participants while demonstrating the need for HCPs to assess phantom pain and teach patients and families about the phenomenon.

Merleau-Ponty (1945/2012) was among the French philosophers who further developed Heidegger's concepts. For example, Colaizzi (1973) and Giorgi (1985, 2010) wrote about phenomenology within psychology. Exploring the various philosophical stances by reading the writings of the philosophers will allow you to ensure that the philosophy, methodology, and research question are congruent (Zahavi, 2019). The nurse researcher considering phenomenological research will want to read primary sources for these philosophers and researchers who have refined the methodology based on their own disciplines and beliefs.

Despite the differences with the philosophical tradition, phenomenologists agree that there is no single reality. Each individual's experience is unique and ever changing, according to the person's array of experiences. Reality is a subjective perception—a tenet that requires the researcher to listen, absorb, and elicit without judgment participants' subjective experiences in as much detail as possible. More information on the conduct of phenomenological research is provided in Chapter 12.

Phenomenology's Contribution to Nursing Science

Phenomenology has been the philosophical basis for many studies conducted by nurses; however, no single branch of phenomenology has been the only one used by nurses. Nurse researchers using phenomenology have based their studies on the philosophies and related methods of all the phenomenological philosophies described in the previous sections. Patricia Benner is known widely within nursing for her research (Benner, 1982) that resulted in the book *From Novice to Expert* (1984a). The publications reported the interpretive phenomenology study during which she observed and interviewed 67 nurses across six hospitals. Interestingly, the study that resulted in widely held views of the transition from new graduate to a nursing expert was not her dissertation. For her dissertation, she interviewed 23 midcareer men about their work stress 12 times each, resulting in 276 interviews and extensive transcripts to be analyzed (Benner, 1984b, 1994b). Her experience in listening with openness and interpreting experiences from the perspectives of participants was extensive by the time she edited a book on interpretive phenomenology (Benner, 1994a). For the book, she described interpretive phenomenology methodology (Benner, 1994b) and selected example studies using the methodology within health care (Benner, 1994a).

The thread of interpretive phenomenology can be seen through Benner's research. Her publications have reflected her broad interests in the science of caring, ethical theory, leadership, mentoring, and issues in nursing education and critical care. Her most recent studies have addressed posttraumatic stress disorders among soldiers wounded in the Middle East (Benner, Halpern, Gordon, Popell, & Kelley, 2018; Kelley, Kenny, Gordon, & Benner, 2015).

You may be wondering what phenomenology has contributed to nursing science. One group of scholars provided an example of phenomenology's contribution to science by critically reviewing phenomenological studies of suffering in chronic illness (Al Kalaldeh, Shosha, Saiah, & Salameh, 2018). Through a systematic search of the literature, 26 studies of suffering as a lived experience were identified. The scholars evaluated the rigor of the studies using a 10-item tool from Critical Appraisal Skills Programme (2017). All the studies met the criteria of rigor. The scholars analyzed the studies' findings and formulated three themes.

The first theme was "suffering and its consequences in phenomenology" (Al Kalaldeh et al., 2018, p. 44). The consequences of suffering were described as being negative, individual, and variable over time. The emotional consequences were synthesized to be anger, depression, anxiety, as well as emotional, physical, existential, and spiritual pain. Three studies that addressed coping with suffering resulted in "positive reinforcement outcomes of personal growth, strength, value, and vision" (Al Kalaldeh et al., 2018, p. 45). Al Kaladeh et al. (2018) described the findings of one study that identified positive consequences.

"The findings of the study revealed that these patients with advanced-stage cancer utilized several methods to cope with existential and spiritual suffering. These coping strategies were openness and choosing to face reality; connectedness and the significance of family; pursuit of meaning; the connection of body, mind, and spirit with humor; and a positive outlook. This study demonstrated robust methodology in which a variety of patients' characteristics and conditions were integrated in the study and strengthened the emerged evidence (Bentur, Stark, Resnizky, & Symon, 2014).... Based on these applications, suffering is an experience that affects the entire human functioning. Patients suffering may entail a set of consequences that are interrelated with the therapeutic interventions especially in the prolonged medical plans. In turn, caregivers play the pivotal role in assessing and eradicating the majority of treatment-related suffering, while the patients receive the conventional therapy." (Al Kalaldeh et al., 2018, p. 46)

The second theme was "the applicability of phenomenology in the study of suffering" (Al Kalaldeh et al., 2018, p. 46). Three of the studies examined the suffering of patients with specific diseases that resulted in unique findings. Al Kalaldeh et al. (2018) noted these finding may be limited to those diseases and not as applicable to patients with other diseases. More broadly, phenomenology was used to study the health needs of hospitalized patients.

"The results showed that patients suffered during caregiving when they felt undervalued or mistreated. Suffering was found to increase due to neglecting a holistic and patient-centered care. It can be described as having the following 4 components: to be mistreated, to struggle for one's healthcare needs and autonomy, to feel powerless, and to feel fragmented and objectified." (Berglund, Westin, Svanstrom, & Sundler, 2012)." (Al Kalaldeh et al., 2018, pp. 5–6)

Al Kalaldeh et al. (2018) identified the third theme to be "approaching suffering through nursing research" (p. 47). Descriptive, interpretive, and hermeneutical phenomenology had been used by the researchers conducting the reviewed studies. Al Kalaldeh et al. (2018) clearly stated phenomenology's essential contributions to nursing science.

"...Suffering is one of the phenomena that nursing is concerned with based on its roots in individual's lived experience. Because it is a complex human response affecting physical, psychological, social, and spiritual aspects, it may decrease self-integrity and induces loneliness, withdrawal, feelings of helplessness, and despair. The phenomenological approach is acknowledged as a route to insight into the understanding of human experiences.... This qualitative synthesis unveiled the magnificence of understanding human experience through phenomenology.... It was acknowledged that nurses' involvement in patients' experience is very effective to understand aspects surrounding suffering and complaints. Nurses have to go beyond the conventional spectrum of practice and take into account other factors that influence suffering as a result of illness, life, or even care.... The phenomenological approach is the key to gain an exhaustive meaning of patients' experiences in the chronically ill." (Al Kalaldeh et al., 2018, pp. 47–48)

Phenomenological studies have made a significant contribution to nursing science and, by doing so, have positively affected nursing practice. Nursing practice informed by an understanding of the patient's lived experience has positive patient and nurse outcomes.

Grounded Theory Research

Grounded theory research is an inductive research technique, whose name means that the findings are grounded in the concrete world as experienced by participants and can be linked to the actual data. The data are interpreted, however, at a more abstract theoretical level. The desired outcome of grounded theory studies is a middle-range or substantive theory (Charmaz, 2014; Creswell & Poth, 2018; Glaser & Strauss, 1967/2011). When a theory is not produced, the research product may be a description of a process. However, Glaser (2019) argues that description only is not the goal of the methodology. The goal is discovering theory in the data (Glaser & Strauss, 1967/2011).

Philosophical and Theoretical Perspectives

Grounded theory began as a methodology to develop theory closely tied to the empirical world of data and thus build a bridge between grand theory and quantitative hypotheses (Glaser & Strauss, 1967/2011). Merton (1949/2004) offered his solution, middle-range theory, as a link between grand theory and empirical research,

and Glaser and Strauss (1967/2011) offered a way to discover middle-range theories through grounded theory qualitative research. However, their ideas were based on the work of previous scholars such as Mead and Blumer.

George Herbert Mead (1863–1931), a social psychologist, posited the existence of self-interaction, human social interaction, and the shared makeup of group life (Blumer, 1969). Mead expanded on the mere existence of different types of interactions by developing the principles of interaction theory, which were posthumously published (Mead, 1934). His principles were shaped and refined by other scholars, such as Herbert Blumer (Crossley, 2010). Building on Mead's work, Herbert Blumer (1900–1987) positioned his views within constructivism philosophy (Clarke, 2019). Congruent with Mead's idea, Blumer stated that the mental perceptions of aspects of life were "formed through the process of shared social interaction" (Blumer, 1980, p. 410). Blumer advocated for naturalistic, exploratory observation as the way to understand the relationships and communication patterns within a group. Blumer is credited with developing the symbolic interaction theory.

Symbolic interaction theory explores how your perceptions of your interactions with others shape your view of self. Your view of self becomes the context for subsequent interactions and thus shapes the meanings that are constructed (Crossley, 2010). **Symbolic meanings** are different for each individual. We cannot completely know the symbolic meanings of another individual; however, individuals in the same group or society may hold common meanings, also called shared meanings. Language and symbols are the means through which we form meaning and share that meaning with others (Charmaz, 2014). These shared meanings are embedded in catch phrases, beliefs, colloquialisms, and social behaviors, which present a core of belonging. Interactions among people may lead to redefinition of experiences, new meanings, and possibly a redefinition of self. Because of their theoretical importance, the interactions among the person and other individuals in social contexts are the focus of data collection in grounded theory research.

Glaser and Strauss (1967/2011) coined the term **grounded theory**, meaning the scholarly process for discovering theory in data (Table 4.4). The resultant theory had a greater likelihood of explaining the

TABLE 4.4   Grounded Theory (GT) Terms

Terms	Description
GT	Scholarly process to discovery theory in qualitative data
Substantive or middle-range theory	Desired outcome of GT; less abstract description of concepts and relationships among them
Symbolic interaction theory	A theoretical perspective upon which some GT studies are based; perceptions of interactions with others shape one's view of self
Constructivism	Approach to GT not focused on building theory but on increased understanding of social processes; acknowledges influence of the researcher on GT findings
Situational analysis	Variation of GT that focuses on nonhuman aspects of an experience such as built environment, plants, animals, and technology

empirical world than a theory deduced from grand theories or an a priori set of assumptions. The publication of the *Discovery of Grounded Theory* (1967) was an infusion of new energy into qualitative inquiry (Clarke, 2019). The ideas of Glaser and Strauss diverged, and each wrote articles and methods books alone (Clarke, 2019). Glaser's early research training was within the positivistic philosophy, and some evidence of positivism continued into his later career. His personal philosophy aligned most clearly with pragmatism. Strauss remained true to his early training as well, which was based on constructivism and interpretive symbolic interactionism.

Building on their legacy, other types of grounded theory have emerged from sociology and psychology. One of these is **situational analysis** focuses not on context, but the nonhuman aspects of the phenomenon. The nonhuman elements are within the situation, not surrounding it. The nonhuman elements include the built environment, technologies, plants, and animals (Clarke, 2019). Clarke was and continues to be one of the proponents of situational analysis. For more information on situational analysis, read Clarke's early book on situational analysis (2005) and more recent coauthored publications (Clarke & Charmaz, 2014; Clarke, Friese, & Washburn, 2015).

Clarke and Charmaz (2014) are considered second-generation grounded theory researchers. Charmaz (2014) builds her methods on a constructivism philosophical foundation. She acknowledges that not all researchers using grounded theory have as their goal to develop a theory. Some researchers may use grounded theory methods to understand relationships in greater depth or provide structure to an emerging phenomenon. Consistent with constructivism, (Charmaz, 2014)

states that "we start with the assumption that social reality is multiple, processual, and constructed, then must take the researcher's position, privileges, perspectives, and interactions into account as an inherent part of the research reality" (p. 13). Symbolic interaction theory is a perspective that works well with grounded theory methods. Symbolic interaction theory is not an explanatory theory, but a perspective through which you consider the participant to be an active agent, interpreting his or her situation. To learn more about Charmaz's constructivist grounded theory, read her primary text (Charmaz, 2014), one of Charmaz's articles (2017), or a chapter in a compilation of chapters by current grounded theory researchers (Bryant & Charmaz, 2019).

Grounded Theory's Contribution to Nursing Science

Grounded theory nursing researchers have contributed to nursing science by describing social processes at the heart of nursing care. Through careful analyses of the relationships among aspects of the social process, the researchers may describe an emerging theory through words and possibly a diagram. Grounded theory researchers examine experiences and processes with a breadth and depth not usually possible with quantitative research. The reader of the research report can intuitively verify these findings through her or his own experiences. The findings resonate with the reader. These contributions to nursing science have contributed to our understanding of (1) patient and family experience in different settings, and (2) pivotal events in the lives of human beings. An example of each contribution will be provided.

The effect of the care environment was the focus of a grounded theory study conducted in Australia. Butler,

Copnell, and Hall (2019b) studied how the physical and emotional environment affected the relationships between the HCPs and the parents of children in the pediatric intensive care unit (PICU) who were dying.

"The aim of this study is to explore the impacts of the PICU physical and social environment on the development and quality of the parent–HCP relationship, with findings drawn from a larger study on bereaved parents' experiences when their child dies in PICU....We followed a constructivist grounded theory approach, which aims to develop a theory about human behaviour and interaction directly from the data itself (Charmaz, 2014). The resultant theory explains the core process occurring within a social context, based upon findings co-constructed from the participants' personal experiences and the researcher's interpretations of them (Charmaz, 2014). Given the focus on social interaction and behaviour, grounded theory was the ideal methodology to explore our aim." (Butler et al., 2019b, p. 29)

Butler et al. (2019b) clearly stated the rationale for using grounded theory as the study methodology. They recognized the ethical issues related to recruiting and interviewing bereaved parents and disseminated what they learned about the ethical issues through other publications (Butler et al., 2018, 2019a).

"Participants were recruited from four Australian PICUs across three states. Our recruitment procedures varied between sites, but included phone calls from social workers involved in hospital based bereavement follow-up, mailed opt-in and opt-out letters from both the research team and a hospital-based research nurse, and advertisements at bereavement support groups (Butler et al., 2017)....Twenty-six bereaved parents, representing 18 deceased children, participated in the study 6–48 months after their child's death.... Data collection included both interviews and document analysis.... Bereaved parents participated in audio recorded, semi-structured interviews lasting 90–150 minutes, in a location of the participants' choosing...." (Butler et al., 2019b, pp. 29–30)

Collaborative relationships were more likely to develop when parents had unimpeded access to their children and there were facilities such as bathrooms, places to wait and rest, and kitchens for the parents to use. When the rules of the PICU limited parent

access and there were no provisions made for parent comfort, parents reported feeling like they were watchers of the care, instead being part of the team (Butler et al., 2019b). We will use the Butler et al. (2018, 2019a, 2019b) study as an example again in Chapters 9 and 12.

Grounded theory researchers have also described pivotal moments on the lives of patients and families. Southby, Cooke, and Lavender (2019) conducted a grounded theory study of women over age 35 years who were pregnant with their first child. The significance of the study was established by two facts: (1) the average age of women's first pregnancy was rising, and (2) pregnancy at advanced maternal age (AMA) had been linked to a higher risk of stillbirth and other complications. The researchers identified constructivist grounded theory as "an ideal methodology to identify key processes relating to how older first-time mothers experience pregnancy and prepare for childbirth" (Southby et al., 2019, p. 2).

"In Phase One, a purposive, maximum variation sample was sought in order to gain a broad spectrum of views and identify an emergent theory which could then be tested using a theoretical sample (Phase Two).... Data analysis and collection were simultaneous and data analysis commenced with the first participant's interview.... In Phase One, data were generated from two broad, open ended interview questions.... Participants in Phase Two were asked a series of five questions, which were based on the initial categories generated in Phase One....This enabled the researchers to advance to a theoretical understanding of the data through the generation of a core category." (Southby et al., 2019, p. 2)

Only one of the pregnancies was unplanned and 5 of the 15 mothers who participated in the study had conceived by using assisted reproductive technologies. Ranging in age from 35 to 44 years, all the mothers attended antenatal classes and all but one had completed an educational qualification beyond secondary school.

One of the researchers who was a midwife interviewed AMA mothers in their homes. The researchers analyzed the transcripts independently before meeting to discuss and agree on the coding. The researchers provided a diagram (Fig. 4.1) showing the relationships among the theoretical categories.

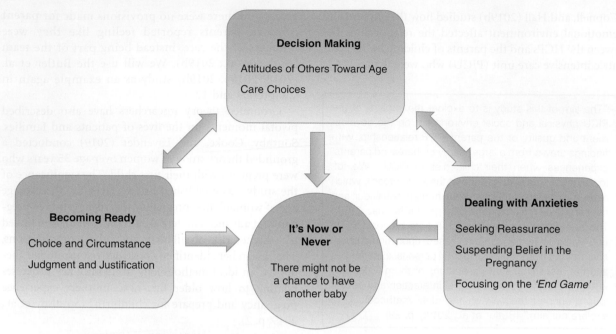

Fig. 4.1 Core category and theoretical categories with theoretical codes. From Southby, C., Cooke, A., & Lavender, T. (2019). 'It's now or never'—nulliparous women's experience of pregnancy at advanced maternal age: A grounded theory study. *Midwifery, 68*(1), 1–8. doi:10.1016/j.midw.2018.09.006

"'It's now or never' is the core category underpinning the interpretive theory of the experience of expecting a first baby after the age of 35 years. Three theoretical categories; 'becoming ready', 'dealing with anxieties' and 'decision making' were formulated from seven theoretical codes.... Our theory is that women's awareness that their age can limit future opportunities to have another baby can affect key aspects of the pregnancy experience, including feelings of readiness to have a baby, perception of risk and decision-making regarding care options." (Southby et al., 2019, pp. 3–4)

The researchers supported each theoretical code with one or more quotations from the mothers. In the discussion and conclusion sections of the study report, Southby et al. (2019) identified ways nurses may influence the mother's experience.

"Our research indicates that women of AMA may feel inadequately supported in the first trimester when they may experience anxiety about miscarriage or having a baby with a chromosomal abnormality. We found that women may be reluctant to share their pregnancy

news with friends and family in the first trimester and may therefore also feel isolated from their social support networks.... The theory... proposes that nulliparous women's experience of pregnancy at AMA may be shaped by awareness that future opportunities to have a baby may be limited. Further research is now needed to test the applicability of this theory with a larger group of women of AMA in their first pregnancy prior to changes in practice being recommended.... Health professionals can play an important role in helping women to feel supported in their pregnancy by understanding and acknowledging issues that are important to women of AMA.... Health professionals have a responsibility to provide women with an evidenced-based understanding of the impact of age upon pregnancy." (Southby et al., 2019, pp. 6–7)

A first pregnancy is a pivotal event in the life of a family, but especially critical when the pregnancy is occurring later in the mother's life. Grounded theory researchers have increased nurses' sensitivity to the experiences of our patients across settings and during pivotal events.

Other grounded theory researchers have studied the perceptions of the communication between healthcare providers and patients with type 2 diabetes (T2D) (Paiva, Abreu, Azevedo, & Silva, 2019), the influence of a clinical instructor's behavior on healthcare student engagement in the clinical area (Knight, 2018), and the process by which a team of multidisciplinary healthcare professionals decide whether a psychiatric patient needs electroconvulsive therapy (Duxbury et al., 2018). As you considered these study topics, did you notice the commonalities of communication, relationships, and perceptions? These commonalities reflect the core of grounded theory, a better understanding of social processes. When this understanding is rich with detail and insight, the researchers may generate a theory, as Southby et al. (2019) did with their study that was described earlier. Their diagram (see Fig. 4.1) displays the relationships among the concepts they identified. Other times, grounded theory researchers may present a description of relationships, communication, and perception as a beginning place for future research and theory generation. The theory that emerges can serve as a framework for understanding and developing nursing interventions acceptable to the persons for whom they were created. Grounded theory researchers interpret their results in terms of social processes; researchers using ethnography, the next qualitative methodology, explore social interactions in the context of culture.

Ethnographical Research

Ethnographical research provides a framework for studying cultures. The word *ethnography* is derived by combining the Greek roots *ethno* (folk or people) and *graphy* (picture or portrait) (Erickson, 2018). The term **culture** refers to a common ancestral heritage, location, and social structure shared by a group of people, or it can be applied to the power structures, roles, and communication patterns of more loosely connected groups such as work cultures or organizational cultures. Therefore the focus of an ethnography is on a culture-sharing group, people who are usually located in the same place, interact often, and share an identity and patterns of behavior, values, language, and power (Creswell & Poth, 2018).

Ethnographies are the written reports of a culture from the perspective of insiders. The insider's viewpoint is referred to as the **emic** perspective, as compared to the **etic** perspective, the views of someone from outside the culture (Marshall & Rossman, 2016). Initially, ethnographical research was limited to anthropology and the study of cultures that were viewed as undeveloped and

remote (Erickson, 2018). The purposes of ethnographical research began to expand, however, beyond description for the sake of description, to description for the sake of promoting social change. Cultures that were proximate, but unknown, were also studied using ethnographical methods, such as DuBois's seminal monograph describing the lives of a Black community living in a specific US census tract in 1899 (Erickson, 2018).

As DuBois demonstrated, ethnography does not require travel to another country or region. Ethnography does require spending considerable time in the setting, studying, observing, and gathering data. **Participant observation**, the primary method of ethnographers (Patton, 2015), is defined as being present and interacting with participants in routine activities while noting what is happening. During these interactions, the researcher maintains the etic perspective and later documents aspects of shared culture, including behaviors, rules, power structures, customs, and expectations. Chapter 12 will provide additional information about methods used in ethnographical research.

Philosophical Orientation

Anthropologists seek to understand people: their ways of living, believing, acquiring information, transforming knowledge, and socializing the next generation. Ethnography is founded on the value of **cultural relativism**, meaning that a culture has to be understood on its own terms (Padgett, 2017). Cultural relativism means that a culture should not be judged by external standards or ideals of more powerful cultures. For example, a nurse ethnographer conducts an ethnographical study of power structures among nurses in an underresourced Ugandan hospital. Cultural relativism would mean that the researcher would avoid describing the Ugandan organization as inferior or lacking because they were different from nursing power structures in hospitals in the United States.

Four schools of thought within ethnography, shown in Table 4.5, have emerged from different philosophical perspectives and social forces (Padgett, 2017). **Classic ethnography**, or realist ethnography, seeks to provide a comprehensive description of a culture (Creswell & Poth, 2018), usually developed by researchers living for extended periods outside their own country in the environment being studied (de Chesnay, 2014). Classic ethnographies are rarely conducted by nurses, but the next type, systematic ethnography, has frequently been conducted by nurses.

TABLE 4.5   **Four Types of Ethnography**

Type	Other Labels	Purpose
Classical	Traditional, realist	Describe a foreign culture through immersion in the culture for an extended period.
Systematic	Focused, institutional	Describe the social organizational structure influencing a specific group of people.
Interpretative	Hermeneutical	Interpret the values and attitudes shaping the behaviors of members of a specific group to promote understanding of the context of culture.
Critical	Disrupted	Examine the life of a group in the context of an alternative theory or philosophy, such as feminism or constructivism.

Systematic ethnography explores and describes the structures of the culture of specific groups, institutions, organizations, and patterns of social interaction. Because the study's scope is limited to a well-defined organizational culture, systematic ethnography is sometimes called **focused ethnography** (Streubert & Carpenter, 2011). For example, nurses in New Zealand conducted a focused ethnography of doctors and nurses providing care to morbidly obese patients in an 18-bed intensive care unit (ICU) (Hales, Coombs, & deVries, 2019). Over 4 months, the first author conducted field work with 80 participants, 8 of whom were patients. The study findings included the challenges of providing care for morbidly obese patients and the need for improvisation, even when using bariatric equipment. An unresolved issue was raised about which term was appropriate to use when referring to the patient (*fat, obese, large*).

Interpretive ethnography has as its goal understanding the values and thinking that result in behaviors and symbols of the people being studied (Streubert & Carpenter, 2011). In contrast to the descriptive goal of classical ethnography, researchers using interpretative ethnography are examining implications of behaviors and drawing inferences (de Chesnay, 2014). Nurses in Finland conducted an interpretive ethnography of intercultural care of immigrant mothers in a maternity unit (Wikberg, Eriksson, & Bondas, 2012). The data from unstructured observations and interviews of 17 mothers from 12 different countries were analyzed using a caring theory. The mothers' expectations for care did not match Finnish maternity care, which was complicated by the nurses' lack of knowledge of traditional care in the countries of origin. Also complicating the care were the differences in the extent to which the mothers were familiar with Finnish culture and health care.

The last type of ethnography, **critical ethnography**, has a political purpose of increasing the awareness of imbalances of power (de Chesnay, 2014), relieving oppression, and empowering a group of people to act on their own behalf. Wolf (2012) calls this type of ethnography disrupted or disruptive and identifies its philosophical foundation to be critical social theory. Bidabadi, Yazdannik, and Zargham-Boroujeni (2019) conducted a critical ethnography of patient dignity in two cardiac surgical ICUs in Iran. The researchers called attention to healthcare professionals' behaviors indicating a lack of respect for the whole person.

"Great focus on patients' bodies instead of viewing them as a unified whole with several biological, psychological, social, cultural, and spiritual aspects was plainly evident in the setting…their care practice was affected by patients' performance and social status. They considered it unpleasant to provide care to addict patients or patients with communicable diseases while felt greater responsibility toward patients with high social status.… This main theme [paternalistic conduct] consisted of two subthemes: 'authoritative behaviors' and 'blaming the patients.' The important point observed during participant observations and approved by the interviews was that most participants forgot that their patients were vulnerable and disabled, hence they were mostly impatient and used imperative words." (Bidabadi et al., 2019, pp. 745–746)

Paternalism and reductionism were found to be two of the prevailing attitudes in the ICU culture that hindered patient dignity. Because ethnography can provide insight into societal issues affecting patients, the qualitative approach has resulted in significant contributions to nursing knowledge.

Ethnography's Contribution to Nursing Science

The knowledge gained by ethnography may not be transferable due to differences in culture across settings. However, the findings of ethnographical studies may lead to innovations in nursing practice in the study setting. For example, the maternity care units that were involved in Wikberg et al.'s (2012) study might benefit from an electronic or printed resource with short descriptions of essential information about the cultures of the countries from which their patients have immigrated. The findings of the study conducted by Bidabadi et al. (2019) indicated ingrained beliefs and values that will be difficult to change, but the first step would be sharing the results and increasing awareness.

The examples of different types of ethnographies conducted by nurses indicate the contributions to nursing science. A discussion of ethnography and nursing would be incomplete, however, without a description of the contributions of Madeline Leininger. Leininger (1970) earned her doctoral degree in anthropology and brought ethnography into nursing science by writing the first book connecting nursing and anthropology. She was not the only nurse researcher who was educated in anthropology and straddled the fence between the two disciplines (Chrisman, 2001); however, she was well known because her writings were widely disseminated. She developed a framework for culture care that became known as the sunrise model with assessment guides that linked the framework to practice (Clarke, McFarland, Andrews, & Leininger, 2009). Chapter 8 contains more information about the theory of culture care developed by Leininger, so this section focuses on the method she developed to be consistent with ethnonursing.

Ethnonursing research values the unique perspective of groups of people within their cultural context that is influenced at the macro level by geographical location, political system, and social structures. Multiple levels of factors affect the culture and, consequently, the care expressions of the people. For example, a Vietnamese family who is the only Asian family in a small rural community in Georgia may have different care practices from those who live in New York City in a predominantly Vietnamese community. Leininger developed enablers, sets of questions to guide the researcher's study of the culture (Leininger, 1997, 2002). The enablers provide a flexible framework for the researcher to use to collect and analyze the qualitative data. For example, one of the enablers is "Leininger's Observation-Participation-Reflection Enabler" (Leininger, 1997, p. 45), which guides the researcher to use the processes of observation, participation, and reflection during a study. The method is naturalistic, meaning that the research is conducted in a natural setting without any attempt to control or alter the context. The researcher is to be open to explore the insider perspective on health and well-being, which was the focus of an ethnonursing study related to malaria.

The Maasai people are a seminomadic people who live in Tanzania and Kenya, countries where malaria is endemic. Although prevention and treatment of malaria in other areas have decreased mortality and morbidity due to the disease, malaria mortality continues to be high among the Maasai people of southern Kenya. Strang and Mixer (2016) found only five studies conducted among the Maasai people related to health care and none specifically focused on malaria. They conducted an ethnonursing study to address this research gap. The theory of culture care diversity and universality (Leininger, 2002) was used to guide the research questions and methods. Interviews were conducted with different members of the community, including general and key informants. Ethnonursing data analysis resulted in detailed patterns supported by the stories and words of the participants that were synthesized into four themes. Related to the theory, three care constructs were revealed: (1) herbs as care, (2) community as care, and (3) praying to/for. Strang and Mixer's (2016) study is an excellent example of following the ethnonursing research method.

Exploratory-Descriptive Qualitative Research

Qualitative nurse researchers have conducted studies with the purpose of exploring and describing a topic of interest but, at times, have not identified or followed a specific qualitative methodology. Descriptive qualitative research is a legitimate method of research that may be the appropriate "label" for studies that have no clearly specified method or in which the method is specified but ends with "a comprehensive summary of an event in the everyday terms of these events" (Sandelowski, 2000, p. 336). Labeling a study as a specific type (grounded theory, phenomenology, or ethnographical) implies fixed categories of research with distinct boundaries, but the boundaries between methods are more appropriately viewed as permeable (Sandelowski, 2010). Benner

(1994b) would agree, as she discussed how critical ethnography and narratives were used within interpretive phenomenology. Many qualitative studies result in descriptions and could be labeled as descriptive qualitative studies, despite the researchers identifying other methodologies. Most of the researchers who do not specify a methodology are in the exploratory stage of studying the subject of interest. To decrease any confusion between quantitative descriptive studies and the discussion of this qualitative approach, we call this approach **exploratory-descriptive qualitative research**. In this book, studies without an identified qualitative method will be labeled as being exploratory-descriptive qualitative research.

Philosophical Orientation

Exploratory-descriptive qualitative studies are frequently conducted to address an issue or problem in need of a solution. One of the worldviews or philosophies that support exploratory-descriptive qualitative studies is the perceived view, a view that is foundational to other methods of qualitative inquiry as well. The perceiver—the person living the experience—is the source and interpreter of information. In addition, exploratory-descriptive qualitative studies are frequently founded on the worldview of pragmatism (Creswell & Creswell, 2018). Nurses who have a problem to solve or a situation for which fresh perspectives are needed will find pragmatism to be a helpful philosophy, because it allows for freedom of choice in the selection of methodologies and methods (Creswell & Creswell, 2018). In addition to exploratory-descriptive qualitative methodology, pragmatism has been linked to grounded theory, phenomenology, case study research, and mixed methods research (Clarke, 2019; Davenport, 2017; Kankam, 2019; Lith, 2014).

Exploratory-Descriptive Qualitative Research's Contribution to Nursing Science

Researchers who value the perspectives of participants may begin a program of research with qualitative methods to (1) develop an intervention, (2) evaluate the appropriateness of an intervention following implementation, or (3) describe participants' definitions of concepts as the first phase in developing an instrument. For example, Currie et al. (2019) explored the bereavement experiences of parents whose child died in the neonatal ICU (NICU) after the implementation of pediatric

palliative care. The researchers gained a better understanding of parents' bereavement experiences and how to better support parents of severely ill infants in the NICU and after the infant's death.

Exploratory-descriptive qualitative research can be applied to a broad range of topics. Ang, O'Brien, and Wilson (2019) interviewed 22 adults caring for older adults at home who were at risk for falls. The caregivers' concerns and strategies identified opportunities for discharge teaching and for support of the caregivers. Another exploratory-descriptive qualitative study was conducted by Chan (2019). Chan conducted 11 focus groups of nursing students ($N = 65$) to explore their perspectives on critical thinking in nursing education. The undergraduate and graduate students described critical thinking as gathering information from multiple sources and then doing your own thinking. The information that was gathered was evaluated for its accuracy and the reliability of the source, called search for truth. Cultural influences were a barrier for critical thinking because the education was designed to provide information with few opportunities for students to ask questions or think independently. The study methods were not complex but were congruent with the study question.

The final example is an exploratory-descriptive qualitative study of emergency personnel's experiences with family presence during resuscitation (FPDR) (Porter, 2019).

> "The aim of this study was to develop an understanding of the experiences and attitudes of emergency personnel immediately post resuscitation events using a descriptive qualitative methodology.... Face to face interviews of key nursing and medical personnel were conducted shortly after resuscitation events to develop an understanding of how, why and when family were permitted to be present during resuscitations." (Porter, 2019, p. 269)

Porter (2019) completed 200 hours of observation in a rural emergency department and an urban emergency department along with interviews ($n = 29$). The method of observation is used more frequently in ethnographical studies, but Porter's focus was not on culture. This is an example of a combination of data sources being appropriate within pragmatism.

> "Following data analysis the author in agreement with two experienced academics organized the data into six themes: care coordinators inconsistently called, gate keepers to implementation, effective communication strategies helping to deliver bad news, life experience generates confidence, allocation of a family support person, family members roles dependent on age of patient." (Porter, 2019, p. 270)

Notice that the themes are not conceptual abstractions of the data but simply descriptive statements. This is a characteristic of most exploratory-descriptive qualitative studies. Porter (2019) found that FPDR occurred more often with pediatric resuscitations than adult resuscitations. The decision of whether to allow FPDR was influenced by the circumstances and age of the patient, the availability of a staff person to support the family members, and the length of the HCPs experience in the emergency department. The members of the emergency team realized their need for additional training about working with the family liaison and the family members of adult patients.

OTHER APPROACHES TO QUALITATIVE RESEARCH

As you search the literature, you will see that qualitative researchers use other approaches in addition to those described in the chapter. We will describe two additional approaches: narrative inquiry and case study method.

Narrative Inquiry

Narrative inquiry focuses on the stories of the participants as told through collaboration with a "story listener," for our purposes, the researcher (Clandinin, Caine, & Lessard, 2018). The stories are situated in time and place, with attention given to the social, emotional, and physical environment (Creswell & Poth, 2018). By analyzing the stories, the researcher learns how the participants recall, construct, and reconstruct their realities. The analysis of the data may be for themes, critical events, plot and conflicts, and chronology. Narrative inquiry has been used in psychological, psychiatric, anthropological, educational, and nursing research (Clandinin & Connelly, 2000). A study conducted by Estefan et al. (2019), introduced earlier in the chapter, is an example of a narrative inquiry study conducted by nurse

researchers. Estefan et al. (2019) spent many years of their nursing careers working with adolescents and young adults (AYA) who had cancer and, at different times, had difficult conversations with AYA about sexuality. The stories of AYA survivorship were hard earned as they lived with cancer. Lost within these stories were other stories of the adolescents' "emergence and development of sexuality" (Estefan et al., 2019, p. 193).

> "An adolescent's story of self as a (developing) sexual being is silenced, or at least refracted, by other more dominant or persuasive stories of the cancer experience…. Something is lost; insights into these silenced stories can teach us—health and social care practitioners—about ways to work helpfully with young people who are experiencing cancer…" (Estefan et al., 2019, p. 193)

With the goal of developing a better appreciation and understanding of sexuality with the life stories of AYA undergoing cancer treatment, the researchers undertook a narrative inquiry with two young adults who were currently cancer free, Anna and Mark. Data collection commenced over 14 months and included formal qualitative interviews, conversations about the interview data, email messages, and telephone conversations (Estefan et al., 2019). As their stories emerged, the researchers and participants reviewed the texts and continued to refine and supplement them. Anna's narrative was titled "Cancer Made Me (Beautiful)" (Estefan et al., 2019, p. 195). Her words are in italics in the following study excerpt.

> "*Cancer was a teacher, and I despised the sympathy. My advantage now. … In my more masculine body, I have complex relationships with women….* In the midst of her early 20s, Anna's forward-looking story was one of possibility and ongoing self-exploration…. She continued to engage in physical relationships with women, and occasionally with men, but did so with more control than she had felt previously." (Estefan et al., 2019, pp. 196–197)

Mark's narrative, "The river, in itself, is benign," began with his description of his life before cancer as a competitive athlete. Cancer had immersed him into a disruption of his masculinity and of his relationships with girls. His words are in italics in the following study excerpt.

"Capacity, ability, appearance, in some relationship with each other... and sometimes taking girls home. I'm past all that now. It's awkward, cancer isn't the first thing I talk about, but I have stretch marks and I have to explain them to girls. They 'friend zone' me now...as a result of his experiences, there were other aspects of his previous life that he was keen to leave behind while he cultivated a different and new way of living in the world.... He felt like he belonged in the world of nature, of retreat, and this was a new version of being a man that he was cultivating.... Although Mark was hopeful for a relationship, he was also aware that he needed to develop relationships with women who understood and could participate in his life the way he was composing it." (Estefan et al., 2019, pp. 197–198)

Estefan et al. (2019) identified two resonant threads from the narratives: (1) inward and outward looking and (2) sexuality and survival. These threads were supported by discussion of relevant aspects of Mark's and Anna's stories.

"Inasmuch as the stories in this inquiry are stories of young people's questions, they are also stories of thriving. In the midst of the tensions and complexities of their stories, Anna and Mark are successful, forward-looking young people. A 'return to normal' is not part of their forward-looking stories. Instead, they are pursuing a revised and evolving sexuality and, as an indicator of well-being, this is something to be supported, sustained, and promoted." (Estefan et al., 2019, p. 203)

Narrative inquiry does not fit every research problem nor is every research team willing to invest the time that Estefan et al. (2019) did. Narrative inquiry, however, is an appropriate method for considering individuals' stories of their experiences of health-illness processes over time. Students wanting to learn more about narrative inquiry refer to books authored and coauthored by Clandinin (Clandinin & Connolly, 2000; Clandinin et al., 2018), Kim (2016), and Dalute (2014).

Case Study

Case studies are frequently used in nursing and in medicine as a teaching strategy. Case studies can also be a methodology for research that may include quantitative or qualitative data, or both. Our focus is on case studies using qualitative data, such as interviews, document reviews, participant observation, and focus groups. Case studies may be exploratory, descriptive, analytical, and/or interpretative, depending on the research question (Yin, 2018). A case study examines closely the recent past and present of an unusual patient, a social phenomenon, or an event (Yin, 2014, 2018). The cases selected for study may be of various types and studied for different purposes. Table 4.6 is provided to describe a few types of case studies that may be helpful in nursing and health care. The unit of analysis for case studies may be a single person or event, a group, or multiple people experiencing the same phenomenon (Padgett, 2017; Schwandt & Gates, 2018). The design and data of case studies may overlap with other types of qualitative methodologies (Schwandt & Gates, 2018), such as a case study of a community's cultural practices (ethnography), a case study of the lived experience of a child with a congenital facial defect (phenomenology), or a case study of adolescents who age out of the foster system that results in a theoretical explanation (grounded theory). Because most case studies are of an exploratory and descriptive nature, there is also a potential overlap with exploratory-descriptive qualitative

TABLE 4.6	**Types of Case Studies**[a]
Type of Case Study	**Description**
Common or typical	An example of what usually happens; used to illustrate or better understand the usual experience
Extreme or unusual	A description of a rare event or an experience that happens infrequently; used to generate discussions of causes and possible responses
Revelatory	A situation or experience providing new and unexpected information; used to stimulate discussion of innovative approaches
Normative or ideal	A real or fictional example of what should happen; used as a description that sets the standard

[a]Adapted and synthesized from Schwandt, T., & Gates, E. (2018). Case study methodology. In N. Denzin & Y. Lincoln (Eds.), *The Sage handbook of qualitative research* (5th ed., pp. 341–358). Thousand Oaks, CA: Sage.

studies. The example that is included is a multiple case study used to generate an initial conceptual framework for factors resulting in detachment in diabetes care.

Significant federal investments were made in studies of diabetic treatment and patient education interventions in the Appalachian region of Tennessee; however, most of the studies were conducted with samples of adults and children. Women were not well represented in the studies, despite Appalachian women having a higher risk for diabetic complications (Abdoli, Wilson, Higdon, Davis, & Smither, 2019). Cost-effective, culturally congruent, self-care interventions were needed for young adult women with T2D. The nurse researchers selected a case study approach along with descriptive qualitative methods to address the research problem and noted that this approach was appropriate for "providing in-depth description of the contextual factors relevant to the experiences of diabetes care in this population" (Abdoli, 2019, p. 33).

The researchers recruited women "with T2D between 20 and 30 years of age…who were born and live in Appalachian Tennessee with an annual income of less than $36,000" (Abdoli et al., 2019, p. 33). The first 9 months of recruitment efforts resulted in no participants contacting the researchers. With institutional review board approval, the researchers mailed 35 flyers to female clinic patients meeting the inclusion criteria.

Three women responded and were eventually interviewed, despite numerous appointments being rescheduled. Interviews lasted 60 to 90 minutes. To enhance the rigor of the methods, Abdoli et al. (2019) independently coded the transcribed interviews before comparison with the other members of the research team. Six months later, they repeated the coding and compared the results. Finally, they shared the "team interpretations with participants and a group of multidisciplinary qualitative researchers" (Abdoli et al., 2019, p. 33).

The experience of each of the women was described in the report and compared across cases to develop a diagram of the overall theme of "detachment from diabetes care." The researchers identified the cultural barriers of food preferences, "obesity-related stigma," and T2D being considered a normal condition and the contextual barriers of "food insecurity" and "poverty and lack of insurance" (Abdoli et al., 2019, p. 34). Personal barriers were also identified and included "resistance to change" and "fear of death and complications" (p. 34). Abdoli et al. (2019) concluded that "the study findings supported the study proposition: 'young women in Appalachia with diabetes face unique challenges that often lead to poor diabetes control'" (p. 35). As a qualitative methodology, case studies offer in-depth focused descriptions and interpretations that may yield clinically important findings.

KEY POINTS

- Qualitative research is a scholarly approach used to describe life experiences, cultures, and social processes from the perspectives of the persons involved.
- The characteristics, purposes, and methods of qualitative research methodologies have been influenced by their disciplinary roots and philosophical foundations.
- Qualitative researchers need to cultivate self-awareness (reflexivity) about how their life experiences may affect data analysis and interpretation (positioning).
- Qualitative researchers use open-ended methods to gather data, such as interviews, focus groups, observation, and examination of documents.
- The goal of phenomenological research is to describe experiences from the perspectives of the participants—to capture the lived experience.

- Phenomenology is the philosophy guiding these studies, a philosophy that began with the writings of Husserl and Heidegger.
- Husserl developed descriptive phenomenology in which researchers bracket their own perspectives on the phenomenon being studied.
- Heidegger believed bracketing was impossible to achieve and developed interpretative phenomenology.
- The goal of grounded theory research is to produce a middle-range or substantive theory about the phenomenon being studied. The label *grounded* indicates the findings of a grounded theory study are connected to the reality of the social processes within the phenomenon.
- Symbolic interactionism is one of the underlying philosophical and theoretical perspectives.

- Ethnographical research is the investigation of cultures through an in-depth study of the members of the culture. Nurse anthropologist Leininger developed the ethnonursing research method.
- Exploratory-descriptive qualitative research elicits the perceptions of participants to provide insights for understanding patients and groups, influencing practice, and developing appropriate programs for specific groups of people.

- Exploratory-descriptive qualitative studies may be guided by the philosophy of pragmatism with a focus on problem solving.
- Narrative inquiry and case study research are examples of other qualitative methods that may be used to answer research questions important to nurses.

REFERENCES

Abdoli, S., Wilson, G., Higdon, R., Davis, A., & Smither, B. (2019). Diabetes detachment: How cultural, contextual, and personal barriers influence low-income young women with diabetes in Appalachia. *Applied Nursing Research, 47*(1), 32–37. doi:10.1016/j.apnr.2019.03.003

Al Kalaldeh, M., Shosha, G., Saiah, N., & Salameh, O. (2018). Dimensions of phenomenology in exploring patient's suffering in long-life illnesses: Qualitative evidence synthesis. *Journal of Patient Experience, 5*(1), 43–49. doi:10.1177/2374373517723314

American Nurses Association (ANA). (2015). *Code of ethics for nurses with interpretive statements.* Silver Springs, MD: Author.

Amos, I. (2016). Interpretive phenomenological analysis and embodied interpretation: Integrating methods to find the 'words that work'. *Counselling and Psychotherapy Research, 16*(4), 307–317. doi:10.1002/capr.12094

Ang, S., O'Brien, A., & Wilson, A. (2019). Understanding carers' fall concern and their management of fall risk among older people at home. *BMC Geriatrics, 19*, Document 144. doi:10.1186/s12877-019-1162-7

Annells, M. (1996). Hermeneutic phenomenology: Philosophical perspectives and current use in nursing research. *Journal of Advanced Nursing, 23*(4), 705–713.

Benner, P. (1982). From novice to expert. *American Journal of Nursing, 82*(3), 402–407.

Benner, P. (1984a). *From novice to expert: Excellence and power in clinical nursing practice.* Reading, MA: Addison-Wesley.

Benner, P. (1984b). *Stress and satisfaction on the job: Work meanings and coping of mid-career men.* New York, NY: Praeger.

Benner, P. (Ed.). (1994a). *Interpretive phenomenology: Embodiment, caring, and ethics in health and illness.* Thousand Oaks, CA: Sage.

Benner, P. (1994b). The tradition and skill of interpretive phenomenology in studying health, illness, and caring practices. In P. Benner (Ed.), *Interpretive phenomenology: Embodiment, caring, and ethics in health and illness* (pp. 99–125). Thousand Oaks, CA: Sage.

Benner, P., Halpern, J., Gordon, D., Popell, C., & Kelley, P. (2018). Beyond pathologizing harm: Understanding PTSD in the context of war experience. *Journal of Medical Humanities, 39*(1), 45–72. doi:10.1007/s10912-017-9484-y

Bentur, N., Stark, D., Resnizky, S., & Symon, Z. (2014). Coping strategies for existential and spiritual suffering in Israeli patients with advanced cancer. *Israel Journal of Health Policy Research, 3*(1), Document 21. doi:10.1186/2045-4015-3-21

Berglund, M., Westin, L., Svanstrom, R., & Sundler, A. (2012). Suffering caused by care-patients' experiences from hospital settings. *International Journal of Qualitative Studies on Health and Well-being, 7*(1), 1–9. doi:10.3402/qhw.v7i0.18688

Betriana, F., & Kongsuwan, W. (2019). Lived experiences of grief of Muslim nurses caring for patients who died in an intensive care unit: A phenomenological study. *Intensive & Critical Care Nursing, 52*(1), 9–16. doi:10.1016/j.iccn.2018.09.003

Bidabadi, F., Yazdannik, A., & Zargham-Boroujeni, A. (2019). Patient's dignity in intensive care unit: A critical ethnography. *Nursing Ethics, 26*(3), 738–752. doi:10.1177/0969733017720826

Blumer, H. (1969). *Symbolic interactionism perspective and method.* Berkley, CA: University of California Press.

Blumer, H. (1980). Mead and Blumer: The convergent methodologies of social behaviorism and symbolic interactionism. *American Sociologist, 43*(3), 409–419. Retrieved from https://www.jstor.org/stable/2095174

Boas, F. (1911). Introduction. In F. Boas (Ed.), *Handbook of American Indian languages: Part I* (Bulletin 40, pp. 1–83). Washington, DC: Government Printing Office.

Brancati, D. (2018). *Social science research.* Thousand Oaks, CA: Sage.

Bryant, A., & Charmaz, K. (Eds.). (2019). *The Sage handbook of current developments in grounded theory.* Thousand Oaks, CA: Sage.

Buetow, S. (2019). Apophenia, unconscious bias, and reflexivity in nursing qualitative research. *International Journal of Nursing Studies, 89*(1), 8–13. doi:10.1016/j.ijnurstu.2018.09.013

Burns, M., & Peacock, S. (2019). Interpretive phenomenological methodologists in nursing: A critical analysis and comparison. *Nursing Inquiry, 26*(2), e12280. doi:10.1111/nin.12280

Butler, A., Copnell, B., & Hall. H. (2017). Ethical and practical realities of using letters for recruitment in bereavement research. *Research in Nursing and Health, 40*(4), 372–377. doi:10.1002/nur.21800

Butler, A., Copnell, B., & Hall. H. (2018). The changing nature of relationships between parents and healthcare providers when a child dies in the paediatric intensive care unit. *Journal of Advanced Nursing, 74*(1), 89–99. doi:10.1111/jan.13401

Butler, A., Copnell, B., & Hall. H. (2019a). Researching people who are bereaved: Managing risks to participants and researchers. *Nursing Ethics, 26*(1), 224–234. doi:10.1177/0969733017695656

Butler, A., Copnell, B., & Hall, H. (2019b). The impact of the social and physical environments on parent–healthcare provider relationships when a child dies in PICU: Findings from a grounded theory study. *Intensive & Critical Care Nursing, 50*(1), 228–235. doi:10.1016/j.iccn.2017.12.008

Bynum, W., & Varpio, L. (2018). When I say…hermeneutic phenomenology. *Medical Education, 52*(3), 252–253. doio:10.1111/medu.13414

Chan, Z. (2019). Nursing students' view of critical thinking as 'own thinking, searching for truth, and cultural influences.' *Nurse Education Today,78*(1), 14–18. doi:10.1016/j.nedt.2019.03.015

Charmaz, K. (2014). *Constructing grounded theory* (2nd ed.). Thousand Oaks, CA: Sage.

Charmaz, K. (2017). The power of constructivist grounded theory for critical inquiry. *Qualitative Inquiry, 23*(1), 34–45. doi:10.1177/1077800416657105

Chrisman, N. (2001). Discussion of Byerly, Kay, and Leininger. *Western Journal of Nursing Research, 23*(9), 807–811. doi:10.1177/01939450122045636

Clandinin, D. (2013). *Engaging in narrative inquiry.* Walnut Creek, CA: Left Coast Press.

Clandinin, D., & Connolly, F. (2000). *Narrative inquiry: Experience and story in qualitative research.* San Francisco, CA: Wiley.

Clandinin, D., Caine, V., & Lessard, S. (2018). *The relational ethics of narrative inquiry.* New York, NY: Routledge.

Clarke, A. (2005). *Situational analysis: Grounded theory after the postmodern turn.* Thousand Oaks, CA: Sage.

Clarke, A. (2019). Situating grounded theory and situational analysis in interpretive qualitative inquiry. In A. Bryant & K. Charmaz (Eds.), *The Sage handbook of current developments in grounded theory* (pp. 3–47). Thousand Oaks, CA: Sage.

Clarke, A., & Charmaz, K. (Eds.). (2014). *Grounded theory and situational analysis.* Sage Benchmark Series (4 vols.). London, England: Sage.

Clarke, A., Friese, C., & Washburn, R. (Eds.). (2015). *Situational analysis in practice: Mapping research with grounded theory.* London, England: Routledge.

Clarke, P. N., McFarland, M. R., Andrews, M. M., & Leininger, J. (2009). Caring: Some reflections on the impact of the culture care theory by McFarland & Andrews and a conversation with Leininger. *Nursing Science Quarterly, 22*(3), 233–239. doi:10.1177/0894318409337020

Colaizzi, P. F. (1973). *Reflection and research in psychology: A phenomenological study of learning.* Dubuque, IA: Kendall Hunt.

Corry, M., Porter, S., & McKenna, H. (2019). The redundancy of positivism as a paradigm for nursing research. *Nursing Philosophy, 2*(1), e12230. doi:10.1111/nup.12230

Creswell, J., & Creswell, J. (2018). *Research design: Qualitative, quantitative, and mixed methods approaches* (5th ed.). Thousand Oaks, CA: Sage.

Creswell, J., & Poth, C. (2018). *Qualitative inquiry & research design: Choosing among five approaches* (4th ed.). Thousand Oaks, CA: Sage.

Critical Appraisal Skills Programme. (2017). CASP qualitative research checklist. Retrieved from http://casp-uk.net.

Crossley, N. (2010). Networks and complexity: Directions for interactionist research? *Symbolic Interaction, 33*(3), 341–363. doi:10.1525/si.2010.33.3.341

Currie, E., Christian, B., Hinds, P., Perna, S., Robinson, C., Day, S., … Meneses, K. (2019). Life after loss: Parent bereavement and coping experiences after infant death in the neonatal intensive care unit. *Death Studies, 43*(5), 333–342. doi:10.1080/07481187.2018.1474285

Dalute, C. (2014). *Narrative inquiry: A dynamic approach.* Thousand Oaks, CA: Sage.

Davenport, L. (2017) Living with the choice: A grounded theory of Iraqi refugee resettlement to the U.S. *Issues in Mental Health Nursing, 38*(4), 352–360. doi:10.1080/01612840.2017.1286531

de Chesnay, M. (2014). Overview of ethnography. In M. de Chesnay, (Ed.), *Nursing research using ethnography* (pp. 1–14). New York, NY: Springer Publishing.

Denzin, N., & Lincoln, Y. (Eds.). (2018). *The Sage handbook of qualitative research* (5th ed.). Thousand Oaks, CA: Sage.

Derico, S. (2017). The use of phenomenology in nursing education: An integrative review. *Nursing Education Perspectives, 38*(6), e7–e11. doi:10.1097/01.NEP.0000000000000216

Dewey, J. (1916/2012). *Essays in experimental logic.* Chicago, IL: University of Chicago Press. [Ebook #40794, Project

Gutenberg]. Retrieved from https://www.gutenberg.org/files/40794/40794-h/40794-h.htm

Duxbury, A., Smith, I., Mair-Edwards, B., Bennison, G., Irving, K., Hodge, S., … Weatherhead, S. (2018). What is the process by which a decision to administer electroconvulsive therapy (ECT) or not is made? A grounded theory informed study of the multi-disciplinary professionals involved. *Social Psychiatry and Psychiatric Epidemiology, 53*(8), 785–793. doi:10.1007/s00127-018-1541-y

Erickson, F. (2018). A history of qualitative inquiry in social and educational research. In N. Denzin & Y. Lincoln (Eds.), *The Sage handbook of qualitative research* (5th ed., pp. 36–65). Thousand Oaks, CA: Sage.

Estefan, A., Moules, N., & Laing, C. (2019). Composing sexuality in the midst of cancer. *Journal of Pediatric Oncology Nursing, 36*(3), 191–206. doi:10.1177/1043454219836961

Fowler, M. (2017). Faith and ethics, covenant and code: The 2015 revision of the ANA Code of Ethics for Nurses with Interpretive Statements. *Journal of Christian Nursing, 34*(4), 216–224. doi:10.1097/CNJ.0000000000000419

Gadamer, H-G. (1992). The expressive power of language: On the function of rhetoric for knowledge. *Publications of the Modern Language Association of American, 107*(2), 345–352. doi:10.2307/462645

Gadamer, H-G. (2011). *Truth and method* (W. Glen-Doepel, Trans.). New York, NY: Continuum International Publishing Group. (Original work published 1960)

Giorgi, A. (1985). *Phenomenology and psychological research.* Pittsburg, PA: Duquesne University Press.

Giorgi, A. (2010). Phenomenological psychology: A brief history and its challenges. *Journal of Phenomenological Psychology, 41*(2), 145–179. doi:10.1163/156916210X532108

Glaser, B. (2019). Grounded description: No no. In A. Bryant & K. Charmaz (Eds.), *The Sage handbook of current developments in grounded theory* (pp. 441–445). Thousand Oaks, CA: Sage.

Glaser, B. G., & Strauss, A. (1965). Discovery of substantive theory: A basic strategy underlying qualitative research. *American Behavioral Scientist, 8* (6), 5–12.

Glaser, B. G., & Strauss, A. (2011). *The discovery of grounded theory: Strategies for qualitative research.* Chicago, IL: Aldine. (Original work published in 1967)

Goodman, R. (2017). William James. In E. Zalta (Ed.), *The Stanford encyclopedia of philosophy.* Retrieved from https://plato.stanford.edu/archives/win2017/entries/james/

Hales, C., Coombs, M., & de Vries, K. (2019). The challenges of caring for morbidly obese patient in intensive care: A focused ethnographic study. *Australian Critical Care, 31*(1), 37–41. doi:10.1016/j.aucc.2017.02.070

Heidegger, M. (2010). *Being and time* (J. Stambaugh, Trans.). Albany, NY: SUNY Press. (Original work published 1927)

Hopkins, R., Regehr, G., & Pratt, D. (2017). A framework for negotiating positionality in phenomenological research. *Medical Teacher, 39*(1), 20–25. doi:10.1080/0142159X.2017.1245854

Horne, C., & Paul, J. (2019). Pain support for adults with a diabetic-related lower limb amputation: An empirical phenomenology study. *Pain Management, 20*(3), 270–275. doi:10.1016/j.pmn.2018.09.007

Husserl, E. (1970). *Logical investigations* (Vol. 1) (N. Findlay, Trans.). New York, NY: Routledge. (Original work published in 1901)

Jackson, A., & Mazzei, L. (2018). Thinking with theory: A new analytic for qualitative inquiry. In N. K. Denzin & Y. S. Lincoln (Eds.), *The Sage handbook of qualitative research* (pp. 717–737). Thousand Oaks, CA: Sage.

James, W. (1890). *The principles of psychology* (Vol. 1). New York, NY: Henry Holt & Co.

James, W. (2007). *Pragmatism and other writings* (Edited with an introduction and notes by G. Gunn). New York, NY: Penguin Books. (Original work published in 1907)

Jansen, J. (2016). Kant's and Husserl's agentive and proprietary accounts of cognitive phenomenology. *Philosophical Explorations, 19*(2), 161–172. doi:10.1080/13869795.2016.1176233

Kankam, P. (2019). The use of paradigms in information research. *Library and Information Science Research, 41*(2), 85–92. doi:10.1016/j.lisr.2019.04.003

Kazdin, A. (2017). *Research design in clinical psychology.* Boston, MA: Pearson.

Kelley, P., Kenny, D., Gordon, D., & Benner, P. (2015). The evolution of case management for service members injured in Iraq and Afghanistan. *Qualitative Health Research, 25*(3), 426–433. doi:10.1177/1049732314553228

Kelly, T., & Kelly, M. (2019). Living with ureteric stents: A phenomenological study. *British Journal of Nursing, 28*(9), 529–537. doi:10.12968/bjon.2019.28.9.S29

Kim, J-H. (2016). *Understanding narrative inquiry for the human sciences.* Thousand Oaks, CA: Sage.

Knight, A. (2018). How clinical instructor behavior affects student clinical engagement from a motivational perspective. *Journal of Nuclear Medicine Technology, 46*(2), 99–106. doi:10.2967/jnmt.118.209320

Ladner, S. (2014). *Practical ethnography: A guide to doing ethnography in the private sector.* Walnut Creek, CA: Left Coast Press.

Lamb, C., Babenko-Mould, Y., Evans, M., Wong, C., & Kirkwood, K. (2018). Conscientious objection and nurses: Results of an interpretive phenomenological study. *Nursing Ethics, 25*(4). Epub. doi:10.1177/0969733018763996

Lamb, C., Evans, M., Babenko-Mould, Y., Wong, C., & Kirkwood, K. (2019). Conscience, conscientious objection, and nursing: A concept analysis. *Nursing Ethics, 26*(1), 37–49. doi:10.1177/0969733017700236

Leininger, M. M. (1970). *Nursing and anthropology: Two worlds to blend.* New York, NY: Wiley.

Leininger, M. M. (1997). Overview of the theory of culture care with the ethnonursing research method. *Journal of Transcultural Nursing, 8*(2), 32–54. doi:10.1177/104365969700800205

Leininger, M. M. (2002). Culture care theory: A major contribution to advance transcultural nursing knowledge and practices. *Journal of Transcultural Nursing, 13*(3), 189–192. doi:10.1177/10459602013003005

Lith, T. (2014). "Painting to find my spirit": Art making as the vehicle to find meaning and connection in the mental health recovery process. *Journal of Spirituality in Mental Health, 16*(1), 19–36. doi:10.1080/19349637.2013.864542

Lynch, M. (2016). Social constructivism in science and technology studies. *Human Studies, 39*(1), 101–112. doi:10.1007/s10746-016-9385-5

Mackey S. (2005). Phenomenological nursing research: Methodological insights derived from Heidegger's interpretive phenomenology. *International Journal of Nursing Studies, 42*(2), 179–186. doi:10.1016/j.ijnurstu.2004.06.011

Marshall, C., & Rossman, G. B. (2016). *Designing qualitative research* (6th ed.). Thousand Oaks, CA: Sage.

Mead, G. H. (1934). *Mind, self, and society.* Chicago, IL: University of Chicago Press.

Melnyk, B. M., & Fineout-Overholt, E. (2019). *Evidence-based practice in nursing and healthcare: A guide to best practice* (4th ed.). Philadelphia, PA: Wolters Kluwer.

Merleau-Ponty, M. (2012). *Phenomenology of perception* (D. Landes, Trans.). London, England: Routledge Classics. (Original work published in 1945)

Merton, R. (1949). On sociological theories of the middle range. In C. Calhoun, J. Gerteis, J. Moody, S. Pfaff, & I. Virk (Eds.) (2004), *Classical sociological theory* (pp. 448–459). Malden, MA: Blackwell Publishing.

Miles, M., Huberman, A., & Saldaña, J. (2020). *Qualitative data analysis: A methods sourcebook.* Thousand Oaks, CA: Sage.

Molzahn, A., Shields, L., Bruce, A., Schick-Makaroff, K., Antonio, M., & White, L. (2019). Living with dying: A narrative inquiry of people with chronic kidney disease and their family members. *Journal of Advanced Nursing, 75*(1), 129–137. doi:10.1111/jan.13830

Morley, J. (2019). Phenomenology in nursing studies: New perspectives–commentary. *International Journal of Nursing Studies, 93*(1), 163–167. doi:10.1016/j.ijnurstu.2019.02.002

Morse, J. (2018). Reframing rigor in qualitative inquiry. In N. Denzin & Y. Lincoln (Eds.), *The Sage handbook of qualitative research* (5th ed., pp. 796–817). Thousand Oaks, CA: Sage.

Munhall, P. L. (2012). *Nursing research: A qualitative perspective* (5th ed.). Sudbury, MA: Jones & Bartlett.

Padgett, D. (2017). *Qualitative methods in social work research* (3rd ed.). Thousand Oaks, CA: Sage.

Paiva, D., Abreu, L., Azevedo, A., & Silva, S. (2019). Patient-centered communication in type 2 diabetes: The facilitating and constraining factors in clinical encounters. *Health Services Research, 54*(3), 623–635. doi:10.1111/1475-6773.13126

Patton, M. (2015). *Qualitative research & evaluation methods* (4th ed.). Thousand Oaks, CA: Sage.

Peirce, C. (1955). *Philosophical writings of Peirce* (Selected and edited with an introduction by J. Buchler). New York, NY: Dover Publications.

Porter, J. (2019). Family presence during resuscitation (FPDR): A qualitative descriptive study exploring the experiences of emergency personnel post resuscitation. *Heart & Lung, 48*(4), 258–272. doi:10.1016/j.hrtlng.2018.09.016

Portes, A., & Rumbaut, R. G. (2001). *Legacies: The story of the immigrant second generation.* Berkeley, CA: University of California Press.

Probst, B. (2015). The eye regards itself: Benefits and challenges of reflexivity in qualitative social work research. *Social Work Research, 39*(1), 37–48. doi:10.1093/swr/svu028

Robson, D. (2013). There really are 50 Eskimo words for 'snow.' Retrieved from https://www.washingtonpost.com

Rockenbach, A., Walker, C., & Luzader, J. (2012). A phenomenological analysis of college students' spiritual struggles. *Journal of College Student Development, 53*(1), 55–75. doi:10.1353/csd.2012.0000

Sandelowski, M. (2000). What happened to qualitative description? *Research in Nursing & Health, 23*(4), 334–340. doi:10.1002/1098-240X(200008)

Sandelowski, M. (2010). What's in a name? Qualitative description revisited. *Research in Nursing & Health, 33*(1), 77–84. doi:10.1002/nur.20362

Schwandt, T., & Gates, E. (2018). Case study methodology. In N. Denzin & Y. Lincoln (Eds.), *The Sage handbook of qualitative research* (5th ed., pp. 341–358). Thousand Oaks, CA: Sage.

Shardonofsky, J., Cesario, S., Fredland, N., Landrum, P., Hiatt, P., & Shardonofsky, F. (2019). The lived experience of fathers caring for a child with cystic fibrosis. *Pediatric Nursing, 45*(2), 87–92.

Sommer, P., Kelley, M., Norr, K., Patil, D., & Vonderheid, S. (2019). Mexican American adolescent mothers' lived experience: Grounded ethnicity and authentic mothering. *Global Qualitative Nursing Research, 6*(1), 1–15. doi:10.1177/2333393619850775

Southby, C., Cooke, A., & Lavender, T. (2019). 'It's now or never'—nulliparous women's experience of pregnancy at advanced maternal age: A grounded theory study. *Midwifery, 68*(1), 1–8. doi:10.1016/j.midw.2018.09.006

Strang, C., & Mixer, S. (2016). Discovery of the meanings, expressions, and practices related to malaria care among the Maasai. *Journal of Transcultural Nursing, 27*(4), 333–341. doi:10.1177/1043659615573841

Streubert, H., & Carpenter, D. (2011). *Qualitative research in nursing: Advancing the humanistic perspective* (5th ed.). Philadelphia, PA: Lippincott Williams & Wilkins.

Vagle, M. (2018). *Crafting phenomenological research* (2nd ed.). New York, NY: Routledge.

van Manen, M. (1990). *Researching lived experience: Human science for an action sensitive pedagogy.* Ontario, Canada: Althouse Press.

van Manen, M. (2007). Phenomenology of practice. *Phenomenology & Practice,1*(1), 11–30.

van Manen M. (2014). *Phenomenology of practice.* Walnut Creek, CA: Left Coast Press.

van Manen, M. (2016). *Phenomenology of practice: Meaning giving methods in phenomenological research and writing.* London, England: Routledge.

van Manen, M. (2017). Phenomenology in its original sense. *Qualitative Health Research, 27*(6), 810–825. doi:10.1177/104973231769938

van Wijngaarden, E., van der Meide, H., & Dahlberg, K. (2017). Researching health care as a meaningful practice: Toward a nondualistic view on evidence for qualitative research. *Qualitative Health Research, 27*(11), 1738–1747. doi:10.1177/104973231771113

Walsh, D., & Evans, K. (2014). Critical realism: An important theoretical perspective in midwifery research. *Midwifery, 30*(1), e1–e6. doi:10.1016/j.midw.2013.09.002

Ward, K., Hoare, K., & Gott, M. (2015). Evolving from a positivist to constructionist epistemology while using grounded theory: Reflections of a novice researcher. *Journal of Research in Nursing, 20*(6), 449–462. doi:10.1177/1744987115597731

White, R. (2004). Discourse analysis and social constructionism. *Nurse Researcher, 12*(2), 7–16. doi:10.7748/nr2004.10.12.2.7.c5935

Wikberg, A., Eriksson, K., & Bondas, T. (2012). Intercultural caring from the perspectives of immigrant new mothers. *Journal of Gynecological and Neonatal Nursing, 41*(5), 638–649. doi:10.1111/j.1552-6909.2012.01395.x

Wolf, Z. (2012). Ethnography: The method. In P. L. Munhall (Ed.), *Nursing research: A qualitative perspective* (5th ed., pp. 285–338). Sudbury, MA: Jones & Bartlett.

Yin, R. (2014). *Case study research: Design and methods.* Thousand Oaks, CA: Sage.

Yin, R. (2018). *Case study research and applications: Design and methods* (6th ed.). Thousand Oaks, CA: Sage.

Zahavi, D. (2019). Getting it wrong: van Manen and Smith on phenomenology. *Qualitative Health Research, 29*(6), 900–907. doi:10.1177/1049732318817547

Zahavi, D., & Martiny, K. (2019). Phenomenology in nursing studies: New perspective: Authors' response to Morley (2019). *International Journal of Nursing Studies, 93*(1), 153–154. doi:10.1016/j.ijnurstu.2019.01.014

5

Research Problem and Purpose

Susan K. Grove

http://evolve.elsevier.com/Gray/practice/

We are constantly asking questions to better understand ourselves and the world around us. This human ability to wonder and ask creative questions about behaviors, experiences, and situations in the world provides a basis for identifying research problems. The problem area chosen by a nurse researcher frequently is the outgrowth of professional observation, such as an awareness of a resurgence in vaccine-preventable diseases in infants and children in the United States (Kubin, 2019). Research is needed to identify effective strategies to improve immunization rates in this country. External opportunities to conduct research may also stimulate thinking about a research problem, such as grant postings, agency calls for internal research, or requirements of graduate nursing programs.

A research problem should be identified from topics of interest to you. **Research topics** are concepts, phenomena of interest, or broad problem areas, such as management of chronic pain that researchers focus on to enhance evidence-based nursing (Kesten, White, Heitzler, Chaplin, & Bondmass, 2019). Research topics contain several potential problems, and each research problem provides the basis for developing many study purposes. The research purpose is the stated reason for conducting a study. Thus the identification of a relevant research topic and a challenging, significant problem can facilitate the development of numerous study

purposes to direct a lifetime program of research. However, the abundance of potential research problems frequently is not apparent to nurses struggling to identify a problem for their first study.

This chapter defines and presents examples of research problems and purposes, identifies potential sources for research problems, and explains the process of formulating a research problem and purpose for a study. In addition, it discusses criteria for determining the feasibility of a proposed study; discusses research topics, problems, and purposes for different methodologies; and provides examples of research problems and purposes from current published studies.

THE RESEARCH PROBLEM

A **research problem** is an area in which there is a gap in nursing's knowledge base. The gap can be one that relates directly to practice, such as the safest and most efficient way for a community emergency department to triage and establish prompt isolation in case of suspected severe acute respiratory syndrome. Because of the scope of what is not known, many studies are required to fill this particular gap in knowledge. Some research problems focus on understanding a phenomenon related to health, such as fathers' perception of social support provision when transitioning their preterm infants from the neonatal intensive care unit to home (Kim, 2018). Research that enhances understanding contributes to nursing's body of knowledge. Other research problems might be related to theory generation. Research that generates theory is qualitative, and only some types of qualitative research generate theory (Creswell & Poth, 2018). (Quantitative research is conducted to test theory.) To some extent, new theory informs practice, such as research that addresses the theory gap about parents' perspective on the quality of life of their children with autism spectrum disorder (ASD) (Epstein et al., 2019), ultimately giving the reader insight and understanding of process but not prescribing practice actions. Epstein and colleagues (2019) conducted a grounded theory qualitative study "to provide an initial framework for understanding quality of life in children with autism spectrum disorder" (p. 71).

Elements That Comprise the Research Problem

The research problem is usually two to three paragraphs in length expressed at the beginning of a research article that focuses on the principal concepts of the study. As demonstrated in Fig. 5.1, the research problem includes significance and background that provide the basis for a problem statement. The **significance of a research problem** indicates the importance of the problem to patients, families, nursing, health care, and society. The **background for the research problem** is a general summary of what is known about the phenomenon of interest. The **problem statement** identifies a gap in nursing knowledge that requires additional research to address. A typical problem statement often begins with wording such as, "Nonetheless, there is inadequate knowledge about" or "limited research related to…." Finally, the research problem identifies a specific

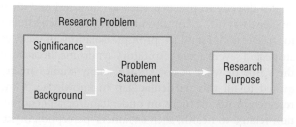

Fig. 5.1 Linking the research problem and purpose.

> ### BOX 5.1 Elements of the Research Problem
>
> - **Significance:** Importance of the problem to nursing and health care that identifies the population studied
> - **Background:** Key knowledge that is known from previous research
> - **Problem statement:** Identified gap in nursing knowledge that provides focus for the research purpose

population and sometimes a general setting for a study. Box 5.1 summarizes the elements of a research problem.

Im and colleagues (2019) conducted a study to examine "racial/ethnic differences in cognitive symptoms during the menopausal transition" (p. 217). This study's research problem discussion is presented as an example, with headers added to facilitate students' identification of the significance, background, and statement of the research problem.

Significance of the Research Problem

"Mainly due to aging process, self-reported memory problems are common in midlife women (Gold et al., 2000; Mitchell & Woods, 2001). Mitchell and Woods (2001) reported that 60% of their research participants noticed memory changes over the last few years. In their study, the participants indicated their problems in remembering words and numbers, interruptions in everyday behavior due to loss of memory, problems in concentrating, and necessity of memory aids. In the Study of Women's Health Across the Nation (SWAN), a significant association of self-reported forgetfulness to peri-menopausal status was also found (Gold et al., 2000). In the SWAN, 31% of pre-menopausal, 44% of early or late peri-menopausal, and 42% of naturally menopausal women reported forgetfulness." (Im et al., 2019, p. 218)

Background of the Research Problem

"Estrogens are reported to have salutary neurophysiologic effects; a decrease in estrogens during menopausal transition would be detrimental to women's cognition (McEwen, 2001, 2002).... Recent studies have supported racial/ethnic differences in hormonal changes (including the decrease in estrogens) during the menopausal transition and subsequent racial/ethnic differences in women's cognitive symptom experience during the menopausal transition....In addition to the hormonal changes, multiple factors have been reported to be associated with cognitive symptoms that are experienced during the menopausal transition, which include employment status, job stress, and multiple life roles (Greendale et al., 2011). Socioeconomic status is one of the most frequently reported factors that are significantly associated with cognitive symptoms (Wee et al., 2012). General health and menopausal status are other factors that are significantly correlated to cognitive symptoms (Greendale et al., 2011)." (Im et al., 2019, pp. 218–219)

Research Problem Statement

"However, the associations of multiple factors to cognitive symptoms in different racial/ethnic groups have rarely been determined, and little is known about the racial/ethnic-specific factors that differently influence cognitive symptoms in different racial/ethnic groups of midlife women." (Im et al., 2019, p. 219)

In this example, the research problem discussion focused on an area of concern: the racial/ethnic differences in cognitive symptoms of midlife women. Im et al. (2019) clearly identified the significance of the problem, which is extensive and relevant to the nursing care of diverse midlife women. The conduct of the research is defensible, based on the identification of the knowledge gap and the size of the population (midlife women) who might benefit from research in this area. The problem background focused on key research that determined hormonal changes during menopause can be detrimental to women's cognition. Studies also supported racial/ethnic differences in hormonal changes. In addition, multiple factors have been reported as related to cognitive symptoms experienced during the menopause transition. The problem statement clearly identifies the gap in nursing knowledge to direct this study.

The research problem in this example gives rise to several concepts or research topics:

- Menopausal transition
- Cognitive symptoms experienced during menopause
- Hormonal changes detrimental to women's cognition during menopausal
- Racial/ethnic differences in cognitive changes during menopause
- Multiple factors associated with menopausal women's cognitive symptoms

- Knowledge needed by nurses for assessment and management of diverse midlife women's cognitive symptoms

Each of these topics includes an array of potential research problems that provide the basis for formulating research purposes for a variety of quantitative, qualitative, mixed methods, and outcomes studies (Creswell & Creswell, 2018).

THE RESEARCH PURPOSE

The **research purpose** is a clear, concise statement of the specific focus or aim of a study, identifying the reason the study was conducted. The research purpose is a short statement, frequently a single sentence. In a research proposal, the purpose statement is couched in the present tense, "The purpose of this research is to investigate…" and in a research report, in the past tense, "The purpose of this study was to determine the effect…." Often the research purpose indicates the principal variables and setting, identifies the population, and hints at both methodology and design of a study. A quantitative purpose statement focuses on identification and description of variables, examination of relationships among variables, or determination of the effects of interventions (Creswell & Creswell, 2018; Shadish, Cook, & Campbell, 2002). A qualitative purpose statement focuses on exploring a phenomenon, such as major depression as it is experienced by pregnant women; developing theories to describe and manage clinical situations; examining the health practices of certain cultures; and describing health-related issues, events, and situations (Creswell & Poth, 2018). Mixed methods research includes both quantitative and qualitative research methodologies (Creswell & Clark, 2018). Outcomes research studies contain purpose statements with similar format to those found in quantitative research and usually focus on safety, quality, and cost outcomes for patients, providers, and healthcare agencies (Moorhead, Swanson, Johnson, & Maas, 2018). (Chapter 2 includes an introduction to the types of research methodologies included in this text.)

Regardless of the type of research, a clear purpose statement is required to indicate what the study was designed to accomplish. Immediately after their research problem summary and identification of the gap in research knowledge, Im et al. (2019, p. 220) reported:

"Purpose
The purpose of this study was to explore racial/ethnic differences in midlife women's cognitive symptoms among four major racial/ethnic groups in the United States, and to determine multiple factors that influenced the women's cognitive symptoms."

The four major racial/ethnic groups included in the Im et al. (2019) study were clearly identified as non-Hispanic (NH) Whites, Hispanic, NH African Americans, and NH Asians. Their study purpose concisely identified the principal study variables (cognitive symptoms, multiple factors influencing these symptoms, and racial/ethnic differences) and population (racial/ethnic diverse women during menopausal transition). This purpose statement suggests that Im et al. (2019) conducted a quantitative descriptive, correlational study to describe racial/ethnic differences in cognitive symptoms of women during midlife and to examine associations of hormonal changes and multiple factors with cognitive symptoms experienced during menopausal transition. The gap in knowledge identified by the problem statement is addressed by their research purpose. Thus this study has a logical flow from the research problem to the research purpose as identified in Fig. 5.1.

SOURCES OF RESEARCH PROBLEMS AND PURPOSES

A nurse researcher who produces a series of related studies within a single problem area is at no loss for identification of a research purpose within that area. The novice researcher, however, especially a master's or doctoral student, may search not only for a purpose statement but also for an entire problem area. Rich sources for generating meaningful research are (1) clinical practice situations, (2) professional literature in one's area of expertise, (3) review of research literature, (4) collaboration with faculty and nurse researchers, and (5) research priorities identified by funding agencies and specialty groups.

Clinical Practice

The practice of nursing must be based on knowledge or evidence generated through research. Thus clinical

practice is an extremely important source for research problems that can evolve from clinical observations. For example, while watching the behavior of a patient and family in crisis, you may wonder how you might intervene to improve the family's coping skills. A review of patient records, treatment plans, and procedure manuals might reveal concerns or raise questions about practices that could be the bases for research problems. For example, you may wonder: "What is the impact of home visits on the level of function, readjustment to the home environment, and rehospitalization pattern of a child with a severe disability?" "What is the best pharmacological agent or agents for treating hypertension in elderly, diabetic patients—diuretic, angiotensin-converting enzyme inhibitor, angiotensin II receptor blocker, beta blocker, calcium channel blocker, or alpha antagonist, or a combination of these drugs?" "What self-care measures improve the health status for patients with serious and persistent mental illnesses?" "What are the cultural factors that promote better birth outcomes in Hispanic women?"

Extensive patient data, such as assessment, diagnoses, treatments, and outcomes, are now computerized. Analyzing this information might generate research problems that are significant to a clinic, community, or national healthcare system. For example, you may ask, "Why has adolescent obesity increased so rapidly in the past 5 years, and what treatments will be effective in managing this problem?" "What are the outcomes (patient health status and costs) for treating chronic illnesses such as type 2 diabetes, hypertension, and dyslipidemia in this practice?" Review of agency patient data often reveals patterns and trends in clinic and hospital settings, which helps nurses and students to identify patient care problems for research. In summary, clinically focused research is essential if nurses are to develop the knowledge needed for evidence-based practice (Hickman et al., 2018; Melnyk et al., 2018; Melnyk & Fineout-Overholt, 2019; Utley, Henry, & Smith, 2018).

Professional Journals in One's Area of Expertise

While reading journals in your area of expertise, you might be captivated by a certain article, either a research report or an essay discussing research reports about patient care or outcomes, in terms of best evidence. In reading a study, you might question the effectiveness of an intervention in terms of quality of care, patient safety, practicality, and/or cost effectiveness. These questions will help you identify possible research problems. For example, Tice, Cole, Ungvary, George, and Oliver (2019) questioned clinicians' accountability for providing a 5-minute rest before taking patients' blood pressure measurements (BPMs). As a result, they studied the effect of a 5-minute rest before BPMs were taken in a primary care clinic setting. Tice et al. (2019) found that the 5-minute rest significantly improved the accuracy of the BPMs and recommended nurses standardize their BPMs in everyday practice.

In reviewing a study of interest, carefully read the conclusion section because it usually contains the authors' recommendations for subsequent research, indicating directions for verification of existent studies' findings or exploration of the problem area in different ways. Designing a study based on these recommendations allows you to build on the work of others and expand what is known.

Review of Research Literature

Having identified a possible problem, you need to do a more extensive review of the research literature to refine the problem area for study. Hundreds of nursing, medical, and health journals are available in print or online. Many of these journals contain a substantial amount of research. For example, *Nursing Research* and *Journal of Psychiatric and Mental Health Nursing* publish 40 to 60 research articles annually, and *Applied Nursing Research* and *Journal of Pediatric Nursing* publish more than 60 studies annually. Reviewing studies in research and clinical journals is helpful in clarifying a research problem area and determining what is already known, versus what is needed for nursing's body of knowledge. You might decide to replicate or repeat one of the studies you reviewed.

Replication Research

Replication involves repeating a study to determine whether its findings are reproducible. Because one or two isolated small-sample studies do not constitute enough evidence on which to base practice, replication of previous research is a respected and essential way to advance the science of nursing. The reason that replication is so important is that even well-conducted research can produce inaccurate findings. This is because statistical testing is based on probabilities, not

certainties. In nursing research, the level of significance typically is set at $p \leq 0.05$ for the hypothesis testing process (Grove & Cipher, 2020). This means that the researcher will allow for a 5% or lower probability of rejecting the null hypothesis when it is indeed true. When this happens, it is called a **Type I error**. The probability of accepting the null hypothesis when it is false is called a **Type II error**. In nursing studies, researchers usually allow a 20% or lower probability of the occurrence of a Type II error. (Chapter 21 provides further information regarding hypothesis testing, Type I error, and Type II error.)

A replication study serves several purposes besides confirmation of previous findings. It can extend generalizability if the replication study's population differs from that of the original research. If findings are similar in the replication study, they can then be applied to both populations. Replication research can improve upon the original study's methods using a more representative sample or an intervention that produces clearer results (Polit & Beck, 2010). Replication of qualitative research can lead to an expanded understanding of the phenomenon of interest, answering some of the questions identified by the original study.

Researchers who conduct replications may do so because the original study's findings resonate with them and they hope to generate supportive evidence. Others are guarded in their enthusiasm, wondering whether replications with different settings or different study participants will affect the strength of the findings and to what degree and in which direction. The career researcher might narrowly identify a research problem area and conduct a series of sequential replication studies to strengthen evidence for generalization to different populations and settings (Polit & Beck, 2010).

Haller and Reynolds (1986) described four types of replication for generating sound scientific knowledge for nursing: (1) exact, (2) concurrent, (3) approximate, and (4) systematic extension. The first, exact replication, is an ideal, not a reality. In an **exact replication,** the replication study is identical to the original and is conducted solely to confirm the original study's results. Haller and Reynolds (1986) stated that "exact replication can be thought of as a goal that is essentially unobtainable" (p. 250) because it demands that everything be the same, including the sample, the site, and the time at which both studies are conducted. A second type, **concurrent** (or internal) **replication**, which is rare in nursing, is closely related because it uses a different site and, obviously, different subjects, but data collection occurs at the same time in both studies. When data collection takes place concurrently at two sites, it is far more common in nursing research for the results to be combined into one larger sample. The researchers analyze the different results in the two samples, including the combined results in one research report.

An approximate (or operational) replication is a common replication strategy implemented in nursing. Different researchers, conducting the original research and the replication study, adhere to the original design and methods as closely as possible. The purpose of an **approximate replication** is to determine whether findings are consistent "despite modest changes in research conditions" (Haller & Reynolds, 1986, p. 250), such as a different site and the subtle changes in distribution of subjects across ranges of age, culture, and gender. If replication results are consistent with the original findings, the evidence gleaned strengthens the likelihood that the results are generalizable (Polit & Beck, 2010).

If the findings generated in an approximate replication are not consistent with those of the original study, there are three possibilities: A Type I error (rejecting the null hypothesis in error) occurred in one or the other study, a Type II error (accepting the null hypothesis in error) occurred in one of the studies, or the changes in research methods such as setting and sample characteristics were responsible for the different findings (Grove & Cipher, 2020). However, the reasons for the inconsistent results may not be immediately apparent. In the case of a Type I error, still another replication should be conducted. In the case of a possible Type II error, a post hoc power analysis should be conducted to determine whether the sample was too small because that is the most common reason a Type II error occurs (see Chapter 21). If so, another replication with a larger sample should be conducted (Cohen, 1988). In the third case, the methods that changed, such as constitution of the sample or nature of the setting, should be scrutinized to determine the reasons the results changed. In any of these cases, additional replication is needed to determine more information.

Systematic (or constructive) **replication**, the other common replication strategy in nursing, is conducted "under distinctly new conditions" (Haller & Reynolds, 1986, p. 250), and its goal is extension of the findings of the original study, most frequently to different settings or to patients with different disease processes. Different methods, such as means of participant selection, are common, and occasionally different research designs are used. Successful systematic replication increases the generalizability of research findings, expanding the population to which results may be applied. An example would be an intervention to decrease anxiety, tested in various settings with diverse clients.

Even though most published nursing research does not consist of replication studies, this is probably a reflection of the limited number of replication studies conducted in nursing. However, the dramatic increase in Doctorate of Nursing Practice (DNP) programs over the last 10 years may influence the conduct of replication studies. In 2019 there were approximately three times as many DNP students as traditional Doctor of Philosophy (PhD) nursing students (American Association of Colleges of Nursing, 2020). Although PhD dissertations usually consist of original research, in DNP programs the culminating projects, many of which include a research component, can be replication studies. This is expected to increase the number of replication studies submitted for publication.

Collaboration With Faculty and Nurse Researchers

For the graduate student searching for a problem area, conversations with nursing faculty members are invaluable, especially when the student cannot think of any problem area that would generate a research purpose with potentially meaningful results. Faculty advisors are adept at identifying areas that matter to students and suggesting those that are most fruitful to pursue. Some faculty members maintain their own programs of research and can suggest parallel research either using existent data or redesigning a proposed study to include an area of inquiry in which the student is interested.

A collaborative relationship is the norm between expert researchers and nurse clinicians. Because nursing research is critical for designation as a Magnet facility by the American Nurses Credentialing Center (ANCC, 2019), hospitals and healthcare systems employ nurse researchers for the purpose of guiding studies conducted by staff nurses. Pintz, Zhou, McLaughlin, Kelly, and Guzzetta (2018) conducted a national study of the nursing research characteristics at Magnet®-designated hospitals and found these hospitals provide most of the needed research infrastructure and have a culture that supports nursing research. In many ways, this is the ideal supportive relationship: The clinician knows the problem area, and the researcher knows how to guide the clinician through the process of proposal writing, approval by nurse manager and medical team, institutional review board (IRB) approval, selection of data collection strategies, and identification of appropriate methods of data analysis. Collaboration between nurse researchers and clinicians, and sometimes with researchers from other health-related disciplines, enhances the potential for generating evidence useful for practice. The opportunity to participate on an interdisciplinary research team is an informative experience and expands the nurse's knowledge of the research process across disciplines.

Research Priorities Identified by Funding Agencies and Specialty Groups

Landmark research by Lindeman (1975) identified several research priorities related to clinical nursing interventions: stress assessment, care of older adults, pain management, and patient education. Generating research evidence in these four areas continues to be a priority for nursing. Since Lindeman's time, various funding agencies and professional organizations have identified nursing research priorities. Most professional organizations display their priorities on their websites. This allows new nurse researchers to use the guidance of their own individual professional organizations when selecting research problem areas.

For instance, the American Association of Critical Care Nurses (AACN) has determined research priorities for the critical care specialty since the early 1980s (Lewandowski & Kositsky, 1983) and revised these priorities based on patients' needs and changes in health care. AACN's (2019) research priorities include (1) effective and appropriate use of technology to achieve optimal patient assessment, management, and/or outcomes; (2) creation of a healing, humane environment; (3) processes and systems that foster the optimal contribution of critical care nurses; (4) effective approaches to symptom management; and (5) prevention and management of complications. In addition, AACN has identified a research agenda calling for nurses to "move away from rituals in practice" with establishment of a work culture that expects "nurses to question their practice," and active broad sharing of research findings

among "key stakeholders," including consumers, industry, and payers (Deutschman, Ahrens, Cairns, Sessler, & Parsons, 2012, p. 23).

A significant funding agency for nursing research is the National Institute of Nursing Research (NINR). A major initiative of the NINR is the development of a national nursing research agenda that involves identifying nursing research priorities, outlining a plan for implementing priority studies, and obtaining resources to support priority projects. In 2018 the NINR's annual budget was $149,252,496, with approximately 65% of the budget allotted for extramural research grants, 3% for the center's programs in specialized areas, 5% for research career development and other research, 7% for predoctoral and postdoctoral training, 10% for research management and support, 3% for research and development contracts, and 7% for its intramural research program (NINR, 2019). Regretfully, the federal annual budget for NINR is $145,842,000 for 2019, which is a reduction of $3,410,496 from the 2018 budget.

Nonetheless, NINR's research priorities are useful for guiding beginning researchers. The NINR (2018) identified the following priority research themes: (1) symptom science, including personalized health strategies; (2) wellness, including promotion of health and prevention of illness; (3) self-management to improve quality of life for persons with chronic illness; (4) end-of-life care, including palliative care; (5) innovative technologies; and (6) training nurse scientists. These differed from previous research priorities in several respects, most notably in the prioritization of symptom science and elimination of health disparity from the listing.

Another federal agency that funds healthcare research is the Agency for Healthcare Research and Quality (AHRQ). Much of AHRQ's budget is earmarked for its internal programs; however, the budget for external grants is approximately half of NINR's total grant budget. Grants are more likely to be awarded to persons connected with academic programs. The AHRQ (2019) research priority areas include (1) research to improve healthcare patient safety, (2) harnessing data and technology to improve healthcare quality and patient outcomes, and (3) research to increase accessibility and affordability of health care by examining innovative market approaches to care delivery and financing.

The World Health Organization's (WHO, 2019) research policy focuses on strengthening health research systems. WHO aims to contribute to health system development and health improvement particularly in poor countries. By 2020, the world's population is expected to increase by 94%, with the elderly population growing by almost 240%. Seven of every 10 deaths are expected to be caused by noncommunicable diseases, such as chronic conditions (heart disease, cancer, and depression) and injuries (unintentional and intentional). The priority areas for research identified by WHO are to (1) improve the health of the world's most marginalized populations; (2) study new diseases that threaten public health around the world; (3) conduct comparative analyses of supply and demand of the health workforce of different countries; (4) analyze the feasibility, effectiveness, and quality of education and practice of nurses; (5) conduct research on healthcare delivery modes; and (6) examine the outcomes for healthcare agencies, providers, and patients around the world. A discussion of WHO's mission and research policies can be found online at https://www.who.int/departments/science-division.

The *Healthy People 2020* website identifies and prioritizes health topics and objectives for all age groups. These health topics and objectives direct future research in the areas of health promotion, illness prevention, illness management, and rehabilitation and can be accessed online at http://www.healthypeople.gov/2020/topicsobjectives2020/default.aspx/. Healthy People 2030 health topics and objectives are in development to be released soon. In summary, funding organizations, professional organizations, and governmental healthcare organizations, both national and international, are sources for identifying priority research problems and offer opportunities for obtaining funding for future research.

FORMULATING A RESEARCH PROBLEM AND PURPOSE

Potential nursing research problems often emerge from real-world situations, such as those in nursing practice. A **situation** is a significant combination of circumstances that occur at a given time. Inexperienced researchers tend to want to study the entire situation, but it is far too complex for a single study. Multiple problems exist in a single situation, and each can be developed into a study. Researchers' perceptions of what problems exist in a situation depends on their research background, clinical expertise, theoretical base, intuition,

interests, and goals (Utley et al., 2018). Some researchers spend years developing different problem statements and new studies from the same clinical situation. For example, the Braden Scales for Predicting Pressure Ulcer Risk in adults, children, and infants have been used in practice for over 40 years and been the focus of numerous studies. A recent study was conducted by Riccioni, Berlanga, Hagan, Schier, and Gordon (2019) to examine the interrater reliability of the Braden and Braden Q scale in assessing pediatric patients' skin. The original Braden scale and other versions of it have been invaluable in the prevention of pressure ulcers in patients.

The exact thought processes used to extract research problems from a clinical situation are abstract, complex, and individual. However, formulating research problems usually involves the following steps: (1) Examine a real-world situation, (2) identify research topics, (3) generate questions, (4) review relevant literature, and (5) ultimately clarify and refine a research problem. When you conduct these steps, you will find that they are not linear but flow back and forth to clarify the focus of study. From the research problem, you will develop a specific focus or research purpose for your study. The flow of these steps is presented in Fig. 5.2 and described in the following sections.

Examining a Real-World Situation and Identifying Research Topics

A clinical nursing situation often includes a variety of research topics or concepts, such as pain, self-care, and social support. Other relevant research topics focus on the healthcare system and providers, such as satisfaction with care, effectiveness of advanced practice nurse roles (nurse practitioner [NP], clinical nurse specialist, midwife, and nurse anesthetist), and redesign of the healthcare system. Outcomes research focuses on topics of health status, quality improvement, satisfaction, accountability, and cost effectiveness (Moorhead et al., 2018). A specific outcome study might focus on a condition, such as terminal breast cancer, and examine the outcomes of nutrition, pain control, and depression for a variety of NP interventions.

Generating Questions and Reviewing the Literature

Situations encountered in nursing stimulate a constant flow of questions. The questions usually fit into

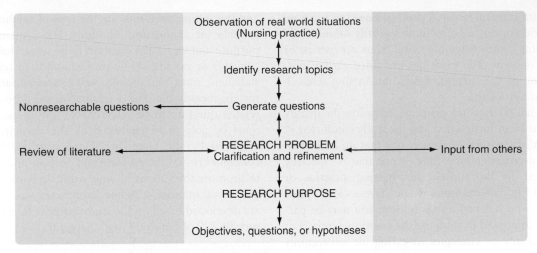

Fig. 5.2 Formulating a research problem and purpose.

three broad categories: (1) philosophical questions, (2) questions answered with problem solving, and (3) research-generating questions (see Fig. 5.2). The first two types of questions are nonresearchable and do not facilitate the formulation of research problems that will generate essential knowledge for nursing. Some questions (such as "What is heaven like?") are not researchable because the answer cannot be known. Some of the questions raised can be answered using problem-solving or evaluation projects. The problem-solving process addresses a specific problem, such as of an adult patient with type 2 diabetes who has uncontrolled blood sugars and nursing care focuses on a positive outcome (i.e., hemoglobin A1c < 7). However, the goal of the research process is the generation of knowledge to be generalized to other similar situations (Polit & Beck, 2010; Shadish et al., 2002).

Many evaluation projects are conducted with minimal application of the rigor and control required for research. These projects do not fit the criteria of research, and the findings are usually relevant only for a specific situation. For example, quality and safety projects involve an evaluation of the patient care implemented by a specific healthcare agency; the results of this evaluation project are usually relevant to just the agency conducting the review.

The type of question that can initiate the research process is one that requires further knowledge to answer it. Some of the questions that come to mind about situations include the following: "Is there a need to explore or describe phenomena, develop theory, understand cultural elements of populations, or explore issues, elements, and situations?" (Creswell & Poth, 2018). This type of knowledge is usually generated through qualitative studies (see Chapter 4). If the problem focuses on description, examination of relationships, or examining the effectiveness of interventions, then quantitative research is the methodology selected (Creswell & Creswell, 2018; Shadish et al., 2002) (see Chapter 3). Research experts have found that asking the right question is frequently more valuable than finding the solution to a problem. The solution identified in a single study might not withstand the test of time or might be useful in only a few situations. However, one well-formulated question can generate numerous research problems with a potential to significantly contribute to nursing's body of knowledge.

Clarifying and Refining a Research Problem

Within your preferred problem area, now, formulate several research questions, ones to which you really would like answers and that are researchable. Imagine prospective studies related to your real-world situation of interest (see Fig. 5.2). You also need to imagine the difficulties likely to occur with each study but avoid being too critical of potential research problems. Which studies seem the most workable? Which problem is the most significant to nursing? Which study is of personal interest? Which problem has the greatest potential to provide a foundation for further research in the field?

Significant nursing research problems need to focus on real-world concerns, be methodologically sound, build on nursing's knowledge base, and focus on current or timely concerns. The priorities identified earlier indicate some of the current, significant nursing research topics and problems.

Personal interest in a problem influences the quality of the problem formulated and the study conducted. A problem of personal interest is one that an individual has pondered for a long time or one that is especially important in the individual's nursing practice or personal life. For example, if you have a close family member who has had a mastectomy, you may be particularly interested in studying the emotional impact of a mastectomy or strategies in caring for mastectomy patients. This personal interest in the topic can become the driving force needed to conduct a quality study.

Answering these questions regarding significance and personal interest can often assist you in narrowing the number of problems. Obtain input from faculty, colleagues, and friends to assist you in narrowing your research problem (see Fig. 5.2). Let them play the devil's advocate and explore the strengths and weaknesses of each idea. Then begin some preliminary reading in the area of interest. Examine literature related to the situation, the variables within the situation, measurement of the variables, previous studies related to the situation, and supportive theories. The literature review often enables you to refine the problem and clearly identify the gap in the knowledge base needed for practice (see Chapter 7 for details of literature review). Once you have identified the problem, you must frame it or ground it in past research, practice, and theory. The discussion of the problem must culminate in a problem statement that identifies the gap in the knowledge base that your proposed study will address. Thus the refined problem has documented significance to nursing practice, is based on past research and theory, and identifies a gap in nursing knowledge that directs the development of the research purpose (Smith & Liehr, 2018; Utley et al., 2018).

Formulating a Research Purpose

Identifying a research purpose begins with review of the research problem. The study purpose should address the problem statement or the gap in nursing knowledge. State the research purpose, including the focus or goal of the study, study variable or concepts, the population,

and the setting; then indicate the type of methodology suitable for conducting the study. For a quantitative purpose and its related question to be researchable, the concepts or variables to be studied and their relational statement must be tangible, well expressed, and ultimately measurable. For a qualitative purpose and its related question to be researchable, the ideas studied must be able to be expressed by the participants or observed by the researcher. Have your faculty and colleagues review the problem and purpose and refine it to promote the success of your study. In some studies, objectives, questions, and/or hypotheses (see Fig. 5.2) are developed based on the study purpose to clarify the specific foci of the study (see Chapter 6).

EXAMPLE OF PROBLEM AND PURPOSE DEVELOPMENT

You might have observed that some children and adolescents receiving care in primary clinics or mental health settings are withdrawn, fearful, depressed, and unable to discuss certain situations in their lives. These children often have difficulty interacting with other children and adults in a variety of settings. Maybe their school performance has recently declined. You think it is important to increase your interactions with these children to assess their needs. Nurses developing a rapport with some children have encouraged them to reveal they are victims of sexual abuse. This situation could lead you to identify research topics and generate searching questions. Research topics of interest include childhood sexual abuse, history and nature of abuse, parental characteristics, physical and psychosocial symptoms, assessment and diagnosis of child sexual abuse (CSA), therapeutic interventions to manage abuse and symptoms, and emotional and psychological adjustment. Possible questions include the following: "Are children of sexual abuse being effectively identified in the current healthcare system?" "What are the physical and psychological problems demonstrated by children who are sexually abused?" "How might a relationship of trust be developed with children who are withdrawn?" "What influences do age, gender, duration, and nature of abuse have on a child's current behavior and psychosocial adjustment?" "How might psychiatric mental health nurses (PMHNs) effectively assess the occurrence, frequency, and impact of CSA?" "What strategies are effective in managing the physical and emotional problems of sexually abused children?" These are the types of questions Güven, Dalgiç, and Erkol (2018, p. 37) might have asked as they developed the problem and purpose for their study focused on CSA. A literature review and consultation with others helped them to clarify their study, titled "Emotional and Psychological Problems Encountered by Children Who Have Been Sexually Abused." The problem and purpose for this study is presented as an example.

Research Problem

"It is estimated that approximately one in 10 children are subject to some form of sexual abuse, including physical contact, before age 8 (Townsend & Rheingold, 2013). Prevalence of sexual abuse in most countries has been confirmed by an international review that reported a prevalence rate of 8% to 31% for female victims and 3% to 17% for male victims (Barth, Bermetz, Heim, Trelle, & Tonia, 2013).... It is believed that most child sexual abuse cases are generally underreported. Therefore, these statistics likely do not reflect the actual number of children who have been abused.... In cases of abuse, it is of utmost importance to provide the child with psychosocial support and rehabilitation services to minimize the effects of the incident and optimize the normality in which the child continues his/her life in a healthy state. Psychiatric–mental health nurses (PMHNs) interact with various patient populations and regularly provide care for many individuals. Any one of these individuals may be a potential or actual victim of child abuse. Therefore, nurses should know the risk factors and symptoms of these types of abuse. PMHNs have important roles in this process, as they are the ones who encounter the victim's families and children first and spend more time with them. The literature indicates a limited number of studies on the emotional and psychosocial problems of children who are exposed to sexual abuse and require professional intervention." (Güven et al., 2018, pp. 37–38)

Research Purpose

"In this context, the current study was planned to contribute to the early identification of the emotional and psychosocial problems of child victims of sexual abuse." (Güven et al., 2018, p. 38)

Güven et al.'s (2018) research problem is significant because the prevalence of CSA is a critical international problem. Sexual abuse cases are underreported and include both girls and boys. Key findings from previous research focused on the number, nature, and duration of the abuse. However, the findings were limited and varied regarding the emotional and psychological problems encountered by children who have been sexually abused. The role of PMHNs needs to be clarified and expanded in providing care to these children. These gaps in nursing's knowledge base provided a basis for the study purpose. Güven et al. (2018) studied 518 children referred to a child advocacy center in Turkey and found 71% of them had been sexually abused. "After-effects reported included despair (46.5%), fear of reoccurrence of the incident (52.8%), distrust of others (36.8%), difficulty sleeping (32.7%), negative expectations about the future (32.1%), and self-blame (31.1%). Nurses have crucial roles and functions in the protection, improvement, treatment, and rehabilitation of the health of children who have been sexually abused" (Güven et al., 2018, p. 37).

FEASIBILITY OF A STUDY

As the research problem and purpose increase in clarity and conciseness, you will have greater direction in determining the feasibility of your study. The **feasibility of a study** is determined by examining (1) the researcher's expertise; (2) availability of study participants, facilities, and equipment; (3) time commitment; (4) money commitment; (5) cooperation of others; and (6) the study's ethical considerations (Creswell & Creswell, 2018; Rogers, 1987; Shadish et al., 2002). These areas are discussed as follows with examples from the Im et al. (2019) study of racial/ethnic differences in cognitive symptoms of menopausal women introduced earlier.

Researcher Expertise

A research problem and purpose should be selected based on the investigator's expertise. Initially you might work with another researcher (mentor) to learn the process and then investigate a familiar problem that fits your knowledge base and experience. Selecting a difficult, complex problem and purpose can only frustrate and confuse the novice researcher. However, all researchers need to identify problems and purposes that are challenging and collaborate with other researchers as necessary to build their research background.

When a team of researchers conducts a study, the team members often have a variety of research and clinical experiences that add to the quality of the study conducted. For example, Im et al. (2019) have research, clinical, and educator expertise in nursing and backgrounds in midlife women's health, technology, biostatistics, and/or biomedical engineering. Dr. Im is the associate dean of research at Duke University and a member of the NINR director's lecture series in midlife women's health with several research publications on this topic. Dr. Hu is affiliated with Duke University and a university in China with national research grants from the United States and China. Dr. Cheng has been a professor of nursing for over 20 years and conducted extensive research in women's health, including biobehavioral studies, with over 30 publications. Dr. Ko is an assistant professor in nursing at Gachon University and is actively involved in research with over 34 publications. Dr. E. Chee has a PhD in bioengineering and biomedical engineering and is currently involved in research with Dr. Im. Dr. W. Chee is an associate professor of nursing at Duke University with research and publications in the area of women's health.

The employment sites and sometimes credentials for the investigators are identified on the first page of the research article. These researchers all appear to have strong backgrounds for conducting research in the discipline of nursing, women's health, and biobehavioral sciences. You can obtain more information about the authors by searching their names online. At the end of a research article, researchers often acknowledge the support of other professionals during their study, such as registered nurses, statisticians, clinical experts, and university colleagues.

Availability of Study Participants, Facilities, and Equipment

In selecting a research purpose, you must consider the type and number of study participants needed. Finding a sample might be difficult if the study involves investigating a unique or rare population, such as quadriplegic individuals who live alone and are currently attending college. The more specific the population selected for study, the more difficult it is to find potential participants. Potential subjects who are stigmatized, such as

persons with human immunodeficiency virus/acquired immunodeficiency syndrome, may be more difficult to access. In addition, the Health Insurance Portability and Accountability Act prevents clinical agencies from sharing lists of potential subjects with a researcher without specific stipulations (see Chapter 9).

Even if you identify a population with many potential subjects, they may be unwilling to participate in the study because of the topic selected. For example, nurses could be asked to share their experiences with alcohol and drug use, but many might fear that sharing this information would jeopardize their jobs and licenses. Researchers need to be prepared to pursue the attainment of study participants at whatever depth is necessary (see Chapter 15). Having a representative sample of reasonable size is critical for generating quality research findings (Cohen, 1988; Grove & Cipher, 2020).

Researchers need to determine whether their studies will require special facilities to implement. Will a special room be needed for an educational program, interview, or observations? If the study is conducted at a hospital, clinic, or college of nursing, will the agency provide the facilities that are needed? Most nursing studies are done in natural settings such as a clinic, hospital unit, conference room, or patient's home.

Nursing studies frequently require a limited amount of equipment, such as a tape or video recorder for interviews or a physiological instrument, such as a scale or thermometer. Often you can borrow equipment from the facility where the study is conducted or you can rent it. Some companies are willing to donate equipment if the study focuses on determining the effectiveness of the equipment and the findings are shared with the company. If specialized facilities or equipment are required for a study, you must be aware of the options available before actively pursuing the study. Im et al. (2019) reported, "The data from two cross-sectional national Internet surveys [Im et al., 2012; Im, Lee, Chee, Brown, & Dormire, 2010] among multi-ethnic groups of midlife women were used in this study" (pp. 220–221). Im et al. (2010, 2012) was the primary author for the two previous internet surveys so this secondary data analysis did not require accessing study participants or using equipment. Duke University was probably the site for the secondary data analysis because Im was the associate dean for research at this institution. The contact information for Dr. Im is provided on the first page of the article if more information is needed.

Time Commitment

Conducting research frequently takes longer than anticipated, making it difficult for any researcher, especially a novice, to estimate the time that will be involved. In estimating the time commitment, the researcher examines the purpose of the study; the more complex the purpose, the greater the time commitment. You can approximate the time needed to complete a study by assessing the following factors: (1) type and number of study participants needed, (2) number and complexity of the variables to be studied, (3) methods for measuring the variables (Are quality instruments available to measure the variables or must they be developed?), (4) methods for collecting data, and (5) the data analysis process. Another factor that can increase the time needed for a study is obtaining IRB approval, especially if more than one clinical agency is used for data collection in a study (see Chapter 9 for additional information on IRBs). Also, researchers often overlook the time commitment necessary to write the research report for presentation and publication. You must approximate the time needed to complete each step of the research process and determine whether the study is feasible.

Most researchers propose a designated time or set a specific deadline for their project. For example, an agency might set a 2-year deadline for studying the turnover rate of nursing staff. The researcher must determine whether the identified purpose can be accomplished by the designated deadline; if not, the purpose could be narrowed or the deadline extended. Researchers are often cautious about extending deadlines because a project could continue for many years. The individual interested in conducting qualitative research frequently must make an extensive time commitment of 2 years or longer to allow for quality collection and analysis of data (Creswell & Poth, 2018; Marshall & Rossman, 2016). Time is as important as money, and the cost of a study can be greatly affected by the time required to conduct it.

Money Commitment

The problem and purpose selected are influenced by the amount of money available to the researcher. Sources for nursing research funding include (1) government funding from such offices as the NINR and AHRQ (previously discussed); (2) professional organizations such as AACN and Oncology Nursing Society; and (3) local clinical agencies, corporations, and universities (see Chapter 29). Potential sources for funding should be considered at the time the problem and purpose are identified. For example, Im et al.'s (2019) study was a secondary analysis of data from two larger studies (Im et al., 2012; Im et al., 2010) that were funded by the National Institutes of Health, including NINR, National Institute on Aging, and National Heart, Lung, and Blood Institute. Federal and private sources of funding greatly strengthen the feasibility of conducting a research project.

The cost of a research project can range from a few dollars for a student's small study to hundreds of thousands of dollars for complex projects, such as multisite clinical trials and complex qualitative studies. In estimating the cost of a research project, the following questions need to be considered, in addition to other areas of expense based on the study being conducted. Study participants and equipment were discussed in an earlier section.

- *Study participants:* How many participants will need to be recruited for the study, and will the subjects have to be paid for their participation in the project?
- *Equipment:* What will the equipment for the study cost?
- *Personnel:* Will assistants or consultants, or both, be hired to collect, computerize, and analyze the data and assist with the data interpretation?
- *Computer time:* Will there be a cost for computer time required to review the literature and analyze the data?
- *Transportation:* What will be the transportation costs for conducting the study and presenting the findings?

Cooperation of Others

A study might appear feasible, but without the cooperation of others, it is not. Some studies are conducted in laboratory settings and require the minimal cooperation of others. However, most nursing studies involve human subjects and are conducted in hospitals, clinics, schools, offices, or homes. Having the cooperation of people in the research setting, the study participants, and the research assistants involved in data collection is essential. People are frequently willing to cooperate with a study if they view the problem and purpose as significant or if they are personally interested. Im et al. (2019) had the support of their universities to conduct their studies with access to the research facilities at Duke University.

Ethical Considerations

The purpose selected for investigation must be ethical, which means that the participants' rights and the rights of others in the setting are protected. If your purpose appears to infringe on the rights of the participants, you should reexamine that purpose; the investigation may have to be revised or abandoned. There are usually some risks in every study, but the value of the knowledge generated should outweigh the risks. Im et al. (2019) reported, "The original studies (Im, 2010, 2012)

got the approvals from the institutional review boards of the institutions where the researchers were affiliated" (p. 221).

EXAMPLES OF RESEARCH TOPICS, PROBLEMS, AND PURPOSES FOR DIFFERENT TYPES OF RESEARCH

Quantitative Research

Quantitative research reports contain problems and purposes that reflect the different foci of each type of quantitative research. Examples from published research of topics, problems, and purposes for the four principal types of quantitative research included in this text (descriptive, correlational, quasi-experimental, and experiment) are presented in Table 5.1. The research

TABLE 5.1 Quantitative Research: Topics, Problems, and Purposes

Type of Research	Research Topic	Research Problem and Purpose
Descriptive research	Environmental contamination, healthcare-associated infection, bacterial pathogens, hospital cleaning, infection prevention, patient safety, hospital roommates	*Title of study:* "Concurrent detection of bacterial pathogens in hospital roommates" (Cohen, Spirito, Liu, Cato, & Larson, 2019, p. 80) *Problem:* "Curtailing the spread of pathogens and preventing healthcare-associated infections (HAIs) are ongoing patient safety challenges. HAI rates are frequently included among the metrics used to measure quality of nursing care.... HAI incidence in U.S. acute care hospitals remains unacceptably high, with estimates in excess of 700,000 per year (Magill et al., 2014). One reason that may account for persistently high infection rates despite improvements in nursing care is that many infection prevention initiatives have focused on patient-level interventions—specifically for high-risk populations, such as those who have indwelling catheters and devices.... These strategies fail to address the patient environment as a potential reservoir for organisms that cause HAIs. Given the demonstrated ability of bacterial pathogens to survive for prolonged periods on hospital surfaces and equipment even after cleaning has occurred (Boyce, Potter-Bynoe, Chenevert, & King, 1997; Dancer, 2009), patient rooms are likely sources of exposure to potentially harmful organisms. There has been limited research characterizing the frequency with which hospital roommates acquire the same organism, which is an important measure for understanding how contamination in patient rooms contributes to HAI incidence.... Examining the role of patient rooms as sources of pathogen exposure is an essential step toward identifying and implementing nursing interventions to break the chain of transmission for all patients." (Cohen et al., 2019, pp. 80–81) *Purpose:* "Hence, the purpose of this study was to determine the incidence of concurrent detection of bacterial pathogens among patients sharing a hospital room." (Cohen et al., 2019, p. 81)

TABLE 5.1   Quantitative Research: Topics, Problems, and Purposes—cont'd

Type of Research	Research Topic	Research Problem and Purpose
Correlational research	Anticipated stigma, health-care utilization, chronic obstructive pulmonary disease (COPD), neurological disorders, Parkinson disease	*Title of study:* "Anticipated stigma and healthcare utilization in COPD and neurological disorders" (Chin & Armstrong, 2019) *Problem:* "Sixty percent of individuals in the United States (U.S.) have one or more chronic health conditions (Buttorff, Ruder, & Bauman, 2017). Chronic illness can lead to long-term disability, reduced health related quality of life (HRQoL) and death. COPD and Parkinson's disease (PD) are currently the 3rd and 14th leading cause of death in the U.S. and along with other neurological disorders have a high morbidity rate (American Lung Association, 2013; Frandsen, Kjellberg, Insen, & Jennum, 2014). … Stigma has been identified in the literature as one reason patients delay, or avoid, using healthcare services (Earnshaw & Quinn, 2011; Weiss et al., 2006) resulting in poor disease management.… A systematic review of stigma-related experiences in individuals with respiratory disease identified negative physical, psychosocial, quality of life, employment, treatment and clinical outcomes (Rose, Paul, Boyes, Kelly, & Roach, 2017). The impact of stigma contributes to the disease burden of chronic illness on many levels, but delay in healthcare seeking is of particular concern for chronic illness management and health outcomes (Quinn & Earnshaw, 2013; Weiss et al., 2006). The literature exploring anticipated stigma in individuals with COPD and neurological disorders is limited. Additionally, the association between anticipated stigma and healthcare utilization has not been described in this population." (Chin & Armstrong, 2019, pp. 63−64) *Purpose:* "The purpose of this study was to explore the experience of anticipated stigma in individuals with COPD and neurological disorders, and examine the relationship between anticipated stigma and healthcare utilization." (Chin & Armstrong, 2019, p. 64)
Quasi-experimental research	Enhanced recovery after surgery (ERAS) intervention, ERAS bundle components, gynecological surgery, length of stay, hospital readmissions, patient satisfaction, randomized controlled trial, Institute of Health Improvement	*Title of study:* "Optimize patient outcomes among females undergoing gynecological surgery: A randomized controlled trial" (Johnson et al., 2019, p. 39) *Problem:* "A hysterectomy is a common gynecological surgical procedure with minimally invasive methods including vaginal or laparoscopic procedures. Studies have shown that preoperative patient education can improve patient outcomes after surgery, including reduced length of hospital stay, decreased post-operative complications, and increased patient satisfaction with the surgical experience (Modesitt et al., 2016; Steiner & Strand, 2017; Wijk, Franzen, Ljungqvist, & Nilsson, 2014). Enhanced recovery programs (ERPs) is a concept that focuses on early patient education, multimodal pain control, early mobility, and alternate diet plans so that the patient can recover faster, with fewer complications, and have a shorter hospital length of stay post-surgical procedure (Kalogera & Dowdy, 2016; Modesitt et al., 2016). The Institute for Healthcare Improvement developed the 'bundle' concept with bundle design guidelines… and 6) compliance with bundles is measured using all or none measurement with a goal of 95% or greater (Institute for Healthcare Improvement-innovations, 2016)." (Johnson et al., 2019, p. 39)

Continued

TABLE 5.1   Quantitative Research: Topics, Problems, and Purposes—cont'd

Type of Research	Research Topic	Research Problem and Purpose
		Purpose: "The purpose of this study was to evaluate whether there was a difference in outcome measures (length of stay, occurrence of readmission, and patient satisfaction) with the addition of a post-operative evidence-based bundle/standard education compared to standard education alone." (Johnson et al., 2019, pp. 39−41)
Experimental research	Biomedical device, intravenous (IV) access, nurse IV skills, pediatric IV, peripheral intravenous catheters (PIVs) insertion, VeinViewer®	*Title of Study:* "Utilization of a biomedical device (VeinViewer®) to assist with peripheral intravenous catheter (PIV) insertion for pediatric nurses" (McNeely, Ream, Thrasher, Dziadkowiec, & Callahan, 2018) *Problem:* "Vascular access presents unique challenges in the pediatric population because peripheral intravenous catheters (PIVs) are difficult to place in children.... Obtaining intravenous access is one of the most frequently performed procedures in hospitals; it is often perceived as routine and the impact on children can be overlooked (Kuensting et al., 2009).... Additional studies have demonstrated the need for increased training and support for staff nurses to build upon their PIV placement skills as well as have highlighted the cost and success rates for insertion.... In another study comparing three different vein visualization devices, the researchers found that suitable veins for cannulation were easily visible with the VeinViewer®; however, the first attempt success rate was not significantly different between groups that utilized each of the different devices (De Graaff et al., 2013).... Furthermore, literature examining pediatric PIV success rates compared with nurse perceived skills/ability and confidence at placing PIVs on pediatric patients is lacking." (McNeely, 2018, pp. 1−2) *Purpose:* "This nurse-driven research study explored time, cost, and resources for intravenous access to determine if a biomedical device, VeinViewer® Vision, would facilitate improvements in pediatric access. In addition, this study looked at nurse perceptions of skills and confidence around intravenous insertion and if the use of the VeinViewer® impacted these perceptions." (McNeely et al., 2018, p. 1)

purpose often hints at the type of quantitative design that was chosen for a study, by use of such words as *identification, description, association,* and *effect.*

Descriptive research is conducted to measure prevalence of a single variable, define variables, identify patterns of variables, examine initial links among variables, and compare and contrast groups on selected variables (Kerlinger & Lee, 2000). For example, Cohen, Spirito, Liu, Cato, and Larson (2019) conducted descriptive research "to determine the incidence of concurrent detection of bacterial pathogens among patients sharing a hospital room" (p. 80). The researchers found that there were multiple scenarios by which patients sharing a room could test positive for newly acquired bacterial pathogens. The furniture, equipment, and surfaces in a hospital room frequently include pathogens, which can

cause hospital-acquired infections. Nurses and environmental service teams need to focus on decontamination of frequently missed surfaces in hospital rooms to decrease infection rates.

Correlational research measures connections or relationships between ideas, and the direction (positive or negative) and strength of those relationships. Chin and Armstrong (2019) conducted a descriptive correlational study "to explore the experience of anticipated stigma in individuals with COPD [chronic obstructive pulmonary disease] and neurological disorders and examined the relationship between anticipated stigma and healthcare utilization" (p. 64). The researchers gathered data from patients receiving follow-up care in pulmonary and neurological offices. The findings from this study described low to moderated anticipated stigma in these patients and significant relationships between higher levels of anticipated stigma and lower levels of healthcare utilization. Chin and Armstrong (2019) recommended implementing strategies to reduce the effects of stigma on healthcare utilization.

Both quasi-experimental and experimental research are conducted to establish evidence for a cause-and-effect relationship: whether the independent variable appears to be effective in causing a change in the dependent variable (Shadish et al., 2002). An example of a quasi-experimental study is Johnson, Razo, Smith, Cain, and Soper's (2019) randomized controlled trial of the effects of an enhanced recovery after surgery (ERAS) intervention on outcomes among females undergoing gynecological surgery. The findings supported the use of the ERAS intervention to enhance early recovery for patients following surgery. The females in the ERAS group were discharged a day earlier, had no 30-day readmissions, and described their overall nursing care as very good to excellent.

An example of experimental research is McNeely, Ream, Thrasher, Dziadkowiec, and Callahan's (2018)

study designed to address the research problem of "utilization of a biomedical device (VeinViewer®) to assist with peripheral intravenous catheter (PIV) insertion for pediatric nurses" (p. 1). The study results "did not demonstrate any clinically significant differences between the VeinViewer® use and standard practice for intravenous catheter insertion in pediatric patients for success of placement, number of attempts, or overall cost" (McNeely et al., 2018, p. 1). The researchers also found no differences between the intervention and control groups for perceived confidence and skills with PIV insertions.

Qualitative Research

Qualitative research reports should contain clearly identified research problems and purposes. Examples from published research of topics, problems, and purposes for the four principal types of qualitative research discussed in this text (phenomenology, grounded theory, ethnography, and exploratory-descriptive qualitative research) are presented in Table 5.2. As with quantitative studies, the qualitative research purpose sometimes hints at the study design. It is not uncommon for the title of a qualitative study to mention the

TABLE 5.2 Qualitative Research: Topics, Problems, and Purposes

Type of Research	Research Topic	Research Problem and Purpose
Phenomenological research	Opioids, pain management, phenomenology, common meanings of opioid-induced sedation, shared practices of sedation assessment	*Title of study:* "The common meanings and shared practices of sedation assessment in the context of managing patients with an opioid: A phenomenological study" (Dunwoody, Jungquist, Chang, & Dickerson, 2019) *Problem:* "Sedation is a challenging concept to assess for several reasons: (a) patient's responses to the sedating effects of opioid medications are individualized and dynamic, (b) patients can easily transition from one level of sedation to another and back, making the necessity of physical assessment and monitoring essential to prevent excessive opioid-induced sedation from advancing to respiratory depression or arrest and (c) there is a complex balance when titrating effective pain management with adverse side effects (Dunwoody & Jungquist, 2018; Jarzyna et al., 2011...). In a 2013 survey of the American Society of Pain Management Nurses members, Jungquist, Willens, Dunwoody, Klingman, and Polomano (2014) found that although 76% of their members endorsed utilizing a sedation scale for patient interventions regarding opioids, only 66% felt that the scales were useful in preventing adverse events suggesting that the scales are missing part of the concept of sedation.... There is a gap in effectively assessing opioid-induced sedation, and this gap could potentially be bridged with the knowledge embedded in expert clinical practice, once captured." (Dunwoody et al., 2019, p. 105)

Continued

TABLE 5.2   Qualitative Research: Topics, Problems, and Purposes—cont'd

Type of Research	Research Topic	Research Problem and Purpose
		Purpose: "The purpose of this study was to describe the expert nurses' experiences and common meanings of advancing sedation for the purpose of informing nursing practice and increasing the knowledge of novice nurses working with patients with acute pain." (Dunwoody et al., 2019, p. 105)
Grounded theory research	Autism spectrum disorders (ASD), children, adolescents, intellectual disability, neuro-developmental disability, qualitative research, grounded theory, quality of life, well-being	*Title of study:* "Parent-observed thematic data on quality of life in children with autism spectrum disorder" (Epstein et al., 2019, p. 71) *Problem:* Population-based estimates of the prevalence of ASD range from 5.1 to 15.5 per 1000 births (Bourke et al., 2016…). The prevalence is increasing in part due to changing diagnostic criteria and assessment practices (Hansen et al., 2015), but the ability to predict and improve individual outcomes has become increasingly vital…. Assessments of quality of life (QoL) are therefore important not only to paint an authentic picture of a child's life, but also to identify areas where support is needed and for evaluating treatment and intervention efficacy to promote successful outcomes,… Having a good QoL is important because it is indicative of positive perceptions of overall health and well-being as well as satisfaction with life experiences (e.g. having meaningful social relationships)… Qualitative methods have previously been used to articulate a framework of QoL domains for children with Rett syndrome…and Down syndrome (Murphy et al., 2017) as observed by their parents…. The QoL domains for children with ASD have not been explored and parent observations could provide a preliminary framework for understanding a child's QoL." (Epstein, et al., 2019, pp. 71–72) *Purpose:* "This study therefore explored parental observations to identify QoL domains important to children with ASD with co-occurring intellectual disability. We also investigated whether different domains would be observed in childhood and adolescence." (Epstein et al., 2019, p. 72)
Ethnography research	Shift reports, patient handoffs, inpatient mental health nursing, psychiatric mental health nurses, psychiatric intensive care unit, qualitative research, focused ethnography	*Title of study:* "Using focused ethnography to explore and describe the process of nurses' shift reports in a psychiatric intensive care unit" (Salzmann-Erikson, 2019, p. 3014) *Problem:* "Shift reports and handoffs are an integral and routine activity among nurses in their everyday work. The tenet in this activity is to pass on and exchange between colleagues' vital information about the patients, health status (… Nasarwanji, Badir, & Gurses, 2016)…. Several studies stress the association between medical errors in hospital environments and the lack of communication between health-care staff…. Psychiatric intensive care units (PICUs) are a well-established concept worldwide and are the level of care in which patients are cared for during the most critical phase of mental illness. Research into acute and intensive psychiatric care has demonstrated that these wards are highly volatile, that patients demonstrate externalizing behavior due to drug and alcohol misuse, that patients demonstrate severe psychiatric symptoms and that threats and violence occur on a regular basis (… Salzmann-Erickson, Lützén, Ivarsson, & Eriksson, 2011). To date, no studies have addressed nursing shift reports in PICUs, hence this study." (Salzmann-Erikson, 2018, pp. 3014–3015)

Type of Research	Research Topic	Research Problem and Purpose
TABLE 5.2	**Qualitative Research: Topics, Problems, and Purposes—cont'd**	
		Purpose: "This study aimed to explore and describe the cultural routine of shift reports among nursing staff in a PICU and further to develop a taxonomic, thematic and theoretical understanding of the process." (Salzmann-Erikson, 2018, p. 3105)
Exploratory-descriptive qualitative research	Diabetes mellitus type 1, newly diagnosed chronic illness, experiences of college students, emerging adult, transitional changes, exploratory-descriptive qualitative study	*Title of study:* "Experiences of college students who are newly diagnosed with type 1 diabetes mellitus" (Saylor, Hanna, & Calamaro, 2019, p. 74) *Problem:* "Emerging adults newly diagnosed with type 1 diabetes (T1DM) and in college are experiencing multiple transitions simultaneously. Transitions, often conceptualized as developmental, health-illness and situational, add complexity to adapting to these changes (Meleis, 2010). Critical transitions for youth with T1DM are the developmental transition of emerging adulthood and the situational transition of college (Hanna, 2012).... Thus, emerging adults in college with a new diagnosis of T1DM must simultaneously adjust to developmental changes, college campus life and the life changing T1DM diagnosis.... Although transitions have the potential to impact health and well-being (Meleis, 2010), little is known about the experience of youth who are in the developmental transitional period of emerging adulthood and the situational transition to college as well as having the added complexity of the health-illness transition of a relatively new diagnosis of T1DM. A greater understanding of the experience of emerging adults who are college students with a relatively new diagnosis of T1DM will help the nursing profession conduct future research of salient factors that predict health outcomes." (Saylor et al., 2019, p. 74) *Purpose:* "Thus, the purpose of this exploratory study was to gain a deeper understanding among emerging adults experiences after being diagnosed with T1DM just prior to or during college." (Saylor et al., 2019, p. 74)

name of the methodology or design that the study utilizes (Creswell & Poth, 2018).

Phenomenological research investigates participants' experiences and often the meaning those experiences hold for them. Problem and purpose statements reflect this emphasis on participants' experiences. Dunwoody, Jungquist, Chang, and Dickerson (2019) conducted a phenomenological study to describe experts' experiences in sedation assessment in the context of managing patients' postoperative pain with an opioid. This study indicated "a deeper complexity in the way opioid-induced sedation is assessed and balanced with pain management by nurses in the Post-Anesthetic Care Unit" (Dunwoody et al., 2019, p. 104). The nurses assessed their patients' level of sedation and incorporated practices of giving small, incremental doses of an opioid drug and changing it as needed.

Grounded theory research investigates a human process within a sociological focus, and some grounded theory research produces theory (Charmaz, 2014; Creswell & Poth, 2018). Problem and purpose statements identify the shared human process and sometimes the intention to generate theory. In their study, entitled "Parent-Observed Thematic Data on Quality of Life in Children With Autism Spectrum Disorder," Epstein et al. (2019) developed an initial framework for understanding quality of life in children with ASD. Data collection was accomplished through interviews with 22 parents who were primary caregivers and spoke on behalf of their child with ASD. Epstein et al. (2019) found the following: "Unique aspects of quality of life included varying levels of social desire, consistency of routines, and time spent in nature and the outdoors" (p. 71).

Ethnographical research examines individuals within cultures, identifying the membership requirements, expected behaviors, enacted behaviors, and rules of the shared culture. The problem and purpose statements identify the culture of interest. These cultures can be actual societal groups, loose associations of persons sharing common experiences, or unconnected individuals who share a common experience (Creswell & Poth, 2018). Salzmann-Erikson (2018) conduced a focused ethnography to describe the cultural routine of nursing shift reports in a psychiatric intensive care unit (PICU). Data were obtained from 20 observational sessions conducted in a PICU over a span of 5 months. Salzmann-Erikson (2018) found the process of shift reports included three phases: "(a) getting settled, (b) giving the report, and (c) engaging in the aftermath" (p. 3014). These phases included different cultural activities, which take place in different areas of the PICU and at varied levels of formality.

Exploratory-descriptive qualitative research is the broad term that includes qualitative descriptive work in which a specific methodology is not mentioned as serving as a foundation for the study. Problem and purpose statements often address the desire to increase knowledge of an issue, process, or situation. Saylor, Hanna, and Calamaro (2019) conducted an exploratory-descriptive qualitative study to gain insight and understanding of the experiences of college students who were newly diagnosed with type 1 diabetes mellitus. Data were collected from 12 college students attending universities in 11 different states who participated in a research focus group conducted at the College Diabetes Network retreat. Through qualitative data analysis, Saylor et al. (2019) identified the following four themes: "1) diabetes affects all aspects of life and complicates college living; 2) college environment affects diabetes management; 3) diabetes diagnosis facilitates growth and maturity; and 4) strategies used for diabetes management in college" (p. 74).

Mixed Methods Research

Mixed methods research reports contain problems and purposes that reflect the combined approach of two methods, quantitative and qualitative research (Creswell & Clark, 2018). In Table 5.3, an example is presented of

TABLE 5.3	**Mixed Methods Research: Topics, Problems, and Purposes**	
Type of Research	**Research Topic**	**Research Problem and Purpose**
Mixed methods research	Patient simulation, anxiety, self-efficacy, nursing knowledge, performance, low-stakes simulation, undergraduate nursing	*Title of study:* "Correlates of student performance during low stakes simulation" (Burbach, Struwe, Young, & Cohen, 2019, p. 44) *Problem:* "Low stakes simulation has been reported to effectively facilitate learning in an environment free from harm to live patients (Kolozsvari, Feldman, Vassiliou, Demyttenaere, & Hoover, 2011), and improve quality of learning, leading to safe and effective patient care (Alexander et al., 2015).... For simulation to be a valid and reliable evaluation tool, simulation performance needs to be correlated with what the student knows (Hauber, Cormier, & Whyte, 2010).... Students often report stress and anxiety during simulation as negatively affecting their performance (Burbach et al., 2016...) but empirical measures of this relationship are needed... Learning what modifiable factors influence simulation performance will make it possible to identify interventions to improve outcomes.... Consequently, the discrepancy in the performance between nursing knowledge- and simulation-based testing makes assessing students' true competency in patient care challenging." (Burbach et al., 2019, pp. 44–45) *Purpose:* "To fill this gap in knowledge, the purpose of this study is to examine the relationship among anxiety, self-efficacy, and nursing knowledge and students' performance during low stakes simulation." (Burbach et al., 2019, p. 45)

the topic, problem, and purpose for Burbach, Struwe, Young, and Cohen's (2019) mixed methods study of student performance during a low-stakes simulation. "Anxiety, self-efficacy, academic achievement, and performance during simulations were measured quantitatively; correlations between principal variables were calculated. Qualitative data were collected during post-simulation debriefing" and used to interpret quantitative findings (Saylor et al., 2019, p. 44). The quantitative part of this study was correlational and the qualitative part was exploratory descriptive. Significant relationships were found between knowledge of nursing care and simulation performance. Qualitative results identified lack of confidence, uncertainty, and heightened anxiety in contrast to quantitative measures. (Chapter 14 provides a detailed discussion of mixed methods research.)

Outcomes Research

Reports of outcomes studies contain problems and purposes that are very similar to those found in quantitative research. The exception is that often the word *outcomes* is included in the purpose statement. In Table 5.4, an example is presented of the topic, problem, and purpose for an outcomes study by Bhatta, Champion, Young, and Loika (2018). This study focused on outcomes of depression among adolescents accessing a school-based pediatric clinic. Routine Patient Health Questionnaires (i.e., Patient Health Questionnaire-9 [PHQ-9]) were used to screen adolescents age 12 to 18 years for potential risk of major depressive disorder (MDD). Implementing the PHQ-9 depression screening protocol was effective in identifying adolescents with MDD so referrals might be made to mental health providers to potentially decrease morbidity and mortality among these adolescents.

TABLE 5.4 Outcomes Research: Topics, Problems, and Purposes

Type of Research	Research Topic	Research Problem and Purpose
Outcomes research (descriptive design)	Adolescents, depression, depression screening, outcomes, school-based pediatric primary care clinic services	*Title of study:* "Outcomes of depression screening among adolescents accessing school-based pediatric primary care clinic services" (Bhatta, Champion, Young, & Loika, 2018, p. 8) *Problem:* "Major Depressive Disorder (MDD) is common in children and adolescents and linked to functional impairment and suicide. Prevalence of major depressive episode among adolescents in the United States was 12.5% in 2015 (National Institute of Mental Health [NIMH], 2015). MDD is higher among adolescent (12–17 years) females (36.1%) than males (13.6%) (Breslau et al., 2017). Suicide is the second leading cause of death among adolescents… Depression in adolescents is under-recognized and undetected (Fallucco, Seago, Cuffe, Kraemer, & Wysocki, 2015). The USPSTF [US Preventative Services Task Force] recommends screening for MDD in adolescents 12–18 years old…. Despite these guidelines, limited screening by primary care providers suggests the opportunity to identify depression is missed (Taliaferro et al., 2013)…. These findings indicate the need for utilization of quality improvement processes for implementation of screening within primary care settings." (Bhatta et al., 2018, pp. 8–9) *Purpose:* "The purpose of this project was to implement routine mental health screening among adolescent ages 12–18 years who were accessing school-based pediatric primary care clinic services for identification of those at risk for depression." (Bhatta et al., 2018, p. 9)

KEY POINTS

- A research problem is an area in which there is a gap in nursing's knowledge base. The typical research problem includes significance, background, and a problem statement in the area of research.
- The major source for nursing research problems is clinical nursing practice. Other good sources are review of professional literature in one's area of expertise, review of research sources, collaboration with faculty and other nurse researchers, and examination of research priorities identified by funding agencies and specialty groups.
- Replication is essential for the development of evidence-based knowledge for practice and consists of four types: exact, approximate, concurrent, and systematic.
- The research purpose is the clear, concise statement of the focus or goal of a study. The purpose usually includes principal variables or concepts, population, and setting for a study and hints at the study methodology.

- In developing a study, you need to examine a real-world situation of interest, identify research topics, generate questions, and ultimately clarify and refine a problem for study.
- From the research problem, a specific aim or research purpose is developed that provides a clear focus for the study.
- The feasibility of the research problem and purpose is determined by examination of the researchers' expertise; availability of subjects, facility, and equipment; time commitment; money commitment; cooperation of others; and the study's ethical considerations.
- Quantitative, qualitative, mixed methods, and outcomes research methods enable nurses to investigate a variety of research problems and purposes.
- The topics, problem, and purpose from a current published study are provided for each type of research method included in this text.

REFERENCES

Agency for Healthcare Research and Quality (AHRQ). (2019). *AHRQ research funding priorities and special emphasis notices.* Retrieved from http://www.ahrq.gov/funding/priorities-contacts/special-emphasis-notices/index.html

Alexander, M., Durham, C. F., Hooper, J. I., Jeffries, P. R., Goldman, N., Kardong-Edgren, S., ... Radtke, B. (2015). NCSBN simulation guidelines for prelicensure nursing programs. *Journal of Nursing Regulation, 6*(3), 39–42. doi:10.1016/S2155-8256(15)30783-3

American Association of Colleges of Nursing (AACN). (2020). *Strategic plan.* Retrieved from https://www.aacnnursing.org/About-AACN/AACN-Governance/Strategic-Plan

American Association of Critical Care Nurses (AACN). (2019). *AACN's research priority areas.* Retrieved from https://www.aacn.org/nursing-excellence/grants/sigma-theta-tau-critical-care/aacns-research-priority-areas

American Lung Association. (2013). *Trends in COPD: Morbidity and mortality.* Retrieved from http://www.lung.org/assets/documents/research/copd-trend-report.pdf.

American Nurses Credentialing Center (ANCC). (2019). *Magnet© program: Overview.* Retrieved from http://www.nursecredentialing.org/Magnet/ProgramOverview

Barth, J., Bermetz, L., Heim, E., Trelle, S., & Tonia, T. (2013). The current prevalence of child sexual abuse worldwide: A systematic review and meta-analysis. *International Journal of Public Health, 58*(3), 469–483. doi:10.1007/s00038-012-0426-1

Bhatta, S., Champion, J. D., Young, C., & Loika, E. (2018). Outcomes of depression screening among adolescents accessing school-based pediatric primary care clinic services. *Journal of Pediatric Nursing, 38*(1), 8–14. doi:10.1016/j.pedn.2017.10.0001

Bourke, J., de Klerk, N., Smith, T., & Leonard, H. (2016) Population-based prevalence of intellectual disability and autism spectrum disorders in Western Australia: A comparison with previous estimates. *Medicine, 95*(21): e3737. doi:10.1097/MD.00000000000003737

Boyce, J. M., Potter-Bynoe, G., Chenevert, C., & King, T. (1997). Environmental contamination due to methicillin-resistant *Staphylococcus aureus*: Possible infection control implications. *Infection Control & Hospital Epidemiology, 18*(9), 622–627. doi:10.2307/30141488

Breslau, J., Gilman, S. E., Stein, B. D., Ruder, T., Gmelin, T., & Miller, E. (2017). Sex differences in recent first-onset depression in an epidemiological sample of adolescents. *Translational Psychiatry, 7*(5), e1139. doi:10.1038/tp.2017.105

Burbach, B. E., Struwe, L. A., Young, L., & Cohen, M. Z. (2019). Correlates of student performance during low stakes simulation. *Journal of Professional Nursing, 35*(1), 44–45. doi:10.1016/j.profnurs.2018.06.002

Burbach, B. E., Thompson, S. A., Barnason, S., Wilhelm, S., Kotcherlakota, S., Miller, C. L., & Paulman, P. M. (2016). Lived experiences during simulation: Student-perceived influences on performance. *Journal of Nursing Education, 55*(7), 396–398. doi:10.3928/01484834-20160615-07

Buttorff, C., Ruder, T., & Bauman, M. (2017). *Multiple chronic conditions in the United States.* Santa Monica, CA: RAND. doi:10.7249/TL221

Charmaz, K. (2014). *Constructing grounded theory* (2nd ed.). Los Angeles, CA: Sage.

Chin, E. D., & Armstrong, D. (2019). Anticipated stigma and healthcare utilization in COPD and neurological disorders. *Applied Nursing Research, 45*(1), 63–68. doi:10.1016/j.apnr.2018.12.002

Cohen, B., Spirito, C. M., Liu, J., Cato, K. D., & Larson, E. (2019). Concurrent detection of bacterial pathogens in hospital roommates. *Nursing Research, 68*(1), 80–83. doi:10.1097/NNR.0000000000000316

Cohen, J. (1988). *Statistical power analysis for the behavioral sciences.* (2nd ed.). New York, NY: Academic Press.

Creswell, J. W., & Clark, V. L. P. (2018). *Designing and conducting mixed methods research* (3rd ed.). Los Angeles, CA: Sage.

Creswell, J. W., & Creswell, J. D. (2018). *Research design: Qualitative, quantitative, and mixed methods approaches* (5th ed.). Los Angeles, CA: Sage.

Creswell, J. W., & Poth, C. N. (2018). *Qualitative inquiry & research design: Choosing among five approaches* (4th ed.). Los Angeles, CA: Sage.

Dancer, S. J. (2009). The role of environmental cleaning in the control of hospital-acquired infection. *Journal of Hospital Infection, 73*(4), 378–385. doi:10.1016/j.jhin.2009.03.030

De Graaff, J. C., Cuper, N., Mungra, R. A. A., Vlaadingerbroek, K., Numan, S. C., & Kalkman, C. J. (2013). Near-infrared light to aid peripheral intravenous cannulation in children: A cluster randomised clinical trial of three devices. *Anaesthesia, 68*(8), 835–845. doi:10.1111/anae.12294

Deutschman, C. S., Ahrens, T., Cairns, C. B., Sessler, C. N., & Parsons, P. E. (2012). Multisociety task force for critical care research: Key issues and recommendations. *American Journal of Critical Care, 21*(1), 15–23. doi:10.4037/ajcc2012632

Dunwoody, D. R., & Jungquist, C. R. (2018). Sedation scales: Do they capture the concept of opioid induced sedation? *Nursing Forum, 54*(1), 1–7. doi:10.1111/nuf.12266

Dunwoody, D. R., Jungquist, C. R., Chang, Y., & Dickerson, S. S. (2019). The common meanings and shared practices of sedation assessment in the context of managing patients with an opioid: A phenomenological study. *Journal of Clinical Nursing, 28*(1), 104–115. doi:10.1111/jocn.14672

Earnshaw, V. A., & Quinn, D. M. (2011). The impact of stigma in healthcare on people living with chronic illnesses. *Journal of Health Psychology, 17*(2), 157–168. doi:10.1177/1359105311414952

Epstein, A., Whitehouse, A., Williams, K., Murphy, N., Leonard, H., Davis, E., … Downs, J. (2019). Parent-observed thematic data on quality of life in children with autism spectrum disorder. *Autism, 23*(1), 71–80. doi:10.1177/1362361317722764

Fallucco, E. M., Seago, R. D., Cuffe, S. P., Kraemer, D. F., & Wysocki, T. (2015). Primary care provider training in screening, assessment, and treatment of adolescent depression. *Academic Pediatrics, 15*(3), 326–332. doi:10.1016/j.acap.2014.12.004

Frandsen, R., Kjellberg, J., Insen, R., & Jennum, P. (2014). Morbidity in early Parkinson's disease and prior to diagnosis. *Brain and Behaviors, 4*(3), 446–452. doi:10.1002/brb3.228

Gold, E. B., Sternfeld, B., Kelsey, J. L., Brown, C., Mouton, C., Reame, N., … Stellato, R. (2000). Relation of demographic and lifestyle factors to symptoms in a multi-racial/ethnic population of women 40-55 years of age. *American Journal of Epidemiology, 152*(5), 463–473. doi:10.1093/aje/152.5.463

Greendale, G. A., Derby, C. A., & Maki, P. M. (2011). Perimenopause and cognition. *Obstetrics and Gynecology Clinics of North America, 38*(3), 519–535. doi:10.1016/j.ogc.2011.05.007.

Grove, S. K., & Cipher, D. J. (2020). *Statistics for nursing research: A workbook for evidence-based practice* (3rd ed.). St. Louis, MO: Elsevier. In press.

Güven, Ş., Dalgiç, A., & Erkol, Z. (2018). Emotional and psychosocial problems encountered by children who have been sexually abused. *Journal of Psychosocial Nursing and Mental Health Services, 56*(2), 37–43. doi:10.3928/02793695-20170929-04.

Haller, K. B., & Reynolds, M. A. (1986). Using research in practice: A case for replication in nursing—Part II. *Western Journal of Nursing Research, 8*(2), 249–252. doi:10.1177/019394598600800214

Hanna, K. M. (2012). A framework for the youth with type 1 diabetes during the emerging adulthood transition. *Nursing Outlook, 60*(6), 401–410. doi:10.1016/j.outlook.2011.10.005

Hansen, S. N., Schendel, D. E., & Partner, E. T. (2015). Explaining the increase in the prevalence of autism spectrum disorders: The proportion attributable to changes in reporting practices. *JAMA Pediatrics 169*(1), 56–62. doi:10.1001/jamapediatrics.2014.1893

Hauber, R. P., Cormier, E., & Whyte, J. (2010). An exploration of the relationship between knowledge and performance-related variables in high-fidelity simulation: Designing instruction that promotes expertise in practice. *Nursing Education Perspectives, 31*(4), 242–246. doi:10.1016/j.ijnurstu.2009.09.001

Hickman, L. D., DiGiacomo, M., Phillips, J., Rao, A., Newton, P. J., Jackson, D., & Ferguson, C. (2018). Improving evidence-based practice in postgraduate nursing programs: A systematic review. Bridging the evidence practice gap (BRIDGE project). *Nurse Education Today, 63*(1), 69–75. doi:10.1016/j.nedt.2018.01.015

Im, E. O., Chang, S. J., Ko, Y., Chee, W., Stuifbergen, A., & Walker, L. (2012). A national internet survey on midlife women's attitudes toward physical activity. *Nursing Research, 61*(5), 342–352. doi:10.109/NNR.0b013e3182.5da85a

Im, E. O., Hu, Y., Cheng, C., Ko, Y., Chee, E., & Chee, W. (2019). Racial/ethnic differences in cognitive symptoms during the menopausal transition. *Western Journal of Nursing Research, 41*(2), 217–237. doi:10.1177/0193945918767660

Im, E. O., Lee, B., Chee, W., Brown, A., & Dormire, S. (2010). Menopausal symptoms among four major ethnic groups in the United States. *Western Journal of Nursing Research, 32*(4), 540–565. doi:10.1177/0193945909354343

Institute for Healthcare Improvement. (2016). *About us: Innovations*. Retrieved from http://www.ihi.org/about/Pages/innovationscontributions.aspx

Jarzyna, D., Jungquist, C. R., Pasero, C., Willens, J. S., Nisbet, A., Oakes, L., … Polomano, R. C. (2011). American Society of Pain Management nursing guidelines on monitoring for opioid-induced sedation and respiratory depression. *Pain Management Nursing, 12*(3), 118–145. doi:10.1016/j.pmn.2011.06.008

Johnson, K., Razo, S., Smith, J., Cain, A., & Soper, K. (2019). Optimize patient outcomes among females undergoing gynecological surgery: A randomized controlled trial. *Applied Nursing Research, 45*(1), 39–44. doi:10.106/j.apnr.2018.12.005

Jungquist, C. R., Willens, J. S., Dunwoody, D. R., Klingman, K. J., & Polomano, R. C. (2014). Monitoring for opioid-induced advancing sedation and respiratory depression: ASPMN membership survey of current practice. *Pain Management Nursing, 15*(3), 682–693. doi:10.1016/j.pmn.2013.12.001

Kalogera, E., & Dowdy, S. (2016). Enhanced recovery pathway in gynecologic surgery: Improving outcomes through evidence-based medicine. *Obstetrics and Gynecology Clinics of North America, 43*(3), 551–573. doi:10.1016/j.ogc.2016.04.006

Kerlinger, F. N., & Lee, H. B. (2000). *Foundations of behavioral research* (4th ed.). Fort Worth, TX: Harcourt College Publishers.

Kesten, K., White, K. A., Heitzler, E. T., Chaplin, L. T., & Bondmass, M. D. (2019). Perceived evidence-based practice competency acquisition in graduate nursing students: Impact of intentional course design. *Journal of Continuing Education in Nursing, 50*(2), 79–86. doi:10.3928/00220124-20190115-07

Kim, H. N. (2018). Social support provision: Perspective of fathers with preterm infants. *Journal of Pediatric Nursing, 39*(1), 44–49. doi:10.1016/j.pedn.2018.01.017

Kolozsvari, N. O., Feldman, L. S., Vassiliou, M. C., Demyttenaere, S., & Hoover, M. L. (2011). Sim one, do one, teach one: Considerations in designing training curricula for surgical simulation. *Journal of Surgical Education, 68*(5), 421–427. doi:10.1016/j.jsurg.2011.03.010

Kubin, L. (2019). Is there a resurgence of vaccine preventable diseases in the U.S.? *Journal of Pediatric Nursing, 44*(1), 115–118. doi:10.1016/j[edm/2018.11.011

Kuensting, L. L., DeBoer, S., Holleran, R., Shultz, B., Steinmann, R. A., & Vanella, J. (2009). Difficult venous access in children: Taking control. *Journal of Emergency Nursing, 35*(5), 419–424. doi:10.1016/j.jen.2009.01.014

Lewandowski, A., & Kositsky, A. M. (1983). Research priorities for critical care nursing: A study by the American Association of Critical Care Nurses. *Heart and Lung: The Journal of Critical Care, 12*(1), 35–44.

Lindeman, C. A. (1975). Delphi survey of priorities in clinical nursing research. *Nursing Research, 24*(6), 434–441.

Magill, S. S., Edwards, J. R., Bamberg, W., Beldavs, Z. G., Dumyati, G., Kainer, M. A. … Emerging Infections Program Healthcare-Associated Infections and Antimicrobial Use Prevalence Survey Team. (2014). Multistate point-prevalence survey of health care-associated infections. *New England Journal of Medicine, 370*, 1198–1208. doi:10.1056/NEJMoa1306801

Marshall, C., & Rossman, G. B. (2016). *Designing qualitative research* (6th ed.). Los Angeles, CA: Sage.

McEwen, B. (2001). Invited review: Estrogens effects on the brain: Multiple sites and molecular mechanisms. *Journal of Applied Physiology, 91*(6), 2785–2801. doi:10.1152/jappl.2001.91.6.2785

McEwen, B. (2002). Estrogen actions throughout the brain. *Recent Progress in Hormone Research, 57*, 357–384.

McNeely, H. L., Ream, T. L., Thrasher, J. M., Dziadkowiec, O., & Callahan, T. J. (2018). Utilization of a biomedical device (VeinViewer®) to assist with peripheral intravenous catheter (PIV) insertion for pediatric nurses. *Journal of Specialists in Pediatric Nursing, 28*(2), 1–8. doi:1111/jjspn.12208

Meleis, A. (2010). *Transitions theory: Middle range and situation specific theories in nursing research and practice.* New York, NY: Springer Publishing Company.

Melnyk, B. M., Gallagher-Ford, L., Zellefrow, C., Tudher, S., Van Dromme, L., & Thomas, B. K. (2018). Outcomes from the first Helene Fuld Health Trust National Institute for Evidence-Based Practice in Nursing and Healthcare Invitational Expert Forum. *Worldviews on Evidence-Based Nursing, 15*(1), 5–15. doi:10.1111/wvn.12272

Melnyk, B. M., & Fineout-Overholt, E. (2019). *Evidence-based practice in nursing and healthcare: A guide to best practice* (4th ed.). Philadelphia, PA: Wolters Kluwer.

Mitchell, S. E., & Woods, N. F. (2001). Midlife women's attributions about perceived memory changes: Observations from the Seattle Midlife Women's Health Study. *Journal of Women's Health & Gender-based Medicine, 10*(4), 351–362. doi:10.1089/152460901750269670

Modesitt, S. C., Sarosiek, B. M., Trowbridge, E. R., Redick, D. L., Shah, P. M., Thiele, R. H., ... Hedrick, T. L. (2016). Enhanced recovery implementation in major gynecologic surgeries: Effect of care standardization. *Obstetrics & Gynecology, 128*(3), 457–466. doi:10.1097/AOG.0000000000001555

Moorhead, S., Swanson, E., Johnson, M., & Maas, M. L. (2018). *Nursing outcomes classification (NOC): Measurement of health outcomes* (6th ed.). St. Louis, MO: Elsevier.

Murphy, N., Epstein, A., Leonard, H., Davis, E., Reddihough, D., Whitehouse, A., ... Downs, J. (2017). Qualitative analysis of parental observations of quality of life in Australian children with Down syndrome. *Journal of Developmental & Behavioral Pediatrics 38*(2), 161–168. doi:10.1097/DBP.0000000000000385

Nasarwanji, M. F., Badir, A., & Gurses, A. P. (2016). Standardizing handoff communication: Content analysis of 27 handoff mnemonics. *Journal of Nursing Care Quality, 31*(3), 238–244. doi:10.1097/NCQ.0000000000000174

National Institute of Mental Health (NIMH). (2015). *Major depression among adolescents*. Retrieved from https://www.nimh.nih.gov/health/statistics/prevalence/ major-depression-among-adolescents.shtml

National Institute of Nursing Research (NINR). (2018). *NIH almanac: National Institute of Nursing Research*. Retrieved from https://www.nih.gov/about-nih/what-we-do/nih-almanac/national-institute-nursing-research-ninr.

National Institute of Nursing Research (NINR). (2019). *Budget & legislation: NINR 2019 Budget*. Retrieved from https://www.ninr.nih.gov/sites/files/docs/NINR-Budget-FY-2019-508c.pdf

Pintz, C., Zhou, Q., McLaughlin, M. K., Kelly, K. P., & Guzzetta, C. E. (2018). National study of nursing research characteristics at Magnet®-designated hospitals. *Journal of Nursing Administration, 48*(5), 247–258. doi:10.1097/NNA.0000000000000609

Polit, D. F., & Beck, C. T. (2010). Generalization in quantitative and qualitative research: Myths and strategies. *International Journal of Nursing Studies, 47*(2010), 14551–1458. doi:10.10106/j.ijnurstu.2010.06.004

Quinn, D. M., & Earnshaw, V. A. (2013). Concealable stigmatized identities and psychological well-being. *Social and Personality Psychology Compass, 7*(1), 40–51. doi:10.1111/spc3.12005

Riccioni, N., Berlanga, R., Hagan, J., Schier, R., & Gordon, M. (2019). Interrater reliability of the Braden and Braden Q by Skin Champion nurses. *Journal of Pediatric Nursing, 44*(1), 9–15. doi:10.1016/j/pedn/2018.09.014

Rogers, B. (1987). Research corner: Is the research project feasible? *AAOHN Journal, 35*(7), 327–328.

Rose, S., Paul, C., Boyes, A., Kelly, B., & Roach, D. (2017). Stigma-related experiences in non-communicable respiratory diseases: A systematic review. *Chronic Respiratory Disease, 14*(3), 199–216. doi:10.1177/1479972316680847

Salzmann-Erikson, M. (2018). Using focused ethnography to explore and describe the process of nurses' shift reports in a psychiatric intensive care unit. *Journal of Clinical Nursing, 27*(15-16), 3104–3114. doi:10.1111/jocn.14502

Salzmann-Erikson, M., Lüzén, K., Ivarsson, A. B., & Eriksson, H. (2011). Achieving equilibrium within a culture of stability? Cultural knowing in nursing care on psychiatric intensive care units. *Issues in Mental Health Nursing, 32*(4), 255–265. doi:10.3109/01612840.2010.549603

Saylor, J., Hanna, K. M., & Calamaro, C. J. (2019). Experiences of college students who are newly diagnosed with type1 diabetes mellitus. *Journal of Pediatric Nursing, 44*(1), 74–80. doi:10.1016/j.pedn.2018.10.020

Shadish, W. R., Cook, T. D., & Campbell, D. T. (2002). *Experimental and quasi-experimental designs for generalized causal inference*. Chicago, IL: Rand McNally.

Smith, M. J., & Liehr, P. R. (2018). *Middle range theory for nursing* (4th ed.). New York, NY: Springer Publishing Company.

Steiner, H. L., & Strand, E. A. (2017). Surgical site infection in gynecologic surgery: Pathophysiology and prevention. *American Journal of Obstetrics and Gynecology, 217*(2), 121–128. doi:10.1016/j.ajog.2017.02.014

Taliaferro, L. A., Hetler, J., Edwall, G., Wright, C., Edwards, A. R., & Borowsky, I. W. (2013). Depression screening and management among adolescents in primary care: Factors associated with best practice. *Clinical Pediatrics, 52*(6), 557–567. doi:10.1177/000992281343874

Tice, J. R., Cole, L. G., Ungvary, S. M., George, S. D., & Oliver, J. S. (2019). Clinician accountability in primary care clinic time-interval blood pressure measurements study: Practice implications. *Applied Nursing Research, 45*(1), 69–72. doi:10.1016/j.apnr.2018.12.006

Townsend, C., & Rheingold, A. A. (2013). *Estimating a child sexual abuse prevalence rate from practitioners: A review of child sexual abuse prevalence studies.* Charleston, SC: Darkness to Light.

Utley, R., Henry, K., & Smith, L. (2018). *Frameworks for advanced practice and research: Philosophies, theories, models, and taxonomies.* New York, NY: Springer Publishing Company.

Wee, L. E., Yeo, W. X., Yang, G. R., Hannan, N., Lim, K., Chua, C., … Shen, H. M. (2012). Individual and area level socioeconomic status and its association with cognitive function and cognitive impairment (low MMSE) among community-dwelling elderly in Singapore. *Dementia and Geriatric Cognitive Disorders Extra, 2*(1), 529–542. doi:0.1159/000345036

Weiss, M. G., Ramakrishna, J., & Somma, D. (2006). Health-related stigma: Rethinking concepts and interventions. *Psychology, Health & Medicine, 11*(3), 277–287. doi:10.1080/13548500600595053

Wijk, L., Franzen, K., Ljungqvist, O., & Nilsson, K. (2014). Implementing a structured enhanced recovery after surgery (ERAS) protocol reduces length of stay after abdominal surgery. *Acta Obstetricia et Gynecologica Scandinavica, 93*(8), 749–756. doi:10.1111/aogs. 12423

World Health Organization (WHO). (2019). *World Health Organization science division.* Retrieved from https://www. who.int/departments/science-division

6

Objectives, Questions, Hypotheses, and Study Variables

Susan K. Grove

http://evolve.elsevier.com/Gray/practice/

Beyond defining the study purpose, some researchers choose to set specific objectives, questions, or hypotheses to guide their study. In quantitative research, objectives, questions, and hypotheses are developed to bridge the gap between the more abstractly stated research purpose and the detailed plan for data collection and analysis. These are merely smaller segments of the overall purpose. The objectives, questions, and hypotheses delineate the study variables, the relationships among the variables, and often the population to be studied. **Study variables** are ideas or concepts at various levels of abstraction that are measured, manipulated, or controlled in a study. Concrete concepts, such as heart rate, blood pressure, and laboratory values, are referred to as variables in a study; abstract ideas, such as resourcefulness, chronic pain, and social support, are usually referred to as concepts.

Qualitative studies are usually guided by the research purpose, but some investigators include research questions or objectives to clarify their study focus. These questions and objectives include concepts, which focus on an experience, situation, culture, or process to be examined in the qualitative study.

In this chapter, you will examine the objectives, questions, and hypotheses reported in published studies. You will also learn how to formulate research objectives, questions, and hypotheses, especially how to test different types of hypotheses through quantitative research. This chapter concludes with a discussion of different types of variables and concepts studied in quantitative, qualitative, mixed methods, and outcomes research.

Guidance is provided for conceptually and operationally defining variables in a quantitative study. Research variables and concepts are conceptually defined using the study framework and are operationally defined to direct their measurement, manipulation, or control in a study.

USE OF RESEARCH OBJECTIVES OR AIMS IN STUDIES

Research objectives or **aims** are clear, concise, declarative statements expressed in the present tense to specify the foci of the study—that is, the reasons for performing the study. There are minimal if any differences between the terms *objective* and *aim*, thus researchers use them interchangeably in studies. Some researchers identify their study purpose as an objective or aim, which can be confusing to readers. In this text, the purpose is the overall focus of the study, and smaller foci of the study are identified in the research objectives/aims or questions. The objectives/aims formulated to guide quantitative and qualitative studies vary in focus, abstractness, and number. The following sections provide guidance for formulating objectives/aims for nursing studies.

Formulating Objectives or Aims in Quantitative Studies

In quantitative research, the objectives or aims usually focus on one or two variables (or concepts) and indicate whether the variables are to be identified or described.

TABLE 6.1   Quantitative Research Objectives/Aims, Focus, and Probable Type of Study

Research Objective/Aim Format	Objective Focus	Type of Quantitative Study
1. Identify the characteristics and incidence of variable X in a selected population.	Identification	Descriptive
2. Describe variable X in a selected population.	Description	Descriptive
3. Determine the difference between existing groups 1 and 2 (such as females and males) or compare groups 1 (females) and 2 (males) on variable X in a selected population.	Group differences	Descriptive
4. Examine the relationship between variables X and Y in a selected population.	Association or relationship	Correlational
5. Determine the independent variables that are predictive of a dependent variable in a selected population.	Prediction	Correlational

Objectives can also focus on relationships or associations among variables, differences between groups or comparison of groups on selected variables, and prediction of a dependent variable with selected independent variables. The formats for developing different types of research objectives/aims for nursing studies are presented in Table 6.1. The focus of each objective is identified followed by the probable type of quantitative study conducted. Often each objective refers to a different part of the study or to a statistical consideration of certain variables and their interrelationships (Kazdin, 2017). The formats in Table 6.1 are essentially the same for objectives/aims developed for the quantitative part of a mixed methods study (Creswell & Creswell, 2018) and outcomes studies, which are usually designed as quantitative studies (Kane & Radosevich, 2011). The objectives in Table 6.1 are placed in order from the least complex to the most complex in generating research evidence for nursing. A study might include one to five objectives/aims based on its complexity, which are usually expressed following the study's purpose.

Objectives/aims are developed based on the research problem and purpose to clarify the study foci, variables, and population. The following excerpts, from a correlational study of the personal and social resourcefulness and spiritual practices of women caregivers of elders with dementia, demonstrate the logical flow from the research problem (including the problem significance, background, and statement) and purpose to research aims (Zauszniewski, Herbell, & Burant, 2019). Specific headers of research problem, research purpose, and research aims are included to clarify the focus of each quote.

Research Problem
"To date, empirical studies suggest that personal (self-help) and social (help-seeking) resourcefulness are important for achieving optimal health and health-related quality of life across various populations.... However, recent literature has also suggested the possibility of additional forms or dimensions of resourcefulness, including academic, entrepreneurial, exercise, sexual, parenting, and spiritual (Zauszniewski, 2016), may exist. Yet the extent to which these additional forms of resourcefulness affect quality of life, particularly spiritual practices, which was recently added to Zauszniewski's theory of resourcefulness and quality of life (Zauszniewski, 2016, 2018), remain unknown.... In addition, studies have not examined the combined effects of resourcefulness and spiritual practices on measures of health outcomes or whether the addition of spiritual practices to resourcefulness in a predictive model has a significant impact on health outcomes." (Zauszniewski et al., 2019, pp. 373–374)

Research Purpose
"This study examined relationships among personal and social resourcefulness and spiritual practices and their associations with perceived stress, depressive symptoms, and self-assessed health in 138 women caregivers of elders with dementia." (Zauszniewski et al., 2019, p. 372)

Research Aims
"The aims of this study were (a) to examine the relationship between personal and social resourcefulness and spiritual practices and their associations with three health outcomes (perceived stress, depressive symptoms, and self-assessed health); (b) to compare

study participants categorized by median splits as high or low on resourcefulness and spiritual practices (i.e., four groups) on the three health outcomes; and (c) to determine the combined and additive effects of resourcefulness and spiritual practices on perceived stress, depressive symptoms, and self-assessed health." (Zauszniewski et al., 2019, p. 375)

In this example, the problem provides a basis for the purpose, and the aims evolve from the purpose to clearly focus the conduct of the study. The problem, purpose, and aims are clearly and concisely expressed. However, the significance of the problem would have been stronger if it had discussed the importance of studying women caregivers of elders with dementia.

The first aim of Zauszniewski et al. (2019) focused on examining relationships or associations among the variables personal and social resourcefulness, spiritual practice, and health outcomes (perceived stress, depressive symptoms, and self-assessed health). The study population (women caregivers of elders with dementia) was clearly identified in the purpose and is not essential in the study aims. The second aim was focused on comparison of high and low resourcefulness and spiritual practice groups. The third aim was focused on using resourcefulness and spiritual practices to predict stress, depressive symptoms, and self-assessed health (see Table 6.1) (Zauszniewski et al., 2019).

This study was conducted to test the resourcefulness theory developed by Zauszniewski (2016). Zauszniewski et al. (2019) found "evidence for relationships among personal and social resourcefulness, spiritual

practices, and outcomes that are consistent with existing theory and support the likelihood that a third dimension of resourcefulness exists—spiritual resourcefulness" (p. 383).

Formulating Objectives or Aims in Qualitative Studies

In qualitative research, objectives/aims also are developed based on the research problem and purpose, to clarify a study's goals. Many qualitative studies are guided by the study purpose and do not include research objectives or questions. However, some qualitative researchers develop objectives to guide selective aspects of their studies. The objectives in qualitative studies usually have a broader focus and include more abstract and complex concepts than those in quantitative studies (Creswell & Creswell, 2018). These objectives include the same major concepts and population identified in the purpose. The format of an objective usually indicates the probable type of qualitative study conducted. Table 6.2 identifies the objective formats for the four types of qualitative research included in this text (phenomenology, grounded theory research, ethnography, and exploratory-descriptive qualitative research) (Creswell & Poth, 2018). The formats in Table 6.2 are the same as would be used for objectives guiding the qualitative part of a mixed methods study (Creswell & Clark, 2018). The following excerpts of research problem, purpose, and objectives are from an exploratory-descriptive qualitative study about registered nurses' (RNs) pediatric pain management experiences in rural hospitals (Marshall, Forgeron, Harrison, & Young, 2018).

TABLE 6.2 Qualitative Research Objectives/Aims and Probable Type of Study

Research Objective/Aim Format	Probable Type of Qualitative Study
Explore and/or describe the lived experience of a phenomenon by persons in a selected population.	Phenomenology
Describe the concepts and processes that characterize the perspectives and experiences of individuals from a selected population for a situation. Objective might indicate that a framework, theoretical model, or theory is being developed.	Grounded theory research
Describe the characteristics or elements of the culture of a selected population and the nature of its members experiencing it.	Ethnography
Explore and/or describe the elements of a concept or the aspects of a situation to increase understanding in a selected population.	Exploratory-descriptive qualitative research

Research Problem

"Pain is a subjective phenomenon that must be prevented and treated, as there are short and long-term negative consequences when left untreated.... These negative consequences of poorly treated pain in children include such things as suffering and fear, future avoidance of healthcare (Twycross & Williams, 2014), and the potential for changes in central nervous system pain processing that predispose a child to increases in pain sensitization.... The need for more attention to children's pain management was marked by the first 'Global Year Against Pain in Children' in 2005..., yet hospitalized children all over the world continue to experience pain.... Linhares et al. (2012) found that although nurses were more likely than medical doctors (MDs) to document their pain assessment using a validated pain assessment tool, most children's charts (74%, $n = 87$) had no documentation on pain, meaning that nurses may not have assessed this parameter and certainly failed to communicate their findings effectively. When pain assessment is not conducted, or the findings are not communicated to other clinicians, children may not receive the appropriate pain treatment.... Understanding of the interplay between rural context and nurses' pediatric pain management practices is limited and is the focus of this study." (Marshall et al., 2018, pp. 89–90)

Research Purpose

"The overall aim [purpose] of this study was to explore rural hospital RN experiences in providing pain care to children in the rural hospital setting in Canada, to understand the challenges and facilitators of providing evidenced-based pediatric pain management within this context." (Marshall et al., 2018, p. 90)

Research Objectives

"This study had four main objectives:

(1) To understand the facilitators RN experience when providing pediatric pain management in the rural setting.

(2) To understand the barriers RN experience when providing pediatric pain management in the rural setting.

(3) To identify and describe RN perception of the challenges and facilitators that are unique to the rural setting.

(4) To describe RN perception of the availability of supportive structures (i.e. policies, procedures, assessment tools, educational opportunities, and pain experts) that may promote successful pain management for children in the rural setting." (Marshall et al., 2018, p. 90)

In this study, the problem significance and background were clearly presented, and the problem statement indicated that there was limited pediatric pain management in rural settings. The purpose, identified as the overall aim of the study, addressed the problem statement by focusing on RN experiences in providing pain care to children and understanding the challenges and facilitators of providing evidence-based pediatric pain management. The objectives focused on specific concepts and aspects of the pediatric pain management situation by RN (population) in the rural setting. Objectives 1 and 2 focused on understanding the concepts of facilitators and barriers to RN experiences in providing pain management. Objective 3 focused on identifying and describing challenges and facilitators unique to pain management in the rural setting. Objective 4 focused on describing RN perceptions of supportive structures to promote successful pain management in children in the rural setting. These objectives focused on identification, understanding, and description of concepts and aspects of a situation, which are typical of exploratory-descriptive qualitative research (see Table 6.2).

Marshall et al. (2019) found resource challenges related to education in pediatric pain management in a rural setting. In addition, pediatric pain was not perceived as a priority in this agency, and RN perceived there were no explicit standards for pain care. The researchers concluded, "Opportunity exists to improve pediatric pain management, however, without a systematic approach that considers the rural context, pain care for children will continue to be based on individual's beliefs and knowledge" (Marshall et al., 2019, p. 89).

FORMULATING RESEARCH QUESTIONS

A **research question** is a concise, interrogative statement that is worded in the present tense and includes one or more of a study's principal concepts or variables. Research questions are actual queries that address variables, and sometimes the relationships among them, within a population. A research question has three parts: (1) a questioning part, such as "what is," "what are," "is there," or "are there"; (2) a word that indicates what the researcher wants to know about the study variables or population; and (3) the naming of the population and the variables or concepts, if appropriate. The format for developing research questions to guide quantitative and qualitative research are discussed in the following sections.

Formulating Questions in Quantitative Studies

In quantitative studies, the research question hints heavily at the type of study conducted, implying incidence, description, connections between ideas, and cause-and-effect relationships, and perhaps even containing the exact words *incidence, prevalence, description, relationship, prediction,* and *cause and effect.* The content of research questions is very similar to objectives, with one being an interrogative statement and the other being a declarative statement. The objective or question format selected is the choice of the research team and what format best directs the implementation of the study.

The formats for developing research questions for different types of quantitative research are presented in Table 6.3. The format for research questions in the quantitative part of a mixed methods study or in an outcomes study are very similar to those in Table 6.3. If a single research question is present in a quantitative, mixed methods, or outcomes research report, it is likely to be a restatement of the research purpose. If more than one research question is present, the questions often relate to the study's different foci. Chin and Armstrong (2019) conducted a predictive correlational study to determine if anticipated stigma is predictive of healthcare utilization by patients with chronic obstructive pulmonary disease (COPD) and neurological disorders. The complete research problem (significance, background, and problem statement) is presented in

Table 5.1. The following excerpts from the Chin and Armstrong (2019) study demonstrate how the research purpose was generated from the problem statement, and the specific foci of the study are identified using research questions. Specific headers are included to clarify the focus of the study excerpts.

Research Problem Statement

"The literature exploring anticipated stigma in individuals with COPD and neurological disorders is limited. Additionally, the association between anticipated stigma and healthcare utilization has not been described in this population." (Chin & Armstrong, 2019, pp. 63–64)

Research Purpose

"The purpose of this study was to explore the experience of anticipated stigma in individuals with COPD and neurological disorders and examine the relationship between anticipated stigma and healthcare utilization." (Chin & Armstrong, 2019, p. 64)

Research Questions

"The research questions were: (a) What are the levels of anticipated stigma by friends and family, coworkers, and healthcare workers experienced by individuals living with COPD or a neurological disorder? (b) What is the relationship between anticipated stigma and healthcare utilization in individuals with COPD or a neurological disorder? (c) What are the predictors of anticipated stigma by friends and family, coworkers, and healthcare workers in individuals with COPD or a neurological disorder? (Chin & Armstrong, 2019, p. 64)

TABLE 6.3 Quantitative Research Questions, Focus, and Probable Type of Study

Research Question Format	Question Focus	Type of Quantitative Study
1. What is the incidence of variable *X* in a selected population?	Identification	Descriptive
2. What are the characteristics or descriptors of variable *X* in a selected population?	Description	Descriptive
3. Is there a difference between existing groups 1 and 2 (such as females and males) for variable *X* in a selected population?	Group differences	Descriptive
4. What is the relationship between variables *X* and *Y* in a selected population?	Association or relationship	Correlational
5. Which independent variables are predictive of a dependent variable in a selected population?	Prediction	Correlational

Chin and Armstrong's (2019) study purpose is clearly focused on the gap in nursing knowledge about the relationship between anticipated stigma and healthcare utilization (variables) by persons with COPD and neurological disorders (populations). The research purpose provides the basis for the research questions that identify the specific foci of the study. The first research question is focused on identification of the levels of anticipated stigma experienced by persons living with COPD and neurological disorders (see Table 6.3). The second question focuses on the relationship between anticipated stigma and healthcare utilization. The third question focuses on determining the predictors of anticipated stigma in individuals with COPD and neurological disorders.

The researchers gathered data from patients receiving follow-up care in pulmonary and neurological offices. The findings from this study described low to moderately anticipated stigma in individuals with COPD and neurological disorders by family and friends, coworkers, and healthcare workers. Significant relationships were found between higher levels of anticipated stigma and lower levels of healthcare utilization. Chin and Armstrong (2019) recommended implementing strategies to reduce these patients' perceptions of anticipated stigma to improve their utilization of health care.

Formulating Questions in Qualitative Studies

Most qualitative nursing studies are guided by the research purpose; very few include stated research questions. In qualitative designs, the research question implies describing the lived experience and possibly the meaning of that experience to the study participants, generating models or theory, understanding human behavior and experience within a social context, understanding the cultural context that acts as a platform for human behavior and experience, or relating basic narrative descriptive information. It may even contain the exact words *lived experience, framework or theoretical development, society, culture,* or *narrative.*

If questions are included in qualitative study, they tend to have a broader and more global phrasing than questions in quantitative reports, underscoring an experience, a feeling, a perception, or a process, and only sometimes mentioning the population of interest. Sometimes the research question hints at a specific type of qualitative study; at other times, the question implies only that the qualitative methodology will be utilized. Sometimes the population is not named in qualitative research purposes and questions, especially if the researcher is attempting to define a concept that transcends one particular population (Creswell & Poth, 2018). Table 6.4 identifies the format for the four types of qualitative research covered in this text. These formats would be the same for the qualitative part of a mixed methods study (Creswell & Clark, 2018).

Anbari, Vogelsmeier, and Dougherty (2019) conducted an exploratory-descriptive qualitative study to "compare the traditional bachelor of science in nursing (BSN) prepared graduates with the associate degree in nursing (ADN) to BSN graduates' communication about patient safety" (p. 174). The following excerpts from this study demonstrate how the research purpose was generated from the stated problem and then phrased as a research question.

TABLE 6.4 **Qualitative Research Questions and Probable Type of Study**	
Research Question Format	**Probable Type of Qualitative Study**
What is the lived experience of a phenomenon by persons in a selected population?	Phenomenology
What are the concepts and processes that characterize the perspectives and experiences of individuals from a selected population for a situation? Questions might indicate that a framework, theoretical model, or theory is being developed.	Grounded theory research
What are the characteristics or elements of the culture of a selected population and the nature of its members experiencing it?	Ethnography
What are the elements of a concept or the aspects of a situation in a selected population?	Exploratory-descriptive qualitative research

Research Problem

"There is a growing body of literature suggesting that an increased percentage of bachelor's degree nurses (BSNs) at the bedside improves patient safety and outcomes, such as decreased patient falls, decreased length of stay, and decreased mortality (Aiken et al., 2011; Aiken, Clarke, Cheung, Sloane, & Silber, 2003; Aiken et al., 2014...). Motivated by this, the Institute of Medicine (IOM), the American Nurses' Association, and other leading nursing organizations recommend increasing the percentage of practicing BSNs to 80% by the year 2020 (The IOM, 2010; Tri-Council for Nursing, 2010).... In 1999, the IOM estimated that between 44,000 and 98,000 people die each year in the United States due to preventable medical errors (National Research Council, 2000).... Since the IOM first placed attention on patient harm in 1999, efforts to improve patient safety and prevent adverse events in hospitals have become a national priority (Agency for Healthcare Research and Quality, 2013; The Joint Commission, 2017; National Research Council, 2000...).... Now, more than 15 years later, the NPSG [National Patient Safety Goals] remain an integral part of patient safety efforts (The Joint Commission, 2017), yet concerns related to safe patient care remain.... Evidence suggests that nurses with a BSN degree are associated with improved patient care and outcomes; however, there is no evidence to distinguish how differences in BSN preparation, either traditional or ADN to BSN completion, might have influenced these outcomes differently." (Anbari et al., 2019, pp. 172–174)

Research Purpose

"Therefore, the purpose of this qualitative study is to begin to address the gap by comparing traditional BSN prepared graduates with ADN to BSN graduates' communication about patient safety." (Anbari et al., 2019, p. 174)

Research Question

"The research question guiding this study was as follows:

Research Question: What are the similarities and differences in the words and descriptors used by traditional BSNs and ADN to BSN graduates to communicate about patient safety?" (Anbari et al., 2019, p. 174)

Anbari and colleagues (2019) provided a detailed research problem that included significance, background, and problem statement. The study purpose addressed the gap in knowledge identified in the problem statement. The focus of the purpose was

understanding communication about patient safety by traditional or prelicensure BSN and ADN to BSN graduates (population). The research question was essentially the purpose reworded as a question according to the language of an exploratory-descriptive qualitative study.

Anbari et al. (2019) concludes, "Findings indicate there are two meaning levels or systems, the local level and the systematic level. At the local level, the meaning of patient safety is focused at the patient's bedside and regulated by the nurse. The systemic level included the notion that health system factors such as policies and staffing are paramount to keeping patients safe. More frequently, ADN to BSN graduates' meaning of patient safety was at the local level, while BSNs' meaning centered at the systemic level" (p. 171).

HYPOTHESES

A **hypothesis** is a stated relationship between or among variables, within a specified population. The hypothesis translates the problem and purpose into a clear explanation or prediction of the expected results or outcomes of the study (Shadish, Cook, & Campbell, 2002). Hypotheses usually include the same variables and population identified in the research purpose. The wording of the hypothesis indicates the study design, through use of phrases such as *over time, associations among variables,* or *intervention effects increase with repeated applications.* Hypotheses also indicate the appropriate statistical tests for a study and are used or organize the study's Results section (Grove & Cipher, 2020). The purpose, sources, and types of hypotheses that are commonly developed by researchers are described in the following sections. In addition, the process for developing and testing hypotheses in nursing studies is detailed.

Purpose of Hypotheses

The purpose of a hypothesis is similar to that of research objectives and questions. A hypothesis (1) specifies the variables you will measure, (2) identifies the population you will examine, (3) indicates the type of research, and (4) directs the conduct of your study. Hypotheses direct the conduct of a study by influencing the study design, sampling technique, data collection and analysis methods, and interpretation of findings. Hypotheses differ from objectives and questions by predicting the outcomes of a study. Hypothesis testing promotes generation of knowledge by testing theoretical statements or relationships identified in previous research, proposed by theorists, or observed in practice (Chinn & Kramer, 2015; Kazdin, 2017).

The scientific method rests on the process of stating a hypothesis, testing it, and rejecting or accepting it. The hypothesis-testing process involves several steps, the first two of which are identification of a research hypothesis and construction of the corresponding null hypothesis. Even if a hypothesis is not identified in a research report, when a study is experimental or quasi-experimental, a hypothesis is implied (Shadish et al., 2002). Most correlational research and some quantitative descriptive research studies use hypotheses as well. Researchers make certain that there is coherency between the hypothesis's posited relationships among variables and the study's identified theoretical framework. If the theoretical framework is not coherent with the hypothesis, a new framework should be chosen, or a framework newly developed, using the hypothesis as a starting point (see Chapter 8) (Smith & Liehr, 2018).

Types of Hypotheses

Hypotheses identify different types of relationships and include different numbers of variables. Studies might have one, three, or more hypotheses, depending on the complexity and scope of the study. The type of hypothesis developed is based on the problem and purpose of a study. The following four categories (Box 6.1) are used to describe types of hypotheses: (1) causal versus associative, (2) simple versus complex, (3) directional versus nondirectional, and (4) null versus research (Creswell & Creswell, 2018; Shadish et al., 2002).

Causal Versus Associative Hypotheses

Relationships in hypotheses may be identified as associative or causal. A **causal hypothesis** proposes a cause-and-effect relationship between variables in which one causes the other. The cause is the independent variable; the result or outcome is the dependent variable. The **independent variable** (intervention, treatment, or experimental variable) is manipulated or varied by the researcher to have an effect on the dependent variable. The **dependent variable** (outcome or response variable) is measured to examine the effect created by the independent variable. (Variables are discussed in more detail later in this chapter.) A format for stating a causal hypothesis is as follows: Subjects in the experimental group receiving the independent variable (intervention) demonstrate greater change in the dependent variable than do the subjects in the control or comparison group. Fig. 6.1 includes a diagram of a causal hypothesis versus an associative hypothesis.

Chen and Hu (2019) conducted a randomized controlled trial (RCT) to determine the effectiveness of a modified stretching exercise program (MSEP) on young women with low back pain during their menstrual period. They stated the following causal hypothesis: "The experimental group treated with a MSEP will score lower on the back pain disability questionnaire (Oswestry Low Back Pain Disability Questionnaire) than the control group" (Chen & Hu, 2019, p. 243). In this hypothesis, the independent variable or

BOX 6.1 Types of Hypotheses Developed to Direct Nursing Studies

Types of Hypotheses	Focus
Causal Versus Associative Hypotheses	Type of relationship presented in the hypothesis
Simple Versus Complex Hypotheses	Number of variables in the hypothesis
Nondirectional Versus Directional Hypotheses	Relationship direction or lack of direction in the hypothesis
Research Versus Null Hypotheses	Relationship expressed in the research hypothesis
	No relationship expressed in a null hypothesis

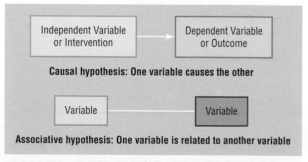

Fig. 6.1 Causal hypothesis versus associative hypothesis. Note the causal arrow points from the independent variable toward the dependent variable. The straight line indicates a relationship between two variables.

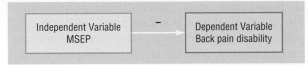

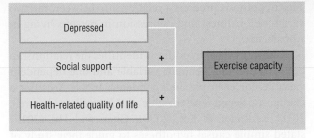

Fig. 6.2 Causal hypothesis: modified stretching exercise program *(MSEP)* reduces back pain disability.

Fig. 6.3 Associative hypothesis of the relationships of depressed, social support, and health-related quality of life with exercise capacity.

intervention MSEP was hypothesized to cause reduction in the dependent or outcome variable back pain disability. As in this example, a causal hypothesis frequently mentions the independent variable first and then the dependent variable(s). Fig. 6.2 includes a diagram of the causal hypothesis formulated for the relationship between MSEP and back pain disability. This is a negative relationship because the implementation of the MSEP is predicted to decrease back pain disability.

An **associative hypothesis** presents a noncausative relationship between or among variables. None of the variables are identified as causing any of the other variables; the variables occur or exist together, and as one variable changes so does the other. Researchers state associative hypotheses when the focus of their study is to examine relationships and not to determine cause and effect (see Fig. 6.1). Variables are positively (+) related when they change in the same direction, increase or decrease together, in a study. Variables are negatively (−) related when they change in opposite or inverse directions, one variable increases as the other decreases, in a study. The formats used for expressing associative hypotheses follow:

1. Variable X is related to or associated with variable Y in a selected population. (Predicts a relationship between two variables but does not indicate the type of relationship)
2. An increase in variable X is related to an increase in variable Y, or variable X is positively related to variable Y in a selected population. (Predicts a positive [+] relationship)
3. A decrease in variable X is related to a decrease in variable Y in a selected population. (Predicts a positive [+] relationship)
4. An increase in variable X is related to a decrease in variable Y, or variable X is negatively related to variable Y in a selected population. (Predicts a negative or inverse [−] relationship)
5. Independent variables X and Y are predictive of a dependent variable in a study. (Predictive correlational study)

Gathright and colleagues (2019) conducted a predictive correlational study to examine the clinical and psychosocial variables associated with improved exercise capacity in those who completed cardiac rehabilitation (CR). These researcher "hypothesized that being less depressed, having more social support, and having better health-related quality of life would be associated with greater improvements in exercise capacity at CR discharge" (Gathright et al., 2019, p. 14). Fig. 6.3 is a diagram of Gathright et al.'s (2019) associative hypothesis that predicts a negative relationship between the variables depressed and exercise capacity and positive relationships for social support and health-related quality of life with exercise capacity.

Simple Versus Complex Hypotheses

Hypotheses may be simple or complex. A **simple hypothesis** predicts the relationship between only two variables and may be either associative or causal. Fig. 6.1 diagrams both a simple casual hypothesis and a simple associative hypothesis, which include two variables. A format for stating a simple associative hypothesis is as follows: Variable X is related to variable Y. Theeke, Carpenter, Mallow, and Theeke (2019) stated eight hypotheses to direct their study examining "gender differences in loneliness, anger, depression, self-management ability (SMA), and biomarkers of chronic illness in chronically ill mid-life adults in Appalachia" (p. 55). (The steps of this study are presented in Chapter 3 with the introduction of the quantitative research process.) These researchers conducted an extensive review of the literature on psychological concepts of persons living in Appalachia and stated the following simple associative hypothesis: "Mean loneliness scores would differ based on diagnosis of depression" (Theeke et al., 2019, p. 56).

This hypothesis predicts a relationship between the two variables loneliness and depression in persons living in Appalachia.

A simple causal hypothesis identifies the relationship between one independent variable and one dependent variable, for example, independent variable *X* causes a change in dependent variable *Y* (Creswell & Creswell, 2018; Kerlinger & Lee, 2000). Chen and Hu (2019) stated simple causal hypotheses to guide their study of the effectiveness of a stretching exercise program on back pain disability, which was expressed in the previous section (see Fig. 6.2). They also stated a simple causal hypothesis focused on exercise self-efficacy: "The experimental group treated with a MSEP will score higher on the exercise self-efficacy (EXSE) scale than the control group" (Chen & Hu, 2019, p. 243). The two variables in this hypothesis were the intervention MSEP (independent variable) and the outcome or dependent variable exercise self-efficacy. The researchers found the experimental group, involved in the MSEP, had significantly lower backpain disability scores and higher exercise self-efficacy than the control group. Chen and Hu recommended that young women with menstrual-related back pain might use the MSEP to reduce their back-pain disability and improve their exercise self-efficacy to enhance their self-care abilities.

A **complex hypothesis** predicts the relationship among three or more variables. It may be either causal or associative. In interventional research, this means one independent variable and two or more dependent variables; in correlational research, this merely indicates that the relationships among three variables or more will be examined. Theeke et al. (2019) also reported a complex associative hypothesis to direct their study of persons living in Appalachia: "In both men and women, loneliness scores would be positively related to depressive symptoms, anger, and chronic control indicators" (p. 56). In this hypothesis, the relationships among four variables (loneliness, depressive symptoms, anger, and chronic control indicators) were examined in a population of men and women living in Appalachia. Gathright et al.'s (2019) hypothesis, presented in the previous section, was also complex and associative predicting the relationships among the following variables: depressed, social support, health-related quality of life, and exercise capacity (see Fig. 6.3).

Vasilevskis and colleagues (2019) conducted an RCT called Shed-MEDS to determine the effects of a patient-centered deprescribing intervention on health outcomes of hospitalized older patients with polypharmacy. The Shed-MEDS trial was conducted "to test the hypothesis that a patient-centered deprescribing intervention initiated in the hospital and continuing through the PAC [post-acute care facility] stay will reduce the total number of medications 90 days following PAC discharge and result in improvements in geriatric syndromes and functional health status" (Vasilevskis et al., 2019, p. 1). This complex causal hypothesis examined the effects of a deprescribing intervention on the number of medications, geriatric syndromes, and functional health status outcomes of hospitalized elders with polypharmacy.

Directional Hypotheses Versus Nondirectional Hypotheses

A **directional hypothesis** states the nature or direction of a proposed relationship between variables. Directional hypotheses are developed from theoretical statements, previous research findings, and clinical experience (Creswell & Creswell, 2018; Smith & Liehr, 2018). As the knowledge on which a study is based increases, the researcher is able to predict the direction of a relationship between the variables being studied. Terms such as *less, more, increase, decrease, positive, negative, greater,* and *smaller* indicate the directions of relationships in hypotheses. Directional hypotheses can be associative or causal and simple or complex. All causal research hypotheses are directional because the independent variable is predicted to cause a specific change (increase or decrease) in the dependent variable. For example, Vasilevskis et al.'s (2019) RCT, introduced in the previous section, was directed by a complex, directional causal hypothesis. A patient-centered deprescribing intervention was implemented to *reduce* the total number of medications and *improve* geriatric syndromes and functional health status in the elderly with polypharmacy following PAC discharge. (The italicized terms indicate the directions in this hypothesis.)

Theeke et al. (2019) stated a directional simple associative hypothesis in their study of persons living in Appalachia. The researchers hypothesized: "In both men and women, higher loneliness scores would be inversely related to self-management ability" (Theeke et al., 2019, p. 56). This hypothesis identifies a negative or inverse relationship where higher loneliness scores would be related to lower SMA. Theeke and colleagues (2019) found, "Loneliness impacts SMA and should be included in the care planning or study of chronically ill adults who struggle with self-management" (p. 55).

A **nondirectional hypothesis**, as the definition implies, does not specify the direction of the relationship between and among variables. If the researcher does not anticipate any particular direction of the proposed relationship from clinical practice, theory, or previous research, the hypothesis will be worded nondirectionally. Rieder, Goshin, Sissoko, Kleshchova, and Weierich (2019) used nondirectional hypotheses to test "the salivary biomarkers of the sympathetic nervous system (SNS) and hypothalamic-pituitary-adrenal (HPA) axis function as predictors of subjective maternal stress" (p. 48) in mothers under criminal justice supervision. These researchers "hypothesized that SNS and HPA axis function, indexed by salivary AA [alpha-amylase] and cortisol levels, would be associated with psychological parenting stress" (Rieder et al., 2019, p. 49). They reported, "Given the exploratory nature of this study and the inconsistencies in the literature, we did not have directional hypotheses regarding the associations between salivary stress biomarkers and parenting stress" (Rieder et al., 2019, p. 49). This is a complex associative hypothesis focused on testing SNA and HPA axis function, using AA and cortisol salivary biomarkers, to predict parenting stress. Rieder et al. (2019) found that the AA and cortisol salivary biomarkers were significantly predictive of maternal stress and might be used to initiate interventions in this population (i.e., mothers under criminal justice supervision).

Null Versus Research Hypotheses

The **null hypothesis** (H_0), also referred to as a **statistical hypothesis**, is used for statistical testing and interpretation of study results. Even if the null hypothesis is not stated, it may be derived by stating the opposite of the research hypothesis (Creswell & Creswell, 2018; Shadish et al., 2002). A null hypothesis can be simple or complex and associative or causal. An associative null hypothesis states that there is no relationship between the variables studied. A causal null hypothesis is usually stated in the following format: There is no difference in the experimental group receiving the study intervention and the control or comparison group receiving standard care for the dependent or outcome variable. Null hypotheses that state no relationships among variables, no difference between study groups, or no effect of an intervention on a study outcome are nondirectional (Grove & Cipher, 2020).

Nowakowski-Grier (2018) studied the effect of an inpatient diabetes nurse mentor (DNM) program on the 30-day readmission rates among diabetic patients. The null hypothesis stated there is "no difference between patient 30-day readmissions between study [patients in the DNM program] and comparison patients" (Nowakowski-Grier, 2018, p. 1). The limited sample size of 74 patients and unequal group sizes (34 patients in the study group and 40 in the comparison group) might have resulted in the null hypothesis being accepted indicating no difference between the two groups for readmissions. Thus further research is needed in this area.

A **research hypothesis** is the alternative hypothesis (H_1 or Ha) to the null, and it represents the researcher's posited results. The research hypothesis states that "there is a relationship" between two or more variables, and that relationship can be simple or complex, nondirectional or directional, and associative or causal (see Box 6.1). As such, it is opposite to the null hypothesis. All of the hypotheses presented previously are research hypotheses, except for the null hypothesis stated by Nowakowski-Grier (2018).

Researchers have different beliefs about when to state a research hypothesis versus a null hypothesis in a research report. Some researchers state the null hypothesis because it is more consistent with the reporting of statistical analyses or is the expected outcome of the study. However, the vast majority of articles present the research hypothesis. This is a matter of style; the reader of a report can easily construct the null hypothesis given the research hypothesis.

Identifying Types of Hypotheses in Published Studies

Study hypotheses can be described in terms of all four of these paired descriptions (causal versus associative, simple versus complex, nondirectional versus directional, and null versus research) (see Box 6.1). Table 6.5 was developed to clarify the types of hypotheses included as examples in this chapter. For instance, Chen and Hu (2019) conducted an RCT to determine the effect of a MSEP on menstrual low back pain. The researchers hypothesized: "The experimental group treated with a MSEP will score higher on the exercise self-efficacy scale (EXSE) than the control group" (Chen & Hu, 2019, p. 243). Of the choices, causal or associative, simple or complex, directional or nondirectional, and null or research, one can identify Chen

TABLE 6.5   Types of Hypotheses From Published Studies

Authors (Year)	Hypothesis	Causal or Associative	Simple or Complex	Directional or Nondirectional	Null or Research
Chen and Hu (2019)	They hypothesized: "The experimental group treated with a MSEP [modified stretching exercise program] will score lower on the back pain disability questionnaire (Oswestry Low Back Pain Disability Questionnaire [ODI]) than the control group" (p. 243).	Causal	Simple	Directional	Research
Gathright et al. (2019)	They "hypothesized that being less depressed, having more social support, and having better health-related quality of life would be associated with greater improvements in exercise capacity at CR [cardiac rehabilitation] discharge" (p. 14).	Associative	Complex	Directional	Research
Theeke, Carpenter, Mallow, and Theeke (2019)	"Mean loneliness scores would differ based on diagnosis of depression" (p. 56)	Associative	Simple	Nondirectional	Research
Vasilevskis et al. (2019)	The Shed-MEDS trial was conducted "to test the hypothesis that a patient-centered deprescribing intervention initiated in the hospital and continuing through the PAC [post-acute care facility] stay will reduce the total number of medications 90 days following PAC discharge and result in improvements in geriatric syndromes and functional health status" (p. 1).	Causal	Complex	Directional	Research
Rieder, Goshin, Sissoko, Kleshchova, and Weierich (2019)	These researchers "hypothesized that SNS [sympathetic nervous system] and HPA [hypothalamic-pituitary-adrenal] axis function, indexed by salivary AA [alpha-amylase] and cortisol levels, would be associated with psychological parenting stress" (p. 49).	Associative	Complex	Nondirectional	Research
Nowakowski-Grier (2018)	There is "no difference between patient 30-day readmissions between study [patients in the diabetes nurse mentor program] and comparison patients" (p. 1).	Causal	Simple	Nondirectional	Null

and Hu's hypothesis as a causal, simple, directional, research hypothesis. The hypothesis is causal because the effect of an intervention (MSEP) is being tested and simple because it includes one independent variable (MSEP) and one dependent variable (exercise self-efficacy). Causal hypotheses are directional; in this example, the experimental group is expected to have higher exercise self-efficacy scores. This is a research hypothesis because the specific outcome of the study is predicted. Review the other hypotheses in Table 6.5 and note the types of hypotheses used as examples.

Testing Hypotheses

A hypothesis should predict a clear, concise relationship between or among variables in a selected population. A **testable hypothesis** contains variables that can be precisely measured or manipulated in a study (Waltz, Strickland, & Lenz, 2017). Formulating a testable hypothesis to guide a study requires several decisions. The research problem and purpose determine whether you will study an associative or a causal relationship. Testing a hypothesis that states a causal relationship requires expertise in implementing an intervention and controlling extraneous variables. You must also decide whether the research problem and purpose are best investigated with the use of simple or complex hypotheses. Complex hypotheses frequently require complex methodology, and the outcomes may be difficult to interpret. Some beginning researchers prefer the clarity of simple hypotheses. Another decision you must make involves the formulation of a research or a null hypothesis based on the most current knowledge of the research problem.

A hypothesis that is clearly and concisely stated gives the greatest direction for conducting a study and interpreting the results. Hypotheses are clearer without identifying methodological points, such as techniques of sampling, measurement, and data analysis (Kerlinger & Lee, 2000). Therefore a statement such as "measured by," "in a random sample of," or "using ANOVA (analysis of variance)" decreases the clarity and conciseness of a hypothesis. For example, the Chen and Hu (2019) study hypotheses would have been clearer and more concise without identifying measurement methods for the study dependent variables.

Hypotheses are evaluated in the hypothesis-testing process using statistical analyses. If the hypothesis states an associative relationship, correlational analyses are usually conducted on the data. Spearman rank-order correlation coefficient is often used to analyze ordinal level data, and Pearson product-moment correlation coefficient is used for interval and ratio level data (see Chapter 23). These correlational analyses determine the existence, type (positive or negative), and degree or strength of the relationship between the variables studied. A hypothesis that states a causal relationship is analyzed using statistics that examine differences, such as the Mann-Whitney U test, the t-test, and ANOVA (see Chapter 25). It is the null hypothesis (stated or implied) that is tested through statistical analysis (Grove & Cipher, 2020).

Following appropriate statistical analyses, hypotheses are used for reporting results, identifying findings, and forming both conclusions and generalizations. The results of hypothesis testing are described with unique wording. Research findings do not "prove" hypotheses true or false: instead, "there is evidence for their support." After a series of studies of the same hypothesis with similar positive findings, the word *proven* is still not used; instead, "there is considerable evidence in support of the hypothesis." When a null hypothesis is tested, it is either "rejected" or "accepted." If a null hypothesis is accepted, that acceptance is always provisional. The same is true for the rejection of a null hypothesis. Rejecting of a hypothesis by a single test, according to Popper (1968), cannot stand, because "non-reproducible single occurrences are of no significance to science" (p. 86). Replication is essential, whether rejection or acceptance is the outcome for a single study.

Selecting Objectives, Questions, or Hypotheses for Different Types of Research

Selecting objectives, questions, or hypotheses for a study is often based on (1) the number and quality of relevant studies conducted on a selected problem (existing knowledge base), (2) the theoretical aspect of the study, (3) the expertise and preference of the researcher, and (4) the type of study to be conducted (quantitative, qualitative, mixed methods, or outcomes research). Commonly, if minimal or no research has been conducted on a problem, investigators usually conduct qualitative or descriptive quantitative studies. These studies are often directed by the study purpose, but researchers might include objectives or questions to clarify the focus of the study (Table 6.6). The theoretical discussion in a study indicates whether the intent is to

TABLE 6.6   Selecting Objectives, Questions, or Hypotheses for Different Types of Research

Type of Research	Objectives, Questions, or Hypotheses Developed to Guide a Study
Qualitative research	Research purpose guides most qualitative studies. Occasionally objectives or questions are stated.
Quantitative research: Descriptive studies	Research purpose guides many descriptive studies. Occasionally objectives or questions are stated.
Correlational studies	Objectives, questions, or hypotheses
Quasi-experimental studies	Usually hypotheses
Experimental studies	Hypotheses
Mixed methods research	Qualitative part of the study might be guided by purpose and an objective or question.
	Quantitative part of the study might be guided by the purpose and objective, questions, or hypothesis based on the type of study.
Outcomes research	Objectives, questions, or hypotheses

develop or to test theory. Objectives and questions are usually stated to guide theory development through qualitative research, and the focus of a hypothesis is to test theory through quantitative or outcomes research (Creswell & Creswell, 2018; Kazdin, 2017).

Researcher expertise and preference can also influence the selection of objectives, questions, or hypotheses to direct a study. The number of nursing studies containing hypotheses continues to grow, and there appears to be a trend away from mainly descriptive quantitative studies toward studies focused on examining relationships between variables and testing hypotheses. Formulating hypotheses to direct quantitative and outcomes research indicates growth of knowledge in selected problem areas and the implementation of more controlled designs (see Chapter 11). However, it is important that researchers explicitly state hypotheses to direct their studies rather than implying them in the text of the article. An explicit statement of a hypothesis is important to provide clear direction for the conduct of a study, analysis of data, interpretation of the findings, and use of the findings in practice (Kazdin, 2017; Melnyk et al., 2018; Melnyk & Fineout-Overholt, 2019; Shadish et al., 2002).

The objectives, questions, or hypotheses designated for a study frequently indicate a pattern that the researcher uses in conducting investigations. Problems can be investigated in a variety of ways. Each study must logically build on the other, as the researcher establishes a pattern for studying a problem area that will affect the quality and quantity of the knowledge generated in that area. In some qualitative research, the investigator uses only a problem and purpose to direct the study (see Table 6.6). The specification of objectives or questions might limit the scope of the study and the methods of data collection and analysis (Creswell & Poth, 2018).

Mixed methods research incorporates two different designs so the study may contain more than one stated purpose (Creswell & Clark, 2018). When only a single purpose is stated, however, two objectives/aims (or research questions) may be identified, clarifying the two distinct parts (quantitative and qualitative) of the inquiry (see Table 6.6). Hypotheses are included only if the quantitative portion of the study involves hypothesis testing as in quasi-experimental and experimental research (Creswell & Creswell, 2018; Shadish et al., 2002).

Researchers often develop hypotheses when the relationships or results of a study can be anticipated or predicted. Hypotheses are typically used in quantitative research to direct predictive correlational, quasi-experimental, and experimental studies and are also important to guide outcomes studies (Creswell & Creswell, 2018; Kane & Radosevich, 2011; Shadish et al., 2002). Outcomes research, because it uses quantitative designs, follows the guidelines presented in this chapter for quantitative research in respect to objectives/ aims, research questions, and hypothesis testing (see

Table 6.6). The exception is that objectives, questions, and hypotheses often contain the word *outcomes* (Moorhead, Swanson, Johnson, & Maas, 2018).

IDENTIFYING AND DEFINING STUDY VARIABLES OR CONCEPTS

The research purpose and objectives, questions, and hypotheses identify the variables or concepts to be examined in a study. **Variables** or concepts are ideas, qualities, properties, or characteristics of persons, things, or situations that are studied in research. Variables are concepts at various levels of abstraction that are concisely defined so they can be measured or manipulated within a study. The concepts examined in research can be concrete and directly measurable in practice, such as heart rate, blood sugar, and weight. These concrete concepts are usually referred to as variables in a study. Other concepts, such as pain, anxiety, and depression, are more abstract and are indirectly observable in the real world. Thus the properties of these concepts are inferred from a combination of measurements. For example, one can infer the properties of anxiety by combining information obtained from (1) observing the signs and symptoms of anxiety (agitated movements, sweating, rapid eye movement, lack of eye contact, and verbalization of anxiety), (2) examining completed questionnaires or scales (state and trait anxiety scales) focused on anxiety, and (3) measuring physiological responses (galvanic skin response). The concept of anxiety might be represented by the variable "reported anxiety" or "perceived level of anxiety" in a study and is operationalized or measured by one or more of the methods previously identified (Bandalos, 2018; Waltz et al., 2017).

At the outset of a qualitative study, abstract concepts are described and sometimes defined but they are not operationalized, because they will not be measured, and they will not necessarily assume more than one value. Because of this, qualitative research does not refer to concepts as variables, except in the special case of grounded theory research in which the sole central concept revealed at the end of the study through data analysis is sometimes called the core variable (Charmaz, 2014; Creswell & Poth, 2018). The following sections discuss demographic variables, the concepts in qualitative research, and the types of variables in quantitative research.

Demographic Variables

Demographic variables are subject or participant characteristics measured during a study and used to describe a sample. Demographic variables are found in all quantitative and most qualitative, mixed methods, and outcomes nursing research reports. Researchers select demographic variables according to the focus of their study, the demographic variables included in previous research, and clinical experience. In nursing research, common demographic variables are age, gender, and race/ethnicity, which define the population represented by the sample. Thorough description of the sample guides the researcher in making appropriate generalizations, conclusions, and recommendations at the study's end. For hospital-based studies, additional demographic variables typically include medical diagnosis, acuity, and length of stay. In nonhospital settings, educational level, income, and occupation may be included as demographics, especially when provision of services is a study focus.

To obtain data about demographic variables, researchers either access existent records or ask subjects to complete an information sheet. After study completion, demographic information is analyzed to provide what are called the **sample characteristics**, or occasionally the sample demographics. In a quantitative research report, sample characteristics are usually presented at the beginning of the Results section in a table accompanied by a brief narrative. Some researchers include clinical characteristics with their demographics that are relevant to the focus of the study. The Chin and Armstrong (2019) study, introduced earlier, focused on the relationship of anticipated stigma and healthcare utilization in patients with COPD and neurological disorders. These researchers presented their study demographic and clinical characteristics in a table with a brief narrative in the article as noted in the following excerpt.

"Demographic and clinical characteristics are presented in Table 1 [Table 6.7]. Thirty-eight participants (49.4%) reported a diagnosis of COPD and 39 (50.6%) participants reported a neurological diagnosis. The sample was predominantly white (n = 73, 95%), married (n = 42, 54.5%) females (n = 53, 68.8%) with a mean age of 61.1 (range 20-91, *SD* [standard deviation] = 16.33)." (Chin & Armstrong, 2019, p. 65)

Chin and Armstrong (2019) provided a quality description of their sample that included the following demographic and clinical variables: age, years with diagnosis, gender, marital status, education, income, and diagnosis. In their study narrative, they identified some key points about the sample characteristics presented in the Chin and Armstrong table (see Table 6.7 in this text).

Concepts in Qualitative Research

There are two types of concepts found in qualitative research. The first is the concept on which the research is focused, which is the topic the researcher explores. The topic of the research is, of course, known to the researcher at the outset and is named in the study purpose and research question. This foundational topic is known in both quantitative and qualitative research as *the phenomenon, the phenomenon of interest, the study focus, the concept of interest,* and *the central issue,* among other terms (Creswell & Poth, 2018; Marshall & Rossman, 2016). In this chapter it is referred to as the **phenomenon of interest**. For example, the phenomenon of interest was "patient safety communication" among differently educated nurses in Anbari et al.'s (2019) exploratory-descriptive qualitative study, introduced earlier. The patient safety communication of traditional or prelicensure BSN and associate (ADN) to BSN graduates was compared.

The second type of concept found in qualitative research is specific to the qualitative inquiry. It is the **emergent concept**, which is what the researcher discovers during the process of studying the phenomenon of interest. Emergent concepts in the Anbari et al. (2019) study, introduced earlier, were reported as the research results. These concepts were two "meaning systems of patient safety communication," one at the local level and the other at the systematic level, that emerged during data analysis: "At the local level, communication about patient safety centered on the phenomenon that patient safety was an event, such as preventing falls and medication errors… [P]atient safety at this level is also more personal, local, and close to the patient," which was the focus of ADN to BSN prepared nurses in this study (Anbari et al., 2019, pp. 180−181). "At the systematic level, nurse communication about patient safety focused on patient safety as a process that had a broad or contextual meaning," which was the focus of traditional or prelicensure prepared BSN nurses (Anbari et al., 2019, p. 183).

TABLE 6.7 Demographic, Clinical Characteristics, and Mean Score of CIASS and HAM (N = 77)

Characteristic	M ± SD (Range)
Age (years)	61.1 ± 16.3 (20–91)
Years with diagnosis	10.7 ± 9.37 (1–39)

Characteristic	n %
Gender	
Male	24 (31.2%)
Female	53 (68.8%)
Marital status	
Single	14 (18.2%)
Married	42 (54.5%)
Widowed	12 (15.6%)
Divorced	9 (11.7%)
Education	
Less than high school	10 (13.0%)
High school	16 (20.8%)
Some college	21 (27.3%)
Associate degree	5 (6.5%)
Bachelor degree	14 (18.4%)
Graduate degree	11 (14.5%)
Income	
<15,000	12 (15.5%)
15,000–35,000	18 (23.4%)
36,000–55,000	17 (22.1%)
56,000–75,000	13 (16.9%)
>75,000	17 (22.1%)
Diagnosis	
COPD	38 (49.4%)
Neurological disorder	39 (50.6%)
Migraine	8
Parkinson	12
Other	19

Scale Scores	M ± SD (Range)
CIASS subscale 1	2.0 ± 0.98 (1–4.75)
CIASS subscale 2 (workers only n-60)	2.6 ± 1.14 (1–5)
CIASS subscale 3	2.2 ± 0.96 (0.75–4.75)
HAM	2.2 ± 0.57 (1–3.5)

From Chin, E. D., & Armstrong, D. (2019). Anticipated stigma and healthcare utilization in COPD and neurological disorders. *Applied Nursing Research, 45*(1), p. 65. https://doi.org/10.1016/j.apnr.2018.12.002
CIASS, Chronic Illness Data Collection Tool; *COPD,* chronic obstructive pulmonary disease; *HAM,* Healthcare Access Measure; *M,* mean; *n,* frequency of a variable; *N,* sample size; *SD,* standard deviation.

Theme is the term most commonly used in qualitative research reports for concepts that emerge during the conduct of a study. Those themes represent the study results, especially in phenomenology and exploratory-descriptive qualitative research, although the words *essences* and *truths* are sometimes seen in phenomenology, as are other terms specific to that type of inquiry. Names for emergent concepts used in grounded theory research are *factors, factors of interest, categories, codes, core variable* or *process,* among others. Ethnography tends to use the word *themes,* and occasionally *factors.* These terms all refer to the emergent concepts— the discoveries—of the research (Charmaz, 2014; Creswell & Poth, 2018; Marshall & Rossman, 2016).

Types of Variables in Quantitative Research
Independent and Dependent Variables

The terms *independent variable* and *dependent variable* are used in two different ways in nursing research. In experimental and quasi-experimental research, they are used to denote the cause and effect of a researcher intervention. In predictive correlational research, they are used to identify potential predictors and their outcome. So an independent variable is either a cause or a predictor, depending on the research design. A dependent variable is the outcome researchers intend to produce, modify, or predict.

Interventional research designs: Independent and dependent variables. Quantitative research is either interventional or noninterventional. Interventional research includes experimental and quasi-experimental designs. In interventional research (see Chapter 11), the researcher enacts an intervention upon the experimental group and not the control group. Interventional research includes two principal types of variables, the independent variable and the dependent variable. As discussed earlier, the independent variable is the intervention or treatment that the researcher applies to the experimental group. Independent variables in true experimental research must be intentionally implemented by the researcher, not by nature, not by chance, for the research to be considered experimental. The dependent variable is so called because it depends on the action of the independent variable. The dependent variable is defined as the result or outcome that is the study's focus.

Johnson, Razo, Smith, Cain, and Soper (2019) conducted an RCT to determine the effects of a postoperative

evidence-based bundle on the main outcomes of "length of stay, occurrence of readmission, and patient satisfaction following all hysterectomies" (p. 42). In this experimental study, an enhanced recovery after surgery educational program (postoperative evidence-based bundle) and standard education packet were provided to the experimental group, and the standard education packet alone was provided to the comparison group. The Institute for Healthcare Improvement (2016) developed the bundle concept, which was the basis for the intervention in this study. The dependent or outcome variables, length of stay, occurrence of readmission, and patient satisfaction were measured during the conduct of the study from women following their hysterectomy.

Predictive correlational design: Independent and dependent variables. Predictive correlational research also uses the terms *independent* and *dependent variables,* but to denote prediction, not causation. The variable whose value the researcher is attempting to predict is the dependent variable, sometimes called the outcome variable. The researcher tests one or more other variables to discover whether they predict the value of the dependent variable, and to what extent they do so. Those predictors are called independent variables. Chin and Armstrong (2019) conducted a predictive correlational study to determine if "the predictors of anticipated stigma by friends and family, coworkers, and healthcare workers" (p. 64) were predictive of healthcare utilization by patients with COPD or a neurological disorder. As described earlier, these sources of anticipated stigma (independent variables) were predictive of lower levels of healthcare utilization (dependent variable) by patients with COPD or a neurological disorder.

Extraneous Variables in Interventional and Correlational Studies

Extraneous variables are those not central to a study's research purpose but have a potential effect on the results, making the independent variable appear more or less powerful than it really is in its effect on the value of the dependent variable. Extraneous variables exist in all studies and can affect the selection of study participants, implementation of the intervention, measurement of study variables, and collection of data. Extraneous variables are of primary concern in quasi-experimental and experimental quantitative studies, because they can obscure one's understanding of the relational or causal dynamics within the studies (Kazdin, 2017; Shadish et al., 2002). An example of an extraneous variable in health research is an unrelated medical condition that makes a study's dependent variables greater or smaller in value. Extraneous variables are classified as (1) recognized or unrecognized and (2) controlled or uncontrolled.

The extraneous variables that are not recognized until the study is in process or that are recognized before the study is initiated but cannot be controlled are referred to as **confounding variables**. Sometimes these variables can be measured during the study and controlled statistically during analysis. In other cases, it is not possible to measure a confounding variable, and the variable thus hinders the interpretation of findings. Such extraneous variables must be identified as limitations or areas of study weakness in the Discussion section of a research report. As control decreases in quasi-experimental and experimental studies, the potential influence of confounding variables increases. As discussed earlier, Johnson et al. (2019) conducted an RCT to determine the effects of a postoperative evidence-based bundle on the outcomes of women following their hysterectomy. They identified the following extraneous variables in their study.

> "**Confounding variables**
> Age can be a confounding factor as older people may be more likely to be inactive and may be at risk of developing complications. The majority of the participants for both groups had an age range of 51–64 years with age distribution similar in both groups reducing the effects of confounding variables. Type of surgical procedure (open, vaginal, or laparoscopic) can be a confounding factor as laparoscopic surgery can reduce postoperative pain, reduce hospital stay, and result in faster return to recovery. The majority of participants for both groups had laparoscopic procedures with similar distributions, the bundle group (20 patients) and the standard group (19 patients) reducing the effect of confounding variables." (Johnson et al., 2019, p. 42)

When conducting your own study, you will be able to identify a number of potentially extraneous variables that might have an effect on your study's findings. As in the Johnson et al. (2019) study, you will need to make adjustments in the research design and methods to attempt to control for the intrusion of the extraneous variables that are most likely to alter the research findings and consequently force an incorrect conclusion. Table 6.8 provides information about the goals of

TABLE 6.8 Controlling for Extraneous Variables

Before and During the Study

Goal	Strategy
Reduce or eliminate extraneous variables' effects on relationships among the study's principal variables.	• Modify the study's inclusion criteria to eliminate potential subjects possessing a specific extraneous variable. • Use a large sample with random assignment to groups, so that subjects with extraneous variables will be equally distributed between groups.[a]
Reduce or eliminate the influence of extraneous variables on calculations that measure relationships.	• Measure the effects of extraneous variables and mathematically remove those effects from statistical calculations.
Establish the magnitude and direction of extraneous variables' effects.	• Treat extraneous variables as predictor variables in statistical calculations.
After Completion of Data Collection Confirm that the effects of potentially extraneous variables were the same in all groups.	• Compare groups to determine whether they demonstrate the same proportion of potentially extraneous variables (post hoc data analysis).[a]

[a]If the groups have approximately the same proportion of subjects with a certain extraneous variable, the researcher can conclude that that particular variable's effects were controlled for by the research design and methods.

Type of Variable	Description
Research variable	Neither an independent nor a dependent variable; the focus of a quantitative research study that is neither causative nor predictive.
Modifying variable	A variable that changes the strength, and possibly the direction, of a relationship between other variables.
Mediating variable	A variable that is an intermediate link in the relationship between other variables.
Environmental variable	A characteristic of the study setting.

TABLE 6.9 Other Variables

controlling for extraneous variables. (For additional information on the effects of extraneous variables and researcher-enacted controls, see Chapters 10 and 11.)

Other Variables Encountered in Quantitative Research

Many other types of variables are named in quantitative research reports. The ones discussed in this section include research variable, modifying variables, mediating variables, and environment variables (Table 6.9). **Research variable** is a default term used to refer to a variable that is the focus of a quantitative study but that is not identified as an independent or a dependent variable. Research variables include those stated in the research purpose and question. The design of a study containing research variables is either descriptive or correlational. Cohen, Spirito, Liu, Cato, and Larson (2019) conducted a descriptive study to "determine the incidence of concurrent detection of bacterial pathogens among patients sharing a hospital room" (p. 80). The research variable was bacterial pathogens, identified in the purpose statement and described using descriptive statistics. (The problem and purpose for this study are presented in Chapter 5, Table 5.1.) The researchers recommended improved environmental decontamination as a comprehensive approach to infection prevention in hospitals.

Environmental variables are those that emanate from the research setting. In a healthcare milieu, they include but are not limited to temperature, ambient noise, lighting, rules regulating certain nursing actions, and actions of other patients and family members. If a researcher is studying humans in an uncontrolled or natural setting, it is impossible and sometimes undesirable to control most of the environmental variables. In qualitative, mixed methods, outcomes, and some quantitative (descriptive and correlational) studies, researchers make little or no attempt to control environmental variables. Their intent is to study participants in their natural environment without controlling or altering it. The environmental variables in quasi-experimental and experimental research can be controlled through the use of a study protocol, precise measurement methods, and/or a laboratory setting or research unit in a hospital. If the researcher assesses an environmental variable as potentially interfering with data collection, the variable should be controlled. For example, the presence of an uncontrolled delusional patient in an intensive care unit (ICU) who interrupts collection of physiological data from subjects should be controlled. The data collection process could be delayed until the ICU is quiet and the participants' physiological variables are stable.

Modifying variables, when present, are those that change the strength and sometimes the direction of a relationship between other variables. **Mediating variables** are intermediate variables that occur as links in the chain between independent and dependent variables. Often they provide insight as to the relationship between the independent and dependent variables, especially in physiological research. For example, in their research of self-efficacy, social support, and other psychosocial variables in patients with diabetes and depression, Tovar, Rayens, Gokun, and Clark (2015) found that self-efficacy was an important link between other variables' relationships, reporting that their findings "suggest complete mediation via self-efficacy and some types of social support" (p. 1405). More information on modifying and mediating variables is presented in Chapter 8.

DEFINING CONCEPTS AND OPERATIONALIZING VARIABLES IN QUANTITATIVE STUDIES

A variable can be defined both conceptually and operationally, revealing both its meaning and its means of measurement in a particular study.

Conceptual Definitions

A **conceptual definition** identifies the meaning of an idea. Regardless of methodology, a study's principal concepts require some amount of conceptual definition, first so that the researcher is clear as to what is being studied, and second so that the eventual audience for the research results will understand what was investigated. A conceptual definition can be derived from a theorist's definition of a variable or developed through concept analysis. However, a definition also may be drawn from the theoretical piece of the literature review (see Chapter 8 for potential sources of conceptual definitions). Alternatively, the conceptual definition may be drawn from previous publications on the same topic, a medical dictionary, and even a standard dictionary, and then synthesized by the researcher so as to encompass the study's intended focus.

In quantitative research, conceptual definitions of the principal variables seldom appear in the published report unless the study focuses on concepts and their interactions, which occurs in a predictive correlational design. If conceptual definitions do appear, they can be found in the Literature Review/Background or Methods section of the report.

Defining Concepts in Qualitative Research

In qualitative research, it is typical for the phenomenon of interest to be conceptually defined quite thoroughly. This definition appears in the Introduction section, in the Review of the Literature section, or (less frequently) in the Results or Conclusions section when definition of the phenomenon of interest is the solitary goal of the research. If a definition is interlaced in discussions of its meaning as revealed in other publications, it is derived from the literature or other sources. If it appears later in the report, the definition emanates from the research data and represents at least part of the study results. The Anbari et al. (2019) study, introduced earlier, defined the two meaning systems (local and systematic levels) of patient safety communication in the Results section of their study. The focus of this qualitative study was the description of patient safety communication among differently educated nurses (traditional BSN and ADN to BSN graduates) in clinical practice.

Operational Definitions in Quantitative Research

Operationally defining a concept converts it to a variable and establishes how it will be measured or manipulated in a particular study. The researcher selects the **operational definition** that results in a measurement of the dependent or research variable that is best for that study. The operational definition for an independent variable or intervention indicates how the intervention will be implemented or manipulated in a study. The variables of focus in quantitative, outcomes, and the quantitative part of mixed methods research must be operationally defined. The Johnson et al. (2019) RCT, introduced earlier, conceptually and operationally defined their independent variable (postoperative evidence-based bundle) and dependent variables (length of stay, occurrence of readmission, and patient satisfaction). The definitions for these variables are presented as examples.

Independent Variable: Postoperative Evidence-Based Bundle
Conceptual definition: The Institute of Healthcare Improvement (2016) developed the bundle concept for delivery of "Enhanced recovery programs (ERP)...that focus on early patient education, multimodal pain control, early mobility, and alternate diet plans so the patient can recover faster... (Kalogera & Dowdy, 2016; Modesitt et al., 2016)." (Johnson et al., 2019, p. 39)
Operational definition: "The chosen components of the post-operative bundle protocol [educational packet] included 1) early mobilization, 2) transitioning to oral pain medications, 3) early feeding, and 4) chewing gum." (Johnson et al., 2019, p. 41) This educational packet was given to subjects in the outpatient physician office during the preoperative period.

Dependent Variables
Length of Stay
Conceptual definition: Reduced length of stay is an optimal patient outcome from an ERP (Kalogera & Dowdy, 2016).
Operational definition: Length of stay was operationally defined "as the numbers of days spent in the hospital from the first post-operative day to the day of discharge, counting the operation day as day zero." (Johnson et al., 2019, p. 42)

Occurrence of Readmission
Conceptual definition: Less than optimal patient outcome from an ERP (Kalogera & Dowdy, 2016).
Operational definition: Occurrence of readmission was operationally defined as follows: "Readmission within 30 days was measured through the EMR [electronic medical record]." (Johnson et al., 2019, p. 42)

Patient Satisfaction

Conceptual definition: Optimal patient outcome from an ERP (Kalogera & Dowdy, 2016).

Operational definition: "Patient satisfaction was measured by the Patient Satisfaction survey consisting of seven questions utilizing a Likert scale from excellent to poor (Kalogera et al., 2013). Permission to use and modify the survey was obtained by the authors with an additional question added; 'did you feel that walking during your hospital stay helped in your recovery'...

Data collected during the study period were stored under lock and key in the PI's [principal investigator's] office and entered into a password protected EMR database by the co-investigator." (Johnson et al., 2019, p. 42)

A succinct format in which to present operational definitions is the general statement: "The variable _____ was operationally defined as _____ measured with _____ ..." and then stating other particulars such as "by the research assistant at 10 a.m." or "in the primary care clinic." More specifics about who will measure, when the measurement will be performed, and where the measurement will be obtained are especially important in physiological studies. Often additional details about the implementation of an intervention and measurement of dependent variables are covered in the Methods section.

KEY POINTS

- Research objectives/aims, questions, and hypotheses are formulated to bridge the gap between the more abstractly stated problem and purpose and the detailed plan for data collection and analysis.
- Studies should have a logical flow from the research problem and purpose to the objectives, questions, or hypotheses formulated to guide the study.
- Research objectives or aims are clear, concise, declarative statements expressed in the present tense following the research purpose.
- A research question is a concise, interrogative statement that is worded in the present tense and includes one or more of the study's principal concepts.
- Qualitative studies are usually guided by the research purpose, but some might include a question or objective.
- A hypothesis is a formal statement of a relationship between or among variables, within a specified population.
- Hypotheses can be described in terms of four categories: (1) associative versus causal, (2) simple versus complex, (3) nondirectional versus directional, and (4) null versus research.
- The selection of objectives, questions, and/or hypotheses to guide quantitative, qualitative, mixed methods, and outcomes researcher are described (see Table 6.6).
- Variables or concepts are ideas, qualities, properties, or characteristics of persons, things, or situations that are studied in research.

- Demographic variables are participants' characteristics measured during a study and analyzed to describe a sample.
- Concepts are the focus of qualitative research and the qualitative part of mixed methods research, which include a phenomenon of interest and emergent concepts.
- Variables are concepts of various levels of abstraction that are concisely defined so they can be measure or manipulated within a quantitative or outcomes study.
- The independent variable is the intervention or treatment that the researcher applies to the experimental group but not to the control group. In predictive correlational research, an independent variable is a predictor of the value of the dependent variable.
- The dependent variable is the result or outcome that is the study's focus.
- An extraneous variable is not central to the study's research purpose but has a potential effect on the results, making the independent variable appear more or less powerful than it really is in its effect on the value of the dependent variable.
- A confounding variable is a special subtype of extraneous variable that is intertwined with the independent variable and needs to be controlled if possible, in quasi-experiment and experimental studies.
- Research variable is a default term used to refer to variables that are the focus of a quantitative study but are not independent or dependent variables.

- Environmental variables are those that emanate from the research setting.
- Modifying variables, when present, are variables that change the strength and sometimes the direction of a relationship between other variables.
- Mediating variables are intermediate variables that occur as links in the chain between independent and dependent variables.

- A conceptual definition makes a concept understandable, revealing its meaning.
- An operational definition described how a variable will be measured or manipulated in a particular study.

REFERENCES

Agency for Healthcare Research and Quality. (2013). *Making health care safer II: An updated critical analysis of the evidence for patient safety practices—Executive summary* (Evidence/Technology Assessment No. 211, p. 16). Retrieved from http://archive.ahrq.gov/research/findings/evidence-based-reports/ptsafetyII-full.pdf

Aiken, L. H., Cimiotti, J. P., Sloane, D. M., Smith, H. L., Flynn, L., & Neff, D. F. (2011). Effects of nurse staffing and nurse education on patient deaths in hospitals with different nurse work environments. *Medical Care, 49*(12), 1047–1053. doi:10.1097/MLR.0b013e3182330b6e

Aiken, L. H., Clarke, S. P., Cheung, R. B., Sloane, D. M., & Silber, J. (2003). Educational levels of hospital nurses and surgical patient mortality. *Journal of the American Medical Association, 290*(12), 1617–1623. doi:10.1001/jama.290.12.1617

Aiken, L. H., Sloane, D. M., Bruyneel, L., Van den Heede, K., Griffiths, P., Busse, R., . . . Sermeus, W. (2014). Nurse staffing and education and hospital mortality in nine European countries: A retrospective observational study. *The Lancet, 383*(9931), 1824–1830. doi:10.1016/S0140-6736(13)62631-8

Anbari, A. B., Vogelsmeier, A., & Dougherty, D. S. (2019). Patient safety communication among differently educated nurses: Converging and diverging meaning systems. *Western Journal of Nursing Research, 41*(2), 171–190. doi:10.1177/0193945917747600

Bandalos, D. L. (2018). *Measurement theory and applications for the social sciences.* New York, NY: The Guilford Press.

Charmaz, K. (2014). *Constructing grounded theory* (2nd ed.). Los Angeles, CA: Sage.

Chen, H., & Hu, H. (2019). Randomized trial of modified stretching exercise program for menstrual low back pain. *Western Journal of Nursing Research, 41*(2), 238–257. doi:10.1177/0193945918763817

Chin, E. D., & Armstrong, D. (2019). Anticipated stigma and healthcare utilization in COPD and neurological disorders. *Applied Nursing Research, 45*(1), 63–68. doi:10.1016/j.apnr.2018.12.002

Chinn, P. L., & Kramer, M. K. (2015). *Knowledge development in nursing: Theory and process* (9th ed.). St. Louis, MO: Elsevier Mosby.

Cohen, B., Spirito, C. M., Liu, J., Cato, K. D., & Larson, E. (2019). Concurrent detection of bacterial pathogens in hospital roommates. *Nursing Research, 68*(1), 80–83. doi:10.1097/NNR.0000000000000316

Creswell, J. W., & Clark, V. L. P. (2018). *Designing and conducting mixed methods research* (3rd ed.). Los Angeles, CA: Sage.

Creswell, J. W., & Creswell, J. D. (2018). *Research design: Qualitative, quantitative, and mixed methods approaches* (5th ed.). Los Angeles, CA: Sage.

Creswell, J. W., & Poth, C. N. (2018). *Qualitative inquiry & research design: Choosing among five approaches* (4th ed.). Los Angeles, CA: Sage.

Gathright, E. C., Goldstein, C. M., Loucks, E. B., Busch, A. M., Stabile, L., & Wu, W. (2019). Examination of clinical and psychosocial determinants of exercise capacity change in cardiac rehabilitation. *Heart & Lung, 48*(1), 13–17. doi:10.1016/j.hrtlng.2018.07.007

Grove, S. K., & Cipher, DJ. (2020). *Statistics for nursing research: A workbook for evidence-based practice* (3rd ed.). St. Louis, MO: Elsevier. In press.

Institute for Healthcare Improvement. (2016). *About us: Innovations.* Retrieved from http://www.ihi.org/about/Pages/innovationscontributions.aspx

Johnson, K., Razo, S., Smith, J., Cain, A., & Soper, K. (2019). Optimize patient outcomes among females undergoing gynecological surgery: A randomized controlled trial. *Applied Nursing Research, 45*(1), 39–44. doi:10.106/j.apnr.2018.12.005

Kalogera, E., & Dowdy, S. (2016). Enhanced recovery pathway in gynecologic surgery: Improving outcomes through evidence-based medicine. *Obstetrics and Gynecology Clinics of North America, 43*(3), 551–573. doi:10.1016/j.ogc.2016.04.006

Kalogera, E., Bakkum-Gamez, J. N., Jankowski, C. J., Trabuco, E., Lovely, J. K., Dhanorker, S., . . . Dowdy, S. (2013). Enhanced recovery in gynecologic surgery. *Obstetrics and Gynecology, 122*(2), 319–328. doi:10.1097/AOG.0b013e31829aa780

Kane, R. L., & Radosevich, D. M. (2011). *Conducting health outcomes research*. Sudbury, MA: Jones & Bartlett Learning.

Kazdin, A. E. (2017). *Research design in clinical psychology* (5th ed.). Boston, MA: Pearson.

Kerlinger, F. N., & Lee, H. B. (2000). *Foundations of behavioral research* (4th ed.). Fort Worth, TX: Harcourt College Publishers.

Linhares, M. B. M., Doca, F. N. P., Martinez, F. E., Carlotti, A. P. P., Cassiano, R. G. M., Pfeifer, L. I., ... Finley, G. A. (2012). Pediatric pain: Prevalence, assessment, and management in a teaching hospital. *Brazilian Journal of Medical and Biological Research, 45*(12), 1287–1294. doi:10.1590/S0100-879X2012007500147

Marshall, C., & Rossman, G. B. (2016). *Designing qualitative research* (6th ed.). Los Angeles, CA: Sage.

Marshall, C., Forgeron, P., Harrison, D., & Young, N. L. (2018). Exploration of nurses' pediatric pain management experiences in rural hospitals: A qualitative descriptive study. *Applied Nursing Research, 42*(1), 89–97. doi:10.1016/j.apnr.2018.06.009

Melnyk, B. M., & Fineout-Overholt, E. (2019). *Evidence-based practice in nursing and healthcare: A guide to best practice* (4th ed.). Philadelphia, PA: Wolters Kluwer.

Melnyk, B. M., Gallagher-Ford, L., Zellefrow, C., Tudher, S., Van Dromme, L., & Thomas, B. K. (2018). Outcomes from the first Helene Fuld Health Trust National Institute for Evidence-Based Practice in Nursing and Healthcare Invitational Expert Forum. *Worldviews on Evidence-Based Nursing, 15*(1), 5–15. doi:10.1111/wvn.12272

Modesitt, S. C., Sarosiek, B. M., Trowbridge, E. R., Redick, D. L., Shah, P. M., Thiele, R. H., ... Hedrick, T. L. (2016). Enhanced recovery implementation in major gynecologic surgeries: Effect of care standardization. *Obstetrics & Gynecology, 128*(3), 457–466. doi:10.1097/AOG.0000000000001555

Moorhead, S., Swanson, E., Johnson, M., & Maas, M. L. (2018). *Nursing outcomes classification (NOC): Measurement of health outcomes* (6th ed.). St. Louis, MO: Elsevier.

National Research Council. (2000). *To err is human: Building a safer health system*. Washington, DC: The National Academies Press. Retrieved from http://www.nap.edu/catalog.php?record_id=9728

Nowakowski-Grier, L. A. (2018). *The impact of implementing an inpatient diabetes nurse mentor program on the 30-day readmission rates among diabetic patients, 1-1*. ISBN: 9780355947588; AN: 131799047.

Popper, K. R. (1968). *The logic of scientific discovery*. New York, NY: Harper & Row, Publishers.

Rieder, J. K., Goshin, L. S., Sissoko, D. R. G., Kleshchova, O., & Weierich, M. R. (2019). Salivary biomarkers of parenting stress in mothers under community criminal justice supervision. *Nursing Research, 68*(1), 48–56. doi:10.109/NNR.0000000000000323

Shadish, W. R., Cook, T. D., & Campbell, D. T. (2002). *Experimental and quasi-experimental designs for generalized causal inference*. Chicago, IL: Rand McNally.

Smith, M. J., & Liehr, P. R. (2018). *Middle range theory for nursing* (4th ed.). New York, NY: Springer Publishing Company.

Theeke, L., Carpenter, R. D., Mallow, J., & Theeke, E. (2019). Gender differences in loneliness, anger, depression, self-management ability and biomarkers of chronic illness in chronically ill mid-life adults in Appalachia. *Applied Nursing Research, 45*(1), 55–62. doi:10.1016/j.apnr.2018.12.001

The Institute of Medicine. (2010). *The future of nursing: Leading change, advancing health*. Author. Retrieved from https://www.nap.edu/catalog/12956/the-futureof-nursing-leading-change-advancing-health/

The Joint Commission. (2017). *Hospital: 2018 national patient safety goals*. Retrieved from https://www.jointcommission.org/hap_2017_npsgs/

Tovar, E., Rayens, M. K., Gokun, Y., & Clark, M. (2015). Mediators of adherence among adults with comorbid diabetes and depression: The role of self-efficacy and social support. *Journal of Health Psychology, 20*(110), 1405–1415. doi:10.1177/1359105313512514

Tri-Council for Nursing. (2010). *Educational advancement of registered nurses: A consensus position*. Retrieved from http://www.aacnnursing.org/Portals/42/ News/5-10-TricouncilEdStatement.pdf?ver=2017-07-27-121244-310

Twycross, A., & Williams, A. (2014). Pain: A biopsychosocial phenomenon. In A. Twycross, S. Dowden, & J. Stinson (Eds.), *Managing pain in children: A clinical guide for nurses and other healthcare professionals* (2nd ed., pp. 36–47). West Sussex, United Kingdom: John Wiley & Sons Ltd.

Vasilevskis, E. E., Shah, A. S., Hollingsworth, E. K., Shotwell, M. S., Mixon, A. S., Bell, S. P., ... Shed-MEDS Team. (2019). A patient-centered deprescribing intervention for hospitalized older patients with polypharmacy: Rationale and design of the Shed-MEDS randomized controlled trial. *BMC Health Services Research, 19*, 1–13. doi:10.1186/s12913-019-3995-3

Waltz, C. F., Strickland, O. L., & Lenz, E. R. (2017). *Measurement in nursing and health research* (5th ed.). New York, NY: Springer Publishing Company.

Zauszniewski, J. A. (2016). Resourcefulness. *Western Journal of Nursing Research, 38*(12), 1551–1553. doi:10.1177/0193945916665079

Zauszniewski, J. A. (2018). Resourcefulness. In J. J. Fitzpatrick (Ed.), *Encyclopedia of nursing research* (pp. 448–449). New York, NY: Springer.

Zauszniewski, J. A., Herbell, K., & Burant, C. (2019). Is there more to resourcefulness than personal and social skills? *Western Journal of Nursing Research, 41*(3), 372–387. doi:10.1177/0193945918790930

7

Review of Relevant Literature

Christy Bomer-Norton

http://evolve.elsevier.com/Gray/practice/

New knowledge is being generated constantly. Fortunately, electronic databases have been developed that can be searched to identify and retrieve publications on a specific topic (Aveyard, 2019). Relevant literature is easily found, but then the challenge lies in selecting the most relevant sources from a very large number of articles. The tasks of reading, critically appraising, analyzing, and synthesizing can become formidable. Tools to manage the complexity of writing a literature review can make the endeavor feasible. The goal of this chapter is to provide basic knowledge and skills about how to write a literature review, beginning with answers to some preliminary questions that the student may have related to that task. The chapter is designed primarily for the nurse with little experience in writing a review of the literature.

GETTING STARTED: FREQUENTLY ASKED QUESTIONS

What Is a Literature Review?

The **literature review** of a research report is an interpretative, organized, and written presentation of what the study's author has read (Aveyard, 2019). The purpose of conducting a review of the literature is to discover the most recent, and the most relevant, information about a particular phenomenon. The literature review provides an answer to the question, "What is known on this topic?" The literature review may be a synthesis of research findings, an overview of relevant theories, or a description of knowledge on a topic (Paré, Trudel, Jaana, & Kitsiou, 2015). Developing the ability to write coherently about what you have found in the literature requires time and planning. You will organize the information you find into sections by themes, trends, or variables. The purpose is not to list all of the material published, but rather to evaluate, interpret, and synthesize the sources you have read. There are four principal reasons a nurse may conduct a literature review. First, for a nursing student, writing a review of the literature is a course requirement, as in "generate a literature review." Second, as an end-program goal, especially at the master's level, some programs assign a capstone project that includes a substantial literature review and summary. The third reason is that a literature review is part of the formal research proposal and subsequent report that represents the summative requirement at the end of a master's or doctoral program. Fourth, nurses in practice may be seeking answers to clinical problems and include their review of the literature as part of a proposal to administrators to implement changes.

What Is the "Literature"?

The **literature** consists of all written sources relevant to the selected topic. It consists of printed and electronic newspapers, encyclopedias, conference papers, scientific journals, textbooks, other books, theses, dissertations, and clinical journals. Websites and reports developed by government agencies and professional organizations are included as well. For example, if you were writing a paper on diabetes mellitus, statistics about the prevalence and cost of the disease could be obtained from publications by the Centers for Disease Control and Prevention and the World Health Organization (WHO). Not every source that you find, however, will prove valid and legitimate for scholarly use. The website of a company that sells insulin may not be an appropriate source for diabetes statistics. Wikipedia and online health encyclopedias may be helpful for gathering preliminary information on a topic such as identifying keywords to use in searching for professional sources. Scholarly papers and graduate course assignments may require that you use exclusively peer-reviewed professional literature as source material, and Wikipedia is not peer reviewed.

Peer review is the process whereby a scholarly abstract, paper, or book is read and evaluated by one or more experts, who make recommendations as to its worth to the professional discipline (Adams & Lawrence, 2019). Peer review is used for many journal submissions and for abstracts submitted for podium or poster presentation at professional conferences. These are accepted or rejected by the journal editor or conference presentation coordinator on the basis of peer review.

What Types of Literature Can I Expect to Find?

You will be able to find a wide variety of literature because of databases. A **database** is a compilation of citations. The database consists of computer data, collected and arranged to be searchable and automatically retrievable. The database may be a broad collection of citations from a variety of disciplines or may consist of citations relevant to a specific discipline or field. Sometimes the latter are called subject-specific electronic databases (Aveyard, 2019). The Cumulative Index to Nursing and Allied Health Literature (CINAHL) is a subject-specific database widely used in nursing.

When searching, you will find two broad types of literature that are cited in the review of literature for a research study: theoretical and empirical. **Theoretical literature** consists of concept analyses, models, theories, and conceptual frameworks that support a selected research problem and purpose. **Empirical literature** is comprised of knowledge derived from research. The quantity of empirical literature depends on the study problem and the number of research reports available. Extensive empirical literature can be found related to common illnesses and health processes: caring for a person with Alzheimer disease, making health promotion and prevention decisions, or coping with cancer treatment. For newer topics or rare diseases, less literature may be available. When searching for empirical literature, you may find seminal and landmark studies. **Seminal studies** are the studies that

prompted the initiation of a field of research. **Landmark studies** are published research that led to an important development or a turning point in a certain field of study. The National Institute of Nursing Research document, *Changing Practice, Changing Lives: 10 Landmark Nursing Research Studies* (2006) provides examples of key landmark studies in nursing. By citing seminal or landmark papers on their topics, authors indicated their awareness of how knowledge has developed as a result of research that has changed their respective fields of study.

Literature is disseminated in several different formats. **Serials** are published over time or may be published in multiple volumes at one time but do not necessarily have recurrent and predictable publication dates. **Periodicals** are subsets of serials with predictable publication dates, such as journals. Periodicals are published over time and are numbered sequentially. This sequential numbering is seen in the year, volume, issue, and page numbering of a journal. The reference for the article by Dale et al. (2019) is as follows:

Dale, J. C., Hallas, D., & Spratling, R. (2019). *Critiquing research evidence for use in practice: Revisited. Journal of Pediatric Health Care 33*(3), 342–346.

The reference indicates that the article was published in volume 33, issue 3, on pages 342 to 346 in the periodical *Journal of Pediatric Health Care*. Next year, the periodical will be identified as volume 34 and the first issue will begin again with page 1. Some journals are published in electronic form only. Because of the high costs of publishing and distributing a printed journal, a publishing company risks losing money unless there is a large market for that journal. Faculty members at some universities have established online journals in particular specialty areas for smaller potential audiences. Online journals may have more current information on your topic than you will find in traditional journals, because the time to review the manuscript is shorter, and accepted manuscripts can be published quickly. Articles submitted to printed journals are usually under review for 8 to 12 weeks and, if accepted, may not be seen in print for up to 1 year. Because of competition from online journals, some print journals are releasing their accepted articles online before publication.

Some online journals are considered open sources. This means that their articles are available online to anyone searching the internet, instead of access being limited to those persons with a subscription to the journal. When you use a journal published online only, be sure to check the journal description to discover whether the journal is peer reviewed. Open-source journals may or may not be peer reviewed.

Monographs, such as books, hardcopy conference proceedings, and pamphlets, are written and published for a specific purpose and may be updated with a new edition as needed. Researchers may present their findings at a national or international conference prior to publishing them, so searching conference proceedings can increase awareness of cutting-edge knowledge in a research area. **Textbooks** are monographs written as resource materials for educational programs. Textbooks and articles that in the past would have been difficult to obtain through interlibrary loan are now available for download to a reading device, cell phone, tablet, laptop, or other computer 24 hours a day.

To develop the significance and background section of a proposal, you might search relevant **government reports** from the United States and other countries. For example, researchers proposing an intervention study related to malaria in Uganda, East Africa, should search the Uganda government's Ministry of Health website for standards and treatment guidelines for malaria. Researchers developing smoking cessation programs for adolescents living in rural communities would do well to consult the *Healthy People 2020* website for the national goals related to smoking cessation among adolescents (and remember that *Healthy People 2030* will be released in 2020 [https://www.healthypeople.gov/]).

Position papers are disseminated by professional organizations, government agencies, and nongovernment organizations to promote a particular viewpoint on a debatable issue. Position papers, along with descriptions of clinical situations, may be included in a discussion of the background and significance of a research problem. For example, a researcher developing a proposal on factors associated with rising cesarean section rates in the United States would benefit from the review of both the WHO website, which has a position paper available online entitled, *WHO Recommendations: Non-clinical Interventions to Reduce Unnecessary Caesarean Sections* (WHO, 2018), and the American College of Nurse-Midwives (ACNM) website, which has a position paper available online entitled, *Elective Primary Cesarean Birth* (ACNM, 2016).

Master's theses and doctoral dissertations are valuable literature as well and are available electronically through ProQuest, a collection of dissertations and theses (https://www.proquest.com/products-services/dissertations/). A **thesis** is a research project completed as part of the requirements for a master's degree. A **dissertation** is the written report of an extensive research project completed as the final requirement for a doctoral degree. Theses (plural for thesis) and dissertations can be found by searching ProQuest and other library databases, such as CINAHL. Most Doctorate of Philosophy (PhD) dissertations represent original research, not replication studies.

The published literature contains primary and secondary sources. A **primary source** is written by the person who originated, or is responsible for generating, the ideas published (Aveyard, 2019). A research publication authored by the person or people who conducted the research is a primary source. A theoretical book or paper written by the theorist who developed that theory or conceptual content is a primary source. A **secondary source** summarizes or quotes content from primary sources (Adams & Lawrence, 2019). Thus authors of secondary sources interpret the works of researchers and theorists, paraphrase the information, and cite the primary articles in their papers. You must read secondary sources with caution, knowing that the secondary authors' interpretations may have been influenced by their own perceptions and biases. Sometimes authors have spread errors and misinterpretations by using secondary sources rather than primary sources (Aveyard, 2019). You should use primary sources as much as possible when writing literature reviews. However, secondary sources are properly used in several instances. Box 7.1 lists situations in which it is appropriate to cite a secondary source. **Citation** is the act of quoting or paraphrasing a source within the body of a paper, using it as an example or presenting it as support for a position taken.

Why Write a Review of the Literature?

Literature reviews require time and energy. Before making that investment, be sure you understand the purpose of the review. You may be reviewing the literature as part of writing a formal paper in a course, or you may be examining published research to discover evidence for use in practice, either to make a change or to oppose a proposed change. At other points in your career, you may be reviewing the literature to write a research proposal. Understanding the purpose for reviewing the

BOX 7.1 **Situations in Which Using Secondary Sources Are Appropriate**

1. The primary source has been destroyed or cannot be accessed.
2. The primary source is in print only and located at such a distance that the cost of travel to review it would be prohibitive.
3. The primary source is written in a language not currently spoken or in one that the researcher has not mastered.
4. The primary publication is written in unfamiliar jargon that is very difficult to decipher, but a secondary source analyzes and simplifies the material.
5. The secondary source contains creative ideas or a unique organization of information not found in the primary source.

literature can guide your efforts and yield a high-quality product. In the next sections, each of these purposes is described.

Writing a Course Paper

While reading the syllabus for a course, you learn one of the course assignments involves a literature review. The professor indicates that you will review published sources on a selected topic, analyze what you read, and write a formal paper that includes those sources. Reviews of the literature for a course assignment vary depending on the level of educational program, the purpose of the assignment, and the expectations of the instructor. The depth, scope, and breadth of a literature review increase as you move from undergraduate courses, to master's level courses, to doctoral courses.

The role for which you are preparing also will shape the review. For a paper in a nurse practitioner course, you might review pharmacology and pathology reference texts in addition to journal articles. In a nursing education course, you may review neurological development, cognitive science, and general education publications to write a paper on a teaching strategy. For a course about clinical information systems in a Doctorate of Nursing Practice program, the review might extend into computer science and hospital management literature. For a theory course in a PhD program, your review may need to include all of the publications of a specific theorist, or you might be expected to write a review of 5 to 10 theories that pertain to one area of nursing inquiry.

For each of these papers, clarify with your professor the publication years and the type of literature to be included. The professor may also indicate the acceptable length of the written review of the literature. Reviews of the literature for course assignments tend to focus on what is known, the strength of the evidence, and the implications of the knowledge. Discussion board postings in a course may also require citations of peer-review literature.

Evaluating Clinical Practice

Another reason to review the literature is to determine whether clinical practice is consistent with the latest research evidence (Dale, Hallas, & Spratling, 2019). In this context, it is necessary to identify all studies that provide evidence of a particular nursing intervention, critically appraise the strength of each individual study's research processes, synthesize the findings of all the studies, and provide an analytical summary. In addition to primary source research reports, any existing systematic literature reviews of the collective evidence for or against a particular intervention should also be included. The search should also include existing evidence-based practice guidelines. Evidence-based practice guidelines are based on prior syntheses of the literature about the nursing intervention in question. Literature syntheses related to promoting evidence-based nursing practice are described in detail in Chapter 19.

Developing a Qualitative Research Proposal

From perusal of the literature, you have identified a research problem and have chosen to address that problem by conducting a qualitative study. The literature also provides information that you may use to establish the significance of the research problem (Marshall & Rossman, 2016). At this point, you need to select the type of qualitative study you plan to conduct, because the purpose and timing of the literature review vary by the type of study (see Chapter 12). In general, phenomenologists believe that no further literature review should be undertaken until after the data have been collected and analyzed so that the knowledge of the results of prior studies in the area does not intrude upon the researcher's interpretation of the text of interviews and other data.

Classical grounded theory researchers begin with tabula rasa, a "blank slate," an attempt to know as little as possible about the area of study before they begin the research. The purpose of a brief literature review prior to beginning the study is to discover whether this particular study has been performed before. As the process progresses, the researchers collect and analyze all data before they return to the literature, so that the entirety of the analysis is grounded in their data, not in the literature (Charmaz, 2014). When the core concept or process has been identified and data analysis is complete, the researcher theoretically samples the literature for extant theories that may assist in explaining and extending the emerging theory (Munhall, 2012).

The role of the literature review for ethnographical research is similar to the role of the literature review for quantitative research. The process of ethnographical research includes extensive preparation before data collection, to familiarize oneself with the culture, and this includes a detailed review of the literature. The literature review provides a background for both conducting the study and interpreting the findings.

Researchers who plan to conduct exploratory-descriptive qualitative study frequently have conducted an extensive review of the literature and found a dearth of research on the topic of interest. The lack of knowledge on the topic supports the need for an exploratory-descriptive qualitative study. Following data collection, the researcher will compare the findings to the literature. Consequently, review of the literature in exploratory-descriptive research usually occurs before and after data collection. Chapter 12 describes in more detail the role of the literature review in qualitative research.

Developing a Quantitative Research Proposal

Quantitative research studies, whether descriptive, correlational, quasi-experimental, or experimental in design, are shaped by the review of literature. Outcomes research and the quantitative portion of mixed methods research are also shaped by the review of the literature in the same way as quantitative research. Based on the review of the literature, you decide a quantitative (or outcomes or mixed methods) study is the best way to address a particular research problem. You plan a study to add knowledge in the area of the identified gap. For example, earlier researchers found that an intervention reduced hospital-acquired infections among postoperative patients who had no history of diabetes mellitus. After a thorough review of the literature, you identify a specific gap in knowledge: The intervention's efficacy has not yet been tested with diabetic, postoperative

patients. You decide to replicate the earlier study with a sample of postoperative diabetic patients. After data collection is complete, you analyze the data and then you again use the literature to compare your findings to those of earlier studies, as well as to other related studies. Your goal is to integrate knowledge from the literature with new information obtained from the study in progress.

Table 7.1 describes the role of the literature throughout the development and implementation of a quantitative study. The types of sources needed and the way you search the literature vary throughout the study. The introduction section uses relevant sources to summarize the background and significance of the research problem. The Review of the Literature section includes both theoretical and empirical sources that document current knowledge of the problem. The researcher develops the Framework section from theoretical literature. If little theoretical literature is found, the researcher may choose to develop a tentative theory to guide the study based on findings of previous research studies (see Chapter 8 for more information) and on the posited relationships in the current study's research hypothesis. In the Methods section, the design, sample, measurement methods, treatment, and data collection processes of the planned study are described. Research texts, describing standards of methodological rigor, and previous studies are cited in this section. In the Results section, the researcher cites sources for the different types of statistical analyses conducted and the computer software used to conduct these analyses. The Discussion section of the research report begins with what the results mean, in light of the results of previous studies. Conclusions are drawn that are a synthesis of the findings from previous studies and from the current study.

PRACTICAL CONSIDERATIONS FOR PERFORMING A LITERATURE REVIEW

How Long Will the Review of the Literature Take?

The time required to review the literature is influenced by the problem studied, the available sources, and the reviewer's goals. The literature review for a topic that is focused and somewhat narrow may require less time than one for a broader topic. The difficulty experienced identifying and locating sources and the number of

TABLE 7.1 Literature in the Quantitative Research Proposal and Report

Phase of the Research Process	How Literature Is Used and Its Role
Research topic	• Narrow topic by reading widely about what is known and what is not known; identify the relevant concepts.
Statement of the research problem, including background and significance of the problem	• Search books and articles to provide an overview of the topic. • Search government reports and other documents to find facts about the size, cost, and consequences of the research problem. • Synthesize literature to identify the specific gap in knowledge that this study will address.
Research framework	• Find and read relevant frameworks. • Develop conceptual definitions of concepts.
Purpose; research questions or hypotheses	• Based on the review of literature and the research problem, state the purpose of the study. • Decide whether there is adequate evidence to state a hypothesis.
Review of the literature	• Find evidence to support why the selected methods are appropriate. • Summarize current empirical knowledge that is related to the topic.
Methodology	• Compare research designs of reviewed studies to select the most appropriate design for the proposed study. • Identify possible instruments or measures of variables. • Describe performance of measures in previous studies. • Provide operational definitions of concepts. • Develop sampling strategies based on what has been learned from studies in the literature.
Findings	• Refer to statistical textbooks to explain the results of the data analysis.
Discussion	• Compare the findings with those of previously reviewed studies. • Return to the literature to find new references to interpret unexpected findings. • Refer to theory sources to relate the findings to the research framework.
Conclusions	• On the basis of previous literature and the current study's findings, draw conclusions. • Discuss implications for nursing clinical practice, administration, and education.

sources to be located also influence the time involved, as does the intensity of effort.

You, as a novice reviewer, will require more time to find the relevant literature than an experienced searcher would require. Consequently, you may underestimate the time needed for the review. Finding 20 relevant sources may take 10 to 15 hours. Usually reading and synthesizing the articles or reports take twice as long as finding the sources (20–30 hours). Graduate students new to the process may need three times as long for reading and developing a detailed synthesis. As searching skills are refined, and the synthesis process becomes more familiar, the required time decreases. Often, performing a literature review is limited by the time that the reviewer can commit to the task. The best strategy is to begin as early as possible and stay focused on the purpose of the review, so as to use time efficiently and prepare the best review possible given the circumstances.

How Many Sources Do I Need to Review?

Many students ask, "How many articles should I have? How many years back should I look to find relevant information?" The answer to both questions is an emphatic, "It depends." Faculty for master's courses commonly require use of full-text articles published in the previous 5 to 10 years that describe studies relevant to the concepts or variables in the proposed study. Seminal and landmark studies should be included, even though they may have been published prior to the time frame the instructor designates. Doctoral students must conduct thorough reviews for course papers, with expectations for increasing analytical sophistication throughout their programs (Wisker, 2015). If you are writing a research proposal for a thesis or dissertation, the literature review will be required to be comprehensive, which means that it will include most or all of the literature that is pertinent to the topic. A comprehensive review includes all of the key papers in a given field of interest. After some initial searches, it is important to discuss what exists in that particular sphere of the literature with the course instructor, thesis chairperson, or dissertation chairperson, who will help you determine a reasonable time period and scope for the review.

Am I Expected to Read Every Word of the Available Sources?

No. If researchers attempted to read every word of every source that is somewhat related to a selected problem, they would be well read but would not complete the course assignment or develop their study proposals. With the availability of full-text online articles, the researcher can easily become lost in the literature and forget the focus of the review. Becoming a skilled reviewer of the literature involves finding a balance and learning to identify the most pertinent and relevant sources. On the other hand, you cannot critically appraise and synthesize what you have not read. Avoid being distracted by information in the article that is not relevant to your topic. Learn to read with a purpose.

STAGES OF A LITERATURE REVIEW

The stages of a literature review reflect a systems model. Systems have input, throughput, and output. The input consists of the sources that you find through searching the literature. The throughput consists of the processes you use to read, critically appraise, analyze, and synthesize that literature. The written literature review is the output of these processes (Fig. 7.1). The quality of the input and throughput will determine the quality of

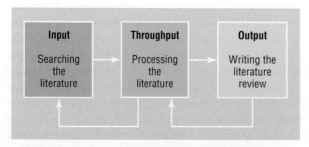

Fig. 7.1 Systems model of the review of the literature.

the output. As a result, attention to detail at each stage is critical to producing a high-quality literature review. Although these stages are presented here as sequential, you will move back and forth between stages. Through an iterative process you expand, refine, and clarify the written review (Wisker, 2015). For example, during the analysis and synthesis of sources, you identify that the studies you cite were conducted only in Europe. You might go back, search the literature again, and specifically search for studies conducted on the topic in other countries. When reading your literature review in progress, you may identify a problem with the logic of the presentation. To resolve it, you will return to the processing stage to rethink and edit the review.

Searching the Literature

Before writing a literature review, you must first perform an organized literature search to identify sources relevant to the topic of interest, keeping in mind the purpose of the review. Whether you are a student, a nurse in clinical practice, or a nurse researcher, the goal is to develop a search strategy to retrieve as much of the relevant literature as possible, given the time constraints of the project (Aveyard, 2019).

Because of the magnitude of available literature, start by setting inclusion criteria. For example, your teacher may have specified that only peer-reviewed or scholarly sources are acceptable. You can set the search engine to retrieve only articles that meet that criterion. As mentioned earlier, other inclusion criteria may be the year of publication or a keyword. A **keyword** is a term or short phrase that is characteristic of a specific type or topic of research (Adams & Lawrence, 2019). For example, keywords for a study of women's adaptation to a diagnosis of multiple sclerosis might include *women, coping,* and *multiple sclerosis.* Consider consulting with an information professional, such as a subject specialist librarian, to develop a literature search strategy (Adams & Lawrence, 2019; Booth, Colomb, Williams, Bizup, & Fitzgerald, 2016; Tensen, 2018). Often these consultations can be performed via e-mail or a Web-based meeting, eliminating the need for travel.

Develop a Search Plan

Before beginning a search, you must consider exactly what information you seek. A written plan helps avoid duplication of effort. Your initial search should be based on the widest possible interpretation of the topic. This

TABLE 7.2	Plan and Record for Searching the Literature			
Database Searched	**Date of Search**	**Search Strategy and Limiters**	**Number and Type of Articles Found**	**Estimate of Relevant Articles**
Cumulative Index to Nursing and Allied Health Literature (CINAHL)				
MEDLINE				
Academic Search Premier				
Cochrane Library				

strategy enables you to envision the extent of the relevant literature. As you see the results of the initial efforts and begin reading the material, you will refine the topic and then narrow the focus for subsequent searches.

As you work through the literature, add selected search terms to the written plan, such as keywords and other words and phrases that you discover while reviewing pertinent references (Aveyard, 2019). For each search, record (1) the name of the database, (2) the date, (3) search terms and searching strategy, (4) the number and types of articles found, and (5) an estimate of the proportion of retrieved citations that were relevant. Table 7.2 is an example of a chart that you can use to record what sources you accessed and how you conducted the search. Some databases allow you to create an account and save a search history online (i.e., the record of what and how you searched). You also may want to export the results of each search to a Word document on a computer, Cloud storage, or external device such as a flash drive.

Select Databases to Search

There are different types of databases. Library electronic databases contain titles, authors, publication dates, and locations for hardcopy books and documents, government reports, and reference books. A library database also includes a searchable list of the journals to which the library maintains a subscription: electronic, paper, or both. Databases typically are comprised of citations that include authors, title, journal, keywords, and usually an abstract of each article (Adams & Lawrence, 2019). For example, nursing's subject-specific electronic database, CINAHL, contains an extensive listing of nursing publications and uses more nursing terminology as subject headings than would a non-nursing journal. With the greater focus on interdisciplinary research, nurse researchers must be consumers of the literature available from the National Library of Medicine

(MEDLINE), government agencies, and professional organizations. Table 7.3 provides descriptions of commonly used databases relevant to nursing.

When two databases are provided by the same company, such as EBSCO Publishing, a simultaneous search of more than one database can be performed to save time. Usually the search engine will combine the results into a single list and automatically delete duplications. You also can change the order in which the results of the search are shown. For example, with EBSCO Publishing databases, you can sort the citations by relevance, date descending (most current first), or date ascending (oldest to more recent).

Search Strategies
Keywords

When a keyword is typed into the search box of an online search engine, such as MEDLINE or CINAHL, each reference on the resultant list contains that keyword. **Subject terms** are standardized phrases and are more formal than keywords. Most databases have a thesaurus for the database in which you can find subject terms. You can also combine subject terms and keywords to expand or focus the literature review. For instance, a search for *heart attack* may yield a few articles. Adding the terms *myocardial infarction, MI,* or *cardiovascular event* may result in a longer list of articles. In contrast, adding the term *women* to the previous search would result in fewer articles, because the search would eliminate studies with samples that were all men.

A simple way to begin identifying a database's standardized subject terms is to search using one of your keywords and display full records of a few relevant citations. The records, in addition to the citations and abstracts of the articles, will include subject terms. The subject terms for the article are listed near the end of the abstract. Examine the terminology used to describe

TABLE 7.3   Databases

Name of Database	Description of the Database by the Publisher[a]
Cumulative Index to Nursing and Allied Health Literature (CINAHL)	"Indexing for more than 5,300 journals, 70 full-text journals… including nursing, biomedicine, health sciences librarianship, alternative/complementary medicine, consumer health and 17 allied health disciplines."
MEDLINE	"Created by the United States National Library of Medicine, MEDLINE is an authoritative bibliographic database containing citations and abstracts for biomedical and health journals." "Citations from over 5,200 worldwide journals…in life sciences with a concentration on biomedicine."
PubMed	"More than 29 million citations for biomedical literature from MEDLINE, life science journals, and online books. Citations may include links to full-text content from PubMed Central and publisher web sites."
PsycARTICLES	"More than 200,000 full-text articles from more than 100 journals…collection from American Psychological Association (APA) provides access to the full spectrum of study in the field."
PsycINFO	"Behavioral and social science research…. Indexing of more than 2,500 journals, 99% of which are peer-reviewed."
Academic Search Complete	"More than 6,300 active full-text journals and magazines. More than 5,700 active full-text peer-reviewed journals…covers a broad range of important areas of academic study, including anthropology, engineering, law, sciences and more."
Health Source Nursing/ Academic Edition	"More than 320 full-text…nursing and allied health journals, many of which are peer-reviewed."
Psychological and Behavioral Sciences Collection	"More than 480 full-text journals." "Subjects include anthropology, emotional and behavioral characteristics, mental processes, observational and experimental methods, psychiatry and psychology."

[a]Direct quotations from EBSCO Publishing descriptions of the databases, available at http://www.ebscohost.com/academic/. Except direct quotation for PubMed database available at https://www.ncbi.nlm.nih.gov/pubmed/.

the major concepts in these articles, and use the same terms to refine additional searches and reveal related articles. Frequently, word-processing programs, dictionaries, and encyclopedias are helpful in identifying synonymous terms and subheadings. Using a combination of keywords and formal subject terms may result in targeted search results.

The format and spelling of search terms can yield different results. Truncating words can allow you to locate more citations related to that term. For example, authors might have used terms such as *intervene, intervenes, intervened, intervening, intervention,* or *intervener.* To capture all of these terms, you can use a truncated term in your search, such as *interven, interven*,* or *interven$.* The form or symbol used to truncate a search term depends on the rule of the search engine you are using. On the other hand, avoid shortening a search word to fewer than four or five letters. If you shorten intervene to *inte** (four letters), the search will contain all articles using the words *internal, interstellar, intestine, integral,*

integrity, intellect, intemperance, intensity, internecine, intervertebral, intern, and *intermittent,* to name a few, taking the searcher far afield from intervene. Also, pay attention to variant spellings. You may need to search, for example, by *orthopedic* or *orthopaedic* (British spelling). For irregular plurals, such as *woman* and *women,* enter both terms into the search.

Authors

If you identify an author who has published on your topic, you can find additional articles written by the same person by including the name as an author term, not a keyword term, during your search. Recognize that some databases list authors only under first and middle initials, whereas others use full first names. Using a general search engine such as Google or Yahoo, search by the author's name, and you may find a personal or university website with a list of their publications.

You may also want to find other researchers who cited the author, and this is especially true for authors who published seminal or landmark studies. Some databases allow you to search the citations and find recent publications in which the author is cited. Web of Science (available at https://clarivate.com/products/web-of-science/) is one such database that combines the *Science Citation Index, Social Science Citation Index, Arts & Humanities Index*, as well as indexes of conference proceedings (Clarivate Analytics, 2019). Indexes such as Web of Science may require that your library subscribe to their services, however. Several other databases, depending on the company, may also have a function for searching the references of articles.

Complex Searches

A complex search of the literature combines two or more concepts or synonyms in one search. There are several ways to arrange terms in a database search phrase or phrases. The three most common ways are by using (1) Boolean operators, (2) locational operators (field labels), and (3) positional operators. **Operators** are words with specific functions that permit you to group ideas, select places to search in a database record, and show relationships within a database record, sentence, or paragraph. Examine the Help screen of a database carefully to determine whether the operators you want to use are available and how they are used.

The **Boolean operators** are the three words *AND, OR*, and *NOT*. In most search engines, the words must be capitalized for them to function in this way. Use AND when you want to search for the presence of two or more terms in the same citation. For example, to find studies in which medication adherence of hypertensive patients has been studied, you might search by "medication adherence AND hypertension." The Boolean operator OR is most useful with synonymous terms or concepts, such as *compliance* and *adherence*. Use OR when you want to search for the presence of either of two terms in the same search. Use NOT when you want to search for one idea but not another in the same citation. NOT is used less frequently because doing so may result in missing relevant publications.

Locational operators (field labels) identify terms in specific areas or fields of a record. These fields may be parts of the simple citation, such as the article title, author, and journal name, or they may be from additional fields provided by the database, such as subject headings, abstracts, cited references, publication type notes, instruments used, and even the entire article. In some databases, these specific fields can be selected by means of a dropdown menu in the database input area. In other databases, specific coding can be used to do the same thing. Do not assume that the entire article is being searched when you are using the default search; the default is usually looking for your terms in the title, abstract, and/or subject fields. You may choose to search for a concept only within the abstract of articles.

Positional operators are used to look for requested terms within certain distances of one another. Availability and phrasing of positional operators are highly dependent on the database search software. Common positional operators are *NEAR, WITH,* and *ADJ;* they also are often required to be capitalized and may have numbers associated with them. A positional operator is most useful in records with a large amount of information, such as those with full-text articles attached. Positional operators may be used simultaneously with locational operators, either in an implied way or explicitly. For example, ADJ is an abbreviation for adjacent; it specifies that one term must be next to another, and must appear in the order entered. ADJ2 commands that there must be no more than two intervening words between the two search terms and that they appear in the order entered. NEAR does not define the specific order of the terms; the command "term1 NEAR1 term2" requires that the first term occur first and within two words of the second term. WITH often indicates that the terms must be within the same sentence, paragraph, or region (such as subject headings) of the record.

Limit Your Search

There are several strategies that will limit a search if, after performing Boolean searches, the list of references is unmanageably long. The limits you can impose vary with the database. In CINAHL, for example, the search may be limited to a single language such as English. You can also limit the years of your search to coincide with an instructor's requirement that publications older than 5 years cannot be cited in a course paper. Searches can be limited to find only papers that are research reports, review papers, or patient education materials. Adding a certain population or intervention to the search strategy is another option that both shortens the list of references and increases their applicability. Fig. 7.2 is a display of the results of a literature search in which the Boolean operator AND was used to combine searches for medication adherence and hypertension. When the search resulted in more references than could be reviewed in the

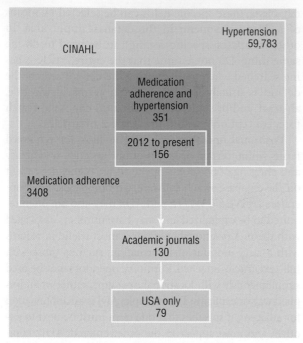

Fig. 7.2 Example of search using operators. *CINAHL,* Cumulative Index of Nursing and Allied Health Literature.

time the reviewer had available (351 citations), the search was further limited by additional characteristics: years of publication, type of journals, and geographical location. This search strategy resulted in 79 articles reporting studies conducted in the USA.

Search the Internet

In some cases, you may have to subscribe to an online journal to gain access to its articles. Some electronic journals are listed in available databases, and you can access full-text articles from an electronic journal through the database. However, many electronic journals are not yet included in databases or may not be in the particular database you are using. Ingenta Connect (http://www.ingenta.com) is a commercial website that allows you to search more than 16,000 publications from many disciplines. Publications available through Ingenta include both those that are free to download and those that require the reader to buy the article. Before purchasing an article, however, check with your library for the journal. If your library does not have the journal, you may request it through interlibrary loan. This may be a good time to request assistance from a librarian or medical information specialist who may be able to locate the article that you have identified.

Metasearch engines, such as Google, also allow you to search the internet. Online documents retrieved within Google are listed based not on relevance to your topic, but on the number of times an individual document has been viewed and the inclusion of specific key words (Hyman & Schulman, 2015). Google Scholar (https://scholar.google.com/) is a specialized tool that allows you to focus your search on research and theoretical publications. Google Scholar also has a reference management software, Google Scholar Citations, which will be discussed later in the chapter. Government reports and publications by professional organizations also may be found by searching the internet.

Prior to using a reference from the internet that has not been subjected to peer review, you must evaluate the accuracy of its information and the potential for bias on the part of its author. Sources may be secondary sources, not written by the original author(s). In general, there is no screening process for information placed on the internet. Thus you may find a considerable amount of misinformation and, for the most part, secondary sources. The accurate information that you find might not be accessed in any other way. It is important to check the source of any information you obtain from the internet so that you can determine whether it is appropriate for inclusion in your literature review.

Locate Relevant Literature

Within each database that you choose to use, conduct your search of **relevant literature** by implementing the strategies described in this chapter. Most databases provide short records that include abstracts of the articles, allowing you to get some sense of their content so you may judge whether the information is useful in relation to your selected topic. If you find the information to be an important reference, save it to a file on your computer or in an online folder maintained by your employer or university, and/or move it to a reference management software (see next section). It is often practical at the end of a search session to use a flash drive for storage of promising articles and for the list of references searched and databases accessed, to avoid duplicating these steps in a subsequent search. At this point in the process, do not try to examine all of the citations listed; merely save them.

It is rare for a scholar to be able to identify every relevant literature source. The most extensive retrievals of literature are funded projects focused on defining evidence-based practice or developing clinical practice guidelines (see Chapter 19). For the most comprehensive of these projects, a literature review coordinator manages the literature review process and has funds to employ several full-time, experienced, professional librarians as literature searchers. When extensive literature reviews are completed, the results are published so that you may have access to synthesis and the citations from the reviewed journal articles.

Systematically Record References

Bibliographical information on a source should be recorded in a systematic manner, according to the format that you will use in the reference list. The purpose for carefully citing sources is that readers can retrieve references for themselves, confirming your interpretation of the findings or gathering additional information on the topic, if they so desire. Many journals and academic institutions use the format developed by the American Psychological Association (APA) (2010). Computerized lists of sources usually contain complete citations for references, which must be saved electronically so you have the information needed in case you decide to cite a particular article, including its publication details in your reference list. The sixth edition of the APA's *Publication Manual* (2010) provides revised guidelines for citing electronic sources and direct quotations from electronic sources. (As this book went to press, the 7th edition of the APA manual was published. For this text, we used the 6th edition.) The APA standard for direct quotations of five or more words is to cite the page of the publication in which the quotation appears. Citing direct quotations from electronic sources has posed unique challenges and may require a paragraph number or a Web address. We present references in this text in APA format, except for modifying how multiple authors are cited. We have included digital objective identifiers (DOIs) when they were available (http://www.doi.org/). A DOI "provides a means of persistent identification for managing information on digital networks" (APA, 2010, p. 188). CrossRef is an example of a registration agency for DOIs that enables citations to be linked to the DOI across databases and disciplines (http://www.crossref.org/).

Each citation on the reference list is formatted as a paragraph with a *hanging indent,* meaning that the first line is on the left margin and subsequent lines are indented. If you do not know how to format a paragraph this way, search the Help tool in your word-processing program to find the correct command to use. When you retrieve an electronic source in portable document format (PDF), you cite the source as if you had made a copy of the print version of the article. Electronic sources available only in hypertext markup language format (Web format) do not have page numbers for the citation. The APA standard is to provide the uniform resource locator (URL) for the home page of the journal from which the reader could navigate and find the source (APA, 2010). Providing the URL that you used to retrieve the article is not helpful because it is unique to the path you used to find the article and reflects your access to search engines and databases.

Use Reference Management Software

Reference management software can make tracking the references you have obtained through your searches considerably easier. You can use such software to conduct searches and to store the information on all search fields for each reference obtained in a search, including the abstract. Within the software, you can store articles in folders with other similar articles. For example, you may have a folder for theory sources, another for methodological sources, and a third for relevant research topics. When you export search results from the database to your reference management software, all of the needed citation information and the abstract are readily available to you electronically when you write the literature review. As you read the articles, you also can insert comments about each one into the reference file.

Reference management software has been developed to interface directly with the most commonly used word-processing software. It organizes the reference information using the specific citation style you stipulate. For instance, you may be familiar with APA format but want to submit a manuscript to a journal that uses another bibliographical style, the term used for different types of citing and referencing sources. Within a reference management program, a reference list or bibliography can be generated in a different format—in this case, the format required by the journal. A mere keystroke or two will insert citations into your paper. Four commonly used reference management software options, along with websites that contain information about them, are as follows:

- EndNote X9 (http://www.endnote.com/) is compatible with Windows and Macintosh computers and allows you to access your saved materials from multiple electronic devices.
- RefWorks (https://refworks.proquest.com/researcher/) operates from the Web and can be accessed free by students and faculty if their respective universities maintain licenses for usage.

- Google Scholar Citations (https://scholar.google.com/citations) operated from the Web and can be accessed for free with the setup of a free Google account.
- Bookends (http://www.sonnysoftware.com/) is a reference manager for Macintosh users that allows users to search databases and download citations and full-text articles. Searches can also be downloaded to other Apple products, such as iPhones and iPads.

Saved Searches and Alerts

When working on a research project in which the literature review may take months or engaged in a field of study that will interest you for years, repeating the same search periodically, using the same strategy, is both necessary and time consuming. Many databases, however, permit you to create an account in which you can save the original search strategy so that the same search will be initiated with just a few clicks without having to enter the entire strategy again. You can also arrange for e-mail notification of any new articles that fit your saved search strategy. Another option available from many journals is to register to have the table of contents of new issues sent automatically by e-mail. Examine the help function of the database or journal home page to determine the available options.

Processing the Literature

The processes of reading and critically appraising sources promote understanding of a research problem. They involve skimming, comprehending, analyzing, and synthesizing content from sources. Skills in reading and critically appraising sources are essential to the development of a high-quality literature review.

Reading

Skimming a source is quickly reviewing a source to gain a broad overview of its content. When you retrieve an article, you quickly read the title, the author's name, and an abstract or introduction. Then you read the major headings and sometimes one or two sentences under each heading. Next, you glance at any tables and figures. Finally, you review the conclusion or summary section. Skimming enables you to make a preliminary judgment about the value of a source, relative to your area of review, and to determine whether the source is primary or secondary. You may choose to review the citations listed in secondary sources to identify primary sources the

authors cited, but secondary sources are seldom cited in a research proposal, review of the literature, or research report.

Comprehension

Comprehending a source requires that you read all of it carefully. This is necessary for key references that you have retrieved. Focus on understanding major concepts and the logical flow of ideas within the source. Highlight the content you consider important or make notes in the margins. Notes might be recorded on photocopies or electronic files of articles, indicating where the information will be used in developing a research proposal, review of the literature, or research report.

The kind of information you highlight or note in the margins of a source depends on the type of study or source. Information that you might note or highlight from the theoretical sources includes relevant concepts, definitions of those concepts, and relationships among them. Notes recorded in the margins of empirical literature might include relevant information about the researcher, such as whether the author is a major researcher of a selected problem, as well as comparisons with other studies by the same author. For a research article, the research problem, purpose, framework, data collection methods, study design, sample size, data collection, analysis techniques, and findings are usually noted or highlighted. You may wish to record quotations with quotation marks (including page numbers) for possible use in the written review. This is essential for avoiding accidental plagiarism. The final decision whether to use a direct quote or paraphrase the information can be made later. You might also record your own thoughts about the content while you are reading a source.

At this point, you will identify relevant categories for sorting and organizing sources. These categories will ultimately guide you in writing the review of literature section, and some may even be major headings in the review.

Appraising and Analyzing Sources for Possible Inclusion in a Review

Through analysis, you can determine the value of a source for a particular review. Analysis must take place in two stages. The first stage involves the critical appraisal of individual studies. The steps of appraising individual studies are detailed in Chapter 18. During

TABLE 7.4 Literature Summary Table							
Author and Year	Purpose	Framework	Sample	Measurement	Treatment	Results	Findings

the critical appraisal process, you will identify relevant content in the articles and evaluate the rigor of the studies.

Conducting an **analysis of sources** to be used in a research proposal, review of the literature, or research report requires some knowledge of the subject to be critiqued, some knowledge of the research process, and the ability to exercise judgment in evaluation (Pinch, 1995, 2001). However, the critical appraisal of individual studies is only the first step in developing an adequate review of the literature. A literature review that is a series of paragraphs in which each paragraph is a description of a single study with no link to other studies being reviewed does not provide evidence of adequate analysis and synthesis of the literature.

Analysis requires not taking the "text at face value" and being able to tolerate the uncertainty (Hyman & Schulman, 2015, p. 64) until you can identify the common elements and contradictions in the text. Analysis involves rewording and reanalyzing the information that you find, literally making it your own (Garrard, 2017). Pinch (1995), a nurse, published a strategy to synthesize research findings using a literature summary table. Pinch (2001) developed a modified table for translating research findings into clinical innovations. We modified this table by adding two columns that are useful in sorting information from studies into categories for analysis (Table 7.4). When using reference management software, tables can be generated from information you entered into the software about each individual study. Cullen et al. (2018) provide examples of other table formats for annotations and for different approaches to analyzing and comparing references during the review.

The second stage of analysis involves making comparisons among studies. This analysis allows you to critically appraise the existing body of knowledge in relation to the research problem. From your appraisal, you will be able to summarize important points that will shape your research proposal (Box 7.2). Different researchers may have approached the examination of the problem from different perspectives. They may have

> **BOX 7.2 Critical Questions to Answer by Synthesizing the Literature**
>
> - What theoretical formulations have been used to identify concepts and the relationships among them?
> - What methodologies have researchers used to study the problem?
> - What methodological flaws were found in previous studies?
> - What is known about the problem?
> - What are the most critical gaps in the knowledge base?

organized the study from different theoretical perspectives, asked different questions related to the problem, selected different variables, or used different designs. Pay special attention to conflicting findings, as they may provide clues for gaps in knowledge that represent researchable problems.

Sorting Your Sources

Relevant sources are organized for inclusion in the different sections of a research proposal or research report. See Table 7.1 to review contributions of the literature to each part of the research process. The sources for a course assignment or review related to a clinical problem can be sorted for different sections of the paper. For example, in the introduction of the assignment, include information from sources that provide background and significance for the study. Research reports can be grouped by concepts that were studied, populations included, or similar findings.

Synthesizing Sources

In a literature review, **synthesis of sources** involves clarifying the meaning obtained from the sources as a whole. Integration refers to "making connections between ideas, theories, and experience" (Hart, 2018, p. 15). Through synthesis and integration, one can cluster and connect ideas from several sources to develop a personal overall view of the topic. Garrard (2017) describes this personal level of knowledge as ownership, as "being so familiar with what has been written by previous researchers that you know clearly how this area of research has progressed over time and across ideas" (p. 7).

Synthesis is the key to the next step of the review process, which is developing the logical argument that supports the research problem you intend to address. Booth et al. (2016) describe the process of constructing an argument as beginning with stating a claim and identifying supporting reasons. The reviewer must also include adequate information so that the reader agrees that the reasons are relevant to the claim. The reviewer provides evidence to support each of the reasons. Thinking at this level and depth prepares you for outlining the written review. Fig. 7.3 provides a visual representation of an argument that can be developed through a written review. The writer/reviewer supports each claim with evidence so that the reader can accept the reviewer's conclusion. For example, the reviewer has synthesized several sources related to medication adherence and is presenting the argument for developing patient-focused medication adherence intervention. The following outline could be developed for this argument.

Claim 1: Interventions to promote medication adherence must incorporate the hypertensive patient's perspective.

Reason 1: Provider-focused interventions have not resulted in long-term improvement in medication adherence.

Evidence 1: Description of studies of provider-focused interventions and their outcomes

Reason 2: Patients who do not adhere to an externally imposed medication regimen (the target population)

may be less likely to use an intervention that is externally imposed.

Evidence 2: Description of studies in which patients failed to return for appointments during a trial of an electronic device to promote adherence

Reason 3: Medication adherence requires behavior change that must be incorporated into the patient's life.

Evidence 3: Theoretical principles of behavior change that recommend individualization of interventions to meet unique patient needs

Conclusion 1: Using a participatory approach to develop individual strategies for promoting medication adherence is an important first step to improving patient outcomes.

Writing the Review of Literature
Writing Suggestions

Clear, correct, and concise are the three Cs of good writing (Curnalia & Ferris, 2014). If you have followed the steps for reviewing the literature in this chapter, you are ready to demonstrate your synthesis and ownership of the literature by clearly presenting your argument. Rather than using direct quotes from an author, you should paraphrase his or her ideas. Paraphrasing involves expressing ideas clearly and in your own words; the ability to paraphrase is an indication of understanding what you have read (Hyman & Schulman, 2015). In paraphrasing, the author of the review connects the meanings of these sources to the proposed study, being careful to present the information correctly. Last, the reviewer combines, or clusters, the meanings obtained

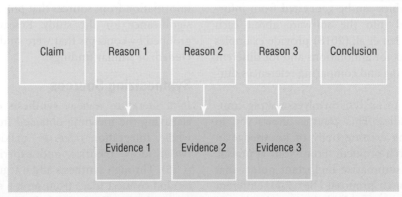

Fig. 7.3 Building the logical argument. (Adapted from Booth, W. C., Colomb, G. G., Williams, J. M., Bizup, J., & Fitzgerald, W. T. [2016]. *The craft of research* [4th ed.]. Chicago, IL: University of Chicago Press.)

from all sources to establish the current state of knowledge for the research problem (Pinch, 1995, 2001).

Each paragraph has three components: a theme sentence, sentences with evidence, and a summary sentence. Start each paragraph with a theme sentence that describes the main idea of the paragraph or makes a claim. Concisely present the relevant studies as evidence of the main idea or claim, and end the paragraph with a concluding sentence that connects to the next claim and next paragraph.

Organization of Written Reviews

The purpose of the written literature review is to establish a context for a research proposal, review of the literature, or research report. The literature review for a research proposal or research report may have four major sections: (1) the introduction, (2) a discussion of theoretical literature, (3) a discussion of empirical literature, and (4) a summary. The introduction and summary are standard sections, but you will want to organize the discussion of sources in a way that makes sense for the topic.

Introduction. By reading the introduction of a literature review, the reader should learn the purpose of the study and the organizational structure of the review. The reader also should gain an appreciation of why the topic is important and significant. You should make clear in this section what you will and will not discuss in the review: the scope of the review. If you are taking a particular position or developing a logical argument for a particular perspective, make this position clear in the introduction.

Discussion of theoretical literature. The theoretical literature section contains concept analyses, models, theories, and conceptual frameworks that support the study. In this section, you will present the concepts, definitions of concepts, relationships among concepts, and assumptions. You will analyze these elements to build the theoretical basis for the study. This section of the literature review may be used to present the framework for the study and may include a conceptual map that synthesizes the theoretical literature (see Chapter 8 for more details on developing frameworks).

Discussion of empirical literature. The presentation of empirical literature should be organized by concepts or organizing topics, instead of by studies. The findings from the studies should logically build on one another so that the reader can understand how the body of knowledge in the research area evolved. Instead of presenting details about purpose, sample size, design, and

specific findings for each study, the researcher presents a synthesis of findings across studies. Conflicting findings and areas of uncertainty are explored. Similarities and differences in the studies should be identified. Gaps and areas needing more research are discussed. A summary of findings in the topic area is presented, along with inferences, generalizations, and conclusions drawn from review of the literature. A conclusion is a statement about the state of knowledge in relation to the topic area. This should include a discussion of the strength of the evidence available for each conclusion.

The reviewer who becomes committed to a particular viewpoint on the research topic must maintain the ethical standard of intellectual honesty. The content from reviewed sources should be presented honestly, not distorted to support a selected problem. Reviewers may read a study and wish that the researchers had studied a slightly different problem or designed the study differently. However, the reviewers must recognize their own opinions and must be objective in presenting information. The defects of a study must be addressed, but it is not necessary to be highly critical of another researcher's work. The criticisms must focus on the content that is in some way relevant to the proposed study and should be stated as possible or plausible explanations, so that the criticisms are more neutral and scholarly than negative and blaming.

Summary. Through the literature review, you will present the evidence and reveal the research problem—what is not known about the particular concept or topic. The summary of the review consists of a concise presentation of the current knowledge base for the research problem. The gaps in the knowledge base are identified. The summary concludes with a statement of how the findings from the current study may contribute to the body of knowledge in this field of research.

Refining the Written Review

You complete the first draft of your review of the literature and breathe a sigh of relief before moving on to the next portion of the assignment or research proposal. Before moving on, you need to read, evaluate, and refine your review. Set the review aside for 24 hours and then read it aloud. In this way, you may identify missing words and awkward sentences that you might overlook when reading silently. Ask a fellow student or a trusted colleague to read your work and provide constructive feedback. Use the criteria and guiding questions in Table 7.5 to evaluate the quality of the literature review.

TABLE 7.5   Characteristics of High-Quality Literature Reviews

Criteria	Guiding Questions
Coverage	Did the writer provide evidence of having reviewed sufficient literature on the topic? Does the review indicate that the writer is sufficiently well informed about the topic and has identified relevant studies?
Understanding	Does the written review indicate that the writer has understood and synthesized what is known about the topic? Have similarities and differences within the synthesized literature been described?
Coherence	Does the writer make a logical argument related to the significance of the topic and the gap to be addressed by the proposed study?
Accuracy	Does the writer's attention to detail give the reader confidence in the conclusions of the review?

Checking References

Sources that will be cited in a paper or recorded in a reference list should be cross-checked two or three times to prevent errors. Questions that will identify common errors are displayed in Box 7.3. To prevent these errors, check all of the citations within the text of the literature review and each citation in the reference list. Typing or keyboarding errors may result in inaccurate information. You may have omitted some information, planning to complete the reference later, and then forgotten to do so. Downloading citations from a database directly into a reference management system and using the system's manuscript formatting functions reduce some errors but do not eliminate all of them. Use your knowledge and skills to enhance your technology use; relying on technology will not ensure a quality manuscript.

BOX 7.3   Checking to Avoid Common Reference Citation Errors

- Does every source cited in the text have a corresponding citation on the reference list?
- Is every reference on the reference list cited in the text?
- Are names of the authors spelled the same way in the text and in the reference list?
- Are the years of publication cited in the text the same as the years of publication that appear on the reference list?
- Does every direct quotation have a citation that includes the author's name, year, and page number?
- Are the citations on the reference list complete so that the reference can be retrieved?

KEY POINTS

- A literature review consists of all written sources relevant to the selected topic. It is an interpretative, organized, and logically written presentation of the sources that have been read.
- Reviewing the existing literature related to a research topic is a critical step in the research process.
- When developing a study proposal, one of the goals of reviewing the literature is to identify a gap in the literature. Information from the literature review guides the development of the statement of the research problem.
- Two types of literature predominate in the review of literature for research: theoretical and empirical.

- Theoretical literature consists of concept analyses, models, theories, and conceptual frameworks that support a selected research problem and purpose.
- Empirical literature is comprised of relevant studies in journals and books as well as unpublished studies, such as master's theses and doctoral dissertations.
- With use of a systems approach, the three major stages of a literature review are searching the literature (input), processing the literature (throughput), and writing the literature review (output).
- Searching the literature begins with a written plan for the review that is maintained as a search history during the first stage of the literature review.

- Searching the literature requires use of bibliographical databases. Using a reference management system may be helpful for organizing retrieved sources and creating reference lists.
- Processing the literature requires the researcher to read, critically appraise, analyze, and synthesize the information that has been retrieved.
- The well-written literature review presents a logical argument for why the research question should be studied and for the specific way of studying it that is being proposed.

REFERENCES

Adams, K., & Lawrence, E. (2019). *Research methods, statistics, and applications* (2nd ed.). Thousand Oaks, CA: Sage.

American College of Nurse Midwives (ACNM). (2016). *Elective primary cesarean birth.* Retrieved from http://www.midwife.org/acnm/files/ACNMLibraryData/UPLOADFILENAME/000000000062/Elective-Primary-Cesarean-Birth-PS-9-12-16.pdf

American Psychological Association (APA). (2010). *Publication manual of the American Psychological Association* (6th ed.). Washington, DC: Author.

Aveyard, H. (2019). *Doing a literature review in health and social care: A practical guide* (4th ed.). New York, NY: Open University Press.

Booth, W. C., Colomb, G. G., Williams, J. M., Bizup, J., & Fitzgerald, W. T. (2016). *The craft of research* (4th ed.). Chicago, IL: University of Chicago Press.

Charmaz, K. (2014). *Constructing grounded theory* (2nd ed.). Thousand Oaks, CA: Sage.

Clarivate Analytics. (2019). *Web of science.* Retrieved from https://clarivate.com/products/web-of-science/

Cullen, L., Hanrahan, K., Farrington, M., DeBerg, J., Tucker, S., & Kleiber, C. (2018). *Evidence-based practice in action: Comprehensive strategies, tools, and tips from the University of Iowa Hospitals and Clinics.* Indianapolis, IN: Sigma Theta Tau International.

Curnalia, R., & Ferris, A. (2014). *CSI: Concepts, sources, integration: A step-by-step guide to writing your literature review in communication studies.* Dubuque, IA: Kendall Hunt Publishing.

Dale, J. C., Hallas, D., & Spratling, R. (2019). Critiquing research evidence for use in practice: Revisited. *Journal of Pediatric Health Care, 33*(3), 342–346. doi:10.1016/j.pedhc.2019.01.005

Garrard, J. (2017). *Health sciences literature review made easy: The matrix method* (5th ed.). Sudbury, MA: Jones & Bartlett.

Hart, C. (2018). *Doing a literature review: Releasing the social science imagination* (2nd ed.). Los Angeles, CA: Sage.

Hatfield, L. A., Murphy, N., Karp, K., & Polomano, R. C. (2019). A systematic review of behavioral of behavioral and environmental interventions for procedural pain management. *Journal of Pediatric Nursing, 44*(1), 22–30. doi:10.1016/j.pedn.2018.10.004

Hyman, G., & Schulman, M. (2015). *Thinking on the page: A college student's guide to effective writing.* Cincinnati, OH: Writer's Digest Books.

Marshall, C., & Rossman, G. B. (2016). *Designing qualitative research* (6th ed.). Los Angeles, CA: Sage.

Munhall, P. L. (2012). *Nursing research: A qualitative perspective* (5th ed.). Sudbury, MA: Jones & Bartlett.

National Institute of Nursing Research (NINR). (2006). *Changing practice, changing lives: 10 landmark nursing research studies.* Retrieved from https://www.ninr.nih.gov/sites/files/docs/10-landmark-nursing-research-studies.pdf

Paré, G., Trudel, M.-C., Jaana, M., & Kitsiou, S. (2015). Synthesizing information systems knowledge: A typology of literature reviews. *Information & Management, 52*(2), 183–199. doi:10.1016/j.im.2014.08.008

Pinch, W. J. (1995). Synthesis: Implementing a complex process. *Nurse Educator, 20*(1), 34–40.

Pinch, W. J. (2001). Improving patient care through use of research. *Orthopaedic Nursing, 20*(4), 75–81.

Tensen, B. L. (2018). *Research strategies for the digital age* (5th ed.). Boston, MA: Cengage Learning.

Wisker, G. (2015). Developing doctoral authors: Engaging with theoretical perspectives through the literature review. *Innovations in Education and Teaching International, 52*(1), 64–74. doi:10.1080/14703297.2014.981841

World Health Organization (WHO). (2018). *WHO recommendations: Non-clinical interventions to reduce unnecessary caesarean sections.* Retrieved from https://www.who.int/reproductivehealth/publications/non-clinical-interventions-to-reduce-cs/en/

8

Frameworks

Christy Bomer-Norton

http://evolve.elsevier.com/Gray/practice/

The interconnection of theory, research, and practice is the foundation of nursing science, and nursing theory and research should guide practice (Peterson & Bredow, 2017). "Research is a source of theory development, and theory is a source of research questions" (Peterson & Bredow, 2017, p. ix). A theoretical **framework** is an abstract, logical structure of meaning that guides the development of a study and enables the researcher to link the findings to the body of knowledge in nursing (Meleis, 2018). Theoretical frameworks are used in quantitative and outcomes research, sometimes in qualitative research, and rarely in mixed methods studies. In quantitative studies, the framework may be a testable theory or may be a tentative theory developed inductively from published research or clinical observation. Most outcomes studies are based on Donabedian's (1987) theory of quality of care. In most qualitative studies, the researcher will identify a philosophical perspective but may not identify a formal theoretical framework (see Chapters 4 and 12). In grounded theory research, concepts and the relationships among them play central roles because the researcher often develops a theory as an outcome of the study.

Almost every quantitative study has a theoretical framework, although some researchers do not identify or describe the framework in the report of the study. Often the theoretical framework can be inferred from research questions or hypotheses. For example, researchers may use their knowledge of anatomy and physiology to guide a study without identifying a framework, although both the language and the reasoning the researcher uses are consistent with known facts of anatomy and physiology. Others may study self-care and not link the concept to Orem's (2001) theory of self-care, despite using terms

from that theory. Ideally, the framework of a quantitative study is carefully structured, clearly presented, and integrated thoroughly with the methodology. One aspect of critically appraising studies is identifying the theoretical framework and evaluating the extent to which the framework is congruent with the study's methodology. Your ability to understand the study findings will depend on your ability to understand the logic within the framework and determine how the findings might be used. In addition, when developing a quantitative study, the theoretical framework should be described.

After introducing relevant terms, this chapter describes processes used to examine and appraise the components of theories and presents approaches to identifying or developing a framework to guide a study.

INTRODUCTION OF TERMS

The first step in understanding theories and frameworks is to become familiar with theoretical terms and their application. These terms are *concept, relational statement, conceptual model, theory, middle-range theory,* and *research framework.* These terms will be introduced and then described more deeply in the following sections.

Concept

A **concept** is a term that abstractly describes and names an object, a phenomenon, or an idea, thus providing it with a distinct identity or meaning. As a label for a phenomenon or a composite of behavior or thoughts, a concept is a concise way to represent an experience or state (Meleis, 2018). Concepts are the basic building blocks of theory (Fig. 8.1). An example of a concept is

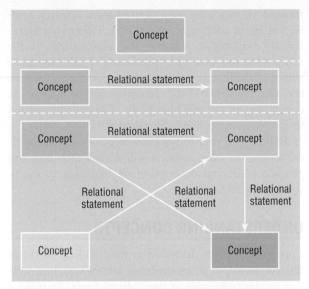

Fig. 8.1 Concepts, relational statements, and theories.

statements are essential for constructing an integrated framework that guides the development of a study's objectives, questions, and hypotheses. The types of relationships described determine the study design and indicate the types of statistical analyses that may be used to answer the research question. Mature theories, such as physiological theories, have measurable concepts and clear relational statements that can be tested through research.

Conceptual Models

A **conceptual model**, one type of which is known as a grand theory, is a set of highly abstract, related constructs. A conceptual model broadly explains phenomena of interest, expresses assumptions, and reflects a philosophical stance. Nurse scholars have expended time and effort to debate the distinctions among definitions of theory, conceptual model, conceptual framework, and theoretical framework (Chinn & Kramer, 2015; Fawcett & DeSanto-Madeya, 2013; Higgins & Moore, 2000; Meleis, 2018). For example, Watson's (1979) theory of caring has been identified as a metatheory (Higgins & Moore, 2000), a theory (Meleis, 2018), a philosophy (Alligood, 2018), and a conceptual model (Fitzpatrick & Whall, 2005). Most of nursing's grand theories, such as Watson's, are global and offer theoretical, almost philosophical, explanations of what nursing should be and what the vital parts of nursing should entail. They are explanations of nursing as a whole. In this textbook, we use the terms *conceptual model* and *conceptual framework* interchangeably. We have deliberately chosen not to contribute to the scholarly debate but to provide the information needed to use concepts, relational statements, and theories.

Theory

A **theory** consists of a set of defined concepts and relational statements that provide a structured way to think about a phenomenon (see the portion of Fig. 8.1 below the lowest dashed line). Theories are developed to describe, explain, or predict a phenomenon or outcome (Goodson, 2015; Walker & Avant, 2019). As discussed earlier, relational statements clarify the relationship that exists between or among concepts. It is the relational statement within a theory that is tested through research, not the entire theory. Thus identifying and categorizing the statements (relationships among the concepts) within the theory are critical to the research

the term *anxiety*. The concept brings to mind a feeling of uneasiness in the stomach, a rapid pulse rate, and troubling thoughts about future negative outcomes. Another example of a concept is *patient*, which denotes a person receiving healthcare services. Think about all the different ways that people receive health care. In many of these settings, the recipients are called patients. The concept of patient encompasses millions of people from widely divergent nationalities, health conditions, and living situations, all of whom share the common characteristic of receiving health care.

Concepts can vary in their levels of abstraction. At high levels of abstraction, concepts that naturally cluster together are called constructs. For example, a construct associated with the concept of anxiety might be emotional responses. Within the same construct, hope, anger, fear, and optimism could be identified. Another construct is health care, which includes the concepts of treatment, prevention, health promotion, palliative care, and rehabilitation, to name a few. Constructs will be discussed more in the next section.

Relational Statements

A **relational statement** is the explanation of the connection between or among concepts (Fawcett & DeSanto-Madeya, 2013; Walker & Avant, 2019). Relational statements provide the structure of a framework (see the middle section of Fig. 8.1). Clear relational endeavor: One or more of these relationships form the basis of the study's framework.

Scientific theories are those for which repeated studies have validated relationships among the concepts (Goodson, 2015). These theories are sometimes called laws for this reason. Although few nursing and psychosocial theories have been validated to this extent, physiological theories have this level of validation through research and can provide a strong basis for nursing studies.

Middle-Range Theories

Middle-range theories present a partial view of nursing reality. Proposed by Merton (1968), a sociologist, middle-range theories are less abstract and address more specific phenomena than do the grand theories (Smith & Liehr, 2018). They apply directly to practice, with a focus on explanation of the specifics of condition, symptom, diagnosis, or process, and on implementation. They differ from grand theories because they are concerned with aspects of nursing, not its totality. Because of the narrower focus, middle-range theories can provide a framework to guide a research study. Ideally middle-range theory developers name their theory, describe the process of theory development, create an illustrated model, describe the theory's connection to nursing research and practice, and remain open to future refinement of the theory (Smith & Liehr, 2018).

Middle-range theories may be developed from grand theories in nursing through substruction. Middle-range theory may also be developed inductively from research findings, such as grounded theory studies. Others emanate from practice or from existent theory in related fields. Whatever their source, middle-range theories are sometimes called **substantive theories** because they are more concrete than grand theories.

Research Frameworks

A **research framework** is the theoretical structure guiding a specific study. One way to describe the research framework is to present a map or diagram of its concepts and relational statements. Diagrams of research frameworks are **conceptual maps** (Fawcett, 1999; Newman, 1979, 1986). A conceptual map summarizes and integrates visually the theoretical structure of a study. A narrative explanation allows us to grasp the essence of a phenomenon in context. A research framework should be supported by references from the literature. The

framework may have been derived from research findings or be an adaptation of a theory. Either way, literature is available to support the explanation. If the framework has emerged from clinical experiences, a search of the literature may reveal supporting studies or theories. Frameworks vary in complexity and accuracy, depending on the available body of knowledge related to the phenomena being described.

Building on your initial knowledge of these theoretical terms, the next sections will revisit each one and provide additional description of analyzing concepts, statements, and theories.

UNDERSTANDING CONCEPTS

Concepts are often described as the building blocks of theory: useful, in an amorphous sort of way, but difficult to clarify because of their abstractness. To make a concept concrete, the researcher must identify how it can be measured. The concept's operational definition is a statement of how it will be measured (see Chapter 6). A concept made measurable is referred to as a **variable**. The word *variable* implies that the values associated with the term can vary from one instance to another. A variable related to anxiety might be palmar sweating, which the researcher can measure by assigning a numerical value to the amount of sweat on the subject's palm. Substruction is linking abstract constructs, concepts, and variables using deductive reasoning. To review this principle and provide examples, Fig. 8.2 shows examples of the links among constructs, concepts, and variables. On the left of the figure is the template of the construct-to-variable continuum. The other two sets of shapes are examples of a construct, concept, and

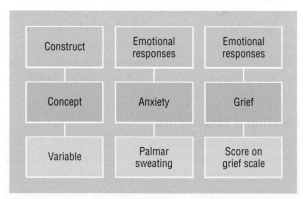

Fig. 8.2 Substruction of constructs, concepts, and variables.

variable. Notice that a concept may have multiple ways of being measured. For example, to measure anxiety, you could assess palmar sweating, ask subjects to complete the State-Trait Anxiety Inventory, or observe subjects and complete a checklist of behaviors such as pacing, wringing of hands, and verbalizing concerns.

Defining concepts allows us to be consistent in the way we use a term in practice, apply it to theory, and measure it in a study. A conceptual definition differs from the **denotative** (or dictionary) **definition** of a word. A **conceptual definition** (connotative meaning) is more comprehensive than a denotative definition because it includes associated meanings the word may have. For example, a connotative definition may associate the term *fireplace* with images of comfort and warmth, whereas the denotative definition would be a rock or brick structure in a house designed for burning wood. Conceptual definitions may be found in theories, but can also be established through concept synthesis, concept derivation, or concept analysis (Walker & Avant, 2019).

Concept Synthesis

In nursing, many phenomena have not yet been identified as discrete entities. Recognizing, naming, and describing these phenomena are critical steps to understanding the process and outcomes of nursing practice. In your clinical practice, you may notice a pattern of behavior or find a pattern or theme in empirical data and select a name to represent the pattern. The process of describing and naming a previously unrecognized concept is **concept synthesis**. Nursing studies often involve previously unrecognized and unnamed phenomena that must be named and carefully defined, so that study readers can understand their meanings and functions. Coyne, Holmström, & Söderbäck (2018) conducted a concept synthesis of family-centered care, person-centered care, and child-centered care. They reviewed 35 articles—including 14 family-centered care, 15 person-centered care, and 6 child-centered care articles—to find common and disparate elements. The findings create a framework for providers to assess centeredness and its three forms.

Concept Derivation

Concept derivation may occur when the researcher or theorist finds no concept in nursing to explain a phenomenon (Walker & Avant, 2019). Concepts identified or defined in theories of other disciplines can provide

insight. In **concept derivation**, a concept is transposed from one field of knowledge to another. If a conceptual definition is found in another discipline, it must be examined to evaluate its fit with the new field in which it will be used. The conceptual definition may need to be modified so that it is meaningful within nursing and consistent with nursing thought (Walker & Avant, 2019). Concept derivation is a creative process that can be fostered by thinking deeply and having a willingness to learn about processes and theories in other disciplines.

Concept Analysis

Concept analysis is a strategy that identifies a set of characteristics essential to defining the connotative meaning of a concept. Several approaches to concept analysis have been described in the nursing and healthcare literature. Because the approaches have varying philosophical foundations and products, nurse theorists and researchers must select the concept analysis approach that best suits their purposes in a specific situation (Table 8.1). A frequently used approach to concept analysis is the process proposed by Walker and Avant (2019). The procedure guides the scholar to explore the various ways the term is used and to identify a set of characteristics that clarifies the range of objects or ideas to which that concept may be applied (Walker & Avant, 2019). These essential characteristics, called *defining attributes* or *criteria,* provide a means to distinguish the concept from similar concepts and provide a foundation for determining whether an instrument has construct validity (see Chapter 16). Nurses may analyze concepts as a means to improve clinical practice. For example, Brooks, Manias, and Bloomer (2019) conducted a concept analysis of culturally sensitive communication in health care. The resulting antecedents, attributes, and consequences are listed in Box 8.1.

Educators may conduct a concept analysis to expand their knowledge of a concept and its implications for their teaching strategies or student development. For example, Mirza, Manankil-Rankin, Prentice, Hagerman, and Draenos (2019) published a concept analysis of practice readiness of new nursing graduates. When researchers are new to a topic or phenomenon, they may analyze both central and related concepts to develop a clear conceptual definition, which is the basis for selecting an appropriate operational definition (see Chapter 6).

TABLE 8.1   Methods of Concept Analysis

Type of Concept Analysis (Author[s], Date)	Unique Characteristics
Principle-based method (Hupcey & Penrod, 2005)	Analysis guided by linguistic, epistemological, pragmatic, and logical principles
Ordinary use approach (Wilson, 1963)	Foci of analysis are exemplars (cases) used to identify criteria, antecedents, and consequences
Evolutionary method (Rodgers, 2000)	Contextual analysis of how the concept has developed over time in different settings
Hybrid method (Schwartz-Barcott & Kim, 2000)	Contextual analysis and data collection in the field leading to conclusions about how concept has developed over time in different settings
Linguistic, pragmatic approach (Walker & Avant, 2019)	Analysis of explicit and implicit concept definitions in the literature to identify criteria, antecedents, and consequences for use in practice and research
Simultaneous analysis method (Haase, Britt, Coward, Leidy, & Penn, 1992)	Examines closely related concepts to distinguish their unique meanings as well as areas of overlap

BOX 8.1   Culturally Sensitive Communication: Antecedents, Attributes, and Consequences

Antecedents
- The environment and culture of the ward
- Organizational structures and policies
- Education and communication experience of clinicians
- Sociocultural characteristics of patients, families, and clinicians
- Personal characteristics and professional experiences of clinicians

Attributes
- Encouraging patients and families to participate in communication and decision making to the degree they feel comfortable
- [Prioritizing] cultural considerations in the planning and provision of care
- Developing a trusting relationship with the patient and family
- The use of a professional interpreter, a best practice recommendation where language differences exist between clinicians, patients, and families

Consequences
- Increased patient and family satisfaction
- Improved adherence to treatment regimens
- Better engagement in patient and family [centered] care
- Improved health outcomes

Data from Brooks, L. A., Manias, E., & Bloomer, M. J. (2019). Culturally sensitive communication in healthcare: A concept analysis. *Collegian, 26*(3), 383–391. doi:10.1016/j.colegn.2018.09.007

EXAMINING STATEMENTS

Understanding the statements in a theory is essential for ensuring consistency among research framework, study design, and statistical analyses. In addition to relational statements that involve two or more concepts, statements can also be nonrelational and involve a single concept. A nonrelational statement indicates a concept exists or defines the concept (Box 8.2). The first two statements are nonrelational statements about concepts in a study of

BOX 8.2   Examples of Nonrelational and Relational Statements

Nonrelational Statements

"According to the Transactional Model of Stress and Coping by Lazarus and Folkman (1984), stress is a specific relationship between a person and the environment that is considered threatening to the individual's well-being by exceeding the limits of their resources" (Jang & Kim, 2018, p. 42).

"The way of coping with stress refers to the response taken to resolve the stress by dealing with internal or external situations or the needs judged to exceed the resources of the individual" (Jang & Kim, 2018, p. 42).

Relational Statements

"Social support had a significant direct negative effect on stress" (Jang & Kim, 2018, p. 45).

"Self-efficacy and stress significantly, directly, and positively affected coping" (Jang & Kim, 2018, p. 45).

psychosocial adjustment in Korean women with breast cancer (Jang & Kim, 2018). Two relational statements derived from the study results are also provided.

Characteristics of Relational Statements

As stated earlier, a relational statement is the explanation of the connection between concepts. Relational statements in a research framework can be described by their characteristics. Relational statements describe the direction, shape, strength, sequencing, probability of occurrence, necessity, and sufficiency of a relationship (Walker & Avant, 2019). One statement may have several of these characteristics; each characteristic is not exclusive of the others. Statements may be expressed as words in a sentence (language form), as shapes and arrows (diagram form), or as equations (mathematical form). In nursing, the language and diagrammatic forms of statements are used most frequently (Figs. 8.3 and 8.4). Fig. 8.3 displays simple statements of relationships among spiritual perspective, social support, and coping, including a dotted arrow to indicate a relationship about which less is known. Fig. 8.4 provides language and diagrammatic forms of a more complex statement among the previous concepts with the addition of perceived stress. Diagrams can be constructed to show how relationships are moderated by another concept, such as the change in the arrow between perceived stress and coping: The arrow is darker and heavier until spiritual perspective and social support modify the relationship. You can infer that the relationship between perceived stress and coping changes due to the influence of spiritual perspective and social support.

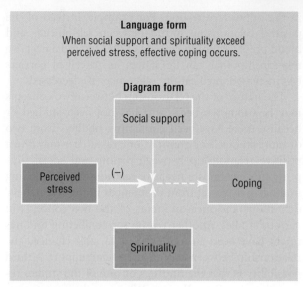

Fig. 8.4 Language and diagram forms of a complex statement.

Direction

The **direction of a relationship** may be positive, negative, or unknown (Fawcett, 1999). The letters A and B in parentheses in the following paragraphs indicate concepts. A **positive linear relationship** implies that as one concept changes (the value or amount of the concept increases or decreases), the second concept will also change in the same direction (Fig. 8.5). For example, in a study of Chinese hypertensive adults 59 years and younger, Ma (2018) found as self-efficacy increases (A), blood pressure monitoring (B) increases, which expresses a positive relationship.

A **negative linear relationship** implies that as a concept changes, the other concept in the statement changes

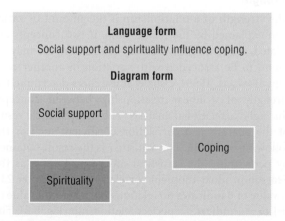

Fig. 8.3 Language and diagram forms of a simple statement.

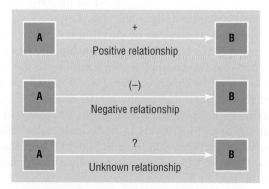

Fig. 8.5 Directions of relational statements.

in the opposite direction. For example, instead of the positive relationship found between self-efficacy and blood pressure monitoring, Ma (2018) found a negative relationship that can be stated: as perceived barriers (A) increased, medication adherence (B) decreased.

The nature of the relationship between two concepts may be unknown because it has not been studied or because there have been conflicting findings from two or more studies. For example, one researcher may find a positive relationship between coping and social support; another finds a negative relationship. Conflicting findings may result from differences in the researchers' definitions and measurements of the two concepts in various studies. Another reason for conflicting findings might have been an unidentified variable changed the relationship between coping and social support. A third possibility is that the findings of one of the studies reflect Type I or Type II error. Whatever the reason, conflicting findings about a relationship between concepts can be indicated diagrammatically by a question mark, the third example shown in Fig. 8.5.

Shape

Most relationships are assumed to be linear, and so initial statistical tests are conducted to identify linear relationships. In a **linear relationship**, the relationship between two concepts remains consistent regardless of the values of each of the concepts. For example, if the value of B increases by 1 point each time the value of A increases by 2 points, then the values continue to increase proportionally whether the values are 2 and 4 or 300 and 600. We can diagram relationships between concepts using a vertical axis and a horizontal axis, with each axis representing the score on one of the concepts. Each subject's paired scores on the two concepts are plotted as a dot on the diagram. If the relationship between the concepts is linear, most of the dots will be clustered around a straight line (Fig. 8.6).

Relationships also can be curvilinear or form some other shape. In a **curvilinear relationship**, the relationship between two concepts varies according to the relative values of the concepts. Wan, Fung, Fong, Chan, and Lam (2016) found that cardiovascular disease (CVD) in patients with type 2 diabetes mellitus was lower when medium or optimal levels of body mass index (BMI) were found. Patients with low and high BMI were found to have more CVD, indicating a curvilinear relationship (Fig. 8.7).

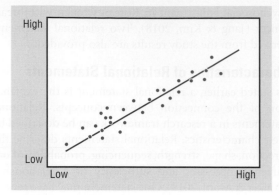

Fig. 8.6 Linear relationship.

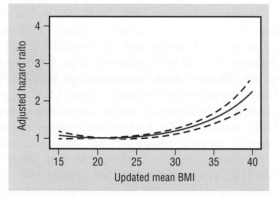

Fig. 8.7 Curvilinear relationship. *BMI,* Body mass index. (From Wan, E. Y. F., Fung, C. S. C., Fong, D. Y. T., Chan, A. K. C., & Lam, C. L. K. [2016]. A curvilinear association of body mass index with cardiovascular diseases in Chinese patients with type 2 diabetes mellitus—A population-based retrospective cohort study. *Journal of Diabetes and Its Complications, 30*[7], 1261–1268. doi:10.1016/j.jdiacomp.2016.05.010.)

Strength

The **strength of a relationship** is the amount of variation explained by the relationship. If two concepts are related, some of the variation in one concept may be found to be associated with variation in another concept (Fawcett, 1999). Usually researchers determine the strength of a linear relationship between concepts through correlational analysis. The mathematical result of the analysis is a correlation coefficient such as the following: $r = 0.35$. The statistic r is the result obtained by performing the statistical procedure known as the Pearson product-moment correlation (see Chapter 23). A value of 0 indicates no relationship, whereas a value of $+1$ or -1 indicates a perfect relationship (Fig. 8.8). The

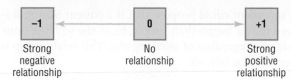

Fig. 8.8 Strength of relationships.

TABLE 8.2 **Characteristics of Relationships**

Type of Relationship	Descriptive Statement
Positive linear	As A increases, B increases. As A decreases, B decreases.
Negative linear	As A increases, B decreases. As A decreases, B increases.
Unknown linear	As A changes, B may or may not change.
Curvilinear	At a specific level, as A changes, B changes to a similar degree. At another specific level, as A changes, B changes to a greater or lesser extent.
Concurrent	When A changes, B changes at the same time.
Sequential	After A changes, B changes.
Causal	If A occurs, B always occurs.
Probabilistic	If A occurs, then probably B occurs.
Necessary	If A occurs, and only if A occurs, B occurs. If A does not occur, B does not occur.
Sufficient	If A occurs, and if A alone occurs, B occurs.
Substitutable	If A_1 or A_2 occurs, B occurs.
Contingent	If A occurs, then B occurs, but only if C occurs.

closer that the correlation is to $+1$ or -1, the stronger the relationship between the variables.

When the correlation is large, a greater portion of the variation can be explained by the relationship; in others, only a moderate or a small portion of the variation can be explained by the relationship. For example, Ma (2018) found a relationship of $r = 0.24$ ($p < 0.01$) between medication adherence and perceived benefits of self-care among Chinese hypertensive adults 59 years and younger ($n = 382$). The strength of the relationship meant that a small portion of the variance in medication adherence was explained by variations in perceived benefits of self-care. Details on statistically determining linear relationships in studies are presented in Chapter 23.

Whether the relationship is positive or negative does not have an impact on the strength of the relationship. For example, $r = -0.24$ is as strong as $r = +0.24$. The closer the r value is to 1 or -1, the stronger the relationship. Stronger relationships are more easily detected, even in a small sample. Weaker relationships may require larger samples to be detected. This idea will be explored further in the chapters on sampling, measurement, and data analysis.

Sequential Relationships

The amount of time that elapses between one concept and another is stated as the sequential nature of a relationship. If the two concepts occur simultaneously or are measured at the same time, the relationship is **concurrent** (Fawcett, 1999). When there is a change in one concept, there is change in the other at the same time (Table 8.2). If a change in one concept now influences changes in a second concept at a later time, the relationship is **sequential**. In a study with 162 Iranian women with breast cancer, Rohani, Abedi, Omranipour, and Languis-Eklof (2015) found that sense of coherence at diagnosis was related positively to health-related quality of life 6 months later, a sequential relationship. These relationships are diagrammed in Fig. 8.9.

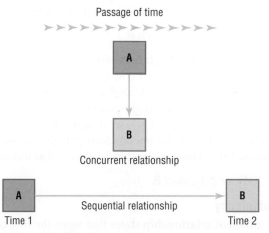

Fig. 8.9 Sequencing of relationships.

Probability of Occurrence

A relationship can be deterministic or probabilistic depending on the degree of certainty that it will occur. **Deterministic** (or **causal**) **relationships** are statements that always occur in a particular situation. Scientific laws are an example of deterministic relationships (Fawcett, 1999). A causal relationship is expressed as follows:

If A, then always B.

A **probability statement** expresses the probability that something will happen in a given situation (Fawcett, 1999). For example, patients who were identified at admission as a high fall risk had a 17% higher probability of falling during the hospitalization than patients identified as a low or medium fall risk (Cox et al., 2015). This relationship is expressed as follows:

If A, then probably B.

This probability could be expressed mathematically as follows:

$p > 0.17$.

The *p* is a symbol for probability. The $>$ is a symbol for greater than. This mathematical statement asserts that there is more than a 17% probability that the second event will occur.

Necessity

In a **necessary relationship**, one concept must occur for the second concept to occur (Fawcett, 1999). For example, one could propose that if sufficient fluids are administered (A), and only if sufficient fluids are administered, the unconscious patient will remain hydrated (B). This relationship is expressed as follows:

If A, and only if A, then B.

In a **substitutable relationship**, a similar concept can be substituted for the first concept and the second concept will still occur (see Table 8.2). For example, a substitutable relationship might propose that if tube feedings are administered (A_1), or if hyperalimentation is administered (A_2), the unconscious patient can remain hydrated (B). This relationship is expressed as follows:

If A_1, or if A_2, then B.

Sufficiency

A **sufficient relationship** states that when the first concept occurs, the second concept will occur, regardless of the presence or absence of other factors (Fawcett, 1999).

A statement could propose that if a patient is immobilized in bed longer than 1 week, he or she will lose bone calcium, regardless of anything else. This relationship is expressed as follows:

If A, then B, regardless of anything else.

A **contingent relationship** will occur only if a third concept is present. For example, a statement might claim that if a person experiences a stressor (A), the person will manage the stress (B), but only if she or he uses effective coping strategies (C). The third concept, in this case effective coping strategies, is referred to as an **intervening** (or **mediating**) **variable**. Intervening variables can affect the occurrence, strength, or direction of a relationship. A contingent relationship can be expressed as follows:

If A, then B, but only if C.

Being able to describe relationships among the concepts is an important first step in identifying, evaluating, and developing research frameworks. Table 8.2 provides a summary of the characteristics of relational statements. Remember that each statement may have multiple descriptive characteristics.

LEVELS OF ABSTRACTION OF STATEMENTS

Statements about the same two conceptual ideas can be made at various levels of abstractness. The relational statements found in conceptual models and grand theories (**general propositions**) are at a high level of abstraction. Relational statements found in middle-range theories (**specific propositions**) are at a moderate level of abstraction. **Hypotheses**, which are a form of statement consisting of an expressed relationship between variables, are at the concrete level, representing a low level of abstraction. As statements become less abstract, they become narrower in scope (Fawcett, 1999).

Statements at varying levels of abstraction that express relationships between or among the same conceptual ideas can be arranged in hierarchical form, from general to specific. This arrangement allows you to see (or evaluate) the logical links among the various levels of abstraction. In Fig. 8.2, abstract constructs were linked to concepts and variables. Linking general propositions to more specific propositions is the same process and links the relationships expressed in the framework with the hypotheses, research questions, or objectives that guide the methodology of the study (McQuiston & Campbell, 1997; Trego, 2009). The following excerpts provide an example of the more abstract theoretical proposition that provided the basis for one of the hypotheses tested in a study by Gillet et al. (2018). The following proposition and hypothesis are provided as an example.

Proposition

"…ethical leaders create an effective unit organizational culture for optimal patient care." (Gillet et al., 2018, p. 2)

Hypothesis

"Hypothesis 1. Ethical leadership is positively associated with patients' perceptions of quality of care." (Gillet et al., 2018, p. 2)

Grand Theories

Most disciplines have several conceptual models, each with a distinctive vocabulary. Table 8.3 lists a few of the conceptual models or grand theories in nursing. Each theory provides an overall picture, or gestalt, of the phenomena they explain. In addition to concepts specific to the theory, nurse theorists include the metaparadigm or domain concepts of nursing: person, health, environment, and nursing (Chinn & Kramer, 2015; Fawcett, 1985). Each theorist may define the domain concepts differently to be consistent with the other concepts and propositions of the theory. For example, Roy (1988) defined health as restoring or maintaining adaptation by activating cognator and regulator systems and using one of four adaptive modes (Roy & Andrews, 2008).

Consistent with her theory of self-care, Orem (2001) defined health as the extent to which persons can meet their own universal, developmental, and health-related self-care requisites. Most grand theories are not directly testable through research and thus cannot be used alone as the framework for a study (Fawcett, 1999; Walker & Avant, 2019). Application of grand nursing theories to research is discussed later in the chapter. For detailed information about grand nursing theories, refer to the primary sources written by the theorist and reference books about nursing theory (Alligood, 2018; Fawcett & DeSanto-Madeya, 2013; McEwen & Wills, 2014).

Middle-Range Theories

Middle-range theories are useful in both research and practice. Middle-range theories are less abstract than grand theories and closer to the day-to-day substance of clinical practice, a characteristic that explains why they can be called substantive theories. As a result, middle-range theories guide the practitioner in understanding the client's behavior, enabling interventions that are more effective. Because of their usefulness in practice, some writers refer to middle-range theories as **practice theories**.

Middle-range theories have been developed from grand nursing theories, clinical insights, and research findings. Mefford and Alligood (2011) combined health promotion principles with Levin's (1967) conservation theory, an older grand nursing theory, to develop a theory of health promotion for preterm infants. Middle-range theories may be developed by combining a nursing and a non-nursing theory. Some middle-range theories have been developed from clinical practice

---

TABLE 8.3 Selected Grand Nursing Theories	
Author (Year)	**Descriptive Label of the Theory**
King, Imogene (1981)	Interacting Systems Theory of Nursing (includes middle-range theory of goal attainment)
Leininger, Madeline (1997)	Transcultural Nursing Care, Sunrise Model of Care
Neuman, Betty (Neuman & Fawcett, 2002)	Self-Care Deficit Theory of Nursing
Newman, Margaret (1986)	Systems Model of Nursing
Orem, Dorothea (2001)	Health as Expanding Consciousness
Parse, Rosemarie (1992)	Human Becoming Theory
Rogers, Martha E (1970)	Unitary Human Beings
Roy, Calista (1988)	Adaptation Model
Watson, Jean (1979)	Philosophy and Science of Caring

guidelines, such as Good and Moore's (1996) theory of acute pain following surgery. Kolcaba's (1994) theory of comfort is an example of a middle-range theory developed over time. Kolcaba's clinical experiences motivated her to analyze the concept of comfort (Kolcaba & Kolcaba, 1991) and continue to refine the theory. Several research instruments have been developed to measure different types of comfort (http://www.thecomfortline.com/). Often grounded theory studies result in a middle-range theory. For example, Sun, Long, Chiang, and Chou (2019) developed a "theory to guide nursing students caring for patients with suicidal tendencies on psychiatric practicum" (p. 159). Through their grounded theory study, Sun et al. (2019) identified 12 key categories and a core category labeled "changing of mindsets towards caring for suicidal patients and promotion of suicidal care competencies" (p. 157). Carr's (2014) theory of family vigilance was developed from the findings of three ethnographical studies the author conducted in hospitals.

Middle-range theories are used more commonly than grand theories as frameworks for research. For example, Mefford and Alligood (2011) tested their middle-range theory of health promotion for preterm infants in their study using clinical data from neonatal units. Another study built upon a middle-range theory was Chism and Magnan's (2009) study of nursing students' perspectives on spiritual care and their expressions of spiritual empathy. Chism (2007) had previously developed the theory upon which the study was based, the middle-range theory of spiritual empathy, as part of her doctoral study. Covell and Sidani (2013a, b) identified empirical indicators for the concepts in Covell's (2008) nursing intellectual capital theory, evaluated the propositions among the concepts, and found mixed support for the relationships.

A specific type of middle-range theory is intervention theory. Intervention theories seek to explain the dynamics of a patient problem and exactly how a specific nursing intervention is expected to change patient outcomes (Wolf, 2015). Using two theories, Peek and Melnyk (2014) developed an intervention theory for a coping intervention to help mothers with the cancer diagnosis of a child. The self-regulation theory of Johnson (1999) was the basis for providing the mothers' anticipatory guidance about the expected behaviors and emotions of a child with cancer. At the same time, the control theory of Carver and Scheier (1982) was used as the basis for equipping the mothers with

"education, information, and behavior skills development of parent behaviors specific to this novel situation" (Peek & Melnyk, 2014, p. 204).

APPRAISING THEORIES AND RESEARCH FRAMEWORKS

Nurses examine and evaluate theories to determine their applicability for practice and usefulness for research. The evaluation of theories is complicated by the availability of several sets of evaluative criteria (Meleis, 2018). From these, we have selected the following for inclusion in the critical appraisal of research frameworks in published studies (Box 8.3).

Critical Appraisal of a Research Framework

During the process of critically appraising a study, the first task related to the research framework is to describe it. This task is easier when the researchers have explicitly identified the framework. For example, Condon et al. (2019) clearly identified the ecobiodevelopmental model by Shonkoff et al. (2012) as the theoretical framework for their study and linked the theoretical framework to their study aim: "The purpose of this study was to describe and examine relationships among maternal caregiving namely, parenting behaviors and PRF [parental reflective functioning] and child indicators of toxic stress in a multiethnic, urban sample of mothers and children of early school age (4–9 years). The ecobiodevelopmental model provides a framework for the study and describes connections among a child's ecology (social and physical environment), biology, and health and development… (Shonkoff et al., 2012)" (p. 426). Table 8.4 includes the conceptual and operational definitions of the three concepts in the research framework.

Other research, such as the Gillet et al. (2018) study previously described in this chapter, did not identify a

---

> ## BOX 8.3 Critical Appraisal of Research Frameworks
>
> - Identify and describe the theory.
> - Examine the logical structure of the framework.
> - Evaluate extent to which the framework guided the methodology of the study.
> - Decide the extent to which the researcher connected findings to the framework.

TABLE 8.4 Conceptual and Operational Definitions for Parenting Behaviors and Parental Reflective Functioning and Child Indicators of Toxic Stress

Concept	Conceptual Definition	Operational Definition
Parenting behavior	"Two aspects of caregiving with important implications for child development are parenting behavior and parental reflective functioning. Parenting behaviors include observable actions that may be supportive (e.g., praising or comforting a child) or hostile (e.g., use of threatening language or corporal punishment)" (Condon et al., 2019, p. 427).	"…measured parenting behaviors using the 20-item self-report Parent Behavior Inventory" (Condon et al., 2019, p. 427).
Parental reflective functioning (PRF)	"PFR, therefore, describes a caregiver's capacity to not only reflect on his or her own mental states but also on the child's internal world and to connect this to the child's behavior in meaningful ways (Slade, 2005)" (Condon et al., 2019, p. 426).	"…measured PRF with the 18-item version of the Parental Reflective Functioning Questionnaire [PRFQ; Luyten et al., 2017]. The PFRQ is a self report measure that includes three subscales" (Condon et al., 2019, p. 428).
Child indicators of toxic stress	"Toxic stress describes chronic activation of the stress-response system, which occurs in response to persistent environmental stressors, such as poverty or community violence, and alters development of the brain and multiple physiologic systems (Johnson, Riley, Granger, & Riis, 2013; Shonkoff et al., 2012)" (Condon et al., 2019, p. 425).	"…neuroendocrine functioning with hair cortisol level…. Immune functioning. We measured salivary C-reactive protein (CRP) level and a panel of four proinflammatory cytokines…. Cardiovascular functioning. We measured children's systolic (SBP) and diastolic (DBP)…. Physical health…measured children's height and weight with a calibrated stadiometer and scale…. Mother's reported on health history…. Behavior and academic performance…using age-appropriate parent-report versions of the 99-item Child Behavior Checklist (CBCL)" (Condon et al., 2019, p. 428).

Data from Condon, E. M., Holland, M. L., Slade, A., Redeker, N. S., Mayes, L. C., & Sadler, L. S. (2019). Associations between maternal caregiving and child indicators of toxic stress among multiethnic, urban families. *Journal of Pediatric Health Care, 33*(4), 425–436. doi:10.1016/j.pedhc.2018.12.002

framework in the study of "ethical leadership, professional caregivers' well-being and patients' perceptions of quality of care in oncology" (p. 1). However, Gillet and colleagues began their research report by presenting related findings from other studies that justified use of the study variables. The relational statements, presented as two hypotheses, were tested and provided the rationale for studying ethical leadership, professional caregivers' well-being, and patients' perceptions of quality of care in this sample.

A diagram of the concepts and relationships among them often makes describing the research framework easier. If a diagram is not provided, you can draw your own (Fig. 8.10). Charette et al. (2015) conducted a pilot study of an intervention to decrease the pain and anxiety experienced by adolescents who had spinal surgery. Fig. 8.10 displays the components of the intervention

in the orange box with a line from the intervention to the relationship between surgery and the effects of pain and anxiety. Charette et al. (2015) did not provide a diagram of the relationships among the concepts. Fig. 8.10 was drawn based on the concepts and relational statements in their research report.

Following your description of the framework, you are ready to examine the logical structure of the framework. Meleis's (2018) criteria for critically appraising theories include assessing the clarity and consistency of the logical structure. When the following questions about clarity and consistency can be answered with yes, the framework has a strong logical structure:

1. Are the definitions of concepts consistent with the theorist's definitions? This question is asked only if the researchers link their framework to a parent theory.

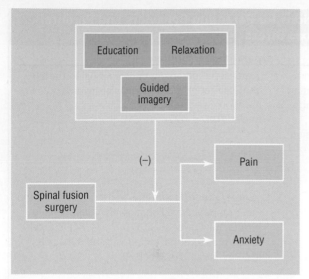

Fig. 8.10 Research framework inferred from Charette et al. (2015).

(The **parent theory** is the theory from which the researchers have selected the constructs for their study.)

2. Do the concepts reflect constructs identified in the framework? Some frameworks may not identify constructs and may be comprised of only concepts.
3. Do the variables reflect the concepts identified in the framework?
4. Are the conceptual definitions validated by references to the literature?
5. Are the propositions (relational statements) logical and defensible?

The next step in critically appraising a study framework is to evaluate the extent to which the framework guided the methodology by asking the following questions:

1. Do the operational definitions reflect the conceptual definitions?
2. Do the hypotheses, questions, or objectives reflect the constructs and/or concepts in the propositions of the framework?
3. Is the design appropriate for testing the propositions of the framework?

When a framework guides the methodology of a study, the answer to these questions will be yes. Some researchers may describe a theory or theories to provide context for their study but fail to use the framework to guide the methodology.

The final step in critically appraising a study framework is to decide the extent to which the researcher connected the findings to the framework by asking the following questions:

1. Did the researcher interpret the findings in terms of the framework?
2. Are the findings for each hypothesis, question, or objective consistent with the relationships proposed by the framework?

Even in studies clearly guided by a research framework, the findings may not be discussed in terms of the framework. Findings that are consistent with the framework are evidence of the framework's validity, and this point should be noted in the discussion. When the findings are not consistent with the research framework, researchers should discuss the possible reasons for this disconnect. One reason may be a lack of construct validity (see Chapters 10, 11, and 16). The instruments used may not have measured the constructs/concepts of the study framework adequately and accurately. Other possible reasons are that the framework was based on assumptions that were not true for the population being studied and that the framework did not represent the reality of the phenomena being studied in this specific sample.

DEVELOPING A RESEARCH FRAMEWORK FOR STUDY

Developing a framework is one of the most important steps in the research process but perhaps also one of the most difficult. A research report in a journal often contains only a brief presentation of the study framework because of page limitations, hardly equivalent to the prolonged work the researchers expended to develop a framework for the study.

As a new researcher, assume you have identified a research problem and are thinking about the proposed study's methodology. You need a research framework, but where do you start? This section presents three basic approaches to beginning the process of constructing a study framework: (1) identify an existing theory from nursing or another discipline, (2) synthesize a framework from research findings, or (3) propose a framework from clinical practice. The final steps of constructing a research framework are discussed after the presentation of the approaches.

Identifying and Adapting an Existing Theory

Take another look at the research reports you have read related to your topic. Which theories have others used when studying this area? In your exploration, include studies on your topic of interest that have been conducted with populations other than your own. For example, researchers have used several health behavior and psychological theories to guide studies related to medication adherence. Existing theories can provide insights into how the topic has been studied and the range of perspectives available on a given research topic.

When trying to find a theory that pertains to your variables and relational statements, you may choose to review theory textbooks and middle-range theory publications to examine the applicability of other nursing theories that might provide insight into your research problem (Alligood, 2018; McEwen & Wills, 2014). Before making a final decision about a theory, you should read primary sources written by the theorists to ensure that your topic is a good fit with the theory's concepts, definitions of concepts, assumptions, and propositions.

Synthesis From Research Findings

Developing a theory or a framework from research findings is the most accepted strategy of theory development (Meleis, 2018). The research-to-theory strategy, an inductive approach, begins by identifying relevant studies. Charette et al. (2015) were concerned about the high levels of pain and anxiety that adolescents reported after surgery to correct scoliosis. The levels and prolonged nature of pain and anxiety following the surgery hindered physical activity and recovery. The researchers reviewed the research literature, identified relevant studies, and found support for the following relationships:

- Spinal fusion, the corrective surgery for scoliosis, is associated with prolonged, severe postoperative pain and anxiety.
- Guided imagery is associated with decreased anxiety and postoperative pain.
- Provision of information and assisting coping through guided imagery and relaxation are more effective in reducing pain and anxiety than either intervention alone (Charette et al., 2015).

Based on these research findings, Charette et al. (2015) developed an intervention that combined "guided imagery, relaxation, and education to decrease postoperative pain and anxiety related to spinal fusion" (p. 212). As mentioned previously, Fig. 8.10 is a visual model of these relationships. The research team tested the intervention in a randomized clinical trial pilot study of its effects on pain, anxiety, coping, and daily activities compared to usual postoperative care. As predicted, the intervention group reported less overall pain at discharge, at 2 weeks postdischarge, and at the 1-month follow-up visit, when compared to the usual care group. The team's next planned steps are to repeat the study with a larger sample over a longer follow-up period. The study findings provided initial support for the proposed relationships among the concepts.

Research findings may support or aid in the modification of existing theoretical frameworks. For example, Jang and Kim (2018) conducted a correlational study of 600 "Korean women with cancer…to examine relationships between stress, social support, self-efficacy, coping, and psychosocial adjustment to construct a model of the effect pathways between those factors, and determine if survivorship stage moderates those effects" (p. 41). The researchers found the "results indicate that the Transactional Model of Stress and Coping accurately models stress, social support, self-efficacy, coping, and psychosocial adjustment in women with breast cancer (Lazarus & Folkman, 1984) and suggests a causal pathway exists from stress, through coping, to psychosocial adjustment" (Jang & Kim, 2018, p. 46). Derived from the study findings, three models for each of the survivorship stages illustrate the relationship between study variables (Fig. 8.11). These models show the direction and strength of the relationships. In the acute survival stage, the strongest relationships were between social support and psychosocial adjustment and between self efficacy and coping. In the extended survival stage (B), the relationship between stress and coping was statistically significant, a difference from the previous model. In the lasting survival stage (C), the relationship between stress and coping was no longer significant. However, the relationship between stress and psychosocial adjustment was stronger than it was in either of the other two stages.

Proposing a Framework From Practice Experiences

As members of a practice discipline, nurses may develop research frameworks from their clinical experiences. Nurses in practice can generalize about patient responses as they provide care to different types of patients. For example, "Patients with increased blood urea nitrogen are impatient and irritable." Nurses who reflect on practice may, over time, realize underlying principles of human behavior that guide their choices of interventions. Meleis (2018) noted that a nurse may have nagging

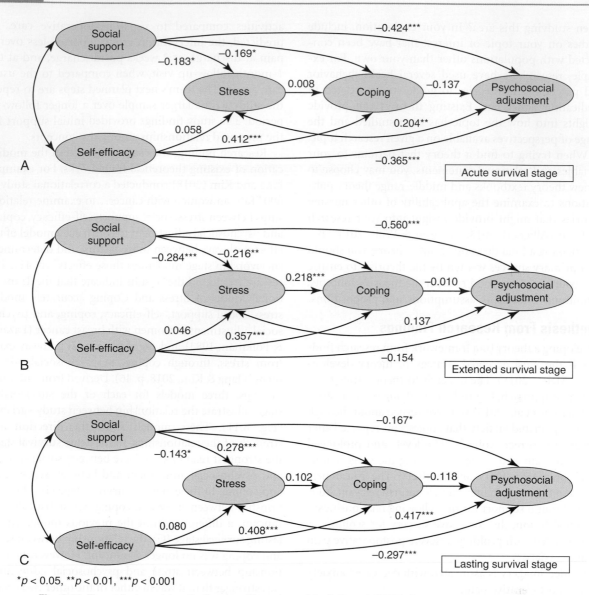

Fig. 8.11 Theoretical model path diagram. (From Jang, M., & Kım, J. [2018]. A structural model for stress, coping, and psychosocial adjustment: A multi-group analysis by stages of survivorship in Korean women with breast cancer. *European Journal of Oncology Nursing, 33*[1], 41–48. doi:10.1016/j.ejon.2018.01.004.)

questions about why certain situations persist, or wonder how to improve patient or organizational outcomes, which can lead to development of tentative theories. For example, a novice researcher who worked in a newborn intensive care unit might become convinced from her clinical experiences that a mother's frequent visits to the hospital might be related to her infant's weight gain. The nurse's ideas could be diagrammed as the lower set of relationships shown in Fig. 8.12C.

The relationship the nurse identified consisted of two concrete ideas: number of mother visits and weight gain. From the perspective of research, these ideas are variables. Instead of starting with a framework and linking the concepts of the framework to possible study variables, she was starting with variables and needed to identify the concepts that the variables represented. The nurse reviewed the literature and looked for explanations for why visits by the mother were important and

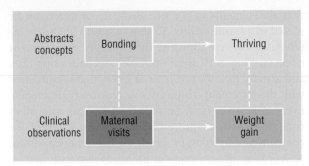

Fig. 8.12 Research framework from clinical practice.

what happened when a mother visited her baby. As she reflected on what she read, she realized that maybe the visits promoted bonding or attachment. The nurse continued to reflect on her experiences and remembered that when babies failed to gain weight or lost weight, they were sometimes labeled as "failing to thrive." Wording that more positively, she decided the concept related to weight gain was thriving. On the basis of her clinical experiences and her thinking processes, the nurse began to learn more about theories of bonding and used what she learned to develop a framework for a study related to bonding and thriving of newborns in neonatal intensive care units (see Fig. 8.12).

Research frameworks rarely develop from only one source of knowledge. Nurse researchers often combine existing theories, research findings, and insights from their clinical experiences into a framework for a study. For example, to study adherence to blood pressure medications among older Chinese immigrants, Li, Wallhagen, and Froelicher (2010) derived their model from four sources: Becker's (1974) health belief model, findings from preliminary studies, hypertension literature, and clinical experience. Rishel (2014) described combining her clinical experience as a pediatric bone marrow transplant nurse with her review of the literature when she began to explore parents' end-of-life decisions. Later in her career as a researcher, she proposed a middle-range theory of the process of parental decision making.

Study frameworks begun in these ways are considered tentative theory until research findings provide evidence to support the relationships as diagrammed. **Tentative theories** are those that are developed from other theories, research findings, and/or clinical practice and that, as yet, do not have evidence to support their relational statements. Whatever your approach to beginning the process, once you can identify possible concepts and relationships, you are ready to move through the remainder of the process to develop the framework that is explicated in the final research report.

Defining Relevant Concepts

Concepts are selected for a framework on the basis of their relevance to the phenomenon of interest. The concepts included in the research framework should reflect the problem statement and the literature review of the proposal. Each concept included in a framework must be defined conceptually. Conceptual definitions may be found in existing theoretical works and quoted in the proposal with sources cited. Conceptual definitions also may be found in published concept analyses, previous studies using the concept, or the literature associated with an instrument developed to measure the concept. Although the instrument itself is an operational definition of the concept, often the writer provides a conceptual definition on which the instrument development was based. (See Chapter 6 for more extensive discussion of conceptual and operational definitions for study variables.) When acceptable conceptual definitions are not available, you should perform concept synthesis or concept analysis to develop them.

Developing Relational Statements

The next step in framework development is to link all of the study concepts through relational statements. If you began with an existing theory, the author may have identified theoretical propositions already. If you synthesized research findings, you have evidence that supports relationships between or among some or all of the concepts. This evidence supports the validity of each relational statement. This support must include a discussion of previous quantitative, qualitative, and mixed methods research that has either examined the proposed relationship or published observations from the perspective of clinical practice.

Extracting relational statements from the written description of an existing theory, published research, or clinical literature can be a daunting task. The following procedure describes how to do so: Select the portion of the theory, research report, or clinical literature that discusses the relationships among concepts relevant to your study. Write single sentences that link concepts. Change each sentence to a diagram of the relationship, similar to those presented earlier in the chapter (see Figs. 8.3 and 8.4). Continue this process until all of the relationships in the text have been expressed as simple diagrams or small maps.

If statements relating the concepts of interest are not available in the literature, statement synthesis is necessary. Develop statements that propose specific relationships among the concepts you are studying. You may gain the knowledge for your statement synthesis through clinical observation and an integrative literature review (Walker & Avant, 2019).

Developing Hierarchical Statement Sets

A **hierarchical statement set** is composed of a specific proposition (relational statement) at the conceptual level and a hypothesis or research question, representing concrete relationships among variables. The specific proposition may be preceded by a more general proposition when an existing theory was the source of the framework (see example earlier in the chapter). The proposition is listed first, with the hypothesis or research question immediately following. In some cases, more than one hypothesis or research question may be developed for a single proposition. The statement set indicates the link between the framework and the methodology. The following is an example:

- Anxiety is intensified by a lack of information about the future (construct level).
- Patient anxiety is reduced when information about a procedure is provided (concept level).
- Preoperative teaching provided several days prior to a procedure and repeated in the preoperative phase produces lower self-rated anxiety than the usual method of preoperative teaching (hypothesis/variable level).

Constructing a Conceptual Map

A conceptual map is the visual representation of a research framework. With the concepts defined and the relational statements diagrammed, you are ready to represent the framework for your study in a visual manner. The resultant map may be limited to only the concepts that you are studying or may be inclusive of other related concepts that are not going to be studied or measured at this time. When the map includes concepts that are not included in the specific study being proposed, you must clearly identify the concepts in the map that will be measured in the study.

From a practical standpoint, first arrange the relational statements you have diagrammed from left to right with outcomes located at the far right. Concepts that are elements of a more abstract construct can be placed in a frame or box. To show a group of closely interrelated concepts, enclose the concepts in a frame or circle (see Fig. 8.10 as an example). Second, using lines and arrows, link the concepts in a way that is consistent with the statement diagrams you previously developed. Every concept should be linked to at least one other concept. Third, examine the framework diagram for completeness by asking yourself the following questions:

1. Are all of the concepts in the study also included on the map?
2. Are all of the concepts on the map defined?
3. Does the map clearly portray the framework and its phenomenon of interest?
4. Does the map accurately reflect all of the statements?
5. Is there a statement for each of the links portrayed by the map?
6. Is the sequence of links in the map accurate?
7. Do arrows point from cause to effect, reflecting direction of relationship?

Developing a well-constructed conceptual map requires repeated tries, but persistence pays off. You may need to reexamine the statements identified. Are there some missing links? Are some of the links inaccurately expressed?

As the map takes shape and begins to seem right, show it to trusted colleagues. Can that person follow your logic? Does that person agree with your links? Can missing elements be identified? Can you explain the map aloud? Seek out individuals who have experienced the phenomenon you are mapping. Does the process depicted seem valid to those individuals? Find someone more experienced than you in conceptual mapping to examine your map closely and critically.

The product of the creative and critical thinking that you have expended in the development of your research framework may provide a structure for one study or become the basis for a program of research. Continue to consider the framework as you collect and analyze data and interpret the findings. While you wait to hear whether your proposal has been funded or while your data are being collected, use the time to expand the written description of the framework and the evidence supporting its relationships into a manuscript for publication (see Chapter 27). When disseminated, your research framework has the potential to make a valuable contribution to nursing knowledge.

KEY POINTS

- A concept is a term that abstractly describes and names an object or a phenomenon, thus providing it with a distinct identity or meaning.
- A relational statement is the explanation of the connection between concepts.
- A conceptual model or grand theory broadly explains phenomena of interest, expresses assumptions, and reflects a philosophical stance.
- A theory is a set of concepts and relational statements explaining the relationships among them.
- Scientific theories have significant evidence, and their relationships may be considered laws.
- Substantive theories are less abstract than grand nursing theories, can easily be applied in practice, and may be called middle-range theories.
- Middle-range theories may be developed from qualitative data, clinical experiences, clinical practice guidelines, or more abstract theories.
- Tentative theories are developed from research findings and clinical experiences, and they have not yet been validated.
- A framework is the abstract, logical structure of meaning that guides the development of the study and enables the researcher to link the findings to the body of knowledge used in nursing.
- Relational statements are the core of the framework; it is these statements that are examined through research.
- Relational statements can be described by their linearity, timing, and type of relationships.
- Almost every study has a theoretical framework, either implicit or explicit.
- The steps of critically appraising a research framework are (1) describing its concepts and relational statements, (2) examining its logical structure, (3) evaluating the extent to which the framework guided the methodology, and (4) determining the extent to which the researcher linked the findings back to the framework.
- The logical adequacy of a research framework is the extent to which the relational statements are clear and used consistently.
- The framework should be well integrated with the methodology carefully structured and clearly presented, whether the study is physiological or psychosocial.
- Research frameworks may start with existing theories, research findings, and/or clinical experiences.
- The remaining steps of the process are (1) selecting and defining concepts, (2) developing statements relating the concepts, (3) expressing the statements in hierarchical fashion, and (4) developing a conceptual map.
- Concepts and relational statements can be diagrammed as a conceptual map to visually represent the research framework.
- Developing a framework for a study is one of the most important steps in the research process.

REFERENCES

Alligood, M. R. (2018). *Nursing theory: Utilization & application* (5th ed.). Maryland Heights, MO: Mosby Elsevier.

Becker, M. (1974). The health belief model and sick role behavior. *Health Education Monographs, 2*(4), 409–462. doi:10.1177/109019817400200405

Brooks, L. A., Manias, E., & Bloomer, M. J. (2019). Culturally sensitive communication in healthcare: A concept analysis. *Collegian 26*(3), 383–391. doi:10.1016/j.colegn.2018.09.007

Butts, J. B., & Rich, K. L. (2018). *Philosophies and theories for advanced nursing practice* (3rd ed.). Burlington, MA: Jones & Bartlett Learning.

Carr, J. (2014). A middle range theory of family vigilance. *Medsurg Nursing, 23*(4), 251–255.

Carver, C., & Scheier, M. (1982). Control theory: A useful conceptual framework for personality-social, clinical, and health psychology. *Psychological Bulletin, 92*(1), 111–135. doi:10.1037/0033-2909.92.1.111

Charette, S., Lachance, J., Charest, M., Villeneuve, D., Theroux, J., … Joncas, J. (2015). Guided imagery for adolescent post-spinal fusion pain management: A pilot study. *Pain Management Nursing, 16*(3), 211–220. doi:10.1016/j.pmn.2014.06.004

Chinn, P. L., & Kramer, M. K. (2015). *Integrated theory and knowledge development in nursing* (9th ed.). St. Louis, MO: Elsevier.

Chism, L. (2007). *Spiritual empathy: A model for spiritual well-being.* Unpublished dissertation, Oakland University, Rochester, MI.

Chism, L., & Magnan, M. (2009). The relationship of nursing students' spiritual care perspectives to their expressions of spiritual empathy. *Journal of Nursing Education, 48*(11), 597–605. doi:10.3928/01484834-20090716-05

Condon, E. M., Holland, M. L., Slade, A., Redeker, N. S., Mayes, L. C., & Sadler, L. S. (2019). Associations between maternal caregiving and child indicators of toxic stress among multiethnic, urban families. *Journal of Pediatric Health Care, 33*(4), 425–436. doi:10.1016/j.pedhc.2018.12.002

Covell, C. (2008). The middle range theory of nursing intellectual capital. *Journal of Advanced Nursing, 63*(1), 94–103. doi:10.1111/j.1365-2648.2008.04626.x

Covell, C., & Sidani, S. (2013a). Nursing intellectual capital theory: Operationalization and empirical validation of concepts. *Journal of Advanced Nursing, 69*(8), 1785–1796. doi:10.1111/jan.12040

Covell, C., & Sidani, S. (2013b). Nursing intellectual capital theory: Testing selected propositions. *Journal of Advanced Nursing, 69*(11), 2432–2445. doi:10.1111/jan.12118

Cox, J., Thomas-Watkins, C., Pajarillo, E., DeGennaro, S., Cadmus, E., & Martinez, M. (2015). Factors associated with falls in hospitalized adult patients. *Applied Nursing Research, 28*(2), 78–82. doi:10.1016/j.apnr.2014.12.003

Coyne, I., Holmström, I., & Söderbäck, M. (2018). Centeredness in healthcare: A concept synthesis of family-centered care, person-centered care and child-centered care. *Journal of Pediatric Nursing, 42*, 45–56. doi:10.1016/j.pedn.2018.07.001

Donabedian, A. (1987). Some basic issues in evaluating the quality of health care. In L. T. Rinke (Ed.), *Outcome measures in home care* (Vol. I, p. 338). New York, NY: National League for Nursing. (Original work published 1976)

Fawcett, J. (1985). Theory: Basis for the study and practice of nursing education. *Journal of Nursing Education, 24*(6), 226–229. doi:10.3928/0148-4834-19850601-04

Fawcett, J. (1999). *The relationship of theory and research* (3rd ed.). Philadelphia, PA: F. A. Davis.

Fawcett, J., & DeSanto-Madeya, S. (2013). *Contemporary nursing knowledge: Analysis and evaluation of nursing models and theories* (3rd ed.). Philadelphia: F.A. Davis.

Fitzpatrick, J. J., & Whall, A. J. (2005). *Conceptual models of nursing: Analysis and application* (4th ed.). Upper Saddle River, NJ: Pearson Prentice Hall.

Gillet, N., Fouquereau, E., Coillot, H., Bonnetain, F., Dupont, S., Moret, L., ... Colombat, P. (2018). Ethical leadership, professional caregivers' well-being, and patients' perceptions of quality of care in oncology. *European Journal of Oncology Nursing, 33*, 1–7. doi:10.1016/j.ejon.2018.01.002

Good, M., & Moore, S. (1996). Clinical practice guidelines as a new source of middle-range theory: Focus on pain. *Nursing Outlook, 44*(2), 74–79. doi:10.1016/S0029-6554(96)80053-4

Goodson, P. (2015). Theory as practice. In J. Butts & K. Rich (Eds.), *Philosophies and theories for advanced nursing practice* (2nd ed., pp. 71–108). Burlington, MA: Jones & Bartlett.

Haase, J., Britt, T., Coward, D., Leidy, N., & Penn, P. (1992). Simultaneous concept analysis of spiritual perspective, hope, acceptance, and self-transcendence. *Image: Journal of Nursing Scholarship, 24*(2), 141–147. doi:10.1111/j.1547-5069.1992.tb00239.x

Higgins, P., & Moore, S. (2000). Levels of theoretical thinking in nursing. *Nursing Outlook, 48*(4), 179–183.

Hupcey, J., & Penrod, J. (2005). Concept analysis: Examining the state of the science. *Research for Theory and Nursing Practice, 19*(2), 197–208. doi:10.1891/088971805780957350

İnan, F. Ş., Günüşen, N., Duman, Z. Ç., & Ertem, M. Y. (2019). The impact of mental health nursing module, clinical practice and an anti-stigma program on nursing students' attitudes toward mental illness: A quasi-experimental study. *Journal of Professional Nursing, 35*(3), 201–208. doi:10.1016/j.profnurs.2018.10.001

Jang, M., & Kim, J. (2018). A structural model for stress, coping, and psychosocial adjustment: A multi-group analysis by stages of survivorship in Korean women with breast cancer. *European Journal of Oncology Nursing, 33*(1), 41–48. doi:10.1016/j.ejon.2018.01.004

Johnson, J. (1999). Self-regulation theory and coping with physical illness. *Research in Nursing & Health, 22*(6), 436–448.

Johnson, S., Riley, A., Granger, D., & Riis, J. (2013). The science of early life toxic stress for pediatric practice and advocacy. *Pediatrics, 131*(2), 319–327. doi:10.1542/peds.2012-0469

King, I. (1981). *A theory for nursing: Systems, concept, and process.* New York, NY: Delmar.

Kolcaba, K. (1994). A theory of holistic comfort for nursing. *Journal of Advanced Nursing, 19*(6), 1176–1184. doi:10.1111/j.1365-2648.1994.tb01202.x

Kolcaba, K., & Kolcaba, R. (1991). An analysis of the concept of comfort. *Journal of Advanced Nursing, 16*(11), 1301–1310. doi:10.1111/j.1365-2648.1991.tb01558.x

Kousoulou, M., Suhonen, R., & Charalambous, A. (2019). Associations of individualized nursing care and quality oncology nursing care in patients diagnosed with cancer. *European Journal of Oncology Nursing, 41*(1), 33–40. doi:10.1016/j.ejon.2019.05.011

Lazarus, R., & Folkman, S. (1984). *Stress, appraisal, and coping.* New York, NY: Springer.

Leininger, M. M. (1997). Overview of the theory of culture care with the ethnonursing research method. *Journal of Transcultural Nursing, 8*(2), 32–54.

Levin, M. (1967). Four conservation principles of nursing. *Nursing Forum, 6*(1), 45–59.

Li, W. W., Wallhagen, M., & Froelicher, E. (2010). Factors predicting blood pressure control in older Chinese immigrants to the United States of America. *Journal of Advanced Nursing, 66*(10), 2202–2212. doi:10.1111/j.1365-2648.2010.05399.x

Luyten, P., Mayes, L. C., Nijssens, L., & Fonagy, P. (2017). The parental reflective functioning questionnaire: Development and preliminary validation. *PloS One, 12*(5), e0176218. doi.org/10.1371/journal.pone.0176218

Ma, C. (2018). An investigation of factors influencing self-care behaviors in young and middle-aged adults with hypertension based on a health belief model. *Heart & Lung, 47*(2), 136–141. doi:10.1016/j.hrtlng.2017.12.001

McEwen, M., & Wills, E. M. (2014). *Theoretical basis for nursing* (4th ed.). Philadelphia, PA: Lippincott Williams & Wilkins.

McQuiston, C., & Campbell, J. (1997). Theoretical substruction: A guide for theory testing research. *Nursing Science Quarterly, 10*(3), 117–123.

Mefford, L., & Alligood, M. (2011). Testing a theory of health promotion for preterm infants based on Levine's conservation model of nursing. *Journal of Theory Construction and Testing, 15*(2), 41–47.

Meleis, A. I. (2018). *Theoretical nursing: Development and progress* (6th ed.). Philadelphia, PA: Wolters Kluwer/Lippincott Williams & Wilkins.

Merton, R. K. (1968). *Social theory and social structure*. New York, NY: Free Press.

Mirza, N., Manankil-Rankin, L., Prentice, D., Hagerman, L. A., & Draenos, C. (2019). Practice readiness of new nursing graduates: A concept analysis. *Nurse Education in Practice, 37*, 68–74. doi:10.1016/j.nepr.2019.04.009

Moore, J., & Pichler, V. (2000). Measurement of Orem's basic conditioning factors: A review of published research. *Nursing Science Quarterly, 13*(2), 137–142.

Neuman, B., & Fawcett, J. (2002). *The Neuman systems model* (4th ed.). Upper Saddle River, NJ: Prentice-Hall.

Newman, M. (1979). *Theory development in nursing*. Philadelphia, PA: F.A. Davis.

Newman, M. (1986). *Health as expanding consciousness*. St. Louis, MO: Mosby.

Orem, D. E. (2001). *Nursing: Concepts for practice* (6th ed.). St. Louis, MO: Mosby Year-Book Inc.

Parse, R. (1992). Human becoming: Parse's theory of nursing. *Nursing Science Quarterly, 5*(1), 35–42. doi:10.1177/089431849200500109

Peek, G., & Melnyk, B. (2014). A coping intervention for mothers of children diagnosed with cancer: Connecting theory and research. *Applied Nursing Research, 27*(3), 202–204.

Pender, N. (1996). *Health promotion in nursing practice* (3rd ed.). Stamford, CT: Appleton & Lange.

Peterson, S. J., & Bredow, T. S. (2017). *Middle-range theories: Application to nursing research*. Philadelphia, PA: Wolters Kluwer/Lippincott Williams & Wilkins.

Rishel, C. (2014). An emerging theory on parental end-of-life decision making as a stepping stone to new research. *Applied Nursing Research, 27*(4), 261–264. doi:10.1016/j.apnr.2014.07.003

Rodgers, B. L. (2000). Concept analysis: An evolutionary view. In B. L. Rodgers (Ed.), *Concept development in nursing: Foundations, techniques, and applications* (2nd ed., pp. 77–102). Philadelphia, PA: W. B. Saunders.

Rogers, M. E. (1970). *An introduction to the theoretical basis of nursing*. Philadelphia, PA: Davis.

Rohani, C., Abedi, H., Omranipour, R., & Languis-Eklof, A. (2015). Health-related quality of life and the predictive role of sense of coherence, spirituality, and religious coping in a sample of Iranian women with breast cancer: A prospective study with comparative design. *Health and Quality of Life Outcomes*, Article 40. doi:10.1186/s12955-015-0229-1

Roy, C. (1988). An explication of the philosophical assumptions of the Roy adaptation model. *Nursing Science Quarterly, 1*(1), 26–34. doi:10.1177/089431848800100108

Roy, C., & Andrews, H. A. (2008). *Roy's adaptation model for nursing* (3rd ed.). Stamford, CT: Appleton & Lange.

Schwartz-Barcott, D., & Kim, H. S. (2000). An expansion and elaboration of the hybrid model of concept development. In B. L. Rogers & K. Knafl (Eds.), *Concept development in nursing: Foundations, techniques, and applications* (pp. 129–159). Philadelphia: W. B. Saunders.

Shonkoff, J., Garner, A., & Committee on Psychosocial Aspects of Child and Family Health. (2012). The lifelong effects of early childhood adversity and toxic stress. *Pediatrics, 129*(1), e232–e246. doi:10.1542/peds.2011–2663.

Slade, A. (2005). Parental reflective functioning: An introduction. *Attachment & Human Development, 7*(3), 269–281. doi:10.1080/14616730500245906

Smith, M. J., & Liehr, P. R. (2018). *Middle range theory for nursing* (4th ed.). New York, NY: Springer Publishing Company.

Sun, F. K., Long, A., Chiang, C. Y., & Chou, M. H. (2019). A theory to guide nursing students caring for patients with suicidal tendencies on psychiatric clinical practicum. *Nurse Education in Practice, 38*, 157–163. doi:10.1016/j.nepr.2019.07.001

Trego, L. (2009). Theoretical substruction: Establishing links between theory and measurement of military women's attitudes toward menstrual suppression during military operations. *Journal of Advanced Nursing, 65*(7), 1548–1559. doi:10.1111/j.1365-2648.2009.05010.x

Walker, L. O., & Avant, K. C. (2019). *Strategies for theory construction in nursing* (6th ed.). Boston, MA: Prentice Hall.

Wan, E. Y. F., Fung, C. S. C., Fong, D. Y. T., Chan, A. K. C., & Lam, C. L. K. (2016). A curvilinear association of body mass index with cardiovascular diseases in Chinese patients with type 2 diabetes mellitus—A population-based retrospective cohort study. *Journal of Diabetes and Its Complications, 30*(7), 1261–1268. doi:10.1016/j.jdiacomp.2016.05.010

Watson, J. (1979). *Nursing: The philosophy and science of caring*. Boston, MA: Little Brown and Company.

Wilson, J. (1963). *Thinking with concepts*. Cambridge, England: Cambridge University Press.

Wolf, L. (2015). Research as problem solving: Theoretical frameworks as tools. *Journal of Emergency Nursing, 41*(1), 83–85. doi:10.1016/j.jen.2014.09.011

9

Ethics in Research

Jennifer R. Gray

http://evolve.elsevier.com/Gray/practice/

Many factors affected your decision to be a nurse but, for most of you, a key motivation was the desire to help others. Nursing as a profession is firmly based on the ethical principles of respect for persons, beneficence, and justice. These ethical principles that guide clinical practice must also be the standards for the conduct of nursing research (Fowler, 2017). In research, the application of ethics begins with identifying a study topic and continues through publication of the study findings.

Ethical research is essential for generating evidence for nursing practice (Lach, 2019), but what does the ethical conduct of research involve? This question has been debated for many years by researchers, politicians, philosophers, lawyers, and even study participants. The debate continues because of the complexity of human rights issues; the focus of research in new, challenging arenas of technology, stem cells, and genomics; the complex ethical codes and regulations governing research; and the various interpretations of these codes and regulations. Unfortunately, specific standards of ethical research were developed in response to historical events in which the rights of participants were egregiously violated or the behavior of research scientists was blatantly dishonest (Grady, 2018). To provide an understanding of the rationale for today's human participant protection requirements, this chapter begins by reviewing five historical events, and the mandates and regulations for ethical research that were generated as a result of them.

In your clinical setting, you are probably familiar with the **Health Insurance Portability and Accountability Act** (HIPAA) and the necessity of protecting the privacy of a person's health information (Department of Health and Human Services [DHHS], 2003). HIPAA, which identified the elements of private health information, has had a significant impact on researchers and institutional review boards (IRBs) in universities and healthcare agencies. The chapter also discusses the actions essential for conducting research in an ethical manner through protection of the rights of human participants. This includes making an unbiased assessment of the potential benefits and risks inherent in a study and ensuring that informed consent is obtained properly. The submission of a research proposal for institutional review is also presented.

An ethical problem that has received increasing attention since the 1980s is researcher misconduct, also called scientific misconduct. **Scientific misconduct** is the violation of human rights during a study, including falsifying results or behaving dishonestly when disseminating the findings. Misconduct has occurred during all study phases, including reporting and publication of studies. Many disciplines, including nursing, have experienced episodes of research misconduct that have affected the quality of research evidence generated and disseminated. A discussion of current ethical issues related to research misconduct and to the use of animals in research concludes the chapter.

HISTORICAL EVENTS AFFECTING THE DEVELOPMENT OF ETHICAL CODES AND REGULATIONS

The ethical conduct of research has been a focus since the 1940s because of mistreatment of human participants in selected studies. Although these are not the only examples of unethical research, five historical experimental projects have been publicized for their unethical treatment of participants and will be described in the order in which the projects began: (1) the syphilis studies in Tuskegee, Alabama (1932–1972); (2) Nazi medical experiments (1941–1946) and resulting trials at Nuremberg; (3) the sexually transmitted infection study in Guatemala (1946–1948); (4) the Willowbrook State School study (1955–1970); and (5) the Jewish Chronic Disease Hospital study (1963–1965). More recent examples are included in the chapter, in relation to specific aspects of research. Although these five projects were biomedical and the primary investigators were physicians, nurses were aware of the research, identified potential participants, delivered treatments to participants, and served as data collectors in all of them. As indicated earlier, these and other incidences of unethical treatment of participants and research misconduct were important catalysts in the formulation of the ethical codes and regulations that direct research today.

Tuskegee Syphilis Study

In 1932, the US Public Health Service (USPHS) initiated a study of syphilis in African American men in the small, rural town of Tuskegee, Alabama (Brandt, 1978; Reverby, 2012; Rothman, 1982). The study, which continued for 40 years, was conducted to observe the natural course of syphilis in African American men. The researcher hired an African American nurse, Eunice Rivers, to recruit and retain participants. The research participants were organized into two groups: one group consisted of 400 men who had untreated syphilis, and the other was a control group of approximately 200 men without syphilis. Most of the men who consented to participate in the study were not informed about the purpose and procedures of the research. Some men were unaware that they were participants in a study. Some were subjected to spinal taps and told the procedure was treatment for their "bad blood" (Reverby, 2012), the colloquial term for syphilis and other diseases of the blood.

By 1936, the group of men with syphilis experienced more health complications than did the control group. Ten years later, the death rate of the group with syphilis was twice as high as that of the control group. The participants with syphilis were examined periodically but were never administered penicillin, even after it became the standard treatment in the 1940s (Brandt, 1978). These results could have been predicted because untreated syphilis was and is the most damaging of the bacterial venereal diseases, with degeneration occurring from cardiac lesions, brain deterioration, or involvement of other organ systems.

The findings of the Tuskegee syphilis study were published beginning in 1936, and additional papers were published every 4 to 6 years. In 1953, Nurse Rivers was the first author on a publication about the study procedures to retain participants (Rivers, Schuman, Simpson, & Olansky, 1953). At least 13 articles were published in medical journals reporting the results of the study. In 1969, the US Centers for Disease Control and Prevention (CDC) reviewed the study and decided that it should continue. In 1972, a story published in the *Washington Star* about the study sparked public outrage. Only then did the US Department of Health, Education, and Welfare (DHEW) stop the study. An investigation of the Tuskegee study found it to be ethically unjustified. In 1997, President Clinton publicly apologized for the government's role in this event (Baker, Brawley, & Marks, 2005; Reverby, 2012).

Nazi Medical Experiments

From 1933 to 1945, the Third Reich in Europe implemented atrocious, unethical activities, some of which they called research (Steinfels & Levine, 1976). Their goal was to produce a population of racially pure Germans, also known as Aryan. Most notably, the Nazis targeted all Jews for imprisonment and systematic genocide, resulting in millions of deaths. Population growth among the Aryans was encouraged. In contrast, Nazi doctors sterilized people regarded as racial enemies, such as the Jews. In addition, Nazis killed people whom they considered racially impure or disabled, such as persons with mental illness, disabilities, and dementia. Almost 0.25 million Germans who were physically or mentally disabled (Jacobs, 2008) and 300,000 psychiatric patients (Foth, 2013) were killed. These same people were also used as research participants.

The medical experiments involved exposing participants to high altitudes, freezing temperatures, malaria, poisons, spotted fever (typhus), new drugs, and unproven surgeries, usually without anesthesia (Steinfels & Levine, 1976). For example, participants were immersed in freezing water to determine how long German pilots could survive if shot down over the North Sea. Identical twins were forced to be participants of experiments in which one would be infected with a disease. Both were later killed for postmortem examination of their organs to determine differences due to the disease. These medical experiments purportedly were conducted to generate knowledge to benefit Aryans at the cost of suffering and death for prisoners in no position to give consent. In addition to the atrocities and coercion, however, the studies were poorly designed and conducted. As a result, little if any useful scientific knowledge was generated.

The Nazi experiments violated ethical principles and rights of the research participants. Researchers selected participants on the basis of race, affliction, or sexual orientation, demonstrating an unfair selection process. The participants also had no opportunity to refuse participation; they were prisoners who were coerced or forced to participate. Frequently, study participants were killed during the experiments or sustained permanent physical, mental, and social damage (Levine, 1986; Steinfels & Levine, 1976). The doctors who propagated the mistreatment of human participants were brought to trial, along with other Nazi soldiers and officers, in Nuremberg, Germany, beginning in 1945.

Nuremberg Code

At the conclusion of the trials of Nazi doctors involved in research, the defense presented 10 guidelines for appropriate research with human participants, which collectively became known as the **Nuremberg Code** (1949). Among the principles were the following: (1) participants' voluntary consent to participate in research; (2) the right of participants to withdraw from studies; (3) protection of participants from physical and mental suffering, injury, disability, and death during studies; and (4) an assessment of the benefits and risks in a study. The Nuremberg Code (1949) forms the basis for protection for all human participants, regardless of a researcher's disciplinary affiliation.

Declaration of Helsinki

The members of the World Medical Organization (WMO) were understandably alarmed by the actions of Nazi researchers during World War II. The World Medical Assembly (WMA) of the WMO drafted a document called the **Declaration of Helsinki** in 1964. The Declaration of Helsinki (WMO, 1996) has subsequently been reviewed and amended, with the last amendment being approved in 2013 (WMA, 2013). The declaration forms the foundation for current research protection practices, such as research ethics committees.

A research ethics committee must review proposed human participant research for possible approval; if the study is approved, the committee is responsible for monitoring its methods and outcomes as well as reviewing and approving any alterations in the research plan before such changes are implemented. The declaration also differentiates therapeutic research from nontherapeutic research. **Therapeutic research** gives the patient an opportunity to receive an experimental treatment that might have beneficial results. **Nontherapeutic research** is conducted to generate knowledge for a discipline: The results from the study might benefit future patients with similar conditions but will probably not benefit those acting as research participants. Box 9.1 contains several ethical principles from the declaration. The complete document is available from the WMA (2018).

Worldwide, most institutions in which clinical research is conducted have adopted the Declaration of Helsinki. It has been revised, with the most recent revision increasing protection for vulnerable populations and requiring compensation for participants harmed by research (WMA, 2018). However, neither this document nor the Nuremberg Code has prevented some investigators from conducting unethical research (Beecher, 1966). Remember that the Tuskegee study continued after the Declaration of Helsinki was first released.

BOX 9.1   Key Ideas of the Declaration of Helsinki

1. Well-being of the individual research participant must take precedence over all other interests.
2. Investigators must protect the life, health, privacy, and dignity of research participants.
3. A strong, independent justification must be documented prior to exposing healthy volunteers to risk of harm, merely to gain new scientific information.
4. Extreme care must be taken in making use of placebo-controlled trials, which should be used only in the absence of an existing proven therapy.
5. Clinical trials must focus on improving diagnostic, therapeutic, and prophylactic procedures for patients with selected diseases without exposing participants to any additional risk of serious or irreversible harm.

From Declaration of Helsinki. (1964, 2013). *WMA declaration of Helsinki—Ethical principles for medical research involving human subjects.* Retrieved from https://www.wma.net/policies-post/wma-declaration-of-helsinki-ethical-principles-for-medical-research-involving-human-subjects/

Guatemala Sexually Transmitted Disease Study

Beginning in 1946, a USPHS employee, Dr. John C. Cutler, conducted a study in Guatemala in which participants were intentionally exposed to syphilis and other sexually transmitted diseases. The participants were "sex workers, prisoners, mental patients, and soldiers" (Reverby, 2012, p. 8). Initially, participants were to be given penicillin or an arsenic compound (the treatment prior to penicillin) between exposure and infection to determine the prophylactic efficacy of each medication. The records for the study are incomplete, and it is not known how many persons developed an infection, died from the infection, or were harmed by the administered treatment (Reverby, 2012). The researchers suppressed information about their interventions and findings because they anticipated negative publicity due to the unethical nature of the study. After Dr. Cutler left in 1948, the USPHS continued to fund researchers to monitor the research participants and conduct serological testing through 1955 (Presidential Commission for the Study of Bioethical Issues, 2011).

In 2010, Reverby (2012) was reviewing the records of researchers who participated in the Tuskegee study and found the papers of Dr. Cutler in which the Guatemala study was described. She shared her discovery with the CDC, and, subsequently, President Obama was informed. A public apology ensued. The Presidential Commission for the Study of Bioethical Issues (2011) investigated and wrote a report confirming the facts of the Guatemala study.

Willowbrook Study

From the mid-1950s to the early 1970s, Dr. Saul Krugman practiced at Willowbrook State School, a large institution for cognitively impaired persons in Brooklyn, New York, and conducted research on hepatitis A infection (Rothman, 1982). The participants, all children, were deliberately infected with the hepatitis A virus. During the 20-year study, Willowbrook closed its doors to new children because of overcrowded conditions. However, the research ward continued to admit new children. To gain a child's admission to the institution, parents were required to give permission for the child to be a study participant. Hepatitis A affects the liver, producing vomiting, nausea, and tiredness, accompanied

by jaundice. The infected children suffered pain and potentially long-term effects.

From the late 1950s to early 1970s, Krugman's research team published several articles describing the study protocol and findings. Beecher (1966) cited the Willowbrook study as an example of unethical research. The investigators defended exposing the children to the virus by citing their own belief that most of the children would have acquired the infection after admission to the institution. They based their belief on the high hepatitis infection rates of children during their first year of living at Willowbrook. The investigators also stressed the benefits that the participants received on the research ward, which were a cleaner environment, better supervision, and a higher nurse-patient ratio (Rothman, 1982). Despite the controversy, this unethical study continued until the early 1970s.

Jewish Chronic Disease Hospital Study

Another highly publicized example of unethical research was a study conducted at the Jewish Chronic Disease Hospital in the 1960s. The USPHS, the American Cancer Society, and Sloan-Kettering Cancer Center funded the study (Nelson-Marten & Rich, 1999). Its purpose was to determine the patients' rejection responses to live cancer cells. Twenty-two patients were injected with a suspension containing live cancer cells that had been generated from human cancer tissue (Levine, 1986).

Most of the patients and their physicians were unaware of the study. An extensive investigation revealed that the patients were not informed they were research participants. They were informed that they were receiving an injection of cells, but the word *cancer* was omitted (Beecher, 1966). In addition, the Jewish Chronic Disease Hospital's IRB never reviewed the study. The physician directing the research was an employee of the Sloan-Kettering Institute for Cancer Research, and there was no indication that this institution had reviewed the study (Hershey & Miller, 1976). The study was considered unethical and was terminated, with the lead researcher found to be in violation of the Nuremberg Code (1949) and the Declaration of Helsinki (WMA, 2013). This research had the potential to cause study participants serious or irreversible harm and possibly death, reinforcing the importance of conscientious institutional review and ethical researcher conduct.

EARLY US GOVERNMENT RESEARCH REGULATIONS

Following World War II, the US government increased funding for research. Federal funding by the National Institutes of Health (NIH) for research grew rapidly from less than $1 million in 1945 to over $435 million in 1965 (Beecher, 1966). This influx of funds along with newly discovered advances in medical treatment raised the potential for increased numbers of research violations. Dr. Henry Beecher (1966) published a paper with 22 examples of experimental treatments implemented without patient consent, raising concerns that the interests of science could override the interests of the patient. The government recognized the need for additional oversight. This section describes three government regulations that were developed as a result.

US Department of Health, Education, and Welfare

In 1973, the DHEW published its first set of regulations intended to protect human participants (Advisory Committee on Human Radiation Experiments, 1995). Clinical researchers were required to be compliant with the new stricter regulations for human research, with additional regulations to protect persons with limited capacity to consent, such as ill, cognitively impaired, or dying individuals (Levine, 1986). All research proposals involving human participants were required to undergo full institutional review, a task that became overwhelming and greatly prolonged the time required for study approval. Even studies conducted by nurses and other health professionals that involved minimal or no risks to study participants were subjected to full board review. Despite the advancement of the protection of participants' rights, the government recognized the need for additional strategies to manage the extended time now required for study approval.

National Commission for the Protection of Human Subjects of Biomedical and Behavioral Research

Because of the problems related to the DHEW regulations, the National Commission for the Protection of Human Subjects of Biomedical and Behavioral Research (1978) was formed. The commission's charge was to identify basic ethical principles and develop guidelines based on these principles that would underlie the conduct of

biomedical and behavioral research involving human participants. The commission developed what is now called the Belmont Report (DHHS, 1979). This report identified three **ethical principles** as relevant to research involving human participants: respect for persons, beneficence, and justice (Grady, 2018; Thakur & Lahiry, 2019). The **principle of respect for persons** holds that persons have the right to self-determination and the freedom to participate or not participate in research. The **principle of beneficence** requires the researcher to do good and avoid causing harm. The **principle of justice** holds that human participants should be treated fairly (Gravetter & Forzano, 2018). The commission developed ethical research guidelines based on these three principles, made recommendations to the DHHS, and was dissolved in 1978. The three ethical principles that the report identified are still followed for all federally supported research, whether implemented in the United States or internationally.

Subsequent to the work of the commission, the DHHS developed federal regulations in 1981 to protect human research participants, which have been revised as needed over the past 35 years (DHHS, 1981). The first of these was the *Code of Federal Regulations* (CFR), Title 45, Part 46, Protection of Human Subjects, with the most recent edition being available online (DHHS, 2018). Box 9.2 lists the types of research governed by DHHS. An arm of the DHHS is the Federal Drug Administration (FDA), and its research activities are governed by CFR Title 21, Food and Drugs, Part 50, Protection of Human Subjects (FDA, 2019b), and Part 56, Institutional Review Boards (IRBs) (FDA, 2019a). Box 9.3 lists the research covered by the FDA regulations.

The DHHS regulations are known as the **Common Rule** because they are applicable across multiple DHHS agencies. The DHHS regulations are interpreted and enforced by the Office for Human Research Protection (OHRP), an agency within the DHHS (2016). In addition to providing guidance and regulatory enforcement, the OHRP develops educational programs and materials, and provides advice on ethical and regulatory issues related to biomedical and social-behavioral research.

STANDARDS FOR PRIVACY FOR RESEARCH DATA

The concern for privacy of patient information related to the electronic storage and exchange of health information resulted in the privacy regulations known as

BOX 9.2 Research Regulated by DHHS: CFR Title 45, Part 46, Protection of Human Subjects

1. Studies conducted by, supported by, or otherwise subject to regulations by any federal department or agency
2. Research conducted in educational and healthcare settings
3. Research involving the use of biophysical measures, educational tests, survey procedures, scales, interview procedures, or observation
4. Research involving the collection or study of existing data, documents, records, pathological specimens, or diagnostic specimens.

Summarized from Department of Health and Human Services (DHHS). (2018). Protection of human subjects. *Code of Federal Regulations,* Title 45 Public Welfare, Department of Health and Human Services, Part 46. Retrieved from https://www.ecfr.gov/cgi-bin/text-idx?SID5ad32ac566ecdb2466df8f06 8b6036a27&mc5true&node5pt45.1.46&rgn5div5

BOX 9.3 Research Regulated by the FDA: CFR Title 21, Parts 50 and 56

- Studies that test
  1. Drugs for humans
  2. Medical devices for human use
  3. Biological products for human use
  4. Human dietary supplements
  5. Electronic healthcare products used with humans
- Responsible for the management of new drugs and medical devices

Data from U.S. Food and Drug Administration. (2019b). Protection of human subjects. *Code of Federal Regulations,* Title 21 Food and Drugs, Department of Health and Human Services, Parts 50 and 56. Retrieved from https://www.ecfr.gov/cgi-bin/text-idx?SID5d494ea202a7a4c40a8f63306fd8b7142&mc5true &node5pt21.1.50&rgn5div5#se21.1.50_11

HIPAA (Bonham, 2018). HIPAA did not require anything that was not required during routine nursing practice before its instigation; however, it addressed both electronic data security and consequences of failure to protect such data. The HIPAA Privacy Rule established the category of protected health information (PHI). The rule allows covered entities, such as health plans, healthcare clearinghouses, and healthcare providers, to use or disclose PHI to others only in certain situations. The

Privacy Rule also applies to research that involves the collection of PHI (DHHS & Office for Civil Rights, 2013; *HIPAA Journal*, 2018). Individuals must provide a signed authorization before their PHI can be used or disclosed for research purposes. This chapter covers these regulations in the sections on protection of human rights, obtaining informed consent, and institutional review of research.

PROTECTION OF HUMAN RIGHTS

Human rights are justifiable claims and demands that are necessary for the self-respect, dignity, and freedom of choice for an individual (Grady, 2018). Our professional code of ethics, the American Nurses Association (ANA) Code of Ethics for Nurses (ANA, 2015), includes protection for the rights of human participants in biological and behavioral research, founded on the ethical principles of beneficence, nonmaleficence, autonomy, and justice. The human rights that require protection in research are (1) the right to self-determination, (2) the right to privacy, (3) the right to anonymity and confidentiality, (4) the right to fair treatment or justice, and (5) the right to protection from discomfort and harm (ANA, 2015; Fowler, 2017). These rights are described as follows, including situations in which they can be violated.

Right to Self-Determination

The **right to self-determination** is based on the ethical principle of respect for persons. Respect for persons means that humans are capable of self-determination or making their own decisions. Because of this right, humans should be treated as autonomous agents who have the freedom to conduct their lives as they choose without external controls. As a researcher, you treat prospective participants as **autonomous agents** when you inform them about a proposed study and allow them to choose voluntarily whether to participate (Thakur & Lahiry, 2019). In addition, participants have the right to withdraw from a study at any time without penalty (Grady, 2018).

A participant's right to self-determination can be violated through covert data collection and deception. The right of self-determination may also be threatened when potential research participants are susceptible to coercion or have diminished capacity to make independent decisions. Specific groups who have been identified as being susceptible to coercion needing additional protection include persons of racial/ethnic minorities, prisoners, pregnant women, fetuses, neonates, and children. Each of these threats and groups requiring additional protection will be described in the following sections.

Covert Data Collection

An individual's right to self-determination can be violated if he or she becomes a research participant without realizing it. Some researchers have exposed persons to experimental treatments without their knowledge, a prime example being the Jewish Chronic Disease Hospital study. With **covert data collection**, participants are unaware that research data are being collected because the investigator's study involves collecting data about normal activity or routine health care (Reynolds, 1979). Studies in which observation is used to collect data, such as ethnographic research, are especially challenging because the researcher does not want to interfere with what would normally happen by identifying that observational data are being collected. Covert data collection can occur if participants' behaviors are public. For example, a researcher could observe and record the number of people walking down a street who are smoking. However, covert data collection is considered unethical when research deals with sensitive aspects of an individual's behavior, such as illegal conduct, sexual behavior, and drug use. In keeping with the HIPAA Privacy Rule (DHHS & Office for Civil Rights, 2013), PHI data collected in any manner can only be used if there is minimal risk of harm to the participants. This means the use of any type of covertly collected data would be questionable and unethical, and illegal if PHI data were being used or disclosed without prior approval.

Deception

The use of deception in research also can violate a participant's right to self-determination. **Deception** is misinforming participants of the study's purpose or withholding some information about the study (Gravetter & Forzano, 2018; Kazdin, 2017). A classic example of deception is the Milgram (1963) study, in which participants thought they were administering electric shocks to another person. The participants did not know the person being shocked was a professional actor who pretended to feel pain. Because of participating in this study, some participants experienced severe mental tension, almost to the point of collapse (Algahtani,

Bajunaid, & Shirah, 2018; Kazdin, 2017). A researcher developing a study involving deception must be prepared to justify the deception by providing evidence that the benefits of the study are greater than the potential risks (Gravetter & Forzano, 2018; Kazdin, 2017). For example, the researcher must argue that deception is the only way the research question can be answered. The research question must be significant, and the researcher will need to specify how debriefing will occur (Gravetter & Forzano, 2018). After data collection is complete, the researcher provides **debriefing** of the participant by presenting the complete, accurate purpose of the study with the goal of minimizing the possible negative effects of the study. The debriefing also includes why the deception was deemed necessary (Kazdin, 2017).

Covert data collection is passive deception. It may be approved by an IRB in situations in which the research is essential, the data cannot be obtained any other way, and the participants will not be harmed. For an example, on a clinical unit, the researcher may indicate that a study is about the number and type of interruptions that occurred during a nurse's day. In reality, the researchers are observing the nurses' compliance with hand hygiene guidelines. Covert direct observation might be approved in such a situation if the results were not going to be linked to individual nurses. In the rare situations in which covert data collection is allowable, participants must be informed of the deception once the study is completed, provided full disclosure of the study activities that were conducted (Gravetter & Forzano, 2018; Kazdin, 2017), and given the opportunity to withdraw their data from the study.

Susceptible to Coercion

Coercion occurs when one person intentionally presents another with an overt threat of harm or the lure of excessive reward to obtain his or her compliance. The older version of the Common Rule (DHHS, 2013) identified specific vulnerable groups, including pregnant women, human fetuses, neonates, children, persons with mental incompetence, and prisoners. Conducting research with members of these groups required additional protection in the conduct of research. The revised Common Rule (DHHS, 2018) does not identify vulnerable populations but describes persons and situations in which persons may be sensitive to coercion or undue influence. The persons sensitive to coercion include some of those who were previously classified as being vulnerable, such as children, prisoners, and persons with diminished decision-making ability. However, persons who are economically or educationally disadvantaged and members of racial and ethnic minorities were included among those susceptible to coercion (DHHS, 2018). This new approach broadens the concept and puts additional responsibility on researchers to consider their inclusion and exclusion criteria and recruitment procedures. However, in many situations, the data needed to determine evidence-based care are dependent on the inclusion of persons who may be sensitive to coercion (Grady, 2018).

Subjects may feel coerced to participate in research because they fear that they will suffer harm or discomfort if they do not participate. Students may feel forced to participate in research to protect their grades or prevent negative relationships with the faculty member conducting the research (Boileau, Patenaude, & St-Ong, 2018). Some patients believe that their medical or nursing care will be negatively affected if they do not agree to be research participants, a belief that may be reinforced if a healthcare provider is the one who attempts to recruit them for a study. **Therapeutic misconception** is the belief that research participation will result in better clinical care (Bailey & Ladores, 2018). Therapeutic misconception has also been defined as participants' failure to distinguish between the therapeutic relationship between a patient and a healthcare provider and the protocol-driven relationship between a participant and a researcher (McConville, 2017). Despite what the clinician-researcher said about the participant's care not being based on their consent, persons with cystic fibrosis (CF) believed their care would be better because they participated in research studies (Christofides, Stroud, Tullis, & O'Doherty, 2017).

Subjects may feel coerced to participate in studies because the study offers a potential treatment and they have exhausted all other treatment options (Grady, 2018). Other participants believe that they cannot refuse the excessive rewards offered, such as large sums of money, specialized health care, special privileges, and jobs. Another example of coercion is what happened at Willowbrook State School. The school offered a specialized education for children with disabilities. The only way that parents could secure admission was to allow their child to be in the study and deliberately infected with hepatitis.

Most nursing studies do not offer excessive rewards to participants. A researcher may offer reasonable payment for time and transportation costs, such as $10 to $30, or a gift certificate for this amount. When participants have a rare disorder and must travel long distances for data collection, the researcher or sponsor of the study should pay travel and lodging expenses (Gelinas, Crawford, Kelman, & Bierer, 2019). An IRB will evaluate whether a proposed payment is coercive compared to the effort and time required to participate in a study (Grady, 2018).

Conducting research ethically requires that persons who are susceptible to coercion have additional protection during the conduct of research (DHHS, 2018). One protective strategy is to have waiting periods between hearing about a study and obtaining informed consent (Grady, 2018). The waiting period allows participants to consult with family and friends or think of questions that they want to ask. Thoughtful planning and open dialogue between researchers and participants can create conditions to ensure informed consent is not coercive.

Diminished Autonomy

Autonomy is the ability to make a voluntary decision based on comprehending information about the study (Kaye, Chongwe, & Sewankambo, 2019). Some persons have **diminished autonomy** because of legal or mental incompetence, terminal illness, or confinement to an institution (Kazdin, 2017). Persons are said to be incompetent if a qualified healthcare provider judges them to be unable to comprehend and voluntarily decide about participation in a study. Incompetence can be temporary (e.g., substance use), permanent (e.g., intellectual disability), or transitory (e.g., delirium or psychosis). Unconscious patients and those with reduced cognitive abilities are seen as legally incompetent to give informed consent because they lack the ability to comprehend information about a study. The concern is that a person who, for whatever reason, is unable to absorb, retain, and evaluate the information about a study cannot protect themselves from possible harm or make an informed decision about whether to participate in a study. However, without finding ways to ethically obtain informed consent and including them in studies, the evidence upon which to base their safe, quality care will continue to be lacking and not grow (Ho, Downs, Bulsara, Patman, & Hill, 2018).

Persons living with psychosis are the logical participants for studies of the safety and efficacy of antipsychotic medications. Nurse researchers conducted a systematic review of 646 clinical trials with participants who had been diagnosed with a psychosis. The purpose of the review was to determine the extent to which the participants were assessed for their capacity to provide informed consent (Weissinger & Ulrich, 2019). They learned that less than 10% of the studies included the capacity to provide informed consent in their inclusion/exclusion criteria. Only 34 studies (5%) reported using a capacity assessment to determine the ability of potential participants to give consent.

Patients with mild to severe dementia or Alzheimer disease may have a compromised capacity to understand the information necessary to giving informed consent. Chester, Clarkson, Davies, Hughes, and Islam (2018) published their study protocol of a pragmatic clinical trial conducted in England comparing caregivers being taught to use memory aids with a person who has early dementia to usual treatment. The researchers elicited input from an advisory group called the Public, Patient, and Carer Reference Group (PPCRG). The process and documents used to recruit potential participants were designed "following guidance from the PPCRG on language and format, to ensure that those with cognitive impairment are fully informed and engaged in the decision to take part" (Chester et al., 2018, p. 4). Using an advisory group such as the PPCRG is a robust strategy for designing appropriate recruitment procedures for any group of persons who may have diminished capacity to provide informed consent.

The use of persons with decreased decision-making ability as research participants is more acceptable if several conditions exist. When the research is therapeutic, there is less concern because the participants have the potential to benefit directly from the experimental process (DHHS, 2018). Samples including persons with diminished autonomy are more acceptable when the researcher is recruiting persons with adequate autonomy as well as those with reduced autonomy as participants. Another positive factor is the availability of preclinical and clinical studies that provide evidence upon which to base the assessment of potential risks for participants. Research with persons with diminished decision-making ability is also more acceptable when risk is minimal and the consent process is strictly followed to protect the rights of the prospective participants (DHHS, 2018).

Other ways to include persons with diminished capacity in studies is to assess their ability to comprehend using a standard instrument. Ho et al. (2018) recommended that researchers develop relationships with potential participants with diminished capacity and their caregivers, observing the potential participant multiple times prior to obtaining consent from the caregiver or the participant. To assess the capacity of the participant to give consent, they used an assessment tool called the "Three-Item Decisional Questionnaire (3-IDQ) adopted from Palmer et al., 2005" (Ho et al., 2018, p. 94). Another assessment, the MacArthur Competency Assessment Tool for Clinical Research (MacCAT-CR), was identified as one of the strongest instruments available for assessing an individual's capacity to give informed consent (Simpson, 2010). The companion tool, the MacArthur Competency Assessment Tool for Treatment (MacCAT-T), has been identified as the gold standard for assessing mental capacity to consent to treatment (Elzakkers, Danner, Grisso, Hoek, & van Elburg, 2018). Evidence has been published for interrater reliability, concurrent validity, and effective use of the tools across a wide range of patients (see Chapter 16) (Elzakkers et al., 2018). For a research study, the persons responsible for recruiting participants and obtaining informed consent would need to be trained in using the MacCAT-CR. Using this instrument or similar tools, researchers can make an objective decision about a participant's ability to consent to research.

If an individual is judged incompetent and incapable of consent, you must seek approval from the prospective participant and his or her legally authorized representative. A **legally authorized representative** means an individual or a group is authorized under law to consent on behalf of a prospective participant to his or her participation in research. The authorized representative is sometimes called a proxy. The legally authorized representative or proxy may be a spouse or close relative, if the potential participant has not designated a power of attorney. If no spouse or close relative can be accessed, a legal representative can be appointed by the state.

Groups Needing Additional Protection

The groups identified as susceptible to coercion require additional protection to participate in research. Five groups requiring additional protection are described in this section: prisoners, terminally ill persons, pregnant women, fetuses and neonates, and children.

Prisoners. Prisoners have diminished autonomy to consent for research because of their confinement. They may feel coerced to participate in research because they fear harm if they refuse (Midwest Nursing Research Society [MNRS], 2018) or because they desire the benefits of special treatment, monetary gain, or relief from boredom. In the past, prisoners were used for drug studies in which the medications had no health-related benefits and, instead, potential harmful side effects. Current regulations regarding research involving prisoners require that "the risks involved in the research are commensurate with risks that would be accepted by nonprisoner volunteers" and "procedures for the selection of participants within the prison are fair to all prisoners and immune from arbitrary intervention by prison authorities or prisoners" (DHHS, 2018, Section 46.305). An IRB that is considering a study that include prisoners must add a prisoner or prisoner representative prior to reviewing the study. When a proposal is reviewed by multiple IRBs, only one of the IRBs must have a member that represents the prisoners.

Terminally ill participants. Two factors need to be considered when designing a study with a sample that includes persons with terminal illness: (1) Who will benefit from the research? and (2) Is it ethical to conduct research on individuals who are unlikely to benefit from the study? Participating in research could have greater risks and minimal or no benefits for these participants. In addition, the dying participant's condition could affect the results, leading to misinterpretation of the findings. Another consideration is persons with terminal illness have limited time remaining in their lives. Is it fair to ask them to spend time on a study instead of spending it with family or engaged in preferred activities? However, unless persons with terminal illness or those receiving palliative care are included in studies, the knowledge base for hospice and palliative care will not grow and be refined (Pereira & Hernández-Marrero, 2019). Some terminally ill individuals are willing participants because they believe that participating in research is a way to contribute to society before they die. Others want to take part in research because they believe that the experimental process may benefit them by slowing their disease process, potentially another example of a therapeutic misconception.

Pregnant women and fetuses. Pregnant women have historically been considered vulnerable participants in regard to research (Ballantyne et al., 2017). Policies to include women, including pregnant women, in studies and policies to exclude women due to potential harm to the fetus contradict each other and result in confusion about how women should be recruited for studies (van der Graaf et al., 2018). Federal regulations define pregnancy as encompassing the period of time from implantation until delivery. "A woman is assumed to be pregnant if she exhibits any of the pertinent presumptive signs of pregnancy, such as missed menses, until the results of a pregnancy test are negative or until delivery" and the fetus is defined as the "product of conception from implantation until delivery" (DHHS, 2018, 45 CFR Section 46.202). Research conducted with pregnant women can occur only after studies have been done with animals and nonpregnant women to assess the potential risks. Table 9.1 lists the conditions under which a pregnant woman can be included, such as the potential for direct benefit to the woman or the fetus. If a study may benefit only the fetus, the consent of the pregnant woman and father must be obtained.

Some researchers did not include pregnant women in their studies because they assumed the women would not want to participate. In New Zealand, Ballantyne et al. (2017) added a qualitative arm to a randomized intervention clinical trial for which the sample was pregnant women. This study was called the Research in Pregnancy Ethics (RIPE) study.

> "The RIPE study set out to ascertain views of pregnant women about research participation, by conducting semi-structured interviews and then analysing the interview transcripts using inductive thematic analysis (Braun & Clarke, 2006). Women were recruited from a pool of participants already participating in the PiP [Probiotics in Pregnancy] study." (Ballantyne et al., 2017, p. 478)
>
> "The main cited benefits of the study by the participants were abstract principles of altruism, playing a valuable civic role and the importance of research. No-one cited personal benefit or gain as a motivation for participating.... The main perceived burdens related to inconvenience and time commitment.... Women wanted to clarify the time commitments and how this would fit into their schedule; they did not want to over-commit given the demands of pregnancy and having a newborn baby." (Ballantyne et al., 2017, pp. 479–480)
>
> "Our results show that at least some pregnant women recognise the value and importance of research during pregnancy. The women we interviewed were deeply invested in the research process and outcomes." (Ballantyne et al., 2017, p. 483)

TABLE 9.1   Conditions That Must Be Present for Pregnant Women to Be Included in a Study

General Condition	Specific Details
Knowledge of potential side effects	Studies with animals and nonpregnant women have been conducted and results indicated safety of the intervention.
Scientifically important information	Woman and fetus may benefit from the intervention. If not, risk is minimal. Knowledge cannot be gained any other way.
Least possible risk	Risk is minimized but study objectives can still be met.
Balance of risks and benefits	If no potential benefit to either mother or fetus, risk must be minimized.
Consent of both parents	Required if fetus is only one to benefit from the study. Father's consent not needed if he is unavailable, incompetent, or pregnancy due to rape or incest.
Fully informed	Potential impact on the mother or fetus is clear in the consent form, before requesting mother to sign.
No incentive or interference to terminate the pregnancy	Mother does not receive any inducement to terminate pregnancy. Research staff not involved in any decision to terminate the pregnancy.
Viability of the fetus	Research staff not involved in any decision about neonate's viability after delivery.

Pregnant women should not be excluded from studies unless an increased risk to the woman or the fetus exists. Ballantyne et al. (2017) provided insight for other researchers considering recruiting pregnant women for a study.

Neonates. A neonate is defined as a newborn and is further identified as either viable or nonviable on delivery. Viable neonates are able to survive after delivery through the use of technology and other therapies. An additional factor in being considered viable is the ability to maintain a heartbeat and respiration. Nonviable neonates may be living after delivery but will not be able to survive (DHHS, 2018). Neonates are extremely vulnerable and require extra protection to determine their involvement in research. However, research may involve viable neonates, neonates of uncertain viability, and nonviable neonates when the conditions identified in Box 9.4 are met. In addition, for the nonviable neonate, the vital functions of the neonate should not be artificially maintained because of the research, and the research should not terminate the heartbeat or respiration of the neonate (DHHS, 2018).

Children and Adolescents. Children are considered vulnerable in the context of research (Singh, Siddiqi, Parameshwar, & Chandra-Mouli, 2019). However, we need more evidence upon which to base pediatric nursing practice. To develop the necessary evidence, children must be recruited for studies and assent or consent obtained (Crane & Broome, 2017).

BOX 9.4   Conditions to Be Met for Approval of Research With Neonates

- Data available from preclinical and clinical study to assess potential risk to neonates
- Potential to provide important biomedical knowledge that cannot be obtained by other means
- No additional risk to the neonate
- Potential to enhance the probability of the neonate's survival
- Both parents fully informed about the research and give consent
- Research team has no part in determining the viability of the neonate

Summarized from Department of Health and Human Services (DHHS). (2018). Protection of human subjects. *Code of Federal Regulations,* Title 45 Public Welfare, Department of Health and Human Services, Part 46. Retrieved from https://www.hhs.gov/ohrp/regulations-and-policy/regulations/45-cfr-46/index.html

The distinction between children and adolescents is not clear. The World Health Organization (WHO, 2018) describes adolescents as being the second decade of life. The age of consenting to participate in a study is usually considered to be 18 years of age, but legal and research experts disagree among themselves (Cherry, 2017; Sade, 2017). Unfortunately, the legal definitions of the minor status of a child are statutory and vary among states and even countries. Neurophysical and psychological evidence supports the premise that adolescents lack the

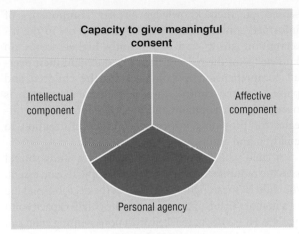

Fig. 9.1 Capacity to give meaningful consent.

BOX 9.5   Sample Assent Form for Children Ages 8 to 12 Years: Weight, Activity, and Eating Habits Before and After Mother-Child Multimedia Intervention

Oral Explanation

We are nurses who want children like you to be strong and have energy to play and go to school. Here at your school, we are doing research on the best ways to teach you and your parents how to eat better and get more exercise using videos and computer games. If you decide to be in the study, we will measure your height and weight in a room with only your mother and the nurse. No one but them will know how much you weigh or how tall you are unless you tell them. We will ask you to answer five questions about what you eat and whether you exercise. Exercise is running, playing games outside, going for a walk, and doing things for fun where you move your body.

After that, you and your mom will play a video game on the computer and watch two videos that are less than 5 minutes long. For the next five Tuesdays, we will be here after school. You and your mom will be asked the same five questions, watch two different videos, and play the video game together. We will have snacks for you and your mom to eat each time. On the sixth Tuesday, we will measure how tall you are and how much you weigh. On that day, we will ask you what you liked and didn't like about the videos and computer games. You can change your mind about being in the study and can stop at any time.

To Child

1. I want to learn about what to eat to make me strong and have energy.
2. I want to answer questions about what I eat and how much exercise I get.
3. I want to watch videos and play a computer game with my mom.

If the child says YES, have him/her put an "X" here:

_____

If the child says NO, have him/her put an "X" here:

_____

Date: _____

Child's signature: _____

cognitive and affective maturity to give consent for themselves.

Cherry (2017) identifies three components that comprise meaningful assent or consent for children and adolescents: intellectual development, affective development, and personal agency (Fig. 9.1). The figure is consistent with the findings of Hein, Troost, Lindeboom, Benninga, and Zwaan (2015), who found that age, followed by intelligence, explained the largest portion of the variance in a child's or adolescent's competence related to consent to research. Grady et al. (2014) studied the perceptions of assent/consent among adolescents enrolled in clinical research and their parents. Approximately 40% of the sample believed that the decision for an adolescent to participate should be jointly made by parents and adolescent. Even among adolescent participants in research, however, understanding their rights and grasping the meaning of the study itself has been found to be less than desired (Cherry, 2017).

Federal regulations contain two stipulations for obtaining informed consent: The research must be of minimal risk, and both the assent of the child (when capable) and the permission of the parent or guardian must be obtained (DHHS, 2018). **Assent** means a child's affirmative agreement to participate in research. Box 9.5 provides an example of an assent form. **Permission to participate in a study** means that the parent or guardian agrees to the participation of the child or ward in research (DHHS, 2018). If a child does not assent to participate in a study, he or she should not be included as a participant even if the parent or guardian gives permission. For therapeutic

research, IRBs can approve studies with children when more than minimal risk is present, provided that potential benefit exists for the child, or when the experimental treatment is similar to usual care and the findings have potential benefit for others. Studies that do not meet these stipulations but have the potential for significant contribution to knowledge that may benefit other children with the same condition can be approved (DDHS, 2018). In all cases, procedures to obtain assent and parental permission must be implemented.

Another point of controversy is the age at which a child can assent to a study. A child's competency to assent is usually governed by age, and research evidence supports the standard of a child over 10 years of age being capable of sufficient understanding to give assent (Crane & Broome, 2017). Children who are developmentally delayed, have a cognitive impairment, suffer an emotional disorder, or are physically ill must be considered on an individual basis. When designing a study in which children will be participants, it is helpful to seek consultation with a child development specialist and the primary IRB to which you will submit the study for approval. Some IRBs have developed assent guidelines or forms specific to their facilities.

Assent and permission require that both the child or adolescent and parents be informed about the study. The information shared with the child about the study should be appropriate for the child's age and culture. In the assenting process, the child must be given developmentally appropriate information on the study purpose, expectations, and benefit-risk ratio (discussed later). Media-enhanced presentations and play activities have been used as a means of providing information about the study. A group of researchers in the Netherlands conducted a participatory study to develop and test comic strips for the purpose of providing information about research participation (Grootens-Wiegers, de Vries, van Beusekom, van Dijck, & van den Broek, 2015). With the input of children at each stage of development, the comic strips evolved and, in their final version, were found to have the potential for increasing children's knowledge about research. Yeh, Chun, Terrones, and Huang (2017) conducted a randomized controlled trial (RCT) comparing the knowledge of children and their parents about pediatric endoscopy. The intervention group ($n = 37$ parent-child pairs) obtained information about the procedure by watching a short, animated video and the control group ($n = 40$ parent-child pairs) received the information by listening to the usual verbal explanation. The 2-minute videos, one for upper endoscopy and the other for lower endoscopy, were developed based on principles of instructional design. Parents and children were interviewed separately and scored on their knowledge of key components of informed consent. The children and parents in the intervention group had significantly higher scores on knowledge of the risks of the procedure and their overall comprehension as compared to the children and parents of the control group. Continued research is needed for development and testing of innovative strategies for providing informed consent information to children and adults.

A child who assents to participate in a study should sign the requisite form and be given a copy. To gain assent, the child is "meaningfully involved in the decision-making in a manner that is appropriate for the child's capacity and age" (WHO, 2018, p. 15). Legally, a nonassenting child can be a research participant if the parents give permission, even if some potential for harm exists. Chwang (2015) argues, however, that including children in a study who have not given assent is every bit as unethical as including nonconsenting adults in a study. A child's willingness to participate in a study should be reassessed throughout a study, reflecting respect for the child's autonomy and dignity (Moore, McArthur, & Noble-Carr, 2018).

Assent becomes more complex with children from various family dynamics and child characteristics. Oulton et al. (2016) conducted a literature review and an anonymous survey of healthcare professionals involved in pediatric research. Combining the findings of the review and the survey with their own experience of conducting pediatric research, Oulton et al. (2016) developed an algorithm that included child-related factors, family dynamics, and the complexity of the study design as components to consider in obtaining assent. A child-related factor might be a child who is bilingual. In this case, the researchers must determine the most appropriate language to use for the assent process for the child and the process to obtain parental permission.

Other children who have no cognitive deficiencies, but are in unusual circumstances, may require the appointment of a legal representative by the legal system. WHO (2018) identifies the need to do this when a child has no living parents, the parents have immigrated and left the child behind, the child lives on the street with no parental supervision, the child who is unaccompanied seeks asylum in the United States, and the child is a member a of child-led household. Children under the age of 18 can give consent for their own participation in research when they have been emancipated by the legal system. In some legal jurisdictions, a girl under the age of 18 who marries is considered an emancipated minor. Other children may have previously be placed in a state's guardianship (wards of the state). When determining the maturity of a child for the purposes of assent and consent, various professions have different standards by which maturity is assessed (WHO, 2018).

Right to Privacy

Privacy is an individual's right to determine the time, extent, and general circumstances under which personal information is shared with or withheld from others. This information consists of one's attitudes, beliefs, behaviors, opinions, and records. The federal government enacted the Privacy Act (1974) to control potential infringement of privacy, related to information collected by the government, or held in federal agencies' records. The act has four important provisions for the researcher: (1) data collection methods must be strategized so as to protect participants' privacy, (2) data cannot be gathered from participants without their knowledge, (3) individuals have the right to access their records, and (4) individuals may prevent access by others to existent federal data (DHHS & Office of Civil Rights, 2013). The intent of this act was to prevent the **invasion of privacy** that occurs when private information is shared without an individual's knowledge or against his or her will.

The HIPAA Privacy Rule expanded the protection of an individual's privacy, specifically his or her PHI that is individually identifiable, extending the protection to data held by private entities. It described the ways in which those entities covered by the rule can use or disclose this information. "**Individually identifiable health information** (IIHI) is information that is a subset of health information, including demographic information collected from an individual, and: (1) is created or received by healthcare provider, health plan, or healthcare clearinghouse; and (2) [is] related to past, present, or future physical or mental health or condition of an individual, the provision of health care to an individual, or the past, present, or future payment for the provision of health care to an individual, and that identifies the individual; or with respect to which there is a reasonable basis to believe that the information can be used to identify the individual" (DHHS, 2013, 45 CFR, Section 160.103).

According to the HIPAA Privacy Rule, IIHI is PHI that is transmitted by electronic media, maintained in electronic media, or transmitted or maintained in any other form or medium. Thus the HIPAA privacy regulations must be followed when a nurse researcher wants to access data from a covered entity, such as reviewing a patient's medical record in clinics or hospitals. Ahalt et al. (2019) defined de-identified data sets as having all PHI removed. **De-identification** consists of removing 18 items from patient records before they are released to other agencies or to researchers. These 18 items include name, contact information, identification numbers, photographs, biometrics, and other elements by which a participant could potentially be identified (Box 9.6). Because de-identification includes removing dates, researchers using de-identified data may not be able to

---

BOX 9.6   **18 Elements That Could Be Used to Identify an Individual to Relatives, Employer, or Household Members**

1. Names
2. All geographical subdivisions smaller than a state
3. All elements of dates (except year) for dates directly related to an individual
4. Telephone numbers
5. Facsimile numbers
6. Electronic mail (e-mail) addresses
7. Social security numbers
8. Medical record numbers
9. Health plan beneficiary numbers
10. Account numbers
11. Certificate/license numbers
12. Vehicle identifiers and serial numbers, including license plate numbers
13. Device identifiers and serial numbers
14. Web universal resource locators (URLs)
15. Internet protocol (IP) address numbers
16. Biometric identifiers, including fingerprints and voiceprints
17. Full-face photographic images and any comparable images
18. Any other unique identifying number, characteristic, or code, unless otherwise permitted by the Privacy Rule for De-identification

Office for Civil Rights, Department of Health and Human Services (DHHS). (2015). *Guidance regarding methods for de-identification of protected health information in accordance with the Health Insurance Portability and Accountability Act (HIPAA) privacy rule.* Retrieved from https://www.hhs.gov/hipaa/for-professionals/privacy/special-topics/de-identification/index.html#standard

answer some research questions such length of hospital stay and seasonal patterns to diseases (Ahalt et al., 2019).

The DHHS (2017) developed the following guidelines to help researchers, healthcare organizations, and healthcare providers determine the conditions under which they can use and disclose IIHI:

- The PHI has been de-identified under the HIPAA Privacy Rule.
- The data are part of a limited data set, and a data use agreement with the researcher(s) is in place.
- The individual who is a potential participant for a study authorizes the researcher to use and disclose his or her PHI.
- A waiver or alteration of the authorization requirement is obtained from an IRB or a privacy board.

The first two items are discussed in this section of the chapter. The authorization process is discussed in the section on obtaining informed consent, and the waiver or alteration of authorization requirement is covered in the section on institutional review of research.

De-identifying Protected Health Information Under the Privacy Rule

Covered entities, such as healthcare providers and agencies, can allow researchers access to health information if the information has been de-identified, either by applying statistical methods (expert determination) or removing information (safe harbor) (Fig. 9.2). The covered entity can apply statistical methods that experts agree render the information unidentifiable. The statistical method used for de-identification of the health data must be documented. **Safe harbor** is certifying that the 18 elements for identification have been removed or revised to ensure the individual is not identified. The covered entity has done what it could to make the information de-identified, but has no information whether the individuals could still be identified (DHHS, 2015a). No matter the method used, you must retain this certification information for 6 years. It is important to note that the element concerning biometrics may be interpreted to include deoxyribonucleic acid (DNA) results and other particularized physiological variants, such as unusual laboratory and histological markers.

Limited Data Set and Data Use Agreement

Researchers can comply with the privacy standards by accessing a limited data set (LDS) that has been de-identified (Ahalt et al., 2019). A HIPAA-limited data set

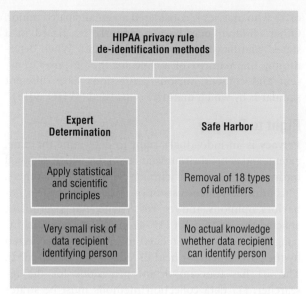

Fig. 9.2 Use of PHI: Two methods of de-identifying data. (Information from the HIPAA Privacy Rule.)

includes clinical patient-specific data combined with some PHI. Patient authorization is not required to use these data sets for "research, public health, or healthcare operations research" as long as the study is approved by an IRB (Ahalt et al. 2019, p. 329). Under certain conditions, researchers and covered entities (healthcare provider, health plan, and healthcare clearinghouse) may use and disclose an LDS to a researcher for a study, without an individual participant's authorization or an IRB waiver. These data sets are considered PHI, and the parties involved must have a data use agreement. The **data use agreement** limits how the data set may be used and how it will be protected, including identification of the researchers who are permitted to use the data set. The researchers receiving the data are not allowed to use or disclose the information in any way that is not permitted by the agreement, is required to protect against the unintended use or disclosure of the information, and must agree not to contact any of the individuals in the LDS (Centers for Medicare & Medicaid Services [CMS], n.d.).

Secondary data analysis reuses data collected for a previous study or for other purposes, such as data in clinical or administrative databases (Wickham, 2019). Duncan, Ahmed, Dove, and Maxwell (2019) used secondary data analysis to study the cost of end-of-life

(EOL) care for Medicare beneficiaries. They selected a sample ($N = 114,028$) from the Medicare Limited Data Set to answer their research questions. The data set was also called the Medicare 5% LDS Analytical file or Medicare 5% file. The file had been de-identified as required by HIPAA and comprised of 5% of the Medicare beneficiaries.

> "For the purpose of understanding cost of care at the EOL, we perform analysis of the Medicare 5% file for the years 2015 and 2016. This file is a random sample of Medicare's claims for the 2 years, containing experience of approximately 2.9 million patients for each year." (Duncan et al., 2019, p. 706)
>
> "Medicare expenditures increase sharply in the last few days of life, particularly for patients who die in hospital. Recent developments in hospice and palliative care offer the possibility of higher quality care at lower cost to Medicare if patients enter hospice earlier. Finding a lower cost site of care that does not jeopardize patients' wishes is a realistic, worthy goal.... Identifying those who will benefit from intensive care from those in which aggressive care is likely to be futile and burdensome is a challenge for providers, patients, and families." (Duncan et al., 2019, p. 709)

The findings of the study conducted by Duncan et al. (2019) provided strategies by which EOL expenditures could be reduced, an important cost savings, without infringing on the desired outcome of a peaceful death.

Right to Anonymity and Confidentiality

On the basis of the right to privacy, the research participant has the right to anonymity and the right to assume that all data collected will be kept confidential. **Anonymity** means that even the researcher cannot link a participant's identity to that participant's individual responses (Adams & Lawrence, 2019). For studies that use de-identified health information or data from a limited data set, participants are anonymous to the researchers.

In most studies, researchers desire to know the identity of their participants and promise that their identity will be kept confidential. **Confidentiality** is the researcher's management of private information shared by a participant that must not be shared with others without the authorization of the participant (Gravetter & Forzano, 2018). Confidentiality is grounded in the premises

that patients own their own information, and that only they can decide with whom to share all or part of it (Kazdin, 2017). When information is shared in confidence, the recipient (researcher) has the obligation to maintain confidentiality. Researchers, as professionals, have a duty to maintain confidentiality consistent with their profession's code of ethics (Gravetter & Forzano, 2018). This section includes breaches in confidentiality that may occur and strategies to maintain confidentiality.

Breach of Confidentiality

A **breach of confidentiality** can occur when a researcher, by accident or direct action, allows an unauthorized person to gain access to a study's raw data. Confidentiality can be breached in the reporting or publishing phases of a study, especially in qualitative studies, in which a participant's identity is revealed by including personal details known to other people (Creswell & Creswell, 2018; Creswell & Poth, 2018). Two other types of research are especially sensitive to breaches in confidentiality. Collecting data through online forums and social media can threaten confidentiality because of the ability to track internet protocol addresses and search the internet participant's quotes (Hunter et al., 2018). Passive data collection also has ethical issues. **Passive data collection** is gathering data without the active involvement of the participant (Maher et al., 2019). The data being gathered are linked to specific participants and are generated by wearable devices such as smartphones or electronic pedometers, by global positioning systems, and by e-mails and text messages.

Breaches of confidentiality can harm participants psychologically and socially as well as destroy the trust they had in the researcher. Breaches can be especially harmful to a research participant when they involve religious preferences, sexual practices, employment, personal attributes, or opinions that may be considered negative, such as racial prejudices (Gravetter & Forzano, 2018). For example, imagine that you have conducted a study of nurses' stressful life events and work-related burnout in an acute care hospital. One of the two male participants in the study describes his anxiety disorder. Reporting that one of the male nurses in the study had an anxiety disorder would violate his confidentiality and potentially cause harm. Nurse administrators might be less likely to promote a nurse who has an anxiety disorder. There are legal limits to confidentiality that occur when a participant reveals current drug use or specific intent to harm oneself or others (Gravetter & Forzano, 2018). For example, in a phenomenological study of the experience of parenting a child with development delays, the informed consent document must describe the specific limitations on confidentiality, such as the researcher being obligated to report a mother who reveals harming her child.

Maintaining confidentiality includes not allowing health professionals to access data the researcher has gathered about patients in the hospital. Sometimes, family members or close friends will ask to see data collected about a specific research participant. Sharing research data in these circumstances is a breach of confidentiality. When requesting consent for study participation, you should assure the potential participant that you will not share individual information with healthcare professionals, family members, and others in the setting. However, you may elect to share a summary of the study findings with healthcare providers, family members, and other interested parties.

Maintaining Confidentiality in Quantitative Research

Researchers have a responsibility to protect the identity of participants and to maintain the confidentiality of data collected during a study. You can protect confidentiality by giving each participant a code number. For example, participant Sarah Young might be assigned the code number 001. All of the instruments and forms that Sarah completes and the data you collect about her during the study will be identified with the 001 code number, not her name. To protect participants' identities, the master list of the participants' names and their code numbers are kept in a locked file and room, separate from the data collected. You should not attach signed consent forms and authorization documents to instruments or other data collection tools, as this would make it easy for unauthorized persons to readily identify the participants and their responses. Consent forms are appropriately stored with the master list of participants' names and code numbers. When entering the collected data into a database, code numbers instead of names should be used for identification. Data should be stored in at least two secure places, such as on a separate storage drive, on the researcher's computer, on web-based or cloud storage, or on a university network. The data files need to be password-protected, and (if possible) have no personal identifiers.

Another way to protect anonymity is to have participants generate their own identification codes when data will be collected over time with multiple data points (Lippe, Johnson, & Carter, 2019). The researcher does not have a master list connecting the codes to the participants' names. You are conducting a study of the role satisfaction of new nurse employees with data collection occurring during the first month, the sixth month, and again at the twelfth month. Each nurse generates an individual code from personal information, such as the first letter of a mother's name, the first letter of a father's name, the number of brothers, the number of sisters, and middle initial. Thus the code would be composed of three letters and two numbers, such as BD21M. This code would be used on each form the participant completes. The premise is that the elements of the code do not change, and the participant can generate the same code each time. However, using participant-generated codes has been found to have mixed results. Although the specific components of the ID number were selected for their stability, the participant may not remember, for example, whether they included half-sisters in the number of sisters or whether they used a parent's legal name or nickname.

In quantitative research, the confidentiality of participants' information must be ensured during the data analysis process. The data collected should undergo group analysis so that an individual cannot be identified by his or her responses. If participants are divided into groups and a group has less than five members, the results for that group should not be reported. For example, a researcher conducts a study with military veterans and collects demographic data. In reporting the results by demographic groups, if only a few women participated, the results by gender should not be reported. In writing the research report, you should describe the findings in such a way that an individual or a group of individuals cannot be identified from their responses.

Maintaining Confidentiality in Qualitative Studies

Maintaining confidentiality of participants' data in qualitative studies often requires more effort than in quantitative research. Participants are known to the data collector, so anonymity is not possible (Cypress, 2019). The smaller sample size used in a qualitative study and the depth of detail gathered on each participant requires planning to ensure confidentiality (Morse & Coulehan, 2015). Informed consent documents should contain details about who will have access to the data and how the findings will be reported. In addition, qualitative researchers should communicate to participants that direct quotes from the interview will be included in both professional publications and presentations. Sometimes qualitative participants inappropriately equate confidentiality with secrecy.

Researchers should take precautions during data collection and analysis to maintain confidentiality in qualitative studies. The interviews conducted with participants frequently are recorded and later transcribed, so participants' names should not be mentioned during the recording. Some researchers ask participants to identify pseudonyms by which they will be identified during the interview and on transcripts. Depending on the methods of the study, the researcher may return descriptions of interviews or observations to participants to allow them to correct inaccurate information or remove any information that they do not want included.

Participants have the right to know whether anyone other than you will be transcribing interview information or whether other researchers will analyze the data. In addition, participants should be reminded on an ongoing basis that they have the right to withhold information. For other researchers to critically appraise the rigor and credibility of a qualitative study, an audit trail is produced. To continue to protect the participants' confidentiality, ensure that the audit trail does not contain information linking the demographic characteristics of participants to the qualitative data. When publishing the findings, researchers must respect participants' privacy as they decide how much detail and editing of private information are necessary to publish a study while maintaining the richness and depth of the participants' perspectives (Morse & Coulehan, 2015). The researcher may choose to amend biographical details, removing identifiers such as cities, healthcare providers' names, and healthcare facilities, and use pseudonyms (Cypress, 2019).

Right to Fair Treatment

The right to **fair treatment** is based on the ethical principle of justice. This principle holds that each person should be treated fairly and should receive what he or she is owed. In research, the selection of participants and their assignment to experimental or control group should be made impartially. In addition, their treatment during the course of a study should be fair.

Fair Selection of Subjects

As discussed earlier, historically, research was conducted on categories of individuals who were thought to be especially suitable as research participants, such as the poor, uninsured patients, prisoners, slaves, peasants, dying persons, and others who were considered undesirable (Reynolds, 1979). Researchers often treated these participants carelessly and had little regard for the harm and discomfort they experienced. The Nazi medical experiments, the Tuskegee syphilis study, and the Willowbrook study all exemplify unfair participant selection and treatment.

In 1986, the NIH implemented a policy requiring the inclusion of women and minorities in federally funded studies. This policy became law in 1993 as part of the NIH Revitalization Act (Office of Research on Women's Health, 2017). Prior to this, concerns had been raised about the exclusion of women from biomedical studies, especially women of childbearing age. From a scientific standpoint, the concern was that "monthly changes in women's hormone levels might affect therapeutic interventions and require more complicated designs" (Clayton & Blome, 2018, p. 177). The exclusion of women to avoid harming a fetus or interfering with childbearing also excluded women from the potential benefits of new medications and treatments, for herself and her fetus.

The selection of a population and the specific participants to study should be fair so that the risks and benefits of the study are distributed appropriately (Shamoo & Resnick, 2015). Subjects should be selected for reasons directly related to the problem being studied. Too often participants are selected because the researcher has easy access to them. Another concern with participant selection is that some researchers select certain people, possibly friends or patients under their care, to participate because they like them and want them to receive the specific benefits of a study. Other researchers included specific participants in study because they received gifts or money.

The Common Rule requires equitable selection of participants (DHHS, 2018). Children, women, minorities, and persons who speak other languages cannot be excluded based solely on their demographic characteristics. Researchers seeking federal funding must describe in their proposals plans to recruit participants from different groups who have been traditionally underrepresented in research. The researchers must remember, if a study poses risk, no demographic group should bear an unfair burden of that risk. Conversely, when a study offers a potential benefit, no demographic group should be deprived of participation solely because of their demographic classification.

Random selection of participants can eliminate some of the researcher bias that might influence participant selection. The researcher should make every effort to include fair representation across demographic characteristics, and increased cost is no longer a valid reason for not doing that. For example, the NIH has implemented stricter policies about the inclusion of women in studies and sex being a required variable in animal studies (Clayton & Blome, 2018). The only exception is when a study involves a condition, such as prostate cancer, that only affects men. Proposals for funding must include specific plans for recruiting and maintaining a diverse sample, and federally funded researchers must include demographic characteristics of participants in their annual reports.

One of the most challenging tasks of a researcher is recruiting an adequate number of participants who meet the inclusion criteria and comprise a sample that includes female participants and participants from racial and ethnic minorities (Leavy, 2017). The HIPAA Privacy Rule requires that individuals give potential authorization before PHI can be shared with others, unless the researcher has IRB approval to access records for the purpose of screening. The Privacy Rule makes it more difficult for researchers to find participants for their studies; however, researchers are encouraged to work closely with their IRBs and healthcare agencies to ensure fair selection and recruitment of adequate-sized samples.

Fair Treatment of Participants

Informed consent is a specific agreement about what inclusion in the study involves and what the role of the researcher will be (Adams & Lawrence, 2019). While conducting a study, you should treat the participants fairly and respect that agreement. If the data collection requires appointments with the participants, be on time for each appointment and terminate the data collection process at the agreed-upon time. You should not change the activities or procedures that a participant is to perform unless you obtain the participant's consent.

The benefits promised the participants should be provided. For example, if you promise a participant a copy of the study findings, you should deliver on your promise when the study is completed. In addition, participants in studies should receive equal benefits, regardless of age, race, and socioeconomic status. When possible, the sample should be representative of the study population and should include participants of various ages, ethnic backgrounds, and socioeconomic levels. Treating participants fairly and respectfully facilitates the data collection process and decreases the likelihood that participants will withdrawal from a study (Clayton & Blome, 2018). Thanking participants is always appropriate; they have given you their time and their honesty.

Right to Protection From Discomfort and Harm

The right to **protection from discomfort and harm** is based on the **ethical principle of beneficence**, which holds that one should do good and, above all, do no harm. Therefore researchers should protect participants from discomfort and harm while ensuring they receive the greatest possible balance of benefits in comparison with harm. Discomfort and harm can be physiological, emotional, social, or economic in nature. This section addresses the level of risk in a study, balancing benefits and risks, and the ethical responsibilities of clinicians to provide the best care possible.

Level of Risk

In his classic text, Reynolds (1979) identified the following five categories of studies based on levels of discomfort and harm: (1) no anticipated effects, (2) temporary discomfort, (3) unusual levels of temporary discomfort, (4) risk of permanent damage, and (5) certainty of permanent damage. Each level is defined in the following discussion.

Studies with **no anticipated effects** are studies without direct involvement of human participants. For example, studies that involve reviewing patients' records, students' files, pathology reports, or other documents have no anticipated effect on the participants. In these types of studies, the researcher does not interact directly with research participants. Even in these situations, however, there is a potential risk of invading a participant's privacy. The HIPAA Privacy Rule requires that the agency providing the health information de-identify the 18 essential elements (see Box 9.6 and Fig. 9.2) that could be used to identify an individual, to promote participants' privacy during a study. Analysis of variables from a data set that has had the 18 elements removed is usually exempt from IRB review.

Participants may experience **temporary discomfort** in low-risk studies. In these studies, the discomfort encountered is similar to what the participant would experience in his or her daily life and ceases with the termination of the study. Many nursing studies require participants to complete questionnaires or participate in interviews, which usually involve minimal risk. Physical discomforts of such research might be fatigue, headache, or muscle tension. Emotional and social risks might entail the anxiety or embarrassment associated with responding to certain questions. Economic harms may consist of the loss of time spent participating in the study or travel costs to the study site.

Most clinical nursing studies examining the impact of a treatment involve minimal risk. For example, your study might involve examining the effects of exercise on the blood glucose levels of patients with noninsulin-dependent diabetes. During the study, you ask the participants to test their blood glucose level one extra time per day. There is discomfort when the blood is obtained and a risk of physical changes that might occur with exercise. The participants might also experience anxiety and fear in association with the additional blood testing, and the testing is an added expense. Diabetic participants in this study would experience similar discomforts in their daily lives, and the discomforts would cease with the termination of the study.

Other studies involve **unusual levels of temporary discomfort** for the participants during the study and after its termination. For example, participants might experience a deep vein thrombosis (DVT), prolonged muscle weakness, joint pain, and dizziness after participating in a study that required them to be confined to bed for 7 days to determine the effects of immobility that severe trauma patients might experience. Studies that require participants to experience failure, extreme fear, or threats to their identity or to act in unnatural ways involve unusual levels of temporary discomfort. In some qualitative studies, participants are asked questions about sensitive topics, which may reopen old emotional wounds or involve reliving traumatic events (Butler, Copnell, & Hall, 2019). For example, asking participants to describe a sexual assault experience could precipitate feelings of extreme fear, anger, and sadness. In studying sensitive topics, you should arrange prior to the study to have appropriate professionals available for referrals should the participants become upset. During the interview, you would need to be vigilant about assessing the participants' discomfort and refer them for appropriate professional intervention as necessary. If a participant appears upset during a qualitative interview, the researcher should ask questions such as, "Do you want to pause for a moment?" or "Do you want to talk about something else for a while?" or "Do you want to stop this interview?" Some participants will want to stop the interview completely. Others will want to continue despite the discomfort because it is important for them to tell their story. Care must also be taken not to reveal a participant's identity inadvertently when disseminating the findings, especially when studying sensitive topics (Turcotte-Tremblay & McSween-Cadieux, 2018).

Studies with a **potential for permanent damage** are more likely to involve biomedical researchers than nurse researchers. For example, medical studies of new drugs and surgical procedures have the potential to cause participants permanent physical damage. However, nurses have investigated topics that have the potential to damage participants permanently, emotionally, spiritually, and socially. Studies examining variables such as human immunodeficiency virus (HIV) diagnosis, sexual behavior, child abuse, or drug use have the potential to cause permanent damage to a participant's personality or reputation. There are also potential economic risks, such as reduced job performance or loss of employment.

Studies in which participants will suffer **certain permanent damage** may be unethical, such as the Nazi medical experiments and the Tuskegee syphilis study. Conducting research that will permanently damage participants is highly questionable and must be scrutinized carefully, regardless of the benefits gained. One exception might be a study that involves participants with a life-threatening disease having the opportunity to have a medical procedure that promises a cure but causes permanent damage to hearing, to peripheral sensation, or to vision. Frequently, in studies that cause permanent damage, other people, not the participants, will receive the benefits of the study. Studies causing permanent damage to participants, without a concomitant gain, violate the Nuremberg Code (1949).

Balancing Benefits and Risks for a Study

Researchers and reviewers of research must compare the benefits and risks in a study. The comparison is called the **benefit-risk ratio**. To begin, you must first predict the most likely outcomes of your study based on previous research findings, clinical experience, and theory. What are the benefits and risks, both actual and potential, of these outcomes? As the researcher, your goal is to maximize the benefits and minimize the risks (Fig. 9.3).

The probability and magnitude of a study's potential benefits must be assessed. A **research benefit** is defined as something of value to the participant whether related to physical health, psychological status, or social gain. Participants may receive the benefit of knowing they have contributed to the acquisition of knowledge for evidence-based practice (EBP). Money and other compensations for participation in research are not benefits but remuneration for research-related inconveniences (DHHS, 2018). In study proposals and informed consent documents, the research benefits are described for the individual participants, participants' families, and society.

The type of research conducted, whether therapeutic or nontherapeutic, affects the potential benefits for the participants. In **therapeutic nursing research**, the individual participant has the potential to benefit from the procedures of the study, such as skin care, range of motion, touch, emotional support, and pain management strategies. The benefits might include improvement in the participant's physical condition, which could facilitate emotional and social benefits. The participant also may benefit from the additional attention of and interaction with a healthcare professional. In addition, knowledge generated from the research may expand the participants' and their families' understanding of health. The conduct of **nontherapeutic nursing research** does not benefit the participant directly but is important to generate and refine nursing knowledge for practice. Subjects who understand the lack of therapeutic benefit for them frequently will participate because of altruism and the desire to help others with their condition (Irani & Richmond, 2015).

To compare the benefits and risks, you must also assess the type, severity, and number of risks that participants might experience by participating in your study. The risks depend on the purpose of the study and the procedures used to conduct it. Studies can have actual (known) risks and potential risks for participants. As mentioned earlier, participants in a study of the effects of prolonged bed rest have the actual risk of transient muscle weakness and the potential risk of DVT. Some studies contain actual or potential risks for the participants' families and society. You must determine the likelihood of the risks and take precautions to protect the rights of participants when implementing your study.

The **benefit-risk ratio** is the term given to a comparison of the benefits and risks of a study and is determined on the basis of the maximized benefits and the minimized risks. The researcher attempts to maximize the benefits and minimize the risks by making changes in the study purpose or procedures, or both (Goldstein et al., 2019). If the risks entailed by your study cannot be eliminated or further minimized, you must justify their existence. If the risks outweigh the benefits, the IRB is unlikely to approve the study and you probably need to revise the study or develop a new one. If the benefits equal or outweigh the risks, you can usually justify conducting the study, and an IRB will probably approve it (see Fig. 9.3).

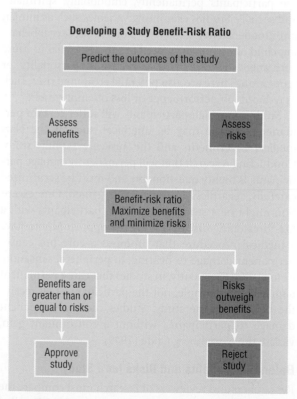

Fig. 9.3 Balancing benefits and risks of a study.

Clinical Equipoise

Clinical equipoise is the responsibility of clinicians to "provide the best possible treatment for their patients"

(Gravetter & Forzano, 2018, p. 90). Studies in which participants are randomly assigned to a treatment (intervention) group or control group may threaten the principle of no harm if the control group receives care that is known to be inferior. For example, in a study of patients with heart failure who have had a myocardial infarction (MI), the intervention group receives a new medication that has been shown in animal studies to be effective with fewer side effects; the control group receives an older medication that has some serious side effects. Some participants are not being protected from harm (Gravetter & Forzano, 2018), because the researchers already know that the older drug potentially can cause serious side effects. To maintain equipoise, researchers who compare clinical treatments must either believe them to be relatively equivalent, acknowledge that it is unknown which is best, or indicate professional disagreement about which is best. The informed consent process for a RCT should include benefits and potential harms of both the intervention and control condition (Kotz, Viechtbauer, Spigt, & Crutzen, 2019).

Some debate exists about clinical equipoise because it implies the objective of clinical care is the same as the objective of research (Thakur & Lahiry, 2019). For valid findings to be available upon which to base clinical care, studies are needed that randomly assign participants to different groups. Chapter 11 provides information about different types of RCTs that address the issue of equipoise, specifically pragmatic clinical trials and cluster RCTs.

HUMAN SUBJECT PROTECTION IN GENOMICS RESEARCH

The Human Genome Project funded by the NIH recognized from the onset the ethical and legal dilemmas of genomic research and allocated 5% of the funding to study these issues (Hammer, 2019). Over $300 million has been invested in studying the ethical and legal issues within genomic research. The funded studies made it "evident that a delicate balance exists between major genomics scientific progress and the challenge of maintaining the ethical tenets of autonomy, beneficence, non-maleficence, and justice" (Hammer, 2019, p. 94).

Several highly publicized cases have increased awareness as well as fear among the public. In 1951, Henrietta Lacks, an African American woman, only 31 years of age, was diagnosed with cervical cancer. She was admitted to the hospital for the standard treatment at the time (Jones, 1997). The specimens collected were taken to the laboratory of a scientist named Dr. Gey. Dr. Gey was trying to identify and reproduce a cell line for research purposes (Jones, 1997). When Mrs. Lacks's cells continued to multiply, Dr. Gey developed methods to produce even more and generously provided the cell line to other researchers free of charge. These researchers, building on Dr. Gey's research, developed a cell line from those especially hardy tumor cells, which were successfully used in research (Bledsoe & Grizzle, 2013; Skloot, 2010). Highly effective treatments, such as the polio vaccine and in vitro fertilization (IVF), were developed using the cell line and were extremely profitable for the researchers and their institutions. Literally billions of dollars were made by selling the cell line to other researchers (McEwen, Boyer, & Sun, 2013). Mrs. Lacks died never knowing her tumor cells were used for research, and her family only learned of her contribution to science in 2010.

In 1990, researchers began collecting blood specimens of members of an isolated Native American Indian tribe, the Havasupai, who lived in the Grand Canyon (Caplan & Moreno, 2011). Diabetes mellitus was a devastating disease among the tribe, and researchers proposed a study to identify genetic clues of disease susceptibility. However, the researchers used the blood specimens to study other topics (McEwen et al., 2013). The publications from the subsequent studies linked schizophrenia to the tribe's DNA and contradicted the tribe's story of their origin. The tribe sued Arizona State University, the employer of the original researcher, and was awarded a financial settlement in 2010. In addition, tribal leaders were given the remaining blood samples to be disposed of in a culturally appropriate way.

Several ethical issues in genomics research have not been resolved. The following section will include issues with de-identification of data, additional studies being conducted with specimens already collected, participants withdrawing from a study, and return of information to the research participant if beneficial to the participant. The second section will identify ethical issues about specific methods such as use of embryonic tissue.

Ethical Issues Related to Genomic Specimens

By its very nature, genomic data cannot be completely de-identified (Quinn & Quinn, 2018; Terry, 2015). Genomic data could be combined with data from publicly available demographic databases and be re-identified. The likelihood of linking genomic data to an individual (re-identification) has increased because genome-wide sequencing and large samples have increased the size of databases, computer processing speeds have dramatically increased, and personal data are available through public internet sources (Quinn & Quinn, 2018). Despite this issue, genomic data that have been de-identified (18 elements removed) can be used by researchers without the notification or authorization of the participants. Without links to individuals, the research is considered nonhuman research (Bledsoe, Russell-Einhorn, & Grizzle, 2018) and not subject to regulation by the Common Rule. Genomic data are being generated from the body tissues and fluids that are left over after specimens are removed during clinical care. For example, a patient has a lung biopsy. The tissue is examined to determine the presence and types of abnormal cells. Not all of the tissue is used, however, and is saved on paraffin blocks. Archival tissue and fluids have been de-identified, studied, and resulted in dramatic and rapid advances in scientific knowledge, including targeted cancer treatments, improved immunotherapy, and genome sequencing of abnormal tissues (Bledsoe et al., 2018).

The issues of whether identified information will be used for future studies was directly addressed in the revised Common Rule (DHHS, 2018). The new rule includes a new type of consent, called broad consent. **Broad consent** asks the patient or potential study participant for permission to store, maintain, and use for future studies private information and biological specimens that are identifiable. Box 9.7 contains the required elements of broad consent. Broad consent addresses whether any profits from commercial processes developed based on participant's biospecimen will be shared with the participant, a statement developed because of the case of Mrs. Lack.

Voluntary participation in research and the possibility of withdrawing are hallmark characteristics of informed consent (Capron, 2018). When biospecimens have been de-identified, withdrawing from a study becomes problematic. How does a researcher delete or remove a participant's data if the data have been de-identified? Researchers must consider this possibility when planning the study. One strategy would be to delay de-identification until data collection is complete. Another would be to de-identify the data over the course of the study but retain a code number linking the data to the participant until the study is completed.

BOX 9.7   Required Elements of Broad Consent

- Potential risks and discomforts
- Possible benefits
- Extent to which private information will be kept confidential
- Participation is voluntary
- Refusal to participate involves no harm or loss of benefits
- May stop participation at any time
- Specimens and information (identifiable and nonidentifiable) may result in commercial products and process
- Whether participant will share any profits
- Whether whole genome sequencing is planned

From Department of Health and Human Services (DHHS). (2018). Basic HHS policy for protection of human subjects. *Code of Federal Regulations,* Sub-Part A of 45, Part 46.

Another pressing question is what happens if the researcher's results include information that would benefit the participants directly? For example, the researchers are studying genetic characteristics of de-identified biospecimens from 20,000 adults who have osteoarthritis and are 61 to 79 years old. They incidentally find that 3% of the 11,000 women in the study have a breast cancer gene *(BRCA)* mutation that is associated with an inherited predisposition to breast cancer. Should the researchers re-identify the 330 specimens with the mutation and inform the women of their results? The ethical principles of beneficence, respect of persons, and justice would support a decision to re-identify the specimens (Bledsoe et al., 2018). However, the researchers need to balance the decision with whether the original study can be completed if funding is diverted to identifying the women and whether harm would occur to women who are informed but do not have breast cancer (Bledsoe et al., 2018). Relative to harm, the researchers would need to know that Black are underrepresented in genetic testing, which means the evidence linking *BRCA* mutations and breast cancer among Black women is weaker than it is for White women. Therefore the researchers would be less confident about notifying Black women about a *BRCA* mutation (Gehlert & Mozersky, 2018). Research teams will need to discuss these issues prior to initiating a study using biospecimens. The revised Common Rule does not require re-identification but does require that a broad consent includes what the researchers would do if this situation occurred (see Box 9.7).

Ethical Issues With Specific Types of Genomic Research

Advanced practice nurses, nurse educators, and nurse administrators are likely to confront the genomic ethical issues in their work. Warren (2016) calls for nurses to be leaders in the policy debate about stem cell and genomic research. Nurse leaders cannot be leaders in the research and policy without understanding physiological and ethical challenges, such as the moral status of embryos and organoids. Specially trained nurses are being utilized to implement the stem cell therapies in clinical trials (Perrin et al., 2018). Stem cells continue to be a controversial source of genetic material and will be discussed first. Much of the related controversy is based on the source of the cells. Ethical issues with embryos are related to the views of researchers and funders on abortion and human cloning. Organoids are produced from stem cells for research and raise some new questions about ethical use of cerebral organoids.

Stem Cell Research

We begin with a few definitions of key terms because the ethical issues are hard to understand without understanding these terms. **Stem cells** are human cells that can reproduce themselves or can develop into specialized cells of other types, such as blood cells or muscle cells. Stem cells have been derived from **somatic cells** of adults and umbilical cord blood of infants (Johnston & Zacharias, 2019). Somatic cells are any cell in the body except those cells used for reproduction, specifically any cells except sperm and eggs. **Pluripotent cells** are master cells and can make cells for any layer of the body. They are important because the cells they produce as they divide are used for tissue repair in the body. Scientific advances have allowed the identification or creation of stem cells from four sources: adult cells, fetal cells, embryos, and reprogrammed human cells. The ethical issues vary based on the source of the cells. For example, stem cells generated from somatic adult and child cells pose no major ethical issues for the majority of the US population. The adults involved can give informed consent to the use their cells, and parents can give consent for use of their infant's blood.

Using the cells from aborted fetuses has been more troublesome because of strong opinions about the morality of terminating a pregnancy. The revised code addresses this issue directly by removing researchers from the decision about the termination of pregnancy and not allowing them to offer any compensation for a woman having an abortion in exchange for use of the fetal tissue (DHHS, 2018). Federal funding is available for research with stem cells generated from fetal tissues or cells; however, researchers involved in fetal stem cell research need to be aware of state regulations because five states have legal bans on using fetal cells (Johnston & Zacharias, 2019).

Stem cells can be extracted from preimplantation human embryos that are 4 to 7 days old because each cell has the potential to develop into all types of human cells. These stem cells are called human embryonic stem cells (hEScs). Based on initial research results, hEScs have the therapeutic potential to repair damaged human organs (Johnston & Zacharias, 2019). The opposition is great, however, because extracting the cells results in the death of the embryo, an embryo that is considered by some to be a potential human being to which ethical principles apply (Hostiuc et al., 2019). The embryos may come from IVF. Reproductive cells that were initially harvested for a future pregnancy may be donated by parents who no longer need them for that purpose. This means of generating hEScs is more acceptable on ethical grounds, because the embryos would have been destroyed anyway (Johnston & Zacharias, 2019). However, the number of donated embryos and the lack of cultural diversity of the embryos do not meet the needs of science.

hEScs can be produced by cloning using a process called somatic cell nuclear transfer (SCNT). SCNT can produce embryos from which stem cells are derived, stem cells that are used for research or therapeutic purposes (Johnston & Zacharias, 2019). The embryos are destroyed after the stem cells are removed, making it ethically unacceptable to some. The hEScs derived from cloned embryo stem cells also have the potential to cause an undesired immune response or abnormal cells in a recipient (Prentice, 2019).

Beginning in 1973, federal funding was not available to study embryos, hEScs, and cloned embryos. Stem cell research continued, however, funded by states, individuals, and foundations. In 1998, a change occurred in federal funding. Once the stem cells were created, federal funds were available to conduct research using the cells (Johnston & Zacharias, 2019). The specifics of funding have varied according to which US president is in office. Stem cell research has become a major political issue, with debate around which ethical principle is stronger: beneficence, nonmaleficence, or respect for persons. Beneficence supports funding and encouraging stem cell research because of its great potential in improving the health of many people suffering with diseases (Warren, 2016). Nonmaleficence supports maintaining the restrictions on any research that produces embryos that will be destroyed. When an individual views an embryo as a human life, respect for persons also supports maintaining the restrictions on destroying embryos produced for research.

Induced pluripotent stem cells (iPSCs) are "human somatic cells reprogrammed to develop into nearly every human cell type, and are believed to be functionally very similar or identical to embryonic stem cells" (Johnston & Zacharias, 2019, p. 1311). Ethical and legal oppositions to iPSCs have been less than the opposition to hESCs. Although iPSCs have some potential for negative side effects, such as immune responses and abnormal cell growth, published studies using iPSCs have increased in number and are outpacing published studies with hESCs (Prentice, 2019).

In 2009, the NIH released *Guidelines for Human Stem Cell Research* (DHHS, 2009). Other guidelines have been released by the National Academies of Science (2005) and the International Society for Stem Cell Research, with the latest revision published in 2016. Nurse researchers who are working in stem cell research will want to be familiar with these guidelines and any relevant state laws, the ethical views of other members of the research team, and the IRBs overseeing the research.

Cerebral Organoids

Organoids are three-dimensional structures created from stem cells to mimic functions of organs (Hostiuc et al., 2019). The organs for which organoids have been generated include the retina, intestines, liver, pancreas, testes, thyroid, heart, kidneys, lungs, and brain (Hostiuc et al., 2019; Lavazza & Massimini, 2018). These miniature organs are different from human organs in that they are less complex and may not exhibit all the desired functions of the full-size organ (Lavazza & Massimini, 2018). However, the similarities to human organs have made organoids an increasingly valuable resource for biomedical research. Cerebral organoids are being used to study autism, Parkinson disease, microcephaly, and

traumatic brain injury. Because human embryonic stem cells are used to make organoids, some researchers would argue against organoids on the same ethical basis as other embryonic research. However, organoids can be generated from iPSCs or hESCs, with the source potentially being the deciding factor in the ethics of creating organoids (see previous section).

Beyond the source of the stem cells, the functions of cerebral organoids are beginning to raise new ethical issues. Research related to developing cerebral organoids has resulted in highly complex structures with neurons specific to each of the six layers of the cortex and others that have been shown to stimulate muscle contractions (Hostiuc et al., 2019). These highly complex cerebral organoids replicate the functions of the brain in an embryo a few months old (Hostiuc et al., 2019). The complexity of these structures gives rise to questions about the extent to which cerebral organoids should be considered human: How long will it be before these tissues are conscious and sentient (Lavazza & Massimini, 2018)? At what point in their development should the ethical principles of human research apply to cerebral organoids? Sancar (2018) reported an interview with Dr. Madeline Lancaster, the scientist whose cultures began to produce the three-dimensional structures that led to the development of organoids. Dr. Lancaster argues that cerebral organoids will not progress to the point of being conscious and sentient. Research conducted with cerebral organoids will continue to be an area of knowledge to monitor. These and other organoid-related ethical questions are likely to generate lively debate in the coming years.

INFORMED CONSENT

Obtaining informed consent from human participants is essential for the conduct of ethical research in the United States (DHHS, 2018) and in other countries. Informing is the transmission of essential ideas and content from the researcher to the prospective participant. Consent is the prospective participant's agreement, after assimilating essential information, to participate in a study as a participant. The phenomenon of **informed consent** was formally defined in the first principle of the Nuremberg Code as follows: "the person involved should have legal capacity to give consent; should be so situated as to be able to exercise free power of choice, without the intervention of any element of

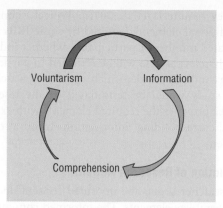

Fig. 9.4 Components of informed consent: information, comprehension, and voluntarism.

force, fraud, deceit, duress, over-reaching, or other ulterior form of constraint or coercion; and should have sufficient knowledge and comprehension of the elements of the participant matter involved, as to enable him to make an understanding and enlightened decision" (Nuremberg Code, 1949, p. 181).

The definition of informed consent from the Nuremberg Code provides a basis for the discussion of consent in all subsequent research codes and has wide acceptance in the research community. Informed consent can only occur when the prospective participant is mentally competent and able to comprehend that information, the researcher discloses essential information, and the prospective participant has the freedom to volunteer to participate (Fig. 9.4) (Thakur & Lahiry, 2019). Fig. 9.4 displays the informed consent process as the related components of information, comprehension, and voluntarism. Informed consent does not meet ethical standards or legal requirements unless all three components are present.

Facilitating Comprehension

Persons with a cognitive impairment may participate in research studies when another person can act on their behalf. To the degree that they are capable, persons with cognitive impairment should have the opportunity to choose whether to participate in research. Previously in this chapter, we discussed persons with limited capacity due to cognitive impairment, psychosis, and dementia. With careful accommodations, a study's participants may include persons with cognitive impairment (Forster & Borasky, 2018), a diagnosis of psychosis (Weissinger & Ulrich, 2019), or dementia (Chester et al., 2018).

To enhance the comprehension of all prospective participants, professional jargon in the consent document needs to be replaced by everyday language. The language of the consent document should be adapted to the expected participants. Healthcare facilities may require that the researcher make the consent form available in the most common languages spoken by their patients. Depending on the geographic area, the consent form may need to be translated into Vietnamese, French, Spanish, or another language. For example, when some of the potential participants are Spanish speakers, the researchers should provide the consent and written instruments in Spanish. However, translating the consent into Castilian Spanish is not helpful if the population is primarily from Central America. Translation of instruments is a complex process, and we recommend the book on measurement by Waltz, Strickland, and Lenz (2017) as a reference (also see Chapter 17).

The reading level of the consent should be adjusted for the expected participants. The recommended reading level for informed consent documents is an eighth-grade reading level (Tamariz et al., 2019). Gehlert and Mozersky (2018) report that half of the US population has a reading level below the eighth grade. When it is likely that some participants may have limited reading ability, the researcher may read the consent aloud to all participants to avoid embarrassment. When study information is not comprehended, there is no *informed* consent. This section describes the information that must be included in the consent document or oral consent and the methods of documenting consent.

Another way to improve comprehension is to provide the consent information in multiple modes and assess the participants' comprehension. Lindsley (2019) conducted a quality improvement initiative that began by assessing the research participants' knowledge of a study to which they had consented to participate. Their knowledge gaps were used as the basis for questions to use in assessing comprehension and developing a multimodal presentation with the required elements of informed consent. The text of the presentation was reduced to a sixth-grade reading level. The presentation was delivered on a touchscreen tablet. Adult volunteers were randomized to receive standard or multimodal format of consent. The comprehension of all participants was assessed. The comprehension of those participants who viewed the multimodal presentation was significantly higher than the comprehension of participants who received the standard method of consent (Lindsley, 2019). Earlier in the chapter, we identified the benefits of using visual and oral methods to enhance comprehension in children and their parents, but Lindsley's results indicated a multimodal approach is appropriate for adults, too.

Information Essential for Consent

Informed consent requires the researcher to disclose specific information to each prospective participant. In addition to the elements that are required by federal regulations (Box 9.8), the IRB or institution where the study will be conducted may have additional elements

BOX 9.8   Required Elements of Informed Consent

- Statement that the study is research
- Purpose of the study
- Expected time the participant will be involved
- Procedures involved and which are experimental
- Reasonable risks and benefits
- Alternative procedures, if applicable
- Extent of confidentiality
- Compensation or treatment if injury occurs
- Who to contact with concerns about study or rights as a study participant
- Voluntary participation; no penalty for not agreeing or discontinuing the study
- Whether de-identified data or specimens will be shared with other researchers
- Additional information to include as applicable
  - Any procedures that would hurt the fetus if a woman is pregnant
  - Circumstances under which participation could be terminated by researchers
  - Any costs related to being in the study
  - Consequences of withdrawal and orderly termination of withdrawing
  - New research findings might influence participant's decision to participate
  - Approximate number of participants in the study
  - De-identified biospecimens may be used for commercial profit
  - Whether and how participant's clinically relevant results will be shared with participant
  - Whether biospecimens will undergo whole genome sequencing

From Department of Health and Human Services (DHHS). (2018). Basic HHS policy for protection of human subjects. *Code of Federal Regulations,* Sub-Part A of 45, Part 46.

that they require (DHHS, 2018). Typical examples of the additional elements required by some IRBs are the anticipated number of participants, whether individual clinically relevant data will be returned to participants, and the conditions under which a person's participation in the study would be terminated by the researcher. Table 9.2 provides the required elements with examples of the corresponding information from a consent document.

Introduction of Research Activities

The researcher begins the informed consent document with several key elements. The informed consent document includes a statement that the prospective participant is being asked to participate in a research study and a description of the purpose of the study, type of data collection, and expected duration of the person's participation (DHHS, 2018; Santos et al., 2017). Prospective participants also must receive a complete description of the procedures to be followed, such as whether assignment to a group will be random if the study includes an intervention and a control group. The researchers must identify the intervention as being experimental (DHHS, 2018; FDA, 2019b). For example, researchers conducting quantitative and outcome studies need to describe the procedures or mechanisms that will be used to examine, manipulate, or measure the study variables. For qualitative studies, the researcher will describe how data will be collected, such as an interview, and the topics to be discussed or observed. Mixed methods studies will include descriptions of the quantitative and qualitative procedures. In addition, they must inform prospective participants about when the study procedures will be implemented, how many times, and in what setting.

Prospective participants must receive a disclosure of alternatives related to their participation in a study. For example, a female hypertensive patient who has uncontrolled blood pressure on a single antihypertensive medication may be recruited for a clinical trial for patients like her who have uncontrolled hypertension on a single drug. The two arms of the trial are following the current EBP guideline of adding a second antihypertensive medication or being prescribed a new experimental antihypertensive medication. She needs to know that, if she decides not to participate, she can continue on her current medication and attend an education program about eating correctly and losing weight. As a prospective participant, the medication plus education is an

TABLE 9.2 Informed Consent Language for a Descriptive Comparative Study

Required Element	Example
Statement that the study is research	You are being asked to participate in a research study about nursing students' attitudes toward poverty.
Purpose of the study	The purpose of the study is to compare junior and senior nursing students' attitudes toward poverty before and after a poverty simulation.
Expected time the participant will be involved	The Attitudes Toward Poverty Short-Form Scale (ATPS) takes 5 to 10 minutes to complete.
Procedures involved and which are experimental	The poverty simulation is a required class activity. You will be asked to complete the ATPS before and after the simulation. The researchers want to know whether the poverty simulation affects your attitudes about poverty.
Reasonable risks and benefits	RISKS: Because the major risk of the study is the potential loss of confidentiality, a faculty not involved in the study will remove only the consent form from the manila envelope. If you said yes to participating, your packet will be retained for the study. If you said no, your packet will be marked that it is not to be included in the study. No other risks have been identified related to participating in this study. BENEFITS: The main benefit to you for participating in this study is knowing you have contributed to expanding the body of knowledge available on nursing student's attitudes toward poverty.
Alternative procedures, if applicable	There are no alternative procedures for this study.
Extent of confidentiality	All information obtained about you in this study is strictly confidential unless the law requires disclosure. The results of this study may be used in reports, presentations, and publications, but the researchers will not identify any individual students.
Compensation or treatment if injury occurs	There are no costs or payments associated with your participation in this study.
Who to contact with concerns about study or rights as a study participant	In the event that you suffer injury as a result of participation in any research project, you may contact Faculty Member at 123-123-1234 or Chair of the IRB at 321-321-4321, who will be glad to review the matter with you.
Voluntary participation; no penalty for not agreeing or discontinuing the study	The poverty simulation is a required class activity, but the researchers want your decision about participating in this study to be absolutely voluntary. If you have questions about the study, please ask the researchers before you agree to participate. It is okay for you to say no. Your decision will not affect your participation or grade in the required poverty simulation activity. Your responses will not be linked to your name.
Whether de-identified data or specimens will be shared with other researchers	The researchers will not share the data with other researchers.

appropriate, alternative course of treatment about which she must be informed (DHHS, 2018).

Research participants also need to know the funding source(s) of a study, such as specific individuals, organizations, or companies (Bonham, 2018). For example, researchers studying the effects of a specific drug must identify any sponsorship by a pharmaceutical company.

Description of Risks and Benefits

Prospective participants must be informed about any foreseeable risks or discomforts (physical, emotional, social, or economic) that might result from the study (Bonham, 2018; DHHS, 2018; FDA, 2019b). Female prospective participants need to know whether the study treatment or procedure involves potential risks to them or their fetuses if they are pregnant or become pregnant during the study (DHHS, 2018). For research involving more than minimal risk, prospective participants must be given an explanation as to whether any compensation or medical treatment, or both, would be available if injury should occur. If medical treatments are available, the person obtaining consent must describe the type and extent of the treatments.

You should also describe any benefits to the participant or to others that may be reasonably expected from the research. The study might benefit the current participants or might generate knowledge that will provide evidence-based care to patients and families in the future (DHHS, 2018; FDA, 2019b). Most critically, prospective participants want to know how the risks of a study were minimized and the benefits maximized. They need time to compare the potential risks and benefits in the context of their lives so they can determine what is best for them without the researcher's influence.

Assurance of Anonymity and Confidentiality

Prospective participants must be assured their research records, including PHI, will be secured during and following the study and remain confidential (DHHS, 2018). All oral or poster presentations and published papers will report only group findings. The exception may be for qualitative studies when participants' quotes may be included in a presentation or publication but will not be linked to an identifiable individual. Any limits to confidentiality, such as the researcher's need to reveal anything the participant reports about ongoing elder abuse, must also be disclosed to the prospective participant before participation begins, if relevant to the study. Depending on the study design, participants' identities may be anonymous to the researchers, which decreases the potential for bias. For example, an internet survey may allow participants to enter their responses and not include their names.

Voluntary and Informed Participation

Despite assessing the capacity of the participant to comprehend the information and providing the consent in the participant's primary language and at the appropriate reading level, some participants may be confused or have additional questions. As a conscientious researcher, you need to offer to answer any questions that the prospective participants may have during the consent process. Study participants also need an explanation of

whom to contact for answers to questions about the research during the conduct of the study and whom to contact in the event of a research-related problem or injury, as well as how to do so (DHHS, 2018). In addition to the researcher who may be contacted, the IRB of the healthcare facility or university IRB to which you are submitting your materials will have specific contact information to include on the consent. A copy of the informed consent should be given to the participant so he or she has this contact information.

Voluntary participation is as critical to the consent process as being informed. A **noncoercive disclaimer** is a statement that participation is voluntary and refusal to participate will involve no penalty or loss of benefits to which the participant is entitled (DHHS, 2018; FDA, 2019b). We do know that participants may agree to participate because they believe their care will be higher quality or they will have improved outcomes (Thakur & Lahiry, 2019). Therapeutic misconception has been documented and may need to be proactively addressed with some participants. For example, CF patients acknowledged that they agreed to participate in research because they believed their care would be better (Bailey & Ladores, 2018). (See previous section for more on therapeutic misconception.)

Researchers may pay participants for their time and effort. However, any payment may be coercive to participants with extremely limited financial means (e.g., $5 may be coercive to a participant who is hungry). Any financial compensation to prisoners to participate in a study has been viewed as coercive. However, Ravi, Christopher, Filene, Reifeis, and White (2018) conducted a study of the attitudes of prisoners ($N = 50$) toward financial compensation for being a study participant. The prisoners overwhelmingly indicated that prisoners who are participants in studies should be compensated (74%) and that payment would not keep prisoners from refusing to participate (88%).

When determining the amount of compensation for a specific study, factors such as transportation expenses, possible childcare costs, and length of participation should be considered. Astute researchers often seek guidance from community representatives and other experts who are familiar with the study population. When compensation is going to be provided, the information should be included in the consent document. Typically, a small financial payment ($10 to $30) is seen as noncoercive and appropriate to compensate participants for time and effort related to study participation (Adams & Lawrence, 2019).

Subjects may discontinue participation in a study at any time without penalty or loss of benefits, meaning that compensation cannot be dependent on completion of the study. There may be circumstances under which the participant's involvement in a study may be terminated by the researcher without regard to the participant's consent (DHHS, 2018). For example, if the intervention being studied becomes potentially dangerous to a participant, you as a researcher have an obligation to discontinue the participant's involvement in the study. The consent needs to include a general statement about the circumstances that could lead to termination of the entire project, such as safety concerns or unexpected risks. This is especially important in therapeutic research.

Consent to Incomplete Disclosure

In some studies, participants experience **incomplete disclosure** of study information, or are not completely informed of the study purpose, because that knowledge would alter their actions. However, prospective participants must know that certain information is being withheld deliberately. You, the researcher, must ensure that there are no undisclosed risks to the participants that are more than minimal and that their questions are truthfully answered regarding the study. Subjects who are exposed to nondisclosure of information must know when and how they will be debriefed about the study. Subjects are **debriefed** by informing them of the actual purpose of the study and the results that were obtained (Shamoo & Resnik, 2015). At this point, participants have the option to have their data withdrawn from the study. If the participants experience adverse effects related to the study, you must make every attempt to compensate or alleviate the effects (DHHS, 2018).

Documentation of Informed Consent

The standard is that informed consent is presented formally and requires the signature of the participant and a witness. There are lower risk studies, however, in which signatures and/or written consent can be waived with the approval of the IRB.

Waivers of Written and Signed Consent

Requirements for written consent or the participants' signatures on their consent forms may be waived in minimal risk research (DHHS, 2018). For example, if you were using questionnaires to collect low-risk data, obtaining a signed consent form from participants might not be necessary. The participant's completion of the questionnaire may serve as consent. The top of the questionnaire might contain a statement such as "Your completion of this questionnaire indicates your consent to participate in this study." In other low-risk studies, data may be collected by mail or online and, after the text of the consent is presented, the participant then signifies consent by completing the questionnaire.

Written consent also is waived when the only record linking the participant and the research would be the consent document, and the principal risk is the harm that could result from a breach of confidentiality. The participants must be given the option of signing or not signing a consent form, and the participant's wishes govern whether the consent form is signed (DHHS, 2018). However, the three elements of consent—information, comprehension, and voluntarism—are essential in all studies (see Fig. 9.4), whether written consent is waived or required.

An example of an alteration of the consent process is found in a study with HIV seropositive African Americans (Coleman, 2017). The descriptive correlational study was designed to test a model of factors related to depression and quality of life. In a private room at an HIV clinic, the researcher described the study purpose and other information about the study. Each set of questionnaires was given a unique identifying number, to protect confidentiality. A "waiver of signature was requested for the consent form from the IRB as it was determined the participant's signature was not needed" (Coleman, 2017, p. 139). In this stigmatized group, confidentiality is especially important. The only link between the data provided and the participants would have been their signatures on the consent form, a valid reason for making this change.

Elements of the Consent Document

The written consent document or **consent form** includes the elements of informed consent required by the DHHS (2018) regulations (see Box 9.8). The IRBs of most healthcare facilities and universities maintain their own templates for the informed consent document with specific requirements, such as detailed headings, suggested wording, and contact information. The participant can read the consent form, or the researcher can read it to the participant; however, the researcher can also explain the study to the participant, using different words, in a conversational manner, which encourages questions. The participant signs the form, and the investigator or research assistant collecting the data witnesses it. This type of consent can be used for minimal-to-moderate-risk studies. All persons signing the consent form must receive a copy. The researcher keeps the original for 3 years in a secure location, such as a locked file cabinet in a locked room.

Studies that involve participants with diminished autonomy require a written consent form. If these prospective participants have some comprehension of the study and agree to participate, they must sign the consent form. However, each participant's legally authorized representative also must sign the form. The representative indicates his or her relationship to the participant under the signature.

The written consent form used in a high-risk study often contains the signatures of two witnesses, the researcher, and an additional person. The additional person signing as a witness must not be otherwise connected with the study and is present to observe the informed consent process and to ensure that it adheres to specifications. The best witnesses are research advocates or patient ombudspersons employed by the institution. Sometimes nurses are asked to sign a consent form as a witness for a biomedical study. They must know the study purpose and procedures and the participant's comprehension of the study before signing the form as a witness. The role of the witness is more important in the consent process if the prospective participant is in awe of the investigator and does not feel free to question the procedures of the study.

Short-Form Written Consent Document

The short-form consent document includes the following statement: "The elements of informed consent required by Section 46.116 have been presented orally to the participant or the participant's legally authorized representative" (DHHS, 2018, 45 CFR, Section 46.117b). The researcher must develop a written summary of what is to be said to the participant in the oral presentation, and the summary must be approved by an IRB. When the oral presentation is made to the participant or to the participant's representative, a witness is required. The participant or representative must sign the short-form consent document. The witness must sign both the short form and a copy of the summary, and the person obtaining consent must sign a copy of the summary. Copies of the summary and short form are given to the participant and the witness; the researcher retains the original documents and must keep these documents for 3 years after the end of the study. Short-form written consent documents may be used in studies that present minimal or moderate risk to participants.

Recording of the Consent Process

A researcher may choose to document the consent process through audio or video recordings. These methods document what was said to the prospective participant as well as record the participant's questions and the investigator's answers. Because recordings can be time consuming and costly, they are rarely used for studies of minimal or moderate risk. If your study is considered high risk, documenting the consent process electronically is recommended. The recording serves as a protection for you and your participants. The researchers and the participant (or representative) will retain a copy of the recording.

Authorization for Research Uses and Disclosure

The HIPAA Privacy Rule provides individuals the right, as research participants, to authorize covered entities (healthcare provider, health plan, and healthcare clearinghouse) to use or disclose their PHI for research purposes. This authorization is regulated by HIPAA and is separate from the informed consent that is regulated by the DHHS (2018). The authorization of the use of information can be included as part of the consent form, but it is probably best to have two separate forms. The authorization focuses on privacy risks and states how, why, and with whom PHI will be shared. The key ideas required on the authorization form when used for research are included in Box 9.9.

INSTITUTIONAL REVIEW

An **institutional review board** (IRB) is a committee that reviews research to ensure that all investigators are conducting research ethically. All hospital-based research must be submitted to the hospital's IRB, which will then determine whether it is high risk, moderate risk, minimal risk, or exempt from review. This is true, as well, of research that does not involve patients. Even though some research clearly falls under the category of

BOX 9.9 **Requirements for Authorization to Release PHI for Research**

- Types of PHI to be used, such as medical diagnosis or assessment data, identified in an understandable way
- Name of researcher who will use the PHI and affiliated institution
- How the PHI will be used in this specific study
- Authorization expiration date, which may be the end of the study or "none" if data will become part of a research database or repository
- Signature of the participant, legal representative if appropriate, and date

From *HIPAA Journal*. (2018). What is HIPAA authorization? Retrieved from https://www.hipaajournal.com/what-is-hipaa-authorization/

"exempt from review" it must, nonetheless, be submitted to the IRB, which then will declare it exempt. Requiring review of all studies is necessary because, in the past, studies that should have been reviewed escaped notice. Universities, hospital corporations, and many managed care centers maintain IRBs to promote the conduct of ethical research and protect the rights of prospective participants at these institutions, as required since 1974. Federal regulations require that the members of an IRB evaluate the study for protection of human participants, including processes for obtaining informed consent. Federal regulations stipulate the membership, functions, and operations of an IRB (DHHS, 2018, 45 CFR, Sections 46.107–46.109).

Each IRB has at least five members of various backgrounds (cultural, economic, educational, professional, gender, racial) to promote a complete, scholarly, and fair review of research that is commonly conducted in an institution (Martien & Nelligan, 2018). If an institution regularly reviews studies with participants susceptible to coercion or with impaired cognition, the IRB should include one or more members with knowledge about and experience in working with these individuals. Any IRB member who has a conflict of interest with a research project being reviewed must excuse himself or herself from the review process, except to provide information requested by the IRB. The IRB also must include members who are not affiliated with the institution and whose primary concern is nonscientific, such as an ethicist, a lawyer, or a minister (DHHS,

2018). IRBs in hospitals are often composed of physicians, nurses, lawyers, scientists, clergy, and community laypersons. The revised Common Rule provides a description of the experience and expertise of the IRB (DHHS, 2018):

"The IRB shall be sufficiently qualified through the experience and expertise of its members (professional competence), and the diversity of its members, including race, gender, and cultural backgrounds and sensitivity to such issues as community attitudes, to promote respect for its advice and counsel in safeguarding the rights and welfare of human subjects. The IRB shall be able to ascertain the acceptability of proposed research in terms of institutional commitments (including policies and resources) and regulations, applicable law, and standards of professional conduct and practice. The IRB shall therefore include persons knowledgeable in these areas." (Section 46.107)

A researcher may first develop a research proposal to obtain funding or approval of a faculty committee, if the researcher is a student. After gaining funding and/or faculty approval, the researcher develops a protocol—a shorter, but detailed description of the proposed study and its methods. The protocol is submitted to the IRB for approval. In addition, the IRB may require a form to gather information specific to the study, such as start and ending dates of the study. The IRB reviews the protocol and form to determine whether the researcher has demonstrated that (1) the benefits of the study outweigh the risks, (2) the risks will be minimized, and (3) the consent process and document are appropriate for the intended participants (Bonham, 2018). The IRB members also protect potential participants by determining the scientific value of the study. The researcher must demonstrate the significance of the research topic and the gap in knowledge that the proposed study will address. If the methods lack rigor or the researcher lacks knowledge and expertise to conduct the proposed study, then the study should not be conducted (Bonham, 2018). For example, a student submitting a protocol will need to document the research experience and professional knowledge of the faculty sponsor relevant to the research topic.

Clinical trials and other large multisite studies funded by the NIH must designate a central IRB. A central IRB is that to which the researchers will submit the study for its ethical review. Facilities that comprise the multiple sites of the study will be expected to accept the central IRB's decision. In the past, each facility's IRB reviewed the protocol, requiring the researchers to submit the protocol, their specific forms, and an informed consent with their facility's contact information. Most IRBs were underresourced and burdened by the increasing paperwork required to review and approve a study (Schnipper, 2017). No single IRB had members with sufficient expertise to review studies in every specialty and type of research. As a result, reviews were inconsistent. When one IRB required a change in the methods or consent form, the change had to be reviewed by all the IRBs. Needless to say, the process delayed the implementation of the study. By requiring a central IRB, multisite, federally funded studies will be implemented more quickly.

The implementation of review by a central IRB faces some barriers, such as failure to consider the local context in which the study will be implemented at a specific site (Schnipper, 2017). Another barrier to central IRBs is concern about the legal liability of a hospital or clinic when a participant at his or her site experiences an adverse event and there was no local review of the study.

Levels of Reviews Conducted by Institutional Review Boards

Federal guidelines identify the levels of reviews required for different types of studies (DHHS, 2018). The functions and operations of an IRB involve the review of research at three different levels of scrutiny: (1) exempt from review, (2) expedited review, and (3) full board review. Researchers cannot determine the level of review their proposed study requires. The IRB chairperson and/or committee, not the researcher, decides the level of the review.

Studies are usually **exempt from review** if they pose no apparent risks for research participants. Studies usually considered exempt from IRB review, according to federal regulations, are identified in Box 9.10. For example, studies by nurses and other health professionals that have no foreseeable risks or are a mere inconvenience for participants may be identified as exempt from review by

BOX 9.10   Research Qualifying for Exemption From Review

1. Conducted in established or commonly accepted educational settings, involving normal educational practices
2. Involving the use of educational tests, survey procedures, interview procedures, or observation of public behavior, *unless*:
   * Recorded in such a manner that human participants can be identified, directly or through identifiers
   * Disclosure of the human participants' responses could reasonably place the participants at risk of criminal or civil liability
   * Disclosure of the human participants' responses could reasonably be damaging to the participants' financial standing, employability, or reputation
3. Research involving the use of educational tests, survey procedures, interview procedures, or observation of public behavior that is not exempt:
   * Exempt if human participants are elected or appointed public officials or candidates for public office
   * Federal statute(s) require(s) without exception that the confidentiality of the personally identifiable information will be maintained throughout the research and thereafter.
4. Involving the collection or study of existing data, documents, records, pathological specimens, or diagnostic specimens if publicly available or recorded by the investigator in such a manner that participants cannot be identified, directly or through identifiers
5. Conducted by or participant to the approval of department or agency heads, and which are designed to study, evaluate, or examine the following:
   * Public benefit or service programs
   * Procedures for obtaining benefits or services under those programs
   * Possible changes in or alternatives to those programs or procedures
   * Possible changes in methods or levels of payment for benefits or services under those programs
6. Taste and food quality evaluation and consumer acceptance studies when:
   * Wholesome foods without additives are consumed
   * Food is consumed that contains a food ingredient at or below the level and for a use found to be safe
   * Food consumed contains an agricultural chemical or environmental contaminant at or below the level found to be safe by the FDA or other federal agency

Adapted from Department of Health and Human Services (DHHS). (2018). Protection of human participants. *Code of Federal Regulations*, Title 45, Part 46. Retrieved from https://www.ecfr.gov/cgi-bin/retrieveECFR?gp5&SID583cd09e1c0f5c6937cd9d7513160fc3f&pitd520180719&n5pt45.1.46&r5PART&ty5HTML#se45.1.46_1104

the chairperson of the IRB committee. In other states or regions, these same studies may be classified as studies appropriate for expedited reviews.

Under **expedited IRB review** procedures, the review may be carried out by the IRB chairperson or by one or more experienced reviewers designated by the chairperson from among members of the IRB. Expedited review procedures can also be used to review minor changes in previously approved research. Studies that have some risks, which are viewed as minimal, are expedited in the review process. **Minimal risk** means that "probability and magnitude of harm or discomfort anticipated in the research are not greater in and of themselves than those ordinarily encountered in daily life or during the performance of routine physical or psychological examinations or tests" (DHHS, 2018, 45 CFR, Section 46.102). In reviewing the research, the reviewers may exercise all of the authorities of the IRB except disapproval of the research. If the reviewer does not believe the research should be approved, the full committee must review the study. Only the full committee can disapprove a study (DHHS, 2018). Box 9.11 identifies research that usually qualifies for expedited review.

A study involving greater than minimal risk to research participants requires a **complete IRB review**, also called a full board review. Any study that does not qualify for exempt or expedited review must undergo a full board review. To obtain IRB approval, researchers must ensure that ethical principles are upheld. Risks must be minimized, and those risks must be reasonable when compared to benefits of participation. Consistent with justice, the selection of participants must be fair and equitable. Informed consent must be obtained from each participant or legal representative and documented appropriately. In addition, the researcher must have a plan to monitor data collection, protect privacy, and maintain confidentiality (DHHS, 2018, 45 CFR, Section 46.111).

Every research report must indicate that the study had IRB approval and whether the approval was from a university and/or clinical agency. For example, nurse researchers Kelechi, Mueller, Madisetti, Prentice, and Dooley (2018) conducted a study of cryotherapy for pain relief among patients with chronic venous disease (CVeD).

> The cryotherapy study was designed as a multicenter randomized controlled trial that compared a 9-month graduated cooling intervention to a placebo control plus usual care among patients with the more severe forms of CVeD. Three wound care centers and an academic medical research center from the south-eastern region of United States (U.S.) participated in the study. The study complied with the Declaration of Helsinki and was approved by the university's Institutional Review Board for Human Research (IRB). (Kelechi et al., 2018, p. 3)

BOX 9.11 Research Qualifying for Expedited Institutional Review Board Review

Expedited review for studies with no more than minimal risk involving:
1. Collection of hair, collection of nail clippings, extraction of deciduous teeth, and extraction of permanent teeth if extraction needed
2. Collection of excreta and external secretions (sweat, saliva, placenta removed at delivery, and amniotic fluid at rupture of the membrane)
3. Recording of data from participants 18 years of age or older using noninvasive procedures routinely used in clinical practice with exception of X-rays
4. Collection of blood samples by venipuncture from healthy, nonpregnant participants 18 years of age or older (amount not > 450 mL in an 8-week period, no more than two times per week)
5. Collection of dental plaque and calculus using accepted prophylactic techniques
6. Voice recordings made for research purposes such as investigations of speech defects
7. Moderate exercise by healthy volunteers
8. The study of existing data, documents, records, pathological specimens, or diagnostic specimens
9. Behavior or characteristics of individuals or groups, with no researcher manipulation. Research will not increase stress of participants.
10. Drugs or devices for which an investigational new drug exemption or an investigational device exemption is not required

Summarized from Department of Health and Human Services (DHHS). (2018). Protection of human participants. *Code of Federal Regulations,* Title 45, Part 46. Retrieved from https://www.ecfr.gov/cgi-bin/retrieveECFR?gp5&SID583cd09e1c0f5c6937cd9d7513160fc3f&pitd520180719&n5pt45.1.46&r5PART&ty5HTML#se45.1.46_1109

Informed consent and IRB approval are necessities for conducting ethical research. With revisions to the Common Rule, researchers will want to communicate early with the IRB from which they will be requesting approval. IRBs will be adapting their procedures to be consistent with the revised Common Rule.

RESEARCH MISCONDUCT

The goal of research is to generate sound scientific knowledge, which is possible only through honest implementation and reporting of studies. Scientific misconduct has been a known problem since the 1980s. In 1992, the DHHS created the Office of Research Integrity (ORI, n.d.). The ORI was instituted to supervise the implementation of the rules and regulations related to research misconduct and to manage any investigations of misconduct. In this section, terms used to describe scientific misconduct will be defined. Cases of scientific misconduct will be described in health care and nursing followed by how the ORI, journal editors, peer reviewers, and researchers can prevent scientific misconduct.

Terms Related to Scientific Misconduct

The most current regulations implemented by the ORI (2019b, 2019c) are CFR 42, Parts 50 and 93, Policies of General Applicability. The ORI was responsible for defining important terms used in the identification and management of research misconduct. **Research misconduct** was defined as "the fabrication, falsification, or plagiarism in processing, performing, or reviewing research, or in reporting research results…. It does not include honest error or differences in opinion" (ORI, 2019b, 42 CFR, Section 93.103). Also from Section 93.103, "**fabrication** is making up data or results and recording or reporting of them" and "**falsification** is manipulating research materials, equipment, or processes or changing or omitting data or results such that the research is not accurately represented in the research record." Fabrication and falsification of research data are two of the most common acts of research misconduct managed by ORI. **Plagiarism** is also research misconduct and is defined as "the appropriation of another person's ideas, processes, results, or words without giving appropriate credit" (ORI, 2019b, 42 CFR, Section 93.103).

Examples of Scientific Misconduct

The ORI's website contains a growing list of persons found to have falsified or fabricated research reports. We have described two completed cases in this section by way of example, but many others are available on the website. In August 2019, Dr. Rahul Agrawal was found to have fabricated data in 59 data files for experiments that were not conducted (ORI, 2019a). Dr. Agrawal was a fellow at the National Cancer Institute at NIH when he fabricated the data. In another case, Brandi Baughman, PhD, acknowledged in 2017 that she had manipulated data for 11 figures in a published paper. At the time, she was a postdoctoral fellow at the University of North Carolina and working on federally funded grants. She signed a letter indicating she had not manipulated data in any other experiments, knowing full well that she and her colleagues had a paper under review in which the findings were based on 14 reused and relabeled Western blot laboratory tests from an unrelated study. The ORI (2018) finding was that she would no longer be eligible to work with a federally funded research team for 2 years.

Research misconduct is a growing concern in nursing (Lach, 2019; Ward-Smith, 2016). Asman, Melnikov, Barnoy, and Tabak (2019) surveyed 119 nurses attending nursing education programs and 32 nurses with graduate degrees about scientific misconduct that they had observed. Among these nurses, 15.5% indicated agreement with one or more items about their inclination to fabricate data, and 26.25% indicated agreement with one or more items about their inclination to select or omit data. Fifty nurses (34.2%) had "knowledge of research misconduct in the workplace" (Asman et al., 2019, p. 864).

When scientific misconduct is identified, the related publications may be retracted. Al-Ghareeb et al. (2018) conducted a systematic review of 37 years of retractions in nursing and midwifery journals. They found 29 articles in nursing journals had been retracted, with the most common reason being duplicate publication (Al-Ghareeb et al., 2018).

Role of the ORI in Promoting the Conduct of Ethical Research

Currently, the ORI applies federal policies and regulations to protect the integrity of the USPHS's extramural and intramural research programs. The extramural programs provide funding to research institutions, and the "intramural programs provide funding for research conducted within Federal government facilities" (ORI, n.d.). Box 9.12 contains a summary of the functions of the ORI.

To be classified as research misconduct, an action must be intentional and involve a significant departure from acceptable scientific practices for maintaining the integrity of the research record. When an allegation is made, it must be proven by a preponderance of evidence. Institutions that received federal research funding must have policies and procedures for investigating any allegations against one of their researchers (ORI, 2017). The institution in which the misconduct occurred gathers the evidence and determines whether research misconduct has occurred. When research misconduct has been found to have occurred, the actions taken against the researchers or agencies have included disqualification to receive federal funding for a specific length of time or lifetime suspension from receiving funds. Other actions taken may be that the researcher can conduct only supervised research and all data and sources must be certified. All publications reporting the findings of the study in question are corrected or retracted (ORI, 2019b, 42 CFR, Section 93.411).

Role of Journal Editors and Researchers in Preventing Scientific Misconduct

Editors of journals also have a major role in monitoring and preventing research misconduct in the published literature (World Association of Medical Editors [WAME], n.d.). WAME has identified data falsification, plagiarism, and violations of legal and regulatory requirements as some types of scientific misconduct. (See Chapter 27 for more information on ethical practices for authorship.)

Preventing the publication of fraudulent research requires the efforts of authors, coauthors, research coordinators, reviewers of research reports for publication, and editors of professional journals (Al-Ghareeb et al., 2018; Asman et al., 2019; Ward-Smith, 2016). Authors who are primary investigators for research projects must be responsible in their conduct and the conduct of their team members, from data collection through publication of research. Coauthors and coworkers should question and, if necessary, challenge the integrity of a researcher's claims. Sometimes, well-known scientists' names have been added to a research publication as coauthors to give it credibility. Individuals should not be listed as coauthors unless they were actively involved in the conduct of the research and preparation of the manuscript (International Council of Medical Journal Editors [ICMJE], 2018). Similarly, supervisors and directors of hospital units should not be included as last author as a "courtesy" for a publication unless they were actively involved in at least one phase of the research.

Principal investigators (PIs) in large, funded studies have a role to promote integrity in research and to identify research misconduct activities (Kovach, 2018). They may have delegated implementation of a study to a research coordinator. These individuals are often the ones closest to the actual conduct of the study, during which misconduct often occurs. The PI should monitor the study closely along with the research coordinator to ensure ethical conduct.

BOX 9.12 Functions of the Office of Research Integrity

- Developing policies, procedures, and regulations related to responsible conduct of research and to the detection, investigation, and prevention of research misconduct
- Monitoring research misconduct investigations
- Making recommendations related to findings and consequences of investigations of research misconduct
- Assisting the Office of the General Counsel (OGC) to present cases before the DHHS appeals board
- Providing technical assistance to institutions responding to allegations of research misconduct
- Implementing activities and programs to teach responsible conduct of research, promote research integrity, prevent research misconduct, and improve the handling of allegations of research misconduct
- Conducting policy analyses, evaluations, and research to build the knowledge base in research misconduct, research integrity, and prevention and to improve the DHHS research integrity policies and procedures
- Administering programs for
  - Maintaining institutional assurances
  - Responding to allegations of retaliation against whistleblowers
  - Approving intramural and extramural policies and procedures
  - Responding to Freedom of Information Act and Privacy Act requests

Summarized from Office of Research Integrity (ORI). (2020). *About ORI.* Retrieved from https://ori.hhs.gov/about-ori

Peer reviewers have a key role in determining the quality of a manuscript and whether it is publishable. They are considered experts in the field, and their role is to examine research for inconsistencies and inaccuracies. Editors must monitor the peer review process and must be cautious about publishing manuscripts that are at all questionable (ICMJE, 2018). Editors also must have procedures for responding to allegations of research misconduct. They must decide what actions to take if their journal contains an article that has proven to be fraudulent. Usually, fraudulent publications require retraction notations and are not to be cited by authors in future publications. However, Al-Ghareeb et al. (2018) found that the retracted articles in their review had been cited an average of seven times *after* being retracted.

The publication of fraudulent research is a growing concern in medicine and nursing (Ward-Smith, 2016). The shrinking pool of funds available for research and the greater emphasis on research publications for retention in academic settings could lead to a higher incidence of fraudulent publications. Dr. Yoshihiro Sato, a Japanese researcher in prevention of bone fractures, committed one of the biggest frauds in scientific history (Kupferschmidt, 2018). His studies came under scrutiny when one researcher found identical means of body mass indexes for patients in the treatment group and control groups of trials conducted in different populations. Researchers in the same area began to question how his team could recruit several hundreds of patients into studies in just a few months (Else, 2019). Sixty of Sato's papers have been retracted and his remaining publications are viewed with skepticism.

Each researcher is responsible for monitoring the integrity of his or her research protocols, results, and publications. In addition, nursing professionals and journal editors must foster a spirit of intellectual inquiry, mentor prospective scientists regarding the norms for good science, and stress quality, not quantity, in publications (Fierz et al., 2014).

ANIMALS AS RESEARCH SUBJECTS

The use of animals as research participants is a controversial issue of growing interest to nurse researchers. A small but increasing number of nurse scientists are conducting physiological studies that require the use of animals. Many scientists have expressed concerns that the animal welfare movement could threaten the future

of health research. For example, a laboratory in Maryland was closed on April 2, 2019, after studying *Toxoplasma gondii* for 37 years. *T. gondii* is a foodborne illness that can lead to death. Although not publicly linked, scientists believe the closure was due to animal welfare activists' protests against the facility (Wadman, 2019). In 2015, the NIH stopped funding studies in which chimpanzees were to be used. NIH has also been advised by lawmakers to continue the reduction in funding for nonhuman primate research by incorporating budget changes in the 2020 US budget (Hou, 2019). Alternative models of investigation have been and continue to be developed, but for now animal research still plays a valuable role in preclinical studies. Studies of new medications and other treatments are based on the findings of preclinical studies done with animals.

The use of animals in research is a complicated issue that requires careful scientific and ethical consideration by investigators. From the scientific perspective, Smith, Clutton, Lilley, Hansen, and Brattelid (2018) developed a guideline for researchers that includes formulating the study, initiating dialogue with the animal facility, and ensuring quality control from the beginning of the experiment until its conclusion. Without attention to detail, the findings of laboratory animal experiments may not be reproducible.

Multiple sets of regulations protect animals in a research environment. Ceremuga et al. (2017) compared the effects of curcumin on anxiety and depression of rats to the effects of typically used medications for anxiety and depression. This team of nurse researchers implemented a study using rats and noted the regulations they used in protecting the animals.

"Fifty-five male Sprague-Dawley rats (Harlan Sprague Dawley Laboratories), each of which weighed between 242 and 298 g, were obtained in 1 shipment.... The animals went through a 14-day adaptation period in a temperature-controlled environment.... The rats were allowed food and water ad libitum. The animals were handled only for the purposes of drug administration, cage cleaning, and obtaining daily weights. All protocols used in this study were performed in accordance with the National Institute of Health Guide for the Care and Use of Laboratory Animals and were approved by the Institutional Animal Care and Use Committee at the US Army Institute of Surgical Research, San Antonio, Texas." (Ceremuga et al., 2017, p. 195)

Ceremuga et al. (2017) found that curcumin did not have a significant effect on the anxiety and depression of rats.

At least five separate sets of regulations exist to protect research animals from mistreatment. Federal government, state governments, independent accreditation organizations, professional societies, and individual institutions work to ensure that research animals are used only when necessary and only under humane conditions. At the federal level, animal research is conducted according to the guidelines of USPHS Policy on Humane Care and Use of Laboratory Animals, which was adopted in 1986 and most recently updated in 2015 (DHHS, 2015b). In addition, more than 1000 institutions in 49 countries have obtained accreditation by the Association for the Assessment and Accreditation of Laboratory Animal Care International (AAALAC International, 2019), which demonstrates the commitment of these institutions to ensure the humane treatment of animals in research. Nurse researchers interested in using animals for research must be trained in their care and appropriate use. They will also need to review the guidelines used by their university, other employers, or funders for conducting research with animals.

KEY POINTS

- The ethical conduct of research begins with the identification of the study topic and continues through the publication of the study to ensure that valid evidence is available for practice.
- Conducting research ethically requires protection of the human rights of participants. Human rights are claims and demands that have been justified in the eyes of an individual or by the consensus of a group of individuals. The human rights that require protection in research are (1) self-determination, (2) privacy, (3) anonymity or confidentiality, (4) fair treatment, and (5) protection from discomfort and harm.
- Two historical documents that have had a strong impact on the conduct of research are the Nuremberg Code and the Declaration of Helsinki.
- US federal regulations direct the ethical conduct of research. These regulations include (1) general requirements for informed consent, (2) documentation of informed consent, (3) IRB review of research, (4) exempt and expedited review procedures for certain kinds of research, and (5) criteria for IRB approval of research.
- HIPAA has affected research recruitment and data collection since it was implemented in 2003.
- The rights of research participants can be protected by balancing benefits and risks of a study, securing informed consent, and submitting the research for institutional review. The responsibility for protection of research participants is borne primarily by the lead or primary researcher.
- To balance the benefits and risks of a study, its type, level, and number of risks are examined, and its potential benefits are identified. If possible, risks must be minimized and benefits maximized to achieve the best possible benefit-risk ratio.
- The sequencing of the human genome has led to advances in how health and disease can be studied. These advances, however, have raised ethical issues about de-identification of genomic records, the reuse of biological specimens, and the appropriateness of using stem cells and organoids.
- Informed consent involves the transmission of essential information, the comprehension of the information, and voluntary consent of the prospective participant.
- In institutional review, a committee of peers (IRB) examines each study for ethical concerns. The IRB conducts three levels of review: exempt, expedited, and full board.
- Research misconduct includes fabrication, falsification, and plagiarism during the conduct, reporting, or publication of research. The ORI was developed to investigate and manage incidents of research misconduct to protect the integrity of research in all disciplines.
- Another current ethical concern is the use of animals as research subjects. The USPHS Policy on Humane Care and Use of Laboratory Animals provides direction along with several other guidelines and regulations on the humane use of animals in research.

REFERENCES

Adams, K., & Lawrence, E. (2019). *Research methods, statistics, and applications* (2nd ed.). Thousand Oaks, CA: Sage.

Advisory Committee on Human Radiation Experiments (ACHRE). (1995). Government standards for human experiments: The 1960s and 1970s. In ACHRE (Ed.), *Final report* (chap. 3). Retrieved from https://bioethicsarchive.georgetown.edu/achre/final/chap3.html

Ahalt, S., Chute, C., Fecho, K., Glusman, G., Hadlock, J., Taylor, C., et al. (2019). Clinical data: Sources and types, regulatory constraints, applications. *Clinical and Translational Science, 12*(4), 329–333. doi:10.1111/cts.12638

Algahtani, H., Bajunaid, M., & Shirah, B. (2018). Unethical human research in neuroscience: A historical review. *Neurological Science, 39*(5), 829–834. doi:10.1007/s10072-018-3245-1

Al-Ghareeb, A., Hillel, S., McKenna, L., Cleary, M., Visentin, D., Jones, M, et al. (2018). Retraction of publications in nursing and midwifery research: A systematic review. *International Journal of Nursing Studies, 81*(1), 8–13. doi:10.1016/j.ijnurstu.2018.01.013

American Nurses Association (ANA). (2015). *Code of ethics for nurses with interpretive statements.* Washington, DC: ANA.

Asman, O., Melnikov, S., Barnoy, S., & Tabak, N. (2019). Experiences, behaviors, and perceptions of registered nurses regarding research ethics and misconduct. *Nursing Ethics, 26*(3), 859–869. doi:10.1177/0969733017727152

Association for the Assessment and Accreditation of Laboratory Animal Care International (AAALAC). (2019). *The AAALAC International accreditation program.* Retrieved from https://www.aaalac.org/accreditation/

Bailey, J., & Ladores, S. (2018). Ethical issues when conducting research in people with cystic fibrosis. *Journal of Nursing Practice Applications & Reviews of Research, 8*(1), 48–52. doi:10.13178/jnparr.2018.0801.0807

Baker, S., Brawley, O., & Marks, L. (2005). Effects of untreated syphilis in the Negro male, 1932–1972: Closure comes to the Tuskegee study, 2004. *Urology, 65*(6), 1259–1262. doi:10.1016/j.urology.2004.10.023

Ballantyne, A., Pullon, S., Macdonald, L., Barthow, C., Wickens, K., & Crane, J. (2017). The experiences of pregnant women in an interventional clinical trial: Research In Pregnancy Ethics (RIPE) study. *Bioethics, 31*(1), 476–483. doi:10.1111/bioe.12361

Beecher, H. K. (1966). Ethics and clinical research. *New England Journal of Medicine, 274*(24), 1354–1360. doi:10.1056/NEJM196606162742405

Bledsoe, M., & Grizzle, W. (2013). Use of human specimens in research: The evolving United States regulatory, policy, and scientific landscape. *Diagnostic Histopathology, 19*(9), 322–330. doi:10.1016/j.mpdhp.2013.06.015

Bledsoe, M., Russell-Einhorn, M. & Grizzle, W. (2018). Shifting sands: The complexities and uncertainties of the evolving US regulatory, policy, and scientific landscape for biospecimen research. *Diagnostic Histopathology, 24*(4), 136–148. doi:10.1016/j.mpdhp.2017.09.004

Boileau, E., Patenaude, J., & St-Ong, C. (2018). Twelve tips to avoid ethical pitfalls when recruiting students as subjects in medical education research. *Medical Teacher, 40*(1), 20–25. doi:10.1080/0142159X.2017.1357805

Bonham, V. (2018). Legal issues in clinical research. In J. Gallin, F. Ognibene, L. Johnson (Eds.), *Principles and practice in clinical research* (4th ed., pp. 161–175). San Diego, CA: Imprint Press.

Brandt, A. M. (1978). Racism and research: The case of the Tuskegee Syphilis Study. *Hastings Center Report, 8*(6), 21–29.

Braun, V., & Clarke, V. (2006). Using thematic analysis in psychology. *Qualitative Research in Psychology, 3*(2), 77–101. doi:10.1191/1478088706qp063oa

Butler, A., Copnell, B., & Hall, H. (2019). Researching people who are bereaved: Managing risks to participants and researchers. *Nursing Ethics, 26*(1), 224–234. doi:10.1177/0969733017695656

Caplan, A., & Moreno, J. (2011). The Havasu 'Baaja tribe and informed consent. *The Lancet, 377*(9766), 621–622. doi:10.1016/S0140-6736(10)60818-5

Capron, A. (2018). Where did informed consent for research come from? *Journal of Law, Medicine, & Ethics, 46*(1), 12–29. doi:10.1177/1073110518766004

Centers for Medicare and Medicaid Services (CMS). (n.d.). *Data disclosures and data use agreements (DUAs).* Retrieved from https://www.cms.gov/Research-Statistics-Data-and-Systems/Files-for-Order/Data-Disclosures-Data-Agreements/Overview.html

Ceremuga, T., Helmrick, K., Kufahl, Z., Kelley, J, Keller, B., Philippe, F, et al. (2017). Investigation of the anxiolytic and antidepressant effects of curcumin, a compound from turmeric (curcuma longa), in the adult male Sprague-Dawley rat. *Holistic Nursing Practice, 31*(3), 193–203. doi:10.1097/HNP.0000000000000208

Cherry, M. (2017). Adolescents lack sufficient maturity to consent to medical research. *The Journal of Law, Medicine & Ethics, 45*(3), 307–317. doi:10.1177/1073110517737528

Chester, H., Clarkson, P., Davies, L., Hughes, J., & Islam, M. (2018). Cognitive aids for people with early stage dementia versus treatment as usual (Dementia Early Stage Cognitive Aids New Trial (DESCANT)): Study protocol for a randomised controlled trial. *Trials, 19,* 546. doi:10.1186/s13063-018-2933-8

Christofides, E., Stroud, K., Tullis, E. D., & O'Doherty, K. (2017). The meaning of helping: An analysis of cystic fibrosis patients' reasons for participating in biomedical research. *Journal of Empirical Research on Human Research Ethics, 12*(3), 180–190. doi:10.1177/1556264617713098

Chwang, E. (2015). Against harmful research on non-agreeing children. *Bioethics, 29*(6), 431–439. doi:10.1111/bioe.12117

Clayton, J., & Blome, J. (2018). National Institutes of Health Policy on the inclusion of women and minorities as subjects in clinical research. In J. Gallin, F. Ognibene, & L. Johnson (Eds.), *Principles and practice in clinical research* (4th ed., pp. 177–188). San Diego, CA: Imprint Press. doi:10.1016/B978-0-12-849905-4.00013-7

Coleman, C. (2017). Health related quality of life and depressive symptoms among seropositive African Americans. *Applied Nursing Research, 33*(1), 138–141. doi:10.1016/j.apnr.2016.11.007

Crane, S., & Broome, M. (2017). Understanding ethical issues of research participation from the perspective of participating children and adolescents: A systematic review. *Worldviews on Evidence-Based Nursing, 14*(3), 200–209. doi:10.1111/wvn.12209

Creswell, J., & Creswell, D. (2018). *Research design: Qualitative, Quantitative, and mixed methods approaches* (5th ed.). Thousand Oaks, CA: Sage.

Creswell, J., & Poth, C. (2018). *Qualitative inquiry & research design: Choosing among five approaches* (4th ed.). Thousand Oaks, CA: Sage.

Cypress. B. (2019). Qualitative research: Challenges and dilemmas. *Dimensions of Critical Care Nursing. 38*(5), 264–270. doi:10.1097/DCC.0000000000000374

Department of Health and Human Services (DHHS). (1979). *The Belmont report.* Retrieved from https://www.hhs.gov/ohrp/sites/default/files/the-belmont-report-508c_FINAL.pdf

Department of Health and Human Services (DHHS). (1981). *Final regulations amending basic HHS policy for the protection of human research subjects.* Code of Federal Regulations, Title 45, Part 46. Retrieved from https://www.hhs.gov/ohrp/regulations-and-policy/regulations/common-rule/index.html

Department of Health and Human Services (DHHS). (2003). *Health information privacy: Summary of the HIPAA Privacy Rule.* Retrieved from https://www.hhs.gov/hipaa/for-professionals/privacy/index.html

Department of Health and Human Services (DHHS). (2009). *National Institutes of Health guidelines for human stem cell research.* Retrieved from https://stemcells.nih.gov/policy/2009-guidelines.htm

Department of Health and Human Services (DHHS). (2013). *Definitions. Common rule.* Code of Federal Regulations, Title 45, Sections 160.103. Retrieved from https://www.govinfo.gov/content/pkg/CFR-2013-title45-vol1/pdf/CFR-2013-title45-vol1-sec160-103.pdf

Department of Health and Human Services (DHHS). (2015a). *Guidance regarding methods for de-identification of protected health information in accordance with the Health Insurance Portability and Accountability Act (HIPAA) privacy rule.* Retrieved from https://www.hhs.gov/hipaa/for-professionals/privacy/special-topics/de-identification/index.html#safeharborguidance

Department of Health and Human Services (DHHS). (2015b). *Public Health Service policy on humane care and treatment of laboratory animals.* Retrieved from https://olaw.nih.gov/sites/default/files/PHSPolicyLabAnimals.pdf

Department of Health and Human Services (DHHS). (2016). *Office for Human Research Protections (OHRP).* Retrieved from https://www.hhs.gov/ohrp/about-ohrp/index.html

Department of Health and Human Services (DHHS). (2017). *HIPAA privacy rule information for researchers: Overview.* Retrieved from https://www.hhs.gov/hipaa/for-professionals/special-topics/research/index.html

Department of Health and Human Services (DHHS). (2018). *Protection of human subjects.* Code of Federal Regulations, Title 45, Part 46. Retrieved from https://www.hhs.gov/ohrp/regulations-and-policy/regulations/45-cfr-46/index.html

Department of Health and Human Services (DHHS) & Office for Civil Rights. (2013). *HIPAA administrative simplification.* Retrieved from https://www.hhs.gov/sites/default/files/hipaa-simplification-201303.pdf

Duncan, I., Ahmed, T., Dove, H., & Maxwell, T. (2019). Medicare cost at end of life. *American Journal of Hospice & Palliative Medicine, 36*(8), 705–710. doi:10.1177/1049909119836204

Else, H. (2019). What universities can learn from epic case of research fraud. *Nature, 570,* 287–288. Retrieved from https://www.nature.com/articles/d41586-019-01884-2

Elzakkers, I., Danner, U., Grisso, T., Hoek, H., & van Elburg, A. (2018). Assessment of mental capacity to consent to treatment in anorexia nervosa: A comparison of clinical judgment and MacCAT-T and consequences for clinical practice. *International Journal of Law and Psychiatry, 58*(1), 27–35. doi:10.1016/j.ijlp.2018.02.001

Fierz, K., Gennaro, S., Dierickx, K., Van Achterbert, T., Morin, K., & De Geest, S. (2014). Scientific misconduct: Also an issue in nursing science? *Journal of Nursing Scholarship, 46*(4), 271–280. doi:10.1111/jnu.12082

Food and Drug Administration (FDA). (2019a). *Institutional review boards.* Code of Federal Regulations, Title 21 Food and Drugs, Department of Health and Human Services, Part 50. Retrieved from https://www.ecfr.gov/cgi-bin/text-idx?SID=8aba8bfe3f42ce78c66cf0bfd1ff22de&mc=true&node=pt21.1.56&rgn=div5

Food and Drug Administration (FDA). (2019b). *Protection of human subjects*. Code of Federal Regulations, Title 21 Food and Drugs, Department of Health and Human Services, Part 50. Retrieved from https://www.accessdata.fda.gov/scripts/cdrh/cfdocs/cfcfr/CFRsearch.cfm?CFRPart=50

Forster, D. & Borasky, D. (2018). Adults lacking capacity to give consent: When is it acceptable to include them in research. *Therapeutic Innovation & Regulatory Science, 52*(3), 275–259. doi:10.1177/2168479018770658

Foth, T. (2013). Understanding 'caring' through biopolitics: The case of nurses under the Nazi regime. *Nursing Philosophy, 14*(4), 284–294. doi:10.1111/nup.12013

Fowler, M. (2017). Faith and ethics, covenant and code. *Journal of Christian Nursing, 34*(4), 216–224. doi:10.1097/CNJ.0000000000000419

Gehlert, S., & Mozersky, J. (2018). Seeing beyond the margins: Challenges to informed inclusion of vulnerable populations in research. *Journal of Law, Medicine, & Ethics, 36*(1), 30–43. doi:10.1177/1073110518766006

Gelinas, L., Crawford, B., Kelman, A., & Bierer, B. (2019). Relocation of study participants for rare and ultra-rare disease trials: Ethics and operations. *Contemporary Clinical Trials, 84*. doi:10.1016/j.cct.2019.105812

Goldstein, C., Weijer, C., Taljaard, M., Al-Jaisha, A., Basile, E., & Garg, A. (2019). Ethical issues in pragmatic cluster-randomized trials in dialysis facilities. *American Journal of Kidney Disease. 74*(5), 659–666. doi:10.1053/j.ajkd.2019.04.019

Grady, C. (2018). Ethical principles in ethical research. In J. Gallin, F. Ognibene, & L. Johnson (Eds.). *Principles and practice in clinical research* (4th ed., pp. 19–31). San Diego, CA: Imprint Press. doi:10.1016/B978-0-12-849905-4.00002-2

Grady, C., Wiener, L., Abdoler, E., Trauernicht, E., Zadeh, S., Diekema, D., et al. (2014). Assent in research: The voices of adolescents. *Journal of Adolescent Health, 54*(5), 515–520. doi:10.1016/j.jadohealth.2014.02.005

Gravetter, F., & Forzano, L-A. (2018). *Research methods for the behavioral sciences* (6th ed.). Boston, MA: Cengage.

Grootens-Wiegers, P., de Vries, M., van Beusekom, M., van Dijck, L., & van den Broek, J. (2015). Comic strips help children understand medical research: Targeting the informed consent procedure to children's needs. *Patient Education and Counseling, 98*(4), 518–524. doi:10.1016/j.pec.2014.12.005

Hammer, M. (2019). Beyond the helix: Ethical, legal, and social implications in genomics. *Seminars in Oncology Nursing, 35*(1), 93–106. doi:10.1016/j.soncn.2018.12.007

Hein, I., Troost, P., Lindeboom, R., Benninga, M., & Zwaan. C. (2015). Key factors in children's competence to consent to clinical research. *BMC Medical Ethics, 16,* Article 74. doi:10.1186/s12910-015-0066-0

Hershey, N., & Miller, R. (1976). *Human experimentation and the law.* Georgetown, MD: Aspen.

HIPAA Journal. (2018). What is protected health information under HIPAA? Retrieved from https://www.hipaajournal.com/what-is-considered-protected-health-information-under-hipaa.

Ho, P., Downs, J., Bulsara, C., Patman, S., & Hill, A. (2018). Addressing challenges in gaining informed consent for a research study investigating falls in people with intellectual disability. *British Journal of Learning Disabilities, 46*(2), 92–100. doi:10.1111/bld.12217

Hostiuc, S., Rusu, M., Negoi, I., Perlea, P., Dorobantu, B., & Drima, E. (2019). The moral status of cerebral organoids. *Regenerative Medicine, 10*(1), 118–122. doi:10.1016/j.reth.2019.02.003

Hou, C.Y. (2019). Lawmakers push NIH to reduce nonhuman primate research. *The Scientist.* Retrieved from https://www.the-scientist.com/news-opinion/lawmakers-push-nih-to-reduce-nonhuman-primate-research-65861

Hunter, R., Gough, A., O'Kane, N., McKeown, G., Fitzpatrick, A., & Kee, F. (2018). Ethical issues in social media research in public health. *American Journal of Public Health, 108*(3), 343–348. doi:10.2105/AJPH.2017.304249

International Council of Medical Journal Editors (ICMJE). (2018). *Recommendations for the conduct, reporting, editing, and publication of scholarly work in medical journals.* Retrieved from http://www.icmje.org/icmje-recommendations.pdf

International Society for Stem Cell Research. (2016). *Guidelines for stem cell research and clinical translation.* Retrieved from http://www.isscr.org/docs/default-source/all-isscr-guidelines/guidelines-2016/isscr-guidelines-for-stem-cell-research-and-clinical-translationd67119731dff6ddbb37cff0000940c19.pdf?sfvrsn=4

Irani, E., & Richmond, T. (2015). Reasons for and reservations about research participation in acutely injured adults. *Journal of Nursing Scholarship, 47*(2), 161–169. doi:10.1111/jnu.12120

Jacobs, S. (2008). Revisiting hateful science: The Nazi "contribution" to the journey of antisemitism. *Journal of Hate Studies, 7*(1), 47–75.

Johnston, J., & Zacharias, R. (2019). US stem cell research policy. In A. Atala, R. Lanza, T. Minkos, & R. Nerem (Eds.), *Principles of regenerative medicine* (3rd ed., pp. 1309–1329). San Diego, CA: Academic Press.

Jones, H. (1997). Record of the first physician to see Henrietta Lacks at the Johns Hopkins Hospital: History of the HeLa cell line. *American Journal of Obstetrics and Gynecology, 176*(6), S227–S228. doi:10.1016/s0002-9378(97)70379-x

Kaye, D. Chongwe, G., & Sewankambo, N. (2019). Ethical tensions in the informed consent process for randomized clinical trials in emergency obstetric and newborn care in low and middle-income countries. *BMC Medical Ethics, 20,* 27. doi:10.1186/s12910-019-0363-0

Kazdin, A. (2017). *Research design in clinical psychology* (5th ed.). Boston, MA: Pearson.

Kelechi, T., Mueller, M., Madisetti, M., Prentice, M. & Dooley, M. (2018). Effectiveness of cooling therapy (cryotherapy) on leg pain and self-efficacy in patients with chronic venous disease: A randomized controlled trial. *International Journal of Nursing Studies, 86*(1), 1–10. doi:10.1016/j.ijnurstu.2018.04.015

Kotz, D., Viechtbauer, W., Spigt, M., & Crutzen, R. (2019). Details about informed consent procedures of randomized controlled trials should be reported transparently. *Journal of Clinical Epidemiology, 109*(1), 133–135. doi:10.1016/j.jclinepi.2019.01.007

Kovach, C. (2018). Editorial: Maintaining trust in science. *Research in Gerontological Nursing, 11*(4), 171–173. doi:10.3928/19404921-20180628-02

Kupferschmidt, K. (2018). Researcher at the center of an epic fraud remains an enigma to those who exposed him. *Science*. Retrieved from https://www.sciencemag.org/news/2018/08/researcher-center-epic-fraud-remains-enigma-those-who-exposed-him. doi:10.1126/science.aav1079

Lach, H. (2019). Research integrity: "Doing the right thing, even when no one is watching." *Clinical Nursing Research, 28*(6), 655–657. doi:10.1177/10547738198572

Lavazza, A., & Massimini, M. (2018). Cerebral organoids: Ethical issues and consciousness assessment. *Journal of Medical Ethics, 44*(9), 606–610. doi:10.1136/medethics-2018-104976

Leavy, P. (2017). *Research design: Quantitative, qualitative, mixed methods, arts-based, and community-based participatory research approaches.* New York, NY: Guilford Press.

Levine, R. (1986). *Ethics and regulations of clinical research* (2nd ed.). Baltimore, MD: Urban & Schwarzenberg.

Lindsley, K. (2019). Improving quality of the informed consent process: Developing an easy-to-read, multimodal, patient-centered format in a real-world setting. *Patient Education and Counseling, 102,* 944–951. doi:10.1016/j.pec.2018.12.022

Lippe, M., Johnson, B., & Carter, P. (2019). Protecting student anonymity in research using a subject-generated identification code. *Journal of Professional Nursing, 35*(2), 120–123. doi:10.1016/j.profnurs.2018.09.006

Maher, N., Senders, J., Hulsbergen, A., Lamba, N., Parker, M., & Broekman, M. (2019). Passive data collection and use in healthcare: A systematic review of ethical issues. *International Journal of Medical Ethics, 129*(1), 242–247. doi:10.1016/j.ijmedinf.2019.06.015

Martien, N., & Nelligan, J. (2018). Organizations with oversight responsibility in clinical research. In N. Marien, & J. Nelligan (Eds.), *The sourcebook for clinical research* (pp. 141–152). Cambridge, MA: Academic Press.

McConville, P. (2017). Presuming patient autonomy in the face of therapeutic misconception. *Bioethics, 31*(9). 711–715. doi:10.1111/bioe.12384

McEwen, J., Boyer, J., & Sun, K. (2013). Evolving approaches to the ethical management of genomic data. *Trends in Genetics, 29*(6), 375–382. doi:10.1016/j.tig.2013.02.001

Midwest Nursing Research Society (MNRS). (2018). *Guidelines for scientific integrity: A handbook for research* (3rd ed.). Brentwood, TN: Author.

Milgram, S. (1963). Behavioral study of obedience. *Journal of Abnormal and Social Psychology, 67*(4), 371–378.

Moore, T., McArthur, M., & Noble-Carr, D. (2018). More a marathon than a hurdle: Towards children's informed consent in a study on safety. *Qualitative Research, 18*(1), 88–107. doi:0.1177/1468794117700708

Morse, J., & Coulehan, J. (2015). Maintaining confidentiality in qualitative publications. *Qualitative Health Research, 25*(2), 151–152. doi:10.1177/1049732314563489

National Academies of Science. (2005). *Guidelines for human embryonic stem cell research.* Washington, DC: National Academies Press. Retrieved from https://www.nap.edu/download/11278

National Commission for the Protection of Human Subjects of Biomedical and Behavioral Research. (1978). *Belmont Report: Ethical principles and guidelines for research involving human subjects* (DHEW Publication No. [05] 78–0012). Washington, DC: US Government Printing Office.

Nelson-Marten, P., & Rich, B. (1999). A historical perspective on informed consent in clinical practice and research. *Seminars in Oncology Nursing, 13*(2), 81–88. doi:10.1016/S0749-2081(99)80065-5

Nuremberg Code. (1949). *Trials of war criminals before the Nuremberg military tribunals under Control Council Law No. 10* (vol. 2, pp. 181–182). Washington, DC: US Government Printing Office. Retrieved from https://history.nih.gov/research/downloads/nuremberg.pdf

Office for Civil Rights & Department of Health and Human Services (DHHS). (2015). *Guidance regarding methods for de-identification of protected health information in accordance with the Health Insurance Portability and Accountability Act (HIPAA) Privacy Rule.* Retrieved from https://www.hhs.gov/hipaa/for-professionals/privacy/special-topics/de-identification/index.html#standard

Office of Research Integrity (ORI). (n.d.). *Historical background.* Retrieved from https://ori.hhs.gov/historical-background

Office of Research Integrity (ORI). (2017). *Checklist: Policies and procedures for handling research misconduct allegations.*

Retrieved from https://ori.hhs.gov/sites/default/files/Policy_Review_Checklist.pdf

Office of Research Integrity (ORI). (2018). *Case summaries—Case summary: Baughman, Brandi.* Retrieved from https://ori.hhs.gov/case-summary-baughman-brandi-m

Office of Research Integrity (ORI). (2019a). *Case summaries—Case summary: Agrawal, Rahul.* Retrieved from https://ori.hhs.gov/content/case-summary-agrawal-rahul

Office of Research Integrity (ORI). (2019b). *Final HHS action with settlement or finding of research misconduct.* Retrieved from https://ecfr.io/Title-42/se42.1.93_1411

Office of Research Integrity (ORI). (2019c). *Part 93: Public Health Service policies on researcher misconduct.* Retrieved from https://www.ecfr.gov/cgi-bin/text-idx?SID=d011527cb366725356718900d2f2a88d&mc=true&node=pt42.1.93&rgn=div5

Office of Research Integrity (ORI). (2020). *About ORI.* Retrieved from https://ori.hhs.gov/index.php/about-ori

Office of Research on Women's Health. (2017). *Report of the Advisory Committee on Research on Women s Health, fiscal years 2015-2016: Office of Research on Women's Health and NIH support for research on women's health* (NIH Publication No. 17OD7995). Bethesda, MD: National Institutes of Health.

Oulton, K., Gibson, F., Sell, D., Williams, A., Pratt, L., & Wray, J. (2016). Assent for children's participation in research: Why it matters and making it meaningful. *Child: Care, Health and Development, 42*(4), 588–597. doi:10.1111/cch.12344

Palmer, B., Dunn, L., Appelbaum, P., Mudaliar, S., Thal, L., Henry, R., et al. (2005). Assessment of capacity to consent to research among older persons with schizophrenia, Alzheimer disease, or diabetes mellitus: Comparison of a 3-item questionnaire with a comprehensive standardized capacity instrument. *Archives of General Psychiatry, 62*(7), 726–733. doi:10.1001/archpsyc.62.7.726

Pereira, S., & Hernández-Marrero, P. (2019). Editorial: Research ethics in palliative care: A hallmark of palliative medicine. *Palliative Medicine.* doi:10.1177/0269216319827178

Perrin, M., Kim, T., Stan, R., Giesie, P., Tabor, J., LeVerche, V., et al. (2018). Role of nursing competencies for accelerating clinical trials in stem cell clinics. *Stem Cells Translational Medicine, 7*(1), 6–10. doi:10.1002/sctm.17-0165

Prentice, D. (2019). Adult stem cells: Successful standard for regenerative medicine. *Circulation Research, 124*(6), 837–839. doi:10.1161/CIRCRESAHA.118.313664

Presidential Commission for the Study of Bioethical Issues. (2011). *"Ethically impossible:" STD research in Guatemala 1946-1948.* Retrieved from https://bioethicsarchive.georgetown.edu/pcsbi/node/5896.html

Privacy Act of 1974, 5 U.S.C. § 552a. The National Archives. Retrieved from https://www.archives.gov/about/laws/privacy-act-1974.html

Quinn, P., & Quinn, L. (2018). Big genetic data and its big data protection challenges. *Computer Law & Security Review, 34*(5), 1000–1018. doi:10.1016/j.clsr.2018.05.028

Ravi, D., Christopher, P., Filene, E., Reifeis, S., & White, B. (2018). Financial payments for participating in research while incarcerated: Attitudes of prisoners. *IRB: Ethics and Human Research, 40*(6), 1–6. doi:10.1002/eahr.406001

Reverby, S. (2012). Ethical failures and history lessons: The US Public Health Service research studies in Tuskegee and Guatemala. *Public Health Reviews, 34,* 1–18. doi:10.1007/BF03391665

Reynolds, P. D. (1979). *Ethical dilemmas and social science research.* San Francisco, CA: Jossey-Bass.

Rivers, E., Schuman, S., Simpson, L., & Olansky, S. (1953). Twenty years of followup experience in a long-range medical study. *Public Health Reports, 68*(4), 391–395.

Rothman, D. J. (1982). Were Tuskegee and Willowbrook "studies in nature"? *Hastings Center Report, 12*(2), 5–7.

Sade, R. (2017). Introduction: Controversies in clinical research ethics. *The Journal of Law, Medicine & Ethics, 45*(3), 291–294. doi:10.1177/1073110517737525

Sancar, F. (2018). For difficult-to-model brain diseases, brain organoids come to the rescue. *Journal of the American Medical Journal, 320*(19), 1966–1968. doi:10.1001/jama.2018.15972

Santos, J., Palumbo, F., Molsen-David, E., Willke, R., Binder, L., Drummond, M., et al. (2017). ISPOR code of ethics 2017 (4th ed.). *Value in Health, 20*(10), 1227–1242. doi:10.1016/j.jval.2017.10.018

Schnipper, L. (2017). Central IRB review is an essential requirement for cancer clinical trials. *Journal of Law, Medicine, & Ethics, 45*(3), 341–347. doi:10.1177/1073110517737532

Shamoo, A., & Resnik, R. (2015). *Responsible conduct of research* (3rd ed.). New York, NY: Oxford University Press.

Simpson, C. (2010). Decision-making capacity and informed consent to participate in research by cognitively impaired individuals. *Applied Nursing Research, 23*(4), 221–226. doi:10.1016/j.apnr.2008.09.002

Singh, J., Siddiqi, M., Parameshwar, P., & Chandra-Mouli, V. (2019). World Health Organization guidance on ethical considerations in planning and reviewing research studies on sexual and reproductive health in adolescents. *Journal of Adolescent Health, 64*(4), 427–429. doi:10.1016/j.jadohealth.2019.01.008

Skloot, R. (2010). *The immortal life of Henrietta Lacks.* New York, NY: Crown Publishing.

Smith, A., Clutton, R., Lilley, E., Hansen, K., & Brattelid, T. (2018). PREPARE: Guidelines for planning animal research and testing. *Laboratory Animals, 52*(2), 135–141. doi:10.1177/0023677217724823

Steinfels, P., & Levine, C. (1976). Biomedical ethics and the shadow of Naziism. *Hastings Center Report, 6*(4), 1–20.

Tamariz, L., Gajardo, M., Still, C., Gren, L., Clark, E., Walsh, S., et al. (2019). The impact of central IRB's on informed consent readability and trial adherence in SPRINT. *Contemporary Clinical Trials Communications, 15*(1). doi:10.1016/j.conctc.2019.100407

Terry, N. (2015). Developments in genetic and epigenetic data protection in behavioral and mental health spaces. *Behavioral Sciences & Law, 33*(5), 653–661.

Thakur, S., & Lahiry, S. (2019). Research ethics in the modern era. *Indian Journal of Dermatology, Venereology, and Leprology, 85*(4), 351–354. doi:10.4103/ijdvl.IJDVL_499_18

Turcotte-Tremblay, A-M., & McSween-Cadieux, E. (2018). A reflection on the challenge of protecting confidentiality of participants while disseminating research results locally. *BMC Medical Ethics, 19*(1), S45. doi:10.1186/s12910-018-0279-0

van der Graaf, R., van der Zande, I., den Ruijter, H., Oudijk, M., van Delden, J., Rengerink, K., et al. (2018). Fair inclusion of pregnant women in clinical trials: An integrated scientific and ethical approach. *Trials, 19*(1), 78. doi:10.1186/s13063-017-2402-9

Wadman, M. (2019). Closure of US *Toxoplasma* lab draws ire. *Science, 364*(6436), 109. doi:10.1126/science.364.6436.109

Waltz, C., Strickland, O., & Lenz, O. (2017). *Measurement in nursing and health research* (5th ed.). New York, NY: Springer Publishing.

Ward-Smith, P. (2016). Evidence-based nursing: When the evidence is fraudulent. *Urologic Nursing, 36*(2), 98–99. doi:10.7257/1053-816X.2016.36.2.98

Warren, H. (2016). Embryonic stem cell research: A policy analysis. *Journal of Plastic Surgical Nursing, 36*(4), 157–161. doi:10.1097/PSN.0000000000000156

Weissinger, G., & Ulrich, C. (2019). Informed consent and ethical reporting of research in clinical trials involving participants with psychotic disorders. *Contemporary Clinical Trials, 84*, 105795. doi:10.1016/j.cct.2019.06.009

Wickham, R. (2019). Secondary analysis research. *Journal of Advanced Practitioner in Oncology, 10*(4), 395–400. doi:10.6004/jadpro.2019.10.4.7

World Association of Medical Editors (WAME). (n.d.). *About WAME*. Retrieved from https://www.wame.org/about

World Health Organization (WHO). (2018). *Guidance on ethical considerations in planning and reviewing research studies on sexual and reproductive health in adolescents*. Geneva, Switzerland: Author.

World Medical Association. (2013). World Medical Association declaration of Helsinki: Ethical principles for medical research involving human subjects. *Journal of the American Medical Association, 310*(20), 2191–2194.

World Medical Association. (2018). *WMA declaration of Helsinki: Ethical principles for medical research involving human subjects*. Retrieved from https://www.wma.net/policies-post/wma-declaration-of-helsinki-ethical-principles-for-medical-research-involving-human-subjects/

World Medical Organization (WMO). (1996). Declaration of Helsinki. *British Journal of Medicine, 313*(7070), 1448–1449. Retrieved from http://www.cirp.org/library/ethics/helsinki/

Yeh, D., Chun, S., Terrones, L., & Huang, J. (2017). Using media to improve the informed consent process for youth undergoing pediatric endoscopy and their parents. *Endoscopy International Open, 5*(1), e41–e46. doi:10.1055/s-0042-121668

10

Quantitative Methodology: Noninterventional Designs and Methods

Jennifer R. Gray

http://evolve.elsevier.com/Gray/practice/

The structure of a study is called the research design. The study design addresses the following questions: How many groups will the study have? Will you collect data one, two, or more times? Do you plan to test an intervention?

Quantitative research may be interventional or noninterventional (Kazdin, 2017), as displayed in Fig. 10.1. Studies using interventional designs test the effect of an intentional action, called an intervention or treatment, on an outcome. An intervention may be an education program, a new medication, or a new procedure, as a few examples. Interventional research includes both experimental and quasi-experimental designs, which will be covered in Chapter 11. This chapter will focus on noninterventional designs, the designs that count and measure characteristics of the phenomenon of interest and the study variables as they exist naturally. As the name indicates, there are no interventions being tested in noninterventional studies. Noninterventional research in this text is divided into descriptive designs and correlational designs (see Fig. 10.1).

This chapter begins by describing concepts important to noninterventional research designs. You will also learn about design validity, the rules that make a noninterventional study a quality study. A set of questions are provided to help you plan and implement a noninterventional study. The chapter concludes by describing specific descriptive and correlational designs.

CONCEPTS IMPORTANT TO NONINTERVENTIONAL RESEARCH DESIGN

To identify a research design and understand the principles of design validity, a working knowledge of a few key concepts are needed. Before delving into other concepts, we will begin with the definitions of research design, methodology, and methods.

Research Design

You may not be aware that the term *research design* is used in two ways in the nursing literature. Some researchers consider research design to be the entire strategy for the study, from identification of the problem to final plans for data collection. Other researchers limit design to clearly defined structures within which the study is implemented. In this text, the first definition refers to the research methodology and the second is a definition of the research design.

A **research design** is the blueprint for conducting a study. It maximizes control over factors that could interfere with the validity of the study findings (Kazdin, 2017; Kerlinger & Lee, 2000). Being able to identify the study design and to evaluate design flaws that might threaten the validity of findings is essential for critically appraising studies. The control achieved through the quantitative study design increases the probability that your study findings are an accurate reflection of reality.

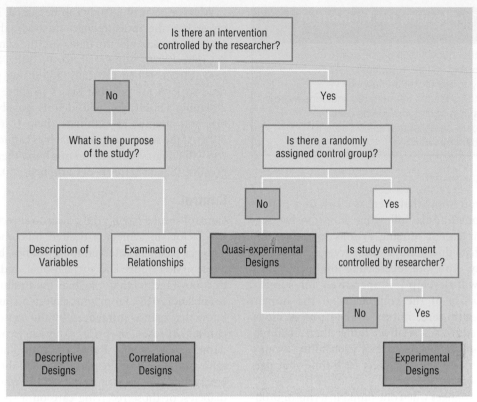

Fig. 10.1 Algorithm to identify a study's design.

A design is not specific to a particular study but rather is a broad pattern or guide that can be applied to many studies. Using the problem statement, framework, research questions, clearly defined variables, and design, you can develop a detailed research plan for collecting and analyzing data.

Research Methodology

Research methodology is the entire strategy of a study, from research problem to the interpretation of the findings. Based on the research problem and the literature, a researcher decides whether the methodology of a study should be quantitative, qualitative, outcomes, or mixed methods. For example, Ang, O'Brien, and Wilson (2019) conducted a study to describe the falls and fears of falling among persons caring for older adults living at home. Ang et al. (2019) used a qualitative methodology (see Chapter 4). Zhang, Li, Li, and Chen (2019) conducted a randomized controlled trial (RCT) of persons treated for cervical cancer who developed insomnia.

Zhang et al. (2019) used a quantitative methodology (see Chapter 3).

Methods

The **methods** are the specific ways in which the researcher chooses to conduct the study, within the chosen design. These are the details of the endeavor, the bare bones of inquiry, and begin by determining how the research site(s) will be selected and concludes with how the data are analyzed. Box 10.1 includes the questions that you need to answer during the planning of a study's methods. The methods of the Zhang et al. (2019) study included randomly assigning 70 participants to the intervention group and the nonintervention group (see Chapter 11). Zhang et al. (2019) implemented a mindfulness intervention and collected data through a sleep diary, self-report questionnaires, polysomnography, and wrist actigraphy. The methods of a study are reported in the Methods section of the proposal or research report.

> ### BOX 10.1   Planning the Methods of a Study
>
> - How will the study site(s) be selected?
> - Which subjects will be included?
> - How many subjects will be needed?
> - How will the subjects be recruited and consented?
> - What data collection tools will be used?
> - How will data be collected?
> - How will data be analyzed?

Probability

As a nurse, you know that there is a risk of a patient developing pneumonia following an extensive surgery. You implement nursing actions to reduce the likelihood that pneumonia will develop. Stated a different way, you are decreasing the probability pneumonia will develop postoperatively for surgical patients. Because of the complexity of the human body and health care, nurses deal in probabilities. **Probability** addresses relative, rather than absolute, causality. From the perspective of probability, a cause will not produce a specific effect each time that particular cause occurs.

Reasoning changes when one thinks in terms of probabilities. The researcher investigates the probability that an effect will occur under specific circumstances. Rather than seeking to prove that A causes B, a researcher would state that if A occurs, there is a 50% probability that B will occur. For example, Lee et al. (2017) conducted a retrospective, descriptive study to determine if the nurse workload/staffing ratio in two intensive care units (ICUs) influenced the probability of patients surviving to hospital discharge. The researchers found that high workload/staffing ratios decreased the probability that ICU patients would survive until hospital discharge.

Bias

The term **bias** means to slant away from the true or expected. A biased opinion has failed to include both sides of the question. A biased researcher may ask participants questions in a way to make the desired answer more likely (Adams & Lawrence, 2019). A biased scale is one that does not provide a valid measurement of a concept (Leedy & Ormrod, 2019). In contrast, using repeatable and transparent methods to synthesize evidence and conduct studies can reduce the risk of bias (Savitz, Wellenius, & Trikalonis, 2019).

Many aspects of a study can be biased, including the researcher, the measurement methods, the individual subjects, the sample, the data, and the statistics (Grove & Cipher, 2020; Stone et al., 2019; Waltz, Strickland, & Lenz, 2017). When critically appraising a study, you need to look for possible biases in these areas. When designing a study, you will identify possible sources of bias and attempt to eliminate them (Mokkink et al., 2018). If the sources of potential bias cannot be avoided, you will design your study to minimize them as much as possible (Shadish, Cook, & Campbell, 2002).

Control

Control means having the power to direct or manipulate factors to achieve a desired outcome. Control is a bigger factor in interventional studies, but also plays a role in descriptive and correlational studies. You want to control factors that may bias the findings (Gravetter & Forzano, 2018). From your experience as a nurse, you know that pain is influenced by the cause of the pain, chronic diseases, or prior experiences with pain, to name a few factors. Based on your knowledge, you may choose to limit the participants to those with non-emergency abdominal surgeries, those who do not have diabetes, or those receiving care on a specific hospital unit or at home. The more control the researcher has over the features of the study, the more credible the study findings. The purpose of research designs is to maximize control factors in the study (Kazdin, 2017; Shadish et al., 2002).

Measurement

Measurement refers to the process by which a number is assigned to a variable. The number indicates the value or quantity of the variable. The tools of measurement, such as questionnaires, online surveys, blood pressure equipment, and laboratory tests, must do their job well. When you as a researcher decide upon a certain measurement for a variable in your study, you want it to be appropriate for that variable's conceptual definition, and you want it to prove both accurate and consistent over time. These attributes of accuracy and consistency refer to that measurement's validity and reliability (Adams & Lawrence, 2019). In addition, precision is essential, so that you can ensure the values obtained are measured with specificity that is adequate for meaningful statistical analysis. Your choice of a measurement method and that method's validity, reliability, and precision all determine the quality of the raw data you so laboriously obtain during the data collection process (Waltz et al., 2017). For example, Zhang et al. (2019) measured several variables using self-report questionnaires and medical devices. They used a seven-item instrument, the Insomnia Severity Index, to quantify the severity of the participants' insomnia. (See Chapters 16 and 17 for further information on measurement.)

Prospective Versus Retrospective

Prospective is a term that means looking forward, whereas **retrospective** means looking backward. Within research, these terms are used primarily to refer to the timing of data collection. Are the measurements being obtained by the research team (prospective)? In contrast, is the study using data collected at a prior time for a different purpose (retrospective)?

In health care, large amounts of data are archived from health and administrative records. Researchers conducting noninterventional studies can use retrospective data, extracted from digital databases. This is especially true of outcomes research (Chapter 13), which examines various aspects of quality of care using predominantly correlational and descriptive designs to analyze preexisting data. Kim, Lyon, Weaver, Keenan, and Stechmiller (2019) conducted a retrospective study using the medical records of 454 patients who were hospitalized for at least 4 days and had a diagnosis of pressure ulcer. The purpose of their correlational design was to determine the influence of demographic variables on the relationships among pressure injuries, pain, and psychological distress. Using the patients' medical records, the researchers extracted variables, such the severity of the pressure ulcer, use of opioids for pain, pain scores, and medications given for depression or anxiety. Kim et al. (2019) concluded patients with pressure ulcers need comprehensive pain management that considered comorbidities, age, and psychological distress. Researchers using retrospective data must examine the raw data and clean it (see Chapter 21) before it is analyzed. The accuracy of retrospective data depends on the meticulousness of those who entered those data originally.

Many nurse researchers choose prospective designed studies so that they can control data collection, with a goal of fewer errors. As a researcher, you can collect the data yourself or encourage the data collectors through training and role-modeling to be rigorous in data collection. Alhurani et al. (2018) conducted a prospective longitudinal descriptive study of stress appraisal, coping, and event-free survival among 88 heart failure (HF) patients with subsequent data collection at 2 weeks, 3 months, and 6 months. Stress appraisal was defined as the way that a person evaluates a stimulus. The three types of appraisal were challenge, threat, or harm/loss. A person might appraise a stimulus to be a threat with the potential to be harmful, while another person might appraise the same stimulus to be a challenge. Each week during the study, trained research assistants searched the participant's medical records and clinic notes for cardiac hospitalizations or all-cause death. Alhurani et al. (2018) described the study variables and explored relationships among these variables. They found that persons who were tended to appraise stressors as harm/loss also had higher levels of stress. Greater use of harm/loss cognitive appraisal predicted shorter event-free survival.

DESIGN VALIDITY

Design validity is the truth or accuracy of the findings of a study. Was the study designed in a way that its findings can be trusted? Questions of validity refer back to the propositions from which the study was developed and address their approximate truth or falsity. Was the study designed in a way to appropriately test the propositions in the study framework? Was the study implemented consistently with sound scientific practices (Kazdin, 2017; Leedy & Ormrod, 2019; Melnyk & Fineout-Overholt, 2019)? Are the findings of the study an accurate reflection of reality?

Validity is a complex idea that is important to nurses reading the study report and considering whether to use the findings in their practice. A factor or condition that decreases the validity of research results is called a **threat to validity**. Critical appraisal of research requires that we think through threats to validity and make judgments about how seriously these threats affect the integrity of the findings. Validity provides a major basis for making decisions about which findings are sufficiently accurate to add to the evidence base for practice (Melnyk &Fineout-Overholt, 2019).

Four types of validity have been identified (Shadish et al., 2002): construct design validity, internal design validity, external design validity, and statistical conclusion design validity. The following sections will define each type and describe threats of validity that occur in noninterventional studies, beginning with construct design validity.

Construct Design Validity

Construct design validity examines the fit between the conceptual definitions and operational definitions of variables (Gravetter & Forzano, 2018). Theoretical constructs or concepts are defined within the study framework (conceptual definitions). These conceptual definitions provide the basis for the operational definitions of the variables. Operational definitions (methods of measurement) must validly reflect the theoretical constructs. Theoretical constructs are discussed in Chapter 8; conceptual and operational definitions of concepts and variables are discussed in Chapter 6.

By examining construct design validity, we can determine if the instrument actually measures the theoretical construct it is intended to measure. Producing evidence to support construct design validity takes years of scientific work by the instrument developers. When selecting the measurement method for a study variable, the researcher must consider the available evidence of construct design validity (Gravetter & Forzano, 2018; Waltz et al., 2017). The threats to construct design validity include inadequate preoperational clarification of constructs, mono-operation bias, and monomethod bias. Table 10.1 summarizes the threats to construct design validity and ways to avoid or minimize these threats.

Inadequate Preoperational Clarification of Constructs

Measurement of a construct stems logically from a concept analysis of the construct, either by the theorist who developed the construct or by the researcher. The conceptual definition should emerge from the concept analysis, and the method of measurement (operational definition) should clearly reflect the conceptual definition (Adams & Lawrence, 2019). A deficiency in the conceptual or operational definition leads to low construct design validity (see Chapters 6 and 8).

Mono-operation Bias

Mono-operation bias occurs when only one method of measurement is used to assess a construct. When only one method of measurement is used, fewer dimensions of the construct are measured. Construct design validity greatly improves if the researcher uses more than one instrument (Waltz et al., 2017). For example, you want to measure physical activity of older adults for a study. You can measure the participants' responses to questions about physical activity on two questionnaires or scales. By using two instruments, you are measuring more dimensions of physical activity and improving the construct design validity of the measurement.

Monomethod Bias

In **monomethod bias**, the researcher uses more than one measure of a variable, but all the measures use the same method of recording participants' responses. Attitude measures, for example, may all be paper and pencil scales, a method that may not capture nuances of the attitude being measured. Participants may omit items about personal, private, or socially unacceptable attitudes. Returning to the study in which you plan to measure physical activity, you could add physiological measures, such as pedometers or actimetry sensors, to increase the construct design validity of the variable. You could also add tests of physical strength and stamina in an exercise laboratory. By using multiple types of measurement, you can avoid monomethod bias.

TABLE 10.1 **Threats to Construct Design Validity for Noninterventional Studies**	
Threat	**How to Avoid or Minimize the Threat**
Inadequate preoperational clarification of constructs	Conduct a concept analysis of primary constructs if not previously done. Compare potential instruments with defining attributes of the construct. Use instruments in a pilot study with participants who meet the study's inclusion/exclusion sampling criteria to ensure meaning is clear for the specific sample.
Mono-operational bias	For research variables, quantify using more than one measurement method.
Monomethod bias	For research variables, use multiple types of measures (not all pencil-paper).
Careless responding	Assess using direct, archival, or statistical methods. Exclude cases that indicate careless responding.

Social Desirability Reponses

Social desirability occurs because human beings want others to think positively about them (Waltz et al., 2017). Construct design validity can be threatened when measuring qualities that are typically viewed as being positive or as being negative. Nurses participating in a study of weekly health behaviors might overestimate the minutes of aerobic exercise and time spent in meditation and underestimate the number of alcoholic beverages consumed and cigarettes smoked. Self-report measures are more likely to be affected by social desirability (Adams & Lawrence, 2019; Esopo et al., 2018). Even when responses are anonymous and confidential, participants may unconsciously select responses that are viewed more positively.

When sensitive or stigmatized topics are being studied, researchers may choose to measure social desirability as part of the study. Kellogg, Knight, Dowling, and Crawford (2018) conducted a predictive correlational study of secondary traumatic stress in a sample of 338 pediatric nurses. Because stigma has been associated with work-related stress and coping processes, Kellogg et al. (2018) chose to include the short version of the Marlowe-Crowne Social Desirability Scale (Crowne & Marlowe, 1960) in their study's measures. The higher the score, the more likely a participant will be to answer other instruments in a socially appropriate manner. Among pediatric nurses, social desirability was negatively correlated with secondary traumatic stress, indicating that secondary traumatic stress may be higher than reported (Kellogg et al., 2018).

Careless Responding

Careless responding occurs when participants lack the motivation to read questions on an instrument closely and mark an answer after thinking about the question (Grau, Ebbeler, & Banse, 2019). Participants may not feel accountable for their answers and may answer randomly. Some participants will select the middle response or one of the extremes on the response set for all the items on the scale. When a scale uses a Likert response set with 1 being "strongly disagree" and 5 being "strongly agree," a participant may select all 1s, 3s, or 5s.

Researchers may choose one of three methods to assess the degree of careless responding in a study: direct, archival, and statistical (Grau et al., 2019). Direct methods include asking a question about data quality, such as "I read every question carefully before I answer" or

"On a questionnaire, I may occasionally answer without reading the question." These transparent methods of assessing careless responding may have the undesired effect of participants believing the researchers do not trust them. This belief may further decrease the motivation to read closely and respond thoughtfully (Grau et al., 2019).

The archival method for assessing careless responding can be used when parallel items or reverse scored items are included on an instrument (Grau et al., 2019). When an instrument has a question with "I enjoy reading research articles" and another with "Research studies provide helpful strategies to address clinical problems," you would expect participants to answer the questions in a similar way. When an instrument has parallel items that are reverse scored, you would expect the participant's response on the second item to be opposite of the response to the first. For example, an instrument has the following items: "My pain is relieved by rest" and "My pain is relieved by moving." A participant who selected the same response of these two items may be responding carelessly (Grau et al., 2019).

Statistical assessment of careless responding can occur by identifying pairs of items with interitem correlations above $r > .60$ (Grau et al., 2019). These items can be used to assess participants' responses. In the archival method, you expected a participant to respond the same way to items that were semantically similar. Items strongly correlated to each other can be considered psychometrically similar and you would expect a participant to have similar responses to both. In contrast, interitem correlations of $r > -.60$ indicate items to which you would expect a participant to respond in opposite ways (Grau et al., 2019). A statistician may be aware of other analyses that can be conducted to assess for careless responding. Refer to Table 10.1 for ways to avoid or minimize the threats to construct design validity.

Internal Design Validity

Internal design validity is the extent to which the relationships or differences detected in the study are a true reflection of reality rather than the result of extraneous variables (Gravetter & Forzano, 2018). Internal design validity is an indicator of quality in all types of studies. Although internal design validity is considered more important when appraising interventional studies (Kazdin, 2017), it should also be evaluated in noninterventional studies. In a correlational study, which is a noninterventional study, you may find a statistically significant relationship between hope and problem-solving coping strategies among patients with obstructive pulmonary disease. However, you do not know whether an unmeasured variable influences the relationship. The unmeasured variable that influences a relationship between two other variables or that influences a difference between groups is an **extraneous variable** (Gravetter & Forzano, 2018). Possibly the patients who are in the early stages in the course of their disease have the energy to use problem solving, or patients with more financial resources have the means to find unique strategies to manage their disease. In these situations, the extraneous variables are the stage of disease and the household income, respectively. Chapters 6 and 8 describe the different types of extraneous variables. Threats to internal design validity for noninterventional studies are described in the following sections. In addition, Table 10.2 includes a list of these threats and strategies to avoid them or minimize their effects.

History

History results when an event that is not directly related to the planned study occurs during the time of the study and changes participants' responses on measurements (Adams & Lawrence, 2019). History can affect any study. For example, you have planned a study of adolescents' sense of safety and well-being at school. You collect the data as scheduled, but unbeknownst to you, a student at the school was found to have a weapon in his locker a couple of days earlier. The event has likely affected the adolescents' sense of safety and well-being.

History is also a potential threat for longitudinal descriptive and correlational studies, studies that are conducted over various lengths of time. In longitudinal designs, data are collected multiple times from the same sample. Stein, Lee, Corte, and Steffen (2019) conducted a 12-month longitudinal correlational study of identity, disordered eating, and weight control among Mexican American college women. The researchers collected data for each participant over a 12-month period, but it took over 5 years for the researchers to recruit a robust sample and complete the study. Although not identified by the researchers as a study limitation, history was a potential threat to internal design validity because changes in public attitudes about obesity or individual events may have affected the participants' behaviors during the year of data collection.

Maturation

In research, **maturation** is defined as internal changes that occur over time (Kazdin, 2017). Examples include growing older, wiser, stronger, hungrier, more tired, or more experienced during the study. Such unplanned and unrecognized changes are a threat to internal design validity and can influence the findings of the study. This threat to validity is more likely to affect longitudinal studies, studies during which each participant provides data multiple times at set intervals. Maturation is not considered a threat to validity when each participant provides data one time, as in a cross-sectional study.

Selection

Selection addresses the process by which subjects are chosen to take part in a study. A selection threat is more likely to occur with nonrandom sampling (Rose, 2019). People selected may be different in some important way from people not selected for the study (Stone et al., 2019). For example, a researcher conducted a study of the attitudes of nurses about spiritual care and collected data during a national conference for Christian nurses. The nurses who attended the conference were likely to have different attitudes about spiritual care than nurses who did not attend the conference.

Hyarat, Subih, Rayan, Salami, and Harb (2019) conducted a descriptive correlational study with 160 persons

TABLE 10.2 **Threats to Internal Design Validity for Noninterventional Studies**	
Threat	**How to Avoid or Minimize the Threat**
History	Avoid seasonal fluctuations or other events that may affect the study.
Maturation	Acknowledge as a potential threat, especially in longitudinal studies.
Selection	Randomly recruit participants if possible. Adjust inclusion and exclusion criteria to represent the target population. Consider effects of environment (social, cultural, type of healthcare setting) that may limit potential subjects.
Subject attrition	Implement strategies to retain subjects in longitudinal studies. Compare those who completed with those who dropped out to determine how the two groups were different.

living with multiple sclerosis (MS) in Jordan. The purpose of the study was to examine relationships between psychosocial adjustment and health-related quality of life (HRQoL) when controlling for the demographic variables. On the HRQoL scale, the participants scored lowest on sexual health. The researchers made these comments about the sample.

> "An important strength point of this study was collecting the data from different institutions, which might increase the possibility of generalization of the findings. In contrast, investigating a sensitive social issue like sexual relationships could provide inaccurate data because this topic has a cultural concern in the Arab world. Willingness to honestly disclose perceptions related to sensitive social issues like sexual relationships in the Arabic culture might represent a threat to internal validity." (Hyarat et al., 2019, p. 16)

The participants reported low HRQoL, which is not surprising considering the impact of MS on activities of daily living (Hyarat et al., 2019). Psychosocial adjustment significantly predicted HRQoL among patients with MS.

Subject Attrition

The **subject attrition** threat to design validity is due to subjects who drop out of a study before completion. Participants' attrition becomes a threat when those who drop out of a study are different types of people from those who remain in the study. Because data collection occurs a single time, subject attrition is not a threat for cross-sectional studies. Cross-sectional designs can be used to study changes over time by recruiting participants who are in different stages of these changes. Subject attrition can occur, however, in longitudinal noninterventional studies. A sample is recruiting at the beginning and then data collection occurs at set times during the study, such as at 1, 2, and 5 years. (Later in this chapter, there is a more thorough explanation of cross-sectional and longitudinal studies.) Returning to the longitudinal study conducted by Stein et al. (2019) with Mexican American college women, data were collected at baseline and at 3, 6, 9, and 12 months. The researchers collected baseline data from 472 women but collected data at 12 months from only 408 women, a 13.5% attrition rate. They did note that 460 women provided data at least two times (4% attrition). The researchers did not identify the attrition

rate as a limitation. Chapter 15 has additional information about attrition and retention rates. Table 10.2 describes each of the threats to internal design validity and provides strategies to minimize the threats.

External Design Validity

External design validity is concerned with the extent to which study findings can be generalized beyond the sample used in the study (Adams & Lawrence, 2019; Porritt, Gomersall, & Lockwood. 2014). When serious threats to external design validity occur, the findings would be meaningful only for the group being studied. To some extent, the significance of the study depends on the number of types of people and situations to which the findings can be applied. Sometimes the factors influencing external design validity are subtle and may not be reported in research reports; however, a nurse must consider these factors when deciding whether the findings are applicable to another setting. Generalization is usually narrower for a single study than for multiple replications of a study using different samples, perhaps from different populations in different settings. The primary threats to the ability to generalize the findings (external design validity) of noninterventional study design are homogeneity of the sample and the interaction of selection and setting (Table 10.3).

Homogeneity of the Sample

When researchers conduct noninterventional studies, they may choose to use narrow sample inclusion criteria to control for extraneous variables. By doing this, the study may have stronger internal design validity. However, the findings of a study may have less external design

TABLE 10.3 Threats to External Design Validity for Noninterventional Studies

Threat	How to Avoid or Minimize the Threat
Homogenous sample	Balance need to control extraneous variables (internal design validity) with the need for a heterogenous sample. Set inclusion and exclusion sampling criteria to be as inclusive as possible.
Interaction of setting and sample	Collect data in multiple sites, if possible, to recruit a more heterogenous sample.

validity (Adams & Lawrence, 2019). To enhance external design validity, the researchers will seek a heterogenous sample that more closely resembles the target population. Researchers often have to decide, for a given study, whether to focus on maximizing internal or external design validity.

Interaction of Setting and Selection

The interaction of the setting and sample selection can occur even when a heterogenous population is found in the setting. You develop a descriptive study of health-related resilience for a target population of patients receiving care at federally qualified health clinics. The clinic where you plan to collect data has a diverse population with patients who were native born and patients who have immigrated from Mexico, Brazil, and Rwanda. The estimated reading level of the clinic patients is grade 5. One of your inclusion criteria is to be able to read and write English. The external design validity of your study's findings will be threatened, because the sample will be literate English speakers, which may limit the study's generalizability. You could minimize this threat by providing the questionnaires and instruments in Spanish, Portuguese, and French and by reading the instruments aloud to the participants.

Shajrawi, Al-Smadi, Al-Shawabkah, Aljribeea, and Khalil (2019) conducted a descriptive comparative study of survivors of an acute myocardial infarction (AMI). They chose as the setting the cardiac clinics affiliated with the Jordan University Hospital (JUH) based on the belief that the sample would be "representative of the general Jordanian population" (Shajrawi et al., 2019, p. 286). Despite this premise, the researchers acknowledged study characteristics that affected external design validity in the following excerpt.

"However, this study also has many limitations, notably its small sample size, which makes it difficult to generalize the findings at a population level. ...In addition, the study sample was recruited from a convenient group of AMI patients admitted to the cardiac centre in Jordan, and more than 50% of screened AMI patients were ineligible. Also, about 30% of eligible AMI patients refused to participate. In addition, it has been implemented in 1 setting, JUH Cardiac Centre, which might also affect the generalisability of the study findings (although this central location is otherwise representative due to the high centralisation of advanced health services in Amman, the most populous city)." (Shajrawi et al., 2019, p. 291)

The study conducted by Shajrawi et al. (2019) compared the participants based on the medical treatment given for the AMI and is discussed in more detail later in this chapter.

Statistical Conclusion Design Validity

Statistical conclusion design validity is the degree to which the researcher makes proper decisions about the use of statistics, so that conclusions about relationships and differences drawn from analyses are accurate reflections of reality (Cook & Campbell, 1979; Shadish et al., 2002). Incorrect decisions produce inaccurate conclusions. To implement valid noninterventional studies, four threats to statistical conclusion design validity must be avoided: (1) low statistical power, (2) violating statistical assumptions, (3) error rate, and (4) unreliable measurements. Table 10.4 includes these threats to statistical conclusion design validity and ways to avoid them.

Low Statistical Power

Low statistical power increases the probability of concluding that there is no significant difference between samples when actually there is a difference, a Type II error. A Type II error is most likely to occur when the sample size is small or when the power of the statistical test to determine differences is low (Aberson, 2019). To avoid this threat, an **a priori power analysis** should be performed before the study is conducted to determine the required number of participants needed to identify relationships and group differences. When sample size is adequate, the significant relationships and/or differences that exist in a study will be revealed through statistical testing (see Chapter 15) (Grove & Cipher, 2020). Then if a statistical test fails to reject the null hypothesis, the researcher can be fairly certain that there was a weak relationship between variables or little difference between the groups studied. However, when nonsignificant statistical result is identified during a study, the researcher should perform a **post hoc power analysis** to determine the power of the statistical result (Grove & Cipher, 2020).

Online applications are available to estimate how large a sample is needed for a study, given the amount of difference between groups or magnitude of the relationship between variables that you expect to find. The group differences and magnitude of relationships can be identified from previous studies in your area of research. In addition, Aberson (2019) and Grove and

TABLE 10.4 **Threats to Statistical Conclusion Design Validity for Noninterventional Studies**

Threat	How to Avoid or Minimize the Threat
Low statistical power	Conduct a priori power analysis to determine the appropriate sample size prior to the conduct of a study. Conduct a post hoc power analysis to determine the power when a statistical result is nonsignificant (Grove & Cipher, 2020).
Violated assumptions of statistical tests	Recruit a random sample. Conduct exploratory analyses to determine the distribution of data for each variable. Use nonparametric analyses as needed (Pett, 2016).
Multiple analyses and error rate	Limit the statistical analysis to those needed to address the research questions or hypotheses (Grove & Cipher, 2020). Use multivariate analyses when appropriate. If multiple comparisons or tests are needed, use an adjusted, more stringent p value.
Unreliable measures	Select measures that have evidence of reliability in other studies. Test internal consistency reliability with your sample.

Cipher (2020) have published texts that provide information on power analysis and demonstrate how to perform power calculations, for use with different types of statistical techniques. If interactions among variables are subtle and small in magnitude, a larger sample is necessary. Statistical power is discussed in greater depth in Chapter 15.

Violated Assumptions of Statistical Tests

Most statistical tests have assumptions about the data collected, such as the following: (1) the data are at least at the interval level, (2) the sample was randomly obtained, and (3) the distribution of scores was normal. When you select the instruments to measure your variables, you determine whether the level of the data are interval or ratio data. In noninterventional studies, the participants are rarely randomly selected and the distribution of the scores may be skewed. If these assumptions are violated, the statistical analysis may provide inaccurate results (Grove & Cipher, 2020). One option is for you to use nonparametric tests that do not require normal distributions (Pett, 2016). The assumptions of statistical tests commonly conducted in nursing studies are provided in Chapters 23, 24, and 25.

Multiple Analyses and Error Rate

A serious concern in research is incorrectly concluding that a relationship or difference exists when it does not (Type I error, rejecting a true null hypothesis). The risk of Type I error increases when the researcher conducts multiple statistical analyses of relationships or differences (Kazdin, 2017). Conducting multiple analyses is

referred to as **fishing**, because a fisherman tries over and over to catch a fish. In a similar way, the researcher may keep analyzing the data to find some significant difference or relationship. When fishing is used during data analysis, a given portion of the analyses may show significant relationships or differences simply by chance (Suter & Suter, 2015). For example, the t-test is commonly used to make multiple statistical comparisons of mean differences in a single sample (Grove & Cipher, 2020). Making multiple comparisons increases the risk of a Type I error because you may identify significant differences when they occurred by chance. These differences are not actually present in the population. Fishing and error rate problems are discussed in Chapter 21.

Reliability of Measures

The technique of measuring variables must be reliable to reveal true differences or true relationships. A measurement method is a **reliable measure** if it gives the same result consistently (Gravetter & Forzano, 2018; Waltz et al., 2017). A measure may be a pencil-paper scale, an online survey or questionnaire, or an evaluation of an activity using a checklist. When the measure is used repeatedly in similar conditions to measure the same construct, the result is approximately the same. You would not expect the measurements to be exactly the same due to measurement error. For example, self-efficacy is a relatively stable construct that is not expected to change dramatically over time. If a scale is used to measure self-efficacy and a person completes the scale repeatedly, any differences in the scores may be due to the scale not being reliable. If an instrument is used that has 20 items, participants' responses to each item are correlated to each other, demonstrating that the items are consistently measuring the same construct. This type of reliability is called internal consistency reliability. Physiological measurement methods that consistently measure physiological variables are considered precise (Grove & Cipher, 2020; Ryan-Wenger, 2017). For example, a thermometer would be considered precise if it showed approximately the same temperature reading when tested repeatedly on the same patient within a limited time (see Chapter 16).

Construct, internal, external, and statistical conclusion design validity are considered when a nonintervention study is appraised for its implications for practice. Validity requires critically appraising the study's design, data collection, and results. Therefore determining the study design is a key decision in the planning of a study.

DECISIONS TO DEVELOP AND IMPLEMENT NONINTERVENTIONAL STUDIES

Developing and implementing a study design requires the researcher to consider multiple details such as those discussed in the sections on design validity and elements of a good design. The more careful consideration given to these details, the stronger the design (Kazdin, 2017). Strong research designs are essential to generate valid research evidence for nursing (Melnyk & Fineout-Overholt, 2019). The elements central to the study design include the presence or absence of a treatment, the number of groups in the sample, the number and timing of measurements, the sampling method, the time frame for data collection, planned comparisons, and the control of extraneous variables.

Box 10.2 contains a list of questions. Finding answers to the questions will help you to develop a noninterventional study design. The first question determines whether you will be conducting a noninterventional study or an interventional study. If describing variables or examining relationships is the study's purpose, you will conduct a noninterventional study. If examination of causality is the study's purpose, you will conduct an interventional study. Chapter 11 describes interventional designs.

The second question is a reminder that designing a study requires attention to ethical issues that may arise.

BOX 10.2   Questions to Guide Development of Noninterventional Study Design

1. Is the primary purpose of the study to describe variables and groups, to examine relationships, or to examine causality within the study situation? (Adams & Lawrence, 2019; Kazdin, 2017)
2. Are there ethical issues to consider when selecting the inclusion and exclusion criteria for the sample or when collecting data? (Chapter 9)
3. Will the sample be randomly or nonrandomly selected? (Chapter 15)
4. Will the sample be studied as a single group or will naturally occurring groups be compared?
5. How many groups will there be?
6. What will be the size of each group? (Aberson, 2019)
7. What instruments will be used to measure the variables? (Waltz et al., 2017)
8. Are the measurement methods valid and reliable or precise and accurate? (Ryan-Wenger, 2017; Waltz et al., 2017)
9. Will data be collected at a single site or at multiple sites?
10. Who will collect the data and how will they be trained? (Chapter 20)
11. Will the variables be measured once (cross sectionally) or multiple times (repeated measures, longitudinal)?
12. Are data being collected on extraneous variables? (Chapter 6)
13. What statistical analyses will be used to describe or compare variables and groups and to examine relationships among the variables? (Grove & Cipher, 2020) (Chapters 23, 24, 25)
14. What strategies are used to ensure consistent collection of data? (Kazdin, 2017; Leedy & Ormrod, 2019; Melnyk & Fineout-Overholt, 2019)

Decisions about the inclusion and exclusion criteria must be based on eliminating potential confounding variables and participants who could not safely complete the study. The ethical principle of justice demands that the criteria be fair and as inclusive as possible (see Chapter 9). The questions are designed to remind you of the steps of the research process. You may not follow the questions in order because the answer to one question affects the answers to other questions. For example, the number of groups and variables will affect the size of the sample. Planning a study is an iterative process.

Notice that question 11 in Box 10.2 asks how many times data will be collected as one of the decisions you make when planning a study. The number of times data are collected and the spacing between the data collection episodes will determine how long each participant is in the study. Although time is a factor in most study designs, the next section includes explanations of how time can affect noninterventional study designs.

NONINTERVENTIONAL DESIGNS THAT CAPTURE CHANGE ACROSS TIME

Time-dimensional designs are used extensively within the discipline of epidemiology to examine change over time in relation to disease occurrence. In nursing research, the change over time that is studied is likely to be the result of a positive change, such as normal development, learning, or self-enacted change in lifestyle, or the result of a negative change such as disease progression, exposure, aging, or other deteriorative process. Time-dimensional designs are useful in establishing patterns and trends in relation to potential precipitating factors and, consequently, can be precursors to developing interventions to be tested.

Nonintervention study designs are more appropriate when interventional research is not ethical for investigating certain health problems. For instance, it would not be ethical to conduct a study to determine the effects of applying potentially harmful substances or treatments. In this case, the information gained from time-dimensional research, when repeatedly replicated, is convincing in implying causation. Examples of this type of cumulative evidence are studies of the effects of human behaviors, such as examining the development of skin cancer in relation to sun exposure, of bronchiolitis in relation to use of electronic cigarettes, of brain changes in relation to nonprescription use of opioid medications, and of deterioration of cognitive and physical capabilities in relation to chronic stress. Even though time-dimensional studies establish a body of descriptive and correlational evidence, their findings only imply causation (Campbell & Stanley, 1963; Shadish et al., 2002). However, the findings of time-dimensional studies can generate evidence for the future, such as interventions to change harmful behaviors or attenuate the effects of harmful behaviors (Kazdin, 2017; Shadish et al., 2002).

Within noninterventional research, there are two principal types of time-dimensional studies: (1) longitudinal research and (2) cross-sectional research. Either of these can be descriptive or correlational in type. Both types of time-dimensional research can be conducted either retrospectively or prospectively.

Longitudinal Designs

Longitudinal designs examine changes in the same subjects over time. In other disciplines, these may be called panel designs or cohort analyses (Fig. 10.2). The purpose of longitudinal designs is to examine changes in a variable over time, within a defined group. In Fig. 10.2, notice that a sample is selected and data are collected from this sample multiple times at designated intervals. For example, a researcher is interested in the bone health of women who were diagnosed with breast cancer that was estrogen receptor positive (ER+) and are receiving an antiestrogen medication. Once a year for 5 years, the women in the study would receive a bone scan to determine changes in bone density. This prospective longitudinal study design could provide valuable information about the long-term effects of antiestrogen medications.

In prospective longitudinal research such as the breast cancer study, samples must be relatively large, because attrition over time is expected. For this reason, if a power analysis is used to calculate optimal sample

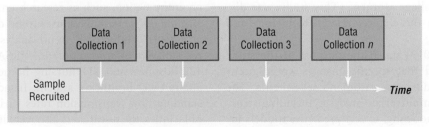

Fig. 10.2 Data collection in a longitudinal study.

size, more subjects should be recruited than needed (Grove & Cipher, 2020). Some samples are recruited in circumstances that support retention in a longitudinal study, such as four consecutive cohorts in an undergraduate nursing program who are strongly committed to finishing the program. You would expect that the attrition rate in a study of nursing students would be lower than a sample of nurse aides working in long-term care. Chapter 15 discusses sampling and retention of subjects.

Longitudinal research that is retrospective involves accessing data and transcribing values that reflect measured increments of time in the past. The researcher interested in bone health of women with ER+ breast cancer could access data from a cancer registry. Data collection for such a study could be collected in less time than a prospective study. With the expansion of the electronic health records, retrospective longitudinal studies have become more feasible on a wide range of health problems.

Consultation with a statistician is recommended for longitudinal research, because data analysis is more complex than it would be in simple descriptive research. Because of the focus on examining changes, many descriptive longitudinal studies employ some correlational statistical methods, such as linear regression or multiple regression analysis (see Chapter 24), as well as descriptive statistics, to describe changes over time. Multiple regression analysis is a statistical procedure that examines many variables from a data set in conjunction with one another, so that their combined effects as well as their individual effects on the principal variable of interest can be understood fully. Other analyses that are commonly used are repeated measures analysis of variance and other more complicated methods addressed in statistical texts (King & Eckersley, 2019; Plichta & Kelvin, 2013). For example, Stein et al. (2019) conducted a 12-month longitudinal study of disordered eating among Mexican American college women. (This study was discussed earlier in the chapter related to history and subject attrition.)

Stein et al. (2019) stated the purpose of the study and hypothesized that specific changes would occur over time depending on a woman's self-schema. The researchers used multivariate analyses, including structured equation modeling, to test predictive models for each type of disordered eating.

"As a preliminary test of the utility of the identity disturbance model in Mexican American women, Stein and colleagues completed a pilot study with a community-based sample of young adult women (Stein, Corte, & Ronis, 2010).... In the current study, we extended this work to determine the ability of the identity disturbance model to predict disordered eating behaviors over a one-year period in a large sample of college-enrolled Mexican American women." (Stein et al., 2019, p. 182)

"We used a 12-month longitudinal design to determine the effects of self-schema properties on disordered eating behaviors in undergraduate Mexican American women. Self-schema properties at baseline were used to predict disordered eating behaviors that were measured at baseline, 3, 6, 9 and 12 months. The study was conducted at two sites, Michigan and Arizona. Data collection occurred between 2006 and 2011. The sample included 484 young adult Mexican American women recruited from universities and community colleges." (Stein et al., 2019, p. 182)

The researchers' hypothesis was partially supported. Women with "fewer positive and more negative schema" endorsed fat as being self-descriptive, which predicted purging and fasting behaviors (Stein et al., 2019, p. 185).

A **trend design**, also called a trend analysis, is a variation of the longitudinal design (Fig. 10.3). Because data are collected repeatedly, trend designs are similar to longitudinal designs. However, in trend designs, a somewhat different sample from the population is selected each time that data are collected. It is used extensively in epidemiology to examine changes across time in incidence, usually incidence of disease. Measurements in trend designs occur at similarly spaced intervals—monthly, yearly, or every 5 years, for instance. Samples usually are large, sometimes entire populations, and the sole aim is to measure incidence of one or more related variables within that population. Research on health of an entire nation, such as research emanating from the *Healthy People* initiatives, uses trend designs. Khader et al. (2019) conducted a trend analysis of methicillin-resistant *Staphylococcus aureus* (MRSA) transmission in 122 hospitals and 111 nursing homes in the veterans affairs (VA) healthcare system. In addition to understanding how transmission rates varied between types of facilities, the researchers also were interested in determining the effects of VA prevention initiatives on MRSA

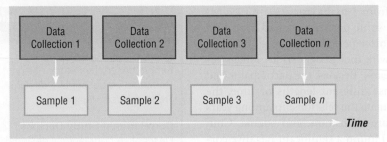

Fig. 10.3 Trend design.

incidence and transmission. Khader et al. (2019) found distinct differences in the transmission dynamics between the group of hospitals and the group of nursing homes, but also found site differences within each group. Although the transmission rate declined in hospitals over the course of the study, the transmission rate stayed stable in nursing homes.

Cross-Sectional Designs

Cross-sectional designs, in their classical form, examine changes over time (Fig. 10.4). Data are collected one time from a sample of participants that are expected to be in various stages of a process. In Fig. 10.4, the arrows starting at different places represent the process being studied. The vertical line "data collection" intersects the

processes at different points. For example, you want to study health behaviors among male survivors of colon cancer. Some of the survivors may be less than 5 years posttreatment, while others are 20 or more years posttreatment for cancer. The purpose of cross-sectional designs is to examine differences in a variable over time by comparing its value across participants who are in various phases of a process. The assumption of the design is that the process for change in that variable is similar across individuals.

Chin and Armstrong (2019) conducted a cross-sectional descriptive correlational study of anticipated stigma and healthcare utilization among persons with neurological disorders or chronic obstructive pulmonary disease (COPD). The 77 participants had lived

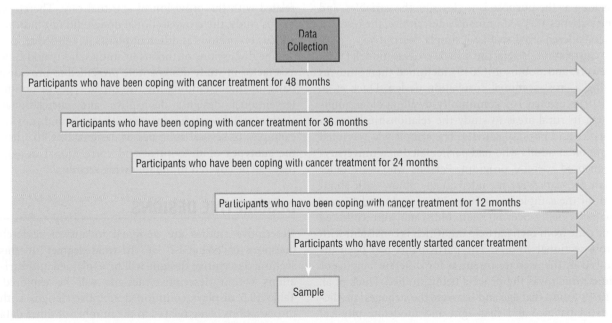

Fig. 10.4 Cross-sectional design.

with their diagnoses from 1 to 39 years ($M = 10.7$, $SD = 9.37$). As expected, some participants had lived with their diagnosis for shorter periods of time (< 5 years) and others had lived with their diagnosis for longer periods of time (> 30 years). Because the participants had lived with their disease different lengths of time, the researchers could calculate the relationship among years with disease, healthcare utilization, and stigma. Chin and Armstrong (2019) found a significant negative correlation between years with diagnosis and anticipated stigma from coworkers. The longer the participants had lived with their diagnosis, the less stigma they anticipated from their coworkers.

Prospective cross-sectional research has the advantage of a fairly rapid time of data collection, as compared with prospective longitudinal research. Its primary disadvantage is that it demands a fairly large sample to increase representation of participants across the trajectory of the process being studied. A large sample increases the potential that measurements truly reflect changes in the characteristics of the phenomenon of interest, not merely differences inherent in individual small groups. As with longitudinal research, because the purpose of the study is tracking changes, many descriptive cross-sectional studies may explore some relationships (correlations) among descriptive variables across different values of the process variable. As long as the purpose is to describe the variables, and the statistics are predominantly descriptive, the research is considered cross-sectional simple descriptive.

Correlation designs can also be cross sectional. Duck, Stewart, and Robinson (2019) identified their study as being a cross-sectional correlation design. Duck et al. (2019) recruited 101 community-dwelling older adults living in rural areas to study the relationship between balance and physical activity. The sample was recruited from older adults who had participated in a university-sponsored exercise program. Persons who were older than 65 years were included in the study, with about half of the sample being 70 to 79 years old and 17 participants being over 80 years old. Data were collected one time from each participant, which is consistent with cross-sectional studies. The participants had been involved in the exercise program for different lengths of time, which was the process being studied. Duck et al. (2019) found that age and sex were the strongest predictors of balance and that light and moderate physical activity did not predict balance as they expected. The

BOX 10.3   Noninterventional Study Designs

Descriptive Study Designs
Simple descriptive study designs[a]
Comparative descriptive designs[a]
Trend analysis designs

Correlational Study Designs
Descriptive correlational designs[a]
Predictive designs[a]
Model-testing designs

[a]Can be cross sectional or longitudinal.

researchers acknowledged the limitations of convenience sampling and the underrepresentation of older persons who were physically inactive.

Researchers may describe their studies as being cross sectional when time is not a focus of the study. In these instances, the label "cross sectional" is used to indicate that data are collected a single time from each participant. For example, Mamier, Taylor, and Winslow (2019) described their study of the prevalence and correlates of spiritual care among tertiary-care nurses as being cross sectional. However, the only considerations of time in the study were the demographic variables of the nurses' ages and years of experience, neither of which were correlated with the provision of spiritual care. Therefore, in this study, the cross-sectional design did not indicate a focus on persons at different points in a process.

The discussions of threats to study validity and time as a factor in study designs were presented to provide a basis for understanding the two broad types of noninterventional designs: descriptive and correlational. Within each broad design, we will identify and provide examples of several subtypes of designs. Box 10.3 lists the subtypes of descriptive and correlational designs that will be covered in the following sections.

DESCRIPTIVE DESIGNS

Descriptive studies are designed to answer research questions of "What is?" or "To what degree?" In this section, descriptive designs will be explained and variations within descriptive designs will be explored. Table 10.5 displays common descriptive designs with the variations being related to the number of times data are collected and whether there is one group or more.

TABLE 10.5 **Descriptive Designs With Time Element**

Type of Design	Purpose	Number of Groups	Data Collection
Simple descriptive, cross sectional	To describe the phenomenon of interest and variables	One	One time
Simple descriptive, longitudinal	To describe the phenomenon of interest and variables over time	One	Two or more times
Comparative descriptive, cross sectional	To describe and compare the phenomenon of interest and variables in naturally occurring groups	At least two, and sometimes more	One time
Comparative descriptive, longitudinal	To describe and compare the phenomenon of interest and variables in naturally occurring groups over time	At least two, and sometimes more	Two or more times

Simple Descriptive Design

The purpose of **simple descriptive design** is to describe the phenomenon of interest and other variables within one single group of participants (Fig. 10.5). This is accomplished through the use of descriptive statistics (see Chapter 22). When a simple cross-sectional descriptive design is conducted, data collection for all subjects occurs within the same time frame, over a span of minutes, hours, days, weeks, or months. Fig. 10.5 displays the events in a simple cross-sectional descriptive study. A sample is recruited and data are collected on the selected variables. Because it is a cross-sectional design, one of the variables being studied is a process (see Fig. 10.4). The researchers expect that participants will be at different points in that process. After the variables are described, the results are interpreted and may result in recognizing the need for replication, in developing a hypothesis, or generating a new research question. Knisely, Conley, and Szigethy (2019) conducted a simple cross-sectional descriptive study with 39 adolescents and young adults with Crohn disease (CD). Using data from a single data collection that was part of a larger study, they described HRQoL "across genotypes of functional single-nucleotide polymorphisms (SNP) in cytokine candidate genes" (Knisely et al., 2019, p. 545). By using a cross-sectional design, the researchers expected the participants to have different genotypes, to have lived with CD for different lengths of time, and to have different levels of HRQoL. Using a snapshot (i.e., a cross-sectional slice) of these variables allowed the researchers to describe the variables and interpret the results (see Fig. 10.5). Based on disease criteria, 66% of the participants were in remission. Despite the large majority

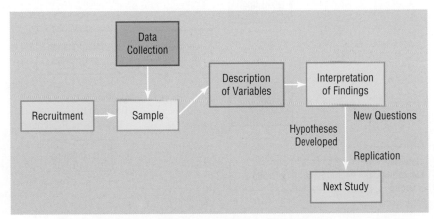

Fig. 10.5 Simple cross-sectional descriptive design.

of the participants being in remission, the mean total HRQoL score was low. The researchers concluded that "variations within cytokine genes can potentially serve as protective or risk factors for poor HRQoL" (Knisely et al., 2019, p. 548). Because of the study's limitations, the researchers did not develop hypotheses or generate research questions for future studies, as shown in Fig. 10.5, but recommended additional studies with larger samples and longitudinal designs.

A simple descriptive longitudinal design (see Table 10.5) would be ideal for a study of HRQoL among persons with CD for the first 3 years following diagnosis. Every 6 months, data would be collected related to hospitalizations, medications, and HRQoL from a large sample of persons living with CD. Fig. 10.2 displays the pattern of data collection. Changes over time could be described with the goals of increasing the understanding of nurse clinicians and of stimulating the development of hypotheses among researchers working with this population.

Comparative Descriptive Design

The purpose of the **comparative descriptive design** is to examine similarities and differences between two naturally occurring groups. It is important to ascertain the

groups were not formed by the researchers as would be appropriate in an interventional study. Fig. 10.6 displays two naturally occurring groups with a single episode of data collection, which indicates a cross-sectional comparative descriptive design. The variables are compared between the groups, the results are interpreted, and the findings are disseminated. For example, you could conduct a study to compare the no-show rate at one clinic to the no-show rate at another clinic. Patients at the first clinic receive a telephone call a week before an appointment as a reminder. Patients at the second clinic receive a text message a week before and the day before an appointment as reminders. You would collect data on the no-show rate for the same month at each clinic and compare the rates. The results of the study would not support inferring that the reminder method caused any difference in the show rate but might lead to the new research questions or hypotheses for future studies.

Longitudinal studies can also be comparative descriptive designs. Fig. 10.7 begins with two naturally occurring groups and the collection of the first set of data to be compared. The process is repeated at least one more time. Shajrawi et al. (2019) used a longitudinal comparative descriptive design to study patients with

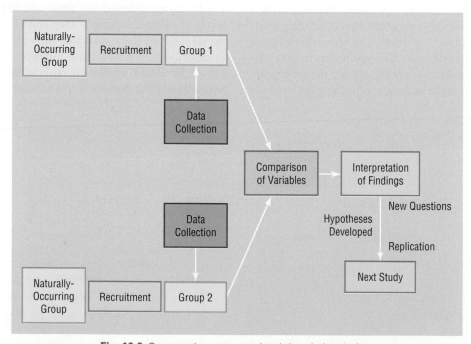

Fig. 10.6 Comparative cross-sectional descriptive design.

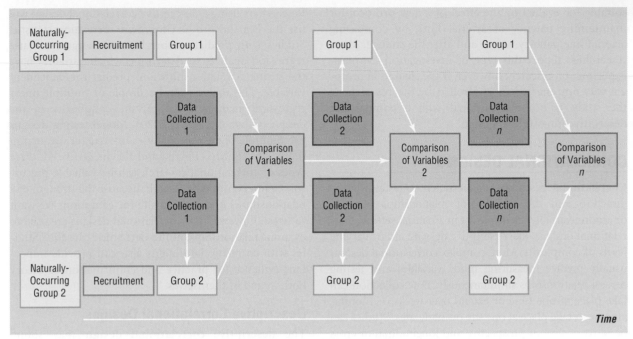

Fig. 10.7 Comparative longitudinal descriptive design.

three groups being formed by the treatment they received for an AMI. The researchers' concern was that these patients did not have access to cardiac rehabilitation but needed physical activity as secondary prevention of future AMIs. The primary variables were sedentary behavior and physical activity as measured by an activity monitoring device.

"The participants were categorized according to type of AMI treatment modalities into 3 groups: ST-elevation myocardial infarction treated by primary percutaneous coronary intervention [PCI], ST-elevation myocardial infarction treated by thrombolytic therapy, and non–ST-elevation myocardial infarction [NSTEMI] treated by medication.... The participants completed the demographic data sheet, whereas clinical data were collected from patients' medical files. The researcher collected the study data from the participants during their visit to the outpatient clinics in the early recovery period, at weeks 2 and 6 after hospitalization. The researcher explained the use of the thigh-worn activity monitor (activPAL3) during the waiting time in the follow-up appointment in the outpatient clinics." (Shajwari et al., 2019, pp. 285, 286)

Shajwari et al. (2019) found that patients treated with PCI had significantly higher mean steps than those treated with thrombolytic therapy. Those treated with thrombolytic therapy had significantly higher mean steps than the patients with NSTEMI who were treated with medication. The same between group differences were also found at Time 2. Between Times 1 and 2, patients treated with PCI also had a higher mean change in steps per day. The researchers noted the study limitations to be a small sample ($N = 94$), 50% of the screened patients were not eligible, and 30% of those who were eligible refused to participate. In addition to these limitations, the researchers did not measure any other risk factors for coronary disease, which certainly could be confounding variables affecting the activity of the participants. The findings of this study provide preliminary information. Therefore the study requires replication before using these findings in practice or as the basis for a policy change.

Researchers also use the comparative descriptive design to compare before and after states related to changes in clinical products, utilization, or protocols, and to other externally driven passive events. For instance, a comparative descriptive longitudinal design would be suitable for evaluating the effect of a new protocol for maintaining patency of arterial lines, by comparing arterial line patency before and after the change. Many researchers report this type of investigation as quasi-experimental research; however, if the change in protocol was not enacted or controlled by the researchers, the study is noninterventional with a comparative descriptive longitudinal design.

CORRELATIONAL DESIGNS

Correlational research is conducted to establish the direction and the strength of relationships between or among variables as they exist in a natural setting. Correlational designs, like descriptive designs, are of varying levels of complexity. More complex correlational designs usually involve measuring many variables and testing several relationships simultaneously. Data collection can take place at one time or extend over weeks or months, and it can take place at one site or many sites. Studies can be retrospective or prospective and longitudinal or cross sectional in their strategies of data collection.

There are three major types of correlational research described in this text: the descriptive correlational design, the predictive correlational design, and the model-testing designs. Table 10.6 displays the three types and the typical purpose of each design. The designs differ in their respective purpose: to describe relationships, to enable prediction, and to confirm theoretical models.

Researchers using a descriptive correlational design will use the Pearson product-moment correlation statistic. Studies with predictive correlational designs may use regression analysis to determine which variables have the strongest relationships and predict the dependent variable. The analysis can be simple or multiple linear regression analysis based on the complexity of the design (Grove & Cipher, 2020). Model-testing designs use multiple regression analyses or structural equation modeling ([SEM], (Plitcha and Kelvin, 2013). All three types of correlational research can be valuable precursors to interventional research, because the strength of a relationship is one prerequisite for causation. We want to stress, however, that correlational designs are used to examine relationships, not to determine causality. Studies with correlational designs also can provide important evidence for practice and confirmation of theory both in and of themselves.

Descriptive Correlational Designs

The **descriptive correlational design** may sound confusing because it includes two types of designs (Fig. 10.8). Descriptive correlational design, however, is a type of correlational research because its primary purpose is to examine relationships between and among variables (Kerlinger & Lee, 2000; Leedy & Ormrod, 2019). Fig. 10.8 shows that, first, the data are collected and the variables are described. Then the bivariate relationships between all possible pairs of the variables are examined and the results are interpreted. Mamier et al. (2019), as mentioned previously in the chapter, conducted a cross-sectional descriptive correlational study. Their accessible population was the 2311 registered nurses (RNs) working in a faith-based hospital. Their purpose and research questions are characteristic of a descriptive correlational design.

TABLE 10.6	Correlational Designs
Type of Design	**Purpose**
Descriptive correlational	To examine the presence and strength of the relationships between and among the variables being described
Predictive correlational	To predict an outcome or dependent variable by examining the presence and strength of relationships among the independent variables used to predict the dependent variable
Model-testing design	To confirm theoretical models by examining the presence and strength of relationships among variables in the model

"The purpose of this study is to describe the types and frequencies of nurse-provided therapeutics intended to support client spiritual well-being and to explore factors associated with these therapeutics.... Research Question 1: How frequently are various types of spiritual therapeutics provided by nurses? Research Question 2: What is the relationship between (a) nurse demographics, (b) nurse work–related characteristics, and (c) nurse spirituality/religiosity measures and frequency of nurse-provided spiritual care?" (Mamier et al., 2019, pp. 539–540)

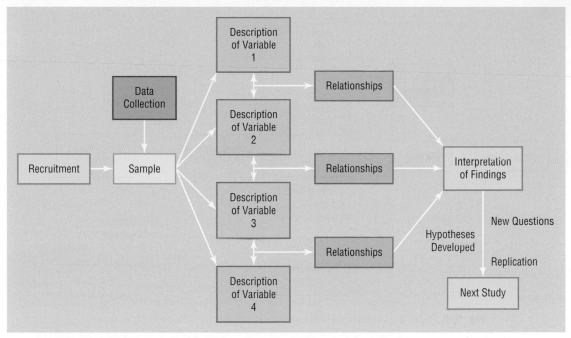

Fig. 10.8 Descriptive correlational design. Note: Bivariate relationships are examined between all possible pairs of variables, such as Variable 1 to Variable 3 and Variable 1 to Variable 4.

In this example, research question 1 focused on description and research question 2 focused on relationships, consistent with a descriptive correlational design. Mamier et al. (2019) identified strengths of their study to be that the participants included male and ethnically diverse nurses, and the nurses worked in different types of acute care units. The researchers used multiple measures of spiritual care and asked nurses to answer the questions based on their most recent care experiences. Unfortunately, spiritual care was rarely documented in the patient's electronic health records, which prevented confirming the frequency of spiritual therapeutics. Another of the study limitations was the possibility that nurses who were more interested in spiritual care were more likely to participate in the study. Statistically significant relationships were found between providing spiritual care and having received spiritual care education, type of unit (spiritual care was less likely to occur on the pediatric unit), higher levels of self-reported spirituality and religiosity, and awareness of patients' spiritual needs (Mamier et al., 2019).

Predictive Correlational Designs

The **predictive correlational design** is used to establish strength and direction of relationships between or among variables, with the intention of predicting the value of one of the variables based on the value(s) of one or more other variable(s) (Fig. 10.9). Predictive correlational research uses the terms *independent* and *dependent* to refer to its principal variables. The **independent variable** (or variables) is also called a predictor. The **dependent variable** is the one whose value or occurrence the researcher wants to be able to predict. When predictive correlational research examines multiple variables and their potential interactions with one another, both linear and multivariate statistical tests are used to determine which predictors are most powerful (Grove & Cipher, 2020). When more than one predictor is tested, a final equation is presented that best explains the change in the value of the dependent variable. The total amount of change in the value of the dependent variable explained by the predictor variables is called the **variance**, and it is represented as R^2. (See Chapter 24 for clarification of the concept of explained variance, R^2.)

Predictive correlational studies can produce findings with theoretical, clinical, and research benefits. Theoretically, the findings of predictive correlational studies are often the prelude to constructing models (see Chapter 8). After construction, the resultant

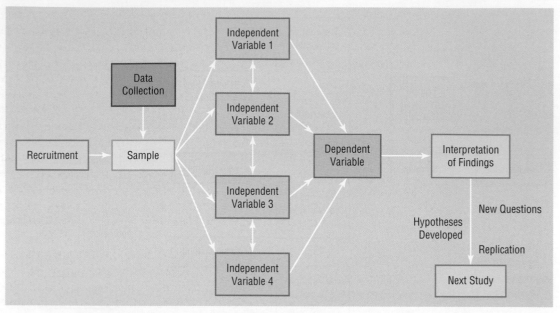

Fig. 10.9 Predictive correlational design with independent and dependent variables.

model would then be evaluated for the statistical strength of the relationships within it, using a model-testing design (see the following section). In the area of clinical benefits, findings can help clinicians facilitate positive health outcomes (Kazdin, 2017; Leedy & Ormrod, 2019). For example, predictive correlational findings identifying behaviors related to relapse would be useful to nurses working with patients who are receiving treatment for opioid addiction. Nurses use the findings to assess patients' behaviors and respond proactively to changes that indicate a higher risk of relapse. From a research standpoint, predictive correlational findings may serve as a precursor to interventional research. For example, in an acute care setting, a bundle of five interventions were implemented to prevent catheter-associated urinary tract infection (CAUTI). Although CAUTIs decreased, implementing the bundle required over 30 minutes three times every day. The labor cost of the bundle of five interventions was unsustainable. Based on these findings and previously published findings, nurse researchers may be able to identify three of the interventions that were more predictive of whether or not a patient develops a CAUTI. With this information, nurse administrators could design a modified bundle consisting of the three interventions most predictive of the absence of CAUTI.

The patient outcomes of the modified bundle could be compared to the patient outcomes of the full bundle to determine whether the modified bundle was harmful. If the two outcomes were not statistically or clinically different, the procedure for urinary catheter care may be changed.

Previously in this chapter, a study by Kellogg et al. (2019) was discussed as an example of researchers testing a sample for social desirability. This study included a predictive correlational design. Certified pediatric nurses ($N = 338$) were the sample for the study of secondary traumatic stress and coping behaviors. The researchers identified the study problem as the lack of evidence related to "how caring for traumatized children and their families' affects the pediatric nurse" (Kellogg et al., 2019, p. 98). The dependent variable was secondary traumatic stress and the independent variables were demographic characteristics of the nurses and coping behaviors used by the nurses. Slightly more than half the participants' scores indicated from moderate to severe secondary traumatic stress. The independent variables of the age of the nurse, years of nursing experience, and years of pediatric nursing experience were not significant predictors of secondary traumatic stress, the dependent variable. However, the types of coping behaviors used by the nurses were statistically significant predictors of secondary traumatic stress. Denial, emotional support, and behavioral disengagement (independent variables) were predictive of higher levels of secondary traumatic stress (dependent variable). The researchers identified a low response rate (5%), self-report measures, and selection as a threat to validity because of the nonrandom sample.

"In this sample of pediatric nurses, emotional support was a positive predictor of secondary traumatic stress. These findings are contradictory to previous research and may be unique to pediatric nurses or the work environments of these nurses. It is possible that this group needs more support than that of family or colleagues to overcome secondary traumatic stress. Professional assistance or more formalized support or programs may help this population.... As expected, negative and possibly dysfunctional coping processes of denial and behavioral disengagement were predictors of secondary traumatic stress in pediatric nurses. Behavioral disengagement does not address a problem, but ignores the stressor.... Secondary traumatic stress impacts many pediatric nurses. Acknowledging the experience in this population through promoting awareness, and educational programs will help to protect nurses' psychological and physical health as they appraise work situations as less stressful leading to psychological wellbeing, and more job satisfaction. This may prevent nurses from leaving the profession due to work-related stress." (Kellogg et al., 2019, p. 102)

Model-Testing Designs

Model-testing designs use correlational research for measurement of proposed relationships within a theoretical model (see Chapter 8). When a theoretical model is described and diagrammed, exogenous and endogenous variables are identified. **Exogenous variables** means literally *grown from outside* and are the variables that affect other variables in the model but are not affected by the other variables in the model (Menard, 2013). Exogenous variables are not explained by the model; their explanations are outside the model. **Endogenous variables** are, conversely, *grown from inside* and influence one or more of the other variables in the model (Menard, 2013). In Fig. 10.10, the variables in the oval shapes, the number of close relationships and prior life experiences, are exogenous variables. Notice that these two variables affect other variables in the model, but the model does not indicate what factors have influenced the variables of number of close relationships and prior life experiences. The variables in the rectangle shapes are the endogenous variables. The model can be tested by measuring the variables in the model and implementing specific statistical analyses (Plichta & Kelvin, 2013).

The primary model-testing analyses used within nursing research are path analyses and SEM, introduced earlier in the chapter. In **path analysis**, the relationship between each pair of variables in a model is tested for its strength and direction without consideration of the other relationships in the model (Maruyama, 2017). The lines drawn between concepts are called paths, hence the name path analysis. Path analysis involves a series of logic regressions in which each endogenous variable is considered to be a dependent variable. **Structural equation modeling** (SEM) is a type of latent variable modeling that tests all the possible theoretical relationships within a model simultaneously (Hallgren,

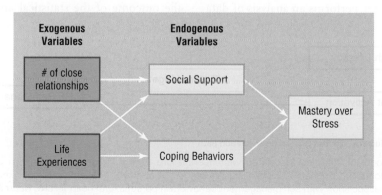

Fig. 10.10 Exogenous and endogenous variables in models.

McCabe, King, & Atkins, 2019; Pourrabi, Babadori, Hosseini, & Ravangard, 2018). Latent variable modeling is a group of analysis techniques that are used to examine relationships among abstract constructs. The constructs are represented by observable indicators and measurement error. SEM's complex calculations allow the researcher to identify the best model that explains interactions among variables and the greatest amount of variance in the dependent variable.

In model-testing designs, the relationships that are statistically significant are retained. Relationships that are weaker than the set point (greater than the p level set by the researcher) are removed from the model. **Residual** refers to effects of unknown variables, some unmeasurable or even unknown, which are not included in the final model (Maruyama, 2017). The residual is equivalent to the total unexplained variance, the amount of change in endogenous variables not explained or accounted for by the terms in the model. The amount of change explained by the model is represented by R^2. The residual is what remains, and it is represented as $(1 - R^2)$.

Because a number of variables may be examined in model-testing studies, samples must be large enough to provide statistical power. The rule of thumb has been that 10 subjects were required for each variable tested, but that is not adequate for model testing. The statistical relationships among the variables are complex, multilevel, and interacting. Because large samples are required, researchers conducting model testing and predictive correlational research frequently use data previously collected during multisite studies or national health surveys. When a researcher reuses data collected for another study, it is called a secondary analysis (see Chapter 17). **Secondary analysis** is a strategy in which a researcher performs an analysis of data collected and originally analyzed by another researcher or agency.

Among patients with HF, self-care was identified by professional organizations as being essential to "improve quality of life and slow disease progression and functional loss" (Jacobson et al., 2018, p. 447). In response to the professional recommendations, the nurse researchers conducted a model-testing study related to self-management of patients living with HF. The concepts in the model were selected based on previous research findings. They also identified a specific gap in the evidence that their study was designed to address.

> "Overall, reports in the literature showed inconsistent relationships among health literacy, HF knowledge and patient activation on self-management and no report studied all 3 factors together for their association with self-management. Specifically, no research was found to learn if higher levels of patient activation and health literacy, mediated by HF knowledge, would increase HF self-management.... The purpose of this study was to test a model of the direct and mediating effects of health literacy, patient activation and HF knowledge on self-management in persons with HF." (Jacobson et al., 2018, p. 448)

Jacobson et al. (2018) tested a model that identified the relationships among the concepts and linked them to HF self-management, the dependent variable. The independent variables in the model were health literacy, HF knowledge, and patient activation (Fig. 10.11). The participants were recruited from four outpatient centers and completed packets of the research instruments while at the center. Table 10.7 displays the hypotheses in the first column. The second column provides the outcome of the statistical analysis related to each

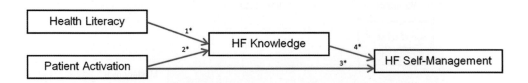

* **Note:** Numeral signifies correlation/mediation path

Fig. 10.11 Model of variables associated with heart failure (HF) self-management. (From Jacobson, A., Sumodi, V., Albert, N., Butler, R., DeJohn, L., Walker, D., et al. (2018). Patient activation, knowledge, and health literacy association with self-management behaviors in persons with heart failure. *Heart & Lung, 47*(1), 448. doi:10.1016/j.hrtlng.2018.05.021.)

TABLE 10.7   Hypotheses From Model-Testing Study: Heart Failure (HF) Self-Management (Jacobson et al., 2018)

Hypotheses	Relationships	Outcome of Hypothesis Testing
Hypothesis 1: HF knowledge and patient activation are positively associated with HF self-management.	Only patient activation was positively associated with HF self-management.	Hypothesis partially supported.
Hypothesis 2: The association of health literacy with HF self-management is mediated through HF knowledge.	Significant association between health literacy and HF knowledge was found. No association of either health literacy or HF knowledge with HF self-management was found.	Hypothesis not supported.
Hypothesis 3: The association of patient activation with HF self-management is partially mediated through HF knowledge.	No significant association between HF knowledge and patient activation was found.	Hypothesis not supported.

hypothesis. Among the demographic variables, age was significantly associated with HF self-management. The researchers used multiple regression to produce a reduced model containing only significant terms.

"In the reduced model, each year increase in age increased the estimate of the HF self-management score by .47 and a 1-level increase in the patient activation level (of 4 possible levels) increased the estimate of the HF self-management score by 5.2.... In this study, patient activation level and patient age, but not health literacy level or HF knowledge, were positively related to HF self-management behaviors. More research is needed to identify strategies for promoting

patient activation and self-management in adults with HF and determine the strength of other factors that influence self-management." (Jacobson et al., 2018, pp. 450, 451)

The sample of 151 patients living with HF was small for a model-testing design. Other limitations were self-report instruments and the exclusion of persons who could not read or write English. Replication of the study in other geographical regions and a larger sample would provide stronger evidence. Models developed from research findings, as Jacobson et al. (2018) did, or from theoretical frameworks can be refined with the findings of model-testing studies.

KEY POINTS

- Research design is a blueprint for the conduct of a study that maximizes the researcher's control over factors that could interfere with the results.
- The purpose of design is to set up a situation that maximizes the possibilities of obtaining valid answers to research questions or testing hypotheses.
- Before planning a noninterventional design, the researcher must understand certain concepts: probability, bias, measurement, and control.
- Study validity is a measure of the truth or accuracy of the research findings and is an important concern throughout the research process.

- The four types of study design validity requiring examination in a noninterventional study are (1) statistical conclusion design validity, (2) internal design validity, (3) construct design validity, and (4) external design validity.
- Statistical conclusion design validity is concerned with if the conclusions about relationships or differences drawn from statistical analyses are an accurate reflection of the real world.
- In noninterventional studies, potential threats to statistical conclusion validity include low statistical power, violating statistical assumptions, error rate

due to multiple analyses, and unreliable measurements (see Table 10.1).
- Internal design validity is the extent to which the effects detected in the study are a true reflection of reality rather than the result of extraneous variables.
- In noninterventional studies, potential threats to internal design validity are history, maturation, selection, and subject attrition (see Table 10.2).
- Construct design validity examines the fit between the conceptual and operational definitions of a variable.
- In noninterventional studies, potential threats to construct design validity are inadequate clarification of constructs, mono-operation bias, monomethod bias, social desirability, and careless responding (see Table 10.3).
- External design validity is concerned with the extent to which study findings can be generalized beyond the sample used in the study.

- In noninterventional studies, potential threats to external design validity are homogeneity of the sample and the interaction of setting and sample (see Table 10.4).
- Questions are provided to guide the reader in developing and implementing a noninterventional study design.
- Description and correlational studies use noninterventional designs.
- Cross-sectional and longitudinal studies examine change over time. Descriptive and correlational studies can be designed to be cross sectional or longitudinal.
- Description designs include simple descriptive, descriptive comparative, and trend analysis.
- Correlational designs include descriptive correlational, predictive correlational, and model-testing designs.

REFERENCES

Aberson, C. L. (2019). *Applied power analysis for the behavioral sciences* (2nd ed.). New York City, NY: Routledge Taylor & Francis Group.

Adams, K., & Lawrence, E. (2019). *Research methods, statistics, and applications* (2nd ed.). Thousand Oaks, CA: Sage.

Alhurani, A., Dekker, R., Ahmad, M., Miller, J., Yousef, K., Abdulqader, B., ... Moser, D. (2018). Stress, cognitive appraisal, coping, and event free survival in patients with heart failure. *Heart & Lung, 47*(1), 205–210. doi:10.1016/j.hrtlng.2018.03.008

Ang, S., O'Brien, A., & Wilson, A. (2019). Understanding carers' fall concern and their management of fall risk among older people at home. *BMC Geriatrics, 19,* 144. doi:10.1186/s12877-019-1162-7

Campbell, D. T., & Stanley, J. C. (1963). *Experimental and quasi-experimental designs for research.* Chicago, IL: Rand McNally.

Chin, E., & Armstrong, D. (2019). Anticipated stigma and healthcare utilization in COPD and neurological disorders. *Applied Nursing Research, 45*(1), 63–68. doi:10.1016/j.apnr.2018.12.002

Cook, T. D., & Campbell, D. T. (1979). *Quasi-experimentation: Design and analysis issues for field settings.* Chicago, IL: Rand McNally.

Crowne, D., & Marlowe, D. (1960). A new scale of social desirability independent of psychopathology. *Journal of Consulting Psychology, 24*(4), 349–354.

Duck, A., Stewart, M., & Robinson, J. (2019). Physical activity and postural balance in rural community dwelling older adults. *Applied Nursing Research, 48*(1), 1–7. doi:10.1016/j.apnr.2019.05.012

Esopo, K., Mellow, D., Thomas, C., Uckat, H., Abraham, J., Jain, P., ... Haushofer, J. (2018). Measuring self-efficacy, executive function, and temporal discounting in Kenya. *Behaviour Research and Therapy, 101*(2), 30–45. doi:10.1016/j.brat.2017.10.002

Grau, I., Ebbeler, C., & Banse, R. (2019). Cultural differences in careless responding. *Journal of Cross-Cultural Psychology, 50*(3), 336–357. doi:10.1177/0022022119827379

Gravetter, F., & Forzano, L. A. (2018). *Research methods for the behavioral sciences* (6th ed.). Boston, MA: Cengage.

Grove, S. K., & Cipher, D. (2020). *Statistics for health care research: A practical workbook* (2nd ed.). St. Louis, MO: Elsevier.

Hallgren, K., McCabe, C., King, K., & Atkins, D. (2019). Beyond path diagrams: Enhancing applied structural equation modeling through data visualization. *Addictive Behaviors, 94*(1), 74–82. doi:10.1016/j.addbeh.2018.08.030

Hyarat, S., Subih, M., Rayan, A., Salami, I., & Harb, A. (2019). Health related quality of life among patients with multiple sclerosis: The role of psychosocial adjustment to illness. *Archives of Psychiatric Nursing, 33*(1), 11–16. doi:10.1016/j.apnu.2018.08.006

Jacobson, A., Sumodi, V., Albert, N., Butler, R., DeJohn, L., Walker, D., ... Ross, D. (2018). Patient activation, knowledge, and health literacy association with self-management behaviors in persons with heart failure. *Heart & Lung, 47*(1), 447–451. doi:10.1016/j.hrtlng.2018.05.021

Kazdin, A. (2017). *Research design in clinical psychology* (5th ed.). Boston, MA: Pearson.

Kellogg, M., Knight, M., Dowling, J., & Crawford, S. (2018). Secondary traumatic stress in pediatric nurses. *Journal of Pediatric Nursing, 43*(1), 97–103. doi:10.1016/j.pedn.2018.08.016

Kerlinger, F. N., & Lee, H. B. (2000). *Foundations of behavioral research* (4th ed.). Fort Worth, TX: Harcourt College Publishers.

Khader, K., Thomas, A., Jones, M., Toth, D., Stevens, V., Samore, M., & CDC Modeling Infectious Diseases in Healthcare Program (MInD-Healthcare). (2019). Variation and trends in transmission dynamics of methicillin-resistant *Staphylococcus aureus* in veterans affairs hospitals and nursing homes. *Epidemics, 28*, 100347. doi:10.1016/j.epidem.2019.100347

Kim, J., Lyon, D., Weaver, M., Keenan, G., & Stechmiller, J. (2019). Demographics, psychological distress, and pain from pressure injury. *Nursing Research, 68*(5), 339–347. doi:10.1097/NNR.0000000000000357

King, A., & Eckersley, R. (2019). *Statistics for biomedical engineers and scientists: How to visualize and analyze data.* London, UK: Academic Press Elsevier.

Knisely, M., Conley, Y., & Szigethy, E. (2019). Cytokine genetic variants and health-related quality of life in Crohn's disease: An exploratory study. *Biological Research for Nursing, 21*(5), 544–551. doi:10.1177/1099800419860906

Lee, A., Cheung, Y., Joynt, G., Leung, C., Wong, W. T., & Gombersall, C. (2017). Are high nurse workload/staffing ratios associated with decreased survival in critically ill patients? A cohort study. *Annals of Intensive Care, 7,* Article 46. doi:10.1186/s13613-017-0269-2

Leedy, P. D., & Ormrod, J. E. (2019). *Practical research: Planning and design* (12th ed.). New York, NY: Pearson.

Mamier, I., Taylor, E., & Winslow, B. (2019). Nurse spiritual care: Prevalence and correlates. *Western Journal of Nursing Research, 41*(4), 537–554. doi:10.1177/0193945918776328

Maruyama, G. (2017). *The basics of structural equations.* Thousand Oaks, CA: Sage.

Melnyk, B. M., & Fineout-Overholt, E. (2019). *Evidence-based practice in nursing & healthcare: A guide to best practice* (3rd ed.). Philadelphia, PA: Lippincott Williams, & Wilkins.

Menard, S. (2013). *Logistic regression: From introductory to advanced concepts and applications.* Thousand Oaks, CA: Sage.

Mokkink, L., deVet, H., Prinsen, C., Patrick, D., Alonso, J., Bouter, L., & Terwee, C. (2018). COSMIN Risk of Bias checklist for systematic reviews of Patient-Reported Outcomes Measures. *Quality of Life Research, 27*(1), 1171–1179. doi:10.1007/s11136-017-1765-4

Pett, M. A. (2016). *Nonparametric statistics for health care research: Statistics for small samples and unusual distributions* (2nd ed.). Thousand Oaks, CA: Sage.

Plichta, S. B., & Kelvin, E. (2013). *Munro's statistical methods for health care research* (6th ed.). Philadelphia, PA: Lippincott Williams & Wilkins.

Porritt, K., Gomersall, J., & Lockwood, C. (2014). Study selection and critical appraisal. *American Journal of Nursing, 114*(6), 47–52. doi:10.1097/01.NAJ.0000450430.97383.64

Pourrabi, P., Babadori, M., Hosseini, S., & Ravangard, R. (2018). The effects of implementing an accreditation process on health care quality using structural equation modeling. *Health Care Manager, 37*(4), 317–324. doi:10.1097/HCM.0000000000000229

Rose, R. (2019). Frameworks for credible causal inference in observational studies of family violence. *Journal of Family Violence, 34*(5), 697–710. doi:10.1007/s10896-018-0011-3

Ryan-Wenger, N. A. (2017). Precision, accuracy, and uncertainty of biophysical measurements for research and practice. In C. F. Waltz, O. L. Strickland, & E. R. Lenz (Eds.), *Measurement in nursing and health research* (5th ed., pp. 427–445). New York, NY: Springer.

Savitz, D., Wellenius, G., & Trikalonis, T. (2019). The problem with mechanistic risk of bias assessments in evidence synthesis of observational studies and a practical alternative: Assessing the impact of specific sources of potential bias. *American Journal of Epidemiology, 188*(9), 1581–1585. doi:10.1093/aje/kwz131

Shadish, W. R., Cook, T. D., & Campbell, D. T. (2002). *Experimental and quasi-experimental designs for generalized causal inference.* Chicago, IL: Rand McNally.

Shajrawi, A., Al-Smadi, A., Al-Shawabkah, G., Aljribeea, H., & Khalil, H. (2019). Impacts of treatment modalities on physical activity after first acute myocardial infarction in Jordan. *Dimensions of Critical Care Nursing, 38*(6), 284–292. doi:10.1097/DCC.0000000000000382

Stein, K., Lee, C., Corte, C., & Steffen, A. (2019). The influence of identity on the prevalence and persistence of disordered eating and weight control behaviors in Mexican American college women. *Appetite, 140*(1), 180–189. doi:10.1016/j.appet.2019.05.008

Stein, K. F., Corte, C., & Ronis, D. L. (2010). Personal identities and disordered eating behaviors in Mexican American women. *Eating Behaviors, 11*(3), 197–200. doi:10.1016/j.eatbeh.2010.02.001

Stone, J., Glass, K., Clark, J., Munn, Z., Tugwell, P., & Doi, S. (2019). A unified framework for bias assessment in clinical research. *International Journal of Evidence-Based Health Care, 17*(1), 106–120. doi:10.1097/XEB.0000000000000165

Suter, W., & Suter, P. (2015). How research conclusions go wrong: A primer for home health clinicians. *Home Health Care Management & Practice, 27*(4), 171–177. doi:10.1177/1084822315586557

Waltz, C. F., Strickland, O. L., & Lenz, E. R. (2017). *Measurement in nursing and health research* (5th ed.). New York, NY: Springer Publishing Company.

Zhang, H., Li, Y., Li, M., & Chen, X. (2019). A randomized controlled trial of mindfulness-based stress reduction for insomnia secondary to cervical cancer: Sleep effects. *Applied Nursing Research, 48*(1), 52–57. doi:10.1016/j.apnr.2019.05.016

11

Quantitative Methodology: Interventional Designs and Methods

Jennifer R. Gray

http://evolve.elsevier.com/Gray/practice/

A **design** is the blueprint for conducting a study that maximizes control over factors that could interfere with the validity of the findings. To select an appropriate research design, you will need to integrate many elements. You will consider these same elements when identifying the design of a published study. Many researchers do not identify their study designs in publications and, as noted in Chapter 10, there is inconsistency among the labels given to study designs (Reeves, Wells, & Waddington, 2017). Determining the design in a published study may require you to put together bits of information from various parts of the research report.

Chapter 10 included questions and an algorithm to help you determine if a study was noninterventional or interventional (see Box 10.1 and Fig. 10.1). This chapter describes the interventional designs most commonly used in nursing research. These designs are broadly categorized as being quasi-experimental and experimental. These two types of designs examine the effects of an intervention by comparing differences between groups that have received the intervention and those that have not received the intervention.

The chapter begins with research terms that you need to understand to critically appraise interventional designs. The distinguishing features of experimental and quasi-experimental designs are the interventions; therefore describing characteristics of interventions that are implemented rigorously is the focus of the next section of this chapter. After the intervention section, threats to validity that are common in experimental and quasi-experimental designs are examined as well as ways to minimize these threats. The chapter concludes with descriptions of interventional designs. Box 11.1 lists the designs included in this chapter. Each of the designs is briefly described and a published example provided. Algorithms are provided at the end of the chapter to help you distinguish the subtypes of interventional designs.

RESEARCH TERMS

Interventional research includes causality, control, and other terms that need to be understood to be able to critically appraise studies of this type. The terms that were defined in Chapter 10 for noninterventional research will not be repeated here, but several of them are also applicable to interventional studies. You might want to review these terms before proceeding.

Causality

Causality can be defined as an action or condition that occurs prior to a specific outcome. The outcome does not occur without the action or condition being present. For causality to occur, there must be a strong relationship between the proposed cause and the effect (Luján & Todt, in press), and the proposed cause must precede the effect in time (Adams & Lawrence, 2019; McBreen, 2018). Another defining characteristic

BOX 11.1   Research Designs Described in Chapter 11

Quasi-Experimental Study Designs
- One-group posttest-only design
- Posttest-only design with comparison group
- One-group pretest-posttest design
- Pretest and posttest design with a comparison group
- Pretest and posttest design with two comparison treatments
- Pretest and posttest design with a removed treatment
- Simple interrupted time series designs
- Interrupted time series design with a no-treatment comparison group
- Interrupted time series design with multiple treatment replications

Experimental Study Designs
- Pretest-posttest control group design
- Solomon four-group design
- Experimental posttest-only control group design
- Within-subjects design
- Factorial design
- Clinical trials
- Randomized controlled trials
- Pragmatic clinical trials

Other Designs
- Comparative effectiveness research
- Methodological designs

BOX 11.2   Defining Characteristics of Causality

- Proposed cause must precede the effect in time.
- Strong relationship must exist between the proposed cause and effect.
- Effect does not occur without the proposed cause (necessary).
- Proposed cause, by itself, is enough for the effect to occur (sufficient).
- No alternative cause can explain the occurrence of the effect.

(Campbell & Stanley, 1963: Cook & Campbell, 1979). The characteristics of causality are listed in Box 11.2.

Causes are frequently expressed within the propositions of a theory, also called relational statements (Walker & Avant, 2019) (see Chapter 8). Propositions from a theory may generate hypotheses that can be tested by research. If the null hypothesis is rejected, the study results provide evidence for the accuracy of the theory. If the study results fail to reject the null hypothesis, the results do not confirm the theory and the theory may need to be revised (Kazdin, 2017). A theoretical understanding of causation is considered important because it improves our ability to predict and, in some cases, control events in the real world. The purpose of an interventional design, such as an experimental design, is to examine cause and effect. The independent variable in a study is the proposed cause, and the dependent variable is expected to reflect the effect of the independent variable (Leedy & Ormrod, 2019).

Multicausality

Multicausality, the recognition that several interrelated variables are involved in causing a specific effect, is a more recent idea related to causality. Because of the complexity of causal relationships, a theory rarely identifies every variable involved in causing an effect to occur. Even well-designed studies are unlikely to include every component influencing a desired change or effect (Kazdin, 2017). In our lives, we use multicausality to explain routine activities and outcomes. Think about the multiple causes of a lamp emitting light. At a system level, the lamp's light can be explained by complex power grids delivering electricity to a neighborhood. You might describe the cause of the lamp emitting light by the conductivity of the wires and the

of causality is the cause must be present whenever the effect occurs (Box 11.2).

A group of philosophers known as essentialists began considering causality during the time of Plato and Aristotle. According to the philosophy of essentialism, two types of relationships characterize causality: necessary and sufficient. **Necessary** means the cause is required before the outcome can occur. In other words, the effect cannot occur unless the cause first occurs. **Sufficient** means that the effect occurs when the cause occurs, without any other factor being present (Gleiss & Schemper, 2019). This leaves no room for a variable that may sometimes, but not always, serve as the cause of an effect. John Stuart Mill, a philosopher, states that in addition to the preceding criteria for causation, there must be no alternative explanations for why a change in one variable seems to lead to a change in a second variable flow of the electrical current or particles, waves, and subparticles. If something as simple as a lamp involves multiple causes, how many causes may be involved in producing human thoughts and behaviors, such as adhering to medications.

Few phenomena in nursing can be clearly reduced to a single cause and a single effect. However, the more causal factors that can be identified and explored, the clearer the understanding of the phenomenon. A clearer understanding improves our ability to predict and control. For example, when patients are prescribed oral hypoglycemic medications or insulin injections for hyperglycemia, we cannot predict whether the medication will effectively lower hemoglobin A1c, the desired long-term effect. We know that a patient's nutritional intake, physical activity, and adherence to the medication affect the outcome. There are also genetic and cellular factors that determine the physiological response of the pancreas and the insulin sensitivity of the body cells. Environmental factors such as the safety of the neighborhood and availability of healthy foods may contribute to whether the patient achieves normoglycemia. Among persons with diabetes, nurse researchers have studied the effects of self-management (Milo & Connelly, 2019), health literacy and patients' self-efficacy (Chen, Hsu, Wang, Lee, & Hsieh, 2019), health-related stigma (Jeong, Quinn, Kim, & Martyn-Nemeth, 2018), and an intervention to prevent cognitive decline (Cuevas, Stuifbergen, Brown, & Ward, 2019). Despite these and many other studies, the causal factors involved are complex and have not been clearly delineated. The research evidence needed to promote adherence to medication, diet, and other healthy behaviors among patients with type 2 diabetes is still being developed, in part due to multicausality.

Manipulation

Manipulation has a negative connotation as a word because it is associated with a person coercing or underhandedly maneuvering someone else to act in ways that benefit the first person. In practice, however, nurses manipulate the environment by dimming the lights in the intensive care unit (ICU) at night, the musculoskeletal system by assisting a patient to ambulate, or the gastrointestinal system by irrigating a nasogastric tube. In practice, a major role of nurses is to implement interventions that involve the manipulation of events related to patients and their environment to improve their health.

Manipulation has a specific meaning when used in experimental or quasi-experimental research: **manipulation** is the implementation of the study treatment or intervention (Creswell & Creswell, 2018; Gravetter & Forzano, 2018). Kim, Gang, Lee, and Park (2019) conducted a quasi-experimental study with older adults who had mild cognitive impairment. The researchers implemented a self-care intervention to decrease the participants' depression and increase their self-efficacy, quality of life (QoL), cognitive function, and dementia-prevention behaviors. In this study, the outcomes of the **treatment group**, comprised of participants who receive the intervention, were compared to those of patients in a **control group**, patients who did not receive the intervention (Leedy & Ormrod, 2019). In nursing research, when quasi-experimental and experimental designs are used to explore causal relationships, the nurse must be free to manipulate the variables under study. For example, in a study of pain management, if the physician is the only healthcare provider able to manipulate the pain medication, a nurse researcher cannot conduct a quasi-experimental or experimental study testing different pain management medications.

Interventions or manipulations may be described as environmental, scenario, instructional, and physiological (Adams & Lawrence, 2019). An environmental manipulation would be determining whether preoperative patients hear their selection of music or normal noise during the preoperative period. The anxiety of the group listening to their choice of music and the group hearing normal noise could be compared. As an example of a scenario interaction, a researcher could randomly assign newly graduated nurses to watch one of three videos of nurse-physician interactions before measuring their confidence in calling the physician. Instructional manipulations consist of delivering patient and family teaching in different formats before measuring the knowledge of the participants. A physiological manipulation occurs in a study when one group receives an existing medication and another group receives a newly developed medication. These categories are not mutually exclusive nor do they represent all the possible interventions that may be tested (Adams & Lawrence, 2019).

Researchers use tables or diagrams to indicate when a treatment (manipulation) occurs during a study. The table format we are using was borrowed from Leedy and Ormrod (2019) because we found it to be

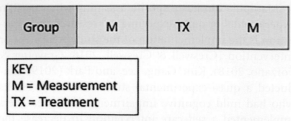

Fig. 11.1 Diagramming interventional designs.

Randomization	Treatment Group	M	TX	M
	Control Group	M		M

KEY
M = Measurement
TX = Treatment

Fig. 11.2 Two-group, pretest-posttest interventional design with randomization.

understandable. Within the columns of the table, you will see TX for treatment, M for measurement, or empty for neither (Fig. 11.1). Rows are used to separate the groups. In Fig. 11.1, the researchers measured the dependent variable, implemented the treatment, and then measured the variable again. The researchers also collected data about other variables, but the emphasis was on the dependent variable that they expected to be changed by the treatment. In Fig. 11.2, the researchers recruited a sample, randomly assigned the participants to a treatment group and a control group before measuring the dependent variable, implementing the treatment to the treatment group only, and measuring the dependent variable. We will use this format to display the interventional designs included in this chapter.

Random Selection

When the intent is to generalize findings to an entire target population, the researcher randomly selects participants to be in the study. **Random selection** means that the researcher chooses elements from the accessible population in a manner that allows each element to have an equal opportunity or chance of being selected (Creswell & Creswell, 2018). As a result, the randomly

selected sample, if large enough, will have the characteristics of the accessible population and in almost the same proportions of those characteristics of the target population. Random sampling may also be called probabilistic sampling (Creswell & Creswell, 2018; Gravetter & Forzano, 2018). (See Chapter 15 for a thorough explanation of populations and samples, and ways in which random sampling may be performed.)

Random sampling is a tactic that increases external design validity—the extent to which results are generalizable to the population (Gravetter & Forzano, 2018). Although a study that uses a random sample has better external design validity than one that does not, an experimental design does not require random sampling.

Random Assignment

Random assignment to groups after participants have been selected and have agreed to be in a study. Whether a study's method of selection is random or nonrandom does not affect the process of random assignment (Kazdin, 2017). The two are different strategies. **Random assignment** is the process of assigning each member of the sample to one of the groups, so that each participant has an equal chance of being in the treatment group (Gravetter & Forzano, 2018). When the sample is large and the participants are randomly assigned to the experimental group and the nonexperimental group, the researcher can expect any extraneous variables to be equally distributed between the groups (Gravetter & Forzano, 2018). You also expect demographic variables to be distributed equally so that the groups are very similar to one another. This allows the researcher to be relatively certain that the group differences in their behaviors, lab values, or clinical course can be attributed to the effects of the experimental intervention, the essence of internal design validity.

Even though the groups are expected to be quite similar, researchers typically compare the experimental group characteristics and control group characteristics. The results usually are displayed as table 1 in the research report, with the percentage distribution in each variable per group, for confirmation of their sameness. In a research report, the information in the first table describes the sample and provides information that helps readers critically appraise the internal and external design validity of a study (Hayes-Larson, Kezios, Mooney, & Lovasi, 2019).

An example would be an examination of the proportion of men versus women in both groups. Instead of expecting the reader to compare the percentages of women in the treatment group and the control group, the researcher will conduct a post hoc test or post hoc analysis. A **post hoc test** is a statistical test to determine if there are statistically significant differences between the groups (Grove & Cipher, 2020). (The term *post hoc* comes from the Latin "after this one.") In table 1, the demographic variables and other known extraneous variables, such as age and medical diagnoses, are described along with the results of the post hoc analyses. For example, El-Deen and Youssef (2018) conducted a quasi-experimental study with patients receiving once-daily subcutaneous anticoagulant injection. They used random assignment to form three groups: a group receiving cryotherapy (ice application) before the injection, a group receiving cryotherapy after the injection, and a control group. In their study report, El-Deen and Youssef (2018) used random assignment to ensure "every patient had an equal probability of being assigned to any of the three groups" and produce "an unbiased representation of the groups" (p. 224). Their table 1 included gender, education, employment status, marital status, and ages, the latter being divided into three categories: 18 to 35 years, 36 to 59 years, and 60 years and older. The table also included the results of the chi-square analyses examining differences in the distributions of the demographic variables across groups, none of which was statistically significant, indicating the similarity of the groups. Random assignment resulted in approximately equivalent groups.

Control

Control in research design means preventing or attenuating the effects of potentially extraneous variables (Cook & Campbell, 1979), a serious issue for interventional research. Exerting control merely means either eliminating the effect of an extraneous variable or measuring its effect on the dependent variable. A **highly controlled setting** almost always implies a research lab or a hospital unit especially designed for the conduct of research. In these environments, intrusion is minimized, and extraneous variables such as sound, light, and temperature are regulated. Basic research usually takes place in a highly controlled environment (Cook & Campbell, 1979).

Random assignment to groups and controlling environmental conditions can prevent many extraneous

variables from affecting the dependent variable. When it is not feasible to control for the effects of known extraneous variables through design (random selection, random assignments, setting), researchers may analyze the relationships between a potential extraneous variable and the dependent variable. The presence of a statistically significant relationship between an extraneous variable and the dependent variable is a threat to internal design validity. A researcher may be able to remove or decrease the threat by statistically controlling the extraneous variable's influence.

Control Groups and Comparison Groups

A **control group** in interventional research is comprised of the participants who do not receive the intervention (Leedy & Ormrod, 2019). Random assignment, described in the previous section, is one strategy for forming control groups. Participants randomly assigned to a control group do not receive the intervention, and these participants are the group to which the experimental group is compared. Therefore these groups are considered independent, and the mean of the dependent variable in the control group will be compared to the treatment group's mean of the dependent variable (Adams & Lawrence, 2019; Grove & Cipher, 2020).

In addition to random assignment, a control group can be selected by matching characteristics of nontreated participants to the characteristics of treated participants (Leedy & Ormrod, 2019) or by using subjects as their own controls. The reason these are considered control groups is that they control, at least to some extent, for the effects of confounding and extraneous variables. The point of differentiation, however, is the extent to which the control group controls for these variables. In addition, these groups are considered dependent or paired so the statistical analyses conducted to identify differences vary from those conducted to identify differences in dependent groups (Grove & Cipher, 2020).

Gregory et al. (2019) conducted a retrospective, quasi-experimental study to examine whether cholesterol testing of obese children would result in weight loss within the next 18 months. From the electronic health records of a large primary care network, the researchers identified children ages 9 to 11 years who attended a well-child visit and had a body mass index (BMI) that was 85% or above. The records for 7765 children met the initial criteria. The 904 children who were tested for cholesterol levels comprised the treatment group. Before matching, the untested group ($n = 6861$) differed from the treatment group on race/ethnicity, Medicaid status, extent of obesity, and clinic sites. From the untested pool, a child was identified who matched each tested child on "sex, race/ethnicity, insurance payer, practice site, time since prior well visit, visit year, modified BMI z-score at the time of testing, and modified BMI z-score at prior well visit" (Gregory et al., 2019, p. 775). After matching, the treatment and control groups had no statistical differences on demographic and weight-related variables.

Because the purpose of a control group is to control for the effect of extraneous variables, a researcher using a nonrandomly selected control group should discuss the characteristics of the control group in the study's limitations. The researcher must argue the extent to which the control group was similar to the treatment group and actually controlled for extraneous variables. Gregory et al. (2019) noted the similarities between the matched groups, but also acknowledged significant study limitations.

> "Our study has several limitations. Even using advanced matching programs, we had difficulty identifying matches for all tested children with regards to BMI.... Our findings addressed only 9- to 11-year olds with elevated BMI in a single health system and may not be generalizable to other populations. Though matching is quasi-experimental, this remains an observational study. We cannot account for unmeasured potential confounders, such as family history, patient preferences, individual motivation, or resources to support change (Stuart, 2010)." (Gregory et al., 2019, p. 778)

The researchers described their study as being quasi-experimental but stated the study was not a test of causality due to the facts that they did not control the treatment and experienced challenges in identifying a matched control group. When a control group is identified through matching and the groups are equivalent, matching is a study strength. However, as in this study, matching did not result in group equivalence and was a limitation. Gregory et al. (2019) found that cholesterol testing as a risk assessment for overweight and obese children was not followed by changes in BMI, as they had hoped.

Comparison groups are groups created for comparison, and they are not products of random assignment. When a researcher identifies one of the groups in a study as a control group, but it does not control for any extraneous variables, the group is by default a comparison group. This is the case in which research data are compared with national norms or averages, or with standard universal values, such as serum sodium levels. When researchers use national norms or averages, they are not creating a control group but using the norms or averages as a comparison group. Comparison groups also may be patients receiving standard care while the treatment group receives the intervention.

Prospective Versus Retrospective

In Chapter 10, prospective and retrospective studies were discussed for noninterventional studies. With interventional designs, studies are more likely to be **prospective**, as in looking forward. Data collection in experimental research is prospective because the researcher enacts the research intervention in real time and then measures its effect. Prospective refers to measurements of the dependent variable that occur after the beginning of the experiment. In a prospective experimental design, a researcher may retrospectively collect demographic data from the medical record but is still said to be conducting prospective experimental research if the intervention and measurements of the dependent variable occur in real time. Researchers, as in the case of Gregory et al. (2019), may use retrospective data with quasi-experimental designs. However, with retrospective studies, the researchers' control of the intervention is possibly limited and the study may have significant threats to validity. For example, because of the threats to validity, Gregory et al. (2019) acknowledged that their study was actually an observational or descriptive design.

Partitioning

Partitioning means dividing a variable into subsets for analysis. The variable being divided may be the independent variable under the control of the researcher or it may be a potentially confounding variable. If the independent variable (the treatment) is partitioned, the researcher may randomly assign participants to the control group and to multiple treatment groups, each of which will receive varying amounts or doses of the independent variable. In healthcare literature, these designs are also called factorial designs. **Factorial designs** allow the researcher to compare different groups of participants with different levels of the independent variable or other variables.

One example of a prospective factorial design would be a quasi-experimental study of adherence to newly prescribed nonsteroidal anti-inflammatory drugs (NSAIDs) among persons with osteoarthritis in one or more joints. After receiving the prescription, the participants are scheduled for a follow-up clinic visit in 8 weeks and asked to bring their pill bottles with them. As you enroll the participants in the study, they are randomly assigned to different frequencies of reminder text messages. Treatment group 1 receives a weekly text message reminder, treatment group 2 receives a text message reminder every other week, and treatment group 3 receives a text message reminder during the third and sixth weeks. The control group receives no text messages. At the follow-up visit, all participants complete a self-report medication adherence scale and their remaining pills are counted. Fig. 11.3 provides a diagram of the design. The statistical analysis will determine whether there are differences in medication adherence among the groups.

Partitioning may occur during the data analysis stage when no differences are found between a treatment group and a control group, but the researcher identifies differences among the participants on another variable. What if, in the osteoarthritis study, your results indicated that adherence varied by age? Because the intervention is text messaging in the osteoarthritis study, you wonder if the age of the participants affects the effectiveness of text messaging. Fig. 11.4 displays this design. The treatment and control groups were originally formed by random assignment. During data analysis, each group can be partitioned by age (<60 years old and ≥60 years old) to create a factorial design.

Factorial designs are complex. Research teams designing studies that include partitioning and factorial designs will need a statistical consultant during the design and analysis phases. The sample size for factorial design (partitioned) studies will need to be larger to ensure an adequate number of participants in each subgroup.

		Week 1	Week 2	Week 3	Week 4	Week 5	Week 6	Week 7	Week 8
Randomization	Treatment Group 1	TX	TX	TX	TX	TX	TX	TX	M
	Treatment Group 2		TX		TX		TX		M
	Treatment Group 3			TX			TX		M
	Control Group								M

KEY
M = Measurement
TX = Treatment

Fig. 11.3 Partitioning a treatment with three treatment groups.

	Week 1	Week 2	Week 3	Week 4	Week 5	Week 6	Week 7	Week 8
Treatment Group 1 <60	TX	TX	TX	TX	TX	TX	TX	M
Treatment Group 1 60 or >	TX	TX	TX	TX	TX	TX	TX	M
Treatment Group 2 <60		TX		TX		TX		M
Treatment Group 2 60 or >		TX		TX		TX		M
Treatment Group 3 <60			TX			TX		M
Treatment Group 3 60 or >			TX			TX		M
Control Group <60								M
Control Group 60 or >								M

KEY
M = Measurement
TX = Treatment

Fig. 11.4 Postanalysis using partitioning of treatment and age with three treatment groups.

STUDY INTERVENTIONS

The intervention is obviously a key component of interventional designs. A rigorous interventional design requires careful planning of the intervention, training of the persons who will be implementing the intervention, and ensuring the reliability and fidelity of the intervention. Intervention mapping is a methodological strategy that is useful in translating evidence from prior research into researchable interventions (Eldredge et al., 2016; Kienen, Wiltenburg, Bittencourt, & Scarinci, 2019). Table 11.1 includes the six steps of intervention mapping with application to the research process. Steps 1 and 2 of intervention mapping involve clarifying the statement of the research problem and concepts that you want to measure. This section will incorporate steps 3 through 6 as an outline. The steps are numbered consecutively but are iterative (Eldredge et al., 2016). As you complete later steps, you may need to edit the results of an earlier step to ensure congruence.

Selecting or Developing an Intervention

There are several sources of interventions for a prospective study. In this section, three sources will be described: study frameworks, research evidence, and previously classified nursing interventions. As an example of the first source, Singelis, Garcia, Barker, and Davis (2018) tested Mexican mothers' perceptions of two oral health pamphlets and the behavioral intentions related to their messages. They developed the pamphlets, the intervention, based on a two-dimensional theory of cultural sensitivity in health communication (Resnicow, Braithwaite, Ahluwalia, & Baranowski, 1999). In the article, the researchers described in detail how the pamphlets incorporated the concept of the theory. In another study, Oertle, Burrell, and Pirollo (2016) identified their study framework to be a nursing theory, the Neuman Systems Model (Neuman & Fawcett, 2011). Oertle et al. (2016) conducted a quasi-experimental study with early cancer survivors to test an exercise intervention designed to

TABLE 11.1	**Intervention Mapping and Application to Developing an Interventional Study**	
Steps in Intervention Development	**Application to Research Process**
1. Needs assessment What is the specific need of the target population to be addressed by the study?	During literature review, identify the research problem for the target population. Explore the study with members and leaders of the proposed population. This study is more likely to be completed when researchers are using community-based participatory research.
2. Performance objectives As a result of the intervention, who and what is expected to change?	Define/refine the inclusion and exclusion sampling criteria for the study to reduce potential confounding variables. Identify the dependent variable.
3. Theory-based intervention How does the intervention link to the concepts of the study framework?	Conceptually and operationally define the dependent variable. Define and describe the intervention as part of the study framework.
4. Intervention plan What are the concrete steps in implementing the intervention?	Develop the intervention protocol. Include as many details as possible: location, materials needed, who will implement, length of the intervention, content of an educational intervention, steps of an action-oriented intervention.
5. Implementation What are the organizational details that combine the unique characteristics of the intervention and the organization?	Who needs to be aware of the study and its intervention? In what clinical areas will participants be recruited? Identify space where the intervention will be implemented.
6. Evaluation How will the intervention be evaluated?	How will the researchers ensure the intervention is implemented consistently? Who will evaluate the intervention's fidelity? How will it be evaluated?

Adapted from Kienen, N., Wiltenburg, T., Bittencourt, L., & Scarinci, I. (2019). Development of a gender-relevant for tobacco cessation intervention for women in Brazil—an intervention mapping approach to planning. *Health Education Research*, 34(5), 505–520. doi:10.1093/her/cyz025

decrease cancer-related fatigue (CRF). The Neuman Systems Model views the human being as having a core of basic structures and resources surrounded by concentric circles called lines of resistance, normal lines of defense, and flexible lines of defense. Nursing actions are categorized as primary, secondary, or tertiary prevention. The human being's flexible and normal lines of defense attempt to protect the core from stressors. If these lines are penetrated, the lines of resistance are the last level of protection. Oertle et al. (2016) described the exercise program in the language of the model as being "a tertiary intervention to promote health and improve QoL by reducing CRF and strengthening the patient's flexible lines of defense" (p. 10).

The second source of interventions is research evidence. Evidence-based guidelines or a synthesis of research findings may provide interventions or evoke ideas for potential interventions. Mathew and Thukha (2018) reviewed the literature related to the role of education

in cardiac rehabilitation following a hospitalization for heart failure among older adults. Based on the findings of several studies and scientific statements of national professional organizations, Mathew and Thukha (2018) developed a nurse-led, patient-centered heart failure education intervention. They conducted a pilot study in a postacute unit, where older adults may be admitted for cardiac rehabilitation. White-Lewis, Johnson, Ye, and Russell (2019) reviewed the research related to equine-assisted therapy (EAT) and found significant evidence of its benefits in meta-analyses and systematic reviews. The research problem was that EAT had not been tested among adults and older adults with arthritis. White-Lewis et al. (2019) conducted a randomized controlled trial (RCT) of 20 participants, basing the sample size on 31 other studies of EAT with an average of 18 participants. Despite the small size, the researchers found significant improvement in QoL and in the pain and range of joint motion.

TABLE 11.2	Classifications of Nursing Interventions: Source of Interventions for Research
System	**Related Resources**
Clinical Care Classification (CCC)	https://www.sabacare.com/
International Classification for Nursing Practice (ICNP)	https://www.icn.ch/what-we-do/projects/ehealth-icnp/about-icnp
Nursing Interventions Classification (NIC)	http://www.nursing.uiowa.edu/cncce/nic-publications

Nursing intervention classification systems can be another source of interventions for studies. There are three primary nursing intervention classification (NIC) systems: One was developed by nurse informaticists for use in electronic health records (Clinical Care Classification); another was developed as a logical companion to nursing diagnoses (NIC); and the last one was developed by the International Council of Nursing to classify nursing phenomena, actions, and outcomes for nurses around the world (International Classification for Nursing Practice). These classification systems are a source of interventions for studies. Table 11.2 contains these classification systems for nursing interventions with their related websites. Sampaio, Araújo, Sequeira, Canut, and Martins (2018) conducted an RCT of the interventions for anxiety, included in the NIC, with a sample of Portuguese participants diagnosed with anxiety. The control group received usual care (psychopharmacotherapy) and the treatment group received psychopharmacotherapy plus nursing interventions. During the first session, nursing diagnoses were identified so that selected nursing interventions could be implemented in subsequent sessions. The treatment group experienced a significantly greater decrease in anxiety than did the control group.

Preparing for Implementation

In a well-designed experimental study, the researcher has complete control of any treatment that is provided. The first step in achieving control is to develop a detailed description of the treatment to ensure standardization of the treatment. The detailed description of the treatment to be implemented in a study is often called an **intervention protocol**. The researchers' thoughts and intents related to the intervention must be delineated into the components that are hypothesized to cause the effect (Crawford, Freeman, Huscroft-D'Angelo, Fuentes, & Higgins, 2019). The study conducted by Sampaio et al. (2018) with adult psychiatric outpatients living with anxiety included a detailed protocol for the intervention.

"The individual-based intervention was provided by a mental health nurse (FS). A total of five sessions were delivered over five consecutive weeks (i.e. one 45–60-minute weekly session). This psychotherapeutic intervention model in nursing recommends delivering 3–12 sessions. It was yet our decision to set an equal number of sessions for all the participants to avoid bias related to the length of the intervention.... Intervention took place at a consultation room located in the psychiatry outpatient ward.... The protocol of this study (prospectively registered in the United States of America Clinical Trials Registry Platform) was methodically designed and the process was meticulously documented to ensure its potential reproduction." (Sampaio et al., 2018, p. 118, 119).

A clear, detailed protocol is needed for intervention studies to support their internal design validity. As Sampaio et al. (2018) noted, the goal is to document the intervention protocol with adequate detail so that other researchers can reproduce the intervention. Sequencing the interventions and other strategies may be part of the protocol.

Sequencing Interventions

In some studies, each subject receives several different treatments sequentially (e.g., relaxation, distraction, and visual imagery) or various levels of the same treatment (e.g., different doses of a drug or varying lengths of relaxation time). Sometimes the application of one treatment can influence the response to later treatments, a phenomenon referred to as a **carryover effect** (Adams & Lawrence, 2019). The carryover effect may also be called the **order effect**, labeled as such because the order of the interventions may influence the dependent variable (Gravetter & Forzano, 2018). If a carryover effect is known to occur, the researcher may be able to minimize its effect by allowing for washout or using a counterbalanced design.

Washout is scheduling time between interventions to allow the effect of the first to dissipate before initiating the next one (Handley, Lyles, McCulloch, & Cattamanchi, 2018). Washout is especially pertinent to the effects of medications, when each participant is going to receive each medication being tested in the study but can also apply to nonmedication studies. For example, Kako et al. (2018) conducted a pilot study to determine the washout period for a fan-to-face intervention for dyspnea among persons with advanced cancer. They learned that 1 hour was an insufficient washout period, which was the information the researchers needed to design a larger study comparing this intervention to other interventions.

The second strategy is **counterbalancing**, administering the various treatments in random order rather than providing them in the same sequence (Adams & Lawrence, 2019; Kazdin, 2017). Ward et al. (2019) published the protocol for a crossover design study of the effects of sleep deprivation on eating behaviors of children. The participants will be randomized to two groups. One group will be exposed to a baseline week, a sleep-deprivation week, a washout week, and a sleep extension week. The second group will also begin with a baseline week, followed by a sleep-extension week, a washout week, and a sleep-deprivation week. "Use of a cross-over design reduces confounders, as each participant receives the same number of experimental manipulations over the same amount of time" (Ward et al, 2019, p. 3). Another critical element of the protocol is the timing and conditions of the measurements.

Measurements Relative to Interventions

The conditions under which the measurements occur and when they occur relative to the intervention should be decided during protocol development. White-Lewis et al. (2019) conducted a RCT of equine-assisted treatment, as described earlier in the chapter. The researchers provided details of the equine intervention, but also provided details of the measurements in this excerpt.

"Pain and active range of motion in the back, knees, hips, and shoulders, and quality of life measurement occurred at baseline and post intervention at weeks three and six. Active range of motion (ROM) was measured with a hand-held goniometer that measures the joint angle in degrees. The participant bent the joint until stiffness began. Measurements included shoulder range of motion (abduction and flexion), back range of motion (forward and bilateral flexion), knee (flexion), and hip (abduction and flexion with knee flexed and extended).... Pain was measured using the 1–100mm Visual Analog Scale (VAS) (Ferreira-Valente, Pais-Ribeiro, & Jensen, 2011), which has moderate to good reliability in measuring musculoskeletal pain.... Quality of life (QOL) was measured using the Arthritis Impact Measurement Scale 2 (AIMS 2) short form using a five-point Likert scale. The AIMS2 has content, construct, and convergent validity...." (White-Lewis et al., 2019, p. 7)

The most detailed protocol will not ensure the credibility of a study's findings unless the persons implementing the intervention and measurements follow the protocol.

Training of Research Assistants

A researcher is fortunate when financial support is available to hire research assistants to complete study-related tasks, which may include implementing the intervention and collecting the data. Research assistants can provide practical support if the researcher is willing to invest the time and effort to properly train them (French, Diekemper, & Irwin, 2015). They need to understand the purpose of the study, how to complete the tasks they will be assigned, and the ethical principles guiding the study (Chang, Chao, Jang, & Lu, 2019). When research assistants will be responsible for obtaining informed consent, the researchers may choose to video record the description and procedures of the study to ensure consistency and accuracy (Kazdin, 2017). Most institutional review boards (IRBs) will require that all members of the research team complete research ethics training. See Chapter 9 for more information about research ethics.

One component of the preparation of research assistants is the necessity to follow the protocol for the intervention, an important component of intervention fidelity (Von Visger et al., 2019). Research assistants are often assigned to collect data from a study's participants relative to the intervention. Preparing and using a script when giving instructions to the participants can reduce variability between data collectors and experimenter bias. **Experimenter bias** occurs when a measurement is affected by the data collector's beliefs about outcomes of the study (Kazdin, 2017). The data collector's personal beliefs are less likely to have an influence on the intervention and data collection when a script is followed for the interaction with participants. Another way to decrease the potential for experimenter bias is to blind the data collectors to group membership.

Blinding

Experimenter expectancies and participants knowing their group assignment are threats to construct design validity. Blinding is a strategy to minimizing these threats. **Blinding** (or masking) is the strategy of not revealing to subjects whether they are experimental or control subjects. They do not know their group assignment. **Double-blinding** is the strategy of withholding information about group assignment from both subjects and data collectors (Cook & Campbell, 1979). This is a common practice in trials of new medications, in which participants receive either the experimental drug or a placebo. It is customary for one member of the research team, usually the pharmacist in medication studies, to know the group assignments of all subjects. Depending on the study design and the intervention, blinding may not be possible but is used when feasible.

Planning for Evaluation

The final step in intervention planning (see Table 11.1) is to plan strategies to ensure consistency in implementing the treatment. Consistency, or intervention fidelity, may involve elements of the treatment such as equipment, time, intensity, sequencing, and staff skill.

Fidelity of the Intervention

Intervention fidelity requires a protocol to standardize the elements of the treatment and a plan for training to ensure consistent implementation of the treatment protocol (Chang et al., 2019). Intervention reliability is another term often used interchangeably with intervention fidelity. **Intervention reliability** ensures that the research treatment is standardized and applied consistently each time it is administered in a study. If the method of administering a research intervention varies from one person to another, the effect size is decreased (Kazdin, 2017) and the risk of Type II error increases.

Monitoring the Intervention

The researcher cannot assume that the intervention will be administered correctly to the appropriate participants. It is recommended that the treatment's fidelity be monitored (Adams & Lawrence, 2018; French et al.,

2015). Several options for evaluating the intervention's implementation have been used. Some researchers have obtained permission from participants to video record the intervention. The researcher watches the recording and completes a checklist of key elements to assess the intervention. A researcher (or an observer) may evaluate the fidelity of an intervention as it is being implemented through observing and documenting the assessments. The researchers may include in the study proposal to evaluate the implementation of the intervention a set number of times. Monitoring should continue over the course of the study. The research assistant may become relaxed and less attentive to detail as the study progresses. The researcher may choose to evaluate the fidelity of an intervention a set number of times per research assistant early and late in the study.

Mapping the intervention during the planning of a study provides the structure for ongoing evaluation and refinement of the intervention. The more consistently the intervention is implemented, the greater the potential effect size and study quality.

THREATS TO VALIDITY IN INTERVENTIONAL STUDIES

Designs are developed to reduce threats that might invalidate the study's results. Although a single study cannot mitigate all threats to validity (Gravetter & Forzano, 2018), some designs are more effective in reducing threats than others. It may be necessary to modify the design to reduce a specific threat. Before selecting a design, you must identify the design validity threats that are most likely to reduce the credibility of your study. These threats are related to construct design validity, internal design validity, external design validity, and statistical conclusion design validity.

Construct Design Validity

Construct design validity is the congruence between the conceptual definition of a variable and the operational definition (Gravetter & Forzano, 2018). Even with closely aligned definitions, incongruence can emerge when measurements are implemented without attention to the study conditions. Table 11.3 includes threats to construct design validity. Construct design validity of interventional studies share five threats to validity with noninterventional studies, marked by a superscript a in Table 11.3. However, interventional studies may have four additional threats to construct design validity.

TABLE 11.3	Threats to Construct Design Validity for Interventional Studies	
Threat	**Definition**	**How to Avoid or Minimize the Threat**
Inadequate preoperational clarification of constructs[a]	Unclear conceptual definitions result in being unable to determine the congruence between the conceptual and operational definitions.	Conduct a concept analysis of primary constructs if not previously done. Compare potential instruments with defining attributes of the construct. Use instruments in a pilot study with participants who meet the study's inclusion/exclusion sampling criteria to ensure meaning is clear for the specific sample. Ensure that the control condition incorporates potentially confounding variables, such as positive social contact.
Confounding levels of constructs	The intensity or abstractness of constructs are not accurately measured.	Extract from research reports the operational definitions of similar interventions. Pilot test the sensitivity of the measurements and the effect of treatments.
Mono-operational bias[a]	The use of a single measurement does not capture the construct completely.	For research variables, quantify using more than one measurement method.
Monomethod bias[a]	The use of a single type of measurement fails to capture the construct completely.	For research variables, use multiple types of measures (not all pencil-paper).
Social desirability[a]	Participants provide data they believe will conform to attitudes and behaviors of which others approve.	Include in data collection directions that there are no right or wrong answers and that all questions must be answered honestly. Measure social desirability and analyze its relationship with the dependent variable. If correlated, may need to control the effects of social desirability statistically.
Other social interaction threats	The communication between the researchers and participants may cause desired effect even without the intervention.	Minimize these threats by delivering a control intervention that is comparable to the treatment intervention in social interaction. Create a safe environment for performance of skills and measurement of variables.
Careless responding[a]	Participants are not engaged in carefully and thoughtfully completing measurements.	Assess using direct, archival, or statistical methods. Exclude cases that indicate careless responding.
Interaction of study components	The measurements and treatments have effects on each other that are unintended.	Include time in protocol for effect of one treatment to washout before initiating the second treatment. Separate pretesting from the intervention by a week or more to decrease testing effects.
Guessing the hypothesis or group assignment	Participants figure out the hypothesis or the group they are in and act differently than they would have otherwise have acted.	Use blinding to group assignment for participants and most of the research team.

[a]Threats to construct design validity for noninterventional studies as well as interventional studies.

Inadequate Preoperational Clarification of Constructs

Construct design validity is important in any quantitative study but is especially important in interventional research. Not only is a complete and detailed operational definition needed for the dependent variables,

but the same is needed for the primary independent variable, the treatment. The content in the previous section on intervention mapping lays the groundwork for a well-defined and consistently implemented treatment. However, interventions may contain a confounding variable. Especially in nursing research, the researchers delivering the treatment (independent variable) possess social skills. Interaction with them is pleasant for research subjects. Positive social contact can be a confounding variable, one that can be mitigated by including positive social contact to the control condition. For example, the research design may include a member of the research team spending an equal amount of time with each member of the control group.

Confounding Constructs and Levels of Constructs

A threat to construct design validity is being uncertain or unclear about the level of constructs that are being implemented, especially the independent variable. When nonlinear relationships exist between the independent variable and dependent variable, the level of the construct being measured must be known by the researcher. For example, you are conducting a study of the effect of diabetic education (independent variable) on intention to adopt the prescribed diet (dependent variable). If the independent variable is defined as a factual educational message with limited persuasive content that lasted 20 minutes, no effect may be detected in participants' intention to adopt the prescribed diet. Participants learn no new content and are not motivated to make a change in behavior. However, if the independent variable is defined as a highly persuasive message with limited factual content that lasts 2 hours, a negative effect on participants' intention to adopt the prescribed diet may be detected. Participants may become angry when they perceive the message to be coercive and intimidating. The educational intervention in the first case would have been reported as being ineffective and in the second case, harmful. If the independent variable had been defined as a message with an equal balance of facts and persuasion that lasted 45 minutes, the study results may have been different. Pilot testing the intervention at different levels of intensity is one way to minimize this threat. Another way is to examine prior research using the same type of intervention more carefully. Extract the operational definitions of the independent and dependent variables or contact the researchers to obtain details about the intervention or measurement tools.

Mono-Operation Bias

One of the construct design validity threats related to measurement is mono-operation bias. **Mono-operation bias** occurs when only one method of measurement is used to quantify a variable. Complex constructs have many dimensions, which are not captured adequately by one measurement. Using multiple instruments to measure the construct or concept improves the construct design validity (see Chapter 16) (Waltz, Strickland, & Lenz, 2017).

Monomethod Bias

Monomethod bias is using a single method of recording participants' responses. Even when multiple measures are used to measure a variable, monomethod bias may still occur when all measurements are the same type, such as pencil-paper instruments (see Table 11.3). For example, when measuring sleep quality, you might use three pencil-paper instruments. Construct design validity would be improved by using a pencil-paper self-report instrument and a wrist-worn device that measures time to fall asleep, uninterrupted sleep, and total sleep time.

Social Desirability Reponses

Social desirability is wanting others to think well of you during a study (Waltz et al., 2017). As a result, when reporting behaviors or attitudes viewed with positive or negative connotations, you may unconsciously answer in ways to appear better than you are. Instruments that use self-report are more susceptible to social desirability (Adams & Lawrence, 2019; Esopo et al., 2018).

Social desirability can be measured during a study. The most commonly used instrument is the Marlowe-Crowne Social Desirability Scale (Crowne & Marlowe, 1960).

Other Social Interaction Threats

Positive social contact and social desirability have already been described as threats to construct design validity. Other threats to construct design validity are closely related to social desirability. The first is called the Hawthorne effect. The **Hawthorne effect** is participants altering their normal behavior because they know they are being scrutinized (Kerlinger & Lee, 2000). The name comes from a study in which workers at the Hawthorne factory were told that a group was coming to do a study of workers' productivity. The research team was unable to test their hypothesis because the workers increased their productivity and became model employees. The Hawthorne effect is like social desirability among individual participants but tends to exert its effect on a group. Some researchers may choose to use deception when the Hawthorne effect is a concern, by informing the participants the study's purpose is different than it is. Refer to Chapter 9 to review the ethical challenges of using deception.

Evaluation apprehension shares some characteristics with social desirability. **Evaluation apprehension** occurs when participants are anxious because they perceive they are being judged on their attitudes or behaviors. Evaluation apprehension may be intensified when participants already have anxiety, such as the participants in Sampaio et al.'s (2018) study. The study sample was selected because they had anxiety. Evaluation apprehension may also be intensified when the dependent variable involves the performance of a skill such as changing a colostomy bag or giving an injection.

Another threat that may occur because of interaction with the researchers is the novelty effect. The **novelty effect** is when participants respond to measurements differently at the beginning of a study. The participants may be enthusiastic when a study first begins but become less so as the study continues. This threat is more likely in studies with measurements repeated over the course of the study. Participants may become bored or less interested and respond differently to self-report instruments than they did at the beginning of the study. The risk for careless responding increases.

Most social interaction threats are related to the beliefs and personality of the participants. However, experimenter biases are related to the beliefs and personality of the researcher or data collector. Experimenter biases or expectancies were defined in the section on developing scripts as part of the treatment protocol. Experimenter expectancies, also called the Rosenthal effect, expectancy effect, self-fulfilling prophecy, and the Pygmalion effect, are defined as participants tending to perform at the levels the researchers expect (Persaud, 2012). The researcher or data collector, who knows the participant's group assignment or admires some characteristic of the participant, may unconsciously influence the participant's responses to support the hypothesis or to present the participant in a favorable light. The Rosenthal effect can be minimized by using a script for data collectors or video recording instructions so that each participant sees the same person deliver the information. Blinding is also another effective way to minimize the Rosenthal effect.

Careless Responding

Careless responding occurs when participants mark answers or select options without thinking about the question (Grau, Ebbeler, & Banse, 2019). Participants who respond carelessly may have a pattern to their responses, such as marking the highest or lowest option on a Likert scale. Grau et al. (2019) identify three methods to assess whether careless responding occurred: direct, archival, and statistical (see Chapter 10).

Interaction Among Study Components

Study components, such as multiple interventions, can interact so that the operationalization of the variable is altered, threatening construct design validity. When two or more interventions are being tested, the researcher must carefully consider how to deliver the interventions in a way that minimizes possible interactions. The **interaction of different treatments** is defined as the relationships among two or more independent variables being tested in the same study. Partitioning, factorial designs, and counterbalancing are methods to minimize this threat to construct design validity. Refer to prior content in this chapter on partitioning and counterbalancing.

Another threat is the **interaction of testing and treatment**, meaning one element of a study inadvertently influences the construct design validity of another element. For example, in a pretest-posttest design, the pretest may increase the posttest's measured effect. Another way this occurs is that the pretest sensitizes the participant to the intervention so that the intervention's effect may be overestimated. To minimize this threat, separate the pretest and the intervention by 1 week or more (see Table 11.3). This decreases the likelihood that the two elements affect each other.

Guessing Hypotheses or Group Assignment

Participants may be astute and recognize cues in the informed consent document, baseline measurements, and the intervention to guess the hypothesis of the study. **Hypothesis guessing within experimental conditions** is a participant guessing what the study is about and modifying his or her behavior to support the hypothesis. Even when group assignment is blinded to the data collectors and others involved in the study, these persons may be aware of the benefits of the intervention and attempt to provide the benefits to all participants. **Compensatory equalization of treatment** occurs when staff, and even family members, provide the social interaction, extra attention, or other benefits to participants identified as being in the control. Another way that guessing group membership or the hypothesis threatens construct design validity is through compensatory rivalry. **Compensatory rivalry** occurs when participants know they are in the control group and exert additional effort to demonstrate that the treatment from which they were excluded is of no value. Blinding participants and most members of the researcher team to group membership is an effective way to minimize these threats. Another way is to design the study so that the control group is wait-listed. Being **wait-listed** means that a participant will not participate in the first implementation of the intervention but will receive the intervention in the second wave. When participants are informed before the study begins that some participants will receive the intervention in 3 months while others will receive it immediately, the threat of compensatory rivalry may be minimized.

Internal Design Validity

Internal design validity is the degree to which changes in the dependent variable occur as a result of the action of the independent variable (Campbell & Stanley, 1963). Internal design validity is an essential component of the logic of how a dependent variable is changed by an independent variable. With strong internal design validity, the researcher can make a "valid causal inference" (Kenny, 2019, p. 1018). How confident can I be that the treatment made a difference in the dependent variable in this study? This is the question that inspires the researcher in the construction phase of a study to eliminate or control for variables that might alter the treatment delivery, confound the results, or produce a rival hypothesis (Adams & Lawrence, 2019; Kazdin, 2017). Internal design validity reflects design-embedded decisions that control for the effects of extraneous variables. An example of this type of decision in interventional research would be random assignment of a large sample to treatment and control groups, so that proportions of potentially extraneous variables would be similarly distributed between groups.

Table 11.4 lists eight threats to internal design validity, compiled from Campbell and Stanley (1963), Kerlinger and Lee (2000), and Shadish, Cook, and Campbell (2002). Four of the listed threats to internal design validity are also threats for noninterventional studies. We will include these threats in our discussion because they have some unique characteristics in interventional studies.

History

History is an event external to the study that occurs and affects the implementation of the intervention or the value of the dependent variable. An example of history exists in a quasi-experimental study in which a researcher collects data about the effect of an online educational program teaching evidence-based urinary catheter care on daily catheter care being provided and documented. The researcher collects data for 2 weeks, followed by opening the online educational program for the nurses. After the intervention, the researcher collects data for an additional 2 weeks. As the second data collection begins, social media begins reporting a story about the life-threatening blood infection of a famous female athlete. The infection was attributed to a surgery she had to repair a sports injury and the fact that she was hospitalized for a week with a urinary catheter. If quality and frequency of catheter care improve during the second data collection, the researcher cannot be sure whether (1) the extraneous variable of the breaking news story affected the dependent variable, or (2) the educational program was effective.

One way to minimize the threat to internal design validity is random assignment to two groups. With a randomly assigned control group, an external event that is a history threat would affect both groups. Another way to minimize the history threat is to keep the study as short as possible. The longer the study, the more opportunities exist for an event to affect the participants.

Maturation

Another threat to internal design validity is **maturation**, which is defined as normal changes that may occur over the course of a study, such as fatigue, hunger, growth, development, and aging. These changes are due to the passing of time, not because of the independent variable. These normal changes may affect the value of the dependent variable. Longitudinal studies and studies conducted with children and adolescents have a great risk of maturation being a threat to internal design validity. For example, the maturation threat to internal design validity would be an issue in a 3-year study of adolescents' decision making. For this one-group, pretest-posttest study, the adolescents provide responses on two instruments measuring their decision-making abilities as the study begins. During the study, the adolescents receive short messages about their decision making on their preferred social media platform. Every 6 months, the adolescents complete the instruments

TABLE 11.4   Threats to Internal Design Validity for Interventional Studies

Threat	Definition	How to Avoid or Minimize the Threat
History[a]	An event before or during the study alters the participants' responses to the treatment or measurement.	Avoid seasonal fluctuations or other events that may affect the study. Maintain a journal during the study of current events relevant to the study. This log may help researchers assess the extent to which history may have been a threat.
Maturation[a]	Participants continue to grow or develop during the study.	Acknowledge as a potential threat, especially in longitudinal studies. For studies with children and adolescents, select a homogenous sample that is randomly assigned to treatment and control groups.
Selection[a]	People who are recruited or agree to participate are different than people who are not recruited or decided not to participate.	Randomly recruit participants, if possible. Adjust inclusion and exclusion sampling criteria to represent the target population. Consider effects of environment (social, cultural, type of health-care setting) that may limit potential subjects. Provide study materials in the languages used by the target population to allow inclusion of more participants.
Selection-maturation interaction	People who are in the study change in unique ways because of time and of being in the study.	Select a homogenous sample, so that the likelihood of selection-maturation is relatively similar across the groups. Randomly assign participants to the treatment and control groups.
Testing	Initial and repeated measurements affect subsequent measurements.	Use multiple forms of measurement (self-report, physiological measures). Random assignment to treatment and control group.
Instrumentation	Measurements are not consistently or accurately implemented.	Train research assistants and data collectors to calibrate equipment per manufacturer's instruction. Monitor implementation of measurements to ensure they are done correctly and consistently
Statistical regression toward the mean	Extreme pretest measurements tend to become average on subsequent measurements.	Avoid selecting participants based on an extreme value of screening variable that is also the dependent variable. Repeated measures will tend to be closer to the mean than the initial extreme values.
Subject attrition[a]	Participants do not complete the study for personal or other reasons.	Implement strategies to retain subjects in longitudinal studies, such as reminder messages and monetary incentives. Compare those who completed with those who dropped out to determine how the two groups were different.

[a]Internal design validity threats for noninterventional studies as well as interventional studies.

again. At the end of the study, any changes in decision-making abilities may be due to normal growth and development, not the messages they received. To reduce this threat, a two-group, pretest-posttest study could be conducted with adolescents randomly assigned to groups (see Table 11.4). The control group would receive messages on sports every week so that they are also receiving attention from the researchers. The one group study has a significant threat to internal design validity and would not provide valuable information.

Selection

Selection is a threat to internal design validity when the treatment and control groups are dissimilar (see Table 11.4).

Sometimes this occurs because of how the researcher makes group assignments. For example, a researcher decides to place all clinic patients recruited on Wednesday in the treatment group. Think of the implications for the study results if Wednesday appointments are reserved for Medicaid patients. Medicaid patients may have access to care at the clinic but may lack other resources such as reliable housing and healthy food. At other times, the selection threat is introduced when patients may choose whether to be members of the treatment group or the control group. Their decision as to group membership might represent a basic difference between types of subjects, which could affect the value of the dependent variable and nullify the study results.

Selection-Maturation Interaction

Threats to internal design validity can interact with one another, producing new threats. One of the more common is the **selection-maturation interaction**. The interaction can be defined as a threat to internal design validity due to changes over time occurring at different rates in two groups. Nonrandom assignment to the treatment and control groups is a selection threat to internal design validity, because the two groups will have fundamental differences. When the nonrandom groups are participating in a longitudinal study, fatigue, developmental changes, or aging may affect the two groups differently, hence the term selection-maturation interaction. For instance, in a study with nonrandom group assignment, selection-maturation interaction can be a threat if the naturally occurring attributes in one group change due to the passage of time, independent of the study treatment.

Testing

The **testing** threat occurs when completing the pretests changes participants' responses to the posttests taken over the course of a study (see Table 11.4). If the same instrument or scale serves as both the pretest and the posttest of knowledge, participants may learn the answers to the questions because they want to do better on the next test. Completing a different version of the same test, or even a different test, may minimize the threat but does not eliminate it. Using different types of measurement for both the pretest and posttest may minimize this threat in some situations. An example would be using a sphygmomanometer to measure blood pressure, a pencil-paper inventory of exercise and diet, and a VAS of intent to change for a study of hypertension control. A better way to attenuate the threat of testing is to randomly assign participants to the treatment group and the control. Participants in both groups complete the tests. Comparing changes in the control group's scores (received testing) to those in the treatment group (received testing and the intervention) allows the researcher to detect differences due to the intervention.

Instrumentation

Instrumentation, a threat to internal design validity, occurs when changes occur in the instrument or its calibration during a study (Kerlinger & Lee, 2000). Instrumentation can occur when a researcher is studying fluid intake and output of infants who have been prescribed a diuretic while in the neonatal intensive care unit (NICU). One task during the study is weighing the infant's diapers on a small portable scale as a measure of urine output. If this is a multisite study, is the same brand of scales used in all sites? Were data collectors trained on the weighing protocol? Are the scales being recalibrated as recommended by the manufacturer over the course of the study? A negative answer to any of these questions means that instrumentation is a threat to validity.

Instrumentation can also be a threat when using a psychological pencil-paper instrument. For example, your study is being conducted with grandmothers who are parenting one or more grandchildren. The study is a one-group, pretest-posttest study with an intervention targeting developmental stages of children. Following the pretest, you notice that several grandparents omitted questions on the pencil-paper instrument. You consider this as you notice that most of the participants have less than a high school education. You realize that the reading level of the instrument may be too high for this sample. You decide to read the questions aloud to each participant on the posttest. Although you are likely to obtain more complete data, you have now added the threat of instrumentation (Shadish et al., 2002).

Statistical Regression Toward the Mean

The threat of **statistical regression toward the mean** is present when subjects are selected for study participation because they display extreme levels of a screening variable (see Table 11.4). In a large sample, statistical regression toward the mean is the tendency of the extreme values of a variable to be closer to the mean on subsequent measurements. From a large clinical database, the statistician identifies all patients whose low-density lipoprotein (LDL) cholesterol value is at least three times higher than the norm. The researcher randomly selects 200 persons from the high cholesterol group to be recruited for a new medication for persons with extremely high cholesterol values. For some of the subjects, the cholesterol readings represent their normal values, but for others the cholesterol is unusually high due to a transient cause such as a temporary change in diet, an infection, or an illness. The latter subjects would be less likely to demonstrate extreme levels at their next lab draw, regardless of intervention; scores regress toward the mean value. When the medication trial is over, the medication may be found to be effective, based on the decrease in the cholesterol levels after 6 months. However, the researchers should exercise caution because a portion of the decrease may be due to statistical regression to the mean.

The example was a situation in which extremely high screening values became lower on repeated measurements. However, the same can occur in studies for which participants are selected for extremely low values of self-esteem, cognitive function, or a physiological variable. With extremely low values, the repeated measures are likely to rise because of statistical regression to the mean. This threat can alter the mean of the dependent variable and result in the conclusion that the intervention was effective. Exploratory data analysis is a way for researchers to examine their data for outliers, ranges, median, and mode (Grove & Cipher, 2020). Examining the results of this analysis will allow the researchers to identify possible careless responding, extreme levels of variables, and unexplained changes in pretest and posttest data. See Chapter 21 for more information on exploratory and other types of data analysis.

Subject Attrition

Subject attrition is the number and percentage of participants who do not complete a study. The credibility of an interventional study can be severely threated if the attrition rate is different between the treatment and control groups. When attrition is proportionately higher in one group than the other, randomly assigned groups become less alike (Kerlinger & Lee, 2000). The difference in the value of the dependent variable may be due to the researcher's intervention or to dissimilarity between the remaining participants in the groups. Researchers may provide a comparison of the characteristics

of the participants who withdrew and who completed the study, to minimize this threat to internal design validity. Chapter 15 provides more information on subject attrition and retention. Table 11.4 includes the threats to internal design validity with strategies to eliminate or minimize the effects of the threats.

External Design Validity

External design validity is the extent to which research results may be generalized back to the population being studied. We typically think about generalizing the findings to similar members of the population. However, methods and settings can also be generalized (Adams & Lawrence, 2019). The findings of studies with heterogenous samples studied in natural settings have increased external design validity. However, heterogenous samples in less controlled settings may not have controlled for confounding variables and have reduced internal design validity.

There is no perfect balance of internal and external design validity. Internal design validity may be emphasized with a homogenous sample, with inclusion sampling criteria that attempt to eliminate individual characteristics that may be confounding variables. Emphasizing internal design validity is important to establish initial evidence of the effects of an intervention. However, as the evidence supporting the intervention grows, the emphasis may shift to external design validity (Shadish et al., 2002). The researchers need to know to whom the intervention can be generalized.

When a target population has been carefully defined before a study begins and the study sample reflects the characteristics of the target population, the findings can be generalized to the target population (Cook & Campbell, 1979). For example, you conduct a quasi-experimental study with women ages 51 to 70 years to improve their recognition of signs and symptoms of an acute myocardial infarction (AMI). The setting is a church with an active women's program, located in a southern US state. The sample is predominantly White, married, and not employed. The study's significant findings can be generalized to women in groups who are like the sample. How similar do the groups have to be? Can these findings be generalized to Black women who are married, not employed, and active in a church group? The challenge of generalizing becomes more difficult when attempting to generalize across populations. Can these findings be generalized across populations to

Hispanic women who are employed and not affiliated with a religious group?

A factor that limits generalization is a threat to external design validity. Threats are typically based on differences between the conditions of the study and the conditions of persons, settings, or treatments in the target population. Threats to external design validity sometimes have as their basis unusual interactions between the treatment and other study components, such as the setting and sample. These interactions may cause the researcher to draw conclusions that are not true for the general population. Table 11.5 includes threats to external design validity with strategies for attenuating or eliminating the threats.

Homogenous Sample

A homogenous sample is desirable when trying to improve internal design validity. However, a homogenous sample limits generalizability because it is not like the target population. In the United States, women and minority groups have been underrepresented in research (Kazdin, 2017). One of the strategies being used to recruit more diverse and heterogenous samples is forming patient and family advisory councils to engage patients as research partners (Harrison et al., 2019). **Patient and family advisory councils** are representatives of the community who agree to collaborate with academic researchers to propose and implement studies on topics that are concerns for the community. The members of the councils may be able explain a proposed study to others in the community and assist with recruitment. These councils can be viewed as a specific example of community-responsive research approaches.

Community-responsive research approaches are recognizing community members as collaborators in studying problems that are concerns in the community (Shaw, Korchmaros, Torres, Totman, & Lee, 2019). For example, you have developed an intervention to promote healthy eating among adults. The intervention has been found to be effective in selected groups of people, and you have received funding to conduct a large study ($N = 1000$) in your state. How will you recruit a sample that includes the diversity of the state's population? Enhancing relationships with the community, recruiting participants in multiple settings, locating data collectors of different race/ethnicities, and performing media-based recruitment strategies may promote a more heterogenous sample that reflects the population of the state. Patient-family advisory councils and other community groups would be ideal for providing advice on which strategies are most likely to produce a heterogenous, diverse sample.

Differential Subject Attrition

High attrition during a longitudinal or repeated measures study is a threat to external design validity, especially when the attrition rate differs across groups. Attrition can result in differences in the characteristics of the treatment and control groups. In interventional studies, participants who realize they are in the control group may be less committed to completing the study. When the problem being studied is relevant to the target population, participants may be more likely to remain engaged in the study. For example, if you are recruiting for a study of hypertension in Black men, you may want to provide information to potential participants about the number of Black men affected by hypertension and the complications of the disease. A study facilitator who is a Black man may be an asset in retaining the participants. Chapter 15 provides information about sampling and recruiting strategies and calculating attrition rates.

High Refusal Rate

When recruiting for a study, potential subjects have the right to refuse participation, a right that should be protected. However, a high refusal rate may be a threat to external design validity if the resulting sample does not reflect the characteristics of the target population. Participants are more likely to agree to participate if they understand how the findings will be used to improve care for their community (Melnyk & Fineout-Overholt, 2019). Researchers can work closely with community representatives, such as a patient and family advisory committee, to identify potential barriers to participation and strategies to eliminate these barriers. Barriers to participation are often logistical concerns, such as childcare and travel expenses. Other barriers may be that data are being collected during the day when potential participants are working. Experienced researchers will often incorporate childcare, travel expenses, and evening or weekend data collection into their proposals for funding.

Interaction of Setting and Sample

The demographic characteristics and behaviors of potential participants vary across settings. A setting may offer a limited range of patient types. For example, you are proposing an interventional study among persons with

TABLE 11.5 Threats to External Design Validity for Interventional Studies

Threat	Definition	How to Avoid or Minimize the Threat
Homogenous sample[a]	Sample that is unique in its characteristics and response to the intervention because of narrow sampling criteria may be unlike the target population.	Balance the need to control extraneous variables (internal design validity) with the need for a heterogenous sample. Set inclusion and exclusion sampling criteria to be as inclusive as possible. Use stratified random sampling to recruit a more heterogenous sample.
Differential subject attrition	Treatment groups have a higher or lower attrition than the control or comparison group; participants who complete the study may vary in some characteristics that make them different from the target population.	Implement strategies to retain participants. Increase the diversity of the research team and data collectors. Ensure that educational materials or other documents are at an appropriate reading level. Remove as many barriers to participation as possible. For example, provide subway cards if transportation is an issue.
High refusal rate	More people choose not to participate in the study; people who agree to participate vary on characteristics that make them different from the target population.	Engage members of the target population to gain their perspectives on recruitment strategies. Provide clear, nonthreatening information during recruitment. Make participation simple and worthwhile. Maintain detailed records of the number of persons approached, number who met eligibility criteria, and number who consented.
Interaction of setting and sample[a]	People who participate in a specific setting are different from the participants in other settings.	Collect data in multiple sites (different types of sites) if possible, to recruit a more heterogenous sample.
Interaction of selection and treatment	People who are recruited or choose to participate have characteristics that may cause them to respond to the intervention differently than persons in the target population would.	Use random sampling, if feasible. Collect data in multiple sites, if possible, to recruit a more heterogenous sample. Analyze for relationships of participants that are correlated with the dependent variable.
Interaction of setting and treatment	The characteristics of a setting have effects on how the treatment is delivered or how participants respond to the treatment.	Collect data in multiple sites (different types of sites), if possible, to recruit a more heterogenous sample.
Interaction of history and treatment	An event or group of events affects the sample or individual participants so that they respond differently to the treatment than persons in the target setting would at a different time.	Maintain journal or other record of events occurring within the organizational and national environment that may relate to the study's topic.

[a]External design validity threats for noninterventional studies as well interventional as studies.

acquired immuneodeficiency syndrome (AIDS). One of the settings is a transitional care unit that provides shelter for persons with AIDS who have been homeless. Another setting is an outpatient clinic affiliated with a government-funded hospital. Another is the office of an infectious disease physician, whose practice is largely comprised of persons living with AIDS. The participants recruited from the first two settings are more likely to be unemployed or earning lower incomes. Participants recruited from the physician's practice are more likely to be employed and have health insurance. Recruiting participants from all three settings would comprise a more diverse sample than participants recruited from any one of the settings. Collecting data from participants in one setting may be a threat to external design validity because of the interaction of the setting and sample. As described in Chapter 10, researchers wishing to minimize the threat of setting and sample interaction will collect data in multiple settings if resources permit.

Interaction of Selection and Treatment

Treatments may interact with the participants recruited into a study. For example, researchers with limited resources may recruit a convenience sample of persons who tend to volunteer, persons who are retired, or patients who keep their appointments. Random assignment to groups may create groups that are similar, but external design validity remains limited by the characteristics of the sample. Consider the group of patients who keep their appointments. Patients may keep their appointments because they value communication with their healthcare providers or believe in carefully following instructions. These patients may respond more favorably to a medication adherence intervention than patients who do not consistently keep appointments. In this case, the interaction between selection and treatment is a threat to external design validity.

Interaction of Setting and Treatment

Characteristics of a setting may interact with a treatment in ways that limit external design validity. You plan an intervention study to motivate nurses to teach patients about their disease processes. You select four hospital units and randomly assign them to receive the treatment or serve as the control. When the study is completed, the results indicate no statistical differences in frequency of patient teaching between the treatment and control units. As you discuss the results with the hospital's nurse leaders, they mention a shortage of nurses that is requiring the hospital to use supplemental staffing. The effectiveness of the intervention may not have been demonstrated because of the involvement of nurses who had no long-term commitment to the hospital.

Unique characteristics of any setting may interact with the treatment being tested. Experienced researchers will investigate potential settings carefully when planning a study. Conducting studies in dedicated clinical research units increase the control to minimize the threats to

internal design validity, but the findings may not be generalizable to other units in the same hospital or to units in rural hospitals or privately owned hospitals.

Interaction of History and Treatment

Researchers who conducted a quasi-experimental, longitudinal study among adolescents rejected the directional hypothesis that an educational treatment about marijuana increases knowledge about the substance's risks and benefits and decreases the participants' intent to use marijuana. Instead the participants in the treatment group had no significant increase in their knowledge and an increase in their intent to use the substance. However, during the study, the voters in the state where the study was conducted legalized the use of medical marijuana. The interaction of history (legal medical marijuana use) and the treatment (educational intervention about marijuana) posed a threat to external design validity, because the findings could not be generalized to other time periods. Were the study results due to events external to the study that interacted with the treatment?

This threat to validity is about generalizing results over time. An event or prevailing assumption has the potential to alter whether or not a treatment is effective and, if so, to what extent. In some situations, the event is on a state or national level. The treatment can also interact with local events or situations, such as the demotion of a nurse manager who was scheduled to be a member of a team implementing a leadership intervention for graduate nurses.

Statistical Conclusion Design Validity

Statistical conclusion design validity refers to correctness of the decisions the researcher makes regarding statistical tests used in the study. A **threat to statistical conclusion design validity** is a factor that produces a false conclusion when data are analyzed (Shadish et al., 2002). Establishing the validity of statistical testing begins by ensuring the assumptions of the statistical tests are met (Table 11.6). Chapters 23, 24, and 25 discuss the use of correct statistical tests and the assumptions of each related to the variables' level of measurement, distribution of values, and interaction with other variables.

Low Statistical Power

One of the most pervasive threats to statistical conclusion design validity in nursing is **low statistical power** due to small samples. The smaller the effect of an intervention,

TABLE 11.6 Threats to Statistical Conclusion Design Validity for Interventional Studies

Threat	Definitions	How to Avoid or Minimize the Threat
Low statistical power[a]	The study did not have enough participants to minimize the risk of a Type II error.	Conduct a priori power analysis to determine the appropriate sample size prior to the conduct of a study. Conduct a post hoc power analysis to determine the power when a statistical result is nonsignificant (Grove & Cipher, 2020). Recruit more participants than projected to allow for attrition.
Violated assumptions of statistical tests[a]	The characteristics of the data were not adequate to use parametric tests and inaccurate results may have been produced.	Recruit a random sample. Conduct exploratory analyses to determine the distribution of data for each variable. Use nonparametric analyses as needed (Pett, 2016).
Multiple analyses and error rate[a]	With multiple analysis, there is increased likelihood that a result will be significant by chance.	Limit the statistical analysis to those needed to address the research questions or hypotheses (Grove & Cipher, 2020). Use multivariate analyses when appropriate. If multiple comparisons or tests are needed, use an adjusted, more stringent p value.
Unreliable measures[a]	The analyses of the data generated by unreliable instruments are more likely to produce results that include errors.	Select measures that have evidence of reliability in other studies. Test internal consistency reliability with your sample.
Unreliable implementation of the treatment	Without intervention fidelity, analyses are more likely to produce results that include errors.	Develop detailed protocol for implementation of the intervention. Invest time and effort in training research assistants. Monitor the consistency of the treatment during implementation.
Environmental extraneous variables	The analysis of data may produce results that include the effects of these variables, resulting in errors.	Select highly controlled settings when appropriate. Include environmental conditions in protocol, such as data collection in a private room.
Random heterogeneity of participants	The analysis of data may produce results that include the effects of the characteristics of the participants, resulting in errors.	Use random assignment to groups to disburse variations across groups. Set inclusion and exclusion sampling criteria to eliminate known confounding variables.

[a]Statistical conclusion design validity threats for noninterventional studies as well as interventional studies.

the larger the sample must be to generate enough power to demonstrate significance. An inadequately sized sample increases the risk that the effectiveness of an intervention is not revealed, resulting in a **Type II error** (previously explained in Chapters 15 and 21). When the power of a study is low and there is the potential of a Type II error, the researcher cannot use negative results as evidence against causality. No conclusions about the interventional portion of the study can be made. Only the descriptive results of a study can be used, and the effort involved in conducting an interventional study is wasted.

To avoid the threat of low statistical power in interventional research, the researcher should perform a power analysis to estimate the number of subjects needed (Aberson, 2019; Grove & Cipher, 2020). A power analysis estimates the sample size that will be required, based on the **effect size**, which means the amount of change in the dependent variable that is expected, as well as to the strength of the relationship between variables. You can review the effect sizes in studies in which similar interventions (or the same intervention) have been used. Frequently, however, the effect size of an intervention in a specific study is unknown until you have collected data. For this reason, you may want to conduct a pilot test to determine effect size. Chapters 15 and 21 discuss statistical power.

Violated Assumptions of Statistical Tests

Most inferential statistical tests have assumptions about the data being analyzed, including that the data are at least interval level and normally distributed (Grove & Cipher, 2020). In human studies, a frequently violated assumption is that the sample was randomly selected. As you select an instrument for a study, consider the level of measurement of the data produced by the instruments. Will the data be interval or ratio level? Exploratory analyses are conducted first to determine whether the data are normally distributed and meet the assumptions of the inferential analyses selected to address the hypotheses (Grove & Cipher, 2020) (see Chapters 21, 22, 23, 24, and 25).

Multiple Analyses and Error Rate

Another threat to statistical conclusion design validity is conducting multiple statistical tests—that is, fishing for statistically significant results (Suter & Suter, 2015). The risk for a Type I error increases when multiple analyses are conducted. For each inferential test conducted at the $p < 0.05$ level of significance, there is 5% possibility of a Type I error (explained in Chapter 21). Type I error means concluding that something is statistically significant when it is not (Grove & Cipher, 2020). Researchers who conduct 20 or more analyses on the same data increase the likelihood of a significant result that is due to chance. The statistical tests you conduct and report should emanate from the research questions or hypotheses. You should decide upon these tests before data are collected. Occasionally, an unanticipated finding will emerge, but you should focus primarily on the planned analyses and their meanings.

Faulty Measurements

Faulty measurements may not detect differences that exist and thus are a threat to statistical conclusion design validity (Shadish et al., 2002). A measurement method is a **reliable measure** if it gives the same result consistently (Gravetter & Forzano, 2018; Grove & Cipher, 2020; Waltz et al., 2017). Imprecise or unreliable measurements, especially of the dependent variable, may lead a researcher to conclude an intervention did not work. For example, when the dependent variable is being measured by

trained observers, one observer may tend to rate the participant's skill higher while another observer tends to rate the skill performance lower. The researcher may conclude the intervention had no effect on skill performance when the lack of consistency may have attenuated any potential effects (see Chapter 16).

Unreliable Implementation of the Intervention

As noted previously in this chapter, intervention fidelity is a necessity when conducting quasi-experimental and experimental studies. The protocol for the intervention must explicitly describe each step and (ideally) be implemented in a pilot study to refine the instructions. Training for the persons implementing the intervention and monitoring the consistency of the implementation are essential.

Environmental Extraneous Variables

Even in highly controlled settings, such as a clinical research unit, it is difficult to eliminate all extraneous variables. Unexpected events, such as the medical director leaving the hospital or participants losing health insurance, can interfere with the effects of the intervention (Shadish et al., 2002). As a study begins, the researchers need to monitor the study environment and observe for any events or conditions potentially affecting the dependent variable.

Random Heterogeneity of Participants

During data collection or data analysis, the researcher may notice unexpected participant characteristics that are correlated with the dependent variable. The inclusion and exclusion sampling criteria for an intervention study are designed to minimize the influence of known confounding variables (Shadish et al., 2002). A homogenous sample allows the effect of the intervention to be clearly seen, which supports the internal design validity of the study. When the sample is more heterogenous and the researchers fail to reject the null hypothesis, one possible explanation is that confounding factors may have attenuated the effect of the intervention (Adams & Lawrence, 2019). Refer to Tables 11.3, 11.4, 11.5, and 11.6 to review ways to minimize the threats to design validity affecting interventional studies.

INTERVENTIONAL DESIGNS

Interventional designs are those designs in which the researcher introduces an environmental condition, educational program, or different medication to determine its effect. Unfortunately there is no universal standard for categorizing designs. Two scholars may review the same study: One scholar labels the study design as experimental and the other labels the study as a quasi-experimental design. To further complicate assigning labels to a study, researchers sometimes merge elements of several designs to meet the methodological needs of a study. From these developments, new designs sometimes emerge. If researchers clearly identified their study design in reporting their research, this would probably improve students' and nurses' understanding of the types of designs used in nursing research.

Quasi-experimental and experimental designs examine causality. The power of an interventional design depends on the extent to which the actual effects of the experimental treatment (the independent variable) can be detected by measuring the dependent variable. Obtaining an understanding of the true effects of an experimental treatment or intervention requires action to control threats to the validity of the findings (see Tables 11.3, 11.4, 11.5, and 11.6). Threats to design validity are controlled through selection of subjects, control of the environment, manipulation of the treatment, and reliable and valid measurement of the dependent variables. In this section we provide an explanation for the differences between experimental and quasi-experimental designs. For these two major categories of designs, specific designs will be diagrammed and explained.

Distinguishing Between Experimental and Quasi-Experimental Designs

Experimental study designs are the most powerful method of examining causality. Researchers who adhere to a logical positivistic philosophy argue that six conditions are necessary for a true experimental design. These conditions are listed in Box 11.3. Researchers who are

---

BOX 11.3 Logical Positivistic Criteria for Experiments

- Random selection of subjects
- Random assignments to control and treatment groups
- Use of control group rather than comparison group
- Rigorous implementation of the intervention
- Highly controlled setting
- Elimination or attenuation of threats to validity

BOX 11.4 Required Elements of Experiments

- Rigorously implemented intervention
- Control group
- Randomized assignments to groups
- Attenuation of threats to design validity

---

social constructivists or pragmatists would argue that all six conditions are not needed for an experimental study. For example, you may randomly select potential participants but not all may agree to participate. Or, a highly controlled setting may not be consistent with the study's purpose. For ethical and logistical reasons, you may not be able to use an experimental design (Handley et al., 2018). In this textbook, an experimental design must have (1) a rigorously implemented intervention, (2) a control group, (3) random assignment to groups, and (4) attenuation of threats to design validity as much as possible (Box 11.4). When one of these conditions is missing, the study is a quasi-experimental design. Fig. 11.5 is an algorithm for distinguishing between experimental and quasi-experimental designs. The algorithms in this chapter use a standard format. The questions to ask as you consider a design are in blue boxes. The answers to the questions are identified as no (*red box*) and yes (*green box*). Follow the line from the no and yes answers to either another question or the appropriate study design. The study designs are labeled in light orange boxes. For example, in Fig. 11.5, the first question is whether the study had an intervention. If the answer is no, the study design is a descriptive or correlational design (see Chapter 10). If the answer is yes, the next box is blue and contains a question about whether the researcher controlled the intervention. The no answers after the next questions lead to quasi-experimental being the study's design.

Quasi-experimental study designs were developed to provide alternative means of examining causality in situations not conducive to experimental controls. Quasi-experimental designs facilitate the search for knowledge, especially in the social sciences, by balancing internal and external design validity (Handley et al., 2018). Fig. 11.6 is an algorithm using the same format as Fig. 11.5; questions are in blue boxes, no answers in red boxes, yes answers in green boxes, and designs in orange boxes. We will refer to the algorithm as we describe quasi-experimental designs.

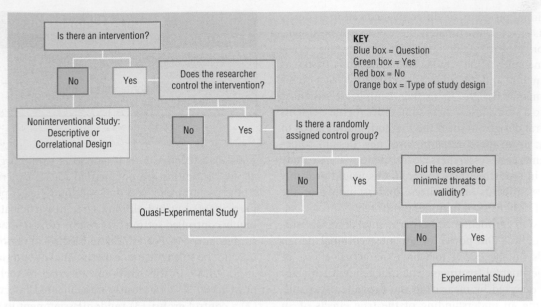

Fig. 11.5 Algorithm to decide whether a study is quasi-experimental or experimental.

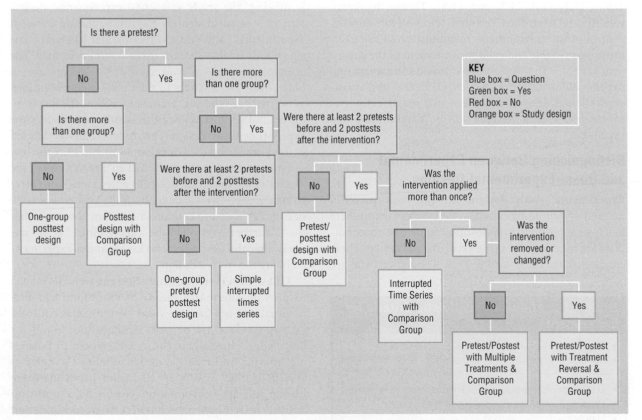

Fig. 11.6 Algorithm to decide which quasi-experimental design was used.

Quasi-Experimental Study Designs

The first two designs are posttest-only designs and have several threats to design validity. Cook and Campbell (1979) and Shadish et al. (2002) describe these designs as pre-experimental. This section will also include descriptions of quasi-experimental designs, such as different pretest-posttest designs and interrupted time series designs.

One-Group Posttest-Only Design

The **one-group posttest-only design**, one of the pre-experimental designs, does not allow the researchers to make causal inferences (Fig. 11.7). One group is selected because of its availability to receive the treatment or intervention. Following the treatment, the dependent variable is measured. The group is not pretested; thus there is no direct way to measure change. The researcher cannot claim that posttest scores were a consequence (effect) of the treatment if scores before the treatment are unknown. Because there is no comparison group, one does not know whether groups not receiving the treatment would have similar scores on the dependent variable. Using the design could be justified, however, if the dependent variable's prevalence or incidence is known in the population. In this case, the researcher could argue that any difference in the dependent variable in the sample and the dependent variable in the population is due to the treatment. The one-group posttest-only design is rarely reported in the literature because of its weaknesses.

Posttest-Only Design With a Comparison Group

The **posttest-only design with a comparison group** is slightly stronger than the one-group posttest-only design (Fig. 11.8). A researcher might use this design to determine the effects of a nurse-directed intervention on prevention of catheter-associated urinary tract infection (CAUTI). The researcher identifies two similar skilled nursing facilities. The nurses in one facility receive the intervention, but the nurses in the other facility do not. Two months following the intervention, the incidence of CAUTI is measured in both facilities. However, the researcher has little to no ability to infer causality.

Treatment Group	TX	M
Comparison Group		M

KEY
M = Measurement
TX = Treatment

Fig. 11.8 Quasi-experimental two-group posttest-only design.

The design has numerous threats to validity, including the threat of selection for both groups. The addition of a comparison group can lead to a false confidence in the validity of the findings. The lack of a pretest remains a serious impediment to knowing whether or not the intervention caused any differences in incidence of CAUTI between the two facilities. Differences in posttest scores between groups may be caused by the treatment or by differences that preceded the intervention.

One-Group Pretest-Posttest Design

The **one-group pretest-posttest design** is one of the more commonly used quasi-experimental designs (Fig. 11.9). The group is selected based on availability or convenience. Participants complete a pretest, are exposed to the treatment, and then complete the posttest. Despite the addition of a pretest, the design has serious weaknesses that may make findings uninterpretable. Pretest scores cannot adequately serve the same function as a comparison group. Events can occur between the pretest and posttest that alter responses to the posttest. Posttest scores might be altered by history, maturation, administration of the pretest, and changes in instrumentation. When participants have high pretest scores, the instrument may not be sensitive enough to measure improvement or the scores may regress toward the mean. In the latter situation, the participants' posttest scores may be lower than the pretest scores. Participants who score low on the pretest may improve on the posttest; however, the improvement may also be due to regression toward the mean. The effort of adding a comparison or control group to this design would improve the researcher's ability to infer causality.

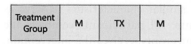

Fig. 11.7 Quasi-experimental one-group posttest-only design.

Fig. 11.9 Quasi-experimental one-group pretest-posttest design.

Mathew and Thukha (2018) conducted a study with a one-group pretest-posttest design. The intervention that they tested was nurse-guided, patient-centered heart failure education, which was described earlier in the chapter as an intervention based on evidence from the literature. The researchers hypothesized that the educational intervention would increase older adults' knowledge of heart failure and related self-care and reduce the likelihood of readmission. The participants were older adults ($N = 26$) who had been hospitalized for heart failure. Data were collected before and after the intervention. Mathew and Thukha (2018) found a statistically significant increase in the participants' knowledge and self-care. Only one participant was readmitted to the hospital for heart failure. The results were promising, but the researchers were forthright about the study's limitations as noted in the following excerpt.

"The limitations of this pilot project include its small sample size, non-randomized convenience sampling design, predominance of female participants, and poor control on various factors that might have influenced the intervention's effectiveness, such as time-since diagnosis or type of service available from the cardiologist or primary care provider. It should also be remembered that the sample for this pilot project consisted exclusively of older adults in a skilled nursing facility. This means that the results, though promising, are not yet generalizable to a larger population." (Mathew & Thukha, 2018, p. 379)

One of the goals of the study conducted by Mathew and Thukha (2018) was to examine the effectiveness of the intervention. The one-group pretest-posttest design was an appropriate design for a pilot study to provide initial support for the intervention before undertaking a larger study with a more controlled design.

Pretest and Posttest Design With a Comparison Group

The **pretest and posttest design with a comparison group** is a commonly used quasi-experimental design (Fig. 11.10). The researcher identifies a group to whom the treatment will be administered and then identifies another group with similar characteristics to serve as the comparison group. All participants complete the pretest, the treatment group receives the intervention, and all participants complete the posttest. Ideally, the

Treatment Group	M	TX	M
Comparison Group	M		M

KEY
M = Measurement
TX = Treatment

Fig. 11.10 Quasi-experimental pretest-posttest with a comparison group.

groups' mean scores on the pretest are not significantly different. The researcher will also compare the groups' demographic characteristics and other variables that might influence the posttest scores, such as disease status or time since diagnosis. When the treatment and comparison groups are similar, the researcher can argue that any difference in posttest scores is due to the intervention that the treatment group received.

This design allows the researcher to make a stronger argument that changes in the treatment group's posttest scores are due to the intervention. However, the design is weakened by several threats to internal design validity. Because participants are not randomly selected or randomized into the treatment group and comparison group, differences in the treatment group's posttest scores could be due to an unmeasured confounding variable. Between the pretest and posttest, external events or changes unrelated to the intervention may positively affect the dependent variable of the comparison group or attenuate positive changes in the dependent variable of the treatment group.

Hinic, Kowalski, Holtzman, and Mobus (2019) conducted a quasi-experimental study with hospitalized children to test a pet therapy intervention ($n = 50$), measuring state anxiety before and after the intervention. Children in the comparison group ($n = 43$) received a puzzle intervention. The researchers provided the reasons why they used a comparison group, instead of a control group, in this excerpt.

"Participants were assigned to either the pet therapy or comparison group based upon the day on which data collection was occurring. Randomization was not feasible due to the open nature of the pediatric unit and the general excitement among the children when the therapy dog and handler teams enter the unit. Instead, data collection was scheduled for 2 days of each week: 1 day when pet therapy visits were scheduled and the other where no pet therapy visits were scheduled and participants were grouped accordingly. The parent was present for all study related activities, including the consent process, the duration of the pet therapy visit and puzzle completion, and completion of questionnaires.... The findings from this study need to be interpreted in the context of several limitations. This was a convenience sample and it is not known how families who chose to participate in the study may have differed from children and families who did not participate. Also, while there were no significant differences between the pet therapy and puzzle groups in relation to age, gender, chronic disease, pet ownership, and baseline anxiety, because we did not use randomization, it is possible that other biases could have been introduced since participants knew which group they were assigned upon enrollment." (Hinic et al., 2019, pp. 57, 60)

	Group	Pretest	Intervention	Posttest
Randomization	G1 Control Group	M	RHC	M
	G2 Treatment 1	M	RHC + Cryotherapy before SCAI	M
	G3 Treatment 2	M	RHC + Cryotherapy after SCAI TX	M

KEY
M = Measurement of pain and hematomas
SCAI = Subcutaneous anticoagulant injection
RHC = Routine hospital care

Fig. 11.11 Quasi-experimental randomized two-treatment groups with a control group. (From El-Deen, D., & Youssef, N. [2018]. The effect of cryotherapy application before versus after subcutaneous anticoagulant injection on pain intensity and hematoma formation: A quasi-experimental design. *International Journal of Nursing Sciences, 5*[3], 223–229. doi:10.1016/j.ijnss.2018.07.006.)

Anxiety decreased in both groups between the pretest and posttest. Between groups, Hinic et al. (2019) found no significant difference on pretest state anxiety and a statistically significant difference on posttest state anxiety, indicating the effectiveness of the intervention. However, the study weaknesses identified by the researchers limit the generalizability of the findings. The researchers also noted that most studies of pet therapy with hospitalized children assessed only short-term outcomes. They recommended future research include outcomes beyond the immediate postintervention period.

Researchers have used variations of this design. One variation is to avoid the threat of instrumentation and use different, but correlated, instruments for the pretest and posttest. Using different tests, however, weakens the design. Another variation is to use retrospective data as the comparison group. This approach may be appropriate when all current patients are to receive a new treatment. The researcher extracts data from the electronic health record about patients who received care prior to the new treatment being initiated. The strength of the study is dependent on how carefully the archived data have been collected and recorded. Measuring the dependent variable more than once prior to the intervention is a variation that strengthens the design.

Pretest and Posttest Design With Two Comparison Treatments

The two-treatment design (Fig. 11.11) is used when two experimental treatments are being compared to determine which is the more effective. In most cases, this design is used when one treatment is the current treatment of choice and the researcher has identified a treatment that may lead to even better outcomes. This design is strengthened by the addition of one or more of the following: a no-treatment group, a placebo-treatment group, or a routine or standard care group (Fig. 11.11). Earlier in the chapter, a study conducted by El-Deen and Youssef (2018) was introduced related to conducting post hoc comparisons of the demographic characteristics of the treatment and control groups. Their design is a strong example of two treatment groups with a control group of routine hospital care (RHC). El-Deen and Youssef (2018) identified their study purpose, the composition of the groups, and implementation of the intervention in the following excerpts.

"...this study aimed to investigate the effect of cryotherapy application before versus after SCAI [subcutaneous anticoagulant injection] on pain intensity and hematoma formation.... Out of 133 patients who were invited and met the inclusion criteria, 128 accepted to participate with a response rate of 96.24% at the baseline phase. Only 105 patients participated three times (response rate 82.03%) and were involved in the data analysis. Based on this sample ($n = 105$), three groups were investigated in this study: (1) Control group [G1, $n = 35$], who received routine hospital care (RHC) and (2) two intervention groups [G2, $n = 35$ & G3, $n = 35$], who followed RHC alongside 5 min cryotherapy application. G2 received 5 min cryotherapy before SCAI, and G3 received cryotherapy after SCAI...." (El-Deen & Youssef, 2018, p. 224)

"For controlling confounders that have been shown in previous studies as factors for increasing pain sensation and hematoma formation...the two study and control groups received the same injection technique. For instance, the anticoagulant dose was slowly injected over a period of 30 s using a syringe ready for injection, with insertion angle of 90°, with no aspiration before the injection, and by holding the skin of the injection site between the thumb and index finger, since these techniques can reduce pain intensity and hematoma formation.... After injection, a piece of cotton was placed on the injection site and was then removed without rubbing. A Kenko sports chronometer was used to measure the duration of the injection. A circle was drawn around the injection site (at the selected arm) on all participants in order to ensure it will not be selected again for the following injection, and to assess the occurrence and size of the hematoma." (El-Deen & Youssef, 2018, p. 225)

El-Deen and Youssef (2018) found that all participants reported only mild to moderate pain, a finding they attributed to the injection technique. The two treatment groups reported lower scores on pain intensity than the control group, but there was no difference in pain intensity between the application of ice before the injection and the application of ice after the injection. At 48 and 72 hours after the injection, there was as statistically significant difference in the number of hematomas between groups, with the participants in the treatment groups having fewer hematomas develop than the control group. The hematomas that did develop were significantly smaller in the cryotherapy after the injection group than the cryotherapy before the injection group. The size of hematomas in the treatment groups were significantly smaller than those in the control group. Although the findings were promising, El-Deen and Youssef (2018)

acknowledged that replication was needed with larger samples and in multiple locations.

Pretest and Posttest Design With a Removed Treatment

Designs in which the treatment is removed are used with caution because of the ethical issue of removing a treatment that may be effective. Researchers may choose this design, however, when gaining access to a comparison or control group is not possible. The removed-treatment design with pretest and posttest creates conditions that approximate the conceptual requirements of a control group receiving no treatment. The design is basically a one-group pretest-posttest design. The pretest data are collected (time 1) and the treatment is begun (Fig. 11.12). The data for the first and second posttests are collected at time 2 and time 3 while the treatment is continuing. After time 3, the treatment is removed. Following an equal period of time, data for the final posttest are collected. The periods between measures must be equivalent. Even if doing so is ethically acceptable, the response of subjects to the removal may make interpreting changes difficult.

Researchers may also choose this design when they are interested in testing how long a treatment is effective. For example, nurses in a large outpatient clinic are aware of the evidence supporting the use of weekly nurse phone calls to improve medication adherence among patients on daily medications. However, it is not known whether the effects of continuing the intervention diminish over time and if the effects of the intervention continue when it is removed. The cost of the intervention (the nurse's time) may prevent the integration of the nurse phone calls into routine care. The nurses develop a study to test the effects of the intervention on medication adherence among 200 persons prescribed antihypertensive medications over time and to measure the effects of the intervention after it is removed. Fig. 11.13 provides a diagram of the proposed study's treatment and observations. The pretest data are

	Time 1	Time 2	Time 3	Time 4	KEY
Treatment Group	M	M	M	M	M = Measurement TX = Treatment
		TX			

Fig. 11.12 Quasi-experimental one-group pretest and posttest design with treatment removed after third observation.

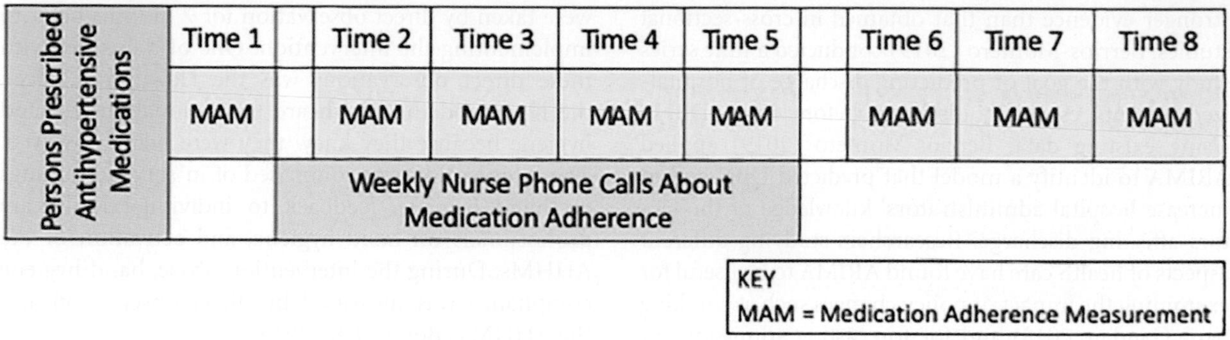

Persons Prescribed Antihypertensive Medications	Time 1		Time 2	Time 3	Time 4	Time 5		Time 6	Time 7	Time 8
	MAM		MAM	MAM	MAM	MAM		MAM	MAM	MAM
			Weekly Nurse Phone Calls About Medication Adherence							

KEY
MAM = Medication Adherence Measurement

Fig. 11.13 Example of quasi-experimental one-group pretest and multiple posttest design to test effects of weekly phone calls on medication adherence over time and after stopping the weekly phone calls.

collected at time 1. The posttests (medication adherence measurements) at time 2 through time 5 will be used to test the initial and continuing effects of the intervention. The posttests at time 6 through time 8 will be used to test whether medication adherence is maintained after the treatment is removed. Although the study as designed may answer the questions of the clinic nurses, the design would be strengthened by a comparison or control group that received usual care. Because multiple measurements of the dependent variable were taken after the intervention, this design shares some similarities with the interrupted time series design, the next design to be described.

Interrupted Time Series Designs

The **interrupted time series designs** are similar to descriptive trend designs except that a treatment is applied at some point in the observations. These designs are longitudinal studies that include repeated measurements of the dependent variable followed by the introduction of the treatment. The treatment is followed by additional measurements of the dependent variable. The term *interrupted* is used to indicate that if the treatment is effective there will be an interruption, a change, in the value of the dependent variable. After describing some of the advantages and challenges of interrupted time series designs, three variations of the design will be explained and examples provided.

Time-series analyses designs can minimize some threats to validity and potentially increase other threats to validity. The repeated pretest observations can be used to minimize the internal design validity threats of history, maturation, and statistical regression toward the mean. By keeping records of events that occur during a time series study, researchers can assess the effect of history on the dependent variable by comparing subsequent measurements to the pretest observations (Shadish et al., 2002). However, the best way to control for the threat of history is to add a control or comparison group. The repeated pretest observations also allow researchers to assess trends indicating maturation before the treatment (Campbell & Stanley, 1963). Assessing trends in the scores before the treatment also decreases the risk of statistical regression, which would lead to misinterpretation of findings.

Some threats, however, are particularly problematic in time series designs. Instrumentation can become a threat if the measurements are not obtained using consistent procedures. Construct design validity can be threated if the definition of the construct for the dependent variable changes over time. Thus maintaining consistency can be a problem. The length of the study and the treatment can result in attrition so that the sample before treatment may be different in important ways from the posttreatment group. Seasonal variation or other cyclical influences may be interpreted as treatment effects. Therefore identifying cyclical patterns and controlling for them are critical to the analysis of study findings (Shadish et al., 2002).

The statistical analyses needed to assess differences in the pattern of pretest scores and the pattern of posttest scores can be complex (Kerlinger & Lee, 2000). One such analysis is called the autoregressive integrated moving average (ARIMA) statistical model, developed by Box and Jenkins (1976). For adequate statistical analysis, at least 50 measurement points are needed; however, Cook and Campbell (1979) believe that ARIMA, even with small numbers of measurement points, can provide stronger evidence than that obtained in cross-sectional studies. Berrios-Montero (2019) conducted a time series study with the goal of predicting discharge of hospitalized patients, especially discharge before noon (DBN). Using existing data, Berrios-Montero (2019) applied ARIMA to identify a model that predicted DBN and to increase hospital administrators' knowledge of the factors affecting discharge. Researchers studying different aspects of health care have found ARIMA to be useful for examining the impact of policy changes such as smoking bans (Linden, 2018) and for forecasting admissions of inpatients and other health system events (Zhou, Zhao, Wu, Cheng, & Huang, 2018).

Simple interrupted time series design. The **simple interrupted time series design** includes repeated pretest measurements, introduction of the intervention, and repeated posttest measurements. Fig. 11.14 displays the design. The treatment, which in some cases is not completely under the control of the researcher, must be clearly defined. There is no control or comparison group in this design. Threats that are well controlled by this design are maturation and statistical regression. The use of multiple methods to measure the dependent variable greatly strengthens the design.

An example of a simple interrupted time series design is a study conducted by Boyce, Cooper, Yin, Li, and Arbogast (2019) related to hand hygiene compliance. The researchers conducted a simple interrupted times series study to assess the effect of automated hand hygiene monitors (AHHMs) in a surgical intensive care unit (SICU) and general medical ward (GMW). Baseline measurements of hand hygiene compliance were taken by direct observation for 7 months prior to implementing the intervention. One of the issues with these direct observations was the Hawthorne effect, the likelihood the healthcare professionals used hand hygiene because they knew they were being observed. The intervention was comprised of in-service trainings on hand hygiene, feedback to individual healthcare professionals on hand hygiene, and activation of the AHHMs. During the intervention phase, hand hygiene compliance was measured by direct observation and the AHHMs (Boyce et al., 2019).

The intervention significantly increased the compliance rate for room entry on both units (SICU from 30.9 to 63.5%, $p < 0.001$; GMW from 21.4 to 45.5%, $p < 0.001$), as measured by direct observation (Boyce et al., 2019). However, the intervention did not improve the compliance rate for room exit (SICU from 76.1 to 80.7%, $p = 0.45$; GMW from 71.1 to 72.7%, $p = 0.86$). The healthcare professionals ($N = 74$) who participated in the evaluation of the AHHMs wore badges that were read by infrared sensors in the rooms and halls. The compliance rates recorded by the AHHMs were less than 40%. The lower compliance rates measured by the AHHMs were attributed to challenges with wireless connectivity, the locations of sensors, and changes in the software, but could also be due the unobtrusiveness of the AHHMs that may have decreased the Hawthorne effect. Boyce et al. (2019) concluded that additional technology refinements were needed to increase the accuracy of the compliance rates and acceptability of AHHMs among healthcare professionals.

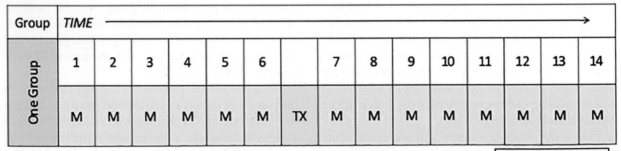

Fig. 11.14 Quasi-experimental simple interrupted time series design with no comparison group.

	1	2	3	4	5	6		7	8	9	10	11	12	13	14
Treatment Group	M	M	M	M	M	M	TX	M	M	M	M	M	M	M	M
Comparison Group	M	M	M	M	M	M		M	M	M	M	M	M	M	M

KEY
M = Measurement
TX = Treatment

Fig. 11.15 Quasi-experimental interrupted time series design with a comparison group.

Interrupted time series design with a no-treatment comparison group. The addition of a comparison group to the interrupted time series design greatly strengthens the internal design validity of the study. The comparison group allows the researcher to examine the differences in trends between groups after the treatment and the persistence of treatment effects over time (Fig. 11.15). When the treatment continues, the initial response to the change may differ from later responses. Hsu et al. (2018) conducted an interrupted time series design study to examine the effect of the elimination of Medicaid payments in 2012 for mediastinitis following coronary artery bypass graft (CABG) surgery. Hsu et al. (2018) described the study design in the following excerpts.

"We used a quasi-experimental interrupted time-series design with comparison group to examine the impact of the Medicaid HAC POA [healthcare-associated condition, Present on Admission] program on reported rates of mediastinitis and deep-space SSI [surgical site infection] after knee replacement before and after the program, adjusting for secular trends. Inclusion of a comparison condition that affects a similar population but is not anticipated to change in response to program implementation is an accepted method in quasiexperimental study design to combat threats to study validity" (Shadish, Cook, & Campbell, 2002). (Hsu et al., 2018, p. 695)

"The risk of mediastinitis remained constant throughout the study period; the odds ratios for the time trend were 0.98 (95% confidence interval [CI], 0.94–1.03) during the preprogram period and 0.99 (95% CI, 0.97–1.02) during the postprogram period. When we examined deep-space SSIs after knee replacement..., we similarly found no measurable change in trend in the postprogram versus preprogram periods (odds ratio [OR], 1.00; 95% CI, 0.95–1.05).... Our results were robust to multiple sensitivity analyses, including adjustment for hospital characteristics, restriction of hospitals to those with more consistent participation in the NHSN [National Healthcare Safety Network] during the study period, and incorporation of a policy implementation roll-in period". (Hsu et al., 2018, p. 697)

The rigorous study conducted by Hsu et al. (2018) found that the Medicaid HAC POA program had no significant effect on the prevalence rate of mediastinitis following CABG when compared to mediastinitis following knee replacement. Most cases of mediastinitis were identified on readmission, rather than during the initial hospitalization, which was the target of the changed policy. Mediastinitis occurred rarely so that incidence of the outcome during a specific period was not an accurate representation of the quality of a hospital's care (Hsu et al., 2018).

Interrupted time series design with multiple treatment replications. The **interrupted time series design with multiple treatment replications** is a powerful design for inferring causality. The design requires that the

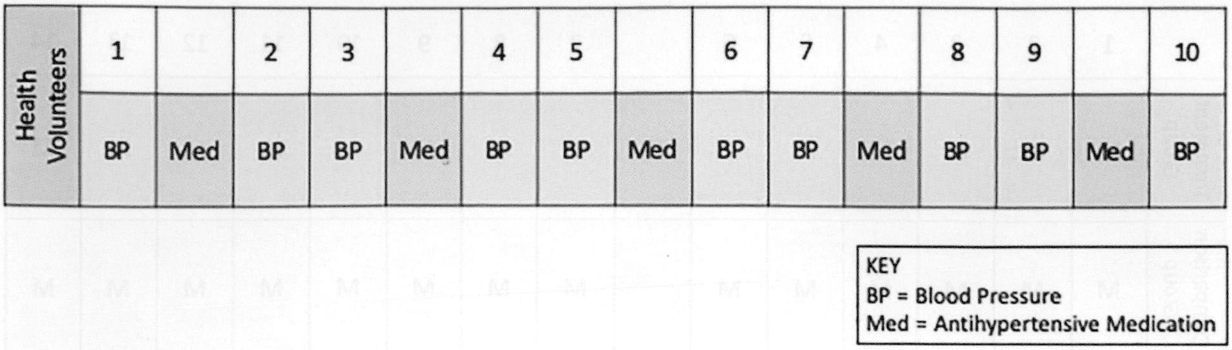

Fig. 11.16 Interrupted time series design with multiple treatment replications: Example of antihypertensive medication effects on blood pressure.

researchers "introduce a treatment, remove it, reintroduce it, remove it again, and so on" (Cook & Campbell, 1979, p. 222). This level of control is rarely possible in social science research outside of laboratories and clinical research units. This design is only appropriate when the effect of the treatment dissipates quickly (Shadish et al., 2002). For significant differences to be interpretable, the pretest and posttest scores must be in different directions with the introduction and removal of the treatment. Within this design, treatments can be modified by substituting one treatment for another or combining two treatments and examining interaction effects. For example, an interrupted times series design study could be designed to examine the expected effects of an antihypertensive medication on blood pressure among healthy volunteers in a laboratory setting. Fig. 11.16 provides a diagram of the study components. One variation of the design could be switching treatments, such as using one antihypertensive medication between measurements 1 and 2 and a different antihypertensive medication between measurements 3 and 4. Other variations could include using one antihypertensive medication for all treatments, but at different dosage levels and using one antihypertensive medication alone for some intervention points and two antihypertensive medications in combination for others. The variations are only limited by the researcher's imagination and control of the testing situation.

Experimental Study Designs

Experimental study designs provide the greatest amount of control possible to examine causality more closely. To examine cause, the researchers attempt to eliminate all factors potentially influencing the dependent variable other than the cause (independent variable) being studied. Some factors cannot be eliminated and may be statistically controlled. The study is designed to focus on the connection between the cause and the effect that the researchers are investigating.

Experiments can be identified by four essential components: (1) random assignment to groups, (2) rigorously implemented intervention, (3) control group, and (4) attenuation of threats to design validity (see Box 11.4) (Adams & Lawrence, 2019; Campbell & Stanley, 1963; Leedy & Ormrod, 2019; Shadish et al., 2002). The steps of the research process must be congruent with each other from the statement of the research process through the interpretation of the results. Researchers who implement experimental studies must recognize that additional effort is needed to eliminate or attenuate the threats to validity.

Threats to design validity can be minimized by identifying explicit inclusion and exclusion criteria for the sample and selecting reliable and valid instruments to measure the variables. Participants are randomly assigned to the treatment or control group. The fidelity of the intervention is monitored during the experiment. Ideally, the study is conducted in a highly controlled environment to prevent the possibility that unstudied factors might modify the dynamics of the process being studied (Adams & Lawrence, 2019; Shadish et al., 2002).

Fig. 11.17 is an algorithm that provides the questions to ask when you review an experimental study to determine its specific design. The first question is whether the study has multiple interventions. If the answer is no, you continue down the left side of the algorithm. As we describe specific experimental designs, we will refer back to this algorithm.

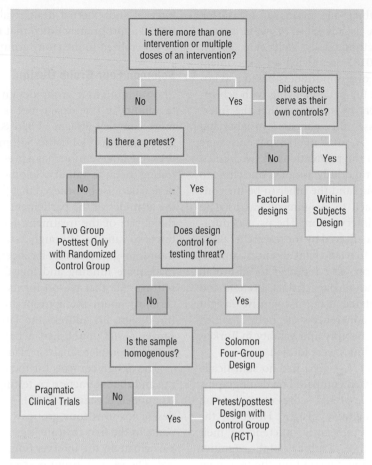

Fig. 11.17 Algorithm to decide which experimental design was used. *RCT,* Randomized controlled trial.

Classic Experimental Design

The **classic experimental design**, or **pretest-posttest control group design** (see Fig. 11.2), continues to be the most commonly used experimental design. In Fig. 11.17, the first question is answered with no because a single intervention is being tested. The presence of a pretest and posttest leads to the question of whether the testing threat to validity was controlled. In the classic experimental design, the answer is no because a pretest was used with both groups. The inclusion and exclusion sampling criteria were used to create a homogenous sample. The yes response leads to design being identified as the pretest-posttest design with control group. The participants were randomly assigned to one of two groups: the treatment group or the control group. Potentially confounding characteristics of the participants should be relatively equal across the groups because of random assignment. The dependent variable is measured in both groups. By comparing pretest scores and the groups' demographic characteristics, a researcher can evaluate the effectiveness of randomization in providing equivalent groups. The intervention is implemented with rigor for the treatment group. The control group receives usual care, no treatment, or a placebo treatment. The dependent variable is measured a second time in both groups (Adams & Lawrence, 2019; Leedy & Ormrod, 2019). As in all well-designed studies, the dependent and independent variables are conceptually linked, conceptually defined, and operationalized. Instruments used to measure the dependent variable must clearly reflect the conceptual meaning of the variable and have good evidence of reliability and validity. Often more than one means of measuring the dependent variable is advisable to avoid mono-operation and monomethod biases (Waltz et al., 2017).

Çetin and Aylaz (2018) conducted an experiment to test the effectiveness of a mindfulness-based psychoeducation intervention for patients living with schizophrenia. The researchers hypothesized that the intervention would increase the patients' insight and medication adherence. A total of 188 patients were randomly selected from the populations of two clinics. Çetin and Aylaz (2018) randomly assigned one clinic to be the intervention group and the other to be the control group. This approach to assignment was used to avoid diffusion of the intervention. The psychoeducational intervention was delivered by the researcher twice a week for 4 weeks. Due to participant absences, components of the intervention were repeated to ensure all content was delivered to all participants. Pretests and posttests were administered using a cognitive insight scale and a medication adherence scale, both of which had been assessed for reliability and validity in Turkey, the country where the clinics were located.

The group members ($N = 135$) had no statistically significant differences when compared on demographic characteristics and on the pretest scores of medication adherence and total cognitive insight. However, the group members were significantly different on their pretest self-confidence scores, a subscale of the cognitive insight scale. Following the intervention, the treatment group's posttest scores were significantly higher on medication adherence ($t = -3.44$, $p = 0.00$) and on cognitive insight ($t = 3.13, p = 0.00$) when compared to the control group's posttest scores. The primary finding of the study was that a mindfulness-based psychoeducational intervention had positive effects on medication adherence and cognitive insight (Çetin & Aylaz, 2018).

Çetin and Aylaz (2018) noted several limitations of the study, including the treatment and control groups being in different provinces. The original plan had been to collect data twice after the intervention, but they were only able to collect posttest data once. The limitations not mentioned were that the primary researcher delivered the intervention and collected the data and that no information was provided about intervention fidelity between the regularly scheduled intervention sessions and the makeup sessions. Finally, subject attrition was high (28.2%) and unequal (41.5% treatment group; 14.9% control group), which was a threat to

internal and external design validity. Çetin and Aylaz (2018) appropriately noted that the findings could only be generalized to the study group.

Solomon Four-Group Design

The Solomon four-group design addresses most threats to validity in one design but is considered one of the more complex designs (Phan & Ngu, 2017; Solomon, 1949). In Fig. 11.17, the Solomon four-group design tests one intervention, has a pretest, and controls for the testing threat to validity. Solomon (1949) proposed this design because he believed that the pretest itself changed the attitudes of the participants and sensitized them to the effects of the treatment. He identified testing as a threat to validity. Although a stringent design, the Solomon four-group design has been underused because of inadequate funding and logistical challenges in some settings. Another reason for its underuse has been uncertainty about the appropriate statistical analyses for the design. To address the latter reason, Braver and Braver (1988) published a paper in which they presented a complete analysis plan for the design.

The design controls for the potential threats of testing and the interaction of testing with the intervention (Campbell & Stanley, 1963). As you would expect, the design involves four groups (Fig. 11.18). The participants in the first treatment group complete the pretest, participate in the intervention, and complete the posttest. The second group is essentially the control group for the first group. The participants in the second group complete the pretest and posttest. The participants in the third group are not pretested but receive the

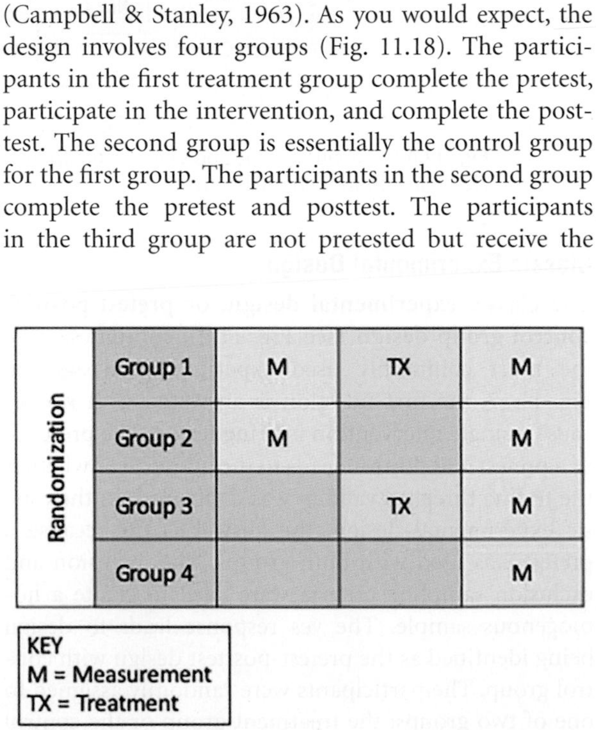

Randomization	Group 1	M	TX	M
	Group 2	M		M
	Group 3		TX	M
	Group 4			M

KEY
M = Measurement
TX = Treatment

Fig. 11.18 Solomon four-group design: Experimental design.

intervention and complete the posttest. The participants in the fourth group only complete the posttest (Kazdin, 2017). One challenge of the design is having a large enough sample to ensure adequate power when the participants are randomly assigned to groups.

Solomon four-group design has not been used extensively in nursing, but Williams and Spurlock (2019) used the design to test the effects of high-fidelity simulation on 98 African American junior nursing students' knowledge of respiratory care. All students received a lecture on respiratory care before two groups received the intervention. The measurement of knowledge was a Health Education System Incorporated (HESI) exam especially prepared for the study. The HESI exam was used as the pretest and posttest. The groups who received the pretest had significantly higher scores on the posttests than those groups who only took the posttest. The main effect of the intervention and the interaction effect of testing and the intervention were not statistically significant. High-fidelity simulation as an intervention did not have an effect on knowledge acquisition in this study. Several limitations were identified: a single site; two-day period between the pretest, intervention, and posttest; and potential contamination of the treatment between groups (Williams & Spurlock, 2019). Conducting a post-priori power analysis would have identified whether the study lacked adequate power due to the sample size.

Knowing whether a pretest activates or potentiates an intervention is important information that affects external design validity (Leedy & Ormrod, 2019). Based on the findings of quasi-experimental and experimental studies, nurses may decide to use an intervention in practice that has been shown to be effective. However, if the intervention only works following a specific pretest, the nurses will be disappointed when the intervention does not work and will have wasted time and money implementing an ineffective intervention. The Solomon four-group design can be used to answer important questions essential for building nursing knowledge.

Experimental Posttest-Only Control Group Design

In some studies, the dependent variable cannot be measured before the treatment. For example, before the beginning of treatment, it is not possible to measure, in a meaningful way, participants' responses to interventions designed to control nausea from chemotherapy or postoperative pain. Additionally, in some cases,

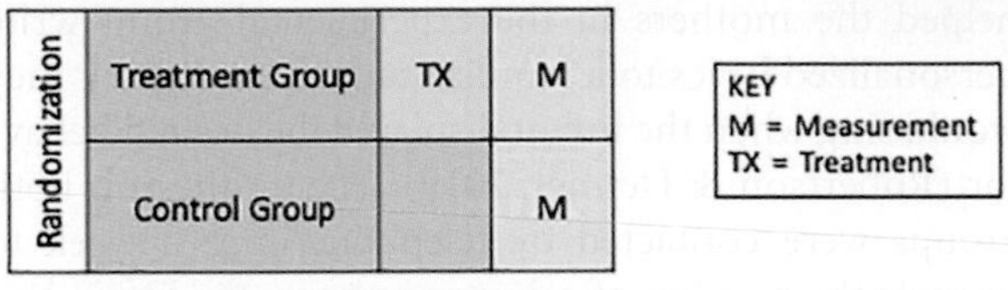

Fig. 11.19 Two-group posttest-only design with randomization and control group.

participants' responses to the posttest can be due, in part, to learning from or having a subjective reaction to the pretest (pretest sensitization or the testing threat to validity). If this issue is a concern in your study, you may opt to eliminate the pretest and use an **experimental posttest-only design with a control group** (Fig. 11.19). The absence of a pretest prevents you, however, from using more powerful statistical analysis techniques within the study and from evaluating the effectiveness of randomization in obtaining equivalent experimental and comparison groups. Answering the first two questions in Fig. 11.17 leads to this design. One intervention is tested and no pretest is used.

Robertson and Detmer (2019) used this design to test the effects of the mother singing a lullaby to reinforce calm infant behavior. In this excerpt, the researchers describe the gap in knowledge and the design.

> "There is little research on the effect of contingent music in the first weeks of life on infant crying behaviors and parent-infant interaction.... Contingent music is a common strategy used in music therapy; it is a behaviorism technique in which music either starts or stops when a behavior is exhibited. For example, if the desired infant behavior is a calm state, music may be provided until the infant becomes fussy or is crying, at which point the music stops until the infant returns to a calm state.... It has been demonstrated that infants as well as parents benefit from the use of music in the early stages of development. To date, there is no such study that analyzes the effects of live, parental contingent singing on attachment and crying behaviors in healthy newborn infants.,,,. This study utilized a posttest-only experimental/no-contact control group design with random assignment to measure mother-infant interactions, and infant crying behaviors." (Robertson & Detmer, 2019, pp. 34–35)

The mothers were randomly assigned to groups, and the demographic and maternal characteristics of the mothers were similar between groups. The researchers helped the mothers in the experimental group write personalized lyrics to a familiar tune as the lullaby they would sing when the infant displayed the desired behavior (Robertson & Detmer, 2019). The mothers in both groups were contacted by telephone once a week to provide the number of minutes or hours the infant had cried the day before. Mothers in the experimental group were also asked how many times they used the lullaby on the same day. At 6 weeks, the researcher met with all the mothers and recorded a 4-minute video of the mother playing with the infant. The recordings were coded independently by three board-certified music therapists who were blind to the group assignment. The coding produced scores for maternal warmth and responsiveness (Robertson & Detmer, 2019).

Infants in the experimental group spent significantly fewer minutes crying over the 6 weeks. Their mothers scored higher on responsiveness and warmth. Infants in both groups experienced less crying over time. This and other findings are described in the following excerpt.

"Mothers in the contingent music group reported significantly shorter infant crying periods than mothers in the control group, but interestingly, mean crying time per day decreased after the fourth week for both groups, which contradicts existing literature. The standard crying curve for newborns consists of an average crying time of 42.7 min for the first couple of weeks of life and peaks at 120 min at six weeks of age.... In the current study, mothers were taught to sing a personalized lullaby or play song that they helped create specifically for their infant as a reinforcement tool for quiet, alert behavior. Results indicated that experimental mothers used the music intervention an average of four to five times a day per week to reinforce calm behavior.... Overall, experimental mothers displayed a higher frequency of interaction behaviors with their infants than did mothers in the control group during the observational period. Look, talk, singing and infant response were all significantly different between groups.... In summary, mothers in the experimental group experienced significantly less infant crying time by using the contingent music interaction which helped to produce more enriching mother-infant interactions." (Robertson & Detmer, 2019, pp. 36, 37)

Robertson and Detmer (2019) acknowledged several limitations of the study, including mothers estimating the time the infant was crying (threat to construct design

validity) and mothers' prior experience with music (threat to internal design validity). Mothers who were experienced or educated in regard to music were able to more easily implement the intervention. Because mothers were enrolled in the study the first day after giving birth, it was not possible to measure baseline behaviors due to maternal fatigue. The demographic characteristics of mothers who refused to participate were similar to the characteristics of those who enrolled; however, other unknown characteristics may have influenced the decision to enroll. Other limitations were not noted by the researchers, such as experimenter expectancy, social desirability, attrition, and differential attrition. The combination of experimenter expectancy and social desirability may have resulted in the mothers providing lower estimates of the time the infant spent crying. Of the 66 mother-infant dyads who were enrolled in the study, only 45 completed the study (31.8% overall attrition; 36.3% experimental group; 27.3% control group). Despite these limitations, Robertson and Detmer (2019) demonstrated the feasibility of a low-cost, effective intervention that could promote maternal-infant bonding and alleviate maternal stress and depression. Researchers replicating the study with larger samples would need to implement strategies to minimize the threats to design validity that were identified.

Within-Subjects Design

Within experimental designs, the usual approach is to randomly assign participants to a treatment group or a control group to test the independent variable and analyze the difference between the groups' scores on the dependent variable. Despite random assignment, characteristics of the participants may be confounding variables that affect the study's outcome. Greenwald (1976) suggested an alternative study design, called the within-subjects design, that allows each participant to serve as his or her own control. The within-subjects design exposes each participant to all the treatment and control conditions in a random order. The design, also called a repeated measures design (Adams & Lawrence, 2019), can achieve adequate power to avoid a Type II error with a smaller sample (Greenwald, 1976).

When reading a report of a study with a within-subjects design and referring to Fig. 11.17, you would answer the first question with a yes. Within-subject designs test at least two interventions. Answering the second question of whether participants serve as their own controls with yes leads you to this study design. Within-subjects designs with two treatments can be simple with a sequence for the participants experiencing the control condition first and a sequence for participants experiencing the treatment condition first. However, within-subjects designs can also be complex with multiple treatments (Fig. 11.20).

Before discussing the complexities of multiple treatments, three terms that were defined in this chapter are important when designing within-subjects designs. The terms are *counterbalancing, carryover effect,* and *washout period.* Counterbalancing is exposing a participant to different treatments in different sequences. When a treatment has a carryover effect (the effect of a treatment persists after the treatment stops), a washout period will be required between treatments to allow the effects of the prior treatment to dissipate. In addition, two other terms (*practice effect* and *fatigue effect*) often appear when these designs are described. A practice effect occurs when the participant's performance improves because of repeating the measurement multiple times (Adams & Lawrence, 2019). A practice effect is essentially the same as the testing threat to internal design validity. A fatigue effect occurs when the participant's performance declines because the participant is tired or bored with being exposed to multiple treatments or conditions (Adams & Lawrence, 2019). The fatigue effect is similar to the maturation threat to internal design validity.

Fig. 11.20 displays a within-subjects design that could be used to test the relative effectiveness of four treatments. When four treatments are being compared, the researcher will randomly assign each participant to receive the treatments in a specific sequence. The researcher will develop four possible sequences because of the four treatments. Fig. 11.20 provides an example of four sequences. Participants will be randomly assigned to receive the treatments in one of these sequences. Measurement of the dependent variable occurs before each treatment and again after each treatment. The second treatment is offered following a washout period (if needed) and another pretest measurement. This pattern continues until the participant has experienced all four treatments. Instead of comparing the means of the posttests across the groups, the researcher will compare the means of the *difference scores* between the pretest and posttest relative to each treatment. In this way, each participant serves as his or her own control.

Previously in the chapter, a study conducted by Ward et al. (2019) was described. These physician researchers used a crossover counterbalanced design to study the effects of sleep deprivation on obesity. They used a within-subjects design by comparing each participant's posttest scores to his or her pretest scores. Golino et al. (2019) implemented a different type of within-subjects design, one in which each participant experienced one intervention. They developed a single group, pretest-posttest study to test the effects of a music intervention

Randomization	Participants-Sequence 1	M	TX-A	M	M	TX-B	M	M	TX-C	M	M	TX-D	M
	Participants-Sequence 2	M	TX-D	M	M	TX-C	M	M	TX-B	M	M	TX-A	M
	Participants-Sequence 3	M	TX-C	M	M	TX-D	M	M	TX-A	M	M	TX-B	M
	Participants-Sequence 4	M	TX-D	M	M	TX-C	M	M	TX-B	M	M	TX-A	M

KEY
M = Measurement
TX-A = Treatment A
TX-B = Treatment B
TX-C = Treatment C
TX-D = Treatment D

Fig. 11.20 Within-subjects experimental design.

on vital signs, pain, and anxiety among patients in an ICU. In this study, there was no crossover because each participant received only one intervention. Data were collected from the 52 participants before and after a 30-minute intervention of either relaxation/guided imagery or a song choice intervention. Heart rate, respiratory rate, and oxygenation level were measured along with the patients' self-reported pain and anxiety. The goal of the two versions of the intervention was the same: to reduce pain perception, decrease anxiety, and promote relaxation. The music therapist decided which intervention would be used based on the immediate needs of the patient. In keeping with the within-subjects design, the pretest and posttest scores were compared using paired *t*-tests. Then additional within-subjects (repeated measures) analyses were done, dividing the group by intervention, age, sex, and presence of family during the intervention to compare difference scores.

> "The purpose of this study was to investigate the effects of 2 music therapy interventions on 3 physiological measures (heart rate, respiratory rate, and oxygen saturation level) and self-reported pain and anxiety among patients in an ICU. After participating in a single music therapy session, patients reported lower pain and anxiety and had decreases in both heart rate and respiratory rate, with no changes in oxygen saturation level detected. Examining each intervention individually, a similar responsiveness profile emerged, with the only difference being in heart rate: participants who received the relaxation intervention had a greater decrease in heart rate than did those who received the song choice intervention.... As ICU treatment teams seek to reduce reliance on medications to address patients' needs (Gelinas, Arbour, Michaud, Robar, & Cote, 2013), nonpharmacological interventions, including music-based interventions, are being more widely implemented. Although findings from studies of music-based interventions in the ICU are mixed, the results of this study indicate that reductions in pain, anxiety, heart rate, and respiratory rate can be achieved after a single music therapy session." (Golino et al., 2019, pp. 52, 54)

Golino et al. (2019) identified limitations of the study to include the lack of a comparison or control group and the inability to determine the duration of the interventions' effects. They also acknowledged the

potential for bias with a single study site and the music therapist collecting data. Golino et al. (2019) clearly outlined their sampling inclusion and exclusion criteria, which resulted in 129 potential participants being ineligible, but they created a more homogenous sample. The ICU had only 12 beds. As a result, it took 18 months for the team to recruit an adequately sized sample. Of 106 patients who were approached, 54 refused to participate (50.9%). The high refusal rate was a threat to external design validity. Within-subjects designs allow researchers to control for potentially confounding variables, such as previous experience with music, by using each participant as his or her control. Factorial designs are another type of design that allows researchers to test different aspects of an intervention with participants divided by their characteristics.

Factorial Design

Factorial designs are not a single design, but a family of designs (Kazdin, 2017). In a **factorial design**, two or more different characteristics, treatments, or events are independently varied within a single study (Gravetter & Forzano, 2018). This design is a logical approach to examining multicausality. We are going to explain how factorial designs can be used in experimental research. It is important to note that factorial designs can also be used in noninterventional studies, such as a correlational factorial design (Adams & Lawrence, 2019). Fig. 11.17 shows this design tests multiple interventions, but participants usually do not serve as their own controls.

The simplest version of this design is one in which two treatments or factors are involved, and within each factor two levels are tested. For example, you are testing a behavioral change intervention with a sample of primary care patients. You want to compare an interactive, online learning game being played once a week or three times a week with patients diagnosed with type 2 diabetes and with chronic obstructive pulmonary disease (COPD). There are four possible combinations of the two frequencies of the intervention and two diagnoses; this is referred to as a 2 × 2 factorial design. This design is illustrated in Fig. 11.21, in which the two independent variables are the learning game once per week and the learning game three times per week, shown in the columns, and the two disease diagnoses are shown in the rows. The dependent variable is self-management confidence, or how confident the patient is to manage

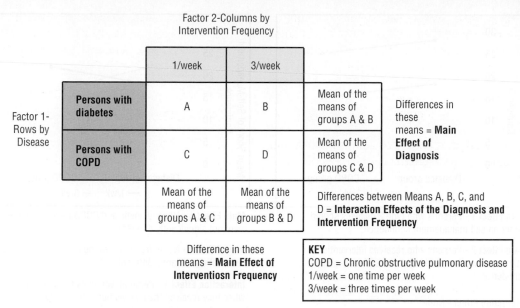

Fig. 11.21 Diagram of a 2 × 2 factorial design.

his or her chronic disease. In the simplest form of this design, you have patients with both diseases who have consented to participate in the study. Then you randomly assign them to receive either the once-a-week intervention or the three-times-a-week intervention. Each person is in only one cell of the study (A, B, C, D) as shown in Fig. 11.21. When each person is in only one cell, the design is a between-subjects design. A **between-subjects design** means that each person will be exposed to one set of experimental conditions, and the focus is on the differences between groups of participants. You want to have approximately the same number of persons in each cell.

Following data collection, the statistical analyses begin by testing for main effects. **Main effects** are the differences found between the two rows (diagnosis) and between the two columns (frequency of the intervention). The first analysis would be testing for a difference between self-management confidence of the persons with diabetes and the persons with COPD. The second analysis would be testing for a difference in self-management confidence between the once-a-week intervention and the three-a-week intervention. You also will test for interaction effects. **Interaction effects** are differences that are due to the combination of the

factors. For example, did persons with diabetes who played the game once a week have significantly different scores than the persons with COPD who played the game three times a week? Did persons with COPD who played the game once a week have significantly different scores than persons with diabetes who played the game three times a week? Frequently researchers will use a line graph such as in Fig. 11.22 to demonstrate main effects and interaction effects. On the graph, the mean score for each cell is plotted. When the lines are relatively parallel, there is no interaction effect (see Fig. 11.22A). However, when the lines intersect, there is an interaction effect (see Fig. 11.22B).

Within-subjects designs can be used with factorial designs. Each participant is exposed to the two or more levels of the intervention in different sequences with data collected between each intervention level. The advantage of a within-subjects factorial design is that a smaller sample is needed than when conducting a between-subjects factorial design (Gravetter & Forzano, 2018). Within-subjects and between-subjects designs can be combined with factorial designs, even having one factor studied within subjects and the other studied between subjects. Factorial designs also become more complex when they are extended to have three levels or

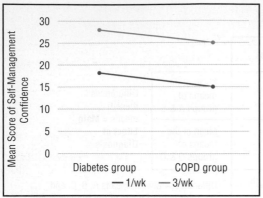

Main Effect 1 - Persons with type 2 diabetes scored higher on self management confidence.

Main Effect 2 - Persons who received intervention 3 times per week scored higher on self-management confidence

Interaction Effect - None

Main Effect 1 - None, diabetic and COPD patients' scores were not significantly different

Main Effect 2 - None, frequency of the intervention scores were not significantly different.

Interaction Effect 1 - Persons with diabetes scored higher when they received the intervention 3 times a week.

Interaction Effect 2 - Persons with COPD scored higher when they received the intervention 1 time per week.

Fig. 11.22 Types of effects in factorial designs. *COPD,* Chronic obstructive pulmonary disease.

types of interventions presented to four age groups (3 × 4 design). When researchers want to use more than two levels of variables, the numbers are adjusted to reflect the design. Note that a 3 × 4 design involves 12 cells and requires a much larger sample size. These designs are limited only by imagination and feasibility.

Factorial designs are not limited to two independent variables; however, interpretation of larger numbers becomes more complex and requires greater knowledge of statistical analysis. Factorial designs do allow the examination of theory-proposed relationships among and between multiple independent variables. However, very large samples are required (Adams & Lawrence, 2019; Gravetter & Forzano, 2018; Shadish et al., 2002). For more information about factorial designs, we recommend the books by Adams and Lawrence (2019) and Gravetter and Forzano (2018).

Clinical Trials

Clinical trials have been used in medicine since 1945 and are described as "research performed on human subjects for the purpose of assessing the safety and/or effectiveness of an intervention" (Klimberg, Shyr, & Wells, 2018, p. 364). A **clinical trial** is defined as an experiment conducted to determine whether a new treatment or medication works for patients with a specific illness or condition. Not only does a clinical trial determine effectiveness, but it also provides a description of side effects and safety concerns. There are several different types of clinical trials based on the specific purpose, the study design, and sponsorship. In this book, we are limiting our discussion of clinical trials to those designed to test medications and interventions. The studies we describe use the pretest-posttest design with control group (see Fig. 11.17).

The phase I, II, III, and IV clinical trial categories were developed specifically for testing experimental drug therapy and devices regulated by the US Food and Drug Administration (FDA). Table 11.7 provides a summary of the purposes of the different phases of clinical trials. Phase I clinical trials, the initial testing of a new drug, focuses on understanding the biochemical processes of absorption, metabolism, and excretion as well as determining the minimally effective dose and identifying initial safety concerns (Klimberg et al., 2018). The sample for phase I trials is usually comprised of healthy

TABLE 11.7 Samples and Phases of Clinical Trials

Phase	Purpose	Typical Sample
Phase I	Understand the biochemical properties of a new drug, such as absorption, metabolism, and excretion; identify optimal doses and scheduling	Healthy volunteers
Phase II	Builds on phase I findings to understand drug's effectiveness and side effects	Persons who may benefit from the drug and meet tight inclusion and exclusion sampling criteria
Phase III	Compares the new drug to the available drugs to determine is relative efficacy compared to the older drugs	Persons who may benefit from the drug are recruited and the sample is accrued over time with frequent comparisons among the groups
Phase IV	Follows regulatory approval of the new medication or device and monitors drug effectiveness and side effects that may increase or decrease over time	Larger samples of persons who may benefit from the drug; their care is overseen in multiple locations

adult volunteers. The samples for phase II trials are the patients who may potentially benefit from the new drug. Phase II studies are designed to seek preliminary evidence of efficacy and side effects of the drug dose based on the findings of the phase I trial (Korn & Freidlin, 2020). Phase II trials may have small samples and rules to stop the trial early if less than 10% of the participants have a positive response to the drug. In some situations, a phase II trial may have a placebo arm to begin comparing the effectiveness of the new drug to the current drug.

Phase III trials are comparative definitive studies in which the new drug's effects are compared with those of the drug that is considered standard therapy. Phase III trials are the most critical, because their results determine if the drug will become available to all patients. The trials are designed to determine whether the experimental drug is more effective than standard treatment. In some phase III clinical trials, the sample size is not determined before initiation of data collection. Rather, data are analyzed at intervals to test for significant differences between groups. If a significant difference is found, data collection may be discontinued. Otherwise the data collection will continue, and retesting is initiated after the accrual of additional subjects (Meinert & Tonascia, 1986).

Phase IV trials occur after regulatory approval of the drug and are designed to monitor patients over time to determine drug safety, side effects, and long-term consequences in a larger population (Klimberg et al., 2018; Zhang et al., 2016). Zhang et al. (2016) reviewed 4722 phase IV clinical trials that were designed to test the

safety and efficacy of a new medication. Based on the analysis of these trials, they were concerned that many of the trials had samples of less than 300 participants, a number that may be too small to identify rare but dangerous adverse drug effects. Over half of the studies were open label, which meant the participants knew whether they were taking the new medication. Participants knowing which drug they are taking may influence their responses to the drug. For example, participants who know they are taking the new medication may expect it to work more effectively or may be more aware of possible side effects.

Randomized Controlled Trials

Currently in medicine and nursing, the **randomized controlled trial design** is noted to be the strongest methodology for testing the effectiveness of a treatment. In fact, RCTs are considered to be the gold standard when appropriately conducted (Bickman & Reich, 2015). Several characteristics of RCTs are designed to limit the potential for bias and eliminate or attenuate threats to internal design validity. Subjects are randomly assigned to the treatment and control groups to reduce selection bias (Shadish et al., 2002). An adequate sample size is critical to be able to detect differences of clinical interest (Klimberg et al., 2018). In addition, blinding or withholding of study information from data collectors, participants, and their healthcare providers can reduce the potential for bias. For example, data collectors may interact with the participants without knowing which participants are in the treatment group and which are in the control group. Rarely can a large enough sample be recruited in one location. For that reason, often RCTs are conducted simultaneously in multiple locations dispersed across geographic regions. The primary researcher is responsible for coordinating activities among the sites, ensuring consistent data collection and fidelity of the intervention (Moher et al., 2010).

RCTs have specific, narrow inclusion and exclusion sampling criteria. To support internal design validity, a homogenous sample and controlled environment are desired. However, the same design elements that support internal design validity may be threats to external design validity (Bickman & Reich, 2015). When one treatment is clearly beneficial, participants cannot be ethically denied access to that treatment. Because of concerns about denying access to a beneficial treatment, participants who are randomly assigned to the control group may be wait-listed. **Wait-listing** participants means that they will serve as the control group during the treatment phase of the study. When the initial study is completed, these participants will be offered the treatment (Adams & Lawrence, 2019).

Another strategy for attenuating bias and calculating effects conservatively is to analyze the data of all participants using an intention to treat approach. An **intention to treat** (ITT) approach compares the outcomes of all participants even if they were not compliant with the protocol or did not complete the study (Gupta, 2011). ITT retains a study's sample size, which maintains the power of the study. The recommended approach is to use the last available data for a participant who withdraws as that participant's outcome data. Even though it underestimates the treatment effect, ITT is considered more responsible than overestimating the treatment effect. The goal is to ensure safety for future patients (Gupta, 2011).

Editors of peer-reviewed scientific journals have agreed on a set of standards for reporting critical information about the design and the results of RCTs. These standards are the Consolidated Standards of Reporting Trials (CONSORT) that were first developed in 1996 (Ghosn, Boutron, & Ravaud, 2019) and most recently updated in 2010 (Antes, 2010). The CONSORT standards were developed first for a two-parallel group RCT (Bickman & Reich, 2017). The CONSORT documents include a flow chart (Fig. 11.23), a checklist, and an explanation of the items on the checklist (CONSORT, n.d.).

Additional CONSORT versions and adaptations, called extensions, have been published for cluster RCTs, herbal medicine intervention RTCs, pragmatic RCTs, and other variations of RCTs. Ghosn et al. (2019) noted that the CONSORT extensions cover almost all types of RCTs but cautioned that compliance with the extensions requires researchers to become familiar with standards from multiple documents.

The study conducted by White-Lewis et al. (2019) was introduced earlier in this chapter. More information is provided here about the study as an example of an RCT. The study was described by White-Lewis et al. (2019) as being a "two-armed parallel single blinded RCT approach" (p. 6). Fig. 11.23 is the CONSORT flow chart they included in their study report. These researchers tested the effects of EAT on pain and mobility among adults with arthritis. The control group received an attention-control intervention, an exercise education program that provided information about arthritis and how to improve mobility and reduce pain. The EAT intervention and the control intervention were delivered each week for 1 hour for 6 weeks. An independent observer was present during the treatment sessions and control sessions to ensure intervention fidelity.

Data from physiological measurements of joint flexibility, self-reports of pain on a VAS, and an arthritis QoL instrument were collected preintervention and at the third week and the sixth week of the study (White-Lewis et al., 2019). Ten participants in each arm completed the study and provided data as scheduled (see Fig. 11.24). The participants in the treatment group had improved pain and ROM at 6 weeks but not at 3 weeks. At the end of the study, QoL scores had improved among the participants in the treatment group. The researchers acknowledged the limitations of a small sample, a lack of ethnic diversity, and the underrepresentation of men in the study (White-Lewis et al., 2019). The study's validity could have been strengthened by having data collected by a data collector blinded to group assignment.

Pragmatic Clinical Trials

RCTs are frequently criticized for their lack of external design validity because of the homogeneity of the sample and the controlled setting. The controls that enhance the internal design validity of an RCT are the

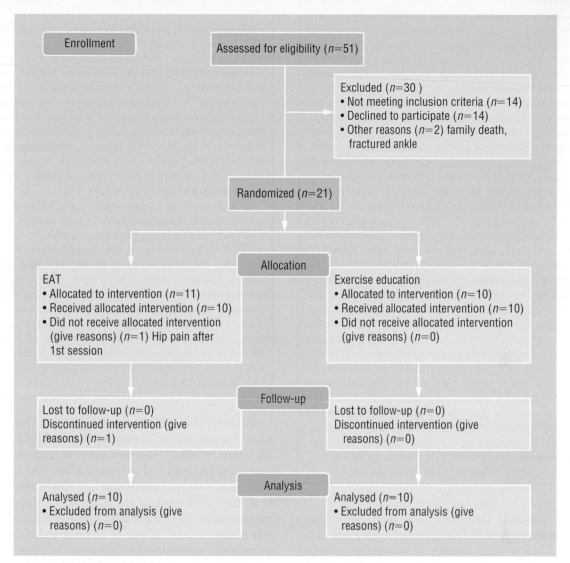

Fig. 11.23 CONSORT flow chart from White et al. (2019). (From White-Lewis, S., Johnson, R., Ye, S., & Russell, C. [2019]. An equine-assisted therapy [EAT] intervention to improve pain, range of motion, and quality of life in adults and older adults with arthritis: A randomized controlled trial. *Applied Nursing Research*, 49[1], 5–12. doi:10.1016/j.apnr.2019.07.002.)

same characteristics that reduce its external design validity. Pragmatic clinical trials have been proposed as an alternative design that balances internal and external design validity (Eckardt & Erlanger, 2018). Pragmatic trials have been recommended to compare the efficacy of two interventions among participants in usual clinical practice. The exclusion criteria are

minimal with the goal that heterogenous samples will be recruited (Littleton-Kearney, 2018).

Pickham et al. (2018) conducted a pragmatic RCT to test an innovative approach to preventing hospital-acquired pressure injuries (HAPI) among ICU patients. The following excerpt includes the study purpose and intervention.

"The purpose of this randomized clinical trial was to assess whether the use of a wearable patient sensor, to promote optimal turning practices, is effective in increasing turning compliance and preventing Hospital Acquired Pressure Injuries in patients admitted to an Intensive Care Unit.... This is an investigator-initiated, pragmatic, single site, open label, two arm, parallel, randomized clinical trial...for patients admitted to either of two Intensive Care Units at a large Academic Medical Center.... Randomization was performed by the investigators and concealment achieved using individual opaque envelopes. Permuted sizes of blocks of two, four, and six were used to approximate equal sample sizes for each stratum (ICU unit [A and B] and treating service team [medicine and surgery]). A wearable patient sensor was applied to the chest below the suprasternal notch. Once enrolled, group allocation was revealed and the patient monitoring system was selected to function in either a control or treatment mode. For patients allocated to the control group, their sensor was recording but data did not feedback to bedside clinicians. Clinicians caring for patients in the control group relied on standard care practices relying on traditional turning reminders, unaided by sensor data. Patients allocated to the treatment group had their sensor data relayed back to a point-of-care dashboard, offering the clinician real-time data on the quality of the turn performed, the patient's current position, and the time-to-next turn.... Patients were blinded to group allocation. Clinicians were not blinded but were independent to the study team." (Pickham et al., 2018, pp. 12, 13)

The clinicians continued with their normal skin assessments every shift that included staging and documenting any pressure injuries. A wound care specialist assessed pressure injuries that were found during the ICU admission and stay. Among the 1312 patients enrolled in the study, 46 pressure injuries were identified; however, only 30 were determined to be HAPIs. Pickham et al. (2018) described their study findings in the following excerpt.

"In this pragmatic randomized clinical trial, optimal patient turning with adults admitted to an Intensive Care Unit was greatest using a wearable patient sensor; improving the total time with turning compliance and significantly reducing the odds for developing Hospital Acquired Pressure Injuries. The intervention was associated with a significant increase in the total time with turning compliance for patients at high risk for pressure injuries.... The pragmatic nature of our study and the comprehensive data obtained from continuous monitoring allows us to make a series of novel observations. It is important to note, as the wearable sensor is placed on the trunk of a patient, it will only detect changes in trunk position and not the off-loading of the heels or other body parts. Notwithstanding, to our knowledge this is the first study to use wearable patient sensors to report data on turning magnitude." (Pickham et al., 2018, p. 16)

"In addition to the novelty of this study, the pragmatic nature has many advantages over prior studies. First, this study used a wearable patient sensor to capture detailed measurements of the frequency and for the first time, the dose of patient turning. No other study has been able to record dosing data, such as turning angle and tissue depressurization time in hospitalized patients. The finding that only 36% of patient turns reach a minimum turn angle threshold of 20° and only 39% of patients maintain their new position for at least 15 min of tissue depressurization, are the first quantitative data on turn dosing in Intensive Care Units." (Pickham et al., 2018, p. 18)

Pickham et al. (2018) clearly identified the advantages of pragmatic RCTs over the standard RCT design. They used stratified random assignment related to ICU admission (A or B) and to type of admission (medical or surgical). Because randomization was at the patient level, they acknowledged the potential for diffusion of the treatment. Pickham et al. (2018) also acknowledged that documentation of type of mattress and surface was incomplete. Replications of the study in other critical care settings are warranted to enhance the generalizability of the findings.

ALGORITHMS FOR IDENTIFYING AND SELECTING INTERVENTIONAL DESIGNS

As mentioned earlier in this chapter, the labels for study designs are not consistent across researchers. You may read the report of a study and note that the researchers identified the design as being experimental. However, as you dig deeper into the article, you find participants were not randomly assigned to the treatment and control groups and the researcher was not in control of the intervention—characteristics that lead you to categorize the study as quasi-experimental. We have provided algorithms or decision trees for you to use in identifying the design of published study according to how we have categorized study designs in this and the previous chapter.

To take the first step in identifying a study design, refer to Fig. 10.1 to identify the major category into which the study fits. When a study has an intervention under the control of the researcher, you know the study is either quasi-experimental or experimental. Use Fig. 11.5 to help you identify which type of interventional study you are reviewing: quasi-experimental or experimental. Two additional algorithms are provided to further specify the type of design of the quasi-experimental (see Fig. 11.6) or experimental (see Fig. 11.17) study. Identifying a design is not a rigid, rule-guided task because the researchers may have chosen to blend two designs together in their study.

Selecting a design for a potential study is a more complicated task. To select a research design, the investigator must follow paths of logical reasoning. You need a calculating mind to explore all the possible consequences of using a particular design in a study. Keep the study purpose and research problem in mind as you consider the consequences of each option. The research design organizes all the components of the study in a way that is most likely to lead to valid responses to the hypotheses that are posed. Each component of a study has to be congruent with all the other components and linked together logically. As a researcher, you have considerable flexibility in choosing a design. Because the pathways within the algorithms are not absolute, they are to be used as guides. You may decide to combine different types of designs to address your study purpose and their research objectives, questions, or hypotheses. You want to implement the most rigorous design you can based on feasibility and cost. You also have to consider how potential participants will respond to being asked to volunteer for the study. You may have difficulty recruiting participants for a study in which data will be collected eight times with each data collection lasting an hour. However, studies with high-quality research designs implemented over time are needed because they can provide evidence applicable to practice (Melnyk & Fineout-Overholt, 2019).

OTHER DESIGNS

As you read the literature, you may notice some studies that do not fit in any of the categories that we have described in this and the previous chapter. More and more studies are being published in which the researchers used quantitative and qualitative methods in the same study. These are mixed methods studies, which are described in Chapter 14. There are two additional types of studies that do not fit well into the categories of descriptive, correlational, quasi-experimental, and experimental research; these are comparative effectiveness research and methodological designs.

Comparative Effectiveness Research

RCTs continue to be the gold standard for establishing cause-and-effect relationships among variables. However, RCTs are expensive to implement. Observational studies using existing data are being conducted more frequently to answer clinical questions (Soni & Spratt, 2019). Observational and other types of studies to determine which treatments and medications have the best outcomes in clinical practice comprise a category of studies called **comparative effectiveness research** (CER) (Martinez, Brouwer, & Moga, 2019). A more comprehensive definition is "the scientific search for and quantification of differences in the full range of benefits and harms of two or more approaches to preventing, diagnosing, treating, or managing disease" (Selby, Whitlock, Sherman, & Slutsky, 2018, p. 270). For example, CER addresses questions such as, "Which medication has the fewest adverse side effects?" and "Which of these treatments has resulted in the most favorable clinical outcomes?" A CER study generates evidence that can be used to guide clinical decisions in the future (Selby et al., 2018). CER studies are frequently retrospective studies, using existing data from administrative and claims databases (Brown & Pham, 2018; Sun & Lipsitz, 2018). CER studies, however, may be prospective studies in which participants are randomly assigned to one of two medications or treatments. Studies conducted for comparing treatments' effectiveness typically have more diverse samples than RCTs. In contrast to the ideal environmental conditions created for RCTs, CER studies reflect how the intervention is being used in clinical practice with the general population (Martinez et al., 2019; Sands, 2019).

Prospective CER studies share some of the characteristics of pragmatic RCTs. A pragmatic RCT may have a similar purpose as a CER study. CER also overlaps with patient-centered outcomes research (PCOR), a type of outcomes research that is guided by the needs and preferences of patients and their families. Since 2012, the Patient-Centered Outcomes Research Institute (PCORI) has been funded by the federal government to conduct CER. PCORI provides formal avenues for patients and families to set priorities for funded CER (PCORI, 2019). PCOR studies are CER that consider clinical outcomes as well as the outcomes that matter to patients and families.

A recent example of CER is a study in which Hines et al. (2019) evaluated the relationship between posttreatment surveillance and long-term survival of colon cancer patients, ages 66 to 84 years, who were diagnosed as being stages II and III. In this observational, retrospective study, researchers used the combination of a surveillance database and a Medicare database to create a sample of persons diagnosed between 2002 and 2009 ($N = 17, 860$). The patients were classified as "more adherent" or "less adherent" based on whether they had completed recommended surveillance testing following treatment. Patients who had not undergone any surveillance testing were not included. The primary result was that patients who were less adherent with surveillance testing had a slightly better 5-year cancer-specific survival and a worse 5-year noncancer-specific survival. However, there was no difference in overall survival between the groups. Based on the results, researchers advocated for providers and patients to make decisions about posttreatment surveillance testing together, using the patient's age, risk for reoccurrence, and other morbidities as considerations. Hines et al. (2019) supported using a CER observational design for this study because an RCT study of whether posttreatment surveillance contributed to survival would be unethical. Hines et al. (2019) also acknowledged the limitations of an observational study, such as unmeasured prognostic factors.

Several scholars have noted the limitations of CER studies, such as the selection bias and the missing data of existing databases. Cancer registries are examples of existing databases that are used frequently but may have missing data (Soni, 2019; Soni & Spratt, 2019). For example, registries and some other databases may lack data on functional status, self-reported health status, and socioeconomic characteristics. These factors have been shown to be confounders when considering outcomes. Sun and Lipsitz (2018) argue that these limitations can be overcome by "rigorous study designs and methodologies, austerity in handling data, and careful use of statistical techniques" (p. 174). If you want to know more about CER, the Sun and Lipsitz (2018) article is an excellent resource. Also Chapter 13 covers outcomes research, including additional information about PCOR.

Methodological Designs

Methodological studies may be conducted to ensure the feasibility of an intervention, compare statistical analyses, or determine the cost/yield ratio for different recruitment strategies. **Methodological designs** are used to test selected methods in studies designed for that purpose. In nursing and healthcare research, the most common methodological studies are those testing the validity and reliability of new and revised instruments to measure psychosocial and functional variables. The process to develop or revise an instrument is lengthy and complex. The average time required to develop a research tool to the point of appropriate use in a study is 5 years (Waltz et al., 2017). Before an instrument is published, the developers have conducted methodological studies to assess content validity, the conceptual structure of the scale, construct design validity, and reliability (see Chapter 16).

Bruckenthal and Gilson (2019) conducted a methodological study to develop an instrument to measure the perceptions of advanced practice registered nurses (APRNs) related to pain management, prescription opioid regulations, and effective pain management. Bruckenthal and Gilson (2019) developed an initial set of 33 items from pain management competencies, model opioid prescribing policies, and a focus group of APRNs. The tool was sent to five experts for content validity testing and then revised based on their input. The revised instrument was sent to members of a state APRN association who were asked to participate by completing the instrument. The instrument was found to have acceptable or near acceptable internal consistency for a new instrument based on the responses of 23 APRNs. Before widespread use, the instrument needs additional psychometric testing with larger samples and in different states.

Quasi-experimental and experimental designs usually require more time and resources than noninterventional designs. Because of this, methodological designs play key roles in determining the validity and reliability of instruments and the feasibility of interventions prior to investing in quasi-experimental and experimental studies.

KEY POINTS

- Researchers have developed designs to meet unique research needs as they emerge.
- Manipulation is the implementation of the study's treatment or intervention.
- Random selection results in a sample such as the accessible population and increases external design validity.
- Random assignment to groups increases the similarity between the treatment and control groups.
- Partitioning is dividing a variable into subsets for analysis.
- Factorial designs allow the researcher to compare different groups of participants with different levels of the independent variable.
- Intervention mapping is a methodological strategy that is useful in translating evidence into researchable interventions.
- An intervention protocol is a detailed implementation plan to rigorously conduct an interventional study.
- Double blinding is hiding participants' group assignments from the participants and data collectors.
- Obtaining an understanding of the true effects of an experimental treatment requires action to control threats to the validity of the findings.
- Threats to validity are controlled through random assignment of participants to groups, intervention fidelity, valid and reliable measurements of variables, blinding participants and data collectors to group assignments, and using strategies to increase retention of participants throughout the study.
- Experimental designs have random assignment to groups, rigorously implemented interventions, control groups, and attenuation of threats to validity. Quasi-experimental designs lack one or more of these characteristics.
- Posttest-only designs are weaker designs and are labeled pre-experiments by some scholars.
- Quasi-experimental designs include pretest-posttest one-group designs, pretest-posttest with treatment and comparison groups, pretest-posttest designs with two or more treatments, pretest-posttest with multiple groups and removed treatments, and interrupted time series designs with and without comparison groups.
- Experimental designs include pretest-posttest control group designs, Solomon four-group design, posttest-only control group, within-subjects design, factorial designs, clinical trials, pragmatic clinical trials, and RCTs.
- Currently in medicine and nursing, the randomized controlled trial design is noted to be the strongest methodology for testing the effectiveness of a treatment because of the elements of the design that limit the potential for bias.
- The CONSORT 2010 Statement clarifies the steps for conducting and reporting an RCT.
- Comparative effectiveness research is similar to pragmatic clinical trials because heterogenous samples are desirable to compare two or more treatments.
- Methodological studies are designed to develop the validity and reliability of instruments to measure constructs used as variables in research.
- Algorithms for design identification and selection are provided in Figs. 11.5, 11.16, and 11.24.

REFERENCES

Aberson, C. L. (2019). *Applied power analysis for the behavioral sciences* (2nd ed.). New York, NY: Routledge Taylor & Francis Group.

Adams, K., & Lawrence, E. (2019). *Research methods, statistics, and applications* (2nd ed.). Thousand Oaks, CA: Sage.

Antes, G. (2010). The new CONSORT statement. *BMJ, 340,* 1432. doi:10.1136/bmj.c1432

Berrios-Montero, R. (2019). Choice of a short-term prediction model for patient discharge before noon: A walk-through of ARIMA model. *The Health Care Manager, 38*(2), 116–123. doi:10.1097/HCM.0000000000000262

Bickman, L., & Reich, S. (2015). Randomized trials: A gold standard or gold plated? In S. Donaldson, C. Christie, & M. Mark (Eds.), *Credible and actionable evidence: The foundation for rigorous and influential evaluations* (2nd ed.), Thousand Oaks, CA: Sage. doi:10.4135/9781483385839

Box, G., & Jenkins, G. (1976). *Time-series analysis: Forecasting and control.* San Francisco, CA: Holden-Day.

Boyce, J., Cooper, T., Yin, J., Li, F. Y., & Arbogast, J. (2019). Challenges encountered and lessons learned during a trial of an electronic hand hygiene monitoring system. *American Journal of Infection Control, 47*(1), 1443–1448. doi:10.1016/j.ajic.2019.05.019

Braver, M., & Braver, S. (1988). Statistical treatment of the Solomon four-group design: A meta-analytic approach. *Psychological Bulletin, 104*(1), 150–154. doi:10.1037/0033-2909.104.1.150

Brown, J., & Pham, P. (2018). The need for deliberate and thorough design and critique of observational comparative effectiveness research. *Research in Social and Administrative Pharmacy, 14*(11), 1085–1087. doi:10.1016/j.sapharm.2018.07.012

Bruckenthal, P., & Gilson, A. (2019). Development and validation of the achieving effective & safe opioid prescribing—advanced practice registered nurse (AESOP-APRN) survey: A pilot study. *Pain Management Nursing, 20*(3), 214–221. doi:10.1016/j.pmn.2019.02.013

Campbell, D. T., & Stanley, J. C. (1963). *Experimental and quasi-experimental designs for research.* Chicago, IL: Rand McNally.

Çetin, N., & Aylaz, R. (2018). The effect of mindfulness-based psychoeducation on insight and medication adherence of schizophrenia patients. *Archives of Psychiatric Nursing, 32*(5), 737–744. doi:10.1016/j.apnu.2018.04.011

Chang, P. S., Chao, A., Jang, M., & Lu, Y. (2019). Intervention fidelity in Qigong randomized controlled trials: A method review. *Geriatric Nursing, 40*(1), 84–90. doi:10.1016/j.gerinurse.2018.07.001

Chen, S., Hsu, H., Wang, R., Lee. Y., & Hsieh, C. (2019). Glycemic control in insulin-treated patients with type 2 diabetes: Empowerment perceptions and diabetes distress as important determinants. *Biological Research in Nursing, 21*(2), 182–189. doi:10.1177/1099800418820170

CONSORT. (n.d.). *Welcome to the CONSORT.* Retrieved from http://www.consort-statement.org/

Cook, T. D., & Campbell, D. T. (1979). *Quasi-experimentation: Design and analysis issues for field settings.* Chicago, IL: Rand McNally.

Crawford, L., Freeman, B., Huscroft-D'Angelo, J., Fuentes, S., & Higgins, K. (2019). Implementation fidelity and the design of a fractions intervention. *Learning Disability Quarterly, 42*(4), 217–230. doi:10.1177/0731948719840774

Creswell, J. W., & Creswell, J. D. (2018). *Research design: Qualitative, quantitative, and mixed methods approaches* (5th ed.). Thousand Oaks, CA: Sage.

Crowne, D., & Marlowe, D. (1960). A new scale of social desirability independent of psychopathology. *Journal of Consulting Psychology, 24*(4), 349–354.

Cuevas, H., Stuifbergen, A., Brown, S., & Ward, C. (2019). A nurse-led cognitive training intervention for individuals with type 2 diabetes. *Research in Gerontological Nursing, 12*(4), 203–212. doi:10.3928/19404921-20190612-01

Eckardt, P., & Erlanger, A. (2018). Lessons learned in methods and analyses for pragmatic studies. *Nursing Outlook 66*(5), 446–454. doi:10.1016/j.outlook.2018.06.012

El-Deen, D., & Youssef, N. (2018). The effect of cryotherapy application before versus after subcutaneous anticoagulant injection on pain intensity and hematoma formation: A quasi-experimental design. *International Journal of Nursing Sciences, 5*(3), 223–229. doi:10.1016/j.ijnss.2018.07.006

Eldredge, L., Markham, C., Ruiter, R., Fernandez, R., Kok, G., & Parcel, G. (2016). *Planning health promotion programs: An intervention mapping approach* (4th ed.). San Francisco, CA: Jossey-Bass.

Esopo, K., Mellow, D., Thomas, C., Uckat, H., Abraham, J., & Haushofer, J. (2018). Measuring self-efficacy, executive function, and temporal discounting in Kenya. *Behaviour Research and Therapy, 101*(2), 30–45. doi:10.1016/j.brat.2017.10.002

Ferreira-Valente, M., Pais-Ribeiro, J., & Jensen, M. (2011). Validity of four pain intensity rating scales. *Pain, 152*(10), 2399–2404. doi:10.1016/j.pain.2011.07.005

French, C., Diekemper, R., & Irwin, R. on behalf of the CHEST Expert Cough Panel. (2015). Assessment of intervention fidelity and recommendations for researchers conducting studies on the diagnosis and treatment of chronic cough in the adult: CHEST Guideline and Expert Panel Report. *CHEST, 148*(1), 32–54. doi:10.1378/chest.15-0164

Gelinas, C., Arbour, C., Michaud, C., Robar, L., & Cote, J. (2013). Patients and ICU nurses' perspectives of non-pharmacological interventions for pain management. *Nursing Critical Care, 18*(6), 307–318. doi:10.1111/j.1478-5153.2012.00531.x

Ghosn, L., Boutron, I., & Ravaud, P. (2019). Consolidated standards of reporting trials (CONSORT) extensions covered most types of randomized controlled trials, but the potential workload for authors was high. *Journal of Clinical Epidemiology, 113*(9), 168–175. doi:10.1016/j.jclinepi.2019.05.030

Gleiss, A., & Schemper, M. (2019). Quantifying degrees of necessity and of sufficiency in cause-effect relationships with dichotomous and survival outcomes. *Statistics in Medicine, 38*(23), 4733–4748. doi:10.1002/sim.8331

Golino, A., Leone, R., Gollenberg, A., Christopher, C., Stanger, D., Davis, T., ... Friesen, M. (2019). Impact of active music therapy intervention on intensive care patients. *American Journal of Critical Care, 28*(1), 48–55. doi:10.4037/ajcc2019792

Grau, I., Ebbeler, C., & Banse, R. (2019). Cultural differences in careless responding. *Journal of Cross-Cultural Psychology, 50*(3), 336–357. doi:10.1177/0022022119827379

Gravetter, F., & Forzano, L. A. (2018). *Research methods for the behavioral sciences* (6th ed.). Boston, MA: Cengage.

Greenwald, A. (1976). Within-in subjects designs: To use or not to use? *Psychological Bulletin, 83*(2), 314–320. doi:10.1037/0033-2909.83.2.314

Gregory, E., Miller, J., Wasserman, R., Seshadri, R., Rubin, D., & Fiks, A. (2019). Routine cholesterol tests and subsequent change in BMI among overweight and obese children. *Academic Pediatrics, 19*(7), 773–779. doi:10.1016/j.acap.2019.05.131

Grove, S. K., & Cipher, D. (2020). *Statistics for health care research: A practical workbook* (3rd ed.). St. Louis, MO: Elsevier.

Gupta, S. (2011). Intention-to-treat concept: A review. *Perspectives in Clinical Research*, 2(3), 109–112. doi:10.4103/2229-3485.83221

Handley, M., Lyles, C., McCulloch, C., & Cattamanchi, A. (2018). Selecting and improving quasi-experimental designs in effectiveness and implementation research. *Annual Review of Public Health, 39*(1), 5–25. doi:10.1146/annurev-publhealth-040617-014128

Harrison, J., Anderson, W., Fagin, M., Robinson, E., Schnipper, J., Symczak, G., ... Auerbach, A. (2019). Patient and family advisory councils for research: Recruiting and supporting members from diverse and hard-to-reach communities. *Journal of Nursing Administration, 49*(10), 473–479. doi:10.1097/NNA.0000000000000790

Hayes-Larson, E., Kezios, K., Mooney, S., & Lovasi, G. (2019). Who is in this study, anyway? Guidelines for a useful Table 1. *Journal of Clinical Epidemiology, 114*(1), 125–132. doi:10.1016/j.jclinepi.2019.06.011

Hines, R., Jiban, M., Specogna, A., Vishnubhotla, P., Lee, E., & Zhanang, S. (2019). The association between post-treatment surveillance testing and survival in stage II and III colon cancer patients: An observational comparative effectiveness study. *BMC Cancer, 19*, 418. doi:10.1186/s12885-019-5613-5

Hinic, K., Kowalski, M., Holtzman, K., & Mobus, K. (2019). The effect of a pet therapy and comparison intervention on anxiety of hospitalized children. *Journal of Pediatric Nursing, 46*(1), 55–61. doi:10.1016/j.pedn.2019.03.003

Hsu, H., Kawai, A., Wang, R., Jentzsch, M., Rhee, C., Horan, K., ... Lee, G. (2018). The impact of the Medicaid health-care-associated condition program on mediastinitis following coronary artery bypass graft. *Infection Control & Hospital Epidemiology, 39*(6), 694–700. doi:10.1017/ice.2018.69

Jeong, Y., Quinn, L., Kim, N., & Martyn-Nemeth, P. (2018). Health related stigma in young adults with type 1 diabetes mellitus. *Journal of Psychosocial Nursing and Mental Health Services, 56*(10), 44–51. doi:10.3928/02793695-20180503-01

Kako, J., Morita, T., Yamaguchi, T., Sekimoto, A., Kobayashi, M., Kinoshita, H., ... Matsushima, E. (2018). Evaluation of the appropriate washout period following fan therapy for dyspnea in patients with advanced cancer: A pilot study. *American Journal of Hospice & Palliative Medicine, 35*(2), 293–296. doi:10.1177/1049909117707905

Kazdin, A. (2017). *Research design in clinical psychology* (5th ed.). Boston, MA: Pearson.

Kenny, D. (2019). Enhancing validity in psychological research. *American Psychologist, 74*(9), 1018–1028. doi:10.1037/amp0000531

Kerlinger, F. N., & Lee, H. B. (2000). *Foundations of behavioral research* (4th ed.). Fort Worth, TX: Harcourt College Publishers.

Kienen, N., Wiltenburg, T., Bittencourt, L., & Scarinci, I. (2019). Development of a gender-relevant for tobacco cessation intervention for women in Brazil: An intervention mapping approach to planning. *Health Education Research, 34*(5), 505–520. doi:10.1093/her/cyz025

Kim, M., Gang, M., Lee, J., & Park, E. (2019). The effects of self-care intervention programs for elderly with mild cognitive impairment. *Issues in Mental Health Nursing, 40*(11), 973–980. doi:10.1080/01612840.2019.1619202

Klimberg, S., Shyr, Y., & Wells, T. (2018). Design and conduct of clinical trials for breast cancer. In K. Bland, E. Copeland, S. Klimberg, & W. Gradishar (Eds.), *The breast: Comprehensive management of benign and malignant diseases* [E-version] (5th ed., pp. 362–376). Philadelphia, PA: Elsevier.

Korn, E., & Freidlin, B. (2020). Clinical trial designs in oncology. In. J. Niederhuber, J. Armitage, J. Doroshow, M. Kastan, & J. Tepper (Eds.), *Abeloff's clinical oncology* (6th ed., pp. 296–307). Philadelphia, PA: Elsevier.

Leedy, P. D., & Ormrod, J. E. (2019). *Practical research: Planning and design* (12th ed.). New York, NY: Pearson.

Linden, A. (2018). Using forecast modelling to evaluate treatment effects in single-group interrupted time series analysis. *Journal of Evaluation in Clinical Practice, 24*(4), 695–700. doi:10.1111/jcp.12946

Littleton-Kearney, M. (2018). Pragmatic clinical trials at the National Institute of Nursing Research. *Nursing Outlook, 66*(5), 470–472. doi:10.1016/j.outlook.2018.02.001

Luján, J., & Todt, O. (in press). Standards of evidence and causality in regulatory science: Risk and benefit assessment. *Studies in History and Philosophy of Science Part A*, doi:10.1016/j.shpsa.2019.05.005

Martinez, A., Brouwer, E., & Moga, D. (2019). Comparative effectiveness research. In Z. Babar (Ed.), *Encyclopedia of pharmacy practice and clinical pharmacy* (pp. 409–419). Philadelphia, PA: Elsevier. doi:10.1016/B978-0-12-812735-3.00209-0

Mathew, S., & Thukha, H. (2018). Pilot testing of the effectiveness of nurse-guided, patient-centered heart failure education for older adults. *Geriatric Nursing, 39*(4), 376–381. doi:10.1016/j.gerinurse.2017.11.006

McBreen, B. (2018). The asymmetry of causality: A realist solution. *Philosophical Investigations, 41*(1), 3–21. doi:10.1111/phin.12174

Meinert, C. L., & Tonascia, S. (1986). *Clinical trials: Design, conduct, and analysis.* New York, NY: Oxford University Press.

Melnyk, B. M., & Fineout-Overholt, E. (2019). *Evidence-based practice in nursing & healthcare: A guide to best practice* (4th ed.). Philadelphia, PA: Lippincott Williams, & Wilkins.

Milo, R., & Connelly, C. (2019). Predictors of glycemic management among patients with type 2 diabetes. *Journal of Clinical Nursing, 28*(9/10), 1737–1744. doi:10.1111/jocn.14779

Moher, D., Hopewell, S., Schultz, K., Montori, V., Gøtzsche, P., Devereaux, P., ... Altman, D. (2010). CONSORT 2010 explanation and elaboration: Updated guidelines for reporting parallel group randomised trials. *BMJ, 340,* 869. doi:10.1136/bmj.c869

Neuman, B., & Fawcett, J. (2011). *The Neuman systems model* (5th ed). Upper Saddle River, NJ: Pearson.

Oertle, S., Burrell, S., & Pirollo, M. (2016). Evaluating the effects of a physician-referred exercise program on cancer-related fatigue and quality of life among early cancer survivors. *Journal of Oncology Navigation & Survivorship, 7*(2), 9–15.

Patient-Centered Outcomes Research Institute (PCORI). (2019). *Research funding.* Retrieved from https://www.pcori.org/sites/default/files/PCORI-Research-Funding.pdf

Persaud, I. (2012). Rosenthal effect. In N. Salkind (Ed.), *Encyclopedia of research design.* Retrieved from https://methods.sagepub.com/reference/encyc-of-research-design

Pett, M. A. (2016). *Nonparametric statistics for health care research: Statistics for small samples and unusual distributions* (2nd ed.). Los Angeles, CA: Sage.

Phan, H., & Ngu, B. (2017). Undertaking experiments in social sciences: Sequential, multiple time series designs for consideration. *Educational Psychology Review, 29,* 847–867. doi:10.1007/s10648-016-9368-0

Pickham, D., Berte, N., Pihulic, M., Valdez, A., Mayer, B., & Desai, M. (2018). Effect of a wearable patient sensor on care delivery for preventing pressure injuries in acutely ill adults: A pragmatic randomized clinical trial (LS-HAPI study). *International Journal of Nursing Studies, 80*(1), 12–19. doi:10.1016/j.ijnurstu.2017.12.012

Reeves, B., Wells, G., & Waddington, H. (2017). Quasi-experimental study designs series-paper 5: A checklist for classifying studies evaluating the effects on health interventions—a taxonomy without labels. *Journal of Clinical Epidemiology, 89*(9), 30–42. doi:10.1016/j.jclinepi.2017.02.016

Resnicow, K., Braithwaite, R., Ahluwalia, J., & Baranowski, T. (1999). Cultural sensitivity in public health: Defined and demystified. *Ethnicity and Disease, 9*(1), 10–21.

Robertson, A., & Detmer, M. (2019). The effects of contingent lullaby music on parent-infant interaction and amount of infant crying in the first six weeks of life. *Journal of Pediatric Nursing, 46*(1), 33–38. doi:10.1016/j.pedn.2019.02.025

Sampaio, F., Araújo, O., Sequeira, C., Canut, M., & Martins, T. (2018). A randomized controlled trial of a nursing psychotherapeutic intervention for anxiety in adult psychiatric outpatients. *Journal of Advanced Nursing, 74*(5), 114–1126. doi:10.1111/jan.13520

Sands, B. (2019). Comparative effectiveness research in inflammatory bowel disease: The VARSITY study and beyond. *Gastroenterology & Hepatology, 15*(12), 682–684.

Selby, J., Whitlock, E., Sherman, K., & Slutsky, J. (2018). The role of comparative effectiveness research. In J. Gallin, F. Ognibene, & L. Johnson (Eds.), *Principles and practice of clinical research* (4th ed., pp. 269–292). Philadelphia, PA: Elsevier.

Shadish, W., Cook, T., & Campbell, D. (2002). *Experimental and quasi-experimental designs for generalized causal inference.* Boston, MA: Houghton Mifflin.

Shaw, S., Korchmaros, J., Torres, C., Totman, M., & Lee, J. (2019). The RxHL study: Community-responsive research to explore barriers to medication adherence. *Health Education Research, 34*(6), 556–568. doi:10.1093/her/cyz029

Singelis, T., Garcia, R., Barker, J., & Davis, R. (2018). An experimental test of the two-dimensional theory of cultural sensitivity in health communication. *Journal of Health Communication, 23*(4), 321–328. doi:10.1080/10810730.2018.1443526

Solomon, R. (1949). An extension of control group design. *Psychological Bulletin, 46*(2), 137–150. doi:10.1037/h0062958

Soni, P. (2019). Selection bias in population registry-based comparative effectiveness research. *International Journal of Radiation Oncology, Biology, & Physics, 103*(5), 1058–1060. doi:10.1016/j.ijrobp.2018.12.011

Soni, P., & Spratt, D. (2019). Population-based observational studies in oncology: Proceed with caution. *Seminars in Radiation Oncology, 29*(4), 302–305. doi:10.1016/j.semradonc.2019.05.011

Stuart, E. (2010). Matching methods for causal inference: A review and a look forward. *Statistical Science, 25*(1), 1–21. doi:10.1214/09-STS313

Sun, M., & Lipsitz, S. (2018). Comparative effectiveness research methodology using secondary data: A starting user's guide. *Urologic Oncology: Seminars and Original Investigations, 36,* 174–182. doi:10.1016/j.urolonc.2017.10.011

Suter, W., & Suter, P. (2015). How research conclusions go wrong: A primer for home health clinicians. *Home Health Care Management & Practice, 27*(4), 171–177. doi:10.1177/1084822315586557

Von Visger, T., Thrane, S., Klatt, M., Dabbs, A., Chlan, L., & Happ, M. (2019). Intervention fidelity monitoring of

Urban Zen Integrative Therapy (UZIT) for persons with pulmonary hypertension. *Complementary Therapies in Medicine, 45,* 45–49. doi:10.1016/j.ctim.2019.03.008

Walker, L., & Avant, K. (2019). *Strategies for theory construction in nursing* (6th ed.). New York, NY: Pearson.

Waltz, C. F., Strickland, O. L., & Lenz, E. R. (2017). *Measurement in nursing and health research* (5th ed.). New York, NY: Springer.

Ward, A., Galland, B., Haszard, J., Meredith-Jones, K., Morrison, S., McIntosh, D., ... Taylor, R. (2019). The effect of mild sleep deprivation on diet and eating behaviour in children: Protocol for the Daily Rest, Eating, and Activity Monitoring (DREAM) randomized cross-over trial. *BMC Public Health, 19,* 1347. doi:10.1186/s12889-019-7628-x

White-Lewis, S., Johnson, R., Ye, S., & Russell, C. (2019). An equine-assisted therapy intervention to improve pain, range of motion, and quality of life in adults and older adults with arthritis: A randomized controlled trial. *Applied Nursing Research, 49*(1), 5–12. doi:10.1016/j.apnr.2019.07.002

Williams, T., & Spurlock, W. (2019). Using high fidelity simulation to prepare baccalaureate nursing students enrolled in a historically Black college and university. *ABNF Journal, 30*(2), 37–43.

Zhang, X., Zhang, Y., Ye, X., Guo, X., Zhang, T., & He, T. (2016). Overview of phase IV trials for postmarket drug safety surveillance: A status report from the ClinicalTrials.gov registry. *BMJ Open, 6,* e010643. doi:10.1136/bmjopen-2015-010643

Zhou, L., Zhao, P., Wu, D., Cheng, C., & Huang, H. (2018). Time series model for forecasting the number of new admission inpatients. *BMC Medical Informatics and Decision Making, 18,* 39. doi:10.1186/s12911-018-0616-8

12

Qualitative Research Methods

Jennifer R. Gray

http://evolve.elsevier.com/Gray/practice/

Qualitative researchers are motivated to know more about a phenomenon, a social process, or a culture from the perspectives of the people who are experiencing the phenomenon, involved in the social process, or living in the culture (Creswell & Poth, 2018). When a qualitative methodology is appropriate, the researcher determines the best qualitative methodology for the study (see Chapter 4). The early steps of the qualitative research process, which are similar to the early steps of the quantitative research process, are explored in Chapters 5 and 6. Other steps in the research process are implemented differently or have unique characteristics in qualitative studies, such as the literature review. In this chapter, qualitative methods for data collection and analysis are described so that you can understand the process and envision what the experience will be like when you conduct a qualitative study.

The purpose of this chapter is to provide examples of the qualitative methods used to gather, analyze, and interpret data. This chapter begins by sharing basic principles of qualitative methods and steps of the research process that are implemented differently in various qualitative methodologies. The chapter also includes information relative to qualitative sampling, in addition to the information provided in Chapter 15. The data collection methods of observation, interviews, focus groups, photovoice, and electronically mediated data are described with examples from the literature. Data analysis is also included in the chapter with specific emphasis on coding, thematic analysis, and use of computer-assisted qualitative data analysis software (CAQDAS) in developing findings. The chapter concludes with a presentation

of methods that are used primarily with only one methodology, such as phenomenology or ethnography.

PRINCIPLES SUPPORTING QUALITATIVE METHODS

Conducting qualitative studies with rigor require certain beliefs and actions on the part of researchers. In Chapter 4, the research-related beliefs held by qualitative researchers, such as valuing the unique perspective of the individual, were described. The actions congruent with these beliefs are described in this section. This section also builds on the discussion of deductive and inductive thinking from Chapter 1. We will add abductive thinking and describe how these thinking processes are used in qualitative studies. These thinking processes are critical to being flexible (introduced in Chapter 4) and maintaining rigor during study implementation. We will describe methods that allow the qualitative researchers to be flexible and rigorous, such us reading primary sources, working with a research mentor, documenting the study with an audit trail, and implementing member checking. To persevere while developing, implementing, and disseminating qualitative studies, researchers must be highly motivated and believe that findings of the studies will make a difference in the lives of patients.

Researcher Commitment

All research requires a commitment of time and energy to design and implement a study using rigorous methods. Qualitative methods, however, may require additional time. Qualitative researchers must develop relationships of trust and vulnerability with participants. The researcher's relationship with the participants and the collection of data may elicit emotional reactions that are inspiring, disturbing, and certainly thought provoking. Creswell and Poth (2018) identify what is required of qualitative researchers related to implementing studies, beginning with being willing to "commit to extensive time in the field" (p. 47) (Box 12.1). These actions are necessary to produce quality findings that are credible and dependable.

The first of these behaviors has already been mentioned: the requirement for an extensive time commitment. Time is needed to read and understand primary sources about the methodology you are using. To identify primary sources, review the reference lists for Chapter 4 and this chapter. We have used primary sources when possible.

In addition to reading primary sources, a researcher new to qualitative methods should identify a research mentor, especially one who has more experience with the specific methods or topic of interest (Corbin & Strauss, 2015). By sharing their personal experiences with the mentees, research mentors can guide less experienced researchers as they become scholars (Block & Florczak, 2017), including planning the study's procedures and timeline in a realistic manner (Marshall & Rossman, 2016). Hafsteinsdóttira, van der Zwaaga, and Schuurmansa (2017) conducted a systematic review of studies related to research mentoring. They found evidence that mentored researchers had increased research knowledge and productivity.

Data collection and data analysis usually occur concurrently in qualitative studies. The data may be collected by one or more of the methods we have previously identified. These methods will be explored in detail later in this chapter. The text of journals and reflective writing will also be analyzed. Creswell and Poth (2018) note the need to write lengthy passages (see Box 12.1). Writing is one way for the researcher to process his or her responses during data collection and insights during data analysis.

Creswell and Poth (2018) also identify the need for flexibility with their statement, "Embrace divergent and emergent procedures" (p. 47). We describe flexibility with rigor later in this section. The last of Creswell and Poth's (2018) behaviors relates to the unique ethical challenges that may arise during a qualitative study, which are discussed in Chapter 9.

Several of the behaviors identified by Creswell and Poth (2018) are documented by Pool (2019), who conducted an interpretive phenomenological study collaboratively with nurses who had experience in providing cancer care to American Indian (AI) patients. As you read the passage, see how many of the behaviors described in this section you can identify.

BOX 12.1 What Qualitative Studies Are Required of Researchers

Are you willing to do the following?
- "Commit to extensive time in the field."
- "Engage in the complex, time-consuming process of data analysis."
- "Write lengthy and descriptive passages."
- "Embrace dynamic and emergent procedures."
- "Attend to anticipated and developing ethical issues." (Creswell & Poth, 2018, p. 47)

From Creswell, J., & Poth, C. (2018). *Qualitative inquiry & research design: Choosing among five approaches* (4th ed.). Thousand Oaks, CA: Sage.

"Participants were recruited via e-mail and word-of-mouth using professional and academic networks and in collaboration with two research mentors, one of whom identifies as AI.... Data collection and analysis procedures for the study intersected and were largely dependent upon one another, thus are concurrently described. An exploratory and hermeneutical interviewing strategy was utilized during repeated one-on-one interviewing with the participants. Interviews lasting approximately 1 hour were conducted in chronological order for each individual participant and not for the sample as a whole.... Following the first and all subsequent interviews, the following procedures were undertaken: (a) immediate reflective writing in a journal to capture first impressions and to note embodied responses that were not captured by the audio-recording; (b) during the interim between interviews, engagement in a period of contemplative dwelling with repeated exposure to the transcribed interviews and the creation of reflective memos exploring potential structures buried within the text; and (c) tentative coding of the emic data utilizing Van Manen's (1990) wholistic/sententious, selective, and detailed approaches. For example, entire passages, short phrases, and single words were all coded for potential significance or for further exploration in future interviews; (d) conscious refrainment from assigning any meaning to the participants' recollections in an effort to remain open and accessible to their individual experiences. Instead, continued reflective journaling was employed to attenuate for the researcher's own inevitable musings; (e) regular debriefing with a research mentor in order to explore tentative coding patterns and to address assumptions and bias in an effort to prevent premature closure; and (f) preparation of the next line of questioning for each individual participant utilizing the emic coding and reflective text from each previous interview" (Pool, 2019, pp. 3–4)

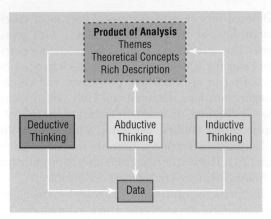

Fig. 12.1 Inductive, deductive, and abductive thinking in qualitative studies.

Our intent in sharing why commitment is needed is not to deter you from qualitative studies, but to ensure you can make an informed decision. We encourage you to conduct qualitative studies because of the knowledge and insights that may be generated. The findings of phenomenological studies can improve relationships with patients and families by expanding nurses' understanding of their perspectives. Grounded theory studies may result in a substantive theory to guide practice. Ethnographical studies may identify injustices or social inequities. Actions can be identified that solve problems as the result of exploratory-descriptive qualitative studies. Our conclusion is that qualitative studies expand our body of knowledge and enhance our relationships with patients, families, communities, and other nurses.

Thinking Processes

Qualitative analysis is the reasoning process that flows from the images, documents, or words provided by the participants toward more abstract concepts and themes. **Themes** are patterns in the data, ideas that are repeated by more than one participant. This inductive reasoning process enables qualitative researchers to see the commonalities among individual, disparate datum (Fig. 12.1) (Miles, Huberman, & Saldaña, 2020). **Inductive thinking** is shown as the arrow on the right side of the figure pointing from the data toward more abstract theoretical concepts, themes, and rich descriptions. While you conduct qualitative data analysis, you will be thinking inductively as you see patterns and move from the specific to the abstract.

As data collection continues, the researcher may compare the generalizations (theoretical concepts, themes, rich descriptions) to the new data to see if the generalization remains consistent or helps to organize the data

(Miles et al., 2020). Can the generalization help the researcher understand the new data? Moving from generalizations to more concrete data is **deductive thinking**, shown by the arrow on the left in Fig. 12.1. Imagine you are conducting an exploratory-descriptive qualitative study with patients who have chronic renal failure. After the first two interviews, as you analyze the data, you tentatively identify the themes of "roller-coaster ride" and "forgetfulness." As you continue to interview, you are thinking deductively when you apply these two themes to new data to see if they remain a good fit.

Abductive thinking is the label for the middle arrow in Fig. 12.1. Charmaz, Thornberg, and Keane (2018) link abductive thinking to grounded theory methodology, but do not limit its use to one methodology. We are defining **abductive thinking** to be the back-and-forth and in-between thinking (two-way arrow) that is influenced by the researchers' knowledge and experiences, as shown by the smaller, dotted line arrows pointing from the thinking processes and beyond. Abductive thinking is often stimulated when researchers are puzzled or surprised by newly collected data (Charmaz et al., 2018; Miles et al., 2020). Abductive thinking may lead to a sudden insight, a seemingly random connection, or a question. During a qualitative study, multiple types of reasoning are used. In other words, the researcher thinks holistically, much like you do when assessing a patient being admitted for care.

Flexibility and Rigor of Methods

To achieve the goal of describing and understanding participant perspectives, qualitative methods of sampling, data gathering, and analysis may shift during the study (Creswell & Poth, 2018). Insights from early data collection and analysis may suggest additional questions that might be asked or other modifications to the study methods (Moser & Korstjens, 2018). For example, suppose a researcher conducts a grounded theory study with persons who lost a limb because of traumatic injury. During the interviews, a participant mentions feeling guilty. Her injury occurred while she was driving too fast. She caused a crash, and passengers in another car were injured. The planned interview questions did not include a question about feelings of guilt and regret. However, the researcher may choose to ask a question on this topic during subsequent interviews. Creswell and Poth (2018) state that evolving designs are a fundamental characteristic of qualitative research.

Qualitative research requires rigorous methods to ensure that the perspectives of the participants are described accurately and interpreted empathetically. Many variations of criteria for qualitative rigor have been developed, because considerable disagreement exists among qualitative researchers on the topic of rigor (Creswell & Poth, 2018; Morse, 2018). Some criteria to evaluate the rigor of a qualitative study violate the assumptions of qualitative research. Other evaluative criteria apply principles of quality used in quantitative research to qualitative studies, such as judging the extent to which the researchers adhered to a preset plan for the study.

Creswell and Poth (2018) compare the language used in 11 different sets of evaluation criteria; Morse (2018) explores the development of standards for qualitative rigor from the 1960s to present day. These experts in qualitative research came to a similar conclusion of ensuring rigor by focusing on validation and verification. Methods that support the rigor of the study should be incorporated into the study plan (Morse, 2018).

We concur and describe methods that are incorporated into qualitative study design to ensure rigor (Box 12.2). Some methods to ensure rigor are specific to one qualitative methodology, such as phenomenology, and are presented later in this chapter. We have already described four methods or principles that support rigor. Rigor with flexibility begins with reflexivity and positioning (see Chapter 4). We also previously introduced the importance of maintaining consistency to the philosophical foundation of the selected methodology and building respectful, trusting relationships with participants.

BOX 12.2 Methods Used to Ensure Rigor in Qualitative Studies

Reflexivity
Positioning
Consistency of the methods to the philosophy and the methodology
Respectful, trusting relationships
Audit trail
Member checking
Triangulation
Research debriefing

Flexibility allows for adapting the data collection and analysis strategies during a qualitative study; however, the changes are not impulsive. The changes must be supported with a clear rationale and documented as part of the study records. One way to document the changes (flexibility) and provide evidence of rigor is to maintain an audit trail. The **audit trail** is the record of events, issues, and decisions during the study to ensure the rigor of the study (Creswell & Poth, 2018). Marshall and Rossman (2016) describe audit trails as a transparent way to provide "evidence and trace the logic leading to the representation and interpretation of findings" (p. 230). An audit trail may include, but is not limited to, the date and location of data collection episodes (interviews, observations, focus groups), location of original recordings and electronic transcription files, team meeting minutes, journals, memos, and decisions about code definitions and analyses. Schumacher, Hussey, and Hall (2018) conducted a grounded theory study of patients with heart failure living at home. Because of shorter hospital stays, patients frequently returned to the home environment unprepared to assess and manage their symptoms. The participants in this grounded theory study had a hospitalization for heart failure in the past 3 months. The researchers used several strategies to increase rigor of the study, one of which was maintaining an audit trail.

"An audit trail of data collect[ion] and analysis procedures was kept to provide evidence of trustworthiness and dependability. Credibility was established through respondent validation during and after interviews, triangulation of data using qualitative software queries, intensive interviews, comparison with a discrepant case, and use of direct quotes to support themes. All interviews were conducted by one person using an interview guide to provide consistency. A researcher journal was kept by (N1) to document self-reflection and address potential researcher bias, thus providing confirmability and impartiality." (Schumacher et al., 2018, p. 299)

Three additional methods are commonly used to ensure rigor: member checking, triangulation, and researcher debriefing. Validation includes the process of confirming descriptions by member checking. **Member checking** is sharing a written description of an interview with the participant (Creswell & Poth, 2018) or scheduling a second interview with a participant to confirm data from the first interview (Morse, 2018). Shumacher et al. (2018) used the term "respondent validation during and after interviews" (p. 299).

Wardlaw and Shambley-Ebron (2019) conducted an ethnographical study with African American women who were depressed and seeking health care. The following quote from their study identifies how they used member checking to increase the credibility of their findings.

"Nineteen African American women between the ages of 30 and 70 years being treated for depression participated in the study. The sample was recruited from community mental health centers in a medium-sized city in the Midwest. Two 1-hour, semi-structured interviews were conducted with each participant. The first interview was to gather data to answer the research questions. The second interview served as a member check to clarify data and ensure its veracity. Categories and patterns that were derived from the data were presented to informants for confirmation." (Wardlaw & Shambley-Ebron, 2019, p. 174)

Member checking allows the participant to revise or confirm that the researcher has accurately represented his or her perspective. You will hear more about Wardlaw and Shambley-Ebron's (2019) study later in the chapter.

Another way to validate or verify the findings of a qualitative study is to triangulate the data. **Triangulation** is using multiple types and sources of data as corroborating evidence for a theme, insight, or perspective (Creswell & Poth, 2018; Flick, 2019; Miles et al., 2020).

An example from clinical practice may help you understand the method. A man enters the emergency department (ED) complaining of chest pain. As the cardiac clinical nurse specialist on call, you direct the team to follow the HEART Pathway (i.e., history, echocardiogram, age, risk factors, and troponin level) (Byrne, Toarta, Backus, & Holt, 2018). According to the pathway, you conduct a patient history, determine the patient's age, and ask about risk factors. Another team member obtains a blood specimen for a stat troponin level, while another obtains a 12-lead electrocardiogram (ECG). This clinical example of triangulation combines data of different types (subjective, objective) and from different sources (patient, echo, ECG, laboratory). What do the data mean when combined? In this case, the 72-year-old patient had no history of cardiac problems but reported being on insulin and taking an antihypertensive medication. The patient reports that his weight is 243 pounds and his height is 5 feet, 5 inches. His troponin was in the dangerous range and his ECG was not normal. The conclusion was that he was having a myocardial infarction and needed immediate intervention. You used triangulation to reach the conclusion. The same method has a great value in research.

For a research example, Crouch (2019) conducted a grounded theory study of nursing and midwifery students who had dyslexia. She described her data analysis to include methods to enhance rigor.

"Transcribed data from the taped interviews were analyzed using the constant comparative method (Glaser & Strauss, 1999) during when themes were generated through substantive, selective and theoretical coding (Stern & Storr, 2011). Content analysis of relevant aspects of students' files and practice portfolios was carried out. Evidence from that data and the qualitative comments from the mentors to help answer research questions 3ii were then compared with the transcribed data collected from the students, using the constant comparative method. This allowed theme generation and theory building. Data triangulation provided 'multiple measures of the same phenomena' to help enhance…the overall trustworthiness of the research (Yin, 2009, p. 116)." (Crouch, 2019, p. 92)

Crouch (2019) identified triangulation as one method for ensuring trustworthiness of the findings. Data were triangulated from transcripts of interviews, student files and practice portfolios, and comments by the mentors. She also included a matrix identifying other studies of dyslexia in health care whose findings supported the different coping strategies identified by participants in her study. The data analysis strategies mentioned in the study excerpt will be explained later in the chapter in the section on grounded theory methods.

The last validation/verification method we are covering in this section is researcher debriefing. **Researcher debriefing** with a mentor or a peer may range from questioning the researcher's analysis of the data, pointing out possible biases, and listening empathetically when the researcher needs to process the emotional impact of the data being collected (Creswell & Poth, 2018). As described earlier, Pool (2019) conducted a phenomenological study of the perspectives of nurses who worked with AIs receiving cancer care. Pool provided a list of several methods of promoting rigor that were used in the study, including debriefing.

"Following the first and all subsequent interviews, the following procedures were undertaken: (a) immediate reflective writing in a journal to capture first impressions and to note embodied responses that were not captured by the audio-recording; (b) during the interim between interviews, engagement in a period of contemplative dwelling with repeated exposure to the transcribed interviews and the creation of reflective memos exploring potential structures buried within the text; (c) tentative coding of the emic data utilizing Van Manen's (1990) wholistic/sententious, selective, and detailed approaches...; (d) conscious refrainment from assigning any meaning to the participants' recollections in an effort to remain open and accessible to their individual experiences. Instead, continued reflective journaling was employed to attenuate for the researcher's own inevitable musings; (e) regular debriefing with a research mentor in order to explore tentative coding patterns and to address assumptions and bias in an effort to prevent premature closure; and (f) preparation of the next line of questioning for each individual participant utilizing the emic coding and reflective text from each previous interview." (Pool, 2019, pp. 3–4)

In summary, member checking, triangulation, and researcher debriefing are methods that can be used in multiple types of qualitative studies to ensure rigor (see Box 12.2).

RESEARCH PROCESS IN QUALITATIVE STUDIES

In this section, literature reviews, theoretical frameworks, study purposes, and research questions or objectives are described in the context of various qualitative approaches, because these are steps in the research process that are implemented somewhat differently in qualitative studies.

Literature Review for Qualitative Studies

Literature reviews in qualitative studies may occur during planning of the study, interpretation of the results, or both. In exploratory-descriptive qualitative studies, the literature review usually occurs while the study is being planned. Marshall, Forgeron, Harrison, and Young (2018) conducted an exploratory-descriptive qualitative study of nurses' pain management practices for hospitalized pediatric patients in rural Northern Ontario, Canada. The researchers began their report by establishing the negative consequences of pain and identifying studies reporting ineffective pain management for hospitalized children. Selected excerpts from their literature review are presented, culminating in the statement of the research problem.

"One factor that has been found to influence the use of research into practice is context (Kitson, Harvey, & McCormack, 1998), which is defined as the environment or setting in which nurses' work (Kitson et al., 1998). Evidence suggests that context can positively or negatively influence nurses' practice behaviours (Cummings, Hutchinson, Scott, Norton, & Estabrooks, 2010; Latimer et al., 2010; Squires et al., 2013), and therefore may play a critical role in nurses' use of evidence in practice.... However, the types of context resources available within the rural context to support RNs [registered nurses] pain care practices have received little attention.... The impact of rural context on Canadian nurses' pediatric pain management practices have only been previously explored in one study (Caty, Tourigny, & Koren, 1995).... Other studies conducted in rural contexts which focused on low and middle-income countries (i.e. Thailand) also found that clinicians held myths and misconceptions about children's pain management and that continuing educational opportunities are limited (Forgeron et al., 2009).... Although these studies have been conducted in rural settings these results may not be transferable to a rural Canadian context where resources are known to differ from the studies mentioned above. Understanding of the interplay between rural context and nurses' pediatric pain management practices is limited and is the focus of this study." (Marshall et al., 2018, p. 90)

Marshall et al. (2018) presented a logical argument for the study's significance and the gap in knowledge the researchers were addressing. Most qualitative proposals and reports include a literature review for these purposes (Creswell & Creswell, 2018) and for providing guidance for the development of data collection methods. A more thorough review of published research findings and theories may occur during data analysis and interpretation to compare the emerging themes, rich descriptions, or theory to published studies and theoretical literature (Charmaz et al., 2018).

Phenomenological studies may have a literature review to heighten the researcher's awareness of particular concerns or experiences of their participants. Pool's (2019) study, introduced earlier, was conducted in the context of cancer care. She recognized that her participants' history as individuals and groups affected relationships with healthcare professionals.

"Literature Review

Effective cancer care requires caring patient–provider relationships, yet the literature suggests that AIs [American Indians] describe significant issues specifically related to providers throughout the health-care experience including ineffectual communication tactics, cultural insensitivity, perceived discrimination, and aggressive or dominating approaches.... Over a third of AIs report experiencing some form of racially based microaggression from a health-care provider, resulting in chronic health condition symptom exacerbation and increased hospitalizations (Walls et al., 2015).

For providers such as nurses, care of AIs presents language and other types of nonverbal communication challenges coupled with conflict surrounding treatment philosophies and discordant interpretations of wellness and disease (Guadagnolo et al., 2009; Koithan & Farrell, 2010; Lowe & Struthers, 2001). ...there is a dearth of literature describing nurses' interpretations or perceptions of caring for AI patients. The unique relationships that develop while providing cancer care to AI patients and the underlying meaning that nurses ascribed to these experiences remain unexplored." (Pool, 2019, p. 2)

Notice the concepts that were identified in the literature review: communication, cultural sensitivity, discrimination, dominating or aggressive behaviors, racially based microaggression, and cancer care inequities. Through the literature review, Pool (2019) prepared herself for the interviews she conducted with the nurses caring for AI patients.

Grounded theory is a methodology for which the purpose and timing of the literature review has generated debate (Charmaz et al., 2018; Thornberg & Dunne, 2019). Early grounded theory researchers argued for delaying the literature until after the initial data collection and analysis to allow the researcher to remain open to the perspectives of the participants (Charmaz et al., 2018; Gilgun, 2019; Thornberg & Dunne, 2019). Glaser and Strauss were adamant that theory should fit the data, rather than data fit the preconceived theory (Thornberg & Dunne, 2019). For example, Crouch's (2019) grounded theory study of dyslexia in nursing and midwifery students contains literature supporting the premise that the study is needed but did not describe different theories that might have been relevant to the research problem. At the end of the research report, however, she included a table with other studies in which the same coping strategies had been identified, a type of triangulation to strengthen the trustworthiness of what she found.

Glaser and Strauss grew to differ on several issues, one of which was when to conduct the literature review. Strauss acknowledged that researchers have prior knowledge and professional experience. He recommended that the researchers be familiar with the literature on the research topic (Thornberg & Dunne, 2019). This familiarity may sensitize the researchers to nuances in the data. The researcher is still expected to return to the literature during and after data analysis.

Among constructivist grounded theory researchers, theory is co-constructed with participants within the social and historical setting. The researcher "maintains an ongoing relationships with the extant literature" (Thornberg & Dunne, 2019, p. 211), beginning with an initial review. The recommended initial stance of the researcher is theoretical agnosticism (Charmaz et al., 2018). The researcher who is a **theoretical agnostic** (1) considers theory fallible and provisional, (2) takes "a critical view toward extant theoretical explanations," and (3) remains "open to all kinds of theoretical possibilities" (Charmaz et al., 2018, p. 414). As a tentative theory begins to develop during data analysis, the researcher returns the literature to see if other evidence supports or contradicts the theory. When the theory is developed, a final review is conducted to locate studies in the existing literature of the discipline (Thornberg & Dunne, 2019).

The literature review serves different purposes in the different grounded theory methodologies but has two common elements. The literature is used initially to support the need for the study by articulating the research problem and, during the interpretation of the findings, to position the findings in contrast to or in support of previous research and theories.

Theoretical Frameworks

Most qualitative researchers do not identify specific theoretical frameworks during the design of their studies, as is expected for quantitative studies. The concern is that designing a study in the context of a theory will influence the researcher's thinking and result in findings that are meaningful in the theoretical context but may not be true to the participants' perspectives on the topic. However, the philosophical bases for the qualitative methodologies may allow a theoretical grounding for a study without predisposing the data analysis to a single interpretation (Flick, 2019).

Theory is an explicit component in some qualitative research designs. The theory may be explicit in the findings of the study, such as a grounded theory study in which the inductive analysis allows an emerging theory to emerge (Charmaz, 2014). Pool (2019) analyzed the data in her grounded theory study and generated a diagram to reflect the substantive theory that resulted.

> "Several themes were generated and grouped into three core categories (Glaser & Strauss, 1999), each with their sub-categories and properties. The core categories namely, I) 'Perceptions of the impact of dyslexia on the student'; II) 'Strategies/resources used to manage perceived impact of dyslexia'; and III) 'Very good, helpful, useful tool; useful strategies' are shown diagrammatically in Fig. 1. [Fig. 12.2]." (Pool, 2019, p. 92)

Ethnographical researchers, at the beginning of a study, may identify a theory by which they will structure the data collection, such as Leininger's (1997, 2007) classic ethnonursing research methods. They may, however,

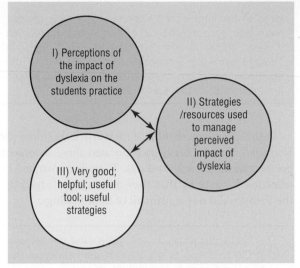

Fig. 12.2 Core categories to which themes were assigned. (From Crouch, A. [2019]. Perceptions of the possible impact of dyslexia on nursing and midwifery students and of the coping strategies they develop and/or use to help them cope in clinical practice. *Nurse Education in Practice, 35*[1], 90–97. doi:10.1016/j.nepr.2018.12.008.)

articulate a critical social theory to position themselves in regard to the culture to be studied as Wardlaw and Shambley-Ebron (2019) did for their study of depression among African American women.

> "Two theoretical frameworks were used to guide this study, the Co-Cultural Theory of Communication (Orbe, 1998) and Black Feminist Thought (Collins, 2000). The Co-Cultural Theory of Communication elucidates the processes by which individuals from traditionally marginalized groups communicate within dominant societal structures. The use of the term 'co-culture' indicates that all cultures in American society exist without hierarchy in value (Orbe, 1998).... With the dominance of 1 co-cultural group, other co-cultural groups such as African American women are marginalized in societal structures such as politics, corporate business, the legal system, and the health care system (Orbe, 1998). As a result, individuals from marginalized groups make decisions about how to communicate when engaging with dominant societal structures." (Orbe, 1998)
>
> "Black Feminist Thought, a critical theory, encourages empowerment and self-definition of African American women's standpoint (Collins, 2000). The purpose of Black Feminist Thought is to resist the practice and

ideas of the intersecting oppressions of race, gender, and class encountered by African American women (Collins, 2000). In the current study, Black Feminist Thought provided a theoretical lens specific to the standpoint of African American women (Collins, 2000)." (Wardlaw & Shambley-Ebron, 2019, p. 174)

In the discussion section of their article, Wardlaw and Shambley-Ebron (2019) incorporated these theoretical perspectives into their findings. They demonstrated intellectual honesty in that they also acknowledged that the theories did not explain all of their findings.

"The intersectionality of race, class, and gender provided the backdrop of the lives of the women in this study. According to Collins (2000), this intersectionality has shaped the realities of women of African descent in America since US slavery. This includes their interaction with systems of health care...their communicative practices were influenced by the intersecting oppressions and were used strategically to navigate the system to obtain the care they needed.... Several of the women indicated that during the initial part of the relationship, they were reluctant to share information about their symptoms with the provider. Co-cultural communication is often strategic communication (Orbe, 1998). Therefore, it is not surprising that African American women would be selective with the information shared within a setting such as the health care system." (Wardlaw & Shambley-Ebron, 2019, pp. 180–181)

"The framework provided by the Co-Cultural Theory of Communication was useful in determining the communicative practices of the women in this study.... The findings in this study were consistent with this theory but suggest that there are additional influences on the communicative practices as well, as indicated by the domains and themes." (Wardlaw & Shambley-Ebron, 2019, p. 182)

Qualitative researchers who use frameworks during study development must prevent the theoretical perspective from obscuring the perspectives of the participants. Your decision about whether to identify a theoretical perspective should be consistent with the research approach you have chosen. If a theoretical perspective has shaped your views of a research problem, you should acknowledge that influence and indicate explicitly the study components that were shaped by the theory.

Purpose of the Study

Purposes should clearly identify the goal or aim of the study that has emerged from the research problem and literature review. The purposes of qualitative studies include the phenomenon of interest, the population, and often the setting (see Chapter 5). After determining the purpose for a study, ask yourself, "Can I achieve this purpose with a qualitative study?" Study purposes such as testing an intervention and measuring the effectiveness of a program are not consistent with qualitative approaches. When the term *measuring* is used, the data collected will be numbers and the analysis would involve statistics. However, a qualitative researcher could address participants' experiences with the intervention or their perceptions about a program. The purpose of qualitative studies will vary slightly depending on the qualitative approach that is being used. Table 12.1 includes a purpose statement consistent with each study's identified philosophical approach. Chapter 4 provides a more detailed discussion of the philosophical approaches for the four types of qualitative research included in this textbook. These are the studies used throughout the chapter as examples of the methods for each qualitative methodology. As you will notice with these examples, the methodology to be used is not explicit. The purpose of Pool's (2019) study of the nurses' perspectives of their relationships with AI cancer patients was congruent with the phenomenological methodology but could have also been studied using an exploratory-descriptive qualitative or an ethnographical methodology. Marshall et al.'s (2018) exploratory-descriptive qualitative study of pediatric pain management of rural RNs could have also been studied with an ethnographical methodology. However, the methods for an ethnographical study with this purpose would have been different than the interviews conducted by Marshall et al. (2018).

Research Objectives or Questions

Qualitative researchers identify research objectives or questions to connect the purpose of the study to the plan for data collection and analysis. Because qualitative research is more open ended and the focus is on participants' perspectives, qualitative researchers may not specify research objectives or research questions to avoid prematurely narrowing the topic.

Table 12.2 continues with our four example studies and contains excerpts of their research questions or objectives. Pool (2019) clearly identified research

TABLE 12.1 Examples of Purpose Statements in Qualitative Studies

Qualitative Methodology	Purpose Statement
Phenomenological research	"The purpose of this study was to describe the meaning of the AI [American Indian] patient–cancer care nurse relationship from nurses' perspectives" (Pool, 2019, p. 2).
Grounded theory research	"The study aimed to explore the perceived impact of dyslexia on nursing and midwifery students and on the coping strategies they used to help them cope with issues related to dyslexia in clinical practice" (Crouch, 2019, p. 90).
Ethnographical research	"The purpose of this study was to identify and describe the communicative practices African American women use when seeking care for depression in health care settings" (Wardlaw & Shambley-Ebron, 2019, p. 173).
Exploratory-descriptive qualitative research	"The overall aim of this study was to explore rural hospital RNs' experiences in providing pain care to children in the rural hospital setting in Canada, to understand the challenges and facilitators of providing evidenced based pediatric pain management within this context" (Marshall et al., 2018, p. 90).

TABLE 12.2 Examples of Research Questions or Objectives in Qualitative Studies

Qualitative Methodology	Research Questions or Objectives
Phenomenological research	"The study included three objectives: (a) to describe the immediate experiences of nurses that have engaged in cancer care relationships with AI [American Indian] patients, (b) to identify the underlying structures of the AI patient–cancer care nurse relationship as described by nurses, and (c) to interpret the meaning of the patient–nurse relationship within the context of AI cancer experiences." (Pool, 2019, p. 2)
Grounded theory research	"1. What is the perceived impact of dyslexia on the nursing and midwifery student in clinical practice? 2. How are any difficulties associated with dyslexia managed by the nursing or midwifery student? 3i. What strategies can help and support dyslexic nursing and midwifery students? 3ii. What are the students' and mentors' perceptions of the poster guidelines used by mentors to support nursing and midwifery students with dyslexia in the clinical practice?" (Crouch, 2019, p. 91)
Ethnographical research	"1. How do African American women describe their use of co-cultural communicative practices with their health care provider when receiving care for depression? 2. How do the cultural experiences of African American women influence their selection of co-cultural communicative practices when receiving care for depression? 3. What is the influence of race, class, and gender on the co-cultural communicative practices of African American women during the health care encounter while receiving care for depression?" (Wardlaw & Shambley-Ebron, 2019, p. 174)
Exploratory-descriptive qualitative research	"This study had four main objectives: (1) To understand the facilitator RNs' experience when providing pediatric pain management in the rural setting. (2) To understand the barriers RNs experience when providing pediatric pain management in the rural setting. (3) To identify and describe RNs' perception of the challenges and facilitators that are unique to the rural setting. (4) To describe RNs' perception of the availability of supportive structures (i.e. policies, procedures, assessment tools, educational opportunities, and pain experts) that may promote successful pain management for children in the rural setting" (Marshall et al., 2018, p. 90).

objectives. Her first and third objectives linked very clearly with phenomenology's focus on lived experiences and their meaning. Interestingly, her second objective targeted the structures of a relationship (social processes and structures) and could have also been studied using a grounded theory methodology. The research questions of Crouch's (2019) study of the perceived impact of dyslexia on the clinical practice of nursing and midwifery students was consistent with her selected methodology (i.e., grounded theory).

> "Research on coping strategies developed by students and on the perceptions of their effectiveness was almost non-existent at the time of this study. The Glasarian grounded theory (Glaser & Strauss, 1999) was thus used to collect and analyse the data to give new perspectives on the chosen topic." (Crouch, 2019, p. 91)

QUALITATIVE SAMPLING

"Sampling is the key to rigorous research" (Morse & Clark, 2019, p. 145). Qualitative researchers seek participants who have experienced the phenomenon of interest (Creswell & Poth, 2018), are willing to participate, and are able to share their experiences or perspectives. Sampling

in qualitative research continues throughout the study as needed to expand the understanding of the culture, phenomenon, social process, or the problem to be solved (Morse & Clark, 2019). The selection of participants is nonrandom and may not be totally specified in terms of number, group members, or characteristics before the study begins.

Chapter 15 addresses sampling for quantitative and qualitative studies. Convenience sampling is the most common type of sampling used in nursing studies. In addition, three qualitative sampling strategies described in Chapter 15 are purposeful, theoretical, and network sampling. These three types of sampling are included in Table 12.3 along with other types of sampling and their definitions. When considering Table 12.3, it is important to remember that the lines between the types of sampling are not distinct (Creswell & Poth, 2018). For example, theoretical sampling could be considered a subtype of purposeful sampling. Another example is that you are conducting a grounded theory study of adherence to antihypertensive medication. As a tentative theory begins to emerge, you realize that all of the participants in the study to this point have been on their medication for less than 1 year and have achieved blood pressure control. You decide to recruit additional

TABLE 12.3   Sampling Strategies Used by Qualitative Researchers

Sampling	Definition
Purposive sampling	Recruiting participants because they can provide in-depth information needed to achieve the study's purpose (see Chapter 15)
Snowball sampling	Asking each participant to refer someone else to participate who has also experienced the study phenomenon; also called chain sampling or network sampling (see Chapter 15)
Theoretical sampling[a]	Recruiting participants whose knowledge and experience will facilitate generating a theory; additional participants may be recruited to validate or expand upon emerging concepts; associated with grounded theory approaches (see Chapter 15)
Criterion sampling[a]	Recruiting participants who do or do not have certain characteristics deemed relevant to the study topic
Maximum variation sampling[a]	Recruiting participants who represent potentially different experiences related to the research topic
Critical case sampling[a]	Recruiting participants whose experiences with the research topic are expected to be very different and whose input may support or not support the emerging results
Deviant case sampling[a]	Recruiting participants who may be outliers or represent extreme cases of the domain of interest; may be called a negative case

[a]Considered by some authors to be subtypes of purposive sampling.
From Creswell, J., & Poth, C. (2018). *Qualitative inquiry & research design: Choosing among five approaches* (4th ed.). Thousand Oaks, CA: Sage; Miles, M., Huberman, A., & Saldaña, J. (2020). *Qualitative data analysis: A methods sourcebook* (4th ed.). Thousand Oaks, CA: Sage.

participants who may have been on their medication for over 1 year or who have not achieved blood pressure control. Depending on which qualitative reference book you consult, the sampling strategy used to select additional participants could be called theoretical, maximum variation, or critical case sampling.

One type of qualitative sampling is criterion sampling. Taylor (2018) conducted a descriptive phenomenological study of African American couples who had experienced infertility. She described her sampling in the following excerpt.

> "…criterion sampling was used. Creswell (2007) indicates that for a phenomenological study, it is imperative that all participants have experience of the phenomenon being studied. The use of 'criterion sampling works well [if] all individuals studied represent people who have experienced the phenomenon' (p. 128). For this study, all 12 participants (a total of six couples) experienced infertility and self-identified as African American." (Taylor, 2018, p. 361)

Taylor (2018) conducted telephone interviews with each spouse separately and then together. Open-ended questions were used. We will return to this study later in the chapter.

Ghahari, Forwell, Suto, and Morassaei (2019) conducted a grounded theory study of successful self-management among persons with multiple sclerosis (MS). The researchers interviewed 18 persons with MS twice, either face-to-face or by telephone. They clearly stated their rationale for using maximum variation sampling and the impact of the sampling methods on their model.

> "People with confirmed diagnosis of MS were included if they had lived with the condition for three years or more, self-identified as successfully managing it at the time of study, and had sufficient English skills to provide informed consent and complete an interview. Having participants self-identify as successful in their management of MS grounds our model in their own understandings and experiences…. In order to build a model of self-management that is applicable to a wide range of people with MS, maximum variation sampling was used (Charmaz, 2006) and participants were not limited to a specific type of MS or level of disability because it is known that, despite differences in needs, people with different types of MS and levels of disability use a

> combination of skills and strategies to manage their condition (Audulv, Ghahari, Kephart, Warner, & Packer, 2019)." (Ghahari et al., 2019, p. 1014)

> "The aim of this study was to examine the strategies used by people with MS in order to develop a model of successful self-management. The results revealed that managing MS successfully meant to participate in life while taking care of oneself, listening to one's body, and making allowances for the limitations. Since the recruited participants had a variety of types of MS and levels of disability, the strategies that emerged can be considered generally relevant to people with MS, regardless of stage or type. Further study could examine more closely how these strategies are affected by the type or stage of MS." (Ghahari et al., 2019, p. 1019)

Ghahari et al. (2019) found that persons with MS used a range of self-management behaviors to live their lives and "be able to do what they want to do" (p. 1019). The participants described using combinations of behaviors to manage challenges such as exacerbations.

In Chapter 15, you will learn more about sample size and how qualitative researchers know when the sample is an adequate size. The sample for a rigorous qualitative study is not as large as the sample for a rigorous quantitative study. You will learn about reaching **saturation**, the point at which new data begin to be redundant with what has already been found, and no new themes can be identified. The researcher has the data needed to answer the research question and remain true to the principles of the study design. Marshall and Rossman (2016) indicate that a better term for data saturation is theoretical sufficiency, because one can never completely know all there is to know about a topic. The researcher stops collecting data when enough rich, meaningful data have been obtained to achieve the study aims. When applying for approval of an institutional review board (IRB), the researcher will be asked the maximum sample size. Morse and Clark (2019) recommend that the researchers overestimate the sample size in IRB documents, including allowing for potentially adding participants further in the study.

Studies in which focus groups will be used typically have larger samples. **Focus groups**, or group interviews, are composed of similar participants to encourage interaction among the participants. The similarity may be diagnosis, age, ethnicity, or having gone through the same experience such as losing a spouse (Quinn & Fantasia,

2018). The researcher plans one or more focus groups and estimates each will have 5 to 10 participants. The actual number of groups conducted may depend on how soon data saturation is achieved.

DATA COLLECTION METHODS

Collecting qualitative data is not a mechanical process that can be completely planned before it is initiated. Because data collection occurs simultaneously with data analysis in most qualitative studies, the process is complex. For a particular study, the researcher may need to respond to ethical issues; reflect on the meanings obtained from the data; address data collection problems related to relationships between the researcher and the participants; and organize, manage, and synthesize large volumes of data. Qualitative researchers are not limited to a single type of data or collection method during a study. For example, Crouch (2019) collected data by interviewing nursing and midwifery students who had dyslexia, reviewing mentors' responses to open-ended questions on an electronic discussion board, and recording relevant information from students' files and students' practice portfolios.

Observations, interviews, focus groups, documents, and media and internet materials are the most common methods of gathering qualitative data, and each is described here in detail, followed by an example from the literature. These data may be collected in face-to-face meetings or by electronic means. Following the general types of data collection, methods specific to each qualitative approach are discussed.

Observations

In many qualitative studies, the researcher observes social behavior and may interact with those being studied. Miles et al. (2020) identify "intense and/or prolonged contact with participants in a naturalistic setting" (p. 21) as a characteristic of qualitative research. Their phrase is especially applicable to observation. **Observation in qualitative research** is collecting data through listening, smelling, touching, and seeing, with an emphasis on what is seen (Creswell & Poth, 2018). Even when other data collection methods are being used, such as interviews, your awareness of the interactions between the participant and other people in the surrounding environment can provide rich data to supplement the other methods being used. Your observations may be recorded during or immediately following the interview.

> **BOX 12.3   Establishing Boundaries for Observation as a Data Collection Method**
>
> Based on the purpose statement and research questions (or objectives), answer the following questions:
> 1. What is the setting?
> 2. Who are the actors, the people to be observed?
> 3. What events are directly related to the study purpose?
> 4. What processes are directly related to the study purpose?

Observation, however, is more than simply being in a situation with participants and having social conversations. Although observations may seem fluid and unpredictable, they can be demarcated by the research question and the unit of analysis. Box 12.3 displays four questions researchers may use to establish boundaries around observation as a data collection method (Creswell & Creswell, 2018). The setting is **naturalistic**, meaning that it is not changed or controlled for the study. The actors in the setting are the people being observed, who may be patients, family members, nurses, or leaders in a community. The activities or events that are of interest to the researchers involved the actors in the setting. The last component to be considered is the processes that are occurring among the actors or behaviors of the actors. In Chapter 4, we described a study of patient dignity in Iran as an example of ethnography (Bidabadi, Yazdannik, & Zargham-Boroujeni, 2019). In the following excerpt, the researchers described observation as one component of their data collection.

> "The organizational culture of CSICUs [cardiac surgery intensive care units] is a subculture of hospital, nursing, and social cultures, and thus, all these cultures can affect patient's dignity.... This study was conducted to uncover the cultural structures of power that hindered maintaining patients' dignity in CSICU." (Bidabadi et al., 2019, p. 740)
>
> "Participants included nurses, physicians, internal medicine specialists, cardiac surgeons, anesthesiologists, auxiliary nurses, radiology and laboratory technicians, physical therapists, clinical supervisors, as well as all patient education, quality improvement, and infection control staffs.... Participant observation was the primary method of data collection and conducted by the main researcher.... Informal interviews [were]

designed to illuminate the information gained through observation, shortly after a period of observation. The tone and body language were considered during observations and interviews.... Observations were immediately documented while brief field notes were also written during observations." (Bidabadi et al., 2019, p. 741)

In this excerpt, the four questions of Box 12.3 can be answered. The setting is cardiac surgery ICUs in Iran and the actors are the nurses, physicians, and other caregivers for the patients in these units. The researchers were interested in caregivers who acted in a way that affected patient dignity.

Observations can be viewed on a continuum from unstructured observations to structured observations (Fig. 12.3). The observations described by Bidabadi et al. (2019) were unstructured observations. **Unstructured observation** involves spontaneously observing and recording what one sees (Creswell & Creswell, 2018). Although unstructured observations give the observer freedom, there is a risk that the observer may lose objectivity or may not remember all the details of the event. Collecting data through unstructured observation may evolve later into structured observations. The researcher may begin with few predetermined ideas about what will be observed. As the study progresses, the researcher clarifies the situations or areas of focus that are most relevant to the research questions and begins to structure the observations. A researcher observing parent behavior in an ambulatory pediatric care clinic may initially focus on the interaction of parents with their children in the waiting area and in the room with the provider. During data collection, the researcher begins to notice common nurturing behaviors of the parents and, from these observations, develops a checklist to use while observing. In this way, the researcher has structured the observations that might be the focus of this or future studies. Other researchers may enter the setting with a checklist or tool for documenting a parent's nurturing behaviors, revising the tool as needed (see Chapter 17 for details on structured observation).

Observers may be participants as well as observers; the researcher's role can be viewed on a continuum also from complete participant to complete observer (see Fig. 12.3). Different combinations of participation and observation are described in Table 12.4. The first combination of participation and observation is complete participation. The people in the situation may not be aware that the participant is a researcher (Creswell & Creswell, 2018). In public settings, such as hospital lobbies, online chat rooms, and coffeeshops, a researcher can ethically observe people and interactions without obtaining permission (Brancati, 2018; Bratich, 2018). In less public settings, the researcher may observe others who learn later that he or she is a researcher. When the researcher's role is unknown to the study participants, they need to have consented to incomplete disclosure before the study is conducted. After the study, they must be debriefed regarding the undisclosed aspects of the study (see Chapter 9). The participants have the option as to whether the data the researcher collected about them are included in the study.

Full engagement in the situation may interfere with the researcher's ability to note important details and move within the setting to follow an evolving situation. In these situations, the role of observer as participant may be more appropriate. As the term indicates, the researcher's observer role takes priority and is the focus of the data collection.

Complete observation occurs when the researcher remains passive and has no direct social interaction in the situation (Brancati, 2018). Although this stance allows the observer to focus on the participants, the environment, and behaviors, the observer's role may be seen as intrusive. Participants may alter their behavior to be more socially desirable or politically correct. Technology has changed observation as a research methodology. Bratich (2018) raises ethical and epistemological issues about the extent to which persons in societies with highly developed technologies live in a world of constant surveillance. In the natural sciences, drones, which are unmanned small aircraft that can be controlled remotely, produce videos of remote areas. Their technology-mediated observations could also be used for observation of human behavior in public settings. Nurse

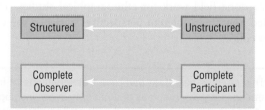

Fig. 12.3 Continuums of structured to unstructured observations and of complete observer to complete participant research roles.

TABLE 12.4   Degree of Participation in Observation

Label	Description	Benefits	Concerns
Complete participant	• Researcher involved in activities with participants • Participants do not know the researcher's purpose for being there	• Researcher may gather rich data without pretense of participants trying to impress the researcher • May have access to more private activities	• Ethical threat due to deception • Participants must be informed of the researcher's role at the end of the study • They may refuse to allow data to be used • Researcher's participation may change what occurs • Potential loss of objectivity
Participant as observer	• Researcher is more participant than observer, with participation as the priority • Researcher's role is known	• Researcher's participation may help participants be less self-conscious • May allow increased access to some activities	• Researcher may miss details of the observation • Researcher's participation may change what occurs
Observer as participant	• Researcher participates to some extent, but observer role is priority • Researcher's role is known	• Researcher may gather rich data and develop honest relationships with participants • Can take field notes during observation	• Initially, participants may be self-conscious and change behavior • Participants usually forget that someone is observing
Complete observer	• Researcher's role is observation only and is overt • Often researcher is at the perimeter of the activity being observed	• Researcher can focus on one role and capture details in the situation • Field notes are taken during the observation	• Participants may be self-conscious and change behavior • Researcher may be uncomfortable because role is more intrusive

Adapted from Creswell, J., & Creswell, D. (2018). *Research design: Qualitative, quantitative, and mixed methods approaches* (5th ed., table 9.2). Thousand Oaks, CA: Sage; Brancati, D. (2018). *Social science research*. Thousand Oaks, CA: Sage.

researchers seeking innovative ways to collect data may want to obtain additional information about ways in which technology can be harnessed for qualitative (and quantitative) research purposes such as observation.

The notes of the researcher during or after observations are called **field notes** (Leavy, 2017). While observing, your notes may be simply jotting down key words, entering phrases on a document app on your smartphone, or audio-recording things to remember on your phone. These cues need to be typed into an organized format with each observation dated. Ideally, a field note identifies the people in the situation, environmental factors, and actions taken by those in the situation. When you are unable to take notes during an observation, it is essential to write a description of what occurred as soon as possible. Field notes include more than the objective aspects of the observation; they also include the researcher's reactions and immediate responses to what has just transpired.

Prip et al. (2019) conducted an exploratory-descriptive qualitative study in an outpatient clinic in which oncology patients received chemotherapy. The purpose of the study was to explore the verbal and nonverbal communication between the nurses and patients, with the desired outcome being increased understanding of how the setting affected the communication. Observation was the primary means of data collection. Two of the nurse researchers were the data collectors; one was an oncology nurse and the other had no oncology experience but had previously done field work for ethnographical studies. They noted how their different perspectives enriched the data they collected.

"This study is based on participant observations of interactions between nurses and patients in an oncology outpatient clinic supplemented with ad hoc interviews with nurses…. Approximately 70 h [hours] of participant observation was conducted over a period of two months. Five hours of observation were conducted a day including observations of the nurse-patient interactions, talking with patients and nurses, and participating in practical non-clinical tasks.

We followed the nurses' daily routines, which provided insight...and gave opportunity for short ad hoc interviews (lasting between 2 and 10 min) with the nurses during the day.... Approximately six hoc interviews were conducted daily.

Fieldnotes were taken during observations, ...the handwritten fieldnotes were transcribed electronically on the same day as the observations.... All the observations were carried out individually on different days and discussed among [the researchers] three times during the observation period to review methodological aspects and identify patterns and variations in the data.... Investigator triangulation was conducted to ensure study credibility and methodological reflection (Malterud, 2001)." (Prip et al., 2019, p. 121)

Prip et al. (2019) provided sufficient details of the study's observations to evaluate the rigor of their data collection. Field notes were transcribed for analysis and included the ad hoc interviews that occurred during the day. Three of the researchers (the two nurse observers and an anthropologist) conferred during the data collection period to develop a structure for future observations. They explicitly identified what they did to increase the credibility of their findings. In addition, the time they invested in observation was sufficient to produce rich data.

"The analytical process led to the identification of three main themes...treatment-centred communication, efficient communication and spatially-bound communication. Although presented separately, the themes are interrelated and mutually influence each other." (Prip et al., 2019, p. 122)

"The findings in this study show that communication in an outpatient oncology clinic is characterized by its treatment-centred content and effective form. Other important aspects of cancer care, such as the patients' existential, psychosocial and sexual concerns are rarely explored.... Our study demonstrated both the general communicative challenges in the outpatient clinic and how nurses work creatively within the constraints of the setting to address patients' individual needs." (Prip et al., 2019, p. 124)

Because the researchers used observation appropriately and rigorously, they produced meaningful findings with implications for clinical practice. They recommended that adjustments be made to the environment to provide opportunities for the patients and nurses to discuss existential, psychosocial, and spiritual needs. Although short ad hoc interviews were used in Prip et al.'s (2019) study, longer and more involved interviews are a common method of data collection in qualitative studies.

Interviews

Interviews differ from the usual conversations that we have with family and friends (Brinkmann, 2018). Interviews are focused conversations between a participant and a qualitative researcher that may occur in person, over the telephone, or via the internet meeting (Brancati, 2018; Brinkmann, 2018). A researcher as an interviewer seeks information from a number of participants individually, whereas the focus group strategy is designed to obtain the perspective of the normative group, not individual perspectives. Interviews may also be conducted in quantitative studies to assist subjects in the completion of a survey or questionnaire, especially when participants may have limited literacy (see interviews in Chapter 17). These interviews are structured, with the researcher or data collector reading the questions aloud to the participants and documenting their responses to the questions in person or over the phone. The participants' responses are coded as numbers and are analyzed statistically. In contrast, our focus in this section is on interviewing in qualitative studies. In qualitative interviews, a transcript is usually prepared after the interview. The researcher analyzes the phrases and words of the participant. Interviews are a frequently used method of data collection in all the qualitative research methodologies that we have described in this book.

Interviews have a purpose beyond the interaction itself. In most studies, interviews as a data collection method are designed to address the researcher's purpose related to a specific topic or phenomenon. Table 12.5 provides examples of questions or prompts a researcher may use related to the purpose and the other defining characteristics of interviews. A more collaborative interview approach gives space in the dialogue for the participant to interject new ideas that were not part of the researcher's original purpose (Brinkmann, 2018), but

TABLE 12.5   Characteristics of Interviews: Examples of Interview Statements, Questions, or Prompts

Interview Characteristic	Examples Related to Study of Coping With Lung Cancer	Examples Related to Family Histories and Disease Prevention
Purpose	Thank you for agreeing to participate in this study of how people live with a diagnosis of lung cancer. Start by telling me how you learned that you had lung cancer.	This study is about telling the next generation of our family—our children—about health problems that have occurred in the lives of their extended family, such as your parents and grandparents.
Description	Describe what led up to you going to the doctor. What did you do the rest of that day?	How did your son react when you told him that your father and your siblings were all diagnosed with hypertension before age 45?
Social-cultural-physical context (lifeworld)	What else was going on in your life at that time? Tell me a little more about the job you had when diagnosed. How were you introduced to cigarettes when you were growing up?	Tell me more about your family. How many children did you say you had? Describe your family when you were growing up. What did your parents tell you about their health?
Interpretation	What does this diagnosis mean to you? Do you have any regrets? What emotions do you have related to the cancer?	How important is it to you to teach your children about preventing hypertension? How does relaying information about hypertension to your children fit with your view of parenting?

the researcher has a purpose for the interview. Interviews provide an opportunity for the participants to describe the experience in their own words. The description contains concrete details of when or how something occurred and the context in which it occurred. The social-cultural-physical context of the experience needs to be elicited if the participant does not initially include this information. The experience does not exist in a vacuum but in the lifeworld of the participant. The researcher prompts or asks questions to encourage the participant to interpret what the experience means in the context of the participant's lifeworld (Brinkmann, 2018).

The extent to which an interview is structured depends on the purpose of the interview. Interviews can be conceptualized as being on a continuum from structured to unstructured (Leavy, 2017). As described earlier, highly structured interviews are used in quantitative research but also may be used in exploratory-descriptive qualitative studies so that participants' answers are more comparable among themselves (Brancati, 2018). Structured interviews are organized with narrower questions in a specific order. The questions may be asked without follow-up questions, and the researcher responses may be scripted in a structured interview (Marshall & Rossman, 2016).

Unstructured interviews are informal and conversational and may be useful during an ethnographical study or in the early stages of other qualitative studies. Brinkmann (2018) argues, however, that neither extreme occurs. A completely structured interview cannot occur because participants will respond in unexpected ways with comments and questions. A completely unstructured interview would mean that the researcher has no purpose for the interview. The researcher must have an idea of how to the start the interview on the selected topic, even if it is only a single statement or question.

Most qualitative interviews are semistructured or organized around a set of open-ended questions. **Semistructured interviews** are rich sources of data because they are flexible; the researcher is free to improvise or alter the wording of a prompt based on how the participant responded to a previous question (Brancati, 2018). The degree of guidance may be as minimal as having a few initial questions or prompts or as structured as multiple predefined questions to narrow the interview to specific aspects of the phenomenon being studied. In either case, the researcher remains open to how the participant responds and carefully words follow-up questions or prompts to allow the **emic view** (the participant's perspective) to emerge. Having this level of structure may decrease the anxiety of less experienced interviewers but may result in findings that reflect the **etic view** (the outsiders' perspective) more than they reflect the emic view. As a best practice, consider testing your interview guide with one participant. In addition to determining the degree of structure for the interviews, the researcher must make several other pragmatic decisions.

What Will I Say and How Will I Respond?

As the researcher, you have the power to shape the interview agenda. Participants have the power to choose the level of responses they will provide. You might begin the interview with a broad request such as, "Describe for me your experience with…" or "Tell me about…." Ideally, the participant will respond as though she or he is telling a story. Madison (2020) describes different types of questions and prompts that may be used in an interview. Table 12.6 was developed to identify categories of questions, with examples, that are used in qualitative research interviews (Madison, 2020). You will not use all of these types of questions in a single interview. The types of questions also have overlap so that one

question could be two types. Seidman (2019) recommends starting with more general questions and moving toward more narrow questions on the topic, a strategy called the funnel approach to interviewing.

You respond nonverbally with a nod or eye contact to convey your interest in what is being said. Try to avoid agreeing or disagreeing with what the participant is saying (Seidman, 2019). Being nonjudgmental allows the participants to share their experiences more freely. When it seems appropriate, encourage your subject to elaborate further on a particular dimension of the topic. Use of nonthreatening but thought-provoking questions is often called probing. Seidman (2019) notes that **probing** sounds intrusive. He prefers the word *exploring* for the process of asking thoughtful questions to gain additional insights into what the participant is sharing. Participants may need validation that they are providing the needed information. Some participants may give short answers, so you may have to encourage them to elaborate. When the participant stops talking, ask a follow-up question that reflects back on what you have heard. Interviewer responses should be encouraging and supportive without being leading. Listening more

TABLE 12.6 Types of Interview Questions

Type of Question	Example
Behavior or experience questions	"I noticed that you use a pill organizer for your medications. What other things do you do to remember to take your pills?"
Opinion or value questions	"In your opinion, which technique for eating out as a person with diabetes is the most helpful?"
Feeling questions	"How did you feel after your clinic appointment last week? Sad, relieved, angry, or some other emotion?"
Knowledge questions	"How were you taught about the rites of passage within your culture?"
Sensory questions	"When you had your first round of chemotherapy, how did your body, your senses, react? What did you taste, hear, see, or smell?
Background/demographic questions	"When was your child diagnosed with autism?"
Descriptive questions	"How do you prepare for dialysis appointments?"
Structured or explanation questions	"Can you help me understand why older people in this community are cared for by their family, instead of moving them to an institutional setting?"
Contrast questions	"How did your wife being diagnosed with cancer compare to you being diagnosed with diabetes?"
Advice questions	"What advice would you give to the person newly diagnosed with high blood pressure?"
Quotation questions	"Someone once said, 'The color of your skin and the thickness of your pocketbook determine the quality of your healthcare.' What do you think?"
Once-upon-a-time or story questions	"Tell me the story of how you and your family moved from Ghana to Montana."

and talking less is a key principle of effective interviews (Seidman, 2019), a principle that requires tolerating silence. If the participant is not talking but seems to be thinking or considering the topic, stay quiet. Silence can be a powerful invitation that allows the participant to show deeper emotions and thoughts.

How Many Interviews Are Needed With Each Participant?

Depending on the research question, the qualitative researcher conducts a single interview or more than one. Instead of a single interview, the researcher may conduct multiple interviews with each participant. Other times, the researcher may collect data during an initial interview and schedule a second clarification interview. During the second interview, the participant can review the researcher's description of the first interview, confirming or correcting the researcher's perceptions and interpretations. As described earlier, Wardlaw and Shambley-Ebron (2019) conducted a study with African American women seeking care for depression. In this study, a second interview was conducted for clarification and to offer the women an opportunity to confirm or revise the categories and patterns found by the researchers. Some researchers have provided a typewritten transcript of the first interview for participants to review during a second interview; others have e-mailed participants a copy to review.

Seidman (2019) recommends that the researcher interview each participant three times for phenomenological studies. The first interview is focused on a life history, the second on details of the phenomenon, and the third on reflection on the experience. Using multiple interviews allows the relationship between the researcher and the participant to develop. Over time, the participant may learn to trust the researcher more and reveal insights about his or her experiences that contribute to the study's findings. Follow-up interviews may be used to share the results of the ongoing data analysis with participants and ask additional questions for clarification. Multiple interviews also may be required to study an ongoing process, such as parenting a child with leukemia.

Will the Interviews Be in Person, by Telephone, or Mediated Through Technology?

Face-to-face interviews are considered best practice because of the nonverbal cues and nuances that may enrich the data. It may be easier for the researcher to develop rapport with the participant and respond more sensitively. The researcher is also able to observe more of the participant's mannerisms or physical conditions. Face-to-face interviews of participants over long distances or in different countries may be too expensive, both in time and money. For example, you are conducting a grounded theory study of the leadership of nurse managers of hemodialysis centers. You may be able to interview a few nurse managers within a 100-mile radius, but they all work for the same company. You want to ensure leadership perspectives in other dialysis centers are included in the study, but the next dialysis center beyond the initial group is 500 miles away. When in-person interviews are not feasible, Web-based meetings through Skype, Zoom, or Facetime provide an excellent alternate, allowing the researcher and participant to see each other (Creswell & Poth, 2018; Seidman, 2019). Not all participants will have access to the internet or the technical skills to use Web-based meetings. Telephone interviews are another alternative and may be a way to communicate that more participants have available. Remember, however, depending on your sample, some participants may not have a telephone. When your participants do not have access to a telephone, in-person meetings may be your only choice.

Ideally, you will have previously contacted the participant and scheduled an appointed time to meet whether in person, by internet, or by telephone. Whatever medium is used for the interview, start with obtaining informed consent. You may have previously e-mailed the consent form and the participant has e-mailed or faxed it back to you. You may obtain verbal consent if that has been approved by your IRB. Often researchers obtain consent after starting the recording and have the recording for verification that consent was obtained ethically.

Where Will I Conduct the Interviews?

Interviews might be conducted in a room in a public library, a fast-food restaurant at an off-peak time, an exam room in a clinic, a public park or garden, or the participant's home. The selected location should be a neutral place that has private areas and is convenient for the participant (Seidman, 2019), with consideration for the safety of both participant and researcher. Accessibility and confidentiality should also be considerations. An exam room may not be a neutral site for a study exploring the patient-provider relationship.

During a community-based study, the researcher's appearance may become associated with a stigmatized topic, such as human immunodeficiency virus (HIV) infection, substance use, or domestic violence. A public place may not protect the participant's identity and confidentiality. A participant's home may not be safe for the researcher to visit at certain times of day. However, a participant's home can offer a sense of comfort and familiarity for the participant and provide the researcher insight into the participant's experience. When preparing for an interview, establish an environment that encourages an open, relaxed conversation (Seidman, 2019). Be sensitive to the physical surroundings. Sit in comfortable chairs and orient the chairs so that neither you nor the participant is facing windows with direct sunlight. Sitting at a table may be more comfortable and provides a surface for the participant to sign the consent form or complete a demographic form. You may want to offer water or another beverage as a way to provide time for a social connection prior to beginning the interview.

What Should I Wear to Conduct the Interviews?

What the researcher should wear to a research interview seems to be a simple question. However, dress is one way that we communicate status, consciously or unconsciously. By virtue of their roles in the interview, the researcher is placed in a power position to direct the interview (Seidman, 2019). To minimize the differences between researcher and participants, the researcher needs to consider how the participant is likely to be dressed. Dressing in formal business attire or a nursing uniform may emphasize the power differences in the relationship with participants from communities with higher rates of poverty. On the other hand, you may be interviewing company executives about workplace stress and business attire is appropriate. Dressing too casually may be viewed as disrespectful of the participant or as an indication that the interaction is not important to the researcher (Brancati, 2018). Power issues may affect the effectiveness of the interview. Visual neutrality is important, as well, in clothing colors. Remember, it is not about you; it is about the participant. Emphasize that by deemphasizing yourself. Olfactory neutrality is important, for the same reason. As nurses do for patient care, researchers should avoid cologne, perfume, and other strong smells when interviewing.

How Will I Record the Interviews?

The words spoken and the nonverbal communication during an interview are the data. Most qualitative researchers audio-record or video-record the interview to allow their focus to be on the interaction and relationship with the participant during the interview (Seidman, 2019). The participant must be aware that the interview is being electronically recorded, but the less obtrusive the equipment, the more quickly the participant will forget its presence, relax, and speak more freely. Logistically, the researcher needs to plan ahead to have the power cords or batteries needed for the recording device. Using batteries may make the device less obtrusive. A sensitive microphone will allow you to pick up even faint or distorted voices, thereby increasing your ability to make an accurate transcription later. Placing the microphone closer to the participant than to the researcher also may result in a better recording. The majority of recording devices are digital, but if using an older model that uses tape, ensure that the length of the tape is adequate to record the entire interview with few interruptions to change the tape. Recording with a digital device that can be saved on a computer can make transcription easier. Voice recognition software has become more sophisticated and may allow conversion of the audio-recording directly to text.

In some situations, recording devices may not be appropriate or the participant may prefer that the interview not be recorded. During the unrecorded interviews, the researcher may take notes and set aside time immediately following the interview to document the interview with as much detail as possible. Check all recordings as soon as possible after the interview, to confirm that they are completely audible. If a recording is not perfectly audible, make notes about the interview content immediately while the words are fresh in your memory. This is also a perfect time to make field notes about content, context, metacommunication, and one's initial reactions and responses.

How Do I Enhance My Interview Skills?

Preparing to interview is critical because interviewing is a skill; some call it a craft that can only be developed through practice (Miles et al., 2020). Interviewing directly affects the quality of the data produced (Creswell & Poth, 2018; Marshall & Rossman, 2016). The challenge for researchers is to be responsive and create a social situation where participants feel comfortable enough to share their stories and perspectives (Brinkmann, 2018). Interviewing skills can be learned (Seidman, 2019); however, researchers must give themselves the opportunity to develop this skill before they start interviewing study participants. A skilled interviewer can elicit higher quality data than an inexperienced interviewer by allowing a silent pause or asking a probing follow-up question without alienating the participant. Unskilled interviewers may not know how or when to intervene, when to encourage the participant to continue to elaborate, or when to divert to another subject.

The researcher begins by developing rapport through active listening (Leavy, 2017; Seidman, 2019). The rapport allows the researcher and participant to be friendly, without developing a friendship (Seidman, 2019). On the whole, qualitative researchers need to learn to be perfectly quiet: to be still, without moving, and to make no sound while the participant speaks. An interview, although interactive, is not a social conversation. The focus is not on the researcher. Rather the focus is on the participant and the participant's experience. Practice looking empathetic and communicating without words. For example, nod instead of saying yes, and chuckle without laughing aloud at humor. More neutral responses allow the interviewee to share good and bad information and events, including socially undesirable feelings and thoughts.

Researchers often underestimate the time needed for an interview. Allow yourself enough time so that you can conduct the interview without feeling rushed. Be sensitive to time-related concerns of the participants, however, and offer the option of stopping if an interview is going longer than expected. Participants may need to catch a bus to get home, pick up children from childcare, or stop to take a dose of medication.

Before beginning data collection, practice interviewing a friend or colleague, possibly about grocery shopping or other noncontroversial or unemotional topic. Record the conversation. Listen to it and listen to the total number of words you say, and how many the interviewee says. Try to limit what you say to phrases or questions that facilitate the interviewee's story. About 90% of the words on the tape should be those of the participant. Continue your practice by conducting interviews with colleagues with experience in interviewing (Munhall, 2012). These rehearsals will help you identify problems before initiating the study. You may want to conduct one or more trial interviews with individuals who meet the sampling criteria to allow you to try out the proposed questions.

How Can I Prevent or Respond to Common Interview Problems?

Difficulties can occur during interviews. Common problems include interruptions such as telephone calls or text messages, "stage fright" that often arises when the participant realizes he or she is being recorded, failure to establish a rapport with your subject, verbose participants, and those who tend to wander off the subject. Turn off or silence your cell phone at the beginning of the interview and ask the participant to do the same. If a participant seems paralyzed by the presence of the recording device, move the device out of his or her line of sight if possible. Ask demographic questions or factual questions to ease into the interview. When the participant moves to a subject that you think is unrelated to the focus of the study, you may want to ask how this new subject is related to previous comments on the topic of interest (Seidman, 2019). You may be surprised to learn that what you perceived to be unrelated is associated with the topic, from the participant's perspective. You may also need to tactfully guide the interview back to the topic. Remind participants that they can decline to answer any question and can end the interview at any time.

When using a series of interview questions, let the participant answer the first question fully. If the topic is an emotional one, the participant will almost always provide a story or example. This sometimes answers one or more of the subsequent interview questions on your list. If this happens, as you proceed down the question list, you can say, "The next question is . . . and you have already told me some things about that. Is there anything else you want to add?"

The physical, mental, and emotional condition of the participant may cause difficulties during the interview. The data obtained are affected by characteristics of the person being interviewed (Seidman, 2019). These include age, ethnicity, gender, professional background, educational level, and relative status of interviewer and interviewee, as well as impairments in vision or hearing, speech impediments, fatigue, pain, poor memory, disorientation, emotional state, and language difficulties. Although IRBs tend to view interviews as noninvasive, interviews are an invasion of the psyche. An interview is capable of producing risks to the health of the participant. Therefore the interviewer must always avoid inflicting unnecessary harm upon the participant. Participants with fatigue or pain related to illness or treatments should be offered the opportunity to stop, take a break, or reschedule the interview for another day.

For some participants, the experience may be therapeutic but that is not the purpose of the interview (Seidman, 2019). Nevertheless, participants in qualitative interviews are often glad for the ability to express their feelings to an interested listener. It is common for participants to say, after a lengthy interview, "Thank you so much for listening to my story. It's not something I can tell everyone."

Emotional expression during an interview may be expected, depending on the topic. Participants who become visibly upset while telling their story should be asked, "Do you want to pause the interview for a few minutes while you take a deep breath and compose yourself?" or even, "You seem upset. Do you want to end this interview, or do you want to proceed?" When the participant becomes distressed or overcome with emotion, however, you may choose to turn off the recording device and stop the interview completely for a few minutes. You may be able to continue if the participant is able to become composed. Stay with the individual; offer a tissue. Recognize topics that are more likely to be distressing, and have a plan developed for emergency assistance, if needed, or a list of mental health professionals available if support or a referral is needed. For example, you might schedule interviews in collaboration with a hospital chaplain or psychiatric mental health nurse practitioner to ensure that one of them is available for consultation when you will be interviewing family members whose spouses are receiving hospice care. Recognize that you, the researcher, may also need emotional and psychological support. The researcher may be strongly affected by the stories of the participants. Arrange to have a mentor or trusted friend available to talk with before or after interviews (Padgett, 2017). Debriefing is more than socioemotional support; the mentor or fellow researcher may suggest different ways to look at the data or a novel way to start the interview. Recognize that interviews are tiring due to the amount of time they require. You leave for an interview so that you can arrive about 30 minutes early. Once you meet the participants, you obtain informed consent, which may take 20 minutes or longer. Then the interview may last for 70 minutes. After the interview, you reserve time to add to your field notes, considering the participant's and your response to the interview. This step may take another hour, meaning that you have spent close to 3 hours on one interview.

Example Study Using Interviews

In this chapter, we have already discussed two studies in which the researchers used interviews. Tables 12.1 and 12.2 may be helpful to review as we consider additional studies. We provided a long excerpt of Pool's (2019) phenomenological study as an example of behaviors that increased rigor. Her study included interviews with nurses who cared for AI cancer patients. Another of the examples in the chapter has been the ethnographical study of African American women with depression conducted by Wardlaw and Shambley-Ebron (2019). They collected data using interviews as well.

"Two 1-hour, semi-structured interviews were conducted with each participant. The first interview was to gather data to answer the research questions. The second interview served as a member check to clarify data and ensure its veracity. Categories and patterns that were derived from the data were presented to informants for confirmation. The interviews were digitally recorded, transcribed, and subjected to a constant comparative analysis." (Wardlaw & Shambley-Ebron, 2019, p. 174)

Focus groups, described in the next section, have been called group interviews. For that reason, several principles of interviewing apply to conducting focus groups, such as building rapport, listening more than talking, and what to wear for a focus group.

Focus Groups

Focus groups began as tools for market researchers (Kamberelis, Dimitriadis, & Welker, 2018). A **focus group** has been defined as a "semi-structured group interview designed to elicit information from participants on a defined topic of interest" (Brancati, 2018, p. 156). Since before pre-World War II, focus groups have evolved from a series of scripted questions asked of a group into free-flowing dialogues that produce creative ideas (Kamberelis et al., 2018). Many different communication forms occur in focus groups, including teasing, arguing, joking, anecdotes, and nonverbal clues, such as gesturing and facial expressions. The different forms of communication and the interactions among participants in a focus group can help individuals clarify their views while generating new thoughts because of comments made by other participants (Brancati, 2018).

Focus groups, as a means of data collection, serve a variety of purposes in nursing research. These groups have been used to understand the experiences of people who are receiving care or may need care. Researchers have conducted focus groups to study mothering in women with ovarian cancer (Arida et al., 2019), quality of life with trauma patients (Kruithof et al., 2018), self-care management of older persons with heart failure (Son, Lee, & Kim, 2019), and communication about hypothermia with parents of neonates in intensive care (Craig, Gerwin, Bainter, Evans, & James, 2018). Collecting data with focus groups is a flexible and efficient method.

The first step in planning a focus group is determining the characteristics of the participants you want in the study (Brancati, 2018). Recruiting appropriate participants for each of the focus groups is critical, because recruitment is the most common source of failure. Selecting participants who are similar to one another in lifestyle or experiences, views, and characteristics is believed to facilitate open discussion and interaction. These characteristics might be age, gender, social class, income level, ethnicity, culture, lifestyle, or health status. For example, for a study of barriers to implementing HIV/acquired immunodeficiency syndrome (AIDS) clinical trials in low-income minority communities, focus groups might be organized by race/ethnicity and gender.

Other researchers have opted to convene focus groups of diverse participants in an effort to trigger new ways of thinking about the research topic. In heterogeneous groups, communication patterns, roles, relationships, and traditions might interfere with the interactions within the focus group. Be cautious about bringing together participants with considerable variation in social standing, education, or authority, because some group members may hesitate to participate fully, whereas others may discount the input of those with perceived lower standing. If a fairly heterogeneous sample is desired, to provide a variety of responses, participants may be selected somewhat randomly from a large group. Although qualitative researchers typically use nonrandom sampling, it is not wrong to use random sampling for focus group research when there is a rationale for doing so.

Preparation is needed to collect data using focus groups beginning with determining how many focus groups and the desired size. Recommendations for the size of focus groups varies among experts. For example, Brancati (2018) recommends 6 to 12 participants and Padgett (2017) recommends 5 to 7 participants. If there are fewer participants, the discussion tends to be inadequate. In most cases, participants are expected to be unknown to one another. However, for a focus group conducted with professional groups such as clinical nurses or nurse educators, such anonymity usually is not possible. You may use purposive sampling to seek out individuals known to have the desired expertise (see Chapter 15). In other cases, you may look for participants through the media, posters, or advertisements.

Another aspect of planning a focus group is determining the location(s), which needs to be carefully selected to ensure privacy, comfort, and safety. Meeting rooms in public facilities such as schools, libraries, or churches may be appropriate community locations for focus groups, depending on the research question and the study aims. For focus groups with specific populations, the facility used for support services may have a quiet room that is accessible and familiar to participants. Nurses or other health professionals may participate in focus groups in a healthcare facility but might be more forthcoming in a location away from the facility. If a focus group is planned for a sensitive topic, indicate on the invitation and on any materials the name by which the group will be identified. For example, instead of identifying the group as the Testicular Cancer Study, a better name might be the Men's Health Study. Also, if a topic is too personal or controversial, participants may be more forthcoming in a one-on-one interview.

Other logistics include the expected length of the meeting, recruiting subjects, and recording the group interactions. Focus groups typically last from 45 minutes to 2 hours. Be clear on the recruitment materials about the expected duration of the focus group. Allow for the time it will take to complete consent and demographic forms in determining the length of the data collection process. Provide a reasonable estimate of the time needed, recognizing that whether people attend may be affected by how long the group meeting is expected to last.

A single contact with an individual who agrees to attend a focus group does not ensure that this person will attend the group session. Overrecruiting may be necessary; a good rule is to invite two more potential participants than you need for the group. You will need to make follow-up phone calls or remind the candidates by mail or e-mail. You may need to offer compensation for their time and effort in the form of cash, phone card, gift card, or bus tokens. Cash payments are, of course, the most effective if the resources are available through funding. Other incentives include offering refreshments at the focus group meeting, T-shirts, coffee mugs, gift certificates, and coupons. The compensation for time and effort needs to be reasonable. Overcompensation may be judged by the IRB to be coercive and delay IRB approval.

The setting for focus groups should be a relaxed atmosphere with space for participants to sit comfortably in a circle or U shape and maintain eye contact with one another. Ensure that the acoustics of the room will allow you to obtain a quality audio-recording of the sessions. As with the one-on-one interview discussed earlier, place your audio or video recorders unobtrusively. Use a highly sensitive microphone. Hiring a court reporter to do a real-time transcription may have advantages over recording the interaction for transcription later. Inaudible voices on the recording or overlapping voices can pose challenges to later transcription.

The facilitator, also called a moderator, is critical to the success of a focus group (Padgett, 2017). Select a facilitator when possible who reflects the age, gender, and race/ethnicity of the group. In contrast, having a facilitator who is dissimilar from the participants may prevent open communication due to a lack of trust. The researcher may be the facilitator of the group or may train another person for the role. Training of the facilitator should be thorough and allow time for practice. The facilitator needs to understand the aims of the focus groups and to communicate these aims to the participants before the group session. Instruct participants that all points of view are valid and helpful and that speakers should not be asked to defend their positions. Make clear to the group that the moderator's role is to facilitate the discussion, not to contribute. In addition to the moderator, you may want to have an observer or assistant moderator who takes field notes (Padgett, 2017), especially of facial expressions or interactions not captured by an audio-recording. Making notes on the dynamics of the group is also useful, including how group members interact with one another.

Carefully plan the questions that are to be asked during the focus group and, if time permits, pilot-test them with people who are similar to the target population. Limit the number of questions to those most essential to allow adequate time for discussion. You may elect to give participants some of the questions before the group meeting to enable them to give careful thought to their responses. Questions should be posed in such a way that group members can build on the responses of others in the group, raise their own questions, and question one another. Probes can be used to elicit richer details, by means of questions such as "How would that make a difference?" or responses such as "Tell us more about that situation." Avoid pushing participants toward taking a stand and defending it. Once rapport has been established, you may be able to question or challenge ideas and increase group interaction.

The researcher and/or moderator may come to the focus groups with preconceived ideas about the topic. Early in the session, provide opportunities for participants to express their views on the topic of discussion. Use probes or questions if the discussion wanders too far from the focus of the study. A good moderator weaves questions into the discussion naturally and clarifies, paraphrases, and reflects back what group members have said. These discussions tend to express group norms, or the majority voice, and individual voices of contrasting viewpoints may be stifled. A participant may be uncomfortable sharing a less acceptable viewpoint, because those with opposing views are listening. However, when a sensitive topic is being discussed, the group format may actively facilitate the discussion because less inhibited members break the ice for those who are more reticent. Participants may also provide group support for expressing feelings, opinions, or experiences. Late in the session, the facilitator may encourage group members to go beyond the current discussion or debate and reflect on differences among the views of participants and inconsistencies within their own thinking.

Example Study Using Focus Groups

Munro et al. (2019) conducted a descriptive qualitative study of the attitudes of pregnant women and their partners toward screening for chromosomal abnormalities. The researchers used focus groups to collect the data.

"Four focus groups were conducted in community locations in the greater Vancouver area (neighborhood houses, community centres, childbirth education centres). Sample sizes for each focus group were as follows: group 1 (*n* = 6); group 2 (*n* = 3); group 3 (*n* = 6); group 4 (*n* = 6). Participants included pregnant persons and their partners or support people.... Participants were recruited by a research assistant and community partners or via poster advertisement in antenatal clinics, community settings, Facebook, and Twitter. Interested individuals contacted a member of the study team, were informed of the purpose of the study, reviewed the consent form by email, and booked a focus group time convenient for their schedule." (Munro et al., 2017, p. 365)

The total sample for the study was 21 people, comprised of 12 mothers and 9 male spouses or common-law partners. Over half of the participants were Asian ethnicity and had a college education. The study findings identified decision points about prenatal chromosomal screening.

"Our findings suggest that women and their partners/support people considered four key decision points when confronted with options for prenatal screening and diagnosis:
(1) Should I/my partner have prenatal screening and diagnostic testing?
(2) Which screening test should I/my partner get?
(3) Which diagnostic test should I/my partner get?
(4) What would I/we do with a positive diagnosis?
Participants expressed a belief that, for the first three choices, the primary decision maker was the pregnant woman, while the partner's role was to provide decision support. The final choice regarding continuing or terminating the pregnancy was considered a shared decision for the couple. The attributes of each decision that were important to pregnant women and their partners included the following: *Time of diagnosis*; *Information acquired*; *Accuracy* (false positives); *Cost*; *Invasiveness*; and *Harm to woman and baby.*" (Wardlaw & Shambley-Ebron, 2019, pp. 366–367)

Wardlaw and Shambley-Ebron (2019) noted that the findings may only be applicable to the similar samples of participants who are primarily Asian ethnicity with university educations and higher household incomes. Also, the participants were not at high risk for chromosomal abnormalities. The study was conducted rigorously as noted in the following excerpt.

"We engaged in verification strategies throughout data collection and analysis to promote rigour, including constant comparison, keeping an audit trail of fieldwork and analysis notes, and sampling to theoretical saturation. Our research team engaged in a number of strategies to enhance reflexivity—being explicitly self-aware of and sensitive to our researcher roles. In focus groups, we sought to attend to participants' comfort and emotional well-being in the context of a topic that may be distressing to some individuals. The interviewer had young children of her own and, where relevant to develop trust, rapport, and minimize power imbalances, she noted her 'insider status' to participants and described that she was also a parent who had been presented with options for prenatal screening and testing." (Wardlaw & Shambley-Ebron, 2019, p. 366)

Focus groups can be an efficient and effective method for data collection, especially when as rigorously implemented as Wardlaw and Shambley-Ebron's (2019) study. The next method of data collection is electronically mediated data collection, including collecting visual and online data.

Visual Data

Anthropologists have included photographs as data in their studies for many years as adjunct to observation (Margolis & Zunjarwad, 2018). However, creating photographic images as part of data collection is not limited to anthropology and ethnography. Creating photographic images is a viable scientific method in different types of qualitative and quantitative studies. Glegg (2019) developed a typology of the ways that visual tools are used in qualitative research, which was adapted for the purposes of this textbook (Box 12.4). Photovoice will be included in this section as a method to collect data.

Visual images can be used to promote validity and quality of the study findings. For example, a researcher may represent data in visual form for member checking, for seeking feedback from the participants (Glegg, 2019). In grounded theory studies, the researchers may develop a diagram to represent the concepts and relationships among them. The diagram could be shared with the participants for their input or verification of the accuracy of the model.

Researchers may use visual images (tables, graphs) in a study report to display aggregated data. This is the most common way that visual images are used in qualitative

BOX 12.4 Purposes for Using Visual Tools in Qualitative Research

1. Rigor of the study: Use figures or photos for member checking
2. Dissemination of the findings: Use graphs and figures to represent data
3. Researcher-participant relationship: Use photos and other images to promote communication
4. Data collection: Use photos taken by participants as data

Adapted from Glegg, S. (2019). Facilitating interviews in qualitative research with visual tools: A typology. *Qualitative Health Research, 29*(2), 301–310.

research and other research methodologies. For example, researchers implementing an intervention to reduce pressure ulcers in patients with low serum albumin may use a line graph showing the trend of pressure ulcers per month before and after the intervention.

Visual images can also be used promote communication and facilitate the relationship between the participant and the researcher. Some potential participants lack verbal or mental capacity to participate in a traditional interview but may be able to select pictures that represent how they feel or their response to a question. Betriana and Kongsuwan (2019) conducted a phenomenological study of the lived experience of Muslim nurses who care for patients who have died in the ICU. It was not known how Muslim nurses experience the death of their patients, because Islam teaches that a person is to accept death and not show grief when a person dies. To enable communication with participants who are not familiar with talking about their grief, the researchers asked the participants to draw a picture of their grief after a patient's death. The interview started with the participants being asked to describe what they drew. Betriana and Kongsuwan (2019) found the pictures were an effective way of overcoming the nurses' reticence to talk about patient deaths. In this study, the pictures themselves were not analyzed as data but were used to start the conversation.

Researcher-generated diagrams and photos may also be used to facilitate the relationship and enable communication. Images with special meaning for the researcher may humanize the researcher and encourage participants to share more of their deeper feelings about the topic. A female researcher who is conducting a qualitative study of the health needs of grandmothers who are raising grandchildren, might start an interview by showing the participant a picture of her own grandchildren. After showing the picture and identifying the grandchildren by name and age, the researcher may ask the grandmother to tell about her grandchildren. In this way, the researcher is building on something she has in common with the participants.

Visual images can also be data for a study. Photovoice is a specific method of using photographs as data in a study. **Photovoice** is a data collection method that asks the participants to take pictures on a selected theme. Photovoice has been closely associated with community-based participatory research, a methodology that begins with the members of a community identifying the research that is needed and conducting the studies to address those needs (Margolis & Zunjarwad, 2018). Photovoice is an appropriate data collection method when participants have limited verbal ability and when the photos may serve as proof of environmental conditions.

Wang and Burris (1997) refined the method for the social sciences and focused on using photovoice as a way for participants with limited verbal abilities to describe or explain their reality. For example, Danker, Strnadová, and Cumming (2019) used photovoice as a means for adolescents with autism spectrum disorder to describe their well-being as well as barriers and assets related to well-being. The adolescents used their phones or digital cameras to take pictures reflective of well-being. If safety or embarrassment was a concern, the adolescent was instructed to use pictures from the internet. The 16 high school students participated in two interviews. During the first interview, the researcher provided instructions about the ethical rules of taking pictures and how to transfer the pictures to a USB drive. The second interview was conducted to allow the students to describe their pictures. Two students used pictures from the internet and three forgot to take the pictures. The photos and images from the internet that were submitted reflected a multidimensional experience of well-being as well as specific barriers and assets. For example, a photo of the school buzzer that sounded when class periods begin and end was described as a barrier to well-being. The noise of the buzzer in addition to all the other noises in the hall was uncomfortable for the participants. Representing assets to facilitate well-being, a photo was submitted of the feet of a group of girls standing in a circle to represent friends as an asset (Danker et al., 2019).

Another reason to use photovoice is that the pictures are evidence of environmental conditions and may help consumers of the research to understand more deeply the context of the participants. Yu, Hope House Men, and Alumni (2018) conducted a grounded theory study with African American men who were reentering the outside world after incarceration or were in recovery from substance abuse. Hope House is a residential rehabilitation project that allows men who are leaving prison or are involved in recovery to live there for 9 months. Photovoice, focus groups, and interviews were sources of data for the study of barriers and resources for reentry and/or recovery.

The study conducted by Yu et al. (2018) was designed to explore how Black adult men reintegrated into their community, specifically the North Lawndale neighborhood. The North Lawndale neighborhood was located on the West Side of Chicago and home to the "largest single site jail in the U.S." (Yu et al., 2018, p. 201). As a result, 57% of the neighborhood's population was persons who had been incarcerated and released. The neighborhood also had high levels of poverty, unemployment, and violent crime. Reentry and recovery were difficult processes in this neighborhood. The members of Hope House and its alumni collaborated with Dr. Yu to understand these processes and identify interventions and resources to overcome the barriers the men experienced.

At the beginning of the study, the men were given digital cameras and taught how to use the camera. Each group completed four photo assignments, which were related to a topic or theme identified by the group. For example, the Hope House members selected as their first assignment photographing challenges and barriers. The alumni group's first assignment was obstacles. After two weeks, the men selected 3 to 4 photographs to show the other participants when they reconvened.

The researcher conducted focus groups and individual interviews with the men to discuss the photos they had taken. During the focus groups, one of the men would share a photograph and identify when and where it was taken. The photographs provided evidence of dilapidated buildings, trash, vacant lots, and gang activity. The men identified themes or groupings of the pictures.

Data analysis of the focus group and interview transcripts resulted in a description of the barriers as being an exploited community characterized by broken relationships. The men described being "locked in the streets" and "between two worlds," each of which was pulling on them (Yu et al., 2018, p. 204). On one side was the street and being pulled back into that environment. The forces pulling in that direction were "stinkin' thinkin'," "guarding emotions," and "conforming behaviors." On the other side was recovery with family, friends, and mentors reaching out and pulling him in that direction. Cultivating recovery involved "internal transformation," "consciousness," "brotherhood," and a "sense of mission." The analysis also revealed opportunities to intervene to improve the community and to provide resources for men during reentry/recovery (Yu et al., 2018).

Photovoice was an effective method for eliciting verbal data in addition to the photos themselves being data. Researchers who are considering photovoice as a research methodology are urged to read primary sources and consult with researchers experienced in the methodology. Photovoice may pose unique ethical considerations because people in photographs can be identified and may not have consented to participation in the study (Marshall & Rossman, 2016). The rights of the research participants must be protected during the conduct and reporting of the research (see Chapter 9).

Internet-Based Data

Internet communication provides a way to collect data from persons separated by distance. Quantitative researchers are regularly using internet-based surveys and instruments to gather data, but qualitative researchers are also using Web-based communities such as online forums and blogs for research purposes. These methods of communication are being used for different reasons by researchers. For example, Nicholas, Bai, and Fiske (2019) identified 41 blogs on research methods in psychology. The blogs provided an avenue for less experienced researchers to learn from those with more expertise in a given area. Facebook, Instagram, and other types of social media have been used to recruit participants but are used less frequently to collect data. The number of participants available for internet-based research is extensive, because such studies provide a unique way to access stigmatized and other hard-to-reach populations (Padgett, 2017). The limitations to the method are that samples include only those who can read and write, are comfortable using a computer, and have access to the internet (Marshall & Rossman, 2016).

Web-based communication can be used as a source of data for secondary analysis. Eddy, Poll, Whiting, and Clevesy (2019) explored blogs, chat rooms, online forums, and websites for data related to fathers' experiences with postpartum depression. Finding sufficient data to analyze, they concluded that paternal postpartum depression does occur. Healthcare professionals need to assess for it just as they do for maternal postpartum depression. In a similar way, Abdoli, Jones, Vora, and Stuckey (2019) collected and analyzed data from blog narratives written by persons with diabetes. The purpose of their study was to explore the experience of diabetic burnout. They found that diabetic burnout began with detachment, could be precipitated by life events, and could be overcome but with great difficulty.

Computer-mediated communication, such as video-conferencing, has been studied as a method for conducting focus groups. Wirtz, Cooney, Chaudhry, Reisner, and the American Cohort Study of HIV Acquisition Among Transgender Women (2019) conducted seven synchronous focus groups ($N = 41$) using an online conferencing system with adult transgendered women in six cities. Because this was a feasibility study, the paper does not report findings from the analysis of the data but described the benefits and barriers of using this method. The online conferencing system allowed access by computer, cell or landline phone, or tablet. With computer and tablet access, the women had the choice of using their built-in web camera. Some women chose not to use the camera to protect their confidentiality. By removing the time and money required to travel to a specific location for a focus group, the researchers were able to recruit a geographically, racially, and ethnically diverse sample, which allowed comparisons by women in different parts of the country. The sample size was sufficient to generate more than an adequate amount of transcribed text for analysis.

In summary, methods for qualitative data collection include observation, interviews, focus groups, visual images, and web-based communication. The data generated by these methods require careful transcription, analysis, and storage.

DATA MANAGEMENT

The data collected by qualitative researchers may include field notes, memos, transcriptions, text-based communication, and digital media. This section will describe how oral recordings and pencil-paper notes are converted to text for analysis and then organized to ensure the researcher can find the documents needed. Preparation of the data for analysis and the organization of the digital files are critical considerations when planning and implementing a study (Miles et al., 2020).

Transcribing Recorded Data

Transcription of verbal data into written data is a routine component of qualitative studies. Transcripts present data in a form that allows the researcher to review the data visually and to share it with team members for analysis and validation. Data collected during a qualitative study may be narrative descriptions of observations, transcripts from audio-recordings of interviews, entries in the researcher's diary reflecting on the dynamics of the setting, or notes taken while reading and reflecting on written documents.

Transcription may require 8 to 10 hours for 90 minutes of interview or focus group time, depending on the equipment used and the transcriber's skill (Padgett, 2017). Audio-recorded interviews are generally transcribed verbatim with different punctuation marks used to indicate laughter, changes in voice tone, or other nuances (Padgett, 2017). Hiring a professional transcriptionist may decrease the time but may be too expensive, depending on the study's budget. When hiring a transcriptionist, be clear about the details, such as whether to correct grammar and how to indicate pauses or laughter (Leavy, 2017; Padgett, 2017). Although some researchers use general transcription or select relevant sections of the recording to transcribe (Seidman, 2019), nurse researchers most frequently report verbatim transcription and link the accuracy of the transcript to the rigor of the study (Rubin & Rubin, 2012).

Transcribing the recordings yourself has the advantage of immediately immersing you in the data. If using tapes, a pedal-operated recorder allows you to listen, stop, and start the recording without removing your hands from the keyboard. With digitalized data, you can start and stop the recording with a click. Even when you hire another person to transcribe the recordings, you will check the transcription by listening to the recording while reviewing the transcript. Voice recognition programs can be of significant benefit as the capacity of the software to learn the voice of the interviewee continues to improve with new versions or updates. For transcription of focus group recordings, voice recognition software may not be as effective. Other software may allow conversion of audio-recording to digital formats ready for analysis within computer analysis software. You also may code the actual recording, negating the need for a word-by-word transcription.

Video-recordings are maintained in their original format. However, the researcher may make notes on sequential segments of the recording, creating a type of field notes. The researcher may also code the recordings directly. When video-recordings are used, you may want to watch and code segments of 15 to 30 seconds. For observational data collection, the researcher may watch 15 seconds of the recording and note whether a specific behavior occurred.

ORGANIZING AND STORING DATA

Because data are frequently collected simultaneously with data analysis, the study manager, who may be the researcher, needs to have a plan developed for how to organize and store data. Label electronic files consistently. For example, the digital files from recordings can be labeled with the date and the code number or pseudonym of the participant. Make copies of all original files on a second computer or external storage device. Similarly, scan or copy all handwritten notes, field notes, or memos and, if possible, store originals in a waterproof and fireproof storage box. When digital files will be transmitted electronically to a transcriptionist or team members, best practices include encrypting the files if they contain personally identifiable information (family member, hospital name, addresses, doctor's name) or de-identifying the file by removing all personal identifiers (see Chapter 9). You may want to keep a Word document or Excel file listing all files by date, file name, and type of document, such as observational memo, transcript, analysis record, or field note. Miles et al. (2020) call this file a data accounting log. The study manager may also want to keep records of who is currently working on which file and whether it

is being transcribed, analyzed, or reviewed by a team member. With Internet-based storage systems (Google drive, cloud storage), researchers can simultaneously analyze files with all input saved quickly and attributed to the contributor.

Some researchers may prefer to make notes, mark text, and label (code) sections of data on a hard copy of a transcript or field note using colored markers, pencil, or pen. If hard copy is used, ensure that each page is clearly identified with the file name in the header or footer of the document. You may want to format the document with large right-hand margins to allow more space for coding and notes. It is recommended that you also include line numbers, not for each page but for the entire document continuously. Having line numbers allows the researcher to note the source of a code by line number within a specific document.

Computer-Assisted Qualitative Data Analysis Software

Many qualitative researchers prefer to work on electronic files within a software program. The simplest software uses tools such the highlight or comment functions on a document within a word-processing file. Visual images, transcripts, field notes, and memos may be analyzed within one of several specialized computer programs, called CAQDAS. The program does not analyze the data but allows the researcher to make notes about tentative themes and record decisions made during the analysis (Miles et al., 2020). CAQDAS can maintain a file directory, allow for annotation of coding decisions, produce diagrams of relationships among codes, and retrieve sections of text that the researcher has identified with the same code (Miles et al., 2020; Padgett, 2017). Using CAQDAS for a small study may not be worth the cost and time to learn the program. However, Miles et al. (2020) state that using CAQDAS is essential for studies with longitudinal designs and multiple sites, types of data, and researchers. Box 12.5 provides a list of the advantages and disadvantages of CAQDAS, extracted from Miles et al. (2020) and Creswell and Poth (2018). Table 12.7 contains descriptions and online suppliers of a selected group of CAQDAS programs. If you are looking for additional information, Creswell and Poth (2018) provide a list of 19 CAQDAS and a list of questions for researchers to consider when selecting which CAQDAS to use.

BOX 12.5   Advantages and Disadvantages of Computer-Assisted Qualitative Data Analysis Software (CAQDAS)

Advantages

Store and organize data files

Provide means for line-by-line analysis

Provide documentation of coding and analysis

Click and drag to merge codes

Have concept-mapping features

Search for related codes and quotations efficiently

Send coded data files to others

Link memos to text

Generate a list of all codes

Retrieve memos related to specific codes

Minimize clerical tasks to allow focus on actual analysis

Support and integrate the work of multiple team members

Decrease paper usage

Disadvantages

Cost of software

Need to allow time and expend energy to learn the software and its functions

Unavailability of understandable instructions for use of the software

Potential that technical/functional aspects will overwhelm thinking about the analysis

Potential for computer problems interfering with the software and causing data and analysis to be lost

Adapted from Creswell, J., & Poth, C. (2018). *Qualitative inquiry and research design: Choosing among five approaches* (4th ed.). Thousand Oaks, CA: Sage; Miles, M., Huberman, A., & Saldaña, J. (2020). *Qualitative data analysis: A methods sourcebook* (4th ed.). Thousand Oaks, CA: Sage; Saldaña, J. (2016). *The coding manual for qualitative researchers* (3rd ed.). Thousand Oaks, CA: Sage.

TABLE 12.7   Selected Examples of Computer-Assisted Qualitative Data Analysis Software (CAQDAS)

Software	Description	Website
ATLAS/ti	Robust CAQDAS functions; large searchable data storage, including audio, video, image, and text files; multiple users allowed; facilitates theory building; flexible; supports use of PDF files.	http://www.atlasti.com/
Ethnograph	Originally developed for use by ethnographers; import and code data files; sort and sift codes; retrieve data and files.	http://www.qualisresearch.com/
HyperRESEARCH	Code and retrieval functions; theory building features; handles media files.	http://www.researchware.com/
MAXQDA	Robust CAQDAS functions, but less powerful search tool; allows integration of quantitative and qualitative analysis; color-based filing; supports different types of text analysis.	http://www.maxqda.com/products
NVivo	Robust CAQDAS functions, including several types of queries; familiar format of file organization system; handles multimedia files; latest version includes compatibility with quantitative analysis and bibliographical software.	https://www.qsrinternational.com/

Synthesized from websites of suppliers.

DATA ANALYSIS

Qualitative data analysis is "both the code and the thought processes that go behind assigning meaning to data" (Corbin & Strauss, 2015, p. 58). The virtual text grows in size and complexity as the researcher reads and rereads the transcripts. Throughout the process of analysis, the virtual text develops and evolves.

Although multiple valid interpretations may occur if different researchers examine the text, all findings must remain trustworthy to the data. Interpretations should be data based, or in the words of a grounded theory researcher, grounded in the data. This trustworthiness applies to the unspoken meanings emerging from the totality of the data, not just the written words of the text. The first step in data analysis is to be familiar with the data.

Becoming Familiar With the Data

Data analysis may start simultaneously with data collection (Creswell & Creswell, 2018), which requires the researcher to continually go back and read previous transcripts and notes. In some studies, more than one researcher is involved in data collection, so the researchers are reading transcripts of interviews or observations made by others. Becoming familiar with the data involves reading and rereading notes and transcripts, recalling observations and experiences, listening to audio-recordings, and viewing videotapes until you begin to have general ideas about what the data may reveal. Recordings contain more than words; they contain feeling, emphasis, and nonverbal communications. These aspects are at least as important to the communication as the words are. As you listen to recordings, look at photographs, or read transcripts, you relive the experiences described and become very familiar with the phrases that different participants used or the images that were especially poignant.

Phenomenological researchers use the phrases "immersed in the data" or "dwelling with the data" to describe this process of spending time coming to know and be familiar with the study's data (Munhall, 2012). **Being immersed** means that you are fully invested in the data and are spending extensive amounts of time reading and thinking about the data.

Coding

The volumes of data acquired in a qualitative study must be reduced by clustering or grouping the data. By doing this, the researcher can more effectively examine them. The reduction of the data occurs as you attach meaning to elements in your data and document that meaning with a word, symbol, or phrase. Codes are "labels that assign symbolic meaning" to "data 'chunks' or units of varying size" (Miles et al., 2020, p. 62). Coding is a means of naming, labeling, and later sorting data elements, which allows the researcher to find themes and patterns. Through coding, the researcher explores the phenomenon of the study. Miles et al. (2020) state "coding is analysis" (p. 63). Coding is more than "technical, preparatory work for higher level thinking about the study…coding is deep reflection about and, thus, deep analysis and interpretation of the data's meanings" (Miles et al., 2020, p. 63).

Organization of data, selection of specific elements of the data for categories, and naming of these categories all reflect the philosophical basis of the study. The type and level of coding vary somewhat according to the qualitative approach being used. Table 12.8 displays types of codes described in the social science literature and used primarily in grounded theory analysis. The terms can be confusing because different writers have given different names to similar types of codes.

Another way to think about codes is to classify them as expected, surprising, or of conceptual interest (Creswell & Creswell, 2018). From your review of the literature, the selection of a theoretical framework, or the wording of your interview questions, you have some codes in mind that you expect to find in the data. For example, you conducted an exploratory-descriptive qualitative study and used Orem's (2004) theory of self-care as the theoretical framework for understanding the home care needs of persons with rheumatoid arthritis who are receiving immunotherapy. The focus group questions you developed for the study fit this theoretical framework. One of your questions for the focus groups was, "What activities can you no longer do for yourself?" You expected to code the descriptions of these activities as "self-care deficits" to be consistent with Orem's theory. Expected codes may be based on either the theoretical framework for the study or your literature review (Saldaña, 2016). During analysis, you also encountered sections of the transcripts in which the participants debated with each other about whether home immunotherapy infusions were better than clinic immunotherapy infusions. Because you did not expect this information, the code of "location of infusions" would be considered a surprise code. When the participants described the activities they could no longer do for themselves, you expected the participants to compare what they could not do now to what they could do prior to the worsening of their illness. Instead the focus group participants compared what they could or could not do with what family and friends who had other illnesses could or could not do. These comparisons to others with other illnesses revealed perspectives of the participants that could affect their satisfaction with home care services, but in terms of coding, "comparisons to others" expanded the concept of self-care deficits in Orem's theory. This is an example of a code of conceptual interest. There are many different strategies and terms used

TABLE 12.8 Types of Coding for Qualitative Data Analysis[a]

Type	Description
Axial coding	Finding and labeling connections between concepts; assigning codes to categories (Belgrave & Seide, 2019); also may be called Level II coding in grounded theory studies
Descriptive coding	Classifying elements of data using terms that are close to the participant's words, also called first-level and primary cycle coding (Miles et al., 2020)
Interpretive coding	Labeling coded data into more abstract terms that represent merged codes; interpretations may be checked with participants; participants may contribute to the actual interpretation (Munhall, 2012)
In vivo coding	Codes are phrases or terms used by the participants (Miles et al., 2020), instead of words selected by the researcher
Open coding	"Breaking apart data into discrete, meaningful pieces" (Belgrave & Seide, 2019, p. 174); also called Level I coding in grounded theory studies
Pattern (explanatory) coding	Grouping of codes from first cycle coding into categories, concepts, or themes (Miles et al., 2020); identifies more abstract commonalities across codes
Selective (focused, theoretical) coding	Second cycle coding that groups codes into categories that create a theme, concept, or process, without extensive focus on describing details or properties of the categories (Saldaña, 2016)
Substantive coding	Using words of participants as codes to group the data; subsumes open coding and selective coding (Belgrave & Seide, 2018)

[a]These terms are not mutually exclusive, because different writers have used different labels for similar analytical processes.

for coding the data. For example, 33 coding methods were described in Saldaña's (2016) coding manual alone.

As data analysis continues, coding may progress to the development of a taxonomy, the emergence of codes into patterns, or, in grounded theory research, to the description of a theoretical framework. For example, you might develop a classification of types of pain, types of patients, or types of patient education. Initial categories should be as broad as possible with minimal overlap. As data analysis proceeds, the codes may be merged and relabeled at a higher level of abstraction. In a study of medication adherence, the initial codes might be "paying attention to time," "counting and recounting," and "remembering to get prescriptions." These codes might be grouped later into the more abstract code "attending to logistics of medication management." The first level of coding is descriptive and uses participant phrases as the label for the code, also called in vivo coding. The label for the merged codes is interpretive and might be called a theme if repeatedly identified in the data.

Arida et al. (2019) conducted a secondary analysis of transcripts from four focus groups with mothers who had ovarian cancer. They extracted text that referenced being a mother and began coding.

"We used an adapted framework analysis to summarize and synthesize qualitative data into major themes and subthemes for each question and for each participant. This iterative process began with a close read of all references to motherhood (coding) and successively summarizing the data to more abstract categories (subthemes, themes, and overarching themes) that encompassed the codes (Gale, Heath, Cameron, Rashid, & Redwood, 2013). Specifically, the primary reviewer (J.A.A.) sent the 5 other reviewers excerpts from the first focus group to review and code using descriptive, axial coding.... All 6 reviewers teleconferenced biweekly to discuss their coding and to develop an initial coding framework, including a codebook with detailed descriptions of each code. Using this coding framework, we then iteratively worked through the additional 3 transcripts.... After the reviewers analyzed and coded the mothering-related excerpts from all 4 focus groups, each reviewer independently organized the final list of codes into higher-order groupings based on their close readings of the original transcripts and codes.... The primary and senior authors (J.A.A. and T.L.H.) compared and contrasted these groupings before arriving at a final integrative coding schema, which was shared with and confirmed by all reviewers. We used Microsoft Word and Excel (Microsoft Corp) for all coding procedures." (Arida et al., 2019, p. E55)

Arida et al. (2019) concluded that the mothers learned to balance the demands of being a cancer patient with those of being a mother. Although the demands increased their stress, the mothers looked to the future as they worked to create a sense of normalcy for their children. Coding is a challenging process, so we have adapted Saldaña's (2016, pp. 79–80) advice for coding and included it in Box 12.6.

Thematic Analysis

While the researchers analyze and code the data, they begin to identify patterns that may be abstract overarching ideas and concepts (Braun & Clarke, 2006). The results of the analysis are frequently "expressed in themes, sub-themes, and categories that require analytical reflection and work" (Connolly & Peltzer, 2016, p. 52). Qualitative researchers may prematurely label a theme with one or two words that are general concepts and could apply to many experiences, such as the concepts of coping and communication. For findings to be meaningful, the researcher must analyze methodically, reflect longer, or possibly repeat the analysis using a different theoretical perspective or heuristic.

Themes are developed by exploring relationships between codes and grouping them by an interpretive statement. For example, you are analyzing the data you collected from interviews with participants on complex medication regimens. You code sections of the transcripts with phrases such as "slipped my mind," "couldn't afford my prescriptions," "too busy to worry about my meds," and "they make me feel bad." You reflect on these phrases and identify a relationship between missing medications and being involved in activities that have a higher priority to the participants. You tentatively identify a theme of "pushed aside" that encompasses the codes of "slipped my mind" and "too busy to worry about my meds." As the analysis continues, you may refine the theme or group it with another preliminary theme. The process is repeated over and over to thoroughly analyze the data. Researchers may leave themes underdeveloped. This may occur because the data lack richness and detail or because too little time and effort are spent on analysis and interpretation (Connolly & Peltzer, 2016).

Currie et al. (2019) conducted an exploratory-descriptive qualitative study with 10 parents whose child had died in the neonatal intensive care unit (NICU). The researchers interviewed the parents individually and wrote field notes after each interview.

BOX 12.6   Coding Advice for Less Experienced Researchers

- Work toward grouping data together, instead of splitting into too many codes.
- Find codes that reoccur within each interview (focus group) and use them repeatedly across participants if possible.
- Tentatively group codes together into more abstract codes. Realize that the abstract codes may evolve during analysis.
- Code only sections of the data that are relevant to the purpose and research questions of the study.
- Document your thinking about the data and codes in analytical memos.

Adapted from Saldaña, J. (2016). *The coding manual for qualitative researchers* (3rd ed.). Thousand Oaks, CA: Sage.

"The interviews and field notes were transcribed verbatim and then verified for accuracy by the first author. All identifying information was replaced with pseudonyms. Data were analyzed using qualitative content analysis methods and involved coding each line of text. In an iterative process of clustering and categorizing similar codes and grouping common categories, a series of themes were identified from the data (Krippendorff, 2004; Miles & Huberman, 1994).... The two major themes identified from the data were (a) living with loss and (b) coping with grief over time...

Living with Loss
Infant loss was described as a profound tragedy in all of these parents' lives. Parents found that living with the loss of an infant was an immense challenge and that their grief was a process that evolved over time. While many of the parents were able to function and continue with their daily lives, they described grief as "always being there." The theme is comprised of five sub-themes—bereavement and grief over time, mental health changes, spiritual suffering, personal growth after loss, and life changes after loss—which serve to provide depth to the primary theme." (Currie et al., 2019, p. 335)

"Coping with Grief Over Time
Parents described the challenges of coping with grief as a process that continually evolved over time. Each

> parent's coping timeline was unique and varied depending on available support resources and prior experiences such as memories with their infant during hospitalization…. Parents appeared to oscillate between focusing on the loss and on living in a world without their infant." (Currie et al., 2019, pp. 336–337)

Thematic analysis is the most common way that qualitative researchers analyze their data. Most often the analysis progresses from smaller meaning units that are clustered into more abstract categories or patterns. Content analysis is another type of analysis used frequently by nurse researchers and other social scientists.

Content Analysis

Content analysis is designed to classify the words in a text into categories. The researcher is looking for repeated ideas or patterns of thought. In exploratory-descriptive qualitative studies, researchers may analyze the content of the text using concepts from a guiding theory, if one was selected during study development. Walker, Lewis, Lin, Zahlis, and Rosenberg (2019) conducted an exploratory-descriptive qualitative study of adolescents following cancer treatment. For their study, they integrated three psychological theories into a framework that illustrated a critical transition period between treatment and posttreatment. They interviewed 29 adolescents over the telephone about being in the early survivorship period. The data from the interviews were analyzed using inductive content analysis.

> "Qualitative data analysis was guided by a multistep process of inductive content analysis…. The coding process involved 5 steps, each maintaining the survivors' exact words: (1) All texts from the transcribed interviews were unitized. Each unit was a direct quotation of a complete idea that included both a noun and verb, whether implicit or explicit. (2) Each unit of data was then open coded using a code that started with a gerund (e.g., feeling confused, being happy). (3) The open codes were then organized into an initial set of categories with descriptions that clearly differentiated each category. (4) Constant comparative analysis was then used to verify the distinctions between the categories and the accuracy of fit between each unit of analysis in each category. (5) The refined set of categories was then

> grouped into higher-order domains that describe the experience of early posttreatment for adolescent cancer survivors (Strauss & Corbin, 1990; Thomas, 2006)." (Walker et al., 2019, pp. e13–e14)

Walker et al. (2019) analyzed movement of the adolescents through this transition and identified 18 categories of meaning within the data. Through further analysis, the categories were integrated into seven domains ranging from "trying to feel normal" to "crossing my fingers." The domains were split between positive and negative aspects of the transition. Because treatment had only recently ended, the adolescents were realistically concerned about relapse. The researchers demonstrated that content analysis was an effective method for deriving meaning from the data. Another analysis strategy is finding the story within the data (i.e., narrative analysis).

Narrative Analysis

Narrative inquiry is a qualitative approach that finds stories in data (Clandinin & Connelly, 2000). Through a series of life experiences, people create their identities in the historical and social context in which they live. "Stories are what keep each of us alive, able to go on with making life in ways that are meaningful" (Clandinin, Caine, & Lessard, 2018, p. 1). A narrative includes a chronological sequence of events that may be shared verbally or visually (Chase, 2018). The stories are socially constructed and influence an individual's identity. Through data analysis, deeper layers of a story may come to light and new dimensions emerge. To identify meaningful stories, the researcher must have gathered detailed data through in-depth interviewing and probing to elicit examples and experiences related to the phenomenon (Connolly & Peltzer, 2016). The data are more likely to describe the participant's emotions and beliefs when the interviewer addresses the existential, psychological, and spiritual aspects of the phenomenon.

In addition to being organized chronologically, you might analyze a story as one would a published novel during a literature course, looking for characters, setting, plot, conflict, and resolution. Peden-McAlpine, Liaschenko, Traudt, and Gilmore-Szott (2015) conducted a narrative inquiry study related to withdrawal of aggressive treatment.

"The aim of this study was to document how experienced ICU [intensive care unit] nurses comfortable with dying patients describe their communication with families to negotiate consensus on withdrawal of aggressive treatment and the shift to palliative care.... This study used a narrative, explanatory approach. Narrative accounts link together actions and events into an understandable plot or story line, which is an organizing scheme that draws together significant actions and events into a schematic whole. The plot highlights the contribution of common actions and events, what we are calling subplots to the overall plot. The results of this type of inquiry represent a retrospective gathering of subplots into an explanation that makes the plot reasonable and believable." (Peden-McAlpine et al., 2015, p. 1148)

"'Constructing the Story' is what the researchers call the communication actions perceived by the experienced nurses who were comfortable working with dying patients and their families who participated in this study.... The overall plot of these narratives, 'constructing the story' specifies nurses' communication actions that help families: (1) follow the patient's declining illness trajectory; (2) understand and accept that their significant other is dying; and (3) accept the withdrawal

of aggressive treatment. When this happens the nurses in our study were able to facilitate a peaceful death for patients and their families. Our work illustrates a trajectory of dying that is constituted by subplots that describe communicative actions that help move the family along the trajectory of their significant others' deteriorating illness." (Peden-McAlpine et al., 2015, p. 1149)

Peden-McAlpine et al. (2015) effectively used narrative analysis to describe the chronological events related to moving the healthcare professionals and family toward consensus on whether to withdraw aggressive treatment. The thematic, content, and narrative analyses covered in this section are only a few of several types of qualitative data analyses. Table 12.9 includes additional types of data analysis with descriptions.

Memos

Some qualitative research experts use the terms *memos* and *research journals* interchangeably (Bazeley, 2013), while others describe them as having different functions. A research journal is usually defined as a record of

TABLE 12.9 Types of Qualitative Data Analysis

Data Analysis	Description
Chronological analysis	Identifying and organizing major elements in a time-ordered description as events and epiphanies (Creswell & Poth, 2018)
Constant comparison	Analyzing new data for similarities to and differences from existing data (Flick, 2019)
Direct interpretation	Identifying a single instance of the phenomenon or topic and drawing out its meaning without comparing to other instances; most frequently used on case studies (Creswell & Poth, 2018)
Dimensional analysis	Describing characteristics of the data without attributing meaning; examining relationships among the dimensions (Bazeley, 2013)
Domain analysis	Categorizing specific aspects of a social situation such as people involved; used in ethnography (Bazeley, 2013)
Narrative analysis	Looking for the story in the data; identifying the characters, setting, plot, conflict, and resolution as an exemplar of the phenomenon being studied (Chase, 2018)
Taxonomic analysis	Identifying categories with a domain (see domain analysis); used in ethnography (Bazeley, 2013)
Thematic analysis	Finding within the data three to six overriding abstract ideas that summarize the phenomenon of interest
Theoretical comparison	Thinking about the properties and characteristics of categories; linking to existing theories and models (Corbin & Strauss, 2015)
Three-dimensional analysis	Thinking about and identifying continuity, interactions, and situations within a story

In addition to the citations in the table, the types of analysis were synthesized from Corbin and Strauss (2015) and Creswell and Poth (2018).

events during a study, thoughts on revisions of questions for the next interview, and clinical or life experiences that may influence the analysis. Miles et al. (2020) defined a **memo** as a "narrative that document the researcher's reflections and thinking processes about the data" (p. 88). During data analysis, the researcher develops memos to record insights or ideas related to notes, transcripts, or codes (Creswell & Poth, 2018). Memos are linked most closely with grounded theory methodology (Charmaz et al., 2018) but can be used with other methodologies as well.

Memos may be written about the methods, the emerging themes, or the commonalities among the perspectives of multiple participants (Corbin & Strauss, 2015). They may link pieces of data together or use a specific piece of data as an example of a conceptual idea. The memo may be written to someone else involved in the study or may be just a note to yourself. The important thing is to value your ideas and document them quickly. Initially you might feel that the idea is so clear in your mind that you can record it later. However, you may soon forget the thought and be unable to retrieve it. As you become immersed in the data, these ideas will occur at odd times, such as when you are sleeping, walking, or driving. Whenever an idea emerges, even if it is vague and not well thought out, develop the habit of writing it down immediately or recording it on a handheld device such as a cell phone (Miles et al., 2020).

REPORTING QUALITATIVE STUDIES

The published reports of qualitative studies are organized similar to reports of quantitative studies. The first sections will introduce the topic, provide the rationale for why the study is needed, and state the study's purpose. Subsequent sections may include a review of the literature, a description of the methodology (including its philosophical orientation), and an explanation of the methods. The final three sections of a qualitative report have some unique characteristics and are covered in this section.

Reporting Results

The first section of a qualitative research report will be a detailed description of the participants. An ethnography report may include descriptions of key informants, the setting, and the environment in which the data were gathered. After the descriptions of the participants and

setting, how the results are presented depends on the methodology of the study.

Phenomenologists provide a thick, rich, and exhaustive description of the phenomenon that was studied. They may include an exemplar such as one participant's story to aid the reader to grasp the meaning of the lived experience. Other phenomenologists include a composite description of the phenomenon in the lives of the participants. Grounded theorists may present their results as either a verbal description of a tentative theory or a verbal description accompanied by a diagram of the concepts and relationships. Ethnographers present findings within the context of a culture, its leaders, normative behaviors, relationships, and other interactive exchanges. Ethnographers may provide photographs to demonstrate key points in the results. Findings of exploratory-descriptive qualitative studies are reported by addressing each research question and providing the pertinent findings.

Including verbatim quotations allows the voices of the participants to be heard (Creswell & Poth, 2018), an expectation of qualitative reports because the philosophical focus is on the perspectives of the participants. The report will include quotations or other evidence to support each theme or pattern that is identified. Some researchers will report the results of the data analysis in the form of a table with the themes in the first column of a table and exemplar quotations in the second column. Using tables in this way increases the transparency of the analysis and interpretation. Other writers will identify, define, and explain each of the study's themes with participants' quotations to support the theme.

Findings and Conclusions

Qualitative findings and conclusions reflect the study's philosophical roots and the data that were collected. The findings and conclusions in a research report, in fact the entire paper, are written with the target audience in mind (Creswell & Poth, 2018). The researchers compare their findings to findings of published studies. For example, a researcher conducting an ethnographical study may have done minimal literature review before implementing data collection. During analysis, the researcher will search the literature more extensively to compare and contrast the data to the findings of other studies conducted with the same culture or studies with similar results (Mannik & McGarry, 2017). Chapter 27 includes additional information about disseminating the findings of studies.

Conclusions are intertwined with the findings in a qualitative study. Conclusions in qualitative research are not generalizable; however, generalization is not the goal of qualitative studies. The findings are specific to the sample. Even though conclusions in qualitative nursing research apply only to the sample, they may be transferable to another group. For example, grounded theory research involves theorizing and serves to inform the nurse or other reader of social forces that may influence outcomes in similar situations. This informing is tantamount to educating the reader or perhaps inspiring the reader. The nurse may gain understanding and sensitivity relative to culturally appropriate behaviors, social forces in play, the experience of a given diagnosis, or common challenges to wellness. In a parallel way, however, qualitative research findings that describe social pressures on a child with spina bifida in Atlanta, Georgia, might resonate, or ring true, with a nurse who works in Tokyo, Japan, with young adult survivors of stroke secondary to aneurism. The nurse may be more sensitive to the clients' needs and concerns and more aware of factors that impact their quality of life, after reading the report on children in Atlanta.

METHODS FOR SPECIFIC METHODOLOGIES

Chapter 4 provides descriptions and examples of four qualitative methodologies. This section is provided to highlight methods used by researchers within a specific methodology, such as bracketing within phenomenology and constant comparison within grounded theory.

Phenomenological Research Methods

Phenomenological researchers have several choices about methods that are related to their specific philosophical views on phenomenology. For example, researchers subscribing to Husserl's views use bracketing, which is consciously identifying, documenting, and choosing to set aside one's own views on the phenomenon (Creswell & Poth, 2018). Heidegger's (1962) view was that researchers could not separate their own perspectives on the phenomenon being studied. Researchers subscribing to Heidegger's view would not bracket but would explicitly describe their experiences and values related to the phenomenon.

In phenomenology, additional philosophical approaches to the analysis and interpretation of data are available. The steps of data analysis described by Giorgi (1970), Colaizzi (1978), and van Kaam (1966) provide structure for researchers conducting descriptive phenomenological studies based on Husserl's stance (Vagle, 2018). The methods of van Manen (1984, 1990) are helpful to researchers conducting interpretive phenomenological studies consistent with Heidegger's philosophy (Vagle, 2018). Reading the primary texts of these more recent phenomenologists would be an excellent first step in deciding which method works best for a particular research question.

Grounded Theory Methodology

Philosophical discussions of grounded theory methodology center on the nuances of the different approaches (Kelle, 2019). Sociologists Glaser and Strauss (1967) worked together during their early years, but eventually their philosophies resulted in at least two variations of grounded theory. The original works provided little detail on data analysis methods. To fill this gap, Corbin and Strauss (2015) described a structured method of data analysis. Researchers considering grounded theory methodology will want to read the primary sources on the different methods and choose the one that is most compatible with the researchers' philosophy.

During grounded theory studies, data analysis formally begins with the first interview or focus group (Corbin & Strauss, 2015). The researchers review the transcript and code each line, constantly comparing the meaning of one line with the meanings in the lines that preceded it. Concepts as abstract representations of processes or entities are named. As the data analysis continues, relationships between concepts are hypothesized and then examined for validity by looking for additional examples within the data (Charmaz, 2014; Corbin & Strauss, 2015). Researchers look for a core category that explains the underlying social process in the experience. Finally, existing theory and literature are reviewed for similarities and parallels to the emergent theory and study findings, including the core category.

During data analysis, Glaser and Strauss (2011) emphasized the constant comparison method. **Constant comparison** is analyzing qualitative data while the data are being collected and coded. The researcher writes memos about possible linkages between concepts, the chronological steps in a process, or any other theoretical insights. These tentative ideas are tested against the analysis of the data from subsequent participants. According to

Glaser and Strauss (2011), another identifying characteristic of grounded theory is the use of comparative groups as a phase of a grounded theory study to increase the credibility of the study findings. **Comparative groups** are samples of participants selected from social groups or systems other than the group or system from which the initial participants were recruited. These participants are asked to provide new data on the research topic; however, the new data are only compared to the categories and potential hypotheses generated by the initial study. For example, you have conducted a grounded theory study of burnout prevention of RNs in two ICUs of a private hospital. You may select comparative groups to be RNs recruited from medical-surgical units of the same hospital, ICUs in public hospitals, or mother-baby units of a hospital in another state. Another example would be an initial sample of parents who have a child with autism. Comparative groups might be foster parents of a child with autism, parents of a child with behavioral issues, older adults raising a grandchild with autism, parents of a child with autism in a support group in another geographical region, and adoptive parents of a child whose mother consumed alcohol during pregnancy. If data collected from parents who are similar to, yet different from, the original sample confirm the categories or relational statements, then the initial grounded theory is verified.

Ethnographical Methods

Ethnography is unique among the qualitative approaches because of its cultural focus. Ethnography requires **fieldwork** (Mannik & McGarry, 2017), which is spending time, being present, observing, and asking questions within the culture. Fieldwork allows the researcher to participate in a wide range of activities (see discussion of levels of observation earlier in the chapter). The observations of the researcher typically focus on patterns of behaviors to understand the ideas and beliefs that become visible through the behavior. The researcher looks below the surface to identify the shared meaning and values expressed through everyday actions, language, and rituals (Creswell & Poth, 2018). Meanings and values may reveal power differences, gender issues, optimism, or views of diversity.

One difficulty in planning an ethnographical study is not knowing in advance how much time will be needed and what will be observed. Enough time in the field is needed to achieve some degree of cultural immersion (Mannik & McGarry, 2017). The resources—money and time—that the researcher has allotted for the project usually limit the length of an ethnographical study. When one is studying a different culture, the time might extend to months or even a year. When studying the culture of a nursing unit or waiting area, the researcher will not live on the unit, but would identify a tentative plan for observing on the unit at different times during the day and night and on different days of the week. The researcher may want to observe unit meetings, change-of-shift reports, or other unit rituals, such as holiday meals or going-away parties. Initial acceptance into a culture may lead to resistance later if the researcher's presence extends beyond the community's expectations or the ethnographer is perceived as prying or violating the community's privacy.

Fieldwork does not always go as expected. For example, the intent of the researcher may be misunderstood, resulting in the researcher being embarrassed or disrespected (Madison, 2020). The researcher needs to blend into the culture but remain in an outsider role. The report written by a researcher who overidentifies with the culture may present only the positive elements of the culture (Creswell & Creswell, 2018). In contrast, a researcher who is ethnocentric may report the findings in a way that is disparaging to the people of that culture. Status and power differences among the researcher and members of the culture can pose unique ethical challenges. The ethnographer is ethically bound to present an accurate report without causing harm. The decisions about how to report the findings can be challenging. Talking to more experienced ethnographers or participants within the culture may help you determine the best approach. Negotiating relationships and roles is a critical skill for ethnographers, who must possess self-awareness and social acumen.

Gatekeepers and Informants

Fieldwork may require identifying members of the culture to assist with gaining access to the site. **Gatekeepers** are people who can provide access to the culture, facilitate the collection of data, and increase the legitimacy of the researcher (Creswell & Poth, 2018). A gatekeeper may be a formal leader, such as a mayor, village leader, or nurse manager, or an informal leader, such as the head of the women's club, the village midwife, or the nurse who is considered the unit's clinical expert. The support of people who are accepted in the culture is key to gaining the access needed to understand that culture. In addition to gatekeepers, you may seek out key informants, individuals who are willing to interpret the culture for you.

Key informants are experts about the culture and also may be gatekeepers. Some key informants are complete insiders in the culture being studied. Others may have an insider-outsider role that spans boundaries. For example, during an ethnographical study of the role of nursing in a hospital in Laos, a nurse administrator who left the country to seek a graduate degree may be a key informant. The nurse administrator has the authority to facilitate access to meetings and some understanding of the researcher's culture. Being on the boundary allows this key informant to translate what the researcher observes into language or explanations that increase the researcher's knowledge and awareness of the culture.

Gathering and Analyzing Data

Observation may be direct as when the researcher is physically present in a setting. Observation can also be mediated through technology, such as viewing a nurse interacting with a family through the video images collected by a security camera (Bratich, 2018) or tracking the participation of computer users in an online forum about chemotherapy. During fieldwork, the researcher makes extensive notes about the setting, time of day, what is observed, and thoughts on possible interpretations. The researcher may seek input on possible interpretations with an informant or a person being interviewed.

Data analysis consists of analyzing field notes and interviews for common ideas and allowing patterns to emerge. Data may also be interpreted through content analysis. The notes themselves may be superficial. However, during the process of analysis, you will clarify, extend, and interpret those notes. The ethnographer compares interview and observation data to find the areas of similarity and contrast. Perspectives of the participants are also compared and analyzed in light of

the participant's standing in the community. Abstract thought processes such as intuition and reasoning are involved in analysis. The data are then formed into categories and relationships developed between categories. From these categories and relationships, the ethnographer describes patterns of behavior and supports the patterns with specific examples.

The analysis process in ethnography produces detailed descriptions of cultures that may be used to increase scientific knowledge. The descriptions may be applied to existing theories of cultures. Although the goal of ethnographical research is not theory, in some cases the findings may lead to the later development of hypotheses, theories, or both. The results may be useful to nurses when members of the community that was described interact with the health system.

In addition to desiring increased cultural knowledge, ethnographers may desire evidence upon which to affect change. On a small scale, the focused ethnography conducted by Bidabadi et al. (2019) is an example of the latter purpose. They observed healthcare professionals caring for the critically ill, cardiac surgery patients to identify behaviors affecting patient dignity. The findings provided the basis for instituting change in these units related to patient dignity. Other ethnographers combine the research with activism to advocate for wider social change, such as Bejarano, Juarez, Garcia, and Goldstein's (2019) work with undocumented immigrants.

Exploratory-Descriptive Qualitative Methodology

Researchers design exploratory-descriptive qualitative studies to make changes in clinical practice, develop an instrument to measure a concept, or simply describe the perspectives of participants related to a specific problem. The researcher selects the methods most likely to gather data relevant to the research problem. Data analysis does not require a specialized method; content and thematic analysis are used most frequently.

KEY POINTS

- Qualitative research requires spending an extensive time in the field with a research mentor, collecting and analyzing data, writing about the analysis and findings, and addressing ethical issues as they arise.

- Qualitative researchers use inductive, deductive, and abductive thinking.
- Qualitative researchers balance flexibility and rigor to produce findings that increase understanding and awareness of patients' perspectives.

- Rigor of qualitative studies are produced with reflexivity, positioning, respectful relationships, audit trails, triangulation, member checking, research debriefing, and consistency of the methods to the philosophy and methodology.
- The theoretical framework, purpose, research questions or objectives, and literature reviews of qualitative studies vary depending on the methodology.
- Sampling for qualitative studies is nonrandom and purposive. Specific types of sampling include criterion, maximum variation, and theoretical and network sampling.
- Data are collected through observation, interview, focus groups, photovoice, and internet interactions.
- Recordings and notes are transcribed into data files prior to analysis.
- Qualitative researchers select coding and analysis strategies consistent with the methodology and philosophical foundation of their studies.
- Data analysis begins by immersing oneself in the data and coding the transcripts, field notes, and other data.
- Coding is identifying key ideas and phrases in the data. As analysis continues, the codes may be merged into themes, incorporated into a narrative, or organized into a taxonomy.

- Qualitative researchers may choose to use a CAQDAS to document coding, memos, and analysis decisions, as well as to combine the analysis of different team members.
- Following coding, researchers may continue by analyzing the content, developing themes, identifying the narrative, or selecting another method of reducing data to the main ideas.
- Phenomenological methods may include bracketing and interviewing to elicit rich descriptions of lived experiences.
- Methods for grounded theory studies include specific types of coding, constant comparison, comparative groups, and the links among the concepts for the purpose of developing a theory.
- Ethnographical methods are characterized by extensive fieldwork that includes observations and interviews to thoroughly describe the culture being studied. Gatekeepers and key informants are part of the culture but work closely with the researcher.
- Researchers using exploratory-descriptive qualitative methodology select methods most likely to answer the research question.
- Qualitative findings are not generalized. They are used to inform the reader and inspire thoughts and actions leading to improvements in health care.

REFERENCES

Abdoli, S., Jones, D., Vora, A., & Stuckey, H. (2019). Improving diabetes care: Should we reconceptualize diabetes burnout? *Diabetic Educator, 45*(2), 214–224. doi:10.1177/0145721719829066

Arida, J., Bressler, T., Moran, S., D'Arpino, S., Carr, A., & Hagan, T. (2019). Mothering with advanced ovarian cancer: "You've got to find that little thing that's going to make you strong." *Cancer Nursing, 42*(4), e54–e60. doi:10.1097/NCC.0000000000000550

Audulv, A., Ghahari, S., Kephart, G., Warner, G., & Packer, T. (2019). The taxonomy of everyday self-management strategies (TEDSS): A framework derived from the literature and refined using empirical data. *Patient Education and Counseling, 102*(2), 367–375. doi:10.1016/j.pec.2018.08.034

Bazeley, P. (2013). *Qualitative data analysis: Practical strategies.* Thousand Oaks, CA: Sage.

Bejarano, C., Juarez, L., Garcia, M., & Goldstein, D. (2019). *Decolonizing ethnography: Undocumented immigrants and new directions in social science.* Durham, NC: Duke University Press.

Belgrave, L., & Seide, K. (2019). Coding for grounded theory. In A. Bryant & K. Charmaz (Eds.), *The Sage handbook of current developments in grounded theory* (pp. 167–185). Thousand Oaks, CA: Sage.

Betriana, F., & Kongsuwan, W. (2019). Lived experiences of grief of Muslim nurses caring for patients who died in an intensive care unit: A phenomenological study. *Intensive & Critical Care Nursing, 52*(1), 9–16. doi:10.1016/j.iccn.2018.09.003

Bidabadi, F., Yazdannik, A., & Zargham-Boroujeni, A. (2019). Patient's dignity in intensive care unit: A critical ethnography. *Nursing Ethics, 26*(3), 738–752. doi:10.1177/0969733017720826

Block, M., & Florczak, K. (2017). Mentoring: An evolving relationship. *Nursing Science Quarterly, 30*(2), 100–104. doi:10.1177/0894318417693312

Brancati, D. (2018). *Social science research.* Thousand Oaks, CA: Sage.

Bratich, J. (2018). Observation in a surveilled world. In N. Denzin & Y. Lincoln (Eds.), *The Sage handbook of qualitative research* (5th ed., pp. 526–545). Thousand Oaks, CA: Sage.

Braun, V., & Clarke, V. (2006). Using thematic analysis in psychology. *Qualitative Research in Psychology, 3*(2), 77–101. doi:10.1191/1478088706qp063oa

Brinkmann, S. (2018). The interview. In N. Denzin & Y. Lincoln (Eds.), *The Sage handbook of qualitative research* (5th ed., pp. 576–579). Thousand Oaks, CA: Sage.

Byrne, C., Toarta, C., Backus, B., & Holt, T. (2018). The HEART score in predicting major adverse cardiac events in patients presenting to the emergency department with possible acute coronary syndrome: Protocol for a systematic review and meta-analysis. *Systematic Reviews, 7,* 148. doi:10.1186/s13643-018-0816-4

Caty, S., Tourigny, J., & Koren, I. (1995). Assessment and management of children's pain in community hospitals. *Journal of Advanced Nursing, 22*(4), 638–645. doi:10.1046/j.1365-2648.1995.22040638.x

Charmaz, K. (2006). *Constructing grounded theory: A practical guide through qualitative analysis.* London, England: Sage.

Charmaz, K. (2014). *Constructing grounded theory* (2nd ed.). Los Angeles, CA: Sage.

Charmaz, K., Thornberg, R., & Keane, E. (2018). Evolving grounded theory and social justice inquiry. In N. Denzin & Y. Lincoln (Eds.), *The Sage handbook of qualitative research* (5th ed., pp. 411–443). Thousand Oaks, CA: Sage.

Chase, S. (2018). Narrative inquiry: Toward theoretical and methodological maturity. In N. Denzin & Y. Lincoln (Eds.), *The Sage handbook of qualitative research* (5th ed., pp. 546–560). Thousand Oaks, CA: Sage.

Clandinin, D., Caine, V., & Lessard, S. (2018). *The relational ethics of narrative inquiry.* New York, NY: Routledge.

Clandinin, D., & Connelly, F. (2000). *Narrative inquiry: Experience and story in qualitative research.* San Francisco, CA: John Wiley & Sons.

Colaizzi, P. (1978). Psychological research as the phenomenologist views it. In R. S. Valle & M. King (Eds.), *Existential phenomenological alternatives for psychology* (pp. 48–71). New York, NY: Oxford University Press.

Collins P. (2000). *Black feminist thought: Knowledge, consciousness, and the politics of empowerment* (2nd ed.). New York, NY: Routledge.

Connolly, L., & Peltzer, J. (2016). Underdeveloped themes in qualitative research: Relationship with interviews and analysis. *Clinical Nurse Specialist, 30*(1), 52–57. doi:10.1097/NUR.0000000000000173

Corbin, J., & Strauss, A. (2015). *Basics of qualitative research: Techniques and procedures for developing grounded theory* (4th ed.). Thousand Oaks, CA: Sage.

Craig, A., Gerwin, R., Bainter, J., Evans, S., & James, C. (2018). Exploring parent experience of communication about therapeutic hypothermia in the neonatal intensive

care unit. *Advances in Neonatal Care, 18*(2), 136–143. doi:10.1097/ANC.0000000000000473

Creswell. J. (2007). *Qualitative inquiry & research design.* Thousand Oaks, CA: Sage.

Creswell, J. W., & Creswell, J. D. (2018). *Research design: Qualitative, quantitative, and mixed methods approaches* (5th ed.). Thousand Oaks, CA: Sage.

Creswell, J., & Poth, C. (2018). *Qualitative inquiry & research design: Choosing among five approaches* (4th ed.). Thousand Oaks, CA: Sage.

Crouch, A. (2019). Perceptions of the possible impact of dyslexia on nursing and midwifery students and of the coping strategies they develop and/or use to help them cope in clinical practice. *Nurse Education in Practice, 35*(1), 90–97. doi:10.1016/j.nepr.2018.12.008

Cummings, G., Hutchinson, A., Scott, S., Norton, P., & Estabrooks, C. (2010). The relationship between characteristics of context and research utilization in a pediatric setting. *BMC Health Services Research, 10,* 168. doi:10.1186/1472-6963-10-168

Currie, E., Christian, B., Hinds, P., Perna, S., Robinson, C., & Meneses, K. (2019). Life after loss: Parental bereavement and coping experiences after infant death in the neonatal intensive care unit. *Death Studies, 43*(5), 333–342. doi:10.1080/07481187.2018.1474285

Danker J., Strnadová, I., & Cumming, T. (2019). Picture my well-being: Listening to the voices of students with autism spectrum disorder. *Research in Developmental Disabilities, 89*(1), 130–140. doi:10.1016/j.ridd.2019.04.005

Eddy, B., Poll, V., Whiting, J., & Clevesy, M. (2019). Forgotten fathers: Postpartum depression in men. *Journal of Family Issues, 40*(8), 1001–1017. doi:10.1177/0192513X19833111

Flick, U. (2019). From intuition to reflexive construction: Research design and triangulation in grounded theory research. In A. Bryant & K. Charmaz (Eds.), *The Sage handbook of current developments in grounded theory* (pp. 127–144). Thousand Oaks, CA: Sage.

Forgeron, P. A., Jongudomkarn, D., Evans, J., Finley, G. A., Thienthong, S., Siripul, P., et al. (2009). Children's pain assessment in northeastern Thailand: Perspectives of health professionals. *Qualitative Health Research, 19*(1), 71–81. doi:10.1177/1049732308327242

Gale, N., Heath, G., Cameron, E., Rashid, S., & Redwood, S. (2013). Using the framework method for the analysis of qualitative data in multi-disciplinary health research. *BMC Medical Research Methodology, 13,* Article 117. doi:10.1186/1471-2288-13-117

Ghahari, S., Forwell, S., Suto, M., & Morassaei, S., (2019). Multiple sclerosis self-management model: Personal and contextual requirements for successful self-management. *Patient Education & Counseling, 102*(5), 1013–1020. doi:/10.1016/j.pec.2018.12.028

Gilgun, J. (2019). Deductive qualitative analysis and grounded theory: Sensitizing concepts and hypothesis-testing. In A. Bryant & K. Charmaz (Eds.), *The Sage handbook of current developments in grounded theory* (pp. 107–122). Thousand Oaks, CA: Sage.

Giorgi, A. (1970). *Psychology as a human science: A phenomenologically based approach.* New York, NY: Harper & Row.

Glaser, B. G., & Strauss, A. (1967). *The discovery of grounded theory: Strategies for qualitative research.* Chicago, IL: Aldine.

Glaser, B. G., & Strauss, A. (1999). *The discovery of grounded theory: Strategies for qualitative research.* New Brunswick, NJ: Aldine Transaction.

Glaser, B. G., & Strauss, A. (2011). *The discovery of grounded theory: Strategies for qualitative research.* New Brunswick, NJ: Aldine Transaction.

Glegg, S. (2019). Facilitating interviews in qualitative research with visual tools: A typology. *Qualitative Health Research, 29*(2), 301–310. doi:10.1177/1049732318786485

Guadagnolo, B. A., Cina, K., Helbig, P., Molloy, K., Reiner, M., Cook, E. F., et al. (2009). Assessing cancer stage and screening disparities among Native American cancer patients. *Public Health Reports, 124*(1), 79–89. doi:10.2307/25682151

Hafsteinsdóttira, T., van der Zwaaga, A., & Schuurmansa, M. (2017). Leadership mentoring in nursing research, career development and scholarly productivity: A systematic review. *International Journal of Nursing Studies, 75*(1), 21–34. doi:10.1016/j.ijnurstu.2017.07.004

Heidegger, M. (1962). *Being and time.* (J. Macquarrie & E. Robinson, Trans). New York, NY: Harper Perennial Modern Thought.

Kamberelis, G., Dimitriadis, G., & Welker, A. (2018). Focus group research and/in figured worlds. In N. Denzin & Y. Lincoln (Eds.), *The Sage handbook of qualitative research* (5th ed., pp. 692–716). Thousand Oaks, CA: Sage.

Kelle, U. (2019). The status of theories and models in grounded theory. In A. Bryant & K. Charmaz (Eds.), *The Sage handbook of current developments in grounded theory.* (pp. 68–88). Thousand Oaks, CA: Sage.

Kitson, A., Harvey, G., & McCormack, B. (1998). Enabling the implementation of evidence based practice: A conceptual framework. *Quality in Health Care, 7*(3), 149–158. doi:10.1136/qshc.7.3.149

Koithan, M., & Farrell, C. (2010). Indigenous Native American healing traditions. *The Journal for Nurse Practitioners, 6*(6), 477–478. doi:10.1016/j.nurpra.2010.03.016

Krippendorff, K. (2004). *Content analysis: An introduction to its methodology* (2nd ed.). Thousand Oaks, CA: Sage.

Kruithof, N., Traa, M., Karabatzakis, M., Polinder, S., de Vries, J., & de Jongh, M. (2018). Perceived changes in quality of life in trauma patients: A focus group study.

Journal of Trauma Nursing, 25(3), 177–186. doi:10.1097/JTN.0000000000000364

Latimer, M. A., Ritchie, J. A., & Johnston, C. C. (2010). Individual nurse and organizational context considerations for better knowledge use in pain care. *Journal of Pediatric Nursing, 25*(4), 274–281. doi:10.1016/j.pedn.2009.03.004

Leavy, P. (2017). *Research design: Quantitative, qualitative, mixed methods, arts-based, and community-based participatory research approaches.* New York City, NY: Guilford Press.

Leininger, M. (1997). Overview of the theory of cultural care with the ethnonursing research method. *Journal of Transcultural Nursing, 8*(2), 32–52.

Leininger, M. (2007). Theoretical questions and concerns: Response from the theory of cultural care diversity and universality perspective. *Nursing Science Quarterly, 20*(1), 9–15. doi:10.1177/0894318406296784

Lowe, J., & Struthers, R. (2001). A conceptual framework of nursing in Native American culture. *Journal of Nursing Scholarship, 33*(3), 279–283. doi:10.1111/j.1547-069.2001.00279.x

Madison, D. S. (2020). *Critical ethnography: Method, ethics, and performance* (3rd ed.). Thousand Oaks, CA: Sage.

Malterud, K. (2001). Qualitative research: Standards, challenges, and guidelines. *Lancet, 358*(9280), 483–488. doi:10.1016/S0140-6736(01)05627-6

Mannik, L., & McGarry, K. (Eds.). (2017). *Practicing ethnography: A student guide to method and methodology.* North York, ON, Canada: University of Toronto Press.

Margolis, E., & Zunjarwad, R. (2018). Visual research. In N. Denzin & Y. Lincoln (Eds.), *The Sage handbook of qualitative research* (5th ed., pp. 600–626). Thousand Oaks, CA: Sage.

Marshall, C., & Rossman, G. B. (2016). *Designing qualitative research* (6th ed.). Los Angeles, CA: Sage.

Marshall, C., Forgeron, P., Harrison, D., & Young, N. (2018). Exploration of nurses' pediatric pain management experiences in rural hospitals: A qualitative descriptive study. *Applied Nursing Research, 42*(1), 89–97. doi:10.1016/j.apnr.2018.06.009

McKean, L., & Raphael, J. (2002). *Drugs, crime, and consequences: Arrests and incarceration in North Lawndale.* Retrieved from https://www.issuelab.org/resource/drugs-crime-and-consequences-arrests-and-incarceration-in-north-lawndale.html

Miles, M., & Huberman, A. (1994). *Qualitative data analysis* (2nd ed.). Thousand Oaks, CA: Sage.

Miles, M., Huberman, A., & Saldaña, J. (2020). *Qualitative data analysis: A methods sourcebook* (4th ed.). Thousand Oaks, CA: Sage.

Morse, J. (2018). Reframing rigor in qualitative inquiry. In N. Denzin & Y. Lincoln (Eds.), *The Sage handbook of qualitative research* (5th ed., pp. 796–817). Thousand Oaks, CA: Sage.

Morse, J., & Clark, L. (2019). The nuances of ground theory sampling and the pivotal role of theoretical sampling. In A. Bryant & K. Charmaz (Eds.), *The Sage handbook of current developments in grounded theory* (pp. 145–166). Thousand Oaks, CA: Sage.

Moser, A., & Korstjens, I. (2018). Series: Practical guidance to qualitative research. Part 3: Sampling, data collection and analysis. *European Journal of General Practice, 24*(1), 9–18. doi:10.1080/13814788.2017.1375091

Munhall, P. L. (2012). A phenomenological method. In P. L. Munhall (Ed.). *Nursing research: A qualitative perspective* (5th ed., pp. 113–175). Sudbury, MA: Jones & Bartlett.

Munro, S., Sou, J., Zhang, W., Mohammadi, T., Trenaman, L., Langlois, S., et al. (2019). Attitudes toward prenatal screening for chromosomal abnormalities: A focus group study. *Birth, 32*(4), 364–371. doi:10.1016/j.wombi.2018.09.006

Nicholas, G., Bai, X., & Fiske, S. (2019). Exploring research-methods blogs in psychology: Who posts, what about, whom, and with what effect. *Perspectives on Psychological Science, 14*(4), 691–704. doi:10.1177/1745691619835216

Orbe, M. (1998). *Constructing co-cultural theory: An explication of culture, power, and communication.* Thousand Oaks, CA: Sage.

Orem, D. (2004). Reflections on nursing practice science: The nature, the structure and the foundation of nursing sciences. *Self-Care, Dependent-Care, and Nursing, 12*(3), 4–11.

Padgett, D. (2017). *Qualitative methods in social work research* (3rd ed.). Thousand Oaks, CA: Sage.

Peden-McAlpine, C., Liaschenko, J., Traudt, T., & Gilmore-Szott, E. (2015). Constructing the story: How nurses work with families regarding withdrawal of aggressive treatment in ICU – A narrative study. *International Journal of Nursing Studies, 52*(7), 1146–1156. doi:10.1016/j.ijnurstu.2015.03.015

Pool, N. (2019). Nurses' experiences of establishing meaningful and effective relationships with American Indian patients in the cancer care setting. *Sage Open Nursing, 5*(1), 1–11. doi:10.1177/2377960819826791

Prip, A., Pii, K., Møller, K., Nielsen, D., Thorne, S., & Jarden, M. (2019). Observations of the communication practices between nurses and patients in an oncology outpatient clinic. *European Journal of Oncology Nursing, 40*(1), 120–125. doi:10.1016/j.ejon.2019.03.004

Quinn, B., & Fantasia, H. (2018). Forming focus groups for pediatric pain research in nursing: A review of methods. *Pain Management in Nursing, 19*(3), 303–312. doi:10.1016/j.pmn.2017.07.002

Rubin, H., & Rubin, I. (2012). *Qualitative interviewing: The art of hearing data* (3rd ed.). Los Angeles, CA: Sage.

Saldaña, J. (2016). *The coding manual for qualitative researchers* (3rd ed.). Thousand Oaks, CA: Sage.

Schumacher, C., Hussey, L., & Hall, V. (2018). Heart failure self-management and normalizing symptoms: An exploration of decision making in the community. *Heart & Lung, 47*(4), 297–303. doi:10.1016/j.hrtlng.2018.03.013

Seidman, I. (2019). *Interviewing as qualitative research: A guide for researchers in education and the social sciences* (5th ed.). New York City, NY: Teachers College Press.

Son, Y. J., Lee, Y. M., & Kim, E. (2019). How do patients develop self-care behaviors to live well with heart failure? A focus group study. *Collegian, 26*(4), 448–456. doi:10.1016/j.colegn.2018.12.004

Squires, J., Estabrooks, C., Scott, S., Cummings, G., Hayduk, L., Kang, S., et al. (2013). The influence of organizational context on the use of research by nurses in Canadian pediatric hospitals. *BMC Health Services Research, 13*(1), 351. doi:10.1186/1472-6963-13-351

Stern, P., & Porr, C. (2011). *Essentials of accessible grounded theory.* Walnut Creek, CA: Left Coast Press.

Strauss, A., & Corbin, J. (1990). *Basics of qualitative research: Grounded theory procedures and techniques.* Newbury Park, CA: Sage.

Taylor, L. (2018). The experience of infertility among African American couples. *Journal of African American Studies, 22*(5), 357–372. doi:10.1007/s12111-018-9416-6

Thomas, D. R. (2006). A general inductive approach for analyzing qualitative evaluation data. *American Journal of Evaluation, 27*(2), 237–246. doi:10.1177/1098214005283748

Thornberg, R., & Dunne, C. (2019). Literature review in grounded theory. In A. Bryant & K. Charmaz (Eds.), *The Sage handbook current developments in grounded theory* (pp. 206–220). Thousand Oaks, CA: Sage.

Vagle, M. (2018). *Crafting phenomenological research* (2nd ed.). New York, NY: Routledge.

van Kaam, A. (1966). *Existential foundations of psychology.* Pittsburgh, PA: Duquesne University Press.

van Manen, M. (1984). *"Doing" phenomenological research and writing.* Alberta, Canada: University of Alberta Press.

van Manen, M. (1990). *Researching lived experience: Human science for an action sensitive pedagogy.* Albany, NY: The State University of New York.

Walker, A., Lewis, F., Lin, Y., Zahlis, E., & Rosenberg, A., (2019). Trying to feel normal again: Early survivorship for adolescent cancer survivors. *Cancer Nursing, 42*(4), e11–e21. doi:10.1097/NCC.0000000000000629

Walls, M. L., Gonzalez, J., Gladney, T., & Onello, E. (2015). Unconscious bias: Racial microaggressions in American Indian health care. *Journal of the American Board of Family Medicine, 28*(2), 231–239. doi:10.3122/jabfm.2015.02.140194

Wang, C., & Burris, M. (1997). Photovoice: Concept, methodology, and use for participatory needs assessment. *Health Education & Behavior, 24*(3), 369–387.

Wardlaw, C., & Shambley-Ebron, D. (2019). Co-cultural communicative practices of African American women seeking depression care. *Advances in Nursing Science, 42*(2), 172–184. doi:10.1097/ANS.0000000000000269

Wirtz, A., Cooney, E., Chaudhry, A., Reisner, S., & American Cohort Study of HIV Acquisition Among Transgender Women. (2019). Computer-mediated communication to facilitate synchronous online focus group discussions: Feasibility study for qualitative HIV research among transgender women across the United States. *Journal of Medical Internet Research, 31*(3), e12569. doi:10.2196/12569

Yin, R. (2009). *Case study research methods* (4th ed.). Thousand Oaks, CA: Sage.

Yu, A., Hope House Men, & Alumni. (2018). "Where we wanna be": The role of structural violence and place-based trauma for street life-oriented Black men navigating recovery and reentry. *Health and Place, 54*(1), 200–209. doi:10.1016/j.healthplace.2018.09.013

13

Outcomes Research

Suzanne Sutherland

http://evolve.elsevier.com/Gray/practice/

Outcomes research has become the predominant mode of inquiry within healthcare institutions. Healthcare professionals and funding agencies now choose this type of research for tracking changes such as survival, hospital-acquired illness, functional status, cost, and patient satisfaction. It is essential for you as an advanced practice nurse to understand the designs and logic upon which it is founded. Outcomes research in health fields is globally defined as research that investigates the outcomes of care, relating them to attributes of care delivery. It has long been an established focus within health care. In outcomes research, the setting may be an individual physician's practice, an agency providing direct care, or the community as a whole. As an advanced practice nurse, you will be evaluated by the outcomes of the patients you see. The research sample is an accessible population, small or large. The research methodology is overwhelmingly quantitative, and designs include a variety of established strategies that establish prevalence, investigate correlates of various outcomes, and occasionally test strategies to measure change for specified outcomes. Correlational designs predominate. Although from time to time outcomes research uses qualitative strategies within mixed methods studies, the qualitative findings are subordinate in importance to the quantitative findings, serving to direct an inquiry, to explain quantitative results, and sometimes to suggest ensuing quantitative investigation.

The bulk of the data for outcomes research is obtained from preexistent sources, such as clinical and administrative databases, and analyzed in the aggregate. You will contribute to these databases as you provide care, whether as a nurse at the bedside or an advanced practice nurse. The application of the findings is to an undefined future population of clients within hospitals, communities, caseloads, or practices rather than to specific clients. Typical research questions address outcomes in terms of practice patterns, attributes of clients, attributes of caregivers, health, efficiency, economics, geography, and specific aspects of care delivery. Within nursing, changes based on findings are not implemented without further testing; rather, they are scrutinized again in subsequent outcomes studies. The outcomes research process is optimally a series of loops centering on the elusive goal of the best possible outcomes.

The roots of outcomes research have existed informally as long as health care has existed and persons delivering health care have been curious enough to count, measure, and hypothesize. More formal inquiry began in the 19th and 20th centuries. In nursing, Florence Nightingale conducted descriptive longitudinal and trend research in the 19th century, documenting morbidity and mortality among soldiers during the Crimean War. She later utilized her data and analyses to argue successfully for reforms in hospitals and hospital barracks, which proved effective in decreasing morbidity and mortality in those settings (Kopf, 1916). In 1910 the Carnegie Foundation chose Flexner (1910/2002) to conduct an evaluation study of the quality of US medical schools. The report made recommendations for medical school control of hospitals in which teaching occurred, use of full-time faculty who did not maintain a separate practice, and increased education for physicians prior to medical school. Better academic and hospital-based preparation for physicians ensued, with improved patient outcomes.

Avedis Donabedian developed the theoretical basis for outcomes research, including its core components and primary elements, 65 years ago (Donabedian, 1980). Concepts foundational to outcomes research overlap those that underlie professional accountability, quality, safety, prevention, competence, patient satisfaction, cost effectiveness, and evidence-based practice (EBP).

This chapter presents an overview of federal agencies currently involved in outcomes research, as well as the current status of outcomes research, including its theoretical basis, three primary elements, relationship to practice, and the research designs and statistical approaches most commonly used in this type of inquiry.

CURRENT STATUS OF OUTCOMES RESEARCH

Researchers conducting outcomes studies do not always state, "This is outcomes research." Although many studies that can be considered outcomes research do not contain the word in their title, most of these can be accessed using the word *outcomes* as a search term.

Although most outcomes studies represent isolated research projects, several authors are notable for their sustained research trajectories on various topics focusing on both patient and nurse outcomes in hospitals and subacute settings. Through the Center for Health Outcomes and Policy Research (CHOPR, 2019) at the University of Pennsylvania, Linda Aiken and Douglas Sloane have coauthored dozens of outcomes research publications (Aiken et al., 2012; Aiken et al., 2018; Ball et al., 2018; Germack, McHugh, Sloane, & Aiken, 2017) over the past 20 years, including investigations of associations among mortality rate, work conditions, hospital staffing patterns, and the educational level of nurses. Their geographical focus has been primarily within the United States, but they have collaborated with authors from many European countries, China, and South Korea over the past decade, extending their findings.

In Belgium, Koen Van den Heede conducted many outcomes research studies (Bruyneel et al., 2013; Li et al., 2013; Van den Heede et al., 2009), examining hospital mortality rates, staffing ratios, nurse burnout,

and readmissions. His current research focus is reorganization of delivery of urgent care and emergency services in Belgian institutions. He has conducted preliminary descriptive and qualitative research that will serve as a foundation for development of trauma centers (Bouckaert, Van den Heede, & Van de Voorde, 2018; De Regge et al., 2018; Van den Heede et al., 2019). It is logical that outcomes research will evaluate the anticipated reorganization of services.

The uptrend in outcomes publications continues, within the current EBP climate. The momentum propelling outcomes research arises from healthcare workers themselves, policymakers, public agencies, and the public. On a more tangible level, insurers and individual healthcare agencies continue to add impetus because of escalating competition for the healthcare dollar (Karim et al., 2018), as do the ongoing changes in Medicare reimbursement (Centers for Medicare and Medicaid Services [CMS], 2018b). The CMS requires healthcare agencies to maintain outcome data, with the intent of reimbursing only for care that does not result in negative outcomes such as hospital-acquired infections and decubitus ulcers. Whatever the cause of the uptrend, everyone is invested in better outcomes.

THE ORIGINS OF MODERN OUTCOMES RESEARCH

Avedis Donabedian was a physician, born in Beirut, and educated there at the American University, where he completed medical school in 1944. He then completed a postgraduate fellowship at University of London in pediatrics and public health. He was a university physician at the American University and taught there, as well, until migrating to America in 1953. He received his master's degree in public health from Harvard University in 1955 and then taught at Harvard, New York Medical College, and the University of Michigan, the latter for over 30 years (Frenk, 2000).

Patterns of Data Collection

Donabedian (2003) developed a theory that was often called the Donabedian paradigm. It focuses on how to assess the quality of health care by examining its structures, processes, and outcomes, each component of which is multifaceted. He envisioned structure as preceding processes and processes as preceding outcomes (Fig. 13.1). Donabedian's (1980) definition of quality of

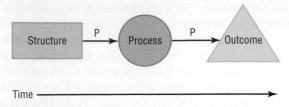

Fig. 13.1 Donabedian's theory of quality. P= Process. (Adapted from Donabedian, A. [2003]. *An introduction to quality assurance in health care.* Oxford, UK: Oxford University Press.)

care stated it is "the balance of health benefits and harm" (p. 27), and many attributes of health care contribute to quality (Box 13.1).

As structures, Donabedian (2003) listed essential equipment of care and qualified healthcare personnel. The processes he identified included expert execution of technical care, "an empathetic, participatory patient-practitioner interaction, prompt institution of care, active patient participation in the process," and standards of care (p. 50). Outcomes were defined as improvement in health and satisfied clients, and described in Donabedian's (1980, 1987, 2003, 2005) various

---

BOX 13.1 The Seven Pillars of Quality

"Seven attributes of health care define its [health care] quality: (1) efficacy: the ability of care, at its best, to improve health; (2) effectiveness: the degree to which attainable health improvements are realized; (3) efficiency: the ability to obtain the greatest health improvement at the lowest cost; (4) optimality: the most advantageous balancing of costs and benefits; (5) acceptability: conformity to patient preferences regarding accessibility, the patient-practitioner relation, the amenities, the effects of care, and the cost of care; (6) legitimacy: conformity to social preferences concerning all of the above; and (7) equity: fairness in the distribution of care and its effects on health. Consequently, healthcare professionals must take into account patient preferences as well as social preferences in assessing and assuring quality. When the two sets of preference disagree the physician faces the challenge of reconciling them."

Reprinted from Donabedian, A. (1990). The seven pillars of quality. *Archives of Pathology and Laboratory Medicine, 114*(11), 1115–1118, with permission from *Archives of Pathology and Laboratory Medicine.* Copyright 1990. College of American Pathologists.

---

publications as clinical end points, satisfaction with care, and general well-being. Donabedian (1987) theorized that the dimensions of health are defined by the subjects of care, not by the providers of care, and are based on "what consumers expect, want, or are willing to accept" (p. 5).

Underlying Donabedian's theory are a sense of fairness and honesty; firm linkage of cause and effect; placing the responsibility for a deficit in structures, processes, or outcomes where it truly belongs; commitment to openly studying healthcare quality and making findings known; and personal accountability. After lifelong pursuit of quality in health care, and his background in epidemiology and systems design, Donabedian still maintained that "to love your profession" is essential to the delivery of high-quality care (Mullan, 2001, p. 140).

Donabedian (1980) presented a "schematic representation of a framework for identifying scope and level of concern as factors in defining the quality of medical care" (p. 17) (Fig. 13.2). This cubic diagram is not a conceptual map of Donabedian's theory or an explanation of the elements of quality. It is, rather, a graphic demonstration of the interactions among human functional levels, care provider levels, and size of consumer network, displaying their interactive breadth and depth. The human functional levels represented are the physical, psychological, and social. Provider levels range from individual through systems. Recipients of care range from the individual through the target population. Essentially, the schematic means that there are several levels of each entity and that analysis can reflect any combination. It is multiplicative: There are 48 possible levels of analysis in the 4 × 4 × 3 cube.

Donabedian's initial work focused on the quality of the physician's practice, using data gained through evaluation of a surgeon's technique and judgment of its outcomes, as revealed by records review, observations, documented behaviors, and opinions (Donabedian, 2005). However, his expanded focus also included care that patients receive within healthcare agencies and contributing factors that are external to the physician's control.

Patterns of Data Collection

Early in his work, Donabedian (1980) stressed the importance of periodic review of data and of paying attention to patterns within the data set. He described this as a continuous loop using the review process,

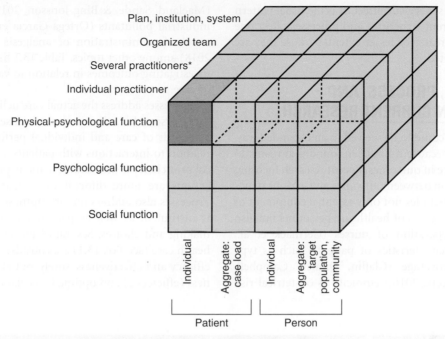

Fig. 13.2 Levels of complexity for provider, recipient of care, and aspect of health.

which later evolved into continuous quality improvement (CQI). This type of periodic review presupposes that agencies, provider groups, and individual providers are motivated to seek CQI, which is now a mainstay of practice in many hospitals. On the practical level, Donabedian encouraged measurement of short-term goals when long-term goals were years in the future, using tracking strategies such as critical pathways and care maps to determine proximate outcomes.

Attribution

Donabedian also emphasized that in the process of evaluation, outcomes must be linked with their true causes, which, in medicine, is especially challenging because so many health-illness problems are multifactorial. For this reason, a healthcare system may not be able to attribute causation to the agency or to the physician unilaterally in all instances in which the patient's condition worsens or new morbidity arises (Donabedian, 1980). Clearly his public health education had broadened Donabedian's view to include the patient, the environment, cultural systems, social conventions, employers, the government, and even insurers as various causes of illness and death.

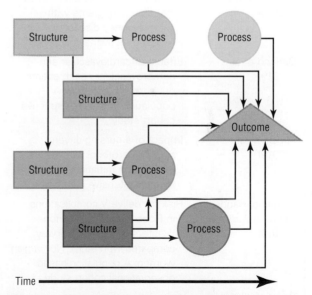

Fig. 13.3 Interactions among structures, processes, and outcomes.

Fig. 13.3 depicts the typical interplay among structures, processes, and outcomes, illustrating the difficulty of attributing definitive cause to any given outcome. Structures may have a direct impact on outcomes and also may foster certain processes that impact those same outcomes, for a synergistic effect. It is the usual pattern that many different structures and processes affect one outcome, to a greater or lesser extent, because they are so very interrelated.

STRUCTURE, PROCESS, AND OUTCOME IN CURRENT RESEARCH

Structures have come to be viewed in an expanded way, over the years, because it has been found that many do make a difference in outcomes. Recent research focusing on the association between outcomes and various structural elements includes not only essential equipment of care and qualifications of healthcare personnel but also educational preparation of nurses (Germack et al., 2017), social characteristics of patients, such as type of insurance coverage (Claflin, Dimick, Campbell, Englesbe, & Sheetz, 2018), ethnicity as obstetrical risk

(Maeland, Sande, & Bing-Jonsson, 2019), proximity of industrial pollutants (Ortega-Garcia et al., 2017), and route of administration of analgesia (Urman et al., 2018) among other topics. Table 13.1 lists recent studies investigating outcomes in relation to various structures of care.

Processes address the actual care delivered by healthcare persons both in a technical sense, as reflected by standards of care and individual performance, and in relation to interactions with patients. Although technical proficiency is measurable, patient-practitioner interactions are more difficult to evaluate quantitatively. Processes also address the promptness with which care is instituted, as well as patient inclusion in decision making and choices. Several of the seven attributes of health care (see Box 13.1) are considered process based: efficacy and effectiveness, surely, but also cost effectiveness (efficiency) and optimality (balancing of costs and

TABLE 13.1	Recent Outcomes Research Focusing Primarily on Structures of Care		
Researcher (Year)	Title	Outcomes	Structures
Campbell et al. (2019)	Screening for latent tuberculosis infection in migrants with chronic kidney disease (CKD): A cost-effectiveness analysis	Calculated cost of screening vs cost of care	Screening for tuberculosis in all migrants from countries with a high incidence of infection
Garland et al. (2019)	Effects of cardiovascular and cerebrovascular health events on work and earnings: A population-based retrospective cohort study	Return to work following a life-threatening health event	Major life-threatening health event
Kaplan et al. (2019)	Impact of a nursing-driven sedation protocol with criteria for infusion initiation in the surgical intensive care unit	Ventilator-free at day 28, total use of opioids and benzodiazepines	Nursing-driven analgesia and sedation protocol
Maeland, Sande, & Bing-Jonsson (2019)	Risk for delivery complications in Robson group 1 for non-Western women in Norway compared with ethnic Norwegian women: A population-based observational cohort study	Emergency cesarean section, postpartum hemorrhage	Ethnicity: Ethnic Norwegian vs women from Asia or Africa
Ro et al. (2019)	Association between county-level cardiopulmonary resuscitation (CPR) training and changes in survival outcomes after out-of-hospital cardiac arrest over 5 years: A multilevel analysis	Survival outcomes after out-of-hospital cardiac arrest	The prevalence of persons in the community with CPR training

TABLE 13.1 Recent Outcomes Research Focusing Primarily on Structures of Care—cont'd

Researcher (Year)	Title	Outcomes	Structures
Seabrook, Smith, Clark, & Gilliland (2019)	Geospatial analyses of adverse birth outcomes in southwestern Ontario: Examining the impact of environmental factors	Adverse birth outcomes: low birthweight and preterm birth	Elevated atmospheric sulfur dioxide levels, due primarily to air pollution from smelters and utilities
Vyas, Kim, & Adams (2019)	Understanding spatial and contextual factors influencing intraregional differences in child vaccination coverage in Bangladesh	Rates of child vaccination coverage	Geographical features, including distance from the home to the vaccination site, quality of the road; maternal age, education, and wealth status; number of microfinance organizations in the area; presence of a community health worker in the area

benefits). Past literature had focused less on processes than structures, but there has been an increase in recent research exploring associations between outcomes and processes of care (Table 13.2), such as the introduction of proactive in-hospital response team rounding as it is related to unplanned escalations in care (Danesh et al., 2019). Other processes that have been studied included the following: surgeons' leadership styles and rates of adverse postoperative events (Shubeck, Kanters, & Dimick, 2019); care protocols (Kaplan et al., 2019); patient and nurse variables and emergency department triage accuracy for myocardial infarction (MI) (Sanders & DeVon, 2016); mutual goal-setting for older adults with chronic illness (Cheng, 2018); and job satisfaction of nursing home employees and quality of nursing home resident care (Plaku-Alakbarova, Punnett, Gore, & Procare Research Team, 2018).

Burnout: Structure of Care or Process of Care?

Sometimes outcomes research that is primarily focused on structures also includes a variable or two that might also be considered processes, such as nurse burnout. Nurse burnout can contribute to patient outcomes by its effect on the interpersonal dimension of patient care. However, burnout also can contribute in a structural sense through increased absenteeism, thereby increasing workload for other nurses.

Outcomes are results, and they are the direct results of health care received. Not all occurrences are necessarily outcomes, though, even if we name them as such. For example, the birth of a healthy full-term infant is usually not the result of a healthcare intervention but a passive and expected occurrence.

Outcomes are clinical end points, satisfaction with care, functional status, and general well-being. They are results of treatment, such as level of rehabilitation, continued or subsequent morbidity, mortality, and total days of hospitalization. It is important to be aware that not every freestanding outcome is necessarily credible. For instance, patient satisfaction may not be the best isolated measurement of quality of care. Fenton, Jerant, Bertakis, and Franks (2012) reported that in a 7-year cohort study, "higher patient satisfaction was associated with less emergency department use but with greater inpatient use, higher overall healthcare and prescription drug expenditures, and increased mortality" (p. 405). The researcher can improve validity by devising multiple ways to measure outcomes.

Like outcomes, functional status can be measured in several ways. For instance, rehabilitation therapists measure the amount of extension at the elbow joint in degrees, as a quantification of recovery of function after surgery, illness, or injury. This provides a numerical rating: fewer degrees, poorer functional status. However, for patients

TABLE 13.2   Recent Outcomes Research Focusing Primarily on Processes of Care

Researcher (Year)	Title	Outcomes	Associated Structures Examined	Processes
Chen et al. (2019)	Procedure-specific volume and nurse-to-patient ratio: Implications for failure to rescue patients following liver surgery	Percentage of failure to rescue patients after liver surgery	Nurse-to-patient ratio	Number of liver surgeries performed in a given institution (marker of physician and staff expertise)
Cheng (2018)	The effects of mutual goal-setting practice in older adults with chronic illness	Achievement of goals related to physical and mental well-being		Mutual goal-setting
Danesh et al. (2019)	Can proactive rapid response team rounding improve surveillance and reduce unplanned escalations in care? A controlled before and after study	Unplanned escalations in care	Rothman Index, generated from patient values in the electronic medical record	Proactive rapid response rounding in response to elevated scores per Rothman Index (risk of deterioration)
Koller, Katz, Charrois, & Ye (2019)	Glucocorticoid-induced osteoporosis preventive (GIOP) care in rheumatology patients	Percentage of patients who received recommended GIOP	Patient characteristics	Physician variation (rheumatologist vs not)
Shubeck, Kanters, & Dimick (2019)	Surgeon leadership style and risk-adjusted patient outcomes	Complications in bariatric surgery patients		Surgeon personality traits and leadership behaviors
Urman et al. (2018)	Improved outcomes associated with the use of intravenous acetaminophen for management of acute postsurgical pain in cesarean sections and hysterectomies	Pain, length of stay, adverse opioid effects, total opioid use		Intravenous vs oral administration of acetaminophen in patients with cesarean section or hysterectomy
Wang, Knight, Evans, Wang, & Smith (2017)	Variations among physicians in hospice referrals of patients with advanced cancer	Length of time in hospice for a patient with advanced cancer (timing of referral, relative to death)		Physician referral

who have sustained traumatic injury and may not elect to undergo further surgeries, what a physical therapist might deem a "poor" ability to extend the arm may be quite acceptable to the patient. As cited previously, it is important to determine "what consumers expect, want, or are willing to accept" (Donabedian, 1987, p. 5).

Because end points often are extremely distant, setting proximate points is recommended for quality assessment purposes. It is difficult to remain focused on a goal that will not be measured until decades later (Box 13.2). Treatment programs can be evaluated after a reasonable increment of time.

BOX 13.2 Proximate Point Versus End Point Outcome Measurement

Strict adherence to diabetes management results in more years of good vision, functional kidneys, patent coronary arteries, and healthy retinal vasculature. Most persons with adult-onset diabetes who maintain moderately good management enjoy 10 to 20 years before they suffer consequences of hyperglycemic episodes. Because the elapsed time from disease diagnosis until first negative consequence may be years, primary healthcare providers concentrate instead on the proximate outcome measure of glycosylated hemoglobin (HbA1c) levels by which average blood sugar over the past 3 to 4 months is tracked in an indirect way.

Evaluating Structures in Relation to Outcomes

Structures of care are elements of organization and administration, as well as provider and patient characteristics, that exist prior to care and that may affect outcomes. The first step in evaluating structure is to identify and describe the characteristics of the structure. Various administration and management theories can be used to identify structural elements within a healthcare agency. Some of these are tolerance of innovativeness, organizational hierarchy, power distribution, financial management, and administrative decision-making patterns. Nurse researchers investigating the influence of structural variables on quality of care and outcomes have studied factors such as nurse staffing, nursing education, nursing work environment, hospital characteristics, and organization of care delivery.

The second step in evaluation is to determine the strength and direction of relationships among one or more structures and selected outcomes. This evaluation requires comparing different structures that provide the same types of care. In evaluating structures, the unit of measurement is the structure. The evaluation requires access to a sufficiently large sample of similar structures with similar functions, which then can be contrasted with a sample of other structures providing the same functions, so as to compare outcomes. An example is a comparison among a metropolitan primary healthcare practice, a primary healthcare practice maintained through a full-service health maintenance organization

(HMO), a rural health clinic, a community-oriented primary care clinic, and a nurse-managed center, with respect to an identified outcome. The focus of the study is calculation of the differing outcome values in different venues.

Federal and state governments require nursing homes, home healthcare agencies, and hospitals to collect and report specifically measured quality variables at periodic intervals (Agency for Healthcare Research and Quality [AHRQ], 2019a; CMS, 2018b; Kleib, Sales, Doran, Malette, & White, 2011). Mandates for reporting were established because of considerable variation in quality of care across facilities (Kleib et al., 2011). Various governmental agencies analyze care provided by healthcare facilities so that they can oversee quality of care provided to the American public. These data are available to the general public so that individuals can inform themselves of the quality of care provided by various nursing homes, home healthcare agencies, or hospitals. Researchers also can access these data for studies of the quality of various structures through a computer search using the phrases *nursing home compare, home health compare,* and *hospital compare.* A specific facility can be selected and considerable general information about outcomes of care accessed. The American Nurses Credentialing Center (ANCC, 2018) provides the current status of individual hospitals seeking Magnet status certification based on excellence in nursing care. (For further information about Magnet status, refer to Chapter 19.)

Evaluating Processes in Relation to Outcomes
Standards of Care

A **standard of care** is a norm by which quality of care is judged. According to Donabedian (1987), a practitioner has legitimate responsibility to apply available knowledge when managing a dysfunction or disease state. This management consists of (1) identifying or diagnosing the dysfunction, (2) deciding whether to intervene, (3) choosing intervention objectives, (4) selecting methods and techniques to achieve the objectives, and (5) skillfully executing the selected techniques or interventions.

Donabedian (1987) recommended the development of criteria to be used as a basis for judging quality of care. These criteria may take the form of clinical guidelines, critical paths, or care maps based on prior validation that the care contributed to the desired outcomes. The clinical guidelines have been refined and published by the National Guideline Clearinghouse (NGC) of the AHRQ (2018a) established norms or standards against which the adequacy of clinical management could be judged. Funding expired in 2018 for continuation of the project. AHRQ will post information as it becomes available. Professional nursing organizations are hosting nurse-specific guidelines on their websites

The core of the problem of identifying quality care, from Donabedian's perspective, is **clinical judgment**, which is the quality of reasoned decision making in healthcare practice. Analysis of the process of making diagnoses and therapeutic decisions is critical to the evaluation of quality of care. The emergence of decision trees and algorithms is partially attributable to Donabedian's work on clinical judgment as it impacts quality.

Practice Styles

The style of a practitioner's practice is another dimension of the process of care that influences quality; however, it is problematic to judge what constitutes goodness of interpersonal style. The Medical Outcomes Study (MOS), described later in this chapter, was designed to determine whether variations in patient outcomes were explained by differences in system of care, clinician specialty, and clinicians' technical and interpersonal styles (Tarlov et al., 1989).

Practice pattern is a concept closely related to practice style. Although **practice style** represents variation in how care is provided, **practice pattern** represents variation in what care is provided. Researchers of variations in practice patterns have found that such variation is not wholly explained by patients' clinical conditions. For instance, patients treated at one major East Coast cancer center experienced a wide variation of timing of referrals for hospice care (Wang, Knight, Evans, Wang, & Smith, 2017), a finding similar to that reported throughout the United States. Variation was related to type of cancer; however, there was a wide range even within areas of physician specialization. For prescribing practices, in their landmark study of all opioid prescriptions dispensed in the United States during one calendar year, McDonald, Carlson, and Izrael (2012) found that prescribing practices differed by region of the country and were influenced, in part, by drug company resources and marketing practices (Zerzan et al., 2006). Because of this type of variation, small area analysis may be suitable for comparisons of practice patterns. These comparisons are described later in this chapter in the section on geographical analyses.

Costs of Care

Donabedian's (1990) **costs of care** refer to costs to the individual or the family. These can be divided into direct and indirect costs. **Direct costs** are those the patient incurs for direct payment for health care, as well as insurance payments and copayments. Direct costs of hospitalization for surgery, for instance, include insurance payments, copayments for the hospitalization or take-home medications not covered by insurance, and supercharges made by the hospital for such amenities as television and newspaper. Direct costs also include the small portion of a publicly funded hospital's budget that arises from the tax base in support of a public institution that provides health care. This public funding applies also to university hospitals and healthcare practices associated with the university system. In comparison with other costs, the latter are almost negligible. **Indirect costs** are hidden or incidental costs incurred by the patient. Indirect costs for surgery include transportation to the facility for the patient and family members, overnight accommodations for the family, parking fees, food purchased at the hospital by the family, and loss of pay for work missed by both patient and family members.

Critical Paths or Pathways

Critical pathways are linear displays, along which common markers of clinical progress are arrayed with anticipated temporal norms for achieving those markers. Critical pathways also are known as **clinical guidelines** or **care maps**. Critical pathways were developed to allow practitioners to identify a number of proximate outcomes or proximate end points, which are a series of clinical goals occurring earlier in the process of treatment, instead of using only the end point to assess quality (Pearson, Goulart-Fisher, & Lee, 1995). Critical pathways may be useful on a shift-to-shift basis for fast-moving in-patient processes, such as recovery from knee replacement surgery, and on a week-to-week basis for slower moving rehabilitative processes, such as stroke recovery. In unknown outcome scenarios, such as recovery from an untimed hypoxic event, use of a

BOX 13.3   Example of Critical Pathways and Proximate End Points

The film *Regarding Henry* (Nichols, Abrams, Greenhut, Rudin, & MacNair, 1991) depicts the lead character after he suffers massive blood loss in an accident, resulting in tissue hypoxia. He eventually regains only some of his personality and some of his mental quickness, most of his ability to walk, and his full ability to speak, but his outcomes cannot be predicted at the onset of his hospitalization. His intensive care unit (ICU) course focuses on Henry's achievement of two event-markers on the critical pathway for ICU patients: the proximate end points of physical stabilization of oxygenation and perfusion, first, and then ability to exist without mechanical support. His acute care after the ICU focuses on gaining the end points of having Henry drink enough fluids to forgo an intravenous (IV) infusion and eat well enough to obtain nourishment independently, establishing his readiness to be discharged to rehabilitation. Henry's brain is essentially a black box—determination of final outcome is impossible, so the end points of circulatory and respiratory stability for exiting the ICU, and independent hydration and nutrition for exiting acute care, are fairly good proximate end points for assessment of quality, as well as very good markers of his progress. Achievement of proximate end points does not represent only quality of care. As with all outcomes, achievement of proximate end points is multifactorial and can be dependent on structures and even processes outside the scope of healthcare provision, as well as on the pathophysiology of the individual patient. In addition, failure to achieve proximate end points does not imply that care was deficient. The inability to achieve the ability to eat and drink independently may be due solely to hypoxic damage and not attributable to care delivery that is anything less than perfect.

Henry's final functional outcome represents confirmation of the extent of his original hypoxia and hypoperfusion. This is modified by structural variables, such as the time of response of the ambulance and the distance from the hospital; how long it takes to begin stabilization procedures in the ambulance and in the emergency department; the educational levels of physicians and nurses; how mentally adept his healthcare workers are at 4:00 a.m., as a function of the length of the shift they work; the fact that he has a family; and his general health, intelligence, determination, abilities, and status in the community prior to his accident. Final outcome also is modified by process variables, such as the attentiveness of individual nurses and respiratory therapists to his pulmonary status; the technical skill of his diagnosticians; standards of care for weaning from mechanical ventilation; the willingness of doctors and nurses to teach and support his wife; and the availability of rehabilitation to him, based on insurance coverage.

---

critical pathway allows an eventual diagnosis to be made as well based on the patient's ability or inability to achieve proximate outcomes (Box 13.3).

FEDERAL GOVERNMENT INVOLVEMENT IN OUTCOMES RESEARCH

Agency for Healthcare Research and Quality

Nurses participated in the initial federal study of the quality of health care. In 1959, two National Institutes of Health study sections, the Hospital and Medical Facilities Study Section and the Nursing Study Section, met to discuss concerns about the adequacy and appropriateness of medical care, patient care, and hospital and medical facilities. As a result of their dialogue, a Health Services Research Study Section was initiated. This study section eventually became the Association for Health Services Research and, subsequently, the Agency for Health Care Policy and Research (AHCPR). A reauthorization act changed the name of the AHCPR to the AHRQ. The AHRQ is designated as a scientific research agency. The new legislation of 1999 also eliminated the requirement that the AHRQ develop clinical practice guidelines. However, the AHRQ (2018a) continued support of those efforts through EBP centers (EPCs) and, until 2018, through the dissemination of evidence-based guidelines through its National Guideline Clearinghouse (NGC) (see Chapter 19 for a more detailed discussion of EPC guidelines).

The AHRQ, as a part of the US Department of Health and Human Services (DHHS), supports research designed to improve both safety and quality of health care, make care both accessible and equitable, reduce costs, and work across services and agencies to achieve these goals (AHRQ, 2018a). The AHRQ website contains information about outcomes research, funding opportunities, and results of research completed recently, including nursing research. In 2018 the budget for AHRQ was $321,800,000 (AHRQ, 2019b). In addition, AHRQ has, in the past, designated about 5% of its budget for research and expansion of projects to help prevent healthcare-associated infections, the most common complication of hospital care. The AHRQ has initiated several major research efforts to examine medical outcomes and improve quality of care.

American Recovery and Reinvestment Act

Funding from the American Recovery and Reinvestment Act (Recovery Act), signed into law in February 2009, allowed AHRQ to expand its work in support of comparative effectiveness research, including enhancing the Effective Health Care Program. A total of $473 million was awarded to AHRQ by DHHS in 2012 and disbursed over a 5-year period, beginning in 2013, for the purpose of funding patient-centered outcomes research (AHRQ, 2019a). This AHRQ program provided patients, clinicians, and others with evidence-based information to make informed decisions about health care, through activities such as comparative effectiveness reviews conducted through the AHRQ's EPCs (see Chapter 19). **Comparative effectiveness research** is descriptive or correlational research that compares different treatment options for their risks and benefits (AHRQ, 2019a). The AHRQ's broad research portfolio touches on nearly every aspect of health care, including clinical practice, outcomes and effectiveness of care, EBP, primary care and care for priority populations, healthcare quality, patient safety/medical errors, organization and delivery of care, use of healthcare resources, healthcare costs and financing, health information technology, and knowledge transfer.

The United States is not the only nation demanding improvements in quality of care and reductions in healthcare costs. Many countries are experiencing similar concerns and addressing them in relation to their particular government structures. Thus the increased focus on outcomes research and the approaches described in this chapter represent a worldwide phenomenon.

NONGOVERNMENTAL INVOLVEMENT IN OUTCOMES RESEARCH

Medical Outcomes Study

The MOS was conducted almost 35 years ago, representing the first large-scale study in the United States to examine factors influencing patient outcomes. The study was designed to identify elements of physician care associated with favorable patient outcomes using a three-city sample of 1681 chronically ill ambulatory patients in 367 medical practices.

The MOS did not control for the effects of nursing interventions, staffing patterns, or nursing practice delivery models upon medical outcomes. Consequently, coordination of care, counseling, and referral activities, which are areas of overlapping responsibility for physicians and nurses, were included as components of medical practice. Kelly, Huber, Johnson, McCloskey, and Maas (1994) suggested modifications to the MOS framework that would reflect collaboration among physicians, nurses, and allied health practitioners and allow analysis of the influence of their separate interactions on patient outcomes. These researchers also suggested adding the domain of societal outcomes to include such outcome variables as cost. They noted the "MOS outcomes framework incorporated areas in which nursing science contributed to health and medical care effectiveness. It also includes structure, process, and outcome variables in which nursing practice overlaps with that of other health professionals" (p. 213). Kelly et al. (1994) further observed that "client outcome categories of the MOS framework that go beyond the scope of physician treatment and intervention alone include functional status, general well-being, and satisfaction with care" (p. 213). A review of the state of the science on nursing-sensitive outcomes published in 2011 confirmed the relevance of these outcomes to nursing practice and suggested several more, including self-care, **therapeutic self-care** (defined as patients' ability to manage their disease and its treatment), symptom control, psychosocial functioning, healthcare utilization, and mortality (Doran, 2011).

Origins of Outcomes/Performance Monitoring

Efforts to collect data systematically did not gain widespread attention in the United States until the late 1970s. At that time, concerns about quality of hospital care prompted the development of the Universal Minimum Health Data Set, which established the minimum data that could be recorded for any patient's hospital stay (Kleib et al., 2011). The Uniform Hospital Discharge Data Set followed. These data sets prescribed the elements to be gathered, providing a database that could be used for assessment of quality of care in hospitals and at the point of discharge. Other countries developed similar data sets. In Canada, the Standards for Management Information Systems (MIS) were developed in the 1980s. Upon the establishment of the Canadian Institute for Health Information in 1994, the MIS designations became a set of national standards used to collect and report financial and statistical data from the day-to-day operations of health service organizations. As in the United States, these data sets did not include data distinct to nursing care (Kleib et al., 2011).

OUTCOMES RESEARCH AND EVIDENCE-BASED PRACTICE

EBP presupposes evidence, a substantial amount of which emanates from outcomes research. Evidence-based care focuses on information that is utilized, sometimes as processes of care, sometimes as structures, to enhance outcomes. Reports of empirical studies explicating the impact of various interventions upon practice, and consequently on patient outcomes, usually name one or the other of the terms *EBP* or *outcome*. However, some explicate both. For example, Danesh et al. (2019) reported the effect of proactive rapid response team rounding on patient outcomes. The team reviewed the patients' individual risk profiles and computed Early Warning scores. Data from the electronic medical record were extracted for the 6 months preceding the proactive rounding intervention, and again for the 6-month trial of the intervention. The intervention was effective in decreasing unplanned intensive care unit transfers ($p < 0.001$). The findings provided evidence to support the intervention. The intervention was also found to improve outcomes, lower hospital costs, and improve the work environment.

Although most research self-identifies as being outcomes research or contributing to EBP, but not both, research that measures outcomes using a strategy confirmed by prior research is clearly evidence based and contributes to further evidence for practice. Conversely, it can be argued that research that is evidence based and designed for application to practice affects outcomes. Trajectories of evidence, some of which emanate from outcomes research, and various paths to the creation of EBP are detailed in Fig. 13.4. As pictured, outcomes research often provides initial evidence of incidence or association through descriptive and correlational research. As Donabedian (1980) recommended, periodic review of data and of paying attention to patterns within the data set reveal incidence and association. After initial evidence is established through either outcomes research or routine data review and if the findings are reproducible, then theoretical modeling may occur. The final step is theory testing through descriptive, correlational, or interventional research. Multiple replications ensue, eventually contributing to evidence for practice, producing the ability to anticipate incidence, to predict, or to intervene.

NURSING-SENSITIVE PATIENT OUTCOMES

Very large studies about the work of individual nurses would be impractical. Such research would be inordinately time consuming and would involve scrutiny that might be construed as workplace harassment. Methodologically, designing such studies would be prohibitive, because patients are cared for by a variety of nurses over a typical hospital stay, compromising the ability to attribute outcomes to any one of them. Consequently, for outcomes research in which nurses and their characteristics function as structures (nursing educational preparation, for example) or as processes (technical capability), aggregates must be used in data analysis.

Formal published outcomes research in which nurses themselves function as processes or structures has been modest in quantity, there is an abundance of ongoing agency-generated quality improvement research that uses data generated from nurses' charting, reflecting task completion relative to nursing-sensitive indicators, using the medical record as data. As Donabedian (1980) recommended, formal quality improvement should function as an ongoing process in which outcomes are scrutinized so as to reveal connections with structures or processes. Hypotheses are formed. Changes in structures and processes are tracked, so as to demonstrate trends. Ultimately, changes in processes are mandated and the results measured. Sometimes structural modifications take place if enough evidence is accrued. Then the results are measured. For instance, research examining correlations between patient outcomes and percentage of nurses in the hospital workforce with a Bachelor of Science

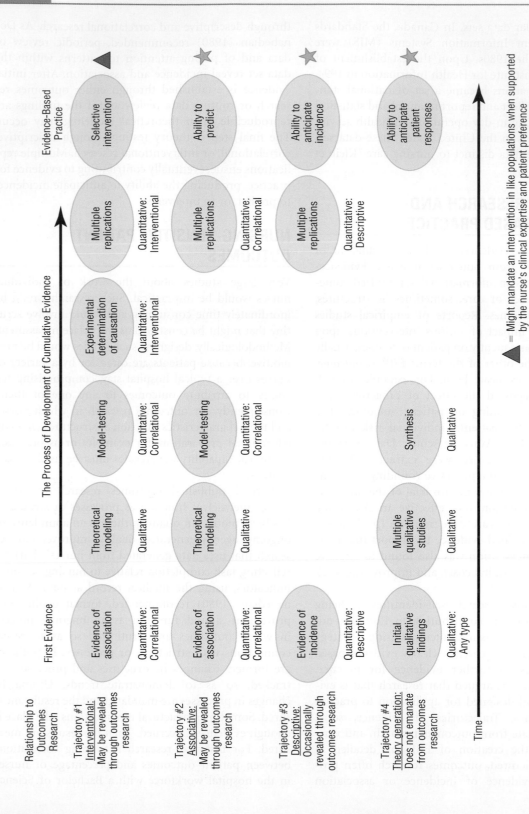

Fig. 13.4 Outcomes research and evidence-based practice (EBP).

degree in Nursing (BSN) has been replicated so often that many hospitals aware of the body of research now offer preferential hiring to BSN graduates. Another example is the ongoing revision of standards of care, instituted in response to the body of evidence.

In current hospital quality improvement research, a **nursing-sensitive patient outcome** (**NSPO**) is one influenced by nursing care decisions, actions, or attributes. It may not be caused by nursing but is associated with nursing. In various situations, the term *nursing* may signify the actions of one nurse, nurses as a working group, an approach to nursing practice, the nursing unit, or the institution. The institution determines numbers of nurses, salaries, educational levels of nurses, assignments of nurses, workload of nurses, management of nurses, and policies related to nurses and nursing practice, all of which can be contributory to NSPOs. Lopez, Blackburn, and Springer (2018) studied the effect of a night-shift intervention to cluster care and, consequently, to interrupt sleep less frequently for acute care patients. This was based on the rationale that sleep contributes to better immune system function, lower stress levels, decreased emotional reactivity, and healthier social interactions.

Two notable changes of the intervention were a unit-wide policy for a default vital sign frequency order of "VS q 4h While Awake" instead of "VS q 4h" and the scheduling of routine lab draws only before 2200 or after 0600. Staff education was provided in advance for all nurses and nursing assistants. The intervention was effective in decreasing the frequency of sleep interruptions.

Professional accountability dictates that nurses identify and document outcomes influenced by care they provide. Efforts to study nursing-sensitive outcomes were initiated by the American Nurses Association (ANA). In 1994, the ANA, in collaboration with the American Academy of Nursing Expert Panel on Quality Health Care, launched a plan to identify indicators of quality nursing practice and to collect and analyze data using these indicators throughout the United States (Mitchell, Ferketich, & Jennings, 1998). The goal was to identify and/or develop nursing-sensitive quality measures. Donabedian's theory was used as the framework for the project. Together, these indicators were referred to as the ANA **Nursing Care Report Card**, which could facilitate setting a desired standard that would allow comparisons among hospitals in terms of their nursing care quality.

At the outset, it was not known which indicators were sensitive to patient outcomes or what outcomes were associated with nurse characteristics and care provided by nurses. Hospitals chose their own ways of measuring the ANA-selected indicators but were ultimately persuaded to change to a standardized measure for each. Nurse researchers within cooperating hospitals conducted multiple pilot studies, tested consistent mechanisms for data collection, resolved problems, agreed on consistent measurement strategies, and continued to amplify indicators and test them (Jennings, Loan, DePaul, Brosch, & Hildreth, 2001).

The ANA proposed that all hospitals collect and report data based on nursing-sensitive quality indicators. To encourage researchers to collect these indicators, ANA-accredited organizations and the federal government helped by sharing selected data and findings with key groups. The ANA also encouraged state nurses associations to lobby state legislatures to include the nursing-sensitive quality indicators in regulations or state law.

In 1998, the ANA provided funding to develop a national database to house data already collected that used nursing-sensitive quality indicators. This became the National Database of Nursing Quality Indicators (NDNQI). In 2019, NDNQI had more than 2000 participating organizations (National Quality Forum [NQF], 2019a). The purpose of the NDNQI is to provide unit-level data for participating organizations, so that those data can be used in quality improvement activities. Participation in NDNQI meets requirements for the ANCC Magnet Recognition Program® (ANCC, 2018), and some database members participate for that reason.

Detailed guidelines for data collection, including definitions and decision guides, are provided by NDNQI. Healthcare organizations submit data electronically. Quarterly and annual reports of structure, process, and outcome indicators are available to participants after each analysis is complete. The database is funded by the ANA, housed at the Kansas University Medical Center School of Nursing, and managed by Press Ganey (2019). The NDNQI nursing-sensitive indicators related to structure include items such as hours of nursing care per patient day, skill mix of nursing providers, nurse turnover rate, registered nurse (RN) education, and certification. Indicators pertaining to process include items related to documentation regarding patient falls and prevention, assessment documentation related to pediatric pain medication, documentation of care provided related to pressure ulcers, nurse practice environment self-assessment, and nurse job satisfaction. Indicators related to outcomes include nosocomial infections, patient falls, pressure ulcer, peripheral intravenous infiltration, and restraint use.

The Collaborative Alliance for Nursing Outcomes California Database Project

Many other organizations currently are involved in the study of nursing-sensitive outcomes. Some of these are the NQF, Collaborative Alliance for Nursing Outcomes California Database, Veterans Affairs Nursing Outcomes Database, the Centers for Medicare and Medicaid Services Hospital Quality Initiative, the American Hospital Association, the Federation of American Hospitals, the Joint Commission, and the AHRQ.

California Nursing Outcomes Coalition (CalNOC) was a statewide nursing quality report card pilot project launched in 1996 (CALNOC, 2019). ANA funded CalNOC as a joint venture of ANA/California and the Association of California Nurse Leaders. Membership is voluntary and is composed of approximately 300 hospitals in the United States. As its membership grew nationally, CalNOC was renamed the Collaborative Alliance for Nursing Outcomes (CALNOC, 2019). It is a not-for-profit corporation, and member hospitals pay a size-based annual data management fee to participate and access the CALNOC benchmarking reporting system.

Hospital-generated unit-level acute care nurse staffing, workforce characteristics, data related to processes of care, and endorsed measurements of nursing-sensitive outcomes are submitted electronically. In addition, the CALNOC database, administered by Press Ganey (CALNOC, 2019), includes unique measures such as the Medication Administration Accuracy metric (CALNOC, 2019), which assesses actual occurrences of medication errors and tracks changes over time. CALNOC data are stratified by unit type and hospital characteristics, and reports can be aggregated by division, hospital, system/group, and geographical location. CALNOC's nursing-sensitive indicators overlap with those of NDNQI, with the addition of utilization of registry personnel, workload intensity, medication administration accuracy, process of insertion of peripherally inserted central catheters, and restraint use.

National Quality Forum

The NQF was created in the United States in 1999 to "promote and ensure patient protections and healthcare quality through measurement and public reporting" (NQF, 2019a). NQF-endorsed standards and recommendations for practice are consensus driven, so they are high-level evidence-based approaches to care delivery (NQF, 2019b). Through its quality improvement priorities and partnerships, it participates in priority-setting by NQF-associated agencies (NQF, 2019a). You can view a complete list of measures included in the NQF portfolio at http://www.qualityforum.org/Field_Guide/List_of_Measures.aspx. Approximately one-third of the measures in NQF's portfolio are of patient outcomes. Examples are mortality, readmissions, depression, and experience of care (NQF, 2019b). The NQF includes in their performance measurement portfolio several nursing-sensitive measures, which are similar to those of the agencies described previously.

Oncology Nursing Society

The Oncology Nursing Society (ONS) is a professional organization of more than 39,000 RNs and other healthcare providers dedicated to excellence in patient care, education, research, and administration in oncology nursing (ONS, 2019). The ONS has taken a leadership role among specialty nursing organizations in maintaining a vast library of information on its website that pertains to EBP. The site provides nurses with a guide to identify, critically appraise, and use evidence to solve clinical problems. It also provides outcome measures, best-practice summaries, and evidence tables related to care of patients with cancer, maintaining an ongoing role in both EBP and outcomes research.

METHODOLOGICAL CONSIDERATIONS FOR OUTCOMES STUDIES

Methodology and Design

We consider outcomes research a distinct methodology because of three attributes: its unique focus upon quality as described by Donabedian (1980), its theoretical framework, and its shared dependent variable cluster (various markers of quality). These and other aspects that distinguish outcomes research are presented here.

Unlike the qualitative and mixed methods methodologies, the outcomes research methodology does not possess its own exclusive array of distinct designs. In terms of methodology and design, outcomes research uses the quantitative methodology and some of the quantitative designs. Within this group, most of the designs are correlational and descriptive. The vast majority of data for outcomes research are obtained retrospectively because of reliance on preexistent databases.

We conducted a focused literature search spanning the years 2015 through 2018, examining three leading nursing journals that publish predominantly research articles. The review revealed no published qualitative studies that produced outcomes research with definitive, measurable results applicable to nursing practice for the designated period. This is because measurable outcomes are not the purview of qualitative studies. However, there is a growing body of qualitative inquiry that contributes preliminary impressions, especially of the patient's experience and of aspects of the phenomenon of interest (Vandermause et al., 2017) that are not well understood by healthcare providers. Qualitative research serves as part of the concept-development process through which researchers generate meaningful definitions of terms and conditions that are topics of outcomes research (Kivelä, Elo, & Kääriäinen, 2018; Sezgin, O'Donovan, Cornally, Liew, & O'Caoimh, 2019). In this manner, or through use of an exploratory mixed methods approach in which qualitative inquiry precedes quantitative (see Chapter 14 for further information), subsequent outcomes research that is accurate and meaningful can be generated. The majority of pilot project investigators who received funding through the Patient-Centered Outcomes Research Institute included some aspect of qualitative research in their proposals (Vandermause et al., 2017). The qualitative aspects of such research provide the patient perspective and lend credibility to choices the researcher makes in designing quantitative research, such as precise problem definition, operationalization of variables, selection of measurement strategies, elimination of ambiguity, and meaningful interpretation. Qualitative metasyntheses and metasummaries often identify one or two themes that characterize all or nearly all of the studies analyzed. Such identification can be powerful in identifying

previously overlooked truths that are fruitful areas for subsequent outcomes studies. An example is the wealth of qualitative work about parenting an autistic child in which a recurrent theme is early parental identification of the child's differentness and failure of the pediatrician to confirm or support that impression (Ahern, 2000; Ryan & Salisbury, 2012). Partially as a result of early qualitative research in this area, quantitative research has supported use of an autism screening tool in the United States, recommended for use at a routine well-child visit between late infancy and mid-toddler age ranges. The originally designed tool, Modified Checklist for Autism in Toddlers (M-CHAT) (Robins, Fein, Barton, & Green, 2001), has now been redesigned as the M-CHAT, Revised, with Follow-Up (M-CHAT-R/F) (Robins et al., 2014).

Philosophical Origins, Theoretical Framework, Overriding Purpose

Like quantitative research, the distant philosophical origin of outcomes research is logical positivism. It relies on what can be measured, and it relies on observed measurements and statistics to identify differences and patterns. Outcomes research reflects the more recent influence of Donabedian's public health–rooted beliefs of fairness and social justice (Mullan, 2001), with the underlying implication that the recipients of health care deserve quality care. Quantitative research in health care shares that same goal of quality care, whether from a humanistic or economic point of view. The goal of quality care is clearly implied in problem statements, in purpose statements, and in recommendations for subsequent research.

The overarching theoretical framework for all outcomes research is Donabedian's paradigm (Lawson & Yazdany, 2012) or a derivative of it. Occasional outcomes studies use a secondary framework, especially when examining a common phenomenon such as pain.

In terms of its general purpose, outcomes research is a type of evaluation research (Dawson & Tilley, 1997), focusing on evaluation of quality/delivery of human health care. Outcomes research shares its focus with public health research; considering Donabedian's background, this is not surprising. Outcomes research overlaps epidemiological research as well, when the focus of epidemiological research is humans (Petitti, 2006). Economic research has some overlap with outcomes research, when the latter focuses on economic resources and outcomes in the context of healthcare delivery (Chelimsky, 1997).

Methods

The overall focus of analysis for outcomes research in healthcare fields is quality reflected as safety, effectiveness, efficiency, system responsiveness, equity of care, timeliness or access to care, and acceptability to the patient. Consequently, the dependent variable cluster in outcomes research is quality of care, operationalized as some tangible outcome such as cost, prevention, patient satisfaction, functional status, resource utilization, clinical end point of care, proximate clinical end point, length of hospital stay, incidence of rehospitalization, or response time to emergencies. The predictor variables are structures and processes of care. For interventional testing, the independent variable is a structure or process.

Samples and Sampling

Donabedian (1980) recommended use of huge databases in outcomes research so that, at the analysis level, connections among variables would be apparent. In contrast to the type of sampling usually found in the quantitative methodology, descriptive or correlational outcomes research tends to use an entire data set for establishment of basic measured values, as well as examination of trends over time. In this case, the sample includes the entire accessible population. Random sampling is used infrequently, primarily for initial testing of interventions designed to impact outcomes. When using an entire database, heterogeneous samples result, enabling generalization to that same accessible population (Kerlinger & Lee, 2000).

Outcomes research is unusual in that when whole databases are used, information emanates retrospectively from the past, and generalization is made to the future situation or population represented by the sample. Because of temporal drift, generalizations are more accurate when recent data are used.

Large Databases as Sample Sources

Two broad categories of databases are used as sources for outcomes research: clinical databases and administrative databases. **Clinical databases** are created by providers such as hospitals, HMOs, and healthcare professionals. Clinical data are generated either as a result of routine documentation of care or in relation to data collection for research purposes. Some databases are data registries that have been developed to gather data related to a particular disease, such as heart disease or cancer (Lee & Goldman, 1989). For instance, the Centers for Disease Control and Prevention (CDC) report information about diseases, treatment, and injuries on the CDC A-Z Index pages of their website (CDC, 2019a). If you wish to access the database, enter *A-Z Disease* into the search bar at the upper right of the CDC homepage. This allows you access to the disease information. A clinical database allows longitudinal analysis. At this time, because of minimum data set regulations for both inpatients and outpatients, clinical data continue to accrue rapidly.

Administrative databases are created by insurance companies, government agencies, and others not directly involved in providing patient care. Administrative databases maintain standardized sets of data for enormous numbers of patients and providers, as part of analyses they perform, relative to cost and expenditures. An example is the Medicare database managed by the CMS. These databases can be used to determine incidence or prevalence of disease, demographic profiles of persons using different types of care, geographical variations in medical care utilization, characteristics of medical care by provider, and outcomes of care. For instance, Gilden et al. (2017) used part of the Medicare database for their study of the cost effectiveness of different modalities in first-line treatment of one type of advanced lung cancer in Medicare patients.

The Specific Designs of Outcomes Research

"Many outcomes studies are retrospective or prospective cohort studies," differing from traditional epidemiological research in that the event or exposure studied may also be an intervention or change in care delivery (Petitti, 2006, p. 210). Those observational designs are what nursing research terms *noninterventional,* and they include both descriptive and correlational research. The interventional designs used in outcomes research usually are quasi-experimental and many adhere to a longitudinal approach that includes periods before and after a change in structure or process.

The noninterventional designs for outcomes research were originally developed by many different disciplines: epidemiology, population studies, medicine, economics, and statistics. Some of these designs are practice pattern profiling (epidemiology and medicine), prospective and retrospective cohort studies (epidemiology), trend studies (epidemiology), geographical designs (epidemiology, surveying, and cartography), meta-analyses (medicine and statistics), and cost-benefit analyses (epidemiology and economics).

Practice Pattern Profiling

Practice pattern profiling is an epidemiological technique that focuses on patterns of care. It was used originally in healthcare research to compare the outcomes of one physician's practice with norms or averages among other physicians. Now researchers use large database analyses to identify the practice pattern of an individual physician, a physician practice group, a combined practice (including nurse practitioners and physician assistants), or a given HMO or hospital, comparing outcomes with those of similar providers or with accepted standards of practice. The technique has been used to determine overutilization and underutilization of services, to examine costs associated with a particular provider's care, to uncover problems related to efficiency and quality of care, and to assess provider performance (Flexner, 1910/2002; Koller, Katz, Charrois, & Ye, 2019). An example of practice profiling is Koller et al.'s (2019) study, conducted for the purpose of determining what percentage of patients under the care of rheumatologists and receiving glucocorticoid therapy were also prescribed medications to prevent glucocorticoid-induced osteoporosis (GIOP). Comparison was made with data collected several years previously and with prescriptions filled by patients not under the care of a rheumatologist. Results indicated that a patient is more likely to receive appropriate GIOP preventive prescriptions when cared for by a rheumatologist. Other factors that favored appropriate coverage were female gender and urban, versus rural, residence.

Profiling does not address methods of improving outcomes, but merely identifies range of performance and outliers. Given existent databases in nursing, profiling nursing care by institution is possible and is now performed by groups such as NDNQI that track nursing-sensitive indicators for purposes of providing benchmarking data to participating database members. Other than tracking by such groups, profiling of nurses' practice patterns has not yet been the focus of formal research.

Prospective Cohort Studies

Prospective cohort studies, which originated in the field of epidemiology, use a descriptive, or occasionally correlational, longitudinal design. The researcher identifies a group of persons at risk for experiencing a particular event and follows that same group over time, collecting data at intervals. This is the strategy used for public health surveillance of diseases that threaten the general welfare (Thacker & Stroup, 2006) and, consequently, involve mandatory reporting, making the sample size the entire population. Sample sizes for other prospective cohort studies must be large, as well, when only a small portion of the at-risk group is expected to experience a disease or event. The entire sample is followed and multiple measurements obtained, often using dichotomous variables. Gradations of outcomes, both before and after confirmation of event occurrence, also can be determined. Weekly reports of seasonal influenza, for instance, are reported as gradations on the CDC website (CDC, 2019b).

The Harvard Nurses' Health Study is an example of a prospective cohort study. In the initial phase, the researchers recruited 100,000 nurses for the purpose of investigating long-term consequences of the use of birth control pills, smoking, and alcohol use in relation to health outcomes such as cancer, cognitive status, and cardiovascular disease (Nurses' Health Study, 2018). Data collection and analyses have been in progress for more than 40 years. Multiple studies reported in the literature have used the same large data set yielded by the study. For instance, Kim et al. (2017) used existing data from the Nurses' Health Study to examine the relationship between optimism and cause-specific mortality in more than 70,000 women. Measurements from 2004, 2006, and 2012 were utilized in the analysis. The relationship with optimism was examined in subgroups for several causes of death, including stroke, heart disease, cancer, infection, and respiratory illness, and the same relationship was found in all of these subgroups as well.

Retrospective Cohort Studies

A **retrospective cohort study** is an epidemiological design in which the researcher identifies a group of people who have experienced a particular event or outcome in the present or the recent past. Data are obtained from existent records or other previously collected data, predating the occurrence of the event. In this way, "the experience of cohorts is constructed through existing records" (Brownson, 2006, p. 78) to establish possible causal relationships for further investigation.

In addition to using a database, researchers can ask patients to recall information relevant to their previous health status. Because some research subjects are quite poor historians, corroboration of the information using records review, or verification by relatives or close friends, is preferable.

Garland et al.'s (2019) study examined the patient outcomes of return to work and yearly income, in the 3 years following MI, cardiac arrest, and stroke. The researchers focused on persons 40 to 61 years of age who had been employed prior to their hospitalizations. Data were drawn from the Canadian Hospitalization and Taxation Database because it contains linked hospital data and income tax data. In comparison with matched controls who did not experience one of the three events of interest during the same time period, the survivors had a lower incidence of returning to work and decreased income. Being unemployed at 3 years postevent was significantly more likely in the cohort of interest than for any of the unaffected controls. Findings were statistically significant for all individual groups but differed by diagnosis: The percentage of unemployment at 3 years was 5% in MI, 12.9% for cardiac arrest, and 19.8% for stroke.

Population-Based Studies

Some **population-based studies** are cohort studies, either prospective or retrospective, undertaken so as to discover information about a population, usually after an event occurs, such as a treatment or an exposure. The sample is derived exclusively from that population, probabilistically whenever possible, allowing generalization of the findings to that specific population. This method enables researchers to understand the natural history of a condition or of the long-term risks and benefits of a particular intervention (Guess et al., 1995). In outcomes research using a large administrative database such as Medicare that spans an entire state or country, the yield is a population-based data set presumed to include the entire population that is 65 years and older.

Maeland et al. (2019) studied the risk of delivery complications in Norway for non-Western low-risk women in comparison with low-risk ethnic Norwegian women. Their abstract explains the study:

"Objectives: To assess the pregnancy outcome of low-risk pregnancies for women originating from non-Western countries compared with ethnic Norwegian women.

Study design: A retrospective population-based observational cohort study with prospectively registered data. Conducted at Stavanger University Hospital, Norway, with approximately 4800 deliveries annually, from 2009 to 2015. We included women with low-risk pregnancies of non-Western origin ($n=1413$), born in Africa ($n=224$), Asia ($n=439$), Eastern Europe ($n=499$), Middle East ($n=138$), South America ($n=85$), Western ($n=979$), and ethnic Norwegian women ($n=7028$).

Main outcome measures: The relative risk of emergency cesarean section or postpartum hemorrhage by country of origin was estimated by odds ratios with 95% confidence intervals using logistic multiple regression.

Results: In total, the pregnancy outcomes of 9392 women were analyzed. Risk of emergency cesarean section was significantly higher for women originating from Asia (aOR: 1.887), followed by Africans (aOR: 1.705). Lowest risk was found in women originating from South America (aOR: 0.480). Risk of postpartum hemorrhage was significantly higher in women originating from Asia (aOR: 1.744) compared to Norwegians.

Conclusion: Even in a low-risk population, women originating from Asia and Africa had an elevated risk of adverse pregnancy outcome compared to the Norwegian group. The elevated risk should be considered by obstetric care providers, and we suggest that women originating from Asia and Africa would benefit from a targeted care during pregnancy and childbirth." (Maeland et al., 2019, p. 42)

Some population-based research is longitudinal, so data collection extends over a period of months or years. A study of this type usually is referred to as having a **trend analysis** design. In addition to trend analysis, population studies are sometimes termed **trend studies**. Trend research measures the prevalence of a variable and its value over time within an entire population, often examining relationships with other variables as well. Because this group of designs uses a whole population instead of a defined cohort, data collected over time do not reflect individual changes, and sequential determination of variable values are based on whichever individuals comprise the population at the time of measurement.

Prevention studies often use trend designs, measuring the occurrence of a disease over time, in response to various interventions. Other undesirable conditions or medical outcomes may be studied using a trend design, as well. In India, Chari, Glick, Okeke, and Srinivasan (2019) studied the association of neonatal mortality with maternal employment in a national workfare program, the Rural Employment Guarantee Scheme, in which approximately 50% of young adults hired were women. The authors performed statistical tests that strongly suggested the worsening trend in neonatal mortality was associated with expectant mothers' participation in the work program. Neonatal mortality was linked to poorer antenatal care due to the time-intensive nature of utilizing this resource. Neonatal mortality was also related to increased rates of prematurity within a context of decreased in-hospital births for program participants.

Geographical Analyses

Another epidemiological strategy is the **geographical analysis**, which examines variations in health status, health services, patterns of care, or patterns of use by geographical area. Geographical analyses are sometimes referred to as **small area analyses**. Variations may be associated with sociodemographic, economic, medical, cultural, or behavioral characteristics. The characteristics of a local healthcare system, such as capacity, access, and convenience, may play a role in explaining variations. Seabrook, Smith, Clark, and Gilliland (2019) performed a geospatial analysis of adverse birth outcomes in southwestern Ontario and their relationship to elevated sulfur dioxide levels in various subregions, due primarily to air pollution from smelters and utilities. Sulfur dioxide level was found to be associated with both low birthweight and preterm birth. Patient data were drawn from existent healthcare system databases, and included both pregnancy outcomes and postal codes. Sulfur dioxide levels were obtained from Canadian climate change studies.

In Bangladesh, Vyas, Kim, and Adams (2019) used multilevel techniques to study differences in child vaccination rates by geographical areas, to explain why some children were not vaccinated despite widely held beliefs in the population regarding the benefits of immunization. Their results indicated that the local geography, including the distance the family had to travel to take the child to be vaccinated, had an impact, as did the quality of the surface route: all-weather road, seasonal road, path, or waterway. However, this interacted with the mother's age, education, and wealth status, as well. In addition, the number of microfinance organizations in the area and the presence of a community health worker in the community also were related to vaccination rates.

Regression analyses are used in geographical analyses to develop models using risk factors and the characteristics of the community. In reports, results often are displayed through the use of maps (Kieffer, Alexander, & Mor, 1992). From a more theoretical perspective, the researcher must then explain the geographical variation uncovered by the analysis (Volinn, Diehr, Ciol, & Loeser, 1994).

Geographical information systems (GISs) are important tools for performing geographical analyses. The GIS is a computer-based modality that supports methodologies for geographical analyses. Interfacing with internet resources, GISs can be used to collect information, provide visual arrays, analyze data, and support the various methodologies for geographical healthcare analysis (Ramani, Mavalankar, Patel, & Mehandiratta, 2007). Relational databases facilitate processing of spatial information. Potential output from GIS-based research includes mapping, summarizing data, and analyzing spatial relationships among datasets. For instance, map-embedded data, such as distance from health care and travel conditions, can be included in a program, allowing an instantaneous calculation of physical access to care (Ramani et al., 2007). In addition, GISs can provide animated models showing change over time, as well as projected change reflecting proposed interventions. This makes GISs especially attractive for presentation of proposals and interim results.

Ortega-Garcia et al. (2017) studied the relationship between childhood cancer and air-polluting industries in the proximity of the diagnosed cases. Global information systems were used to map all cases and identified pollution sources. Using a specialized statistical computer program permitted verification of several high-risk areas in which cases of cancer were clustered around industrial sources. The researchers' abstract provides a description of their use of statistical analysis superimposed on geography:

"We analysed all incidences of pediatric cancer (< 15) diagnosed in a Spanish region during the period 1998–2015. The place of residence of each patient and the exact geographical coordinates of main industrial facilities was codified in order to analyse the spatial distribution of cases of cancer in relation to industrial areas. Focal tests and focused Scan methodology were used for the identification of high-incidence-rate spatial clusters around the main industrial pollution foci." (Ortega-Garcia, 2019, p. 63)

Economic Studies

Donabedian (1980) described efficiency as the "ability to obtain the greatest health improvement at the lowest cost" and optimality as the "most advantageous balancing of costs and benefits" (p. 27). In the field of outcomes research, economic studies often focus on outcomes as they relate to efficiency. The cost here is the cost to the institution, not the cost passed on to the insurance company and consumer. The total cost for health care is the unit of analysis in economic studies, rather than the welfare of the individual.

The most widely used term in the discussion of cost is the cost-benefit analysis. In general, cost-benefit analysis is analogous to Donabedian's concept of optimality, in that it involves comparison of costs and increased benefits, in terms of some single unit of analysis. In financial systems, the unit is money. However, in medical epidemiology, various other units of analysis may be selected, as well as cost, such as lives, disability, missed workdays, number of vials of vaccine used, or extent of visible scarring. A cost-benefit analysis may be actual or it may be hypothetical, emanating from a projection of probable results, based on some kind of factual financial data. When a cost-benefit analysis uses money for the unit of analysis, often it is referred to as a cost-effectiveness analysis.

Sung et al. (2018) performed a cost-benefit analysis to determine whether a smoking cessation treatment strategy of offering modest financial incentive and/or mailed nicotine patches in addition to usual care would result in savings for Medicaid in California (Medi-Cal). A pilot study in that state had previously demonstrated that in 2012-2013 paying Medi-Cal recipients $60 in

addition to providing them nicotine patches and usual care was more effective than were patches or usual care. Sung et al. (2018) calculated the hypothetical expense of providing the cash incentive, as well as patches and usual care to all Medi-Cal smokers aged 35 through 64 in the calendar year 2014. The cost-benefit ratio of 1.30 would yield an eventual net savings of $44 million per year to Medi-Cal when costs of treatments for smoking-related disorders and hospitalizations were considered.

In economics, efficiency refers to the most benefit with the least possible cost. In public health, efficiency has two meanings: technical efficiency and allocative efficiency. **Technical efficiency** refers to whether there is waste-minimum utilization of precious resources, which are usually inadequate for serving an entire population and can be scarce. Technical efficiency is critical for issues such as storage and transportation of scarce vaccines and use of expiration-sensitive items before they are obsolete. **Allocative efficiency** refers to whether resources go to the area in which they will do the most good in terms of delivery of services: effectiveness, usefulness to persons served, number of persons actually reached, and adherence rates (McQuestion et al., 2011). Allocative efficiency addresses such issues as nurse staffing during a shortage and scheduling in clinic settings.

Cost efficiency is merely the cheapest way of delivering a commodity or service. In all business endeavors, cost efficiency means paying the lowest price for an acceptable product or worker. Essentially, a cost-effectiveness analysis provides an assessment of how much was purchased for a given sum, determining cost per unit of commodity. As noted earlier, cost-effectiveness analysis is a subtype of cost-benefit analysis, using money as the unit of analysis. It is used currently within healthcare outcomes research to make decisions based on dollar power. Campbell et al. (2019) performed a cost-effectiveness analysis to determine the cost of one life-year saved by routine tuberculosis (TB) screening for migrants to Canada with chronic kidney disease (CKD). Screening was performed when individuals who were already residing in Canada finally required dialysis for CKD. Identification of TB by blood test, the interferon gamma release assay (IGRA), was found to have better accuracy than a skin test. IGRA testing was found to be cost effective only in patients 60 years or older who had emigrated from countries with an elevated incidence of TB. In these elderly patients, the cost of 1 life-year saved was $48,000, which is less than the medical cost anticipated for an untreated case of TB in this population. In addition, treatment prevents additional cases in the community, so routine IGRA testing of high-risk individuals is well supported from a community health promotion standpoint.

Measurement Problems and Methods

The selection of appropriate outcome variables is critical to the success of a study (Bernstein & Hilborne, 1993), but the method of measurement of those variables is just as important. As in any study, the researcher must evaluate the evidence of validity and the reliability of the measurement methods. However, because so much of the data used for outcomes research are drawn from existent data sources, often the researcher has no control over the method of measurement or its accuracy (see Chapter 17 for discussion of the quality of databases).

As previously discussed, rather than selecting the final outcome of care, which may not occur for months or years, researchers use measures of proximate outcomes, sometimes those that are available in existent databases. The researcher must make a logical argument as to the validity of those proximate outcomes in predicting the final outcome (Freedman & Schatzkin, 1992). Analyses of the degree of correlation between the proximate outcome and the final outcome of care should be included in the research report, when possible.

In most population-based or other large-sample outcome studies, researchers select outcome measures that allow utilization of secondary data sources (e.g., Sung et al., 2018). Secondary analysis is "any reanalysis of data or information collected by another researcher or organization, including analysis of data sets collected from a variety of sources" (Shi, 2008, p. 129). Data collected through NDNQI or CALNOC can be used in nursing outcomes research. Secondary analysis poses problems because, in most cases, data cannot be verified.

In evaluating a particular outcome measure, the researcher should consult the literature for previous studies that have used that same method of measurement, including the publication describing development of the method of measurement. Sensitivity to change is an important measurement property to consider in outcomes research because often researchers are interested in evaluating how outcomes change in response to healthcare interventions. As the sensitivity of a measure increases, statistical power increases, allowing smaller sample sizes to detect significant differences. Chapter 16 provides a more complete discussion of reliability and validity of scales and questionnaires, precision and accuracy of physiological measures, and sensitivity and specificity of diagnostic tools.

Statistical Methods for Outcomes Studies

On a methodological level, Donabedian (1980) stressed that when performing research on healthcare quality, Type I error should be preferred to Type II error: In other words, sample sizes should not be small, and level of significance should be set high enough (0.05–0.10) to achieve possibly erroneous positive results with moderate samples. This was quite divergent from the medical research practices of the time in which levels of significance were set at 0.01 to 0.05.

Because of the huge samples utilized for much of outcomes research, mastery of statistical methods or employment of a statistician is mandatory. In addition, some databases are compiled using weighted sampling, in which persons from underrepresented groups are oversampled. When studies are conducted using weighted databases, sophisticated statistical methods are needed to report the results for a corresponding unweighted sample. Multiple regression analysis is just as much an art as a science, and a good statistician develops an eye for best methods of analysis. Some effects discerned in large-sample database data are subtle, so it is essential to calculate the needed sample size for a given effect size using power analysis (Grove & Cipher, 2020).

Analysis of Change and Analysis of Improvement

Analysis of change is used in trend analysis studies. Analysis of change can be determined by using *t*-tests, percentage comparison, analysis of variance, analysis of covariance, correlational analyses, and chi-square analyses. However, the interpretation of the test must be appropriate, and the test must fit the level of measurement and the research question. To reiterate, careful operationalization of variables is essential. There is much benefit in performing multiple measures and tracking an indicator and an outcome over time. With analysis of change, more data than required are better than not enough.

Analysis of improvement is a directional version of analysis of change. Because statistical tests for analysis of improvement focus on one direction only, statistical significance may be reached with smaller samples than for analysis of change. When possible, quantification of improvement is preferable to a binary "did improve versus did not improve" measure.

Measures of Outcomes That May Be Used Non-Numerically

Variance analysis in outcomes research, in practice, is a lot less like arithmetic than it sounds. It is merely a strategy that defines expected outcomes, and the times they are expected to occur, based on population means, and then tracks delay or nonachievement of these outcomes. Delays and nonachievements are called variances. A critical pathway is a listing of expected short-term and long-term outcomes within a specific problem focus. When a patient fails to achieve an intermediate outcome by the expected time, a variance is said to have occurred. Variance analysis also can be used to identify at-risk patients who might benefit from the services of a case manager. Variance analysis tracking is sometimes expressed through the use of graphics, with the expected pathway plotted on a graph. The care providers plot deviations (negative variances) on the graph.

Longitudinal modeling is a method for analysis of data collected over time (Pretz et al., 2013). Data are obtained from population means and reflect achievement of anticipated outcomes. As with variance analysis, longitudinal models are useful for tracking outcomes that have an indefinite time of appearance because the models reflect repeated measures.

Latent transition analysis (Nylund, Bellmore, Nishina, & Graham, 2007) is a multivariate approach that produces a model based on average change of a phenomenon or occurrence within the group studied. The assumption is that change is continuous and occurs linearly. These analyses are projected probabilities or proportions of expected outcomes, and they track movement over a series of outcomes. They are helpful in keeping perspective about a patient's recovery or progress during an attenuated treatment, providing an idea of how an individual patient responds over time.

Because they are based on an average of actual patient progress within the population, they allow simple quantification of the concept of outcome variance.

Multilevel Analysis

Multilevel analysis is merely use of more than one way to analyze a data set. In outcomes research, an unexpectedly positive outcome may be associated with increases or decreases in certain structural or process variables. Multilevel analysis uses statistical techniques, allowing the researcher to "tease out" various different factors that seem promising in predicting an outcome by using multiple regression analysis. In outcomes research, multilevel analysis is useful for assigning attribution when many factors are involved. It also may be used to determine major predictors of an outcome and to predict the proposed effect of planned changes.

Ro et al. (2019) used multilevel analysis in their nationwide study of the goodness of survival outcomes following out-of-hospital cardiac arrest, after an increase in cardiopulmonary resuscitation training for laypersons in the community. Their results and conclusions are as follows:

"**Results**: A total of 81,250 OHCAs [out-of-hospital cardiac arrests] in 254 counties were analyzed. The risk-adjusted good neurological recovery rates increased from 5.4% in 2012 to 7.1% in 2016 (adjusted rates difference: 1.6% (1.2–2.1)). The OHCAs that occurred in counties with the highest county-level CPR training rates were more likely to survive with good neurological recovery (adjusted rates: 5.2% in 2012 and 7.4% in 2016, difference: 2.2% (1.5–2.9)) than were those occurring in the lowest county-level CPR training counties (adjusted rates: 5.9% in 2012 and 6.0% in 2016, difference: 0.1% (-1.1 to 1.2)). The difference-in-differences was 2.1% (0.8–3.5).

Conclusions: There were moderate associations between county-level CPR training and improvements in good neurological recovery rates over 5 years in the counties." (Ro et al., 2019, p. 1)

In this example, multilevel analysis was a useful technique for determining that the overall degree of cardiopulmonary resuscitation preparedness of the county in which the arrest took place was associated with both survival and end point neurological outcomes.

KEY POINTS

- Outcomes research is quantitative. Qualitative methods may inform concept definition, as well as the direction and interpretation of outcomes research.
- Donabedian developed the theory on which outcomes research is based.
- Quality is the overriding construct of Donabedian's (1980) theory, which he defined as "the balance of health benefits and harm" (p. 27).
- The three major concepts of the theory are structures, processes, and outcomes.
- Some structural variables are attributes of a healthcare facility, such as equipment of care, educational preparation/skill mix of healthcare workers, care protocols, staffing, and workforce size.
- Some process variables are standards of care, individual technical expertise, professional judgment, degree of patient participation, and patient-practitioner interactions.
- Donabedian (1987) defined outcomes as clinical end points, satisfaction with care, functional status, and general well-being. He emphasized that the outcomes were determined by "what consumers expect, want, or are willing to accept" (p. 5).
- Whenever possible, an attempt should be made to clearly link outcomes with the processes and structures with which they are associated.
- A NSPO is influenced by nursing care decisions, actions, or attributes.
- Organizations currently involved in efforts to study NSPOs include the ANA, the NQF, the Collaborative Alliance for Nursing Outcomes, the Veterans Affairs Nursing Outcomes Database, the Centers for Medicare and Medicaid Services Hospital Quality Initiative, the American Hospital Association, the Federation of American Hospitals, the Joint Commission, and the AHRQ.
- Most measurements obtained for outcomes research are retrospective and obtained from existent data sources, such as clinical and administrative databases.
- Statistical approaches used in outcomes studies are usually descriptive or correlational, using very large samples. Levels of significance are most often set at $p < 0.05$ or occasionally at even less stringent levels. In outcomes research, Type I error is preferred to Type II error.

REFERENCES

Agency for Healthcare Research and Quality (AHRQ). (2018a). *Agency for Healthcare Research and Quality: A profile*. Retrieved from https://www.ahrq.gov/cpi/about/profile/index.html#what3

Agency for Healthcare Research and Quality (AHRQ). (2018b). *Clinical guidelines and recommendations*. Retrieved from https://www.ahrq.gov/gam/updates/index.html

Agency for Healthcare Research and Quality (AHRQ). (2019a). *AHRQ health care innovations exchange*. Retrieved from https://innovations.ahrq.gov/node/5009

Agency for Healthcare Research and Quality. (2019b). *Budget estimates for appropriations committees*. Retrieved from https://www.ahrq.gov/cpi/about/mission/budget/2019/index.html

Ahern, K. (2000). "Something is wrong with my child": A phenomenological account for a search for a diagnosis. *Early Education and Development, 11*(2), 187–201.

Aiken, L. H., Sermeus, W., Van den Heede, K., Sloane, D. M., Busse, R., … McKee, M. (2012). Patient safety, satisfaction, and quality of hospital care: Cross-sectional surveys of nurses and patients in 12 countries in Europe and the United States. *British Medical Journal, 2012*(344), 1–14. doi:10.1136/bmj.c1717.

Aiken, L. H., Sloane, D., Barnes, H., Cimiotti, J., Jarrín, O., & McHugh, M. (2018). Nurses' and patients' appraisals show patient safety in hospitals remains a concern. *Health Affairs, 37*(11), 1744–1751. doi:10.1377/hlthaff.2018.0711

American Nurses Credentialing Center (ANCC). (2018). *ANCC magnet recognition program*. Retrieved from https://www.nursingworld.org/ancc/

Ball, J., Bruyneel, L., Aiken, L. H., Sermeus, W., Sloane, D. M., Rafferty, A. M., … Griffiths, P. D. (2018). Post-operative mortality, missed care and nursing staff in nine countries: A cross sectional study. *International Journal of Nursing Studies 78*, 10–15. doi:10.1016/j.ijnurstu.2017.08.004

Bernstein, S. J., & Hilborne, L. H. (1993). Clinical indicators: The road to quality care? *Joint Commission Journal on Quality Improvement, 19*(11), 501–509. doi:10.1016/s1070-3241(16)30031-1

Bouckaert, N., Van den Heede, K., & Van de Voorde, C. (2018). Improving the forecasting of hospital services: A comparison between projections and actual utilization of hospital services. *Health Policy, 122*(7), 728–736. doi:10.1016/j.healthpol.2018.05.010

Brownson, R. C. (2006). Outbreak and cluster investigations. In R. C. Brownson & D. B. Petitti (Eds.), *Applied epidemiology: Theory to practice* (pp. 68–98). New York, NY: Oxford University Press.

Bruyneel, L., Baoyue, L., Aiken, L., Lesaffre, E., Van den Heede, K., & Sermeus, W. (2013). A multi-country perspective on nurses' tasks below their skill level: Reports from domestically trained nurses and foreign trained nurses from developing countries. *International Journal of Nursing Studies, 50*(2), 202–209. doi:10.1016/j.ijnurstu.2012.06.013

Campbell, J. R., Johnston, J. C., Ronald, L. A., Sadatsafavi, M., Balshaw, R. F., Cook, V. J., . . . Marra, F. (2019). Screening for latent tuberculosis infection in migrants with CKD: A cost-effectiveness analysis. *American Journal of Kidney Diseases, 73*(1), 39–50. doi:10.1053/j.ajkd.2018.07.014

Center for Health Outcomes and Policy Research (CHOPR). (2019). *Center leadership.* Retrieved from https://www.nursing.upenn.edu/chopr/center-leadership/

Centers for Disease Control and Prevention (CDC). (2019a). *CDC A-Z index.* Retrieved from https://www.cdc.gov/

Centers for Disease Control and Prevention (CDC). (2019b) *CDC weekly US map: Influenza summary update.* Retrieved from https://www.cdc.gov/flu/weekly/usmap.htm

Centers for Medicare and Medicaid Services (CMS). (2018a). Hospital-acquired conditions. Retrieved from https://www.cms.gov/Medicare/Medicare-Fee-for-Service-Payment/HospitalAcqCond/Hospital-Acquired_Conditions.html

Centers for Medicare and Medicaid Services (CMS). (2018b). IRFS (Inpatient Rehabilitation Facilities) quality reporting program (QRP). Retrieved from https://www.cms.gov/medicare/quality-initiatives-patient-assessment-instruments/irf-quality-reporting/index.html

Chari, A. V., Glick, P., Okeke, E., & Srinivasan, S. V. (2019). Workfare and infant health: Evidence from India's public works program. *Journal of Development Economics, 138,* 116–134. doi:10.2139/ssrn.3149366

Chelimsky, E. (1997). The political environment of evaluation and what it means for the development of the field. In E. Chelimsky & W. R. Shadish (Eds.), *Evaluation for the 21st century: A handbook* (pp. 53–68). Thousand Oaks, CA: Sage Publications.

Chen, Q., Olsen, G., Bagante, F., Merath, K., Idrees, J., Akgul, O., . . . Pawlik, T. (2019). Procedure-specific volume and nurse-to-patient ratio: Implications for failure to rescue patients following liver surgery. *World Journal of Surgery, 43*(3), 910–919. doi:10.1007/s00268-018-4859-4

Cheng, W. L.-S. (2018). The effects of mutual goal-setting practice in older adults with chronic illness. *Geriatric Nursing, 39*(2), 143–150. doi:0.1016/j.gerinurse.2017.07.007

Claflin, J., Dimick, J. B., Campbell, D. A., Englesbe, M. J., & Sheetz, K. H. (2018). Understanding disparities in surgical outcomes for Medicaid beneficiaries. *World Journal of Surgery, 43*(3), 1–7. doi:10.1007/s00268-018-04891-y

Collaborative Alliance for Nursing Outcomes (CALNOC). (2019). *About us.* Retrieved from https://calnoc.org/about-us.

Danesh, V., Neff, D., Jones, T. L., Aroian, K., Unruh, L., Andrews, D., . . . Jimenez, E. (2019). Can proactive rapid response team rounding improve surveillance and reduce unplanned escalations in care? A controlled before and after study. *International Journal of Nursing Studies, 91,* 128–133. doi:10.1016/j.ijnurstu.2019.01.004

Dawson, R., & Tilley, N. (1997). An introduction to scientific realist evaluation. In E. Chelimsky & W. R. Shadish (Eds.), *Evaluation for the 21st century: A handbook* (pp. 405–418). Thousand Oaks, CA: Sage Publications.

De Regge, M., De Pourco, K., Gemmel, P., Van de Voorde, C., Van Den Heede, K., & Eeckloo, K. (2018). Varying viewpoints of Belgian stakeholders on models of inter-hospital collaboration. *BMC Health Services Research, 18*(1), 1–14. doi:10.1186/s12913-018-3763-9

Donabedian, A. (1980). *Explorations in quality assessment and monitoring. Volume I. The definition of quality and approaches to its assessment.* Ann Arbor, MI: Health Administration Press.

Donabedian, A. (1987). Some basic issues in evaluating the quality of health care. In L. T. Rinke (Ed.), *Outcome measures in home care* (Vol. I, p. 338). New York, NY: National League for Nursing. (Original work published 1976)

Donabedian, A. (1990). The seven pillars of quality. *Archives of Pathology and Laboratory Medicine, 114*(11), 1115–1118.

Donabedian, A. (2003). *An introduction to quality assurance in health care.* Oxford, UK: Oxford University Press.

Donabedian, A. (2005). Evaluating the quality of medical care. *Milbank Quarterly, 83*(4), 691–729.

Doran, D. M. (Ed.). (2011). *Nursing outcomes: The state of the science* (2nd ed.). Sudbury, MA: Jones & Bartlett.

Fenton, J. J., Jerant, A. F., Bertakis, K. D., & Franks, P. (2012). The cost of satisfaction: A national study of patient satisfaction, health care utilization, expenditures, and mortality. *JAMA Internal Medicine, 172*(5), 405–411. doi:10.1001/archinternmed.2011.1662

Flexner, A. (1910/2002). Medical education in the United States and Canada: A report to the Carnegie Foundation for the Advancement of Teaching. *Bulletin of the World Health Organization, 80*(7), 594–602. Retrieved from http://www.ncbi.nlm.nih.gov/pmc/articles/PMC2567554/

Freedman, L. S., & Schatzkin, A. (1992). Sample size for studying intermediate endpoints within intervention trials or observational studies. *American Journal of Epidemiology, 136*(9), 1148–1159. doi:10.1093/oxford-journals.aje.a116581

Frenk, J. (2000). Obituary: Avedis Donabedian. *Bulletin of the World Health Organization, 78*(12), 1475.

Garland, A. G., Jeon, S.-H., Stepner, M., Rotermann, M., Fransoo, R., Wunsch, H., . . . Sanmartin, C. (2019). Effects of cardiovascular and cerebrovascular health events on work and earnings: A population-based retrospective cohort study. *Canadian Medical Association Journal, 191*(1), e3–e10.

Germack, H. D., McHugh, M. D., Sloane, D. M., & Aiken, L. H. (2017). US hospital employment of foreign-educated nurses and patient experience: A cross sectional study. *Journal of Nursing Regulation, 8*(3), 26–35.

Gilden, D. M., Kubisiak, J. M., Pohl, G. M., Ball, D. E., Gilden, D. E., John, W. J., . . . Winfree, K. B. (2017). Treatment patterns and cost-effectiveness of first line treatment of advanced non-squamous non-small cell lung cancer in Medicare patients. *Journal of Medical Economics, 20*(2), 151–161. doi:10.1080/13696998.2016.1230550

Grove, S. K., & Cipher, D. J. (2020). *Statistics for nursing research: A workbook for evidence-based practice* (3rd ed.). St. Louis, MO: Elsevier.

Guess, H. A., Jacobsen, S. J., Girman, C. J., Oesterling, J. E., Chute, C. G., Panser, L. A., & Lieber, M. M. (1995). The role of community-based longitudinal studies in evaluating treatment effects. Example: Benign prostatic hyperplasia. *Medical Care, 33*(4), AS26–AS35.

Jennings, B. M., Loan, L. A., DePaul, D., Brosch, L. R., & Hildreth, P. (2001). Lessons learned while collecting ANA indicator data. *Journal of Nursing Administration, 31*(3), 121–129.

Kaplan, J. B., Eiferman, D. S., Porter, K., MacDermott, J., Brumbaugh, J., & Murphy, C. V. (2019). Impact of a nursing-driven sedation protocol with criteria for infusion initiation in the surgical intensive care unit. *Journal of Critical Care, 50*, 195–200.

Karim, S. A., Pink, G. H., Reiter, K. L., Holmes, G. M., Jones, C. B., & Woodard, E. K. (2018). The effect of the magnet recognition signal on hospital financial performance. *Journal of Healthcare Management, 63*(6), e131–e146. doi:10.1097/JHM-D-17-00215

Kelly, K. C., Huber, D. G., Johnson, M., McCloskey, J. C., & Maas, M. (1994). The Medical Outcomes Study: A nursing perspective. *Journal of Professional Nursing, 10*(4), 209–216.

Kerlinger, F. N., & Lee, H. B. (2000). *Foundations of behavioral research* (4th ed.). Fort Worth, TX: Harcourt College Publishers.

Kieffer, E., Alexander, G. R., & Mor, J. (1992). Area-level predictors of use of prenatal care in diverse populations. *Public Health Reports, 107*(6), 653–658.

Kim, E. S., Hagan, K. A., Grodstein, F., DeMeo, D. L., De Vivo, I., & Kubzansky, L. D. (2017). Optimism and cause-specific mortality: A prospective cohort study. *American Journal of Epidemiology, 185*(1), 21–29.

Kivelä, K., Elo, S., & Kääriäinen, M. (2018). Frequent attenders in primary health care: A concept analysis. *International Journal of Nursing Studies, 86*, 115–124.

Kleib, M., Sales, A., Doran, D. M., Malette, C., & White, D. (2011). Nursing minimum data sets. In D. M. Doran (Ed.), *Nursing outcomes: The state of the science* (2nd ed., pp. 487–512). Sudbury, MA: Jones & Bartlett.

Koller, G., Katz, S., Charrois, T. L., & Ye, C. (2019). Glucocorticoid-induced osteoporosis preventive care in rheumatology patients. *Archives of Osteoporosis, 14*(1), 1–7. doi:10.1007/s11657-019-0570-9

Kopf, E. W. (1916). Florence Nightingale as statistician. *Publications of the American Statistical Association, 15*(116), 388–404.

Lawson, E. F., & Yazdany, J. (2012). Healthcare quality in systemic lupus erythematosus: Using Donabedian's conceptual framework to understand what we know. *International Journal of Clinical Rheumatology, 7*(1), 95–107.

Lee, T. H., & Goldman, L. (1989). Development and analysis of observational data bases. *Journal of the American College of Cardiology, 14*(3), SA44–SA47.

Li, B., Bruyneel, L., Sermeus, W., Van den Heede, K., Matawie, K., . . . Aiken, L. (2013). Group-level impact of work environment dimensions on burnout experiences among nurses: A multivariate multilevel probit model. *International Journal of Nursing Studies, 50*(2), 281–291. doi:10.1016/j.ijnurstu.2012.07.001

Lopez, M., Blackburn, L., & Springer, C. (2018). Minimizing sleep disturbances to improve patient outcomes. *MedSurg Nursing, 27*(6), 368–371.

Maeland, S. M., Sande, R. K., & Bing-Jonsson, P. C. (2019). Risk for delivery complications in Robson group 1 for non-Western women in Norway compared with ethnic Norwegian women—A population-based observational cohort study. *Sexual & Reproductive Healthcare, 20*, 42–45. doi:10.1016/j.srhc.2019.02.006

McDonald, D. C., Carlson, K., & Izrael, D. (2012). Geographic variation in opioid prescribing in the US. *The Journal of Pain, 13*(10), 988–996.

McQuestion, M., Gnawali, D., Kamara, C., Kizza, D., Mambu-Ma-Disu, H., . . . Mbwangue, J. (2011). Creating sustainable financing and support for immunization programs in fifteen developing countries. *Health Affairs, 30*(6), 1134–1140.

Mitchell, P. H., Ferketich, S., Jennings, B. M., & American Academy of Nursing Expert Panel on Quality Health Care. (1998). Quality health outcomes model. *Image: Journal of Nursing Scholarship, 30*(1), 43–46.

Mullan, F. (2001). A founder of quality assessment encounters a troubled system firsthand. *Health Affairs, 20*(1), 137–141.

National Quality Forum. (NQF). (2019a). *About us.* Retrieved from http://www.qualityforum.org/About_NQF/

National Quality Forum. (NQF). (2019b). *Improving care through nursing.* Retrieved from http://www.qualityforum.org/improving_care_through_nursing.aspx

National Quality Forum. (NQF). (2019c). *Measures, reports, and tools.* Retrieved from http://www.qualityforum.org/Measures_Reports_Tools.aspx

Nichols, M., Abrams, J. J., Greenhut, R., Rudin, S., MacNair (Producers), & Nichols, M. (Director). (1991). *Regarding Henry* [Motion picture]. Los Angeles, CA: Paramount.

Nurses' Health Study. (2018). *About NHS.* Retrieved from https://www.nurseshealthstudy.org/about-nhs

Nylund, K., Bellmore, A., Nishina, A., & Graham, S. (2007). Subtypes, severity, and structural stability of peer victimization: What does latent class analysis say? *Child Development, 78*(6), 1706–1722. doi:10.1111/j.1467-8624.2007.01097.x

Oncology Nursing Society (ONS). (2019). *Putting evidence into practice.* Retrieved from https://www.ons.org

Ortega-Garcia, J. A., Lopez-Hernandez, F. A., Cárceles-Alvarez, A., Fuster-Soler, J. L., Sotomayor, D. I., & Ramis, R. (2017). Childhood cancer in small geographical areas and proximity to air-polluting industries. *Environmental Research, 156*, 63–73. doi:10.1016/j.envres.2017.03.009

Pearson, S. D., Goulart-Fisher, D., & Lee, T. H. (1995). Critical pathways as a strategy for improving care: Problems and potential. *Annals of Internal Medicine, 123*(12), 941–948. doi:10.7326/0003-4819-123-12-199512150-00008

Petitti, D. B. (2006). Outcomes research. In R. C. Brownson & D. B. Petitti (Eds.), *Applied epidemiology: Theory to practice* (pp. 207–232). New York, NY: Oxford University Press.

Plaku-Alakbarova, B., Punnett, L., Gore, R. J., & Procare Research Team. (2018). Nursing home employee and resident satisfaction and resident care outcomes. *Safety and Health at Work, 9*, 408–415. doi:10.1016/j.shaw.2017.12.002

Press Ganey. (2019). *Resources and research.* Retrieved from https://www.pressganey.com/resourcesDocument26

Pretz, C. R., Kozlowski, A. J., Dams-O'Connor, K., Kreider, S., Cuthbert, J. P., … Corrigan, J. D. (2013). Descriptive modeling of longitudinal outcomes measures in traumatic brain injury: A National Institute on Disability and Rehabilitation Research Traumatic Brain Injury Model Systems study. *Archives of Physical Medicine and Rehabilitation, 94*(3), 579–588. doi:10.1016/j.apmr.2012.08.197

Ramani, K. V., Mavalankar, D., Patel, A., & Mehandiratta, S. (2007). A GIS approach to plan and deliver healthcare services to urban poor: A public private partnership model for Ahmedabad City, India. *International Journal of Pharmaceutical and Healthcare Marketing, 1*(2), 159–173. doi:10.1001/jama.1989.03430070073033

Ro, Y. S., Song, K. J., Shin, S. D., Hong, K. J., Park, J. H., Kong, S. Y., & Cho, S.-I. (2019). Association between county-level cardiopulmonary resuscitation training and changes in survival outcomes after out-of-hospital cardiac arrest over 5 years: A multilevel analysis. *Resuscitation, 139*, 291–298. doi:10.1016/j.resuscitation.2019.01.012

Robins, D., Fein, D., Barton, M., & Green, J. (2001). The modified-checklist for autism in toddlers (M-CHAT): An initial investigation in the early detection of autism and pervasive developmental disorders. *Journal of Autism and Developmental Disorders, 31*(2), 131–144. doi:10.1023/a:1010738829569

Robins, D. L., Casagrande, K., Barton, M. L., Chen, C., Dumont-Mathieu, T., & Fein, D. (2014). Validation of the modified checklist for autism in toddlers-revised with follow-up (M-CHAT-R/F). *Pediatrics, 133*(1), 37–45. doi:10.1542/peds.2013-1813

Ryan, S., & Salisbury, H. (2012). 'You know what boys are like': Pre-diagnosis experiences of parents of children with autism spectrum conditions. *British Journal of General Practice, 62*(598), e378–e383. doi:10.3399/bjgp12X641500

Sanders, S. F., & DeVon, H. A. (2016). Accuracy in ED triage for symptoms of acute myocardial infarction. *Research, 42*(4), 331–337. doi:10.1016/j.jen.2015.12.0

Seabrook, J. A., Smith, A., Clark, A. F., & Gilliland, J. A. (2019). Geospatial analyses of adverse birth outcomes in Southwestern Ontario: Examining the impact of environmental factors. *Environmental Research, 172*, 18–26. doi:10.1016/j.envres.2018.12.068

Sezgin, D., O'Donovan, M., Cornally, N., Liew, A., & O'Caoimh, R. (2019). Defining frailty for healthcare practice and research: A qualitative systematic review with thematic analysis. *International Journal of Nursing Studies, 92*, 16–26. doi:10.1016/j.ijnurstu.2018.12.014

Shi, L. (2008). *Health services research methods* (2nd ed.). Clifton Park, NY: Delmar Cengage Learning.

Shubeck, S., Kanters, A., & Dimick, J. (2019). Surgeon leadership style and risk-adjusted patient outcomes. *Surgical Endoscopy, 33*(2), 471–474. doi:10.1007/s00464-018-6320-z

Sung, H.-Y., Penko, J., Cummins, S. E., Max, W., Zhu, S.-H., Bibbins-Domingo, K. & Kohatsu, N. D. (2018). Economic impact of financial incentives and mailing nicotine patches to help Medicaid smokers quit smoking: A cost-benefit analysis. *American Journal of Preventive Medicine, 55*(6), S148–S158. doi:10.1016/j.amepre.2018.08.007

Tarlov, A. R., Ware Jr., J. E., Greenfield, S., Nelson, E. C., Perrin, E., & Zubkoff, M. (1989). The Medical Outcomes Study: An application of methods for monitoring the results of medical care. *Journal of the American Medical Association, 262*(7), 925–930. doi:10.1001/jama.1989.03430070073033

Thacker, S. B., & Stroup, D. F. (2006). Public health surveillance. In R. C. Brownson & D. B. Petitti (Eds.), *Applied epidemiology: Theory to practice* (pp. 207–232). New York, NY: Oxford University Press.

University of Pennsylvania School of Nursing. (2019). *Center for Health Outcomes and Policy Research (CHOPR).* Retrieved from https://www.nursing.upenn.edu/chopr/

Urman, R. D., Boing, E. A., Pham, A. T., Khangulov, V., Fain, R., Nathanson, . . . Cirillo, J. (2018). Improved outcomes associated with the use of intravenous acetaminophen for management of acute post-surgical pain in Cesarean sections and hysterectomies. *Journal of Clinical Medicine Research, 10*(6), 499–507. doi:10.14740/jocmr3380w

Van den Heede, K., Dubois, C., Mistiaen, P., Stordeur, S., Cordon, A., & Farfan-Portet, M. I. (2019). Evaluating the need to reform the organisation of care for major trauma patients in Belgium: An analysis of administrative databases. *European Journal of Trauma and Emergency Surgery,* 45; 855-892. doi:10.1007/s00068-018-0932-9.

Van den Heede, K., Lasaffre, E., Diya, L., Vleugels, A., Clarke, S. P., . . . Aiken, L. H. (2009). The relationship between inpatient cardiac surgery mortality and nurse numbers and educational level: Analysis of administrative data. *International Journal of Nursing Studies, 46*(6), 796–803. doi:10.1016/j.ijnurstu.2008.12.018

Vandermause, R., Barg, F. K., Esmail, L., Edmundson, L., Girard, S., & Perfetti, A. R. (2017). Qualitative methods in patient-centered outcomes research. *Qualitative Health Research, 27*(3), 434–442. doi:10.1177/1049732316668298

Volinn, E., Diehr, P., Ciol, M. A., & Loeser, J. D. (1994). Why does geographic variation in health care practices matter (and seven questions to ask in evaluating studies on geographic variation)? *Spine, 19*(18), S2092–S2100. doi:10.1097/00007632-199409151-00012

Vyas, P., Kim, D., & Adams, A. (2019). Understanding spatial and contextual factors influencing intraregional differences in child vaccination coverage in Bangladesh. *Asia Pacific Journal of Public Health, 31*(1), 51–60. doi:10.1177/1010539518813604

Wang, X., Knight, L. S., Evans, A., Wang, J., & Smith, T. J. (2017). Variations among physicians in hospice referrals of patients with advanced cancer. *Journal of Oncology Practice, 13*(5), e496–e504. doi:10.1200/JOP.2016.018093

Zerzan, J. T., Morden, N. E., Soumerai, S., Ross-Degnan, D., Roughhead, E., . . . Zhang, F. (2006). Trends and geographic variation of opiate medication use in state Medicaid fee-for-service programs, 1996-2002. *Medical Care, 44*(11), 1005–1010. doi:10.1097/01.mlr.0000228025.04535.25

Mixed Methods Research

Jennifer R. Gray

http://evolve.elsevier.com/Gray/practice/

Quantitative research and qualitative research have different philosophical foundations. Because of these differences in philosophy, researchers do not always agree on the best approach with which to address a research problem. The convergence of technology, health disparities, globalization, and the complex healthcare system has given rise to several research problems that cannot be answered completely with either type of research (Kazdin, 2017; Molina-Azorin & Fetters, 2019; Poth, 2018). To address complex problems, researchers may choose to combine quantitative and qualitative designs into one study using the methodology called **mixed methods research** (Creswell & Clark, 2018). Using mixed methods offers researchers the ability to use the strengths of both qualitative and quantitative research designs to answer different stages or parts of a complex research question (Bazeley, 2018).

This chapter begins with a description of the philosophical foundation of mixed methods research and continues with descriptions of three mixed methods study designs with an example of a published study for each type. A description of different methods of integrating the results from each of the study components also is included. The chapter concludes by describing the challenges of conducting mixed methods research followed by criteria for evaluating mixed methods studies.

PHILOSOPHICAL FOUNDATIONS

Mixed methods are considered by some experts to be a third paradigm for research (Bazeley, 2018). Other experts have found the methodology consistent with blending the worldviews of members of interdisciplinary teams (Creswell & Clark, 2018). The philosophical differences among team members from different disciplines can be challenging (Bazeley, 2018). However, Creamer (2018) offers four assumptions that support using mixed methods. Box 14.1 lists the assumptions that may provide points of agreement for a diverse research team.

The philosophical underpinnings of mixed methods research and the paradigms that best fit these methods continue to evolve. At the foundation of the differences between qualitative and quantitative studies are philosophical differences regarding the question, What is truth? A philosophy's ontology (What is reality?) shapes the epistemology (how we can know the truth), that then influences the methodology (research design) (Bazeley, 2018). Over the last few years, many researchers have departed from the idea that one paradigm or one research strategy is superior, and instead have taken the position that the search for knowledge requires the use of all available strategies. Researchers who hold these views and seek answers using mixed methods may have exchanged the dichotomy of positivism and constructivism for pragmatism (Creswell & Clark, 2018; Leavy, 2017).

Pragmatism refers to a philosophy of making decisions based on solving problems, such as considering the research question and the knowledge needed (desired outcome) and selecting a methodology that addresses the question (Bazeley, 2018; Curry & Nunez-Smith, 2018). As discussed in previous chapters, the process of developing a study design is iterative and reflexive. Decisions are made tentatively about the question and the

BOX 14.1 **Assumptions of Mixed Methods Research**

- Quantitative and qualitative data are not incompatible.
- Combining "qualitative and quantitative approaches produce more robust findings" (p. 5).
- Corroborating findings by using multiple types of data increases the validity of the study.
- Combining methods allows the weaknesses of one to be offset by the strengths of the other.

Adapted from Creamer, E. (2018). *An introduction to fully integrated mixed methods research.* Thousand Oaks, CA: Sage.

design and then reconsidered as each phase is developed. With mixed methods designs, the researcher can allow the strengths of one method to compensate for the possible limitations of the other (Poth, 2018), resulting in the methods being complementary to each other.

OVERVIEW OF MIXED METHODS DESIGNS

The focus on problem solving or answering the research question means that a mixed methods research design is selected based on study purpose, timing of the quantitative and qualitative elements, and emphasis on one element over the other. Table 14.1 provides a description of mixed methods designs classified by the researcher's reasons for combining methods. The reasons range from explaining quantitative findings to integrating different perspectives into the conduct of a study. Another classification of mixed methods design is based on the timing of each type of data collection in the study design (Table 14.2). In Table 14.3, another way to label mixed methods designs is displayed. This classification is based on which element is emphasized. In this classification, the emphasized element is noted in uppercase letters (QUANT or QUAL) and the other element in lowercase font (quant or qual).

Creswell and Creswell (2018) presented three basic designs that are a combination of the purpose and timing of the different types of data collection: (1) convergent concurrent mixed methods, (2) explanatory sequential mixed methods, and (3) exploratory sequential mixed methods. They continue by describing four complex designs that capitalize on the strengths of mixed methods designs for specific purposes. The first type,

TABLE 14.1 **Mixed Methods Studies Classified by Purpose**

Label	Description
Exploratory	Qualitative methods are used to explore a new topic, followed by quantitative methods that measure aspects of what was learned qualitatively.
Explanatory	Quantitative methods are used to establish evidence related to incidence, relationship, or causation. Then qualitative methods provide a more robust explanatory description of the human experience aspect of the quantitative results.
Expansion	Quantitative and qualitative methods are used to provide a wider or deeper understanding of a concept or a sample. Data may be collected in an organization from people at different levels of responsibility.
Evaluation	Quantitative and qualitative methods are used to determine the effectiveness of an intervention or project.
Transformative	Quantitative and qualitative methods are used with a community-based research team to address a social problem in the community.
Advocacy	Quantitative and qualitative methods are used, guided by feminism, disability theory, race/ethnicity theory, or other approaches to raise awareness of the needs of a specific group; aspects of advocacy research may overlap with transformative designs.

Content compiled and adapted from Creamer, E. (2018). *An introduction to fully integrated mixed methods research.* Thousand Oaks, CA: Sage; Creswell, J., & Creswell, D. (2018). *Research design: Qualitative, quantitative, and mixed methods approaches* (5th ed.). Thousand Oaks, CA: Sage; Leavy, P. (2017). *Research design: Quantitative, qualitative, mixed methods, arts-based, and community-based participatory research approaches.* New York, NY: Guilford Press.

mixed methods experimental or interventional designs, is characterized by the researchers seeking participants' perspectives on the usefulness of the intervention being tested or healthcare providers' perspectives on the challenges of implementing the intervention. The mixed methods participatory–social justice design is

TABLE 14.2 Typology of Mixed Methods Designs Based on Timing of Quantitative and Qualitative Elements

Label	Description
Sequential	Either the quantitative or the qualitative phase may be implemented first. Results from the first phase of the study are used to inform the specific methods of the second phase.
Concurrent	Qualitative and quantitative elements are implemented at the same time through the study. Findings are integrated at interpretation.

Data from Creswell, J. W. (2015). *A concise introduction to mixed methods research.* Los Angeles, CA: Sage; Creswell, J. W., & Clark, P. (2018). *Designing and conducting mixed methods research* (3rd ed.). Thousand Oaks, CA: Sage.

the second complex design. This study design is to "give voice to participants and collaborate with them in shaping the research" (Creswell & Creswell, 2018, p. 230). The goal is to use the study findings to make policy changes or community improvements. In mixed methods case study designs, the third complex design, the cases are selected or described using qualitative and quantitative data. Case studies need extensive, detailed information from multiple perspectives, ideally addressed by using both qualitative and quantitative data. The last complex design is the mixed methods evaluation design, the design that incorporates collecting quantitative and qualitative data to produce a broader and deeper assessment of a project or program. For example, a hospital may expand its services to include a mobile clinic that rotates between four underserved neighborhoods. At the end of a year, a comprehensive evaluation is conducted of the mobile clinic that includes quantitative data (numbers of people served, operating expenses [including healthcare providers' salaries]) and qualitative data (perspectives of neighborhood key informants, input from people attending the clinic, stories of people who were referred for additional care). The comprehensive evaluation provides the hospital board with meaningful findings on which to base a decision about continuation of the clinic.

From this discussion, you can see that there are multiple perspectives from which you can describe mixed methods designs (see Tables 14.1, 14.2, and 14.3). For simplicity, we are limiting our discussion to the three approaches usually implemented in nursing and health

TABLE 14.3 Typology of Mixed Methods Designs by Emphasis, Sequence, and Integration

Label	Description
QUANT + qual	Quantitative elements are the primary methods used to answer the research question; at the same time, a supplementary aim or secondary question may be addressed by using qualitative methods.
QUANT → qual	Quantitative methods are implemented first, chronologically, and are emphasized in the analysis and in the reporting of findings.
QUAL + quant	Qualitative elements are the primary methods used to answer the research question; at the same time, a supplementary aim or secondary question may be addressed by using quantitative methods.
QUAL → quant	Qualitative methods are implemented first, chronologically, and are emphasized in the analysis and in the reporting of findings.
quant → QUAL	Quantitative methods are implemented first, chronologically, but qualitative methods are emphasized in the analysis and in the reporting of findings.
qual → QUANT	Qualitative methods are implemented first, chronologically, but quantitative methods are emphasized in the analysis and in the reporting of findings.

Note: Uppercase font indicates the study element that is emphasized with lowercase font indicating the less emphasized element; +, concurrent implementation; →, sequential implementation.
Information from Creswell, J. W. (2015). *A concise introduction to mixed methods research.* Los Angeles, CA: Sage; Creswell, J. W., & Clark, P. (2018). *Designing and conducting mixed methods research* (3rd ed.). Thousand Oaks, CA: Sage.

research and consistent with Creswell and Creswell's (2018) three basic designs: (1) exploratory sequential strategy, (2) explanatory sequential strategy, and (3) convergent concurrent strategy.

To decide which design is appropriate, you should begin by contemplating the purpose for combining the methods. This decision will shape the study. A researcher may implement a sequential study design in which the results of the first phase, either quantitative or qualitative, will determine the specific methods for the second phase. To accomplish this, the findings of the first phase must be completed prior to beginning the second phase. Sequential designs therefore have the disadvantage of taking more time and potentially costing more to implement.

Mixed methods studies in which data are collected concurrently usually involve the qualitative and quantitative data being analyzed independently. Then the independently generated findings are compared, connected, or combined. Concurrent mixed methods designs can also have multiple points of convergence with both types of data being examined throughout data collection and analysis. In this chapter, models of the three mixed methods approaches and examples of each are provided to expand your understanding of these designs.

Exploratory Sequential Designs

The **exploratory sequential design** begins with collection and analysis of qualitative data, followed by collection of quantitative data. Often findings of the qualitative data analysis are used to design the quantitative phase (Fig. 14.1). This approach may be used to design a quantitative tool (Bazeley, 2018). For example, interviews may be conducted with members of a target population, and items

for the quantitative tool may be developed using phrases and content generated qualitatively. Another reason to use this strategy is to collect data about patients' perspectives concerning an issue or problem. With this input, an intervention can be developed or refined, incorporating the patients' perspectives.

Shamsalinia, Masoudi, Rad, and Ghaffari (2019) conducted an exploratory sequential study in Iran to develop an instrument to measure the stigma experienced by persons living with epilepsy. The researchers wanted to study the effects of stigma on their quality of life, but the available instruments had not been developed with their input.

> "In Iran, no study has yet been conducted on the development of research instruments to measure social stigma of epilepsy in adults. ...the development and psychometric evaluation of the questionnaire were performed based on the proposed steps of Schwab (2013). Schwab divided the development and psychometric evaluation of a research instrument into three basic steps, namely, item development, scale development, and evaluation scale. In the present study, the first and second stages of the study comprised the qualitative phase and the third stage was the quantitative phase." (Shamsalinia et al., 2019, p. 142).

Twenty interviews that averaged 45 minutes in length were conducted in the Persian language with persons living with epilepsy. The interviews were conducted in a place convenient to the participant. Data analysis was occurring during the data collection phase and data saturation was reached. Shamsalinia et al. (2019) evaluated the rigor of the qualitative phase

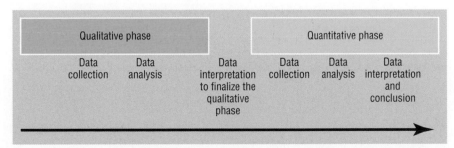

Fig. 14.1 Exploratory sequential mixed methods.

using four aspects of trustworthiness: credibility, dependability, confirmability, and transferability (Trainor & Graue, 2014).

"...maximum variation sampling with respect to age, gender, marital status, occupation, education level, duration of illness, number of seizures per month, etc. was followed to achieve credibility. ...the transcripts of the interviews and the drawn codes were provided to a number of participants so that they could comment on their correctness. ...every attempt was made to provide a comprehensive description of the research procedure, including data collection and analysis, and the formation of themes in order to allow the readers of the article to judge the quality of the study. ...rich and accurate findings, supported by appropriate quotes, were provided to further improve transferability." (Shamsalinia et al., 2019, p. 143)

Shamsalinia et al. (2019) developed 40 items for the questionnaire from the participants' quotes and 36 items from the literature. The researchers reviewed the items, asked 10 persons with epilepsy to review the scale for face validity, asked 10 clinical and methods experts to rate the items for content validity, and calculated the content validity ratio and the content validity index (see Chapter 16). These procedures resulted in the scale being reduced to 54 items. The 54-item scale was given to 450 persons with epilepsy to assess construct validity using principal component factor analysis and to evaluate internal consistency and test-retest reliability.

"Five factors including family consequences, internal emotions, dangerous escape, individual consequences, and

destructive assumptions with eigenvalue[s] of over 1 were drawn from principal component analysis with oblique rotation... At this stage, 5 items were deleted because of [a] factorial load of less than 0.4. Finally, a 49-item instrument with a factorial load of .401–.879 was achieved. ...Cronbach's alpha coefficient was calculated at 0.901. ...Measuring perceived social stigma by using a valid and reliable tool can lead to preventive and timely interventions. Standard research instruments are therefore essential to examine and document the effectiveness of evidence-based programs." (Shamalinia et al., 2019, p. 145)

Shamsalinia et al. (2019) identified the strengths and limitations of their study and concluded that their scale, Perceived Social Stigma Questionnaire for adults with epilepsy, needed additional development. The researchers demonstrated how an exploratory sequential mixed methods design provides a process for developing scales consistent to participants' perspectives. Exploratory sequential mixed methods studies can also be used to explore new research topics during the qualitative phase and to develop research questions or hypotheses to be examined during the quantitative phase.

Explanatory Sequential Designs

When using an **explanatory sequential design**, the researcher collects and analyzes quantitative data and then collects and analyzes qualitative data to explain the quantitative findings (Fig. 14.2). The findings represent integration of the data. Qualitative examination of the phenomenon facilitates a fuller understanding and is well suited to explaining and interpreting relationships.

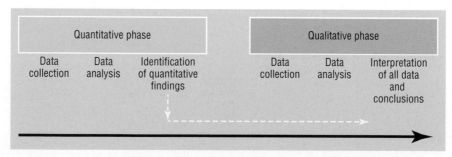

Fig. 14.2 Explanatory sequential mixed methods.

Explanatory sequential designs are easier to implement than are designs in which quantitative and qualitative data are collected at the same time. This type of approach shares the disadvantage of other sequential designs in that it also requires a longer period of time and more resources than would be needed for one single-method study (Creswell & Clark, 2018). Published studies using this strategy may be more difficult to identify in the literature because the two phases sometimes are published separately. Amorim, Alves, Kelly-Irving, and Silva (2019), however, published the findings of their explanatory sequential mixed methods study in one article. In Portugal, Amorim et al. (2019) were concerned that the needs of parents were not being met when their preterm infants were in the neonatal intensive care unit (NICU). They provided the rationale for the study by describing previous research findings based on data collected primarily from mothers and by pointing out that very few studies had included the characteristics of the unit and infant. The researchers collected quantitative data from parents during their child's hospitalization in the NICU. Trained interviewers administered the NICU Family Needs Inventory (Ward, 2001) to parents separately ($N = 207$). Parents were asked to rate each of 56 need statements on a scale of 1 (not important) to 4 (very important). Data about pregnancy complications and the infant's weight and gestation were collected from the medical records. Four months after the birth of the child, the parents who agreed to be contacted were interviewed about their concerns, decisions, and needs. The interviews were conducted with the parents as a couple in their homes or other locations of convenience. Amorim et al. (2019) described their study in the following excerpt.

"By integrating quantitative and qualitative data, this study aims to explore needs of mothers and fathers of very preterm infants hospitalised in NICU according to their socioeconomic position, obstetric history and infant's characteristics.... This observational mixed methods study used a sequential explanatory design, whereby the quantitative data were first collected to provide a general overview of the most valued needs and gender specific differences, followed by an interpretation of qualitative data to refine, explain and expand those statistical results (Creswell, 2015)...." (Amorim et al., 2019, p. 89)

"The sample of young parents (70% under 35 years of age) identified the need for assurance as the most important. The medians for all of the need categories fell between 3.1 and 3.9 on the 1 to 4 scale. Amorim et al. (2019) integrated the quantitative and qualitative data in a table with the first two columns being the need categories and the items that were rated very important by 90% of the participants. The third and fourth columns were key ideas from the interviews matched to the need categories. The researchers were able to draw conclusions using both types of data."

"Quantitative data suggest gender differences in factors associated with the importance attributed to parental needs: mothers valued more information needs than fathers and their overall scores were mainly influenced by age and level of education, while fathers' perception of their needs was mainly influenced by previous children. ...All interviewees mentioned the need for instrumental support from the government for facilitating the presence of both mothers and fathers in NICU, and for regular emotional support from psychologists and social workers.... This knowledge will contribute to...reducing social inequalities and the stress created by financial hardship and dealing with bureaucracy in caring for a very preterm baby. This is particularly significant in the context of the socio-economic situation that parents find themselves in." (Amorim et al., 2019, p. 94)

"This mixed methods study draws attention to family-friendly and gender-equality policies for supporting quality family-centred and integrated healthcare services in Neonatology. ...this study raises awareness for the need of flexibility and sensitivity in developing conceptual frameworks and instruments to assess parental needs that take notice of socioeconomic position and reproductive trajectories of parents, as well as issues of privacy and regular emotional support in NICU." (Amorim et al., 2019, p. 95)

Amorim et al. (2019) noted that the categorization of the items into the need categories was subjective and warrants further review. They noted other limitations to be interviewing the parents together, which may have prevented a parent from discussing sensitive issues in the presence of the other parent. The researchers identified the length of the inventory to be another limitation. The quantitative and qualitative findings complemented each other and provided a deeper understanding of parental needs during a child's hospitalization in the NICU.

Convergent Concurrent Designs

The **convergent concurrent design** is a more familiar approach to researchers. This type of design is selected when a researcher wishes to use quantitative and qualitative methods in an attempt to confirm, cross-validate, or corroborate findings within a single study. Quantitative and qualitative data are collected at the same time, frequently from the same sample. With convergent concurrent designs, the two methods are used to complement each other. This strategy usually integrates the results of the two methods during the interpretation phase, and convergence strengthens the knowledge claims, whereas the lack of convergence identifies areas for future studies or theory development (Fig. 14.3). Researchers must have significant expertise and be willing to exert extensive effort to study a phenomenon with two methods. Because two different methods are used, researchers are challenged with the difficulty of comparing the study results from each arm of the study and determining the overriding findings. It is still unclear how best to resolve discrepancies in findings between methods (Creswell & Clark, 2018).

In 2016, the World Health Organization supported an initiative to reduce maternal and infant death due to sepsis that included an awareness campaign and the Global Maternal Sepsis Study (GLOSS) in 53 countries (Brizuela et al., 2019). The purpose of the study was to determine the burden and management of maternal sepsis. Each country had a coordinator to ensure the study and the awareness campaign were implemented as planned. Brizuela et al. (2019) conducted a convergent

concurrent mixed methods study with a baseline survey of sepsis awareness and interviews of key informants. The researchers reviewed health communication and behavioral theories to develop a framework around which they designed the study.

> "This study sought to understand what factors influence healthcare provider awareness regarding the identification and management of maternal sepsis, including challenges and opportunities to increase awareness.... Qualitative and quantitative data were collected between July and November 2017....We took a purposive sample of GLOSS regional and country coordinators for the interviews because they were respectively in charge of coordinating broad aspects of the study at the regional level and implementing the study on the ground.... All the recorded interviews were transcribed verbatim and corroborated with notes taken during the interviewing.... We developed a 32-question survey to gather information on healthcare provider awareness on maternal sepsis.... The surveys were distributed primarily through an online platform, SurveyMonkey or Qualtrics, allowing us to reach a large audience. Online surveys were administered in eight languages...." (Brizuela et al., 2019, pp. 2–3)

From 13 interviews of regional and country coordinators, 24 subconcepts emerged that were categorized according to the four constructs of the framework: (1) severity of maternal health conditions, (2) determinants of maternal health, (3) barriers to

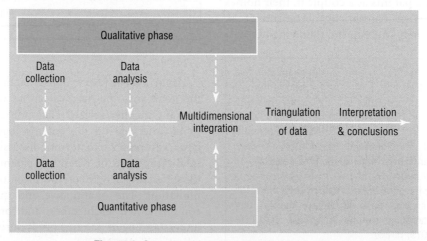

Fig. 14.3 Convergent concurrent mixed methods.

identifying and managing maternal sepsis, and (4) facilitators to identify and manage maternal sepsis. The survey was completed by 1555 healthcare leaders and providers in 48 of the 53 participating countries. Most of the participants (92%) were aware of maternal sepsis but could not identify the diagnostic characteristics.

> "Awareness on maternal sepsis remains low. Correct identification and management of maternal sepsis is deficient and the environments in which healthcare providers work are not optimal for them to accurately understand and respond to maternal sepsis. The factors that mostly influence awareness of healthcare providers on maternal sepsis are training and qualifications.... A campaign aimed at increasing awareness among providers in multiple countries has the potential to improve awareness for sepsis identification and management. This study provided a more in-depth understanding of the factors affecting provider awareness of maternal sepsis allowing for the development of a campaign, as well as a sound basis upon which to evaluate campaign impact and effectiveness." (Brizuela et al., 2019, p. 9)

Brizuela et al. (2019) conducted an international mixed methods study in which they integrated the data according to the structure of their conceptual framework. The data were collected within 5 months, an accomplishment that would not have occurred without adequate funding and staffing. The convergent concurrent design was appropriate for the study purpose and provided a multidimensional description of maternal sepsis that was needed as a baseline for the global awareness campaign.

CHALLENGES OF MIXED METHODS DESIGNS

Throughout the chapter, we have alluded to some of the challenges of implementing mixed methods studies. In this section, we explicitly identify and describe the challenges related to the functioning of the research team, having the resources needed for a mixed methods study, interpreting different types of data, and displaying data integration.

Functioning of the Research Team

Mixed methods studies require a team of researchers with skills in different methods (Creswell, 2015; Poth, 2018).

Effective research teams allow a team member's lack of a specific skill to be balanced by another member's strength in that area (Molina-Azorin & Fetters, 2019). The more complex the research problem, the greater the need for team members to "capitalize on their differences in perspectives, experiences, and assumptions" and to create a synergistic team that multiplies its effectiveness (Poth, 2018, p. 207). Not every member of a team requires specialized skills. A generalist with a wide range of experiences may contribute to the team by promoting harmony (Bazeley, 2018) and being the member of the team with expertise in communication and teamwork. In a study proposal, researchers must provide information about the feasibility of completing the study, which is dependent to a great extent on the expertise of the team members and their ability to work together.

Teams consisting of members from different professions and disciplines are likely to have some conflicts due to contrasting philosophical views about research (Sendall, McCosker, Brodie, Hill, & Crane, 2018). For example, a member with expertise in quantitative methods may not value the contributions of qualitative researchers. The member with qualitative expertise may not understand hypothesis testing and not contribute to the discussion about those results.

Box 14.2 contains characteristics of effective research teams in the top half of the box. Effective research teams are needed for studies in which a single methodology is implemented, such as a

---

BOX 14.2 Characteristics of Effective Teams Implementing Mixed Methods Research

Research Teams
- Clear goals and expectations
- Manageable size
- Specified roles
- Respectful communication
- Members possess expertise needed for the study
- Members willing to collaborate with others
- Members accountable for completing tasks

Mixed Methods Research Teams
- Strong leader who is a role model
- Roles adapted to changing conditions
- Egalitarian communication
- Members willing to innovative
- Members willing to learn new skills

quasi-experimental quantitative study. The lower half of the box includes those characteristics that are especially needed for teams conducting mixed methods studies (Poth, 2018). Mixed methods research teams need many of the same characteristics as any other research team but with more flexibility. Flexible practices and roles are needed for mixed methods research teams to adapt to unforeseen results and conflicts.

Extra time may be required for research teams to come to agreement on the study purpose, design, methods, and findings. Points of disagreement among team members may become a deterrent to study completion. The major challenges of working with a team can be prevented by identifying expectations of team members and being respectful of each person's opinions (Sendall et al., 2018). Expectations of the team members need to be in writing, including order of authors on the planned publications, standards of research integrity, and conflict resolution processes.

Use of Resources

As you can surmise from the examples provided in the chapter, mixed methods studies may require additional resources and more time to complete than single method studies. Amorim et al. (2019) collected data from seven NICUs in the northern region of Portugal. To do that, five members of the team were trained as data collectors to administer a needs inventory during the hospitalization. Between July 2013 and June 2014, the five team members assisted 207 individual parents to complete the needs inventory. Then the team members extracted additional information from the medical record about the pregnancy and characteristics of 122 infants. Approximately 4 months after the initial data collection, the team members selected a purposive sample from the couples who agreed to be contacted for a qualitative follow-up interview. The team interviewed 26 couples in their homes, a conference room at the university, or a private room at the hospital, with the average length of the interview being 39 minutes. A significant resource of time was required to collect the sequential study's data (Amorim et al., 2019). From this information about the data collection, you may realize that the study required extensive resources in the form of time and effort.

Sequential designs require collection and analysis of data amassed during the first phase of the study before moving to the second phase. This lengthens the time required to complete the study. Creswell and Clark (2018) note that the exploratory sequential mixed method design takes the most time to implement. Sequential methods are not recommended when the researcher has limited time to complete a degree or establish a trajectory of research for advancement on tenure track at a university (Creswell & Clark, 2018).

Conducting mixed methods studies, like other complex designs, requires financial resources. Because of the length of time required for sequential designs and the complexity of concurrent designs, funding is usually needed to ensure that the study is completed. Funding may be needed to compensate team members for travel expenses related to attending team meetings, or the principal researcher may need to purchase access to online meeting software to host Web meetings. Individual researchers may need to hire a consultant to provide guidance for the component of the study with which the researcher is less familiar. All of these strategies require additional funding.

Interpreting Quantitative and Qualitative Data

In sequential mixed methods studies, whether exploratory or explanatory, the results from one phase is the basis for the detailed methods of the second phase. For example, in an exploratory sequential mixed methods study, the researchers may analyze the data from interviews to identify key concepts of a phenomenon and select appropriate instruments for the quantitative phase. The dependence of the second phase on the finding of the first phase means that the quantitative and qualitative data are not directly combined. Interpreting the results of quantitative and qualitative data analyses primarily occurs in convergent concurrent mixed methods studies. The proposal for these studies should include a tentative plan for combining the data as part of understanding the results and answering the research questions.

Triangulation

Historically, mixed methods studies were characterized by triangulation. **Triangulation** is drawing conclusions based on multiple points of data, multiple types of data, or multiple research approaches. When the data converge, the results are verified or corroborated (Creamer, 2018). Fig. 14.4 displays triangulation as simple convergence. The researchers identify areas of

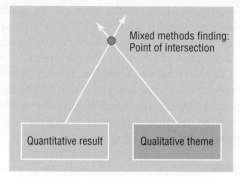

Fig. 14.4 Triangulation with convergence.

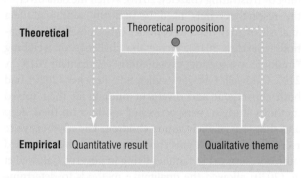

Fig. 14.5 Triangulation of empirical results and theoretical statements.

agreement among the various perspectives and types of data to draw conclusions. For example, a researcher conducts a mixed methods study in which participants complete a quality of life instrument and are interviewed about quality of life. To triangulate, the researcher would compare participants' statements to the instrument items having the highest means. The instances in which the qualitative data and quantitative data agree are areas of convergence.

Another type of triangulation is shown in Fig. 14.5, a visual representation of empirical-theoretical triangulation. For example, a team of researchers plans a series of studies to develop and test an effective intervention or bundle of interventions to improve medication adherence among persons newly diagnosed with hypertension. From their review of relevant theories and research reports, they identified one research problem to be the lack of evidence of whether there are gender differences in factors that influence medication adherence. They state the theoretical proposition as: "Gender, access to care, and self-efficacy influence

medication adherence." In Fig. 14.5, the proposition is represented by the arrows down from the theoretical level toward the empirical level.

The research team designs a mixed methods study to gather data that will either support or fail to support the proposition. Using a concurrent convergent design (see Fig. 14.3), they collect quantitative data about adherence from 120 persons diagnosed with hypertension in the past 6 months and prescribed at least one antihypertensive medication. The quantitative instrument yields a total adherence score and a ranking of possible factors affecting medication adherence. From the quantitative sample, every other person is asked to participate in an interview until at least 40 interviews have been conducted or data saturation occurs. The data collected represent the empirical level in Fig. 14.5. The results of the quantitative and qualitative phases are compared to the theoretical proposition to evaluate whether the results support the proposition. The arrows from the empirical level (quantitative and qualitative results) to the theoretical level indicate that the findings were integrated at the theory level (see Fig. 14.5).

Integration and Convergence

Combining data is also known as integration. **Integration** is the combining and comparing of a study's qualitative and quantitative results and methods. The process may include assimilating one type of data into the other, identifying similarities and differences, and linking the data within a theoretical framework. The goal of integration may be enactment of a policy, stimulating community or individual actions, or simply understanding a phenomenon or situation comprehensively (Steinmetz-Wood, Pluye, & Ross, 2019). Integration of findings is crucial to mixed methods and can be very challenging to accomplish (Lynam et al., 2019).

Similarities across the types of data and the analyses are points of convergence. Tasseff, Tavernier, Watkins, and Neill (2018) conducted a convergent parallel (concurrent) mixed methods study with rural dwelling healthcare providers, nurses, and adults in the community exploring the topic of palliative care. They conducted 25 interviews with providers, nurses, and adults to explore their definitions and knowledge of palliative care. The qualitative data were analyzed for subthemes and themes. The themes that emerged indicated a lack of knowledge about the meaning and purposes of palliative care. Tasseff et al. (2018) also collected quantitative data from 51 rural dwelling providers ($n = 7$) and nurses ($n = 44$) using the Palliative Care Knowledge Test (PCKT) to compare the differences in knowledge between providers and nurses and between those who had received palliative care education and those who had not received such education. The 20-item PCKT was dichotomously scored as correct/not correct, with one point for each correct answer. The mean score on the PCKT for the entire group was 10.73 (*SD* 2.93), reflecting extremely low scores. The researchers included several statements in the discussion and conclusions that indicated convergence of the findings.

> "The low PCKT scores obtained by rural providers and rural nurses, when combined with the key themes that palliative care is perceived as end-of-life care, makes it alarmingly clear that significant changes are needed to improve the quality of provider and nurse academic preparation and continuing education related to palliative care." (Tasseff et al., 2018, pp. 179–180)
>
> "Considering the results of this small-scale study, coupled with the evidence presented by existing research, it can be concluded that the misperceptions and poor knowledge related to palliative care likely prevent the broader application of palliative care in the rural and highly rural areas where this study was conducted...palliative care, when offered as a vital component of comprehensive primary care in rural areas, may provide the best opportunity for rural adults to remain active and age in place." (Tasseff et al., 2019, p. 182)

In this study, the quantitative and qualitative data supported the same conclusions. The researchers cautioned, however, that the sample was small and the study was conducted in only two counties.

Convergence may also be documented by converting qualitative data to quantitative data. Essentially, this means using qualitative data to generate (quantitative) counts of the frequency with which various codes or themes occurred. For example, Cotner et al. (2018) conducted a convergent concurrent mixed methods study (see Fig. 14.3) to assess quality of life among veterans with spinal cord injuries who participated in an individual placement and support program that was designed to help them find competitive employment. The sample ($N = 213$) was divided into three groups based

on employment status at the time of the qualitative interview: the veterans who were employed; those who were not employed but later became employed; and those who did not find employment during the 24-month study. The researchers counted the number of veterans in each group who made comments that fit into the subthemes and themes identified during the qualitative analysis. The differences in frequencies between the three groups confirmed the quantitative findings.

Divergence

Researchers using convergent concurrent mixed method designs may find divergence or dissonance to be unsettling or frustrating (Bazeley, 2018). When the data diverge, the researchers may need to perform additional data analysis or may need to consider other possible explanations (Bazeley, 2018), facing the challenge of weighing "multiple competing explanations" (Creamer, 2018, p. 219). Caldwell, Ordway, Sadler, and Redeker (2020) had both convergent and divergent findings in their mixed methods study of perspectives of mothers on their sleep and the sleep of their young children. The mothers were recruited through a government program that provided nutrition support to families living in poverty. Caldwell et al. (2020) allowed the qualitative methods to determine the sample size, continuing to recruit and interview mothers until data saturation was reached. The mothers ($N = 32$) completed scales measuring their sleep quality, depression, and risk for apnea. They also completed scales describing the child's behavior and sleep habits.

> "Many mothers reported in interviews that their children had no problems sleeping. However, these reports contrasted with the questionnaire data that indicated that many children had shorter than adequate sleep duration relative to normative data, variable sleep onset and offset times.... The discrepancy between some mothers' positive perceptions of sleep and information provided on the Children's Sleep Habits Questionnaire [CSHQ] are consistent with previous reports of discrepancy (Molfese et al., 2015) and suggests that educational and behavioral interventions can help clear misconceptions about sleep. Providing simple information about normative sleep requirements for children's developmental stages may help clarify these possible misconceptions, especially given the findings from the CSHQ that some children had sleep problems." (Caldwell et al., 2020, pp. 8, 10)

The divergence of the quantitative and qualitative data related to mothers' perspectives on the sleep of the children was not totally unexpected because it had occurred in at least one other study. Caldwell et al. (2020) used the discrepancy as the basis for one of their recommendations about educational interventions for mothers living in economical adversity. They recommended that educational interventions include information about the sleep needs of children at different stages of development.

Divergent or dissonant results from the qualitative and quantitative analyses may be explainable through using theory, identifying and comparing extreme cases, and considering the possible effects of social desirability. Researchers who encounter divergence or dissonance are

referred to Bazeley (2018) for additional information and examples.

Displaying Convergence and Divergence

Depending on the purposes of the mixed methods study, presentation of findings can be accomplished using various types of graphs, tables, and figures (Creswell & Clark, 2018; Curry & Nunez-Smith, 2015). Table 14.4 provides possible ways to display the findings of studies with different motivations and strategies. This section will provide examples of how different types of displays might be used to integrate and report findings. Some examples are from the literature, and others were created by the authors to illustrate a type of display.

TABLE 14.4 Integration and Display of Quantitative and Qualitative Results for Different Mixed Method Designs

Strategy	Study Goal	Type of Display	Description
Exploratory sequential	Use qualitative findings to develop a quantitative instrument or intervention	Construction of instrument display	Table: First column with quote or theme; second column has the item(s) developed from the specific finding.
Exploratory sequential	Add quantitative findings to the qualitative findings	Expanding perspective display	Table: First column with qualitative study finding; second column has supportive evidence that may be numerical or textual.
Explanatory sequential	Explain the quantitative results using qualitative results	Follow-up results joint display	Table: First column with quantitative findings; second column has the corresponding additional information from the qualitative component; third column has information articulating the links between the two types of data.
Convergent concurrent	Display findings that converge between the components	Matrix of interpretation of convergence and divergence	Matrix: First column of each row is filled with the qualitative results (themes or patterns); columns are labeled with quantitative variables; cells contain findings that result from the integration of that theme and variable. Not all cells will be filled.
Convergent concurrent	Identify similarities (convergence) and differences (divergence) between the two types of data	Matrix/graph of points of convergence and divergence	Matrix/graph: x-axis is the quantitative findings by question or variable; y-axis is the themes or qualitative findings. Where findings converge, mark the point with a plus sign; where findings diverge, mark the point with a negative sign.

Adapted from Creswell, J. W. (2015). *A concise introduction to mixed methods research*. Los Angeles, CA: Sage; Creswell, J. W., & Clark, P. (2018). *Designing and conducting mixed methods research* (3rd ed.). Thousand Oaks, CA: Sage.

TABLE 14.5 Veteran-Identified Quality of Life Outcomes From Participating in Individual Placement and Support by Type of Participant

Themes	PARTICIPANT EMPLOYMENT STATUS AT TIME OF INTERVIEW		
	Employed ($n = 54$)n (%)	Unemployed, Became Employed ($n = 37$)n (%)	Never Became Employed ($n = 60$)
Productivity			
Contribute to society	33 (61)	19 (51)	18 (30)
Earn an income	14 (26)	16 (43)	12 (22)
Maintain employment: On the job modifications	13 (24)	0 (0)	0 (0)

Table adapted from Table 3 in Cotner et al. (2018). Quality of life outcomes for veterans with spinal cord injury receiving individual placement and support (IPS). *Topics in Spinal Cord Injury Rehabilitation, 24*(4), 325–335. doi:10.1310/sci 17-00046

The study by Cotner et al. (2018) among veterans with spinal cord injuries was described earlier in the chapter as an example of convergence. They displayed the convergence using a table. Table 14.5 is a portion of a table in the Cotner et al. (2018) article. The table divides the participants into three groups based on their employment status and then displays the number of participants in each group whose comments supported the productivity theme's subthemes of contributing to society, earning an income, and maintaining employment. Johnson, Grove, and Clarke (2019) labeled this type of integration as data transformation. **Data transformation**, in the context of mixed methods studies, is changing qualitative data to a quantitative format, usually by counting the number of times a specific theme is noted by the participants. Data transformation may also involve using the wording of highly rated items on a questionnaire as additional qualitative data to be considered during qualitative analysis.

Five tables are provided as examples of integrating qualitative and quantitative data using different types of displays. To allow you to compare the displays across the tables, we use the same data for all of them. Because no published studies were found that used multiple types of tables to display integration of the same data, we chose to use data from a study we invented. The invented study was conducted with adolescents to understand their intent to change their health behaviors.

For Table 14.6, the invented study used an exploratory sequential design to develop an instrument (see Fig. 14.1).

TABLE 14.6 Example of a Display for an Invented Exploratory Sequential Study of Adolescents' Intent to Change Health Behaviors: Developing an Instrument

Quotation From a Participant	Resulting Item on Instrument
"When I looked in the mirror and saw how fat I looked, I knew I had to stop eating junk food and eat healthy food."	My appearance motivates me to eat healthier.
"Some of my friends are real health nuts and it is easier to exercise and eat right around them. Other of my friends think exercising is texting their friends."	My health-related behaviors are influenced by whom I hang out with.
"I tried going to the gym and there wasn't anyone my age who was there. The music they used during classes was really old-school."	I want to exercise in a safe place with other people my age. When I exercise, I want to listen to my favorite music.
"I have a job at a fast-food restaurant. I can eat for free, but there isn't much on the menu that is healthy. I can't afford to bring fruit and healthier snacks."	I eat healthier when in a place with many healthy foods on the menu. The cost influences my food choices.

Data from an invented study to develop an instrument to measure "intent to change health behaviors among adolescents."

Table 14.6 is a display for connecting the qualitative findings to the items of the instrument being developed. For example, in the first row, a participant's quote is included: "When I looked in the mirror and saw how fat I looked, I knew I had to stop eating junk food and eat healthy food." The second column contains an item for an instrument to measure intent to change: "My appearance motivates me to eat healthier." The subsequent rows are similar examples of participants' quotations being translated into instrument items.

For the remaining tables, the invented study's design was changed to a convergent concurrent design (see Fig. 14.3). The participants were interviewed and then asked to complete instruments measuring self-efficacy, body image, healthy food choices, and peer pressure.

Table 14.7 displays the similarities of the participants' quotes from interviews in the first column and the related quantitative findings in the second column. For example, in the first row the participant's quote, "When I looked in the mirror and saw how fat I looked, I knew I had to stop eating junk food and eat healthy food," was compared to the sample's mean score on the body image scale and the relationship found between body image and healthy food choices.

Table 14.8 includes a column for integration in addition to columns for quantitative and qualitative results. The first column contains quantitative results, such as low scores on self-efficacy. Continuing across on the first row of Table 14.8, the second column includes quotes from the interviews that reflect low self-efficacy

TABLE 14.7 Example Display for an Invented Exploratory Sequential Study of Adolescents' Intent to Change Health Behaviors: Expanding Perspectives

Participants' Quotes	Related Quantitative Finding
"When I looked in the mirror and saw how fat I looked, I knew I had to stop eating junk food and eat healthy food."	$M = 4.5$ ($SD = 0.8$) on the Body Image Scale $r = 0.4$ ($p = 0.001$) between body image and healthy food choices
"Some of my friends are real health nuts and it is easier to exercise and eat right around them. Other of my friends think exercising is texting their friends."	$r = -0.28$ ($p = 0.01$) between sensitivity to peer pressure and healthy food choices
"I tried going to the gym and there wasn't anyone my age who was there. The music they used during classes was really old-school."	Response to open-ended question about reasons for not exercising: "No gyms where my age goes"
"I have a job at a fast-food restaurant. I can eat for free, but there isn't much on the menu that is healthy. I can't afford to bring fruit and healthier snacks."	Subjects with lower incomes scored lower on Healthy Food Choice Scale than subjects with higher incomes ($t = 8.3$, $df = 1$, $p = 0.05$)

Data from an invented study to provide an expanded perspective on the intent of adolescents to change their health behaviors.

TABLE 14.8 Example Display for an Explanatory Sequential Study: Follow-Up Results Joint Display

Quantitative Results	Qualitative Results	Integration
Low scores on self-efficacy related to healthy eating	"I never know what to eat at a party." "I usually eat what everyone else is eating."	Lack of knowledge may contribute to low self-efficacy related to healthy eating.
Significant difference in knowledge of healthy foods between adolescents with higher incomes and adolescents with lower incomes	"There is no grocery store in my neighborhood, only a convenience store on the corner." "I've read about nutritious fruits like kiwi and cantaloupe but I don't even know what they are. No one eats that kind of thing where I live."	Adolescents living in lower income neighborhoods may have limited access and exposure to healthy foods.

Integration of data from an invented study to explain adolescents' intent to change their health behaviors using a mixed methods study.

related to healthy food choices. The third column of the first row contains a summary statement of the integration of the previous two columns.

Table 14.9 is an example of a matrix. A matrix display is helpful when there are convergence and divergence of quantitative and qualitative data. In the cell at

the juxtaposition of a column and row, the positive sign is used to show convergence and the negative sign is used to show divergence. For example, in the first row, the theme "desire to fit in" diverged from the quantitative results related to self-efficacy, so a negative sign is displayed. Table 14.10 is another type of matrix, displaying the integration of the findings from the same invented study of adolescents' intent to change health behaviors. Instead of a mathematical symbol in the cell at the juxtaposition of a column and a row, there is a short phrase of the integration.

No matter the specific design of a mixed methods study, articulate your plans to integrate the data in the study proposal (Steinmetz-Wood et al., 2019). It is critical to make at least tentative decisions about integrating the data as you plan the study. The plans may need to be adjusted during the study, but they provide the structure needed to successfully complete the study.

CRITICALLY APPRAISING MIXED METHODS DESIGNS

Over 500 tools have been developed to appraise quantitative, qualitative, and mixed methods studies (Hong et al., 2019). Some researchers have argued for treating mixed methods studies as two separate studies and appraising

---

TABLE 14.9 Example Display for a Convergent Concurrent Study: Matrix Graph of Points of Convergence and Divergence

Qualitative Themes	QUANTITATIVE RESULTS				
	Body image	Self-efficacy	Knowledge	Environment	Behaviors
Desire to fit in		(−)			
Inner beauty	+			(−)	+
Knowing I can do it			+	+	+
Access to healthy foods	(−)		(−)	+	+
"Cool" place to exercise				(−)	+

Note: Convergence noted by positive sign. Divergence noted by negative sign.
Integration of data from an invented study to explain adolescents' intent to change their health behaviors using a mixed methods study.

TABLE 14.10 Example Display for a Convergent Concurrent Study: Matrix of Interpretation of Convergence and Divergence

Qualitative Themes	QUANTITATIVE FINDINGS				
	Body Image	Self-Efficacy	Knowledge	Environment	Behaviors
Desire to fit in				Being accepted in my neighborhood	
Inner beauty	Positive view of self				
Knowing I can do it		Strong belief in self			Healthy behaviors require commitment
Access to healthy foods			Without access, hard to know	Neighborhood makes a difference	
"Cool" place to exercise	No mirrors but great music				Easier to exercise in an adolescent-friendly place

Note: Cells contain findings that result from the integration of that theme and variable.
Integration of data from an invented study to explain adolescents' intent to change their health behaviors using a mixed methods study.

each phase by the appropriate qualitative or quantitative criteria. However, this approach fails to address mixed methods' unique characteristic of combining two types of data. Standards are needed to address the integration of the two types of data. The Mixed Methods Appraisal Tool (MMAT) was developed to appraise the quality of quantitative, qualitative, and mixed methods studies as part of conducting a mixed methods research synthesis (Pluye, Gagnon, Griffiths, & Johnson-Lafleur, 2009). The MMAT has five broad standards by which to appraise

mixed methods studies. Other standards have been developed to appraise the quality of mixed methods studies (Creswell, 2015; Creswell & Clark, 2018; Fábregues, Paré, & Meneses, 2019).

For this text, we have synthesized standards across sources, resulting in a concise set of quality standards for mixed methods research (Table 14.11). Building on the foundation of your knowledge of quantitative and qualitative methods, learning how to critique mixed methods studies extends your capacity as a scholar.

TABLE 14.11   Criteria for Critically Appraising Mixed Methods Studies

Study Characteristic	Questions Used to Guide the Appraisal
Significance	1. Was the relevance of the research question convincingly described?
	2. Was the need to use mixed methods established?
Expertise	3. Did the researcher or research team possess the necessary skills and experience to rigorously implement the study?
	4. Were the contributions or expertise of each team member noted?
Appropriateness	5. Were the study purposes aligned with the mixed methods strategy that was used?
	6. Did the mixed methods strategy fulfill the purpose(s) of the study?
Sampling	7. Was the rationale for selecting the samples for each component of the study provided?
	8. Were study participants selected who were able to provide data needed to address the research question?
Methods	9. Were the data collection methods for each study component appropriate for the philosophical foundation of that component?
	10. Were the methods for each component of the study described in detail?
	11. Were the reliability and validity of quantitative methods described?
	12. Were the trustworthiness, dependability, and credibility of qualitative methods described?
	13. Were the timing of data collection, analysis, interpretation, and integration of the data specified?
	14. Was protection of human subjects addressed in the study?
Findings	15. Was the integration of quantitative and qualitative findings presented visually in a table, graph, or matrix?
	16. Was the integration presented as a narrative?
	17. Were the study limitations noted?
	18. Were the findings consistent with the analysis, interpretation, and integration of the qualitative and quantitative data?
Conclusions and implications	19. Were the conclusions and implications congruent with the findings of the study?
Contribution to knowledge	20. Was the study's contribution to knowledge worth the time and resources of a mixed methods study?

Synthesized from Creswell, J. W. (2015). *A concise introduction to mixed methods research.* Thousand Oaks, CA: Sage; Creswell, J., & Creswell, D. (2018). *Research design: Qualitative, quantitative, and mixed methods approaches* (5th ed.). Thousand Oaks, CA: Sage; Creswell, J., & Clark, V. (2018). *Designing and conducting mixed methods research* (3rd ed.). Thousand Oaks, CA: Sage.

The standards of quality displayed in Table 14.11 provide a systematic method for critically appraising mixed methods studies. Using the quality standards proposed, a critical appraisal of a mixed methods study conducted by Whipple et al. (2019) is provided as an example.

Summary of the Study

Older persons with peripheral artery disease (PAD) and type 2 diabetes mellitus (DM) have several potential barriers to physical activity. Whipple et al. (2019) conducted a study of older adults with PAD and DM using a "concurrent mixed methods multiple-case study design" (p. 94). The effects of PAD and DM on exercise had not been simultaneously assessed along with the effects of geriatric syndromes, such as falls, cognitive impairment, and urinary incontinence. The researchers used the social ecological model (McLeRoy, Bibeau, Steckler, & Glanz, 1988) as theoretical framework for the study. The variation of the social ecological model they used had an inner circle, labeled "Individual Choice," surrounded by increasing larger circles of "Interpersonal," "Community," and "Public Policy." The framework was selected because the researchers wanted to ensure that the effects of others, the community, and policy were considered as they studied physical activity of older adults. They used the framework to guide first-round coding of the qualitative data. The researchers did a second round of coding using inductive processes.

The researchers recruited participants who also had diabetes from a supervised exercise program for persons with PAD. Data were collected at one visit from each of the 10 participants, 8 of whom were men. The researchers uniquely combined data from semistructured interviews; the Exercise Benefits and Barriers Scale (EBBS) (Sechrist, Walker, & Pender, 1987); functional measures and the Short Physical Performance Battery; measures of walking impairment, quality of life, and geriatric syndromes; and accelerometry of physical activity and sedentary time (Whipple et al., 2019). The participants were given an accelerometer to wear for the 2 weeks following the visit.

The semistructured interviews revealed the barriers to physical activity were "lack of accessibility, lack of enjoyment of activity, lack of motivation, and pain and physical health" (Whipple et al., 2019, p. 96). The participants shared that "social support, accessibility and convenience, and enjoyment of the activity" were facilitators

of physical activity whereas the benefits were "energy, mobility and physical health, and sense of accomplishment" (Whipple et al., 2019, p. 99). Each of the themes were supported by quotes from the participants.

A multiple case study design has in-depth data about a small number of cases (Yin, 2018). Because of the smaller number of participants, descriptive analyses of the quantitative data were conducted. Whipple et al. (2019) integrated qualitative and quantitative results using matrices. The first matrix listed the participants by their pseudonyms, one per row. The mean scores for the different quantitative measures were listed on the row as well as the qualitative barriers and facilitators identified by that participant. Two additional tables combined the qualitative and quantitative results in different ways.

Key findings were that the participants who feared falling reported higher barriers to physical activity, had higher levels of sedentary time, and were able to walk shorter distances during the 6-minute walk test. By integrating the qualitative and quantitative data, the researchers found the participants who mentioned increased energy or sense of accomplishment as benefits of physical activity in the interviews had higher scores on the benefit domains of the EBBS. Among the EBBS items for barriers and the interviews, participants who reported lack of enjoyment as a barrier also identified time expenditure as a barrier. Whipple et al. (2019) concluded that the findings of the mixed methods study provided insight and warranted further research. The goal would be to develop interventions to reduce perceived barriers to physical activity among persons with PAD and diabetes. The following sections cover the critical appraisal of the Whipple et al. (2019) study using the criteria in Table 14.11.

Significance

Whipple et al. (2019) established the relevance and significance of physical activity for persons with PAD and diabetes by providing the number of people affected by these conditions and the consequences. The researchers noted 10% to 15% of Americans over age 65 have PAD. In addition to decreasing the person's physical functioning, PAD increases the risk of morbidity and mortality, especially related to cardiovascular disease. The combination of PAD and diabetes increases the likelihood of poor health more than either disease alone (Whipple et al., 2019).

Whipple et al. (2019) linked the significance of the research topic with the rationale for using a mixed methods design.

"...there are no studies that collect and integrate assessments of both perceived barriers to physical activity and actual engagement in physical activity. Both subjectively assessed perceptions and objectively measured activity levels are key to understanding the impact of barriers to physical activity and developing strategies to address those barriers...there are no studies that integrate simultaneous assessment of both perceived barriers to physical activity and the actual degree of engagement in physical activity among older adults with PAD and diabetes. This type of integration is key to understanding the impact of barriers on physical activity and developing strategies to address those barriers. As these issues could not be adequately addressed through the use of only qualitative or only quantitative techniques, we conducted a mixed methods study.... This design was appropriate for the present study because a single method (e.g. qualitative or quantitative) was deemed insufficient to fully evaluate barriers to physical activity and engagement in physical activity among older adults with PAD and diabetes." (Whipple et al., 2019, pp. 92–94)

The researchers highlighted the need for qualitative and quantitative methods to understand barriers, benefits, and facilitators of physical activity in a unique population of persons with both PAD and diabetes.

Expertise

Dr. Whipple's doctoral education was funded by a grant from the National Hartford Center of Gerontological Nursing Excellence. Her dissertation, the study we are appraising, was funded by a predoctoral award from the National Institute of Nursing Research and another grant from the National Center for Advancing Translational Sciences (see Chapter 19), a component in the National Institutes of Health (NIH). At the time the article was written, she was a PhD candidate and working with the Adult and Gerontological Health Cooperative at the University of Minnesota. Her clinical specialty of gerontological nursing along with her developing research skills were supported by her PhD advisor, Dr. Erica Schorr, and her dissertation committee. Dr. Whipple is currently a postdoctoral fellow in the geriatric medicine division at the University of Colorado.

The rest of the research team made various contributions to the study. In addition to her role as Dr. Whipple's advisor, Dr. Schorr contributed her clinical expertise with cardiovascular disease, specifically PAD, and her knowledge of mixed methods as a research methodology. Dr. Kristine Talley, a certified nurse practitioner in gerontology, had conducted studies of urinary continence in older adults, one of the geriatric syndromes included in the study (Talley, Wyman, & Shamliyan, 2011). Dr. Ruth Lindquist is currently the coprimary investigator of an NIH-funded community-based study to reduce heart disease risks among African American men. She is also the lead editor of a textbook about complementary and alternative therapies for nurses (Lindquist, Tracy, & Snyder, 2018). The only non-nurse on the team was Dr. Ulf Bronas, who contributed his expertise in physical activity as an intervention for patients with claudication. Dr. Diane Treat-Jacobson, the last author, is the associate dean for research at the University of Minnesota. She was one of the developers of the Peripheral Artery Disease Quality of Life Questionnaire (Treat-Jacobson et al., 2012) that Dr. Whipple and the team used in the study.

As you may have surmised, the research team for the study had extensive clinical and research expertise as well as the experience of working together on other studies. However, the contributions of each team member to the study were not noted in the publication.

Appropriateness

After establishing the significance of the clinical conditions and identifying the research problem, Whipple et al. (2019) stated the purpose of the study.

"Given the dearth of information related to barriers to and engagement in physical activity among older adults with PAD and diabetes, we conducted a mixed methods study investigating these phenomena.... The purpose of this mixed methods study was to investigate the unique experiences of older adults with PAD and diabetes related to physical activity. We sought to address the following overarching question: How does having PAD and diabetes shape older adults' perceptions of and engagement in physical activity?" (Whipple et al., 2019, pp. 93–94)

The mixed methods methodology fulfilled the study's purpose by providing the researchers the opportunity to address the research problem in a wholistic way. The qualitative aspect of the study allowed the participants' perspectives to be heard. The quantitative aspect of the study measured the physical capacity and actual physical activity of the participants.

Sampling

Collecting quantitative and qualitative data from the same sample was appropriate for the study's convergent concurrent multiple-case study design. The participants were recruited from persons participating in a physical activity program for patients with PAD. The researchers identified those who also had diabetes and approached them about the study. The participants were purposefully selected from an available population because they had the medical conditions addressed by the study, were already involved in physical activity, and were able to provide the data needed to address the research question.

Methods

The quantitative and qualitative data collection methods were appropriate for their specific philosophical foundations. Table 14.12 contains the variables, the specific methods used to collect the quantitative data, and the information provided about the measures'

TABLE 14.12   Reliability and Validity of the Measures: Perceived Barriers, Geriatric Syndromes, and Physical Activity in Persons with Peripheral Artery Disease and Diabetes (Whipple et al., 2019)

Variable(s)	Instrument or Method	Reliability and Validity
Perceived barriers and benefits of physical activity	Exercise Barriers and Benefits Scale (EBBS) (Sechrist, Walker, & Pender, 1987)	"The EBBS has been used in a variety of populations, including older adults, and has good psychometric properties." (Whipple et al., 2019, p. 94)
Standing balance, 4-meter walking velocity, and repeated chair rises	Short Physical Performance Battery (Gularnik et al., 1994)	"This battery has been shown to be effective in characterizing physical function across a broad spectrum of functional status and predictive of mortality and institutionalization across this spectrum (Gularnik et al., 1994)." (Whipple et al., 2019, p. 94)
Disease status	6-Minute walk (6MWT distance) (McDermott et al., 2014)	No information on accuracy, selectivity, and precision
Grip strength	Jamar digital hand dynamometer (Patterson Medical Corp, St. Paul, Minnesota)	"…mean of 3 trials of each hand using a Jamar digital hand dynamometer (Patterson Medical Corp, St. Paul, Minnesota) according to the American Society of Hand Therapists guidelines for measurement of grip strength (Fess, 1992)." (Whipple et al., 2019, p. 95)
Walking impairment	Walking Impairment Questionnaire (Sagar Brown, Zelt, Pickett, & Tranmer, 2012)	"This questionnaire has been shown to correlate well with treadmill walking distance and to be sensitive to change over time (Sagar et al., 2012)." (Whipple et al., 2019, p. 95)
Quality of life	PAD-Specific Quality of Life (PADQOL) Questionnaire (Treat-Jacobson et al., 2012)	No information on reliability and validity
Mental and physical health	Short Form (SF)-36 Health Survey (Ware, 1976, 2000)	"The SF-36 has been used extensively in clinical research (Ware, 2000) and in patients with PAD (Turner-Bowker, Bartley, & Ware, 2002)." (Whipple et al., 2019, p. 95)
Geriatric syndromes related to falling	Question about falls in past month (Lamb et al., 1985)	No information on reliability and validity
Fear of falling	Falls Efficacy Scale-International (FES-I) (Yardley et al., 2005)	No information on reliability and validity
Physical activity and sedentary time	ActiGraph wGTX3-BT (ActiGraph Corp, Pensacola, Florida)	No information about accuracy, selectivity, and precision

psychometric characteristics. The instruments and physical tests used to measure the quantitative variables were described in detail in the narrative. However, limited information was provided about their psychometric characteristics. In contrast, the researchers provided the complete interview guide in the article, which was appropriate for the study emphasis.

> "For this study, priority (emphasis) was given to the qualitative (QUAL) strand. Quantitative (quan) data were used to enhance understanding and contribute to overall completeness.... Each semistructured interview was conducted by the lead author MOW and lasted between 16 and 55 minutes (mean: 37.8 minutes, standard deviation [SD]: 12.1 minutes).... Interviews were audio recorded and transcribed verbatim before analysis. All participants completed the interview before the quantitative survey measures to reduce the potential influence of the measures on the content of the interviews." (Whipple et al., 2019, p. 94)
>
> "Both directed and conventional inductive content analyses were used to identify themes (Hsieh, 2005). After transcription, audio recordings and transcripts were reviewed to ensure the accuracy of transcription...read multiple times to obtain a sense of the interviews as a whole. Interviews were then read individually, and directed content analysis was used to identify themes.... In addition, we used elaborative coding, a second-cycle coding method (Saldana, 2013), to identify additional categories that appeared to represent key concepts or ideas that were not included in the social ecological framework. This second-cycle method was more typical of conventional inductive content analysis (Hsieh, 2005)." (Whipple et al., 2019, p. 96)

Similar to the limited information provided about psychometric properties of the quantitative measures, the researchers also provided limited information about the rigor of the qualitative data collection and analysis. They noted that they produced a detailed audit trail to reduce biases and that each theme was supported by exemplar quotes of the participants.

Whipple et al. (2019) provided a flow chart displaying the concurrent timing of collecting, analyzing, and integrating the quantitative and qualitative data. All data were collected in one session. Each type of data was analyzed independently prior to integration.

Whipple et al. (2019) documented the protection of the study participants' human rights (see Table 14.11) in their research report. The steps taken to protect the rights of the participants were described briefly as follows: "This study was reviewed and approved by the University of Minnesota Institutional Review Board. All participants provided written informed consent. Participants received $50 for the time and inconvenience associated with data collection and were provided with a parking pass for the duration of their visit" (Whipple et al., 2019, p. 94).

You may be thinking that $50 seems like a potentially coercive payment for participating in the study. However, the payment seems reasonable in light of the number of physical and psychological tests (five of each), the time required to complete the tests and interview (over an hour), and the fact that the participants wore the accelerometer for 2 weeks following the data collection session.

Findings

Whipple et al. (2019) presented the integration of the quantitative and qualitative analyses in three matrices or tables (see Table 14.11). One table was identified as a metamatrix with the pseudonyms of the 10 participants listed in the first column. Then for each participant, his or her scores on the accelerometry results, physical measures, and qualitative benefits and facilitators of exercise were provided in the same row. This presentation allowed patterns to be identified. Two additional tables were provided that displayed integration of the interview themes and the quantitative scores on the subscales of the EBBS. The integration was also provided in narrative form.

> "Participants with greater sedentary time and less MVPA [moderate to vigorous physical activity] tended to report greater fear of falling (higher FES-I score) and barriers to physical activity and had slower gait speeds, more difficulty with the chair rise, and lower 6MWT distances.... Some patterns did emerge with respect to scores on the EBBS and qualitative themes. Participants who endorsed increased energy as a benefit of exercise in the interview tended to have higher scores on all the EBBS benefits domains...as did participants who reported that exercise gave them a sense of accomplishment." (Whipple et al., 2019, p. 99)

"The theme "lack of accessibility" from the interviews corresponded most closely to the EBBS domain "exercise milieu," with participants who expressed difficulty with accessibility in their interviews having higher scores on this subscale. Similarly, participants who reported that lack of enjoyment of the activity was a barrier tended to place more importance on the time expenditure involved in exercise as a barrier to activity." (Whipple et al., 2019, p. 101)

The researchers clearly stated one of the study limitations to be the narrow scope of the participants' experiences because they were recruited from current and former PAD patients involved in an exercise program. The small sample included only two women, and saturation was not reached in the interviews. However, even among these participants who had been exercising, the number of and emphasis placed on barriers to exercise were revealing. Whipple et al. (2019) also noted that data about other comorbid conditions were not collected, some participants lacked the physical measure of disease severity in their medical records, and the study was cross sectional. One limitation that was not identified was the lack of data collected about the status of the participants' diabetes, including their glycosylated hemoglobin values and type of medication being used to maintain blood sugar. However, the findings were consistent with the interpretation and integration of the data, the latter being a strength of the study.

Conclusions and Implications

After a thorough discussion of the findings, Whipple et al. (2019) summarized the report of the study with appropriate conclusions and implications for future research.

"In conclusion, this mixed methods study provides rich insight into both the nature of barriers to physical activity and engagement in physical activity among older adults with PAD and diabetes. The integration of both self-reported and objective measures facilitates our understanding of the lived experiences of individuals with these conditions and provides opportunities for future research. The findings of this study can be used to support further investigation into factors that influence engagement in physical activity among individuals with PAD and diabetes and assist in the development of strategies to address perceived barriers, particularly as supervised exercise therapy programs for individuals with PAD become more widely available in clinical care." (Whipple et al., 2019, p. 103)

Contributions to Knowledge

Extensive effort was expended to implement the complicated measures, analyze multiple data points, and integrate the results into the study findings. The effort produced a rigorous study with complex data to be analyzed and interpreted. As a result, the study, despite a small sample, made initial contributions to the evidence needed to improve the care and health outcomes of older adults living in the community with PAD and diabetes.

KEY POINTS

- Mixed methods research designs combine quantitative and qualitative research methods to answer research questions requiring both perspectives.
- Quantitative and qualitative data in mixed methods studies may be collected sequentially or concurrently.
- The philosophical foundation for many mixed methods studies is pragmatism, the philosophy that supports selecting methods for a study based on their ability to address the research problem.
- The three mixed method designs implemented most frequently in nursing research are (1) exploratory sequential designs, (2) explanatory sequential designs, and (3) convergent concurrent designs.

- Exploratory sequential designs may be used when the researcher wants to expand on what is known about a phenomenon and the researcher does not want the content of the quantitative instruments to bias data collected qualitatively.
- When using an exploratory sequential strategy, the researcher collects and analyzes qualitative data before beginning the quantitative component of the study. Results from the qualitative component are used to plan or refine the methods of the quantitative phase.
- Explanatory sequential strategies are used to provide additional qualitative insight into a topic that is initially studied using quantitative data.

- When using the explanatory sequential strategy, the researcher finalizes the questions for the qualitative phase for the purpose of explaining the quantitative findings. These studies are most useful in providing answers to "why" and "how" questions that arise from quantitative findings.
- Convergent concurrent strategies are used when the research question can be addressed using quantitative and qualitative methods, with one method weighted more heavily.
- When using convergent concurrent strategies, the researcher collects quantitative and qualitative data at the same time, analyzes each set of data, and integrates the findings.
- Quantitative and qualitative data usually are combined during analysis or interpretation.

- Mixed methods research strategies require a depth and breadth of research knowledge, as well as a significant commitment of time for completion.
- The challenges of mixed methods research include developing an effective team of researchers with diverse abilities and perspectives and having adequate time and funding to complete all data collection and integration.
- It is critical to determine the method of integration prior to beginning the study. Integration of the data can be displayed in tables, graphs, or matrices.
- Criteria for critically appraising mixed methods studies are identified and applied to a convergent concurrent mixed methods study.

REFERENCES

Amorim, M., Alves, E., Kelly-Irving, M., & Silva, S. (2019). Needs of parents of very preterm infants in neonatal intensive care units: A mixed methods study. *Intensive & Critical Care Nursing, 54*, 88–95. doi:10.1016/j.iccn.2019.05.003

Bazeley, P. (2018). *Integrating analyses in mixed methods research.* Thousand Oaks, CA: Sage.

Brizuela, V., Bonet, M., Souza, J., Tuncalp, O., Viswanath, K., & Langer, A. (2019). Factors influencing healthcare providers on maternal sepsis: A mixed-methods approach. *BMC Public Health, 19*, 683. doi:10.1186/s12889-019-6920-0

Caldwell, B., Ordway, M., Sadler, L., & Redeker, N. (2020). Parent perspectives on sleep and sleep habits among young children living with economic adversity. *Journal of Pediatric Health Care, 34*(1), 10–22. doi:10.1016/j.pedhc.2019.06.006

Cotner, B., Ottomanelli, L., O'Connor, D., Njoh, E., Barnett, S., & Miech, E. (2018). Quality of life outcomes for veterans with spinal cord injury receiving individual placement and support (IPS). *Topics in Spinal Cord Injury Rehabilitation, 24*(4), 325–335. doi:10.1310/sci 17-00046

Creamer, E. (2018). *An introduction to fully integrated mixed methods research.* Thousand Oaks, CA: Sage.

Creswell, J., & Creswell, D. (2018). *Research design: Qualitative, quantitative, and mixed methods approaches* (5th ed.). Thousand Oaks, CA: Sage.

Creswell, J. W. (2015). *A concise introduction to mixed methods research.* Thousand Oaks, CA: Sage.

Creswell, J. W., & Clark, P. (2018). *Designing and conducting mixed methods research* (3rd ed.). Thousand Oaks, CA: Sage.

Curry, L., & Nunez-Smith, M. (2015). *Mixed methods in health sciences research: A practical primer.* Thousand Oaks, CA: Sage.

Fábregues, S., Paré, M. H., & Meneses, J. (2019). Operationalizing and conceptualizing quality in mixed methods research: A multiple case study of the disciplines of education, nursing, psychology, and sociology. *Journal of Mixed Methods Research, 13*(4), 424–445. doi:10.1177/1558689817751774

Fess, E. (1992). *Grip strength.* Chicago, IL: American Society of Hand Therapists.

Gularnik, J., Simonsick, E., Ferrucci, L., Glynn, R., Berkman, L., & Wallace, R. (1994). A short physical performance battery assessing lower extremity function: Association with self-reported disability and prediction of mortality and nursing home admission. *Journal of Gerontology, 49*(2), M85–M94. doi:10.1093/geronj/49.2.M85

Hong, Q., Pluye, P., Fabregues, S., Bartlett, G., Boardman, F., Cargo, M., & Vedel, I. (2019). Improving the content validity of the mixed methods appraisal tool: A modified e-Delphi study. *Journal of Clinical Epidemiology, 111*(1), 49–59. doi:10.1016/j.jclinepi.2019.03.008

Hsieh, H. F. (2005). Three approaches to qualitative content analysis. *Qualitative Health Research, 15*(9), 1277–1288. doi:10.1177/1049732305276687

Johnson, R., Grove, A., & Clarke, A. (2019). Pillar integration process: A joint display technique to integrate data in mixed methods research. *Journal of Mixed Methods Research, 13*(3), 301–320. doi:10.1177/1558689817743108

Kazdin, A. (2017). *Research design in clinical psychology* (5th ed.). Boston, MA: Pearson.

Lamb, S., Jørstad-Stein, E., Hauer, K., & Becker, C. on behalf of Prevention of Falls Network Europe and Outcomes Consensus Group. (1985). Development of a common outcome data set for fall injury prevention trials: The Prevention of Falls Network Europe Consensus. *Journal of the American Geriatric Society, 53*(9), 1618–1622.

Leavy, P. (2017). *Research design: Quantitative, qualitative, mixed methods, arts-based, and community-based participatory research approaches.* New York, NY: Guilford Press.

Lindquist, R., Tracy, M., & Snyder, M. (2018). *Complementary & alternative therapies for nurses* (8th ed.). New York, NY: Springer.

Lynam, T., Damayanti, R., Titaley, C., Suharno, N., Bradley, M., & Krentel, A. (2019). Reframing integration for mixed methods research. *Journal of Mixed Methods Research.* E-pub ahead of print. doi:10.1177/1558689819879352

McDermott, M., Guralnik, J., Criqui, M., Liu, K., Kibbe, M., & Ferrucci, L. (2014). Six-minute walk is a better outcome measure than treadmill walking tests in therapeutic trials of patients with peripheral artery disease. *Circulation, 130*(1), 61–68. doi:10.1161/CIRCULATIONAHA.114.007002

McLeRoy, K., Bibeau, D., Steckler, A., & Glanz, K. (1988). An ecological perspective on health promotion programs. *Health Education & Behavior, 15*(4), 351–377. doi:10.1177/109019818801500401

Molfese, V., Rudasill, K., Prokasky, A., Champagne, C., Holmes, M., Molfese, D. L., & Bates, J.E. (2015). Relations between toddler sleep characteristics, sleep problems, and temperament. *Developmental Neuropsychology, 40*(3), 138–154. doi:10.1080/87565641.2015.1028627

Molina-Azorin, J., & Fetters, M. (2019). Building a better world through mixed methods research. *Journal of Mixed Methods Research, 13*(3), 275–281. doi:10.1177/1558689819855864

Pluye, P., Gagnon, M. P., Griffiths, F., & Johnson-Lafleur, J. (2009). A scoring system for appraising mixed methods research, and concomitantly appraising qualitative, quantitative and mixed methods primary studies in mixed studies reviews. *International Journal of Nursing Studies, 46*(4), 529–546. doi:10.1016/j.ijnurstu.2009.01.009

Poth, C. (2018). *Innovations in mixed methods research: A practical guide to integrative thinking with complexity.* Thousand Oaks, CA: Sage.

Sagar, S., Brown, P., Zelt, D., Pickett, W., & Tranmer, J. (2012). Further clinical validation of the walking impairment questionnaire for classification of walking performance in patients with peripheral artery disease. *International Journal of Vascular Medicine, 2012.* doi:10.1155/2012/190641

Saldana, J. (2013). *The coding manual for qualitative researchers* (2nd ed.). Thousand Oaks, CA: Sage.

Schwab, D. (2013). *Research methods for organizational studies.* East Sussex, UK: Psychology Press.

Sechrist, K., Walker, S., & Pender, N. (1987). Development and psychometric evaluation of the exercise benefits/barriers scale. *Research in Nursing & Health, 10*(6), 357–365. doi:10.1002/nur.4770100603

Sendall, M., McCosker, L., Brodie, A., Hill, M., & Crane, P. (2018). Participatory action research, mixed methods, and research teams: Learning from philosophically juxtaposed methodologies for optimal research outcomes. *BMC Medical Research Methodology, 18,* 167. doi:10.1186/s12874-018-0636-1

Shamsalinia, A., Masoudi, R., Rad, R., & Ghaffari, F. (2019). Development and psychometric evaluation of the Perceived Social Stigma Questionnaire (PSSQ-for adults with epilepsy): A mixed method study. *Epilepsy & Behavior, 96*(1), 141–149. doi:10.1016/j.yebeh.2019.04.055

Steinmetz-Wood, M., Pluye, P., & Ross, N. (2019). The planning and reporting of mixed methods studies on the built environment and health. *Preventive Health, 126,* Article 105752. doi:10.1016/j.ypmed.2019.105752

Talley, K., Wyman, J., & Shamliyan, T. (2011). State of the science: Conservative interventions for urinary incontinence in frail community-dwelling older adults. *Nursing Outlook, 59*(4), 215–220. doi:10.1016/j.outlook.2011.05.010

Tasseff, T., Tavernier, S., Watkins, P., & Neill, K. (2018). Exploring perceptions of palliative care among rural dwelling providers, nurses, and adults using a convergent parallel design. *Online Journal of Rural Nursing and Health Care, 18*(2), 152–188. doi:10.14574/ojrnhc.v18i2.527

Trainor, A., & Graue, E. (2014). Evaluating rigor in qualitative methodology and research dissemination. *Remedial and Special Education, 35*(5), 267–274. doi:10.1177/0741932514528100

Treat-Jacobson, D., Lindquist, R., Witt, D., Kirk, L., Schorr, E., & Regensteiner, J. (2012). The PADQOL: Development and validation of a PAD-specific quality of life questionnaire. *Vascular Medicine, 17*(6), 405–415. doi:10.1177/1358863X12466708

Turner-Bowker, D., Bartley, P., & Ware, J. (2002). *SF-36 health survey & 'SF' bibliography* (3rd ed.). Lincoln, RI: QualityMetric Inc.

Ward, K. (2001). Perceived needs of parents of critically ill infants in a neonatal intensive care unit (NICU). *Pediatric Nursing, 27*(3), 281–286.

Ware, J. (1976). Scales for measuring general health perceptions. *Health Services Research, 11*(4), 396–415.

Ware, J. (2000). SF-36 health survey update. *Spine, 25*(24) 3130–3139. doi:10.1097/00007632-200012150-00008

Whipple, M., Schorr, E., Talley, K., Lindquist, R., Bronas, U., & Treat-Jacobson, D. (2019). A mixed methods study of perceived barriers to physical activity, geriatric syndromes, and physical activity levels among older adults with peripheral artery disease and diabetes. *Journal of Vascular Nursing, 37*(2), 91–105. doi:10.1016/j.jvn.2019.02.001

Yardley, L., Beyer, N., Hauer, K., Kempen, G., Piot-Ziegler, C. & Todd, C. (2005). Development and initial validation of the Falls Efficacy Scale-International (FES-I). *Age and Ageing, 34*(6), 614–619. doi:10.1093/ageing/afi196

Yin, R. (2018). *Case study research and applications: Designs and methods* (6th ed.). Thousand Oaks, CA: Sage.

15

Sampling

Susan K. Grove

http://evolve.elsevier.com/Gray/practice/

Many of us have preconceived notions about sampling techniques and samples acquired from television commercials, public opinion polls, online surveys, and reports of research findings. A medical company boasts that four of five doctors recommend its product; the news reporter announces that John Smith is predicted to win the senate election by a margin of 3 to 1; an online survey identifies the jobs with the highest satisfaction rate; and researchers in multiple studies conclude that taking a statin drug, such as atorvastatin (Lipitor), significantly reduces the risk of coronary artery disease.

All of these examples use sampling techniques. However, some of the outcomes are more valid than others, partly because of the techniques used to recruit a sample. In most instances, news reports and advertisements do not explain their sampling techniques. You may hold opinions about the adequacy of these techniques, but there is not enough information to make a judgment about the quality of the samples. Research reports usually include a detailed description of the sampling process because the nature of the sample is critical to the credibility of the study findings.

The sampling component is an important part of every type of study that needs to be carefully planned and implemented and clearly described in the research report. To accomplish this, you need to understand the techniques of sampling and the reasoning behind them. With this knowledge, you can make intelligent judgments about sampling when you are critically appraising studies or developing a sampling plan for your own study. This chapter examines sampling theory and concepts; sampling plans; probability and nonprobability

sampling methods for quantitative, qualitative, mixed methods, and outcomes research; sample size; and settings for conducting studies. The chapter concludes with a discussion of the strategies for recruiting and retaining participants for studies from various settings.

SAMPLING THEORY

Sampling theory was developed to determine mathematically the most effective way to acquire a sample that would accurately reflect the population under study. The theoretical, mathematical rationale for decisions related to sampling emerged from survey research, although the techniques were first applied to experimental research by agricultural scientists. Some important concepts of sampling theory include sampling, sampling plan, and sample. **Sampling** involves selecting a group of people, events, behaviors, or other elements with which to conduct a study. A **sampling plan** defines the process of making the sample selections; **sample** denotes the selected group of people or elements included in a study. One of the most important surveys that stimulated improvements in sampling techniques was the US census. Researchers have adopted the assumptions of sampling theory identified for census surveys and incorporated them within the research process (Thompson, 2012; Yates, 1981).

Key concepts of sampling theory covered in this text include (1) populations, (2) elements, (3) sampling criteria, (4) representativeness, (5) sampling errors, (6) randomization, (7) sampling frames, and (8) sampling plans. These concepts are described here and later used to critically appraise various sampling methods from published studies. These ideas will guide you in developing a sampling plan for a future study.

Populations and Elements

The **population** is a particular group of people, such as people who have lost a child, or type of element, such as intravenous catheters, that is the focus of the research. Fig. 15.1 shows the relationships among the population, target population, and accessible population. The **target population** is the entire set of individuals or elements meeting the sampling criteria, such as women who have experienced their first myocardial infarction in the past 12 months. An **accessible population** is the portion of the target population to which researchers have reasonable access. The accessible population might be individuals within a country, state, city, hospital, nursing unit, or clinic, such as the adults with diabetes in a primary care clinic in Fort Worth, Texas. The sample is obtained from the accessible population by a particular sampling method, such as simple random sampling. The individual units of the population and sample are called **elements**. An element can be a person, event, behavior, experience, or any other single unit of study. When elements are persons, they are usually referred to as **subjects, participants,** or **informants** (see Fig. 15.1). The term used by researchers depends on

the philosophical paradigm that is reflected in the study and the design. The term *subject,* and sometimes *research participant,* is used within the context of the positivist or postpositivist paradigm of quantitative research (Kazdin, 2017; Shadish, Cook, & Campbell, 2002). The terms *study* or *research participant* and *informant* are used in the context of the naturalistic paradigm of qualitative and often mixed methods research (Creswell & Clark, 2018; Creswell & Poth, 2018).

Generalizing means that the findings can be applied to more than just the sample under study because the sample is representative of the study population (Miles, Huberman, & Saldaña, 2020; Thompson, 2012). Polit and Beck (2010) described two models of generalization in research: analytical generalization and statistical generalization. **Analytical generalization** is most frequently linked to qualitative and mixed methods research. Qualitative researchers develop conceptualizations of human experiences and processes through in-depth analysis of data and higher-order abstraction. In the course of analysis, qualitative researchers distinguish between information that is relevant to many participants in contrast to aspects of the experience that are unique to particular participants: "Through rigorous inductive analysis, together with the use of confirmatory strategies that address the credibility of conclusions, qualitative researchers can arrive at insightful, inductive generalizations regarding the phenomenon under study" (Polit & Beck, 2010, p. 1453) (see Chapter 12).

Statistical generalization, most commonly discussed in the research literature, is linked to quantitative and outcomes research. Quantitative researchers identify the population to which they wish to generalize and then select participants from the population with a goal of achieving a representative sample (Aberson, 2019; Polit & Beck, 2010). Random sampling is thought to be the best strategy for obtaining a representative sample (Tappen, 2016). In quantitative and outcomes research, the findings from a study are generalized first to the accessible population and then, if appropriate, more abstractly to the target population (Kane & Radosevich, 2011) (see Fig. 15.1). The definition of the target and accessible population should be reasonable (i.e., not too narrow or broad). A narrow definition of the accessible population reduces the ability to generalize from the study sample to the target population and diminishes the meaningfulness of the findings. Biases may be introduced with a narrowly defined accessible population

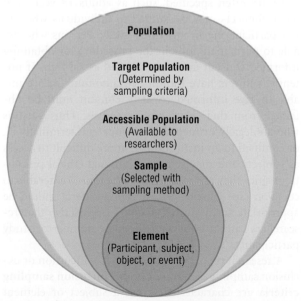

Fig. 15.1 Linking population, sample, and element in research.

that makes generalization to the broader target population difficult to defend. If the accessible population includes individuals in a white, upper-middle-class setting, one cannot generalize to nonwhite or lower-income populations. These biases are similar to those that may be encountered in a nonrandom sample and are threats to external design validity (Borglin & Richards, 2010; Kazdin, 2017; Shadish et al., 2002) (see Chapters 10 and 11).

In some studies, the entire population is the target of the study. These studies are referred to as **population studies**. Many of these studies use data available in large databases, such as the census data or other government-maintained databases. Epidemiologists sometimes use entire populations for their large database studies. In other studies, the entire population of interest might be small and well defined. For example, one could conduct a study in which the target population was all living recipients of heart and lung transplants.

In some cases, a hypothetical population is defined for a study. A **hypothetical population** assumes the presence of a population that cannot be defined according to sampling theory rules, which require a list of all members of the population (Thompson, 2012). For example, individuals who successfully lose weight would be a hypothetical population. The number of individuals in the population, who they are, how much weight they have lost, how long they have kept the weight off, and how they achieved the weight loss are unknown. Some populations are elusive and constantly changing. For example, identifying all women in active labor in the United States, all people grieving the loss of a loved one, or all people coming into an emergency department would be impossible.

Sampling or Eligibility Criteria

Sampling criteria, also referred to as **eligibility criteria**, include a list of characteristics essential for membership or eligibility in the target population. The criteria are developed from the research problem, the purpose, a review of literature, the definitions of study variables, and the design. The sampling criteria determine the target population, and the sample is selected from the accessible population within the target population (see Fig. 15.1). When the study is complete, the findings are generalized from the sample to the accessible population and then to the target population if the study has a representative sample (see the next section) and

the findings are consistent with previous research (Kazdin, 2017).

You might identify broad sampling criteria for a study, such as all adults older than 18 years of age able to read and write English. These criteria ensure a large target population of **heterogeneous** or diverse potential subjects. A heterogeneous sample increases your ability to generalize the findings to the target population. In descriptive, correlational, and outcomes studies, the sampling criteria may be defined to ensure a heterogeneous population with a broad range of values for the variables being studied. However, in quasi-experimental or experimental studies, the primary purpose of sampling criteria is to limit the effect of extraneous variables on the particular interaction between the independent and dependent variables. In these types of studies, sampling criteria are usually specific and designed to make the population as **homogeneous** or similar as possible to control for the extraneous variables (Kazdin, 2017; Shadish et al., 2002). Subjects are selected to maximize the effects of the independent variable and minimize the effects of variation in extraneous variables (see Chapter 6) so that they have a limited impact on the dependent variable scores or values.

Sampling criteria may include characteristics such as the ability to read, to write responses on the data collection instruments or forms, and to comprehend and communicate using the English language. Age limitations are often specified, such as adults 18 years and older. Subjects may be limited to individuals who are not participating in any other study. Persons who are able to participate fully in the procedure for obtaining informed consent are often selected as subjects. If potential subjects have diminished autonomy or are unable to give informed consent, consent must be obtained from their legal representatives. Thus persons who are legally or mentally incompetent, terminally ill, or confined to an institution are more difficult to access as subjects and may require additional ethical precautions since they are considered to be more vulnerable to coercion (see Chapter 9). Sampling criteria should be appropriate for a study but not so restrictive that researchers cannot obtain an adequate number of study participants.

A research report should specify the inclusion or exclusion sampling criteria (or both). **Inclusion sampling criteria** are characteristics that a subject or element must possess to be part of the target population.

Exclusion sampling criteria are characteristics that can cause a person or element to be eliminated or excluded from the target population. Individuals with these characteristics would be excluded from a study even if they met all the inclusion criteria. For example, when studying patients with heart failure, you might exclude all patients with heart failure who are acutely ill because participation in the study might increase their risk for harm. The inclusion and exclusion sampling criteria for a study should be different and not repetitive. For example, you should not have inclusion criteria of individuals 18 years of age and older and exclusion criteria of individuals less than 18 years of age because these criteria are repetitive. Researchers need to provide logical reasons for their inclusion and exclusion sampling criteria, and certain groups should not be excluded without justification. In the past, some groups, such as women, ethnic minorities, elderly adults, and economically disadvantaged people, were unnecessarily excluded from studies (Larson, 1994). Today, federal funding for research is strongly linked to including these understudied populations in studies (National Institutes of Health [NIH], 2019). Exclusion criteria limit the generalization of the study findings and should be carefully considered before being used in a study.

Lee and Park (2019) implemented a randomized controlled trial (RCT) to determine the effects of "auricular acupressure (AA) on pain, pain threshold (PT), disability, and cervical range of motion in adults with chronic neck pain" (p. 12). The study included 50 adults randomized into either the AA experimental group or the sham AA control group. The sham AA intervention was used with the control group so that they perceived they were receiving an intervention but it was not the therapeutic AA provided to the experiment group. Thus the study participants were unaware or blinded to who was receiving the experimental treatment. The sampling criteria implemented in this study are described in the following study excerpt.

"The criteria for participant selection were as follows: (a) adults aged 18 to 65 years, (b) adults with neck pain for at least 6 months, (c) a score of 5 or more on the NDI [Neck Disability Index], (d) no medical history of neck injury, cervical fracture, or cervical surgery, (e) no allergic diseases, such as lesions or atopic dermatitis in both ears, (f) agreed not to receive other treatments for neck pain during the experimental period, and (g) were willing to participate in the study and be randomly allocated into study groups… Eligible participants were assigned, 25 in each of the experimental and control groups, in consideration of a dropout rate of 20%. Two participants dropped out of the control group, so the total number of the participants was 48 (see [Fig. 15.2])." (Lee & Park, 2019, p. 13)

Lee and Park (2019) clearly identified the inclusion and exclusion sampling criteria that were used to screen potential study participants for the target population. Adults 18 to 65 years old with neck pain for at least 6 months, who scored 5 or more on NDI, and were willing to participate were included in the study. Those individuals with a history of neck problems, allergic diseases, and received other treatments for neck pain during the study were excluded. The sampling criteria were appropriate for this study to reduce the effect of possible extraneous variables that might have an impact on the AA treatment or intervention delivery method and the measurement of the dependent variables (neck pain, PT, disability, and cervical range of motion). The controls imposed by the sampling criteria strengthened the likelihood that the study outcomes were caused by the intervention and not by extraneous variables or sampling errors.

Fifty-eight individuals were screened for this study and eight were excluded for not meeting the sampling inclusion criteria. Thus the sample from the accessible population included 50 adults with neck pain who were randomized equally into the experimental and control groups. The sampling process and assignment of participants to groups is documented in Fig. 15.2. This figure is an example of a Consolidated Standards of Reporting Trials (CONSORT) table that is frequently included in RCTs reports. (The CONSORT [2010] statement is an internationally accepted format for reporting RCTs.) Lee and Park (2019) found "that AA leads to improvements on PT, neck disability, and cervical range of motion" (p. 12) but not in reported neck pain. The researchers recommended using AA as an alternative nursing intervention for chronic neck pain, but additional research is needed to document the effectiveness of this intervention (Tappen, 2016).

Sample Representativeness

For a sample to be **representative**, it must be similar to the target population in as many ways as possible. It is

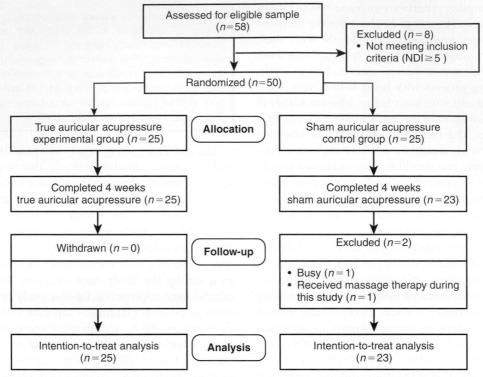

Fig. 15.2 Participant flow chart. *NDI,* Neck Disability Index. (Lee, S., & Park, H. [2019]. Effects of auricular acupressure on pain and disability in adults with chronic neck pain. *Applied Nursing Research,* *45*[1], 14. doi:10.1016/j.apnr.2018.11.005)

especially important that the sample be representative in relation to the variables you are studying and to other factors that may influence the study variables. For example, if you examine attitudes toward childhood immunizations, the sample should represent the distribution of attitudes toward immunizations that exists in the specified population. You would want to include those who did and did not immunize their children and their family and friends that have been shown to influence attitudes. In addition, a sample must represent the demographic characteristics of the target population for such variables as age, gender, race/ethnicity, income, and education, which often influence study variables.

The accessible population must be representative of the target population. If the accessible population is limited to a particular setting or type of setting, the individuals seeking care at that setting may be different from the individuals who would seek care for the same problem in other settings or from individuals who self-manage their problems. Studies conducted in private

hospitals usually exclude economically disadvantaged patients, and other settings could exclude elderly or undereducated patients. People who do not have access to care are usually excluded from health-focused studies. Study participants and the care they receive in research centers are different from patients and the care they receive in community clinics, public hospitals, veterans hospitals, and rural health clinics. Obese individuals who choose to enter a program to lose weight may differ from obese individuals who do not enter a program. These factors limit the sample's representativeness, thus limiting our understanding of the phenomena in practice. Representativeness of a sample is important in quantitative, qualitative, mixed methods, and outcomes research (see Chapters 3, 4, 12, and 13) (Miles et al., 2020; Tappen, 2016).

Representativeness is usually evaluated by comparing the numerical values of the sample (a **statistic** such as the mean) with the same values from the target population. A numerical value of a population is called a **parameter**. We can estimate the **population parameter** by identifying the values obtained in previous studies examining the same variables (Grove & Cipher, 2020). The accuracy with which the population parameters have been estimated within a study is referred to as **precision**. Precision in estimating parameters requires well-developed methods of measurement that have been used repeatedly in several studies (Waltz, Strickland, & Lenz, 2017). You can define parameters by conducting a series of descriptive and correlational studies, each of which examines a different segment of the target population; then you perform a meta-analysis to estimate the population parameter (Kazdin, 2017; Kerlinger & Lee, 2000). Due to a recent outbreak of measles, additional research has been conducted to estimate the population parameters for those who do and do not immunize their children.

Sampling Error

Sampling error is the difference between a sample statistic and the estimated population parameter that is actual but unknown (Fig. 15.3). A large sampling error means that the sample statistic does not provide a precise estimate of the population parameter; it is not representative. Sampling error is usually larger with small samples and decreases as the sample size increases. Sampling error reduces the **power** of a study, or the ability of the statistical analyses conducted to detect differences between groups or to describe the relationships among variables (Aberson, 2019; Cohen, 1988). Sampling error occurs as a result of random variation and systematic variation.

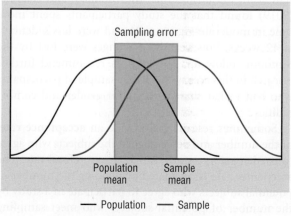

Fig. 15.3 Sampling error.

Random Variation

Random variation is the expected difference in values that occurs when one examines different subjects from the same sample. If the mean is used to describe the sample, the values of individuals in that sample will not all be exactly the same as the sample mean. The difference is random because the value of each subject is likely to vary in value and direction from the previously measured one. Some values are higher and others are lower than the sample mean. The values are randomly scattered around the mean. As the sample size becomes larger, overall variation in sample values decreases, with more values being close to the sample mean. As the sample size increases, the sample mean is also more likely to have a value similar to that of the population mean (Grove & Cipher, 2020; Tappen, 2016).

Systematic Variation

Systematic variation, or **systematic bias**, is a consequence of selecting subjects whose measurement values are different, or vary, in some specific way from the population. Because the subjects have something in common, their values tend to be similar to the values of others in the sample but different in some way from the values of the population as a whole. These values do not vary randomly around the population mean. Most of the variation from the mean is in the same direction; it is systematic. All the values in the sample may tend to be higher or lower than the mean of the population (Thompson, 2012). For example, if all the participants in a study examining knowledge of weight management have an intelligence quotient (IQ) higher than 120, many of their scores will likely be higher than the mean of a population that includes individuals with a wide variation in IQ, such as IQs that range from 90 to 130. The IQs of the participants have introduced a systematic bias. This situation could occur, for example, if all the subjects were college students, which has been the case in the development of many measurement methods in psychology (Kazdin, 2017).

Because of systematic variance, the sample mean is different from the population mean. The extent of the difference is the sampling error (see Fig. 15.3). Exclusion criteria tend to increase the systematic bias in the sample and increase the sampling error, but it is necessary to exclude persons who might be harmed by participating in a study. An example of this problem is the highly restrictive sampling criteria used in some experimental studies that result in a large sampling error that diminishes the representativeness of the sample. If the method of selecting subjects produces a sample with a systematic bias, increasing the sample size does not decrease the sampling error. When systematic bias occurs in an experimental study, researchers may conclude that the treatment has made a difference when, in actuality, the values would be different even without the treatment. This situation usually occurs because of an interaction of the systematic bias with the treatment (Shadish et al., 2002).

Refusal and acceptance rates in studies. Sampling error from systematic variation or bias is most likely to occur when the sampling process is not random. However, even in a random sample, systematic variation can occur if potential subjects decline participation. Systematic bias increases as individuals' refusal rate to participate in a study increases. A refusal rate is the number and percentage of individuals who decline to participate in the study. High refusal rates to participate in a study have been linked to individuals with serious physical and emotional illnesses, low socioeconomical status, weak social networks, and elderly (Gluck, Shaw, & Hill, 2018; Goldman et al., 2018). The higher the refusal rate, the less representative the sample is of the target population.

Ramadi and Haennel (2019) conducted a correlational study to examine the associations among "changes in sedentary behavior, breaks in sedentary time, and physical activity (PA) in CR [cardiac rehabilitation] participants from commencing CR to 6 months after CR entry" (p. 8). A total of 69 individuals declined to participate in this study. The setting and sample are briefly described in the following study excerpt.

"We recruited patients from two centers that offered supervised CR program.... The program involved 1-2 sessions/week of supervised exercise.... A total of 83 patients were recruited. Data from 25 participants who refused follow-up assessments ($n = 15$) or their CR program was terminated due to medical issues ($n = 10$), were excluded. Fifty-eight participants who attended in all the 3 assessment points were included in the analysis" [see Fig. 15.4]. (Ramadi & Haennel, 2019, p. 9)

Ramadi and Haennel (2019) clearly identified the number of patients refusing to participate in their study

using a flow diagram (Fig. 15.4). These researchers approached 152 CR patients in two rehabilitation centers and 69 declined to participate in the study. The refusal rate is calculated by dividing the number of potential subjects refusing to participate by the number of potential subjects meeting sampling criteria and multiplying the results by 100%.

Refusal rate formula

$$= \frac{\text{Number potential subjects refusing to participate}}{\text{Number potential subjects meeting sample criteria}} \times 100\%$$

The refusal rate for the Ramadi and Haennel (2019) study is calculated as:

Refusal rate

$$= \frac{69 \text{ (number refusing)}}{152 \text{ (number meeting sampling criteria)}} \times 100\%$$
$$= 0.4539 \times 100\% = 45.39\% = 45.4\%$$

The refusal rate for the Ramadi and Haennel (2019) study was extremely large at 45.4%. No information was provided about why the CR patients refused to participate. A research report should include the refusal number and rate for potential subjects and their rationale for not participating in a study. The large refusal rate and the small sample size ($n = 83$) decrease the representativeness of this sample and increase the potential for sampling error (Tappen, 2016; Thompson, 2012). These weaknesses have a potential to produce erroneous, nonsignificant findings in this study. Ramadi and Haennel (2019) found that the study participants spent more time in moderate-vigorous PA and were less sedentary at 12 weeks; however, these changes were lost by the 6-month follow-up. The authors recommend further research in this area with a larger sample of participants who had varied characteristics for gender and comorbidities.

Sometimes researchers provide an **acceptance rate**, or the number and percentage of the subjects who agree to participate in a study, rather than a refusal rate. The acceptance rate is calculated by dividing the number of potential subjects who agree to participate in a study by the number of potential subjects who meet sampling criteria and multiplying the result by 100%.

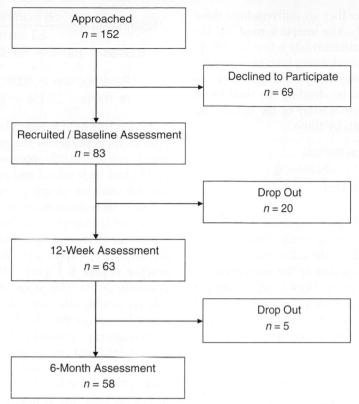

Fig. 15.4 Flow diagram of participants. (Ramadi, A., & Haennel, R. G. [2019]. Sedentary behavior and physical activity in cardiac rehabilitation participants. *Heart & Lung, 48*[1], 10. doi:10.1016/j.hrtlng.2018.09.008)

Acceptance rate formula

$$= \frac{\text{Number potential subjects agreeing to participate}}{\text{Number potential subjects meeting sample criteria}} \times 100\%$$

If you know the refusal rate, you can also subtract the refusal rate from 100% to obtain the acceptance rate. Usually researchers report either the acceptance rate or the refusal rate but not both. In the Ramadi and Haennel (2019) study, 152 potential subjects met the sampling criteria; 83 agreed to participate in the study, and 69 refused (see Fig. 15.4).

Acceptance rate

$$= \frac{83 \text{ (number accepting)}}{152 \text{ (number meeting sampling criteria)}} \times 100\%$$

$$= 0.5461 \times 100\% = 54.61\% = 54.6\%$$

Acceptance rate = 100% − Refusal rate
or 100% − 45.4% = 54.6%

Sample attrition and retention rates in studies. Sampling error can also occur in studies with large sample attrition. **Sample attrition** is the withdrawal or loss of subjects or participants from a study before its completion. Systematic variation tends to increase when a high number of participants withdraw from the study before data collection is completed or when a large number of participants withdraw from one group but not the other in the study (Kazdin, 2017; Thompson, 2012). In studies involving an intervention, participants in the control group who do not receive the intervention may be more likely to withdraw from the study. Sample attrition should be reported in the published study to determine if the final sample represents the target population (Tappen, 2016). Researchers also need to provide a rationale for the participants withdrawing from the study and to determine whether they are different from those who completed the study. The sample is most like the target population if the attrition rate is low (< 10% to 15%) and the subjects withdrawing from the study are similar to the subjects completing the study. Sample attrition rate is calculated by dividing the number of subjects withdrawing from a study by the sample size and multiplying the results by 100%.

Sample attrition rate formula
$$= \frac{\text{Number subjects withdrawing}}{\text{Sample size}} \times 100\%$$

Ramadi and Haennel (2019) reported that 25 participants withdrew from their study. Fifteen of the participants (18.1%) refused the follow-up assessment and no rationale was provided by the researchers for their refusals. Ten participants (12%) had to drop out of CR for medical reasons, which is a common reason for study attrition. The attrition of 25 participants from this study resulted in a large attrition rate of 30.1%.

$$\text{Attrition rate} = \frac{25 \text{ (number withdrawing)}}{83 \text{ (sample size)}} \times 100\%$$
$$= 0.3012 \times 100\%$$
$$= 30.12 = 30.1\%$$

The opposite of the attrition rate is the **retention rate**, or the number and percentage of participants completing the study. The higher the retention rate, the more representative the sample is of the target population and the more likely the study results are an accurate reflection of reality. Often researchers identify either the attrition rate or the retention rate but not both. It is better to provide a rate in addition to the number of participants withdrawing or completing a study. The Ramadi and Haennel (2019) study had a sample size of 83; if 25 subjects withdrew from the study, then 58 subjects were retained or completed the study (see Fig. 15.4). The retention rate is calculated by dividing the number of subjects completing the study by the initial sample size and multiplying by 100%.

Sample retention rate formula
$$= \frac{\text{Number subjects completing study}}{\text{Sample size}} \times 100\%$$

$$\text{Retention rate} = \frac{58 \text{ (number retained)}}{83 \text{ (sample size)}} \times 100\%$$
$$= 0.6988 \times 100\% = 69.88\% = 69.9\%$$

$$\text{Retention rate} = 100\% - \text{Attrition rate}$$
or $100\% - 30.1\% = 69.9\%$

Researchers need to report both refusal and attrition rates in their studies so the representativeness of the sample can be critically appraised. Ramadi and Haennel (2019) had high refusal and attrition rates increasing the potential for sampling error and decreasing the sample's representativeness of the target population. Because of the sampling weaknesses and nonsignificant results, the study findings should not be generalized to the target population and are not ready for use in practice (Grove & Cipher, 2020; Melnyk & Fineout-Overholt, 2019). This study should be repeated with a larger sample size with additional strategies implemented to reduce the refusal and attrition rates.

In quasi-experimental and experimental studies, the experimental and control groups need to be of similar size and have limited attrition. The RCT by Lee and Park (2019), introduced earlier, examined the effects of AA on pain and disability of adults with chronic neck pain. The study included 50 participants who were randomly assigned to the AA experimental group ($n = 25$) and the sham AA control group ($n = 25$; see Fig. 15.2). Two subjects from the control group withdrew from the study because one was busy and the other received massage therapy during the study, which was an exclusion criterion. The withdrawal or attrition rate for the study was very small at 4% ([2 ÷ 50] × 100% = 0.04 × 100% = 4%). In addition, the attrition rate for the experimental group was 0% and for the control group was 8% ([2 ÷ 25] × 100% = 0.08 × 100% = 8%). The experimental and control group sizes were similar ($n = 25$ and $n = 23$, respectively) and the attrition rate was small supporting the representativeness of the sample (Kazdin, 2017; Tappen, 2016).

Randomization

From a sampling theory point of view, **randomization** means that each individual in the population should have a greater than zero opportunity to be selected for the sample. The method of achieving this opportunity is referred to as **random sampling** (Thompson, 2012). In experimental studies, participants are sometimes randomly selected and are usually randomly assigned to either the control group or the experimental group. The term **control group**—the group not receiving the treatment or intervention—is used when study participants are probably randomly selected and are randomly assigned to either the intervention group or control group. If nonrandom sampling methods are used for sample selection, the group not receiving the intervention receives usual or standard care and is generally referred to as a **comparison group**. With a comparison group, there is an increase in the probability of preexisting differences between that group and the intervention group (Shadish et al., 2002).

Random sampling increases the extent to which the sample is representative of the target population. However, random sampling must take place in an accessible population that is representative of the target population (see Fig. 15.1). Exclusion criteria limit true randomness. Thus a study that uses random sampling techniques may have such restrictive sampling criteria that the sample is not truly a random sample of the population. In any case, it is rarely possible to obtain a purely random sample for nursing studies because of informed consent requirements. Even if the original sample is random, persons who volunteer or consent to participate in a study may differ in important ways from persons who are unwilling to participate. All samples with human subjects must be **volunteer samples**, which includes individuals willing to participate in the study, to protect their rights (see Chapter 9). Methods of achieving random samples are described later in this chapter.

Sampling Frame

For each person in the target population to have an opportunity to be selected for a sample, the individuals in the population must be identified. To accomplish this goal, the researcher must acquire a list of every member of the target population through the use of the sampling criteria to define membership. This listing of members of the population is referred to as the **sampling frame**. The researcher selects subjects from the sampling frame using a sampling plan. For example, if you wanted to conduct a study with a population of psychiatric mental health nurse practitioners, the sampling frame of all certified PMHNPs is available through the American Nurses Credentialing Center (ANCC). ANCC is the only agency certifying PMHNPs, so you could request a

random sample of the PMHNPs to include as your study sample.

Sampling Plan

A **sampling plan** describes the strategies that will be used to obtain a sample for a study. The plan is developed to enhance representativeness, reduce systematic bias, and decrease sampling error. Sampling strategies have been devised to accomplish these three tasks and to optimize sample selection (Kazdin, 2017; Tappen, 2016). The sampling plan may use probability (random) sampling methods or nonprobability (nonrandom) sampling methods.

A **sampling method** is the process of selecting a group of people, events, behaviors, or other elements that represents the population being studied. A sampling method is similar to a design; it is not specific to a study. The sampling plan provides details about the application of a sampling method in a specific study. This plan should be described in depth in a research report for purposes of critical appraisal, replication, and future meta-analysis. The sampling method implemented in a study varies with the type of research being conducted. Quantitative and outcomes studies apply a variety of probability and nonprobability sampling methods (Creswell & Creswell, 2018; Kane & Radosevich, 2011; Kazdin, 2017). Qualitative and mixed methods studies usually include nonprobability sampling methods (Charmaz, 2014; Creswell & Clark, 2018; Creswell & Poth, 2018). The probability and nonprobability sampling methods included in this text are identified in Table 15.1 and are linked to the types of research (quantitative, qualitative, mixed methods, and outcomes) that most commonly incorporate them. The representativeness of the sample obtained is discussed for each of the sampling methods.

PROBABILITY (RANDOM) SAMPLING METHODS

Probability sampling methods have been developed to ensure some degree of precision in estimations of the population parameters. The term **probability sampling method** means that every member (element) of the population has a greater than zero opportunity to be selected for the sample. Inferential statistical analyses are based on the assumption that the sample from which data were derived has been obtained randomly

TABLE 15.1   Probability and Nonprobability Sampling Methods Commonly Applied in Nursing Research

Sampling Method	Common Application(s)	Representativeness
Probability		
Simple random sampling	Quantitative and outcomes research	Provides strong representativeness of the target population that increases with sample size (Thompson, 2012).
Stratified random sampling	Quantitative and outcomes research	Provides strong representativeness of the target population that increases with control of stratified variable(s).
Cluster sampling	Quantitative and outcomes research	Is less representative of the target population than simple random sampling and stratified random sampling but representativeness increases with sample size (Innocenti, Candel, Tan, & van Breukelen, 2019).
Systematic sampling	Quantitative and outcomes research	Is less representative of the target population than simple random sampling and stratified random sampling methods, but representativeness increases with sample size (Tappen, 2016).
Nonprobability		
Convenience sampling	Quantitative, qualitative, mixed methods, and outcomes research	There is questionable representativeness of the target population that improves with increasing sample size in quantitative and outcomes research (Kane & Radosevich, 2011; Kerlinger & Lee, 2000; Thompson, 2012). It is used in qualitative or mixed methods research so that an adequate number of participants might be found to promote understanding of the study area (Creswell & Clark, 2018; Creswell & Creswell, 2018).
Quota sampling	Quantitative and outcomes research, rarely qualitative or mixed methods research	Use of stratification for selected variables in quantitative and outcomes research makes the sample more representative than convenience sampling (Thompson, 2012). In qualitative and mixed methods research, stratification might be used to provide greater understanding of the subgroups of the populations to increase the representativeness of the phenomenon, processes, or cultural elements studied (Marshall & Rossman, 2016; Miles, Huberman, & Saldaña, 2020).
Purposeful or purposive sampling	Qualitative and mixed methods research, sometimes quantitative research	Focus is on insight, description, and understanding of a phenomenon, cultural event, situation, or process with specially selected study participants who are representative of the area of study (Creswell & Poth, 2018; Miles et al., 2020).
Snowball or network sampling	Qualitative and mixed methods research and sometimes quantitative research	Focus is on insight, description, and understanding of a phenomenon, cultural element, situation, or process in a difficult to access population. Intent is to identify participants who are representative of the study focus (Creswell & Clark, 2018; Kazdin, 2017; Miles et al., 2020; Tappen, 2016).
Theoretical sampling	Qualitative and mixed methods research	Focus is on obtaining quality participants, with different perspectives, of an adequate number for developing a relevant theory, framework, or model for a selected area of study (Charmaz, 2014; Tappen, 2016).

(Grove & Cipher, 2020). Thus probability sampling methods are often referred to as **random sampling methods**. These samples are more likely to represent the population and minimize sampling error than are samples obtained with nonprobability sampling methods. All subsets of the population, which may differ from one another but contribute to the parameters of the population, have a chance to be represented in the sample. Probability sampling methods are most commonly applied in quantitative and outcomes studies (see Table 15.1). More nursing researchers are using probability sampling methods in their studies with the selection of samples from large administrative and clinical databases. Often national and international survey research is conducted with probability sampling methods (Kazdin, 2017; Tappen, 2016).

There is less opportunity for systematic bias or error when subjects are selected randomly. Using random sampling, the researcher cannot decide that person X would be a better subject for the study than person Y. In addition, a researcher cannot exclude a subset of people from selection as subjects because he or she does not agree with them, does not like them, or finds them hard to deal with. Potential subjects cannot be excluded just because they are too sick, not sick enough, coping too well, or not coping adequately. The researcher, who has a vested interest in the study, could (consciously or unconsciously) select subjects whose conditions or behaviors are consistent with the study hypothesis. Because random sampling leaves the selection to chance and decreases sampling error, the validity of the study is increased (Kandola, Banner, Okeefe-McCarthy, & Jassal, 2014).

Theoretically, to obtain a probability sample, the researcher must develop a sampling frame that includes every element in the population. The sample must be randomly selected from the sampling frame. According to sampling theory, it is impossible to select a sample randomly from a population that cannot be clearly defined. Four commonly implemented probability sampling designs are included in this text: simple random sampling, stratified random sampling, cluster sampling, and systematic sampling.

Simple Random Sampling

Simple random sampling is the most basic of the probability sampling methods. To achieve simple random sampling, elements are selected at random from the sampling frame. This goal can be accomplished in

various ways, limited only by the imagination of the researcher. If the sampling frame is small, the researcher can write names on slips of paper, place the names in a container, mix well, and draw out one at a time until the desired sample size has been reached. Another technique is to assign a number to each name in the sampling frame. In large population sets, elements may already have assigned numbers. For example, numbers are assigned to medical records, organizational memberships, national certification, and professional licenses. The researcher can use a computer to select these numbers randomly to obtain a sample.

There can be some differences in the probability for the selection of each element, depending on whether the name or number of the selected element is replaced before the next name or number is selected. Selection with replacement, the most conservative random sampling approach, provides exactly equal opportunities for each element to be selected (Thompson, 2012). For example, if the researcher draws out names from a hat to obtain a sample, each name must be replaced before the next name is drawn to ensure equal opportunity for each subject.

Selection without replacement gives each element different levels of probability for selection. For example, if the researcher is selecting 10 subjects from a population of 50, the first name has a 1 in 5 chance (10 draws, 50 names), or a 0.2 probability, of being selected. If the first name is not replaced, the remaining 49 names have a 9 in 49 chance, or a 0.18 probability, of being selected. As further names are drawn, the probability of being selected decreases.

Random selection of a sample can also be achieved using a computer, a random numbers table, or a roulette wheel. The most common method of random selection is the computer, which can be programmed to select a sample randomly from the sampling frame with replacement. However, some researchers still use a table of random numbers to select a random sample. Table 15.2 shows a section from a random numbers table. To use a table of random numbers, the researcher, with eyes closed, places a pencil or a finger on the table. The number touched is the starting place. Moving the pencil or finger up, down, right, or left, the researcher identifies the next element to be included and uses the numbers in order until the desired sample size is obtained. For example, the researcher places a pencil on 58 in Table 15.2, which is in the fourth column from the left and fourth row down. If five subjects are to be selected from a population of 100 and the researcher decides to go

TABLE 15.2 Section From a Random Numbers Table

06	84	10	22	56	72	25	70	69	43
07	63	10	34	66	39	54	02	33	85
03	19	63	93	72	52	13	30	44	40
77	32	69	58	25	15	55	38	19	62
20	01	94	54	66	88	43	91	34	28

across the column to the right, the subject numbers chosen are 58, 25, 15, 55, and 38. Table 15.2 is useful only if the population number is less than 100. However, tables are available for larger populations, such as the random numbers table provided in the Thompson (2012) sampling text.

Hurley, Edwards, Cupp, and Phillips (2018) conducted a predictive correlational study "to determine the relationship between nurses' personal health practices and their perceptions of themselves as role models for health promotion and to assess the relationship of selected personal and professional characteristics both on perception of self as role model and on the practice of healthy behaviors" (p. 1135). The simple random sampling method used in this study is described in the following excerpt with the key sampling concepts identified in brackets.

"Participants

The population from which the study sample was drawn included all registered nurses in Tennessee ($n = 61,829$) listed in the Tennessee Board of Nursing 2015 database [sampling frame]. After approval from East Tennessee State University's Institutional Review Board, a simple random sample [sampling method] was drawn from the database. Inclusion criteria were active registered nurse licensed in the state of Tennessee, and a valid e-mail in the database [sampling criteria]." (Hurley et al., 2018, p. 1136)

"Results

Demographics

A total of 1,428 participants responded to the e-mail by following the link to the survey. Questionnaires that were less than 80% complete were excluded from the sample. The final sample consisted of 804 registered nurses [sample size]. There were 716 (89%) females and 86 (10.7%) males [sample characteristics]. The percentage of male nurses in the sample was comparable with male nurses in the national nursing population at 9%." (Hurley et al., 2018, p. 1138)

Hurley and colleagues (2018) clearly identified that a simple random sampling method was used to select study participants from a population of registered nurses (RNs) in Tennessee. The sampling frame was extensive, including all licensed RNs with a valid e-mail in Tennessee. The process for obtaining the random sample was not described but was probably done using a computer program. It is also unclear if the random sampling was done with or without replacement (Thompson, 2012). The researchers did not report how many e-mails were sent to the RNs, but 1428 potential participants responded and 804 participants completed at least 80% of their surveys. The response rate for the surveys was not reported, and inadequate information is provided to calculate it. The researchers reported that the percentage of males (10.7%) in the sample was comparable to the national nursing population (9%). The simple random sampling method, large sample size, and the representative percentages of males and females in the study increased the likelihood that the sample was representative of the target population. The sampling section of the study would have been strengthened by the researchers providing details on the random sampling process and the response rate to the surveys (Thompson, 2012).

Hurley et al. (2018) reported, "Approximately 70% [of the RNs] do not meet the weekly physical activity recommendations of 150 min, and 36.2% follow guidelines for a healthy diet only 50% of the time or less. There were significant correlations between following a healthy diet or physical activity and the Self as a Role Model of Health Promotions (SARMHEP) scores" (p. 1131). The researchers recommended interventions be developed and tested to increase the healthy behaviors among nurses and to increase their awareness of role modeling as a motivator of change in others.

Stratified Random Sampling

Stratified random sampling is used when the researcher knows some of the variables in the population that are critical to achieving representativeness. Variables commonly used for stratification are age, gender, race/ethnicity, socioeconomical status, geographical region, medical diagnosis, site of care, and types of institution, care, and care provider. The variable(s) chosen for stratification are those found in previous studies to be correlated with the dependent variable(s) being examined in the study. Subjects within each stratum are expected to be more similar (homogeneous) in relation to the study variables than they are to be similar to subjects in other strata or the total sample (Tappen, 2016; Thompson, 2012).

Subjects in the population to be studied are partitioned into different strata (such as male or female gender) and are randomly selected on the basis of their classification into either the male stratum or female stratum. For example, you want to select a stratified random sample of 100 adult subjects using age as the variable for stratification. The sample might include 25 subjects in the age range 18 to 39 years, 25 subjects in the age range 40 to 59 years, 25 subjects in the age range 60 to 79 years, and 25 subjects 80 years or older. Stratification ensures that all levels of the identified variable, in this example age, are adequately represented in the sample. With a stratified random sample, you could use a smaller sample size to achieve the same degree of representativeness as that provided by a large sample acquired through simple random sampling. Sampling error decreases, power increases, data collection time is reduced, and the cost of the study might be lower if stratification is used (Thompson, 2012).

One question that arises in relation to stratification is whether each stratum should have equivalent numbers of subjects in the sample (termed **disproportionate sampling**) or whether the numbers of subjects should be selected in proportion to their occurrence in the population (termed **proportionate sampling**). For example, if stratification is being achieved by ethnicity and the population is 45% white non-Hispanic, 25% Hispanic nonwhite, 25% African American, and 5% Asian, your research team would have to decide whether to select equal numbers of each ethnic group or to calculate a proportion of the sample. Good arguments exist for both approaches. Stratification is not as useful if one stratum contains only a small number of subjects. In the aforementioned situation, if proportions are used and the sample size is 100, the study would include only five Asians, hardly enough to be representative or to identify statistical significance. If equal numbers of each group are used, each group would contain at least 25 subjects; however, the white non-Hispanic group would be underrepresented. In this case, mathematically weighting the findings from each stratum can equalize the representation to ensure proportional contributions of each stratum to the total score of the sample. You can conduct proportional or disproportional systematic sampling methods for a study or seek the assistance of a statistician for this process (Levy & Lemsbow, 1980; Thompson, 2012).

Willgerodt, Brock, and Maughan (2018) used a stratified random sampling method to "describe the demographic and school nursing practice patterns among self-reported public school nurses and the number and full-time equivalent positions of all school nurses in the United States" (p. 232). The following study excerpt details the stratified random sampling method used in this study with key sampling terms identified in brackets.

"**Sampling**

The survey sample was drawn proportionally from two NCES [National Center for Educational Statistics] surveys: the annually administered common core data (CCD) and the Private School Survey (PSS), which collect data on public and private schools, respectively (U.S. Department of Education, 2014). The NCES collects CCD data to provide a publicly available database on school demographics and data that are comparable across states. The PSS collects similar data among all private schools in the United States...

The CCD and PSS data sets both collect data at the school level and therefore, we conducted all analyses using the school as the unit of analysis. The most recent public data (2013-2014 school year for CCD and 2011-2012 school year for PSS) were used for this study (U.S. Department of Education, 2014). In 2013-2014, data were available for 102,716 public elementary and secondary schools representing approximately 18,000 school districts in the United States, Washington, DC, and U.S. territories. In 2011-2012, there were 26,983 private schools listed in the PSS database. The total number of schools in the study population was 129,699...

The final data set excluded 7,148 charter schools; 259 schools that were not designated as a public, private, or public charter school; and 1,717 territorial schools (e.g. Guam and the Marshall Islands) [exclusion sampling criteria], leaving a total survey population of 120,575 public and private schools [sampling frame]...

We estimated a conservative response rate (40%) and retrieved a random sample of 2,646 schools. The sample was proportionally stratified [sampling method] by public/private status, elementary/secondary/mixed status, HRSA [Health Resources and Services Administration] regions (Northeast, Midwest, South, and West), and the HRSA Federal Office of Rural Health Policy's, Rural–Urban Commuting Area Codes designation for urban/rural status. Individual strata were then sampled by simple random sampling [part of the stratified sampling method].... A total of 1,283 public and private schools [sample size] responded for an overall response rate of 48.5%." (Willgerodt et al., 2018, pp. 234–235)

The large sampling frame for this study was obtained using the data from two national surveys (CCD and PSS) and the sampling exclusion criteria, which resulted in 120,575 public and privates schools. The sampling method was clearly identified as proportional stratified random sampling, with the sample stratified by public/private status, elementary/secondary/mixed status, HRSA regions, and rural/urban status. The process used to randomly select schools from the different strata is unclear but was probably done using a computer program. The study did have an adequate response rate (48.5%) to the surveys sent to the public and private schools, resulting in a large sample ($n = 1283$). The data obtained from the CCD and PSS surveys were representative of the school nurses in public and private schools throughout the United States. The random stratified sampling method and large sample size increased the representativeness of the sample and decreased the potential for sampling error (Tappen, 2016; Thompson, 2012). However, a description of the initial random sampling of schools and the random selection of schools from the different strata would have strengthened the reported sampling process.

Cluster Sampling

Cluster sampling is a probability sampling method that is similar to stratified random sampling but takes advantage of the natural clusters or groups of population units that have similar characteristics. Cluster sampling is used in the two following situations: (1) A simple random sample would be prohibitive in terms of travel time and cost. Imagine trying to arrange personal meetings with 100 people, each in a different part of the United States. (2) The cases in which the individual elements making up the population are unknown, preventing the development of a sampling frame (Innocenti, Candel, Tan, & van Breukelen, 2019; Kazdin, 2017). For example, there is no list of all the heart surgery patients who complete rehabilitation programs in the United States. In these cases, it is often possible to obtain lists of institutions or organizations with which the elements of interest are associated.

In cluster sampling, the researcher develops a sampling frame that includes a list of all the states, cities, institutions, or organizations with which elements of the identified population would be linked. For example, large cardiac hospitals with 300 or more beds are selected randomly as units or clusters from which to obtain heart transplant patients for a sample. This is an example of two-stage cluster sampling, where the clusters of hospitals and the heart transplant patients within them are randomly sampled. Another important part of cluster sampling is whether the sampling is proportional or equal (nonproportional) for the cluster and the number of individuals in each cluster (see the previous section on proportional sampling). Innocenti et al. (2019) identified three alternatives for two-stage cluster sampling and provided details for accomplishing these sampling methods.

1. "Sampling clusters with probability proportional to cluster size [number of cardiac hospitals in the northeast, southern, central, and west U.S. regions] and then sampling the same number of individuals [heart transplant patients] from each sampled cluster.
2. Sampling clusters with equal probability and then sampling per sampled cluster a number of individuals proportional to cluster size.
3. Sampling clusters with equal probability and then sampling the same number of individuals per cluster." (Innocenti et al., 2019, p. 1818)

In some cases, this random selection continues through several stages and is referred to as **multistage cluster sampling** (Innocenti et al., 2019; Thompson, 2012). For example, the researcher might first randomly select states and next randomly select cities within the sampled states. Hospitals within the randomly selected cities might then be randomly selected. Within the hospitals, nursing units might be randomly selected. At this level, either all of the patients on the nursing unit who fit the sampling criteria for the study might be included, or patients could be randomly selected.

Cluster sampling provides a means for obtaining a larger sample at a lower cost than simple random sampling. However, it has some disadvantages. Data from subjects associated with the same institution are likely to be correlated and not completely independent. This correlation can cause a decrease in precision and an increase in sampling error. However, such disadvantages can be offset to some extent by the use of a larger sample.

McCarthy, Wills, and Crowley (2018) conducted a cross-sectional correlational study to examine how nurses' age and job demands are associated with PA at work and activity at leisure. These researchers described their cluster sampling method in the following study excerpt with key sampling concepts placed in brackets.

"A cross-sectional study was conducted with a sample of qualified nurses recruited from two hospitals in the Southern part of Ireland. The sample was representative of qualified nurses within the target population. Data were collected during 2016. A two-stage sampling approach was taken [sampling method]. The first stage involved the selection of different work areas within two teaching hospitals. The work areas included were; medical, surgical, …emergency departments, intensive care, coronary care…. The second stage involved the random selection of a sample of nurses from each of these work areas.

Respondents

Nurses were randomly selected from the nursing off-duty (work roster) [sampling frame] using a random generator application…. All qualified nurses working part or full-time were eligible to be included in the sample [sampling criteria]. In total 300 nurses [sample size] were invited to participate in the study. This sample size was seen to be representative of nurses working in the teaching hospitals although data on total numbers of nurses working in the sampled hospitals were not available. A response rate of 70% was obtained (n = 210); however, only n = 203 of the returned questionnaires were completed properly and thus included in these analyses." (McCarthy et al., 2018, pp. 117–118)

McCarthy and colleagues (2018) clearly described their use of two-stage cluster sampling to select work areas from two hospitals and to randomly select nurses from these work areas. The authors indicated the sample was representative of the nurses in the target population. The sampling frame was appropriate and a random generator application was used to identify potential study participants. The sample size of $n = 300$ was strong and reported as representative of the nurses working in the teaching hospitals; however, the numbers of nurses working in the hospitals were not available. Data were collected through questionnaires provided at work and a strong 70% response rate was obtained. McCarthy et al. (2018) should have recalculated the response rate based on the 203 completed questionnaires returned. The revised response rate is 67.7% ([203 ÷ 300] × 100% = 0.6767 × 100% = 67.67% = 67.7%). The probability cluster sampling method used in this study has a potential to provide a representative sample. The strong sample size and response rate also increased the representativeness of the sample.

McCarty et al. (2018) found the following: "Older nurses ($\geq$ 40 years) were significantly less likely to report engaging in recommended PA levels at work than younger nurses…. Nurses with high quantitative demands were over twice as likely to engage in recommended levels of PA at work and at leisure" (p. 116). The authors recommended that initiatives be implemented to ensure that older nurses could fulfill their roles within their capabilities. In addition, hospitals could offer PA education to both on-duty and off-duty nurses.

Systematic Sampling

Systematic sampling can be conducted when an ordered list of all members of the population is available. The process involves selecting every kth individual on the list, using a starting point selected randomly. If the initial starting point is not random, the sample is not a probability sample. To use this design in your research, you must know the number of elements in the population and the size of the sample desired. Divide the population size by the desired sample size, giving k, the size of the gap between elements selected from the list. For example, if the population size is $N = 1200$ and the desired sample size is $n = 100$, then you could calculate the value of k:

$$k = \text{Population size} \div \text{Sample size desired}$$

$$\text{Example}: \quad k = \frac{1200 \text{ (population size)}}{100 \text{ (sample size desired)}} = 12$$

Thus $k = 12$, which means that every 12th person on the list would be included in the sample. Some authors argue that this procedure does not truly give each element an opportunity to be included in the sample; it provides a random but unequal chance for inclusion (Thompson, 2012). Researchers must be careful to determine that the original list has not been set up with any ordering that could be meaningful in relation to the study. In systematic sampling, it is assumed that the order of the list is random in relation to the variables being studied. If the order of the list is related to the study, systematic bias is introduced. In addition to this risk, it is difficult to compute sampling error with the use of this design (Floyd, 1993).

Kulig and colleagues (2018) conducted a descriptive study to determine the "perceptions of sense of community and community engagement among rural nurses" (p. 60). Their systematic stratified sampling method is described in the following study excerpt with key sampling concepts placed in brackets.

"Design, setting, and participants
The Rural and Remote Nursing Practice Study II (RRNII) included a survey of Nurse Practitioners (NP), Registered Nurses (RN), Registered Psychiatric Nurses (RPN), and Licensed Practical Nurses (LPN) living or working in rural communities in all Canadian provinces and territories. Rural was defined as communities that are outside the commuting zone of urban areas with 10,000 or more inhabitants.... All nurses working in remote and northern communities were captured by the rural definition.

Participants were recruited through the 29 provincial/territorial nursing regulatory organizations. Eligible participants were all regulated nurses (NP, RN, RPN, LPN) [population] currently registered to practice or on leave for 6 months or less, who were working in a rural community, or in any community in the three northern territories [sampling criteria]. A sampling frame of $N = 9622$ eligible rural RNs, RPNs, LPNs, and NPs was determined through an analysis of the 2010 Canadian Institute for Health Information Nurses Database...with the goal of obtaining statistical significance (confidence level of 95% and a margin of error of 0.05).

A multi-level systematic stratified sample [sampling method] was obtained, with stratification by province and territory, type of nurse, and geographic area. Each provincial nursing organization was provided an excel file with all rural postal codes in their province and a request to select a specific number of nurses (every

k'th nurse) within each type of nurse, matching the nurses' work postal code, until the sample size was reached [systematic sampling method]. Due to the low numbers, all NPs in rural communities were included. In the territories, all nurses were included...

Surveys were distributed in postage paid return envelopes. Nurses had the option to respond by mail or online. A total of 3822 useable responses were obtained, of which 728 (19%) were completed on-line and 3094 (81%) on paper. This translated into a 40% response rate with a 1.5% margin of error. We can say with 100% confidence that the respondents are representative of rural Canada nurses as a whole. The population of rural RNs, the sample of RNs, as well as the number of RN surveys received from the sample, were used to calculate confidence levels and determine the representativeness of the respondents." (Kulig et al., 2018, pp. 61–62)

Kulig et al. (2018) provided a quality description of their population, sampling frame, probability sampling methods, sample size, and response rate to their study survey. A large national sample ($n = 3822$) of NPs, RNs, RPNs, and LPNs was randomly selected using a systematic stratified sample. The researchers determined that the study respondents were representative of rural Canadian nurses as a whole. The sampling section of this study is extremely strong supporting the representativeness of this sample for the population studied, with limited potential for sampling error (Thompson, 2012). The findings from this study provided key variables or traits of nurses that might be used to modify recruitment and retention interventions to encourage nurses to practice in rural areas. Nurses originally from smaller communities are often the best to recruit to rural areas. Another initiative is to match nurses based on their age and stage of their family with community activities in rural areas.

NONPROBABILITY (NONRANDOM) SAMPLING METHODS COMMONLY APPLIED IN QUANTITATIVE AND OUTCOMES RESEARCH

In **nonprobability sampling**, not every element of the population has an opportunity to be included in the sample. Nonprobability sampling methods increase the likelihood of obtaining samples that are not representative of their target populations. In conducting clinical studies in nursing and other health disciplines, limited subjects are available and it is difficult to obtain a random sample. Thus most nurse researchers use nonprobability sampling methods to select their study samples. Researchers often use convenience sampling, where any subjects who meet the eligibility criteria and are willing to participate in the study are included.

There are several types of nonprobability (nonrandom) sampling designs. Each addresses a different research need. The five nonprobability sampling designs described in this textbook are (1) convenience sampling, (2) quota sampling, (3) purposive or purposeful sampling, (4) network or snowball sampling, and (5) theoretical sampling. These sampling methods are applied in both quantitative and qualitative research. Convenience sampling and quota sampling are applied more often in quantitative, outcomes, and mixed methods research than in qualitative studies and are discussed in this section (see Table 15.1). Purposive sampling, network sampling, and theoretical sampling are more commonly applied in qualitative studies and are discussed later in this chapter and in Chapter 12.

Convenience Sampling

In **convenience sampling**, subjects are included in the study because they happen to be in the right place at the right time. Researchers simply enter available subjects into the study until they have reached the desired sample size. Convenience sampling, also called **accidental sampling**, is not considered a strong approach to sampling for interventional studies because it provides little opportunity to control for biases. Multiple biases may exist in convenience sampling; these biases range from minimal to serious. Researchers need to identify biases by carefully thinking through the sampling criteria used to determine the target population and taking steps to improve the representativeness of the sample. For example, in a study of home care management of patients with complex healthcare needs, educational level would be an important extraneous variable. One solution for controlling this extraneous variable would be to redefine the sampling criteria to include only patients with a high school education. Doing so would limit the extent of generalization but decrease the bias created by educational level. Another

option would be to select a population known to include individuals with a wide variety of educational levels. Data could be collected on educational level so that the description of the sample would include information on educational level. With this information, one could judge the extent to which the sample was representative with respect to educational level (Tappen, 2016).

Decisions related to sample selection must be carefully described to enable others to evaluate the possibility of biases. In addition, data should be gathered to allow a thorough description of the sample that can also be used to evaluate for possible biases. Data on the sample can be used to compare the sample with other samples and to estimate the parameters of populations through meta-analyses (Melnyk & Fineout-Overholt, 2019).

Many strategies are available for selecting a convenience sample. A classroom of students might be used. Patients who attend a clinic on a specific day, individuals who attend a support group, patients currently admitted to a hospital with a specific diagnosis, and every person who enters the emergency department on a given day and are willing to participate in a study are examples of convenience samples. Convenience samples are inexpensive, accessible, and usually require less time to acquire than other types of samples. This sampling method allows the conduct of studies on topics that could not be examined through the use of probability sampling. Convenience sampling also enables researchers to acquire information in unexplored areas. According to Kerlinger and Lee (2000), a convenience sample is probably adequate when used with reasonable knowledge and care in implementing a study. Healthcare studies are frequently conducted with patients experiencing various health problems, who may be reluctant to participate in research. Thus nurse researchers often find it difficult to recruit subjects for their studies and must use convenience sampling.

Lee and Park (2019) conducted an RCT focused on the effects of an AA intervention on pain, disability, and cervical range of motion in adults with chronic neck pain. The sampling criteria and the participant flow chart (see Fig. 15.2) for this study were introduced earlier. Participants for this study were obtained using convenience sampling that is described in the following study excerpt with key sampling concepts placed in brackets.

"Study participants were recruited by announcing the study on bulletin boards of three universities and three churches in D city, South Korea [sample of convenience].... Eligible participants were randomly assigned to the experimental and control groups in a 1:1 ratio by drawing lots [group assignment].... The criteria for participants section were as follows: ... (b) adults with neck pain for at least 6 months [population]... (g) willing to participate in the study and be randomly allocated into study groups [sampling criteria].... A total of 48 people [sample size] participated in this study: 25 in the experimental group and 23 in the control group." (Lee & Park, 2019, p. 13)

Lee and Park (2019) clearly described their study population but did not identify their sampling method. However, the recruitment methods and the inclusion of individuals meeting sampling criteria and willing to participate in this study are consistent with convenience sampling. The refusal rate (see Fig. 15.2) for the study was acceptable at 13.8% ($[8 \div 58] \times 100\% = 0.138 \times 100\% = 13.8\%$). The attrition rate for the total sample was small at 4% ($[2 \div 50] \times 100\% = 0.04 \times 100\% = 4\%$) with 0% attrition for the experimental group and 8% (two subjects) for the control group. The use of a nonprobability convenience sampling method decreased the representativeness of this sample. The small sample size ($n = 48$) also increased the potential for sampling error. However, the 13.8% refusal rate, limited attrition rate (4%), and approximately equal group sizes increased the representativeness of this sample and reduced the potential for sampling error (Tappen, 2016; Thompson, 2012).

Quota Sampling

Quota sampling is a nonprobability convenience sampling technique in which the proportion of identified groups is predetermined by the researchers. Quota sampling may be used to ensure the inclusion of subject types or strata in a population that are likely to be underrepresented in the convenience sample, such as women, minority groups, elderly, poor people, rich people, and undereducated adults. This method may also be used to mimic the known characteristics of the target population or to ensure adequate numbers of subjects in each stratum for the planned statistical analyses. The technique is similar to the one used in stratified random sampling, but the initial sample is not

random. If necessary, mathematical weighting can be used to adjust sample values so that they are consistent with the proportion of subgroups found in the population. Quota sampling offers an improvement over convenience sampling and tends to decrease potential biases. In most studies in which convenience samples are used, quota sampling could be used and should be considered (Thompson, 2012).

Kim, Im, Liu, and Ulrich (2019) conducted a model-development correlational study "to explore race/ethnicity-specific dimensionalities of chronic stress before and during pregnancy for non-Hispanic (N-H) White, N-H Black, Hispanic, and Asian women in the United States" (p. 704). This study was "a secondary data analysis using New York City (NYC) and Washington State (WA) Pregnancy Risk Assessment Monitoring System (PRAMS) data between 2004 and 2007" (Kim et al., 2019, p. 706). The original PRAMS project included 34 states, where newly delivered mothers were selected using a stratified random sampling without replacement of the live birth certificates. Only the PRAMS data from NYC and WA were included in this study, because these questionnaires obtained data about the chronic stress experienced by racial/ethnic minorities. The sampling process for this study is described in the following excerpt with key sampling concepts placed in brackets.

"**Sample**
The analytic sample consisted of women who (a) identified themselves as N-H White, N-H Black, Hispanic, or Asian and (b) delivered live singleton birth registered in NYC or WA in 2004-2007 [sampling criteria]. A total of 9,371 women (2,846 N-H White, 2,082 N-H Black, 3,009 Hispanic, and 1,440 Asian) participated in the PRAMS survey. Among them, 2,521 women (26.9%) were excluded due to missing information on the proxy variables of chronic stress before and during pregnancy used for analysis.... The fact that racial/ethnic minorities, relative to N-H Whites, tended to have more missing information in the data (data not shown) might not necessarily produce biased results among the groups because statistical analysis in this study was conducted stratified by race/ethnicity, subsequently, the study participants were 6,850 women [sample size] (2,314 N-H White, 1,476 N-H Black 1,999 Hispanic, and 1,061 Asians) [groups sizes] who recently gave live singleton birth in NYC or WA [settings] in 2004-2007." (Kim et al., 2019, pp. 707–708)

The sampling criteria clearly identified the target population and were relevant to the study purpose focused on race/ethnicity-specific dimensionalities of chronic stress for women before and during pregnancy (Kim et al., 2019). The researchers conducted a secondary data analysis of PRAMS survey data from only one city and one state, and the survey return rates for NYC and WA were not provided. In addition, 26.9% of the sample was excluded due to missing data on chronic stress before and during pregnancy, which decreases the representative and randomness of the sample. Kim et al. (2019) described stratification by race/ethnicity but did not identify the sampling method used. The sample selection seemed like one of convenience with quota sampling for race/ethnicity versus a stratified random sampling (Thompson, 2012; Tappen, 2016). The sample size for this study was extremely strong ($n = 6850$), and the racial/ethnic groups were of adequate size so the findings were probably an accurate reflection of reality.

Kim and colleagues (2019) concluded, "Considering the concurrent exposures and thereby increased vulnerability to multiple chronic stressors among racial/ethnic minority women, both targeted and coordinated approaches should be taken to address physical violence in Black and perceived isolation in Hispanic and Asian communities" (p. 722). The researchers also recommended the development of strategies to help women with chronic stressors cope more effectively before childbirth.

NONPROBABILITY SAMPLING METHODS COMMONLY APPLIED IN QUALITATIVE AND MIXED METHODS RESEARCH

Qualitative research is conducted to gain insights and discover meaning about a particular experience, situation, event, or cultural element. The intent is an in-depth understanding of a selected sample and not the generalization of the findings from a randomly selected sample to a target population, as in quantitative and outcomes research. In qualitative and some mixed methods research, experiences, events, and incidents are more the focus of sampling than people (Charmaz, 2014; Creswell & Poth, 2018; Marshall & Rossman, 2016). Researchers attempt to select participants or informants who can provide extensive information about the experience being studied. For example, if the goal of

your study was to describe the phenomenon of living with chronic pain, you would purposefully select participants who were articulate and reflective, had a history of chronic pain, and were willing to share details about their pain experiences.

The three common sampling methods applied in qualitative nursing research are purposive or purposeful sampling, network or snowball sampling, and theoretical sampling (see Table 15.1). These sampling methods enable researchers to select the specific participants who would provide the most extensive, quality information about the phenomenon, event, or situation being studied (Creswell & Poth, 2018; Tappen, 2016). The sample selection process should be representative of both the area of study and the philosophy underlying the study design and described in enough depth to promote the interpretation of the findings and replication of the study (Miles et al., 2020; Tappen, 2016).

Purposive Sampling

In **purposive sampling**, sometimes referred to as purposeful, judgmental, or selective sampling, the researcher consciously selects certain participants, elements, events, or incidents to include in the study. Qualitative researchers select **information-rich cases**, or cases that can teach them a great deal about the central focus or purpose of the study (Marshall & Rossman, 2016). Efforts might be made to include typical and atypical participants or situations representative of the area of study. Researchers also seek **critical cases**, or cases that make a point clearly or are extremely important in understanding the purpose of the study (Miles et al., 2020; Tappen, 2016). Researchers might select participants or informants of various ages with differing diagnoses or illness severity, or informants who received an ineffective treatment versus an effective treatment for their illness.

Purposive sampling has been criticized by some investigators because it is difficult to evaluate the quality of a researcher's judgment in selecting a study participant. How does one determine that a participant or situation was typical or atypical, good or bad, effective or ineffective? Researchers must indicate the characteristics that they desire in participants and provide a rationale for selecting these types of participants to obtain essential data for addressing their study questions. Purposive sampling is used to gain insight into a new area of study or to obtain in-depth understanding of a complex experience or event.

Epstein and colleagues (2019) conducted a grounded theory study to investigate parents' observations about the quality of life (QoL) domains that are important to their children with autism spectrum disorder (ASD). Purposive, theoretical, and network sampling methods were used to obtain the sample for this study and are discussed in the following excerpt with key sampling concepts placed in brackets.

"Participants

A total of 23 families of children with ASD (aged 6-17 years) who were registered with the Western Australian Autism Biological Registry (WAABR) [sampling criteria] were invited to participate.... Two additional families residing in rural communities were recruited through network sampling [sampling method] and were included in our final sample. We were unable to include families who were not fluent in English. In all, 22 parents (two fathers) [sample size] who were primary caregivers were interviewed and spoke on behalf of their children with ASD diagnosis. Three families declined participation due to other commitments [refusal frequency] and one family withdrew from the study after the interview [attrition frequency] and did not cite a reason. The remaining 21 interviews were used for analysis.

Recruitment was purposive and theoretically [sampling methods] directed until data saturation was reached in order to capture variability within the sample for gender, age, social communication ability, intellectual ability, health comorbidities, other neurodevelopmental problems, and residence by urban or rural location." (Epstein et al., 2019, p. 72)

Epstein et al. (2019) clearly identified the sample size, sampling criteria, and sampling methods used in this qualitative study. The refusal ($n = 3$) and attrition ($n = 1$) frequencies were low promoting an adequate, representative sample. The researchers also provided a rationale for using each type of sampling method that was relevant for collecting essential data for this study (Creswell & Poth, 2018). Purposive and theoretical sampling were the key methods used in this study. The researchers conducted purposive sampling "to capture variability within the sample for gender, age, social communication abilities, ...and residence by urban or rural location" (Epstein et al., 2019, p. 72). Theoretical sampling is commonly used in grounded theory research to develop theoretical findings, such as a framework, model, or theory, and to ensure that the full range of the experience is described (Charmaz, 2014; Creswell & Poth, 2018). The purpose of this study was to develop an initial framework for understanding QoL in children with ASD. Network sampling was used to recruit two additional families from rural locations. Network and theoretical sampling methods are discussed in the next two sections.

Network Sampling

Network sampling, sometimes referred to as snowball or chain sampling, holds promise for locating samples difficult or impossible to obtain in other ways or that had not been previously identified for study. Network sampling takes advantage of social networks and the fact that friends tend to have characteristics in common. The first few participants are often obtained through convenience or purposive sampling methods, and the sample size is expanded using network sampling. Network sampling is an effective strategy for identifying participants who know other potential participants who can provide the greatest insight and essential information about an experience, situation, or event that is identified for study (Marshall & Rossman, 2016). This sampling method is also used to ensure researchers have a representative sample of participants for a study. For example, Epstein et al. (2019) used network sampling to include two more participants from rural communities so the sample was representative of both urban and rural locations.

Network or snowball sampling is particularly useful in both quantitative and qualitative research for finding participants in socially devalued populations, such as alcoholics, child abusers, sex offenders, drug addicts, and criminals. These individuals are seldom willing to identify themselves as fitting these categories. Other groups, such as widows, grieving siblings, or individuals successful at lifestyle changes, can be located using this strategy. These individuals are outside the existing healthcare system and are difficult to find. Biases are built into the sampling process because the participants are not independent of one another. However, the participants selected have the expertise to provide the essential information needed to address the study purpose.

Marshall, Forgeron, Harrison, and Young (2018) conducted an exploratory-descriptive qualitative study to investigate RNs' pediatric pain management experiences in rural hospitals. The study included 10 RNs who were obtained using purposive and snowball sampling methods that are described in the following study excerpt with key sampling concepts placed in brackets.

> **"Participants**
> RNs who worked with children in one of the nine eligible rural hospital sites [settings] were invited to participate. Inclusion criteria were: regularly employed staff RN (full or part-time); employed at one of the eligible sites; worked with inpatient pediatric patients; and were able to communicate (write, read, speak) in English. Exclusion criteria were: RNs with less than three months experience on a unit with inpatient pediatric patients; and RNs who worked on a casual basis [sampling criteria]. Participants working at any of these nine hospitals were invited using a purposeful sampling method to gain a broad understanding of the research subject by those who experience it.... The authors also employed snowball sampling by asking participants to refer other RNs, who work with the pediatric population at their site, to the study [sampling methods]." (Marshall et al., 2018, pp. 90–91)

Marshall et al. (2018) identified the focus of their purposive sampling method, and their rationale for using snowball sampling was to increase the sample size. The study was conducted in multiple rural hospital sites with knowledgeable RNs who provided in-depth information about their experiences in managing the pain of pediatric patients. This study demonstrated a quality sampling process for addressing the study purpose. Marshall et al. (2018) concluded that pediatric pain management in rural areas presents challenges to RNs. They perceived that they lack the resources and the necessary continuing education to provide quality pediatric pain care. Future research is needed to identify strategies to improve resources in rural hospitals and to promote the use of evidence-based pain management to pediatric patients.

Theoretical Sampling

Theoretical sampling is usually applied in grounded theory research to advance the development of a selected theory or model throughout the research process (Charmaz, 2014). The researcher gathers data from any individual or group that can provide relevant data for theory generation. The data are considered relevant if they include information that generates, delimits, and saturates the theoretical codes in the study needed for framework, model, or theory generation. A code is saturated if new participants present similar ideas or concepts and the researcher can see how it fits into the emerging theory. The researcher continues to seek sources likely to advance the theoretical knowledge in progress and to gather data until the codes are saturated and the framework, model, or theory evolves from the codes and the data. Diversity or heterogeneity in the sample is encouraged so that the theoretical themes developed represent a wide range of ideas in varied situations (Charmaz, 2014; Miles et al., 2020).

Epstein and colleagues (2019) conducted a grounded theory study of parents' perspective on the QoL in their children with ASD, which was introduced earlier during the discussion of purposive sampling. These researchers conducted theoretical sampling using a grounded theory approach that is presented in the following excerpt.

> "Recruitment was purposive and theoretically directed until data saturation was reached...
> Grounded theory approach allowed for the assessment and comparison of different themes in order for domains [of QoL] to spontaneously evolve.... Transcripts were sent to participants for first-level member checking (completed by 13/21 [62%]), which gave parents an opportunity to review and edit their responses to confirm accuracy and validate their narrative.... Parents offered further examples of their children's experiences that enriched our understanding of QoL and provided new dimensions to our data.... This feedback enhanced how we had conceptualized some of the concepts, and parents confirmed our overall pattern of domains as important components of QoL for the children." (Epstein et al., 2019, pp. 72–73)

Epstein et al. (2019) identified the use of theoretical sampling to achieve data saturation in their study. The researchers obtained additional reviews by the parents to ensure the data were accurate. The parents' comments were used to expand the study framework about the QoL of children with ASD. The researchers only indicated 21 interviews were used for analysis but did not discuss if any additional participants were interviewed to achieve data saturation (see Chapter 12). Additional information is needed to determine the quality of theoretical sampling in this study (Charmaz, 2014; Miles et al., 2020).

In addition, Epstein et al. (2019) reported the following findings: "Unique aspects of quality of life included varying levels of social desire, consistency of routines, and time spent in nature and the outdoors, which are not comprehensively captured in existing measures. Parent observations provide an initial framework for understanding quality of life in autism spectrum disorder and support the development of a new measure for this population" (p. 71).

SAMPLE SIZE IN QUANTITATIVE RESEARCH

One of the questions beginning researchers commonly ask is, "What size sample should I use?" Historically, the response to this question has been that a sample should contain at least 30 subjects for each study variable measured. Statisticians consider 30 subjects the minimum number for data on a single variable to approach a normal distribution. So if a study includes four variables, researchers would need at least 120 subjects in their final sample. Researchers are encouraged to determine the probable attrition rate for their study to ensure an adequate sample size at the completion of their study. For example, researchers might anticipate a 10% to 15% attrition rate in their study and need to obtain a sample of 132 to 138 subjects to ensure the final sample size after attrition is 120. Currently the best method for determining sample size in quantitative research is a power analysis. However, if information is not available to conduct a power analysis, this recommendation of 30 subjects per study variable might be used (Kerlinger & Lee, 2000).

The deciding factor in determining an adequate sample size for correlational, quasi-experimental, and experimental studies is power. **Power** is the capacity of the study to detect differences or relationships that actually exist in the population. Expressed another way, power is the capacity to reject a null hypothesis correctly. The minimum acceptable power for a study is 0.80 (80%) (Aberson, 2019; Cohen, 1988; Kraemer & Blasey, 2016). You determine the sample size needed to obtain sufficient power by performing a **power analysis**. Power analysis includes four elements: (1) the standard power of 80%, (2) level of significance (usually set at 0.05 in nursing studies), (3) effect size (discussed in the

next section), and (4) sample size (Box 15.1) (Aberson, 2019; Grove & Cipher, 2020).

Many nurse researchers are using power analysis to determine sample size, but it is essential that the details of the power analyses be included in the published studies. Not conducting a power analysis to determine sample size and omitting the power analysis results in the research report are serious problems if the study failed to detect significant differences or relationships. Without this information, you do not know whether the results are due to an inadequate sample size or to a true absence of a difference or relationship. The calculation for power analysis varies with the types of statistical analyses conducted to determine study results (Aberson, 2019; Taylor & Spurlock, 2018). Various statistical programs are available online to conduct a power analysis for a study (see Chapter 21). Grove and Cipher (2020) detail the process for conducting and interpreting power analysis in their text.

The adequacy of sample sizes must be evaluated more carefully in future nursing studies prior to data collection. Studies with inadequate sample sizes should not be approved for data collection unless they are preliminary pilot studies conducted before a planned larger study. If it is impossible for you to obtain a larger sample because of time or numbers of available subjects, you should redesign your study so that the available sample is adequate for the planned analyses. If a sufficient sample size cannot be obtained, Cohen (1988) recommends the studies not be conducted.

Large sample sizes may be costly and difficult to obtain in nursing studies, resulting in long data collection periods. In developing the methodology for a study, you must evaluate the elements of the methodology that affect the required sample size. Kraemer and Blasey (2016) identified the following factors that must be taken into consideration in determining sample size.

1. The more stringent the significance level (e.g., 0.001 vs 0.05), the greater the necessary sample size. Most

nursing studies include a level of significance or alpha (α) = 0.05.

2. Two-tailed statistical tests require larger sample sizes than one-tailed tests. (Tailedness of statistical tests is explained in Chapters 21 and 25.)

3. The smaller the effect size (*ES*), the larger the necessary sample size. The *ES* is a determination of the effectiveness of a treatment on the outcome (dependent) variable or the strength of the relationship between two variables.

4. The larger the power required, the larger the necessary sample size. Thus a study requiring a power of 90% requires a much larger sample than a study with power set at 80%.

5. The smaller the sample size, the smaller the power of the study, which often results in an underpowered study (Aberson, 2019).

6. The factors that must be considered in decisions about sample size (because they affect power) are *ES*, type of study, number of variables, sensitivity of the measurement methods, and data analysis techniques. These factors are discussed in the following sections.

Effect Size

Effect is the presence of a phenomenon. If a phenomenon exists, it is not absent, and the null hypothesis is in error. However, effect is best understood when not considered in a dichotomous way—that is, as either present or absent. If a phenomenon exists, it exists to some degree. **Effect size** is the extent to which a phenomenon is present in a population. In this case, the term *effect* is used in a broader sense than the term *cause and effect*. For example, you might examine the impact of distraction on the experience of pain during an injection. To examine this question, you might obtain a sample of participants receiving injections and measure the perception of pain in the group that was distracted during the injection and the group that was not distracted. The null hypothesis would be: "There is no difference in the level of pain perceived by the experimental group receiving distraction when compared with that of the comparison group receiving no distraction." If this were so, you would say that the effect of distraction on the perception of pain was zero, and the null hypothesis would be accepted. In another study, the Pearson product moment correlation *r* could be conducted to examine the relationship between coping and anxiety. Your null hypothesis would be: "The population Pearson *r*

value is zero, meaning that coping is not related to anxiety" (Cohen, 1988).

In a study, it is easier to detect large differences between groups than to detect small differences. Strong relationships between variables in a study are easier to detect than weak relationships. Thus smaller samples can detect large effect sizes; smaller effect sizes require larger samples. Effect sizes can be positive or negative because variables can be either positively or negatively correlated. A negative effect size exists when an intervention causes a decrease in the study mean, such as an exercise program that decreases the weight of subjects. Broadly speaking, the definitions for effect size strengths may be as follows:

* **Small *ES* would be < 0.3 or < −0.3**
* **Medium *ES* would be about 0.3 to 0.5 or −0.3 to −0.5**
* **Large *ES* would be > 0.5 or > −0.5**

These broad ranges are provided because the effect size definitions of small, medium, and large vary based on the analysis being conducted. For example, the effect sizes for comparing two means, such as the intervention group mean and the comparison group mean (expressed as *d*), are small = 0.2 or −0.2, medium = 0.5 or −0.5, and large = 0.8 or −0.8. The effect sizes for relationships (expressed as *r*) might be defined as small = 0.1 or −0.1, medium = 0.3 or −0.3, and large = 0.5 or −0.5 (Aberson, 2019; Cohen, 1988).

Extremely small effect sizes (e.g., < 0.1) may not be clinically important because the relationships between the variables are small or the differences between the intervention and comparison groups are limited. Knowing the effect size that would be regarded as clinically important allows us to limit the sample to the size needed to detect that level of effect size (Kraemer & Blasey, 2016). A result is clinically important if the effect is large enough to alter clinical decisions. For example, in comparing glass thermometers with electronic thermometers, an *ES* = 0.1° F in oral temperature is probably not important enough to influence selection of a particular type of thermometer in clinical practice. The clinical importance of an effect size varies on the basis of the variables being studied and the population. For example, a decrease in average ambulance transfer time to a trauma center from 15 minutes to 12 minutes would probably have clinical significance for unstable patients. Researchers must determine the effect size for the particular relationship or intervention effect being studied in a population. The most desirable source of this information is evidence from previous studies (Aberson, 2019; Kazdin, 2017; Melnyk & Fineout-Overholt, 2019).

A correlation value r is equal to the effect size for the relationship between two variables. For example, if depression is correlated with anxiety at $r = 0.45$, the $ES = r = 0.45$, a medium effect size.

$$ES \text{ formula for relationships} = r$$
$$\text{Example}: ES = r = 0.45$$

Most effect sizes are calculated using a computer program (Grove & Cipher, 2020). However, in published studies with interventions, means and standard deviations (*SDs*) can be used to calculate the effect size. For example, if the mean weight loss for the intervention group is 5 pounds per month with $SD = 4.5$ and the mean weight loss of the comparison group is 1 pound per month with $SD = 6.5$, you can calculate the effect size, which is usually expressed as d.

Effect size formula for group differences = d = (mean of the treatment group − mean of the control group) ÷ standard deviation of the control group:

$$\text{Example}: ES = d = (5 - 1) \div 6.5$$
$$= 4 \div 6.5 = 0.615 = 0.62$$

This calculation can be used only as an estimate of effect size for a specific study. If the researcher changes the measurement method used, the design of the study, or the population being studied, the effect size will be altered. When estimating effect size based on previous studies, you might note the effect sizes vary from 0.33 to 0.45; it is best to choose the lower effect size of 0.33 to calculate a sample size for a study. As the effect size decreases, the sample size needed to obtain statistical significance in a study increases. The best estimate of a population parameter of effect size is obtained from a meta-analysis in which an estimated population effect size is calculated through the use of statistical values from all studies included in the analysis (Aberson, 2019; Cohen, 1988; Grove & Cipher, 2020).

If few relevant studies have been conducted in the area of interest, a small pilot study can be performed, and data analysis results can be used to calculate the effect size. If pilot studies are not feasible, a dummy power table analysis can be used to calculate the smallest effect size with clinical or theoretical value. Yarandi (1991)

described the process of calculating a dummy power table. If all else fails, effect size can be estimated as small, medium, or large. Numerical values would be assigned to these estimates and the power analysis performed. As mentioned earlier, Cohen (1988) and Aberson (2019) indicated the numerical values for small, medium, and large effects on the basis of specific statistical procedures. In new areas of research, effect sizes for studies are usually set as small (< 0.3). Gaskin and Happell (2014) conducted a study of the statistical practices in nursing research and noted inconsistent reporting and infrequent interpretation of effect sizes, which require improvement by nurse researchers.

Most power analysis discussions are focused on those conducted prior to a study to determine an adequate sample size. However, Aberson (2019) discusses the importance of a post hoc power analysis to determine the power achieved in a study based on the actual sample size achieved in the study with an alpha set at 0.05. If the power is low, the study needs to be replicated with a larger sample to determine if a Type II error occurred. If the power is high, this supports the acceptance of the null hypothesis in the study.

Lee and Park (2019) conducted a power analysis to determine the sample size needed for examining the effect of AA on pain and disability of adults with chronic neck pain. The sampling criteria and methods for this study were discussed earlier, and the power analysis and sample size are described in the following excerpt.

"The sample size for this study was calculated using the G-Power 3.1. According to previous studies (Movahedi et al., 2017; Yeh, Morone et al., 2014), the effect size was 0.75, power (1-ß) was 0.80 [80%]), and the significance level (α) was 0.05. The resulting number of participants required for each group was 23 people. Eligible participants were assigned, 25 in each of the experimental and control groups, in consideration of a dropout rate of 20%. Two participants dropped out of the control group, so the total number of the participants was 48 (see [Fig. 15.2])." (Lee & Park, 2019, p. 13)

Lee and Park (2019) described the essential elements of power analysis (see Box 15.1) conducted to determine an adequate sample size for their study. These elements included a standard power of 80%, α = 0.05, and an *ES* of 0.75, which was calculated based on the effects of the AA intervention in previous studies. The statistical basis for the power analysis was not identified; however, the researchers did report the data were analyzed using independent *t*-test and repeated measures analysis of variance (ANOVA) (see Chapter 25). These statistics are appropriate for determining differences between the experimental and control groups (Grove & Cipher, 2020). The total sample size was $n = 48$, which is larger than the 46 participants (23 participants per group) recommended by the power analysis. The researchers did adjust for sample attrition to maintain an adequate sample size, and the groups were approximately equal. The study results were significant for three variables (pain threshold, disability, and cervical range of motion); but neck pain, as measured by a visual analog scale (VAS), was not significantly different between the experimental and control group. The power needs to be examined for this nonsignificant result to determine if the sample was adequate for the study or there was a Type II error (Aberson, 2019).

Type of Study

The type of study conducted also influences the sample size for a quantitative study. Descriptive case studies tend to use small samples. Groups are not compared, and problems related to sampling error and generalization have little relevance for such studies. A small sample size may better serve the researcher who is interested in examining a situation in depth from various perspectives. Other descriptive studies, measuring study variables with surveys, questionnaires, or scales, and correlational studies require large samples. In these studies, multiple variables may be examined, and extraneous variables are likely to affect subject responses to the variables under study. Statistical comparisons are often made among multiple subgroups in the sample, requiring that an adequate sample be available for each subgroup being analyzed. In addition, subjects are likely to be heterogeneous in terms of demographic variables, and measurement tools are sometimes not adequately refined. Although target populations may have been identified, sampling frames may be unavailable, and parameters have not usually been well defined by previous studies. All of these factors decrease the power of the study and require increases in sample size (Aberson, 2019; Kraemer & Blasey, 2016).

Quasi-experimental and experimental studies often have smaller samples than descriptive and correlational studies. As control in the study increases, the sample size can decrease and still approximate the population. Instruments in these studies tend to be refined, improving precision. However, sample size must be sufficient to achieve an acceptable level of power (0.8) and reduce the risk of a Type II error (indicating the study findings are nonsignificant, when they really are significant) (Aberson, 2019; Kraemer & Blasey, 2016).

The study design influences power, but the design with the greatest power may not always be the most valid design to use. The experimental design with the greatest power is the pretest-posttest design with a historical control or comparison group. However, this design may have questionable validity because of the historical control group. Can the researcher demonstrate that the historical control group is comparable to the experimental group? The repeated measures design increases power if the trait being assessed is relatively stable over time. Lee and Park (2019) conducted an RCT with repeated measures that increased the power of their study.

Designs that use blocking or stratification usually require an increase in the total sample size. The sample size increases in proportion to the number of cells included in the data analysis. Designs that use matched pairs of subjects have greater power and require a smaller sample (see Chapter 11 for a discussion of these designs). The higher the degree of correlation between subjects on the variable on which the subjects are matched, the greater the power (Kraemer & Blasey, 2016).

Kraemer and Blasey (2016) classified studies as exploratory or confirmatory. According to their approach, confirmatory studies should be conducted only after a large body of knowledge has been gathered through exploratory studies. **Exploratory studies** are designed to increase the knowledge in a field of study and often include smaller nonprobability samples. Exploratory studies are not intended for generalization to large populations. For example, pilot or preliminary studies to test a methodology or provide estimates of an effect size often are conducted before a larger study. In other exploratory studies, the variables, not the subjects, are the primary area of concern. Several studies may examine the same variables using different populations. In these types of studies, the specific population used may be incidental. Data from exploratory studies are used to define population parameters and to provide information for conducting confirmatory studies.

Confirmatory studies are expected to have strong designs that include large samples obtained with random sampling techniques. These studies are conducted to test the effects of nursing interventions on patient outcomes or to examine the fit of research findings to a theoretical model. For example, clinical trials are conducted in nursing for the purpose of confirming knowledge in an area of study. The power of these large, complex studies must be carefully analyzed (Leidy & Weissfeld, 1991). For the large sample sizes to be obtained, subjects are acquired in numerous clinical settings, sometimes in different parts of the United States. Kraemer and Blasey (2016) believed that these studies should not be performed until extensive information is available from exploratory studies. This information should include a meta-analysis and the definition of a population effect size.

Number of Variables

As the number of variables under study grows, the needed sample size may also increase. Adding variables such as age, gender, ethnicity, and education to the analysis plan (just to be on the safe side) can increase the sample size by a factor of 5 to 10 if the selected variables are uncorrelated with the dependent variable. In this case, instead of a sample of 50, you may need a sample of 250 to 500 if you plan to include the variables in the statistical analyses. (Using demographic variables only to describe the sample does not cause a problem in terms of power.) If the variables are highly correlated with the dependent variable, however, the effect size will increase, and the sample size can be reduced.

Variables included in the data analysis must be carefully selected. They should be essential to the research purpose or should have a documented strong relationship with the dependent variable (Aberson, 2019; Kraemer & Blasey, 2016). Sometimes researchers have obtained sufficient sample size for the primary analyses but failed to plan for analyses involving subgroups, such as analyzing the data by age categories or by race/ethnic groups, which require a larger sample size. A larger sample size is also needed if multiple dependent variables have been measured in the study. For example, the Lee and Park (2019) study included four dependent variables (neck pain, PT, disability, and cervical range of motion) and probably needed a larger sample size to detect significant differences for all these variables.

Measurement Sensitivity

Well-developed physiological instruments measure phenomena with precision. For example, a thermometer measures body temperature precisely, usually to one-tenth of a degree. Instruments measuring psychosocial variables tend to be less precise. However, a scale with strong reliability and validity tends to measure more precisely than an instrument that is not as well developed. Variance tends to be higher in a less well-developed tool than in one that is well developed. An instrument with a smaller variance is preferred because the power of a test always decreases when within-group variance increases (Kraemer & Blasey, 2016). If you were measuring the phenomenon of anxiety and the actual anxiety score for several subjects was 80, the subjects' scores on a less well-developed scale might range from 70 to 90, whereas a well-developed scale would tend to show a score closer to the actual score of 80 for each subject. As variance in instrument scores increases, the sample size needed to gain an accurate understanding of the phenomenon increases (Waltz et al., 2017).

The range of measured values influences power. For example, a variable might be measured in 10 equally spaced values, ranging from 0 to 9. Effect sizes vary according to how near the value is to the population mean. If the mean value is 5, effect sizes are much larger in the extreme values and lower for values near the mean. If you decided to use only subjects with values of 0 and 9, the effect size would be large, and the sample could be small. The credibility of the study might be questionable, however, because the values of most individuals would not be 0 or 9 but rather would tend to be in the middle range of values. If you decided to include subjects who have values in the range of 3 to 6, excluding the extreme scores, the effect size would be small, and you would require a much larger sample. The wider the range of values sampled, the larger the effect size (Kraemer & Blasey, 2016). In a heterogeneous group of study participants, you would expect them to have a wide range of scores on a stress scale, which would increase the effect size.

A strong measurement method has validity and reliability, and measures variables at the interval or ratio level (see Chapter 16). The stronger the measurement methods used in a study, the smaller the sample that is needed to identify significant relationships among variables and differences between groups. Lee and Park (2019) used a VAS to measure pain in their experimental and control groups. The VAS is a single-item scale 100 mm long that participants in this study marked to indicate their amount of neck pain (see Chapter 17 for a copy of the VAS). The VAS has limited reliability and validity because it is a single-item scale; therefore, the effect size of future studies might be increased with the use of a valid and reliable multiitem pain scale or including two different scales to measure neck pain. Lee and Park (2019) reported the VAS pain scores decreased in both groups, and the participants had positive beliefs about the AA intervention, which might have had a placebo (artificial) or psychological effect on the control group (Kazdin, 2017; Shadish et al., 2002).

Data Analysis Techniques

Data analysis techniques vary in their ability to detect differences in the data. Statisticians refer to this as the power of the statistical analysis. For your data analysis, choose the most powerful statistical test appropriate to the data. Overall, parametric statistical analyses are more powerful than nonparametric techniques in detecting differences and should be used if the data meet criteria for parametric analysis (Grove & Cipher, 2020). However, in many cases, nonparametric techniques are more powerful if your data do not meet the assumptions of parametric techniques. Parametric techniques vary widely in their capacity to distinguish fine differences and relationships in data (see Chapter 21). There is also an interaction between the measurement sensitivity and the power of the data analysis technique. The power of the analysis technique increases as precision in measurement increases. Larger samples must be used when the power of the planned statistical analysis is low (Gaskin & Happell, 2014).

For some statistical procedures, such as the t-test and ANOVA, having equal group sizes increases power because the effect size is maximized. The more unequal the group sizes are, the smaller the effect size. In unequal groups, the total sample size must be larger (Kraemer & Blasey, 2016).

The chi-square test is the weakest of the statistical tests and requires very large sample sizes to achieve acceptable levels of power. As the number of categories (cells in the chi-square analysis) in a study grows, the sample size needed increases. Also, if there are small numbers in some of the categories, you must increase the sample size (Aberson, 2019; Grove & Cipher, 2020).

Kraemer and Blasey (2016) recommended that the chi-square test be used only when no other options are available. In addition, the categories should be limited to those essential to the study.

SAMPLE SIZE IN QUALITATIVE RESEARCH

In quantitative research, the sample size must be large enough to describe variables, identify relationships among variables, or determine differences between groups. However, in qualitative research, the focus is on the quality of information obtained from the person, situation, or culture sampled versus the size of the sample (Marshall & Rossman, 2016; Morse, 2000; Tappen, 2016). The sample size and sampling plan are determined by the purpose and philosophical basis of the study. In addition, the sample size varies with the depth of information needed to gain insight into a phenomenon, develop a framework or theory, examine a cultural element, or explore and describe a concept or situation (Creswell & Poth, 2018; Miles et al., 2020). The sample size can be too small when the data collected lack adequate depth or richness. An inadequate sample size can reduce the quality and credibility of the research findings. Thus qualitative researchers frequently use purposive sampling to obtain an adequate number of participants who can provide the rich data needed to gain insights and discover new meaning in an area of study.

The researchers should justify the adequacy of the sample size in their qualitative study. Often the number of participants is adequate when saturation of information is achieved in the study area. **Saturation of data**, also referred to as informational redundancy, occurs when additional sampling provides no new information, only redundancy of previously collected data. Important factors that must be considered in determining sample size to achieve saturation of data are (1) scope of the study, (2) nature of the topic, (3) quality of the data, and (4) study design (Marshall & Rossman, 2016; Morse, 2000, 2012; Tappen, 2016).

Scope of the Study

If the scope of a study is broad, researchers need extensive data to address the study purpose, and it takes longer to reach data saturation. A study with a broad scope requires more sampling of participants or situations than a study with a narrow scope (Morse, 2000, 2012). A study that has a clear focus and uses focused data collection usually has richer, more credible findings. For example, fewer participants would be needed to detail the phenomenon of chronic pain in adults with rheumatoid arthritis than would be needed to describe the phenomenon of chronic pain in elderly adults. A study of chronic pain experienced by elderly adults has a much broader focus, with less clarity, than a study of chronic pain experienced by adults with a specific medical diagnosis.

Nature of the Topic

If the topic of your study is clear and the participants can easily discuss it, fewer individuals are needed to obtain the essential, rich data. If the topic is difficult to define and awkward for people to discuss, you will probably need a larger number of participants or informants to reach the point of data saturation (Marshall & Rossman, 2016; Miles et al., 2020). For example, a phenomenological study of the experience of an adult living with a history of childhood sexual abuse is a sensitive, complex topic to investigate. This type of topic would probably require a greater number of participants and increased interview time to collect essential data.

Quality of the Data

The quality of information obtained from an interview, observation, focus group, or document review influences the sample size. The higher the quality and richness of the data, the fewer research participants needed to saturate data in the area of study. Quality data are best obtained from articulate, well-informed, and communicative participants. These participants are able to share richer and often more data in a clear and concise manner. In addition, participants who have more time to be interviewed usually provide data with greater depth and breadth. However, researchers should have enough participants so there is not overreliance on one or two key informants (Tappen, 2016).

Qualitative studies require that you critically appraise the richness of communication elicited from the participants, the degree of access provided to events in a culture, or the number and quality of observations obtained in a situation studied. These characteristics directly affect the richness of the data collected and influence the sample size needed to achieve credible study findings (Miles et al., 2020).

Study Design

Some studies are designed to conduct more than a single interview with each participant. The more interviews conducted with a participant, the greater the quantity and probably the quality of the data collected. For example, a study design that includes an interview both before and after an event would produce more varied data than a single interview. Designs that involve interviewing a family or a group of individuals produce more data than an interview with a single study participant. In grounded theory studies, participants are interviewed until a framework, model, or theory is developed for the area of study (Charmaz, 2014). In some qualitative studies, data are best collected with focus groups or observations or a combination of methods (see Chapter 12) (Creswell & Poth, 2018). In critically appraising a qualitative study, determine whether the sample size is adequate for the design of the study.

Marshall et al. (2019) conducted an exploratory-descriptive qualitative study about nurses' pediatric pain management experiences in rural hospitals that was introduced earlier. The sample was obtained with purposive and network sampling methods, and the following study excerpt provides the researchers' rationale for the final sample size of 10 participants.

> "Participants working at any of these nine hospitals were invited using a purposeful sampling method to gain a broad understanding of the research subject by those who experience it…. The authors also employed snowball sampling by asking participants to refer other RNs, who work with the pediatric population at their site, to the study…
>
> Although sample size in qualitative research is not predetermined (Morse, 2000), factors such as the scope of the study, nature of the topic, quality of the data obtained, and the study design all influence how many participants are needed to ensure richness of data (Morse, 2000). Sample sizes of eight (Boström, Magnusson, & Engström, 2012) to 22 (Goldblatt, 2009) have been used for qualitative studies using individual interviews to collect data. A sample size of eight to ten participants was targeted.
>
> A total of 12 RNs from eight of the sites [rural hospitals] contacted the research team, and 10 of these consented to participate. The reasons for declining to participate were that they felt they would be unable to contribute to the study findings although the first author

did clarify that they had relevant experience.... Most of the participants were female, over 40 years of age and their highest level of nursing education was a RN diploma. The length of career as a nurse varied (0–30+ years) and all worked with children at least monthly. In addition to working in a rural hospital most of the RNs had some experience working in urban settings.... Interviews ranged between 30 and 60 min long (median = 48 min), and three of the participants chose to have Skype interviews." (Marshall et al., 2018, pp. 91–92)

Marshall and colleagues (2018) described the relevant sampling methods used to obtain their study participants and provided support for their choices by citing relevant sources. The sample size was influenced by the "scope of the study, nature of the topic, quality of data obtained, and the study design" (Marshall et al., 2018, p. 91). After a review of other qualitative studies, the researchers determined that 8 to 22 participants were needed for studies using individual interviews to collect data. They targeted an adequate sample size (8–10 RNs) with a final sample of 10 RNs from eight rural hospitals. The characteristics of the participants indicated they had a strong background for providing quality, trustworthy data for this study. The discussion of sample size would have been strengthened by a description of the process used to reach data saturation.

RESEARCH SETTINGS

The **research setting** is the location where a study is conducted. There are three common settings for conducting nursing research: natural, partially controlled, and highly controlled. These types of settings are described in the following sections.

Natural Setting

A **natural setting**, or field setting, is an uncontrolled, real-life situation or environment (Creswell & Creswell, 2018; Kerlinger & Lee, 2000). Conducting a study in a natural setting means that the researcher does not manipulate or change the environment for the study. Descriptive and correlational quantitative studies, qualitative, mixed methods, and outcomes nursing studies often are conducted in natural settings. For example, Hurley and colleagues (2019) conducted a correlational study to examine the relationships of nurses' personal

health practices to their perceptions of themselves as role models for health promotion in a natural setting. This study was introduced earlier in the section on simple random sampling, and the study setting is presented in the following excerpt.

"Data were collected through an anonymous, online questionnaire using the Checkbox® survey. The randomly selected participants received an email with an invitation to participate in the study. The email assured the participant of confidentiality and that only aggregate results would be reported. Completion and return of the survey were considered consent to participate; those who did not wish to participate were instructed to simply delete the email invitation. The name or email was not linked to the participant's responses.... Participants' reponses were downloaded directly from the electronic Checkbox® system into the IBM SPSS®v.22 database and reviewed for accuracy." (Hurley et al., 2019, p. 1137)

Studies that involved data collection through online e-mails or mailed surveys (questionnaires or scales) all have a natural setting. Study participants receive an e-mailed version of the survey or are mailed or handed a hard copy of the survey to complete. As indicated in this example, the confidentiality of the participants is protected, and they can complete the survey in any location of their choice, usually their home or work. Hurley et al. (2019) provided a detailed discussion of their collection of data through an online questionnaire that participants could complete when and where they desired. Data were managed confidentially during data collection and analysis and in reporting of study results (Kazdin, 2017; Kerlinger & Lee, 2000; Waltz et al., 2017).

Partially Controlled Setting

A **partially controlled setting** is an environment that the researcher manipulates or modifies in some way while conducting a study. An increasing number of nursing intervention studies are conducted in partially controlled settings (Kazdin, 2017; Shadish et al., 2002). Ramadi and Haennel (2019) conducted a prospective repeated measures study to examine the relationships among the variables sedentary behavior, breaks in sedentary time, and PA for participants progressing through a CR program. This study was introduced earlier with the discussion of refusal and attrition rates in sampling, and the study's partially controlled setting is highlighted in the following excerpt.

"Exercise Program
We recruited patients from two centers that offered supervised CR program.... Participants attended 8-12 weeks of CR program. The program involved 1-2 sessions/week of supervised exercise. Participants were given activity logs and were encouraged to supplement their exercise program with 1-4 additional sessions/week independently. Exercise training regimen included aerobic training..., steady-state exercise (20-60 min), and a cool-down (5 min). During steady-state exercises, participants exercised at a perceived exertion level of 12-14 (on the Borg 6-20 scale). During the program, participants had access to a variety of education classes including a session on exercise and leading an active life style...

Daily PA and sedentary behavior were assessed objectively using the SenseWear Mini Armband (SWA...). The SWA uses multiple sensors... to estimate energy expenditure (EE)... We used minute by minute EE data to obtain information on sedentary time and time spent in different PA intensities." (Ramadi & Haennel, 2019, p. 9)

The setting for the Ramadi and Haennel (2019) study was partially controlled because it was conducted in two CR centers that offered a structured CR program. The CR exercise program was highly structured by the number of sessions per week, the types of exercises performed, and the exertion level during the exercises. The study variables were measured with objective, precise physiological devices to increase measurement accuracy and reduce error. The CR centers provided a quality partially controlled setting for implementing this study.

Highly Controlled Setting

A **highly controlled setting** is a structured environment that often is artificially developed for the purpose of conducting research. Laboratories, research or experimental centers, and highly structured units in hospitals or other healthcare agencies are examples of highly controlled settings. Often experimental and sometimes quasi-experimental studies are conducted in these types

of settings. A highly controlled setting reduces the influence of extraneous variables, which enables researchers to examine accurately the effect of an intervention on an outcome.

Leng and colleagues (2018) conducted an RCT to determine if "electroacupuncture reduces weight in diet-induced obese rats" (p. 1). The study was conducted in a laboratory setting that is briefly described in the following study excerpt.

"Animals and Animal Care. All experimental procedures were approved by Institutional Animal Care and Use Committee...for animal research. SPF-grade SD male rats that had weights of 70~90 g and had just been weaned (three to four weeks of age) were chosen.... After arrival, the experimental animals were fed at a density of five rats per cage, during the first week with standard laboratory water and chow ad libitum, and then allowed to take food and drink water freely under a 12 h natural light-dark cycle at a temperature in the range of 22°C–24°C, and ventilation was conducted on a regular time basis. The relative humidity was 50%–70%. Rat cages were cleaned and drinking flasks were rinsed every day, and the feeds were ensured to be clean and fresh. Animals were divided into high-fat (HF) and normal feed group (chow group) randomly. The HF group of rats were fed with the high-fat feed (fat 20%, glucose 10%, dry powder of yolk 10%, standard chow 60%, 492.8 kcal/100 g) in enough amount for 14 weeks, while the chow group of rats (*n* = 18) were fed with normal feeds in enough amount for 14 weeks." (Leng et al., 2018, p. 2)

Leng et al. (2018) detailed the laboratory setting they used for their experimental study with rats. The care of the rats was according to national standards, and their environment was highly controlled. The process for inducing obesity in the rats through HF diet (experimental group) was detailed; the rats in the control group received a normal diet. All animal research and some complex physiological studies are conducted in highly controlled settings. This is a type of basic or bench research that is often conducted prior to applied research with humans (Kazdin, 2017; Kerlinger & Lee, 2000; Waltz et al., 2017).

RECRUITING AND RETAINING RESEARCH PARTICIPANTS

After the research team makes decisions about the sample size and setting, the next step is to develop a plan for **recruiting research participants**. This plan involves identifying, accessing, and communicating with potential study participants who are representative of the target population. Recruitment strategies differ, depending on the type of study, population, and setting. Special attention should focus on recruiting study participants who tend to be underrepresented in studies, such as minorities, women, children, adolescents, elderly, the critically ill, the economically disadvantaged, and the incarcerated (Chhatre et al., 2018; Gluck et al., 2018; Goldman et al., 2018; Goshin & Byrne, 2012; NIH, 2019).

The sampling plan, initiated at the beginning of data collection, is almost always more difficult than expected. In addition to participant recruitment, retaining acquired subjects is critical to achieve an acceptable sample size and requires researchers to consider the effects of the data collection strategies on sample attrition. **Retaining research participants** involves the participants completing the required behaviors of a study to its conclusion. The problems with retaining participants increase as the data collection period lengthens. Some researchers never obtain their planned sample size, which could decrease the power of the study and potentially produce nonsignificant results (Aberson, 2019; Cohen, 1988).

With an increasing number of studies being conducted in health care, recruiting and retaining study participants have become very complex issues for nurse researchers to manage. An increasing number of articles examining the effectiveness of various strategies for participant recruitment and retention are appearing in the literature focused on such populations as pregnant adolescents (Wise & Cantrell, 2019), young adult cancer patients (Leuteritz et al., 2018), elderly adults (NIH, 2019), African Americans (Gluck et al., 2018), and the acutely ill (Irani & Richmond, 2015). This chapter concludes with a discussion of strategies for recruiting and retaining research participants to guide you in conducting your own study.

Recruiting Research Participants

The effective recruitment of study participants is crucial to the success of a study. Table 15.3 was developed to identify the steps for recruiting potential subjects and the strategies used to promote success in these steps. The initial step is the identification of settings for accessing potential study participants. The settings for obtaining subjects might include healthcare agencies, nurse practitioner or physician offices, professional meetings, churches, universities, or social events. You might also obtain a list of potential participants with their contact information and send them a letter, text, or e-mail about the study. Some researchers develop fliers and hand them to potential participants or post them on selected bulletin boards. Your research team could also place posters in public places such as churches, universities, supermarkets, drugstores, and laundries.

Researchers and their team members might advertise in a community through radio public service announcements and social media or in newsletters and local papers. If the study is funded, money might be available to advertise on television. Researchers could speak to groups relevant to the study population. Many individuals with chronic illnesses or other health conditions attend support groups or educational programs and might be contacted through these meetings. For example, Wise and Cantrell (2019) recruited pregnant adolescents for their nutrition intervention study from a local teen parenting program. With permission, you and your research team can set up tables in shopping malls to recruit subjects. Plan for possible challenges in recruitment and include multiple methods and two to three locations in your application for human subject approval for your study. Otherwise you would need to submit a modified protocol to the institutional review board (IRB) if a method or site for recruitment is added. However, obtaining access to additional locations is time consuming due to the IRB process (see Chapter 9).

Social media, such as Facebook and Twitter, have become successful ways to contact potential subjects. Marshall et al. (2018) used a variety of recruitment strategies to identify participants for their qualitative study focused on nurses' pediatric pain management experiences in rural hospitals. This study was introduced earlier in the sections focused on sampling methods and sample size. These researchers' strategies for identifying potential study participants are presented in the following excerpt.

TABLE 15.3 Reasons for Participation in Clinical Research After Minor Physical Injury

Recruitment Steps	Strategies
1. Identification of potential participants	• Contact healthcare agencies, providers' offices, professional organizations, support groups, churches, or community leaders • Review healthcare records • Mail-out strategy, texting, or e-mailing requests for participation • Handing out fliers in person or posting them at key sites • Placing posters at public locations • Presentations to selected groups • Social media campaign by Twitter and Facebook • Community advertising by radio, newsletter, local papers, or television
2. Initial communication with potential participants	• Recruiter's approach (positive, polite, and unrushed) by the best method for the population (in person, phone, e-mail, text, or letter) • Cultural competence • Provision of information about the study in an understandable way • Clear, concise response to questions
3. Promoting participation	• Personal benefits to potential participants • Interest in the study • Contributing to knowledge development • Helping others • Increased healthcare information • Being regularly monitored

Retention Steps	Strategies
1. Consent to participate	• Clarify the focus of the study • Clarify time, energy, behaviors for study • Clear presentation of the consent form and process • Obtain the required consent
2. Retention during the study	• Frequent personal contact by meetings, phone calls, texts, or e-mails • Remember birthdays or other events with a card or e-mail • Group communication by Facebook, Twitter, text, or e-mail • Appointments scheduled based on participants' needs • Participants provided transportation to the research site • Respect the participants' time • Communicate the value of the participant completing the study • Financial compensation for time and effort, if possible • Results provided to participants at the completion of the study

"Participants were recruited through a combination of efforts: a mail out strategy; a social media campaign, and community advertisement. The mail out strategy was based on a list of RNs who authorized the provincial licensing board to release their names and contact information for research purposes.... Initially, the RNs were mailed an information cover letter, and consent form, if there was no response they received a one-page reminder letter two weeks, later, and lastly a few weeks later if there was still no response, they were sent a last letter of invitation and consent.... Additional recruitment efforts included social media campaign (using Twitter and Facebook) and community advertisement." (Marshall et al., 2018, p. 91)

Marshall et al. (2018) provided a detailed description of the various strategies they used to identify potential study participants. They tried contacting potential participants at least three times by mail, which is supported in the literature. Goldman et al. (2018) conducted a study of the "recruitment and retention of hardest-to-reach families in community-based asthma interventions" (p. 543) and found that participants required 3.1 contact attempts before they were enrolled into the studies. Marshall et al. (2018) might have expanded on their community advertisement strategies.

The next step in the recruitment process is the initial communication with potential study participants (see Table 15.3). This communication usually strongly affects the individual's decision about participating in the study. Therefore the approach must be pleasant, positive, informative, culturally sensitive, and unrushed. The researcher needs to explain the importance of the study and clarify exactly what the individual will be asked to do, how much time will be involved, and what the duration of the study will be. You also need to address potential subjects' questions in a clear, concise manner in terms they understand (Chhatre et al., 2018). Study participants are valuable resources, and researchers must communicate this value to them. High-pressure, aggressive techniques, such as insisting that the potential subject make an instant decision to participate in a study, usually lead to resistance and a higher rate of refusals.

When an individual refuses to participate in your study, you must accept the refusal gracefully—in terms of body language as well as words. Your actions can influence the decision of other potential participants who observe or hear about the encounter. Studies in which a high proportion of individuals refuse to participate have a serious validity problem (see the earlier discussion of acceptance and refusal rates). The sample is likely to be biased because only a certain type of individual has agreed to participate. You should keep records of the numbers of persons who refuse, and their reasons for refusal. With this information, you can include the refusal frequency, rate, and rationales for refusal in the published research report. It would also be helpful if you could determine whether the individuals who refused to participate differed from those who agreed to participate in the study, in terms of demographics, reasons for seeking health care, course of medical treatment, or other pertinent factors. This information will help you determine the representativeness of your sample (Chhatre et al., 2018; Kazdin, 2017).

Recruiting minority subjects for a study can be particularly problematic. Minority individuals may be difficult to locate and might be reluctant to participate in studies because of their negative feelings about research or possible distrust of the medical community. When conducting studies with minorities, researchers must be culturally competent or knowledgeable and skilled in relating to the particular ethnic group being studied. If the researcher is not of the same culture as the potential subjects, he or she may employ a data collector who is of the same culture. Effective strategies for recruiting minorities include developing partnerships with target groups, community leaders, and potential participants in the community; using active face-to-face recruitment in nonthreatening settings; and using appropriate language to communicate clearly the purpose, benefits, and risks of the study.

Promoting the participation of individuals in research often requires implementing many strategies, such as providing increased access to health information and care, supporting individuals' desire to help others in a community, or receiving financial compensation (see Table 15.3). Gluck et al. (2018) described their recruitment of "older African Americans to brain health and aging research through community engagement" (p. 78). This area of research is extremely important because African Americans have two to three times the prevalence of Alzheimer disease than Caucasians. These researchers identified the following strategies for recruitment and retention of their study participants.

- "Build trust through long-term relationships that bring value to the community. . . .
- Communicate health information through known and trusted community leaders. . . .
- Recruit older black men through targeted efforts. . . .
- Cultivate research participants as ambassadors for brain research." (Gluck et al., 2018, pp. 79-80)

Gluck et al. (2018) reported, "Community participants recruited to our research have come primarily from long-standing partnerships with local churches, senior centers; city, county, and state offices for health and aging; as well as from outreach to public and other low-income housing sites" (p. 80). Through these recruitment and retention strategies, the researchers were able to recruit over a 1000 older African Americans for their short health and lifestyle survey and many agreed to participate in additional studies.

If you collect data by mailed or online surveys, you may never have personal contact with the subjects. Thus researchers use a variety of strategies to encourage individuals to participate in their study with the initial contact. Researchers use attention-getting techniques, persuasively written materials, and strategies for following up on individuals who do not respond to the initial written or e-mail communication. The strategies need to be appropriate for the potential participants; mailed surveys are probably still the best way to obtain information from elderly adults. The NIH (2019) considered the elderly a very understudied population and mandated that older adults be included in all NIH-supported research involving human subjects when scientifically appropriate.

Currently, researchers use the internet to recruit participants and to collect survey data. This method makes it easier for you to contact potential participants and for them to provide the requested data. However, an increased number of surveys are being sent by the internet, which can decrease the response rate of potential participants who are frequently surveyed but increase the participation of potential participants not accessible by traditional recruitment measures.

Most internet questionnaires or scales are going to an e-mail list of potential study participants or are posted on a website. The letter encouraging potential participants to take part in the study must be carefully composed. It may be your only chance to persuade them to invest the time needed to complete the study questionnaire or scale. You must sell the reader on the importance of both your study and his or her response. The tone of your letter will be the potential subject's only image of you as a person; yet, for many subjects, their response to the perception of you as a person most influences their decision about completing the questionnaire. Seek examples of letters sent by researchers who have had high response rates, and save letters you received to which you responded positively. You also might pilot-test your letter on potential research participants who can give you feedback about their reactions to the letter's tone.

The use of follow-up e-mails, letters, or cards has been repeatedly shown to raise response rates to surveys. The timing is important. If too long a period has lapsed, the potential subject may have deleted the questionnaire from his or her e-mail inbox or discarded the mailed copy. However, sending the follow-up too soon could be offensive. A bar graph could be developed to record the return of the questionnaires as a means of suggesting when the follow-up mailing or e-mailing should occur. The cumulative number and percentage of responses over time would be logged on the graph to reflect the overall data collection process (Goldman et al., 2018). When the daily or weekly responses decline, a follow-up e-mail or first-class letter could be sent encouraging individuals to complete the study questionnaire. Often a third follow-up, with a modified cover letter, is sent to participants with a final request that they complete the study questionnaires or scales.

The factors involved in the decision of whether to respond to a questionnaire are not well understood. One factor is the time required to respond; this includes the time needed to orient oneself to the directions and the emotional energy necessary to deal with any threats or anxieties generated by the questions. There is also a cognitive demand for making decisions. Subjects seem to make a judgment about the relevance of the research topic and the potential for personal application of findings. Previous experience with questionnaires is also a deciding factor.

Because of the serious problems of analysis and interpretation posed by low response rates with surveys, using strategies to increase the response rate is critical. In some cases, small amounts of money ($1–$5) are enclosed with the letter, which may suggest that the recipient buy a soft drink or that the money is a small gift for completing the questionnaire. This strategy imposes some sense of obligation on the recipient to complete the questionnaire, but it is not thought to be coercive. Also, you should plan e-mailing or mailings to avoid holidays or times of the year when activities are high for potential subjects, possibly reducing the return rate. For example, if you were conducting a study with mothers of school-age children, you would want to avoid the beginning of a new school term.

If researchers use data collectors in their studies, they need to verify that the data collectors are following the sampling plan, especially in studies using random samples. For instance, when data collectors encounter difficult subjects or are unable to make contact easily, they may simply shift to the next available person without informing the principal investigator. This behavior could violate the rules of random sampling and bias the sample. If data collectors do not understand, or do not believe in, the importance of randomization, their decisions and actions can undermine the intent of the sampling plan. Thus data collectors must be carefully selected and thoroughly trained. A plan for the supervision and follow-up of data collectors to increase their accountability should be developed (see Chapter 20).

Traditionally, subjects for nursing studies have been sought in the hospital setting. However, access to these subjects is becoming more difficult—in part because of the larger numbers of nurses and other healthcare professionals now conducting research. The largest involvement of research subjects within a healthcare agency usually occurs in the field of medical research and is primarily associated with clinical trials that include large samples. Chhatre et al. (2018) identified three successful recruitment methods to use in healthcare agencies: (1) identifying potential participants using administrative or clinical databases, (2) developing trust and obtaining referrals of potential participants through healthcare providers and other sources, and (3) effectively communicating when approaching a potential subject. An initial phase of recruitment may involve obtaining community and institutional support and approval for the study. Support from other healthcare professionals, such as nurses, physicians, and clinical agency staff, is usually crucial for the successful recruitment of study participants in healthcare agencies.

Recruitment of subjects for clinical trials requires a different set of strategies because the recruitment may occur simultaneously in several sites (perhaps in different cities). Many of these multisite clinical trials never achieve their planned sample size. The number of participants meeting the sampling criteria who are available in the selected clinical sites may not be as large as anticipated. Researchers must often screen twice as many patients as are required for a study to obtain a sufficient sample size. Screening logs must be kept during the recruiting period to record data on patients who met the criteria but were not entered into the study. Researchers commonly underestimate the amount of time required to recruit study participants for a clinical trial. In addition to defining the number of participants and the time set aside for recruitment, it may be helpful to develop short-term or interim recruitment goals designed to maintain a constant rate of patient entry (Chhatre et al., 2018; Friese et al., 2017).

Retaining Participants in a Study

A serious problem in many studies is participant retention, which sometimes cannot be avoided. Subjects move, die, or withdraw from a treatment. If you must collect data at several points over time, subject attrition can become a problem. Study participants who move frequently or are without phones pose particular problems. Several strategies have been identified to effectively maintain participants in studies (see Table 15.3) (Friese et al., 2017; Gluck et al., 2018; Goldman et al., 2018; Moss, Still, Jones, Blackshire, & Wright, 2019). It is a good idea to obtain the names, e-mail addresses, and phone numbers (cell and home numbers if possible) of at least two family members or friends when you enroll the participant in the study. Ask whether the participant would agree to give you access to unlisted phone numbers in the event of changes in his or her number.

In some studies, subjects are reimbursed for time and expenses related to participation. For example, subjects might be provided transportation to the research site and home. A bonus payment may be included for completing a certain phase of the study. Gifts can be used in place of money. Researchers have found that money was more effective than gifts in retaining subjects in longitudinal studies. However, some people think this strategy can compromise the voluntariness of participation in a study and particularly has the potential of exploiting low-income persons. When the monetary gift is small ($20–$50) and consistent with the responsibilities of the participants, most consider these acceptable (Goldman et al. 2018). It is important that the incentives used to recruit and retain research participants be documented in the published study.

Collecting data takes time. The participant's time is valuable and should be used frugally. During data collection, it is easy to begin taking the participant for granted. Taking time for social amenities with participants may also pay off. However, take care that these interactions do not influence the data being collected. Beyond that, nurturing subjects participating in the study is critical. In some situations, providing refreshments and pleasant surroundings are helpful. During the data collection phase, you also may need to nurture others who interact with the participants; these may be volunteers, family, staff, students, or other professionals. It is important to maintain a pleasant climate for the data collection process, which pays off in the quality of data collected and the retention of study participants (Friese et al., 2017; Goldman et al., 2018; Leuteritz et al., 2018; Wise & Cantrell, 2019).

Qualitative studies with more than one data collection point and longitudinal quantitative studies require extensive time commitments from participants. They are asked to participate in detailed interviews or to complete numerous forms at various intervals during a study (Creswell & Creswell, 2018; Marshall & Rossman, 2016; Miles et al., 2020). Sometimes data are collected with diaries that require daily entries over a set period of time. These studies face the greatest risk of participant attrition. Chapters 12 and 14 provide more details on the recruitment and retention of research participants for qualitative and mixed methods studies.

Moss and colleagues (2019) conducted an exploratory-descriptive qualitative study focused on hypertension self-management from the perspectives of older African Americans adults. Their strategies that promoted success with retention of participants in their study are presented in the following excerpt.

> "Refreshments were available for participants at each of the focus group sessions. Each participant was given a US$50 gift card and provided taxicab transportation service or a US$10 gas card for each of the two focus group sessions they attended. At the close of the study, participants were each mailed a personal-sized copy of the graphic recording image along with a thank-you note for participating." (Moss et al., 2019, p. 671)

In summary, research participants who have a personal investment in a study are more likely to complete the study. This investment occurs through interactions with and nurturing by the researcher. A combination of the participant's personal belief in the significance of the study, the perceived altruistic motives of the researcher in conducting the study, the ethical actions of the researcher, and the nurturing support provided by the researcher during data collection can greatly diminish participant attrition (Gluck et al., 2018; Goldman et al., 2018; Wise & Cantrell, 2019). Recruitment and retention of study participants will continue to be significant challenges for researchers, and creative strategies are needed to manage these challenges.

KEY POINTS

- Sampling involves selecting a group of people, situations, behaviors, or other elements with which to conduct a study. Sampling denotes the process of making the selections; sample denotes the selected group of elements (see Fig. 15.1).
- A sampling plan is developed to increase representativeness and reduce sampling error; there are two main types of sampling plans: probability and nonprobability.
- Sampling error includes random variation and systematic variation. Refusal and attrition rates are important to calculate in a study to determine potential systematic variation or bias.
- The probability or random sampling designs commonly used in nursing studies include simple random sampling, stratified random sampling, cluster sampling, and systematic sampling (see Table 15.1).
- In nonprobability (nonrandom) sampling, not every element of the population has an opportunity for selection in the sample. The common nonprobability sampling designs used in quantitative and outcomes studies include convenience and quota sampling. Occasionally network or snowball sampling and purposive sampling might be used.
- The nonprobability sampling designs used in qualitative and mixed methods research include convenience sampling, purposive or purposeful sampling, network sampling, and theoretical sampling.
- Convenience sampling is the most common sampling method used in all types of nursing studies.
- In quantitative studies, sample size is best determined by a power analysis, which is calculated using the level of significance (usually $\alpha = 0.05$), standard power of 0.80 (80%), and ES. Factors important to sample size in quantitative research include (1) type of study, (2) number of variables studied, (3) measurement sensitivity, and (4) data analysis techniques.
- The number of participants in a qualitative study is adequate when saturation of information is achieved

in the study area, which occurs when additional sampling provides no new information, only redundancy of previously collected data. Important factors that must be considered in determining sample size needed to achieve saturation of data are (1) scope of the study, (2) nature of the topic, (3) quality of the data, and (4) study design.

- The three common settings for conducting nursing research are natural, partially controlled, and highly controlled. A natural (or field) setting is an uncontrolled, real-life situation or environment. A partially controlled setting is an environment that the researchers have manipulated or modified in some way for conducting their study. A highly controlled setting is often an artificially constructed environment, such as a laboratory or research unit in a hospital, developed for the sole purpose of conducting research.

- Recruiting and retaining research participants have become significant challenges in research; some strategies to assist researchers with these challenges are provided so that their samples might be more representative of their target population (see Table 15.3).

REFERENCES

Aberson, C. L. (2019). *Applied power analysis for the behavioral sciences* (2nd ed.). New York, NY: Routledge Taylor & Francis Group.

Borglin, G., & Richards, D. A. (2010). Bias in experimental nursing research: Strategies to improve the quality and explanatory power of nursing science. *International Journal of Nursing Studies, 47*(1), 123–128. doi:10.1016/j.ijnurstu.2009.06.016

Boström, M., Magnusson, K., & Engström, Å. (2012). Nursing patients suffering from trauma: Critical care nurses narrate their experiences. *International Journal of Orthopaedic and Trauma Nursing, 16*(1), 21–29. doi:10.1016/j.ijotn. 2011.06.002

Charmaz, K. (2014). *Constructing grounded theory: A practical guide through qualitative analysis* (2nd ed.). Thousand Oaks, CA: Sage.

Chhatre, S., Jefferson, A., Cook, R., Meeker, C. R., Kim, J. H., Hartz, K. M., … Jayadevappa, R. (2018). Patient-centered recruitment and retention for a randomized controlled study. *Trials, 18*(1), 205. doi:10.1186/s13063-018-2578-7

Cohen, J. (1988). *Statistical power analysis for the behavioral sciences* (2nd ed.). New York, NY: Academic Press.

Consolidated Standards of Reporting Trials (CONSORT). (2010). *The CONSORT statement.* Retrieved from http://www.consort-statement.org/.

Creswell, J. W., & Clark, V. L. P. (2018). *Designing and conducting mixed methods research* (3rd ed.). Los Angeles, CA: Sage.

Creswell, J. W., & Creswell, J. D. (2018). *Research design: Qualitative, quantitative, and mixed methods approaches* (5th ed.). Los Angeles, CA: Sage.

Creswell, J. W., & Poth, C. N. (2018). *Qualitative inquiry & research design: Choosing among five approaches* (4th ed.). Los Angeles, CA: Sage.

Epstein, A., Whitehouse, A., Williams, K., Murphy, N., Leonard, H., Davis, E., … Downs, J. (2019). Parent-observed thematic data on quality of life in children with autism spectrum disorder. *Autism, 23*(1), 71–80. doi:10.1177/1362361317722764

Floyd, J. A. (1993). Systematic sampling: Theory and clinical methods. *Nursing Research, 42*(5), 290–293.

Friese, C. R., Mendelsohn-Victor, K., Ginex, P. McMahon, C. M., Fauer, A. J., & McCullagh, M. C. (2017). Lessons learned from a practice-based, multisite intervention study with nurse participants. *Journal of Nursing Scholarship, 49*(2), 194–201. doi:10.1111/jnu.12279

Gaskin, C. J., & Happell, B. (2014). Power, effects, confidence, and significance: An investigation of statistical practices in nursing research. *International Journal of Nursing Studies, 51*(5), 795–806. doi:10.1016/j.ijnurstu.2013.09.014

Gluck, M. A., Shaw, A., & Hill, D. (2018). Recruiting older African Americans to brain health and aging research through community engagement. *Journal of the American Society on Aging, 42*(2), 78–82.

Goldblatt, H. (2009). Caring for abused women: Impact on nurses' professional and personal life experiences. *Journal of Advanced Nursing, 65*(8), 1645–1654. doi:10.1111/j.1365-2648.2009.05019.x

Goldman, H., Fagnano, M., Perry, T. T., Weisman, A., Drobnica, A., & Halterman, J. S. (2018). Recruitment and retention of the hardest-to-reach families in community-based asthma interventions. *Clinical Trials, 15*(6), 543–550. doi:10.1177/1740774518793598

Goshin, L. S., & Byrne, M. W. (2012). Predictors of post-release research retention and subsequent reenrollment for women recruited while incarcerated. *Research in Nursing & Health, 35*(1), 94–104. doi:10.1002/nur.21451

Grove, S. K., & Cipher, DJ. (2020). *Statistics for nursing research: A workbook for evidence-based practice* (3rd ed.). St. Louis, MO: Elsevier.

Hurley, S., Edwards, J., Cupp, J., & Phillips, M. (2018), Nurses' perceptions of self as role models of health. *Western Journal of Nursing Research, 40*(8), 1131−1147. doi:10.1177/0193945917701396

Innocenti, F., Candel, M. J. J. M., Tan, F. E. S., & van Breukelen, G. J. P. (2019). Relative efficiencies of two-stage sampling schemes for mean estimation in multilevel populations when cluster size is informative. *Statistics in Medicine, 38*, 1817−1834. doi:10.1002/sim.8070

Irani, E., & Richmond, T. S. (2015). Reasons for and reservations about research participation in acutely injured adults. *Journal of Nursing Scholarship, 47*(2), 161–169. doi:10.1111/jnu.12120

Kandola, D., Banner, D., Okeefe-McCarthy, S., & Jassal, D. (2014). Sampling methods in cardiovascular nursing research: An overview. *Canadian Journal of Cardiovascular Nursing, 24*(3), 15–18.

Kane, R. L., & Radosevich, D. M. (2011). *Conducting health outcomes research.* Sudbury, MA: Jones & Bartlett Learning.

Kazdin, A. E. (2017). *Research design in clinical psychology* (5th ed.). Boston, MA: Pearson.

Kim, S., Im, E., Liu, J., & Ulrich, C. (2019). Factor structure for chronic stress before and during pregnancy by racial/ethnic group. *Western Journal of Nursing Research, 41*(5), 704−727. doi:10.1177/0193945918788852

Kerlinger, F. N., & Lee, H. B. (2000). *Foundations of behavioral research* (4th ed.). Fort Worth, TX: Harcourt College Publishers.

Kraemer, H. C., & Blasey, C. (2016). *How many subjects? Statistical power analysis in research.* Newbury Park, CA: Sage.

Kulig, J. C., Townshend. I., Kosteniuk, J., Karunanayake, C., Labrecque, M. E., & MacLeod, M. L. P. (2018). Perceptions of sense of community and community engagement among rural nurses: Results of a national survey. *International Journal of Nursing Studies, 86*(1), 60−70. doi:10.1016/j.ijnurstu.2018.07.018

Larson, E. (1994). Exclusion of certain groups from clinical research. *Image: Journal of Nursing Scholarship, 26*(3), 185–190. doi:10.1111/j.1547-5069.1994.tb00311.x

Lee, S., & Park, H. (2019). Effects of auricular acupressure on pain and disability in adults with chronic neck pain. *Applied Nursing Research, 45*(1), 12−16. doi:10.1016/j.apnr.2018.11.005

Leidy, N. K., & Weissfeld, L. A. (1991). Sample sizes and power computation for clinical intervention trials. *Western Journal of Nursing Research, 13*(1), 138–144. doi:10.1177/019394599101300111

Leng, J., Xiong, F., Yao, J., Dai, X., Luo, Y., Hu, M., … Li, Y. (2018). Electroacupuncture reduces weight in diet-induced obese rats via hypothalamic Tsc1 promoter demethylation and inhibition of the activity of a mTORC1 signaling pathway. *Evidence-based Complementary and Alternative Medicine, 3039783.* doi:10.1155/2018/3039783

Leuteritz, K., Friedrich, M., Nowe, E., Sender, A., Taubenheim, S., Stoebel-Richter, Y., & Geue, K. (2018). Recruiting young adult cancer patients: Experiences and sample characteristics from a 12-month longitudinal study. *European Journal of Oncology Nursing, 36*(1), 26−31. doi:10.1016/j.ejon.2018.05.001

Levy, P. S., & Lemsbow, S. (1980). *Sampling for health professionals.* Belmont, CA: Lifetime Learning.

Marshall, C., Forgeron, P., Harrison, D., & Young, N. L. (2018). Exploration of nurses' pediatric pain management experiences in rural hospitals: A qualitative descriptive study. *Applied Nursing Research, 42*(1), 89−97. doi:10.1016/j.apnr.2018.06.009

Marshall, C., & Rossman, G. B. (2016). *Designing qualitative research* (6th ed.). Los Angeles, CA: Sage.

McCarthy, V. J., Wills, T., & Crowley, S. (2018). Nurses, age, job demands and physical activity at work and at leisure: A cross-sectional study. *Applied Nursing Research, 40*(1), 116−121. doi:10.1016/j.apnr.2018.01.010

Melnyk, B. M., & Fineout-Overholt, E. (2019). *Evidence-based practice in nursing and healthcare: A guide to best practice* (4th ed.). Philadelphia, PA: Wolters Kluwer.

Miles, M. B., Huberman, A. M., & Saldaña, J. (2020). *Qualitative data analysis: A methods sourcebook* (4th ed.). Los Angeles, CA: Sage.

Morse, J. M. (2000). Determining sample size. *Qualitative Health Research, 10*(1), 3–5. doi:10.1177/104973200129118183

Morse, J. M. (2012). *Qualitative health research: Creating a new discipline.* Walnut Creek, CA: Left Coast Press.

Moss, K. O., Still, C. H., Jones, L. M., Blackshire, G., & Wright, K. D. (2019). Hypertension self-management perspectives from African American older adults. *Western Journal of Nursing Research, 41*(5), 667−684. doi:10.117/0193945918780331

Movahedi, M., Ghafari, S., Nazari, F., & Valiani, M. (2017). The effect of acupressure on fatigue among female nurses with chronic back pain. *Applied Nursing Research, 36*(1), 111–114. doi:10.1016/j.apnr.2017.06.006

National Institutes of Health (NIH). (2019). *Examining diversity: Recruitment and retention in aging research.* Bethesda, MD: NIH. Retrieved from https://grants.nih.gov/

Polit, D. F., & Beck, C. T. (2010). Generalization in quantitative and qualitative research: Myths and strategies. *International Journal of Nursing Studies, 47*(2010), 14551−1458. doi:10.10106/j.ijnurstu.2010.06.004

Ramadi, A., & Haennel, R. G. (2019). Sedentary behavior and physical activity in cardiac rehabilitation participants. *Heart & Lung, 48*(1), 8−12. doi:10.1016/j.hrtlng.2018.09.008

Shadish, W. R., Cook, T. D., & Campbell, D. T. (2002). *Experimental and quasi-experimental designs for generalized causal inference.* Chicago, IL: Rand McNally.

Tappen, R. (2016). *Advanced nursing research: From theory to practice* (2nd ed.). Burlington, MA: Jones & Bartlett Learning.

Taylor, J., & Spurlock, D. (2018). Statistical power in nursing education research. *Journal of Nursing Education, 57*(5), 262−264. doi:10.3928/0148434-20180420-02

Thompson, S. K. (2012). *Sampling* (3rd ed.). New York, NY: John Wiley & Sons.

U.S. Department of Education, National Center for Education Statistics. (2014). *Common core data 2013-2014.* Washington, DC: NCES. Retrieved from https://nces.ed.gov/ccd/ccdata.asp

Waltz, C. F., Strickland, O. L., & Lenz, E. R. (2017). *Measurement in nursing and health research* (5th ed.). New York, NY: Springer Publishing Company.

Willgerodt, M. A., Brock, D. M., & Maughan, E. D. (2018). Public school nursing practice in the United States. *Journal of School Nursing, 34*(3), 232−244. doi:10.1177/105840517752456

Wise, N. J., & Cantrell, M. A. (2019). Research methodology: Effectiveness of recruitment and retention strategies in pregnant adolescent nutrition intervention study. *Journal of Advanced Nursing, 75*, 215−223. doi:10.1111/jan.13840

Yarandi, H. N. (1991). Planning sample sizes: Comparison of factor level means. *Nursing Research, 40*(1), 57–58.

Yates, F. (1981). *Sampling methods for censuses and surveys.* New York, NY: MacMillan.

Yeh, C. H., Morone, N. E., Chien, L. C., Cao, Y., Lu, H., Shen, J., … Suen, L. K. (2014). Auricular point acupressure to manage chronic low back pain in older adults: A randomized controlled pilot study. *Evidence-based Complementary and Alternative Medicine, 2014*(1), 1–11. doi:10.1155/2014/375173

Quantitative Measurement Concepts

Susan K. Grove

http://evolve.elsevier.com/Gray/practice/

Measurement in quantitative and outcomes research is the process of assigning numbers to elements, events, or situations in accord with some rule (Kaplan, 1963). The numbers assigned can indicate numerical values or categories for the physiological variables, such as weight and urine output, or psychosocial concepts, such as pain and anxiety, being measured. The rules of measurement were developed so that the assigning of values or categories might be done consistently from one subject (or event) to another and eventually, if the measurement method is found to be meaningful, from one study to another. The rules of measurement established for research are similar to the rules of measurement implemented in nursing practice. For example, when you measure the urine output from patients, you use an accurate measurement device, observe the amount of urine in the device or container in a consistent way, and precisely record the urine output in the electronic health record. Measurement of urine output in clinical practice or research requires precision and accuracy (Ryan-Wenger, 2017). If physiological variables are accurately and precisely measured, the potential for measurement error is decreased, resulting in a quality assessment of reality (Waltz, Strickland, & Lenz, 2017).

When measuring a subjective concept such as pain experienced by a child, researchers and nurses in practice need to use an instrument that captures the pain the child is experiencing. A commonly used scale to measure a child's pain is the Wong-Baker FACES Pain Rating Scale (Wong-Baker FACES Foundation, 2019). When you use a reliable and valid scale to measure a child's pain, any change in the measured value can be attributed to a change in the child's pain rather than

measurement error. **Instrumentation** is a component of measurement that involves the rigorous application of specific rules to develop a measurement instrument (Bandalos, 2018). Quality scales and questionnaires take years to develop to ensure that trustworthy data are collected on relevant nursing concepts in research.

Understanding the logic within measurement theory is necessary for you to critically appraise the quality of measurement methods used in research and practice (Waltz et al., 2017). This knowledge will also assist you in selecting and using existing instruments in nursing studies. Measurement theory, as with most theories, uses terms with meanings that can be best understood within the context of the theory. The following explanation of the logic of measurement theory includes definitions of directness of measurement, measurement error, levels of measurement, and reference of measurement. The reliability and validity of measurement methods, such as scales and questionnaires, are detailed. The accuracy, precision, and error of physiological measures are also described because of their increased use in nursing research. The chapter concludes with a discussion of sensitivity, specificity, and likelihood ratios (LRs) examined to determine the quality of diagnostic tests and instruments used in healthcare research and practice (Melnyk & Fineout-Overholt, 2019).

DIRECTNESS OF MEASUREMENT

Measurement begins by clarifying the characteristic, element, or factor to be measured. Only then can one identify or develop strategies or methods to measure it. In some cases identification of the measurement element and measurement strategies can be objective, specific, and straightforward as when we are measuring concrete factors, such as a person's weight or waist circumference (WC); this is referred to as **direct measurement**. Healthcare technology has made direct measures of many physiological variables—such as height, weight, vital signs, and oxygen saturation—familiar to us. Technology is also available to measure many biological and chemical characteristics, such as laboratory values, pulmonary functions, and sleep patterns (Stone & Frazier, 2017). Nurses are also experienced in gathering direct measures of demographic variables, such as age, gender, ethnicity/race, marital status, income, and education.

However, in nursing, the characteristic or element we want to measure often is an abstract idea or concept, such as pain, stress, depression, anxiety, caring, or coping. If the concept to be measured is abstract, it is best clarified through a conceptual definition (see Chapters 6 and 8). The conceptual definition can be used to select or develop appropriate means of measuring a concept in a study. For example, you are implementing a study comparing two methods of diabetic education, and the outcome you want to measure is diabetic self-management. The instrument or measurement strategy selected must match the conceptual definition of self-management developed for the study. An abstract concept is not measured directly; instead, indicators or attributes of the concept are used to represent the abstraction. This is referred to as **indirect measurement**. For example, the complex concept of coping might be defined by the frequency or accuracy of identifying problems, the creativity in selecting solutions, and the speed or effectiveness in resolving the problem. A single measurement strategy rarely, if ever, can completely measure all aspects of an abstract concept. Multi-item scales have been developed to measure abstract concepts, such as the Spielberger State-Trait Anxiety Inventory developed to measure individuals' innate anxiety trait (personal level of anxiety) and their anxiety in a specific situation, such as prior to surgery (Spielberger, Gorsuch, & Lushene, 1970). Many sources for scales are older because the process of instrumentation is extremely complex and rigorous (Bandalos, 2018; DeVellis, 2017).

MEASUREMENT ERROR

There is no perfect measure because error is inherent in any measurement strategy. **Measurement error** is the difference between what exists in reality and what is measured by an instrument. Measurement error exists in both direct and indirect measures and can be random or systematic. Direct measures are considered highly accurate in the measurement of variables, but they are still subject to error. For example, the weight scale may not be accurate, laboratory equipment may be precisely calibrated but may change with use, or the tape measure may not be placed in the same location or held at the same tension for each measurement of a patient's WC.

Indirect measures usually have more error than direct measures (Bandalos, 2018). Efforts to measure concepts usually result in capturing only part of the concept, but they also contain other elements that are not part of the concept. Fig. 16.1 shows a Venn diagram of the concept A measured by instrument A-1. In this figure, A-1 does not measure all of concept A. In addition, some of what A-1 measures is outside the concept of A. Both situations are examples of errors in measurement that are shaded in Fig. 16.1.

Types of Measurement Errors

Two types of errors are of concern in measurement: random error and systematic error. To understand these types of errors, we must first understand the elements of a score on an instrument or an observation. According to measurement theory, there are three components to a measurement score: true score, observed score, and error score (Bandalos, 2018; Cappelleri, Lundy, & Hays, 2014). The **true score** (T) is what we would obtain if there was no error in measurement. Because there is always some measurement error, the true score is never known. The **observed score** (O) is the measure obtained

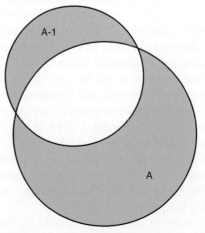

Fig. 16.1 Measurement error when measuring a concept.

for a subject using a selected instrument during a study. The **error score** (E) is the amount of random error in the measurement process. The theoretical equation of these three measures is as follows:

Observed Score (O) = True Score (T) + Error Score (E)

This equation is a means of conceptualizing random error and not a basis for calculating it. Because the true score is never known, the random error is never known but only estimated. The desired goal is to reduce the error; with smaller error scores, the observed score more closely reflects the true score, at least in theory. Therefore using instruments that reduce error improves the accuracy of measurement (Bandalos, 2018; Cappelleri et al., 2014; Waltz et al., 2017).

Several factors can occur during the measurement process that can increase random error. Transient personal factors (e.g., fatigue, hunger, attention span, health, mood, mental status, motivation) and situational factors (e.g., a hot stuffy room, distractions, the presence of significant others, rapport with the researcher, the playfulness or seriousness of the situation) can increase random error. You as the researcher can increase random error by varying how a measurement method is administered. For example, in interviews, the wording or sequence of questions is varied; questions are added or deleted; or researchers code responses differently. During data processing, errors in accidentally marking the wrong column, hitting the wrong key when entering data into the computer, or incorrectly totaling instrument scores will increase random error (DeVon et al., 2007; Waltz et al., 2017).

Random error causes individuals' observed scores to vary in no particular direction around their true score. For example, with random error, one subject's observed score may be higher than his or her true score, whereas another subject's observed score may be lower than his or her true score. According to classical measurement theory, "the mean of the [random] errors for a population of respondents is expected to be zero, and the correlation between the true scores (T) and error scores (E) for a population of respondents is zero" (Bandalos, 2018, p. 161). Random error does not influence the mean to be higher or lower; rather, it increases the amount of unexplained variance around the mean. The increased unexplained variance around the mean results in the estimation of the true score being less precise.

If you were to measure a variable for three study participants and diagram the random error, it might appear as shown in Fig. 16.2. The difference between the true score of participant 1 (T_1) and the observed score (O_1) is two positive measurement intervals. The difference between the true score (T_2) and observed score (O_2) for participant 2 is two negative measurement intervals. The difference between the true score (T_3) and observed score (O_3) for participant 3 is zero. The random error for these study participants is zero ($+2 - 2 + 0 = 0$). In considering his example, you need to remember this is only a means of conceptualizing random error (Bandalos, 2018).

Measurement error that is not random is referred to as systematic error. A scale that measures all study participants as weighing 3 pounds more than their true weights is an example of systematic error. All the measurements of body weights would be higher than the true scores and, as a result, the mean based on these measurements would be higher than the true mean. **Systematic error** occurs because something else is being measured in addition to the concept. A conceptualization of systematic error is presented in Fig. 16.3.

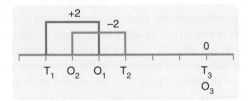

Fig. 16.2 Conceptualization of random error.

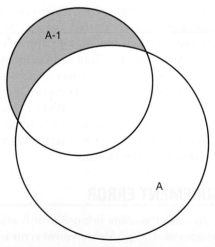

Fig. 16.3 Conceptualization of a systematic error.

Systematic error (represented by the shaded area in the figure) is due to the part of A-1 that is outside of A. This part of A-1 measures factors other than A and biases scores in a particular direction.

Systematic error is considered part of true score and reflects the true measure of A-1, not A. Adding the true score (with systematic error) to the random error (which is zero) yields the observed score, as shown by the following equations:

$$\text{(True Score With Systematic Error) T} +$$
$$\text{(Random Error of 0) E} = \text{(Observed Score) O}$$

Or

$$T + E = O$$

Some systematic error is incurred in almost any measure; however, a close link between the abstract theoretical concept and the development of the instrument that measures it can greatly decrease systematic error. Because of the importance of this factor in a study, researchers spend considerable time and effort in selecting and developing quality measurement methods to decrease systematic error (Bandalos, 2018; Cappelleri et al., 2014).

Another effective means of diminishing systematic error is to use more than one measure of an attribute or a concept and to compare the measures. To make this comparison, researchers use various data collection methods, such as scale, interview, and observation. Campbell and Fiske (1959) developed a technique of using more than one method to measure a concept, referred to as the **multimethod-multitrait technique**. More recently, the technique has been described as a measurement version of mixed methodology (Creswell & Clark, 2018). This technique allows researchers to measure more dimensions of abstract concepts, which decreases the effect of the systematic error on the composite observed score. Fig. 16.4 illustrates how various dimensions of concept A are captured through the use of four instruments, designated A-1, A-2, A-3, and A-4.

For example, a researcher could decrease systematic error in measures of anxiety by (1) administering the Spielberger State-Trait Anxiety Inventory (Spielberger et al., 1970), (2) recording blood pressure (BP) readings, (3) asking the subject about anxious feelings, and (4) observing the subject's behavior. Multimethod measurement strategies decrease systematic error by combining the

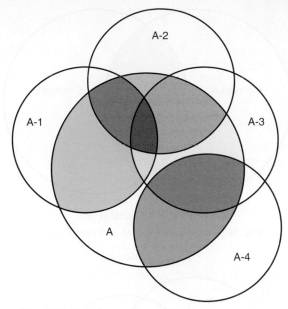

Fig. 16.4 Multiple measures of an abstract concept.

values in some way to give a single score of anxiety for each subject. However, sometimes it may be difficult logically to justify combining scores from various measures, and a mixed methods research design might be the most appropriate to use in the study (see Chapter 14). A mixed methods study, previously referred to as triangulation, uses two quantitative research designs to better represent truth. However, the vast majority of mixed methods studies use one quantitative and one qualitative design (Creswell & Clark, 2018).

In some studies, researchers use instruments to examine relationships. Consider a hypothesis that tests the relationship between concept A and concept B. In Fig. 16.5, the shaded area enclosed in the dark lines represents the true relationship between concepts A and B, such as the relationship between anxiety and depression. For example, two instruments, A-1 (Spielberger State-Trait Anxiety Inventory) (Spielberger et al., 1970) and B-1 (Center for Epidemiological Studies of Depression Scale [CES-D]) (Radloff, 1977), are used to examine the relationship between concepts A and B. The part of the true relationship actually reflected by A-1 and B-1 measurement methods is represented by the colored areas in Fig. 16.6. The darkest color of the relationship is measured by instrument A-1 only, a lighter color of the relationship (to the right) is measured by

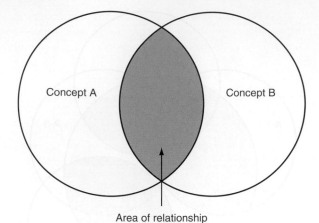

Fig. 16.5 True relationship of concepts A and B.

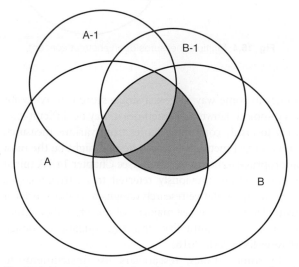

Fig. 16.6 Examining a relationship using one measure of each concept.

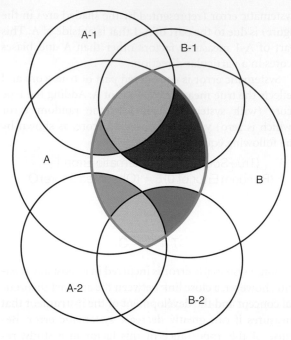

Fig. 16.7 Examining a relationship using two measures of each concept.

instrument B-1 only, and the lightest color is the part of the relationship measured by A-1 and B-1. Because two instruments provide a more accurate measure of concepts A and B, more of the true relationship between concepts A and B can be measured. So, if additional instruments (A-2 and B-2) are used to measure concepts A and B, more of the true relationship is reflected. Fig. 16.7 demonstrates with different colors the parts of the true relationship (outlined in blue) between concepts A and B that is measured when concept A is measured with two instruments (A-1 and A-2) and concept B is measured with two instruments (B-1 and B-2). In this

example, the majority of the relationship between A and B is examined by these four instruments.

LEVELS OF MEASUREMENT

In 1946, Stevens organized the rules for assigning numbers to objects so that a hierarchy in measurement was established, which is called the **levels of measurement**. Fig. 16.8 provides a summary of the rules for the levels of measurement—nominal, ordinal, interval, and ratio. These levels of measurement are described in the following sections.

Nominal Level of Measurement

Nominal level of measurement is the lowest of the four measurement levels. Nominal level data are also referred to as categorical data, where the values are names, not real numbers. Table 16.1 describes some of the different types of concepts or terms used in the literature that pertain to measurement. Nominal data can be organized into categories of a defined property, but the categories cannot be ordered. For example, diagnoses of chronic diseases are nominal data with categories such as hypertension, type 2 diabetes, and dyslipidemia. One cannot say that one category is higher than another or

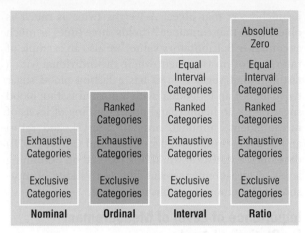

Fig. 16.8 Summary of the rules for levels of measurement.

that category A (hypertension) is closer to category B (diabetes) than to category C (dyslipidemia). The categories differ in quality but not quantity. One cannot say that subject A possesses more of the property being categorized than does subject B. (Rule: The categories must be unorderable.) Categories must be established so that each datum fits into only one of the categories. (Rule: The categories must be exclusive.) For example, you would not want a category of cardiovascular disease and another of heart failure because the datum for a person with heart failure could be placed in either or both of these categories. All the data must fit into the established categories (see Fig. 16.8). (Rule: The categories must be exhaustive.) For example, the datum for a person with chronic obstructive pulmonary disease would not be included if the categories were cardiovascular disease, metabolic disease, and neurological disease. A category for respiratory disease would be needed to include the person's datum.

Data obtained from measuring the demographic variables ethnicity/race, gender, marital status, religion, and diagnoses are examples of nominal or categorical data. When data are coded for entry into the computer, the categories are assigned numbers. For example, gender may be classified as $1 =$ male and $2 =$ female. The numbers assigned to categories in nominal measurement are used only as labels and cannot be used for mathematical calculations.

Ordinal Level of Measurement

Data that can be measured at the **ordinal level of measurement** can be assigned to categories of an attribute that can be ranked. As with nominal scale data, the categories must be exclusive and exhaustive. In addition, with ordinal level data, the ranking an attribute possesses can be identified. However, it cannot be shown that the intervals between the ranked categories are equal (see Fig. 16.8). Ordinal data are considered to have unequal intervals. Scales with unequal intervals are referred to as **metric ordinal scales** or **ordered metric scales**.

Many scales used in nursing research are ordinal levels of measure. For example, one could rank intensity of pain, level of mobility, ability to provide self-care, or daily amount of exercise on an ordinal scale. There are rules for how one ranks data. For daily exercise, the scale could be $0 =$ no exercise; $1 =$ moderate exercise, no sweating; $2 =$ exercise to the point of sweating; $3 =$ strenuous exercise with sweating for at least 30 minutes per day. This type of scale is an example of a metric ordinal scale because the different levels for measuring daily exercise are numbered in order from a low of 0 to a high of 3. Variables measured with metric ordinal scales are considered **discrete** because they represent specific numerical values without

Measurement Concept	Other Name	Description
Dichotomous	Binary	The variable has only two possible values.
Nominal[a]	Categorical	Values are names or categories, not real numbers.
Discrete	Ordinal level data or metric ordinal scale	Numerical values used are not continuous.
Continuous	Interval level data or ratio level data	Values include the real number scale, where higher numbers are indicative of more of something and lower numbers are indicative of less of something.

TABLE 16.1 Types of Measurement Concepts

[a]From the Latin *nomina*, which means "name."

an underlying continuum of equal values (see Table 16.1) (Bandalos, 2018).

Interval Level of Measurement

In **interval level of measurement**, distances between intervals of the scale are numerically equal. Such measurements also follow the previously mentioned rules: mutually exclusive categories, exhaustive categories, and rank ordering. Interval scales are assumed to represent equal interval categories (see Fig. 16.8). With interval level data, the researcher can identify the magnitude of the attribute much more precisely. However, it is impossible to provide the absolute amount of the attribute because of the absence of a zero point on the interval scale that signifies an absence of the concept being measured (Waltz et al., 2017).

Fahrenheit and Celsius temperatures are commonly used as examples of interval scales. A difference between a temperature of 70° F and one of 80° F is the same as the difference between a temperature of 30° F and one of 40° F. We can measure changes in temperature precisely for the human body and the environment. However, it is impossible to say that a temperature of 0° C or 0° F means the absence of temperature because it still exists. Therefore temperature has no absolute zero (Waltz et al., 2017).

All interval scales, such as the Spielberger State-Trait Anxiety Inventory (Spielberger et al., 1970), are artificial measurement methods. These scales have been created by humans for indirect measurement of complex abstract concepts, such as anxiety, depression, and quality of life (QoL). Many of these are Likert scales with multiple items to measure a select concept and are considered by most researchers to be interval level measurement (Bandalos, 2018; Waltz et al., 2017).

Ratio Level of Measurement

Ratio level of measurement is the highest form of measurement and meets all the rules of the lower forms of measures: mutually exclusive categories, exhaustive categories, rank ordering, equal spacing between intervals, and continuous values. In addition, ratio level measures have absolute zero points (see Fig. 16.8). Weight, height, and volume are common examples of ratio scales. Each has an **absolute zero point** at which a value of zero indicates the absence of the property being measured. For example, zero weight means the absence of weight. In addition, because of the absolute zero point, one can

justifiably say that object A weighs twice as much as object B, or that container A holds three times as much as container B. Laboratory values are also an example of ratio level of measurement where the individual with a fasting blood sugar of 180 has a fasting blood sugar twice that of an individual with a normal fasting blood sugar of 90. To help expand understanding of levels of measurement (nominal, ordinal, interval, and ratio) and to apply this knowledge, Grove and Cipher (2020) developed a statistical workbook focused on examining levels of measurement, reliability, and validity of measurement methods in published studies.

Importance of Level of Measurement for Statistical Analyses

An important rule of measurement is that one should use the highest level of measurement possible. For example, you can collect data on age in a variety of ways: (1) You can obtain the actual age of each subject based on year, month, or day of birth (ratio level of measurement); (2) you can ask subjects to indicate their age by selecting from a group of categories, such as 20 to 29, 30 to 39, and so on (ordinal level of measurement); or (3) you can sort subjects into two categories of younger than 65 years of age and 65 years of age and older (nominal level of measurement). The highest level of measurement in this example is the actual age of each subject, which is ratio level of data (Grove & Cipher, 2020). If age categories are to be used for specific analyses in your study, the computer can be instructed to create age categories (ordinal level data) from the initial age data. Data are **dichotomous** if the variable, such as age, has only two possible values (e.g., < 65 years of age and ≥ 65 years of age) (see Table 16.1).

The level of measurement is associated with the types of statistical analyses that can be performed on the data. Mathematical operations are limited in the lower levels of measurement. With nominal levels of measurement, only summary statistics, such as frequencies, percentages, and contingency correlation procedures, can be conducted. Variables measured at the interval or ratio level can be analyzed with the most powerful statistical techniques available, which are more effective in identifying relationships among variables and determining differences between groups (King & Eckersley, 2019). Therefore researchers need a compelling reason for categorizing a continuous variable such as age because this limits the statistical techniques that can be conducted on the data (Bandalos, 2018; Knapp & Brown, 2014; Waltz et al., 2017).

Controversy Over Measurement Levels

Controversy exists over the system that is used to categorize measurement levels, dividing researchers into two factions: fundamentalists and pragmatists. Pragmatists regard measurement as occurring on a continuum rather than by discrete categories, whereas fundamentalists adhere rigidly to the original system of categorization (Nunnally & Bernstein, 1994; Stevens, 1946). The primary focus of the controversy relates to the practice of classifying data into the ordinal and interval categories. This controversy developed because, according to the fundamentalists, many of the current statistical analysis techniques can be conducted only with interval and ratio data (see Fig. 16.8). Therefore the fundamentalists insist that the analysis of ordinal data, including data from psychosocial scales, be limited to nonparametric statistical procedures designed for ordinal data.

Many pragmatists believe that if researchers rigidly adhered to rules developed by Stevens (1946), few, if any, measures in the social sciences would meet the criteria to be considered interval level data. They also believe that violating Stevens's criteria does not lead to serious consequences for the outcomes of data analysis. Pragmatists often treat summed ordinal data from multi-item scales as interval data. Therefore the data from multi-item scales are analyzed with parametric statistical techniques, such as the Pearson product-moment correlation coefficient, t-test, and analysis of variance (ANOVA) (Bandalos, 2018; Knapp, 1990).

The Likert scale, as previously discussed, is an example of a multi-item scale that uses points such as "strongly disagree," "disagree," "uncertain," "agree," and "strongly agree." Numerical values (e.g., 1, 2, 3, 4, and 5) are assigned to these categories. Fundamentalists claim that equal intervals do not exist between these categories. It is impossible to prove that there is the same magnitude of feeling between "uncertain" and "agree" as there is between "agree" and "strongly agree." Therefore they hold that these are ordinal level data, and parametric analyses cannot be used. Pragmatists believe that many measures taken at the ordinal level, such as scaling procedures, have an underlying continuum that justifies the use of parametric statistics (Knapp, 1990; Nunnally & Bernstein, 1994).

Our position agrees more with the pragmatists than with the fundamentalists. Many nurse researchers analyze data from Likert scales and other rating scales as though the data were interval level (Bandalos, 2018; Grove & Cipher, 2020; Waltz et al., 2017). However, some of the data in nursing research are obtained through the use of crude measurement methods that can be classified only into the lower levels of measurement (ordinal or nominal). Therefore we have included the nonparametric statistical procedures needed for analyses at those levels (see the chapters on statistics: [23, 24, and 25]).

REFERENCE TESTING MEASUREMENT

Reference testing involves comparing a subject's score against a standard. Norm-referenced testing and criterion-referenced testing are two common types of testing that involve referencing. Norm-referenced testing is a type of evaluation that yields an estimate of the performance of the tested individual in comparison to the performance of others in a well-defined population. This testing involves standardization of scores for an instrument that is accomplished by data collection over several years, with extensive reliability and validity information available on the instrument. Evidence of the reliability and validity of an instrument can also be evaluated through the use of methods described later in this chapter. Standardization involves collecting data from thousands of subjects expected to have a broad range of scores on an instrument. The means and standard deviations calculated from these scores can be used to predict population parameters (see Chapter 15).

Many college entrance exams use norm-referenced tests. For example, the Graduate Record Examination (GRE) compares an individual's performance with the performances of a normative sample of potential graduate students. GRE scores have been standardized over many years and used for admission by some graduate programs. Norm-referenced tests can also be used in research and clinical practice (see Waltz et al. [2017] for a detailed discussion of norm-referenced and criterion-referenced testing).

Criterion-referenced testing involves deciding whether an individual or research participant has demonstrated mastery in an area of content and competencies. It involves comparing an individual's score with a criterion of achievement that includes the definition of target behaviors. When individuals master these behaviors, they are considered proficient in the behaviors (Waltz et al., 2017). The criterion might be a level of knowledge and clinical performance required of students in a course. For example, a criterion-referenced clinical evaluation form could include the critical behaviors a nurse practitioner student is expected to demonstrate in a pediatric course to be considered clinically competent to care for pediatric patients at the end of the course. Many certification and licensure examinations are criterion-referenced tests.

Criterion-referenced measures have been used for years to examine the outcomes of healthcare agencies, nurse providers, and patients. For example, Magnet status for hospitals is achieved when agencies and personnel have accomplished the criteria designated by the American Nurses Credentialing Center (2019) for the Magnet Recognition Program®. Criterion-referenced measures are also used in nursing research, such as tests to measure the clinical expertise of a nurse or the self-care ability of a cardiac patient after cardiac rehabilitation (Waltz et al., 2017).

RELIABILITY

The **reliability** of an instrument denotes the consistency of the measures obtained of an attribute, concept, or situation in a study or in clinical practice. An instrument with strong reliability demonstrates consistency in the participant scores, resulting in less measurement error (Kazdin, 2017; Waltz et al., 2017). For example, if you use a scale to measure depression levels of 10 individuals at two points in time a day apart, you would expect the individuals' depression levels to be relatively unchanged from one measurement to the next if the scale is reliable. If two data collectors observe the same event and record their observations on a carefully designed data collection instrument, the measurement would be reliable if the recordings from the two data collectors were comparable. The equivalence of their results would indicate the reliability of the measurement technique and the data collectors. If responses vary each time a measure is performed, there is a chance that the instrument is unreliable (inconsistent), meaning that it yields data with a large random error. The **psychometric characteristics** of an instrument or scale includes both reliability and validity (Bannigan & Watson, 2009; Kazdin, 2017). An instrument is valid to the extent that it adequately measures what it was developed to measure (see the validity discussion later in this chapter). An instrument must be both reliable and valid to limit measurement error.

Reliability Testing

Reliability testing examines the amount of measurement error in the instrument being used in a study. All measurement techniques contain some random error, and the error might be due to the measurement method used, the study participants, or the individuals gathering the data (Bandalos, 2018; Waltz et al., 2017). Researchers should report the reliability obtained for each of the instruments used in a study.

Reliability exists in degrees and is usually expressed as a correlation coefficient, with 1.00 indicating perfect reliability and 0.00 indicating no reliability (Bialocerkowski, Klupp, & Bragge, 2010; Grove & Cipher, 2020). Reliability coefficients of 0.80 or higher would indicate strong reliability for a psychosocial scale such as the State-Trait Anxiety Inventory by Spielberger et al. (1970). With test-retest, the closer a reliability coefficient is to 1.00, the more stable the measurement method is over time. Reliability coefficients vary based on the aspect of reliability being examined. The three main aspects of reliability are stability, equivalence, and internal consistency (Kazdin, 2017; Waltz et al., 2017). Table 16.2 summarizes the common types of reliability included in nursing research reports.

Stability Reliability

Stability reliability is concerned with the consistency of repeated measures over time of the same attribute or concept with a given instrument. **Test-retest reliability** is conducted to examine instrument stability, which reflects the reproducibility of a scale's scores on repeated administration over time when a subject's condition has not changed (Cappelleri et al., 2014). This measure of reliability is generally used with physical measures, technological measures, and psychosocial scales. Test-retest reliability of scales can be applied to both single-item and multi-item scales. The technique requires an assumption that the factor to be measured remains essentially the same at the two testing times and that change in the value or score is due to measurement error.

The optimal time period between test-retest measurements depends on the variability of the variable being measured, complexity of the measurement process, and characteristics of the participants (Kazdin, 2017). Physical measures can be tested and then immediately retested to determine reliability. For example, in measuring BP, researchers often take two to three BP readings 5 minutes apart and average the readings to

TABLE 16.2 Determining the Reliability and Validity of Measurement Methods

Quality Indicator	Description
Reliability	**Stability reliability:** Consistency of scores with repeated measures of the same concept or attribute from one administration of an instrument or scale to another after a particular time interval has elapsed. Stability is usually examined with test-retest reliability.
	Equivalence reliability: Involves examining the consistency of scores between two forms of the same measure or instrument (alternate forms reliability) or two observers measuring the same event (interrater reliability).
	Alternate forms reliability: The correlation between different or parallel forms of the same measure to determine their equivalence in measuring a concept.
	Interrater reliability: The extent to which different observers, assessors, or raters agree on the scores they provide in assessing or rating subjects' performance in a study. Determining the equivalence of the scores varies based on the measures used and might include percent agreement, Pearson correlations, and Cohen kappa (Bandalos, 2018; Kazdin, 2017).
	Internal consistency: The degree of homogeneity or consistency of the items within a multi-item scale. Each item on a scale is correlated with all other items by calculating a coefficient alpha (Cronbach alpha) for interval and ratio level data. If the data are dichotomous, the Kuder-Richardson (KR) 20 or KR 21 formulas are conducted to determine the consistency of a scale in measuring a concept (Bandalos, 2018; Waltz et al., 2017).
Validity	**Face validity:** Refers to the extent that a measure or instrument appears to assess the construct of interest. Face validity is often considered a precursor of or an aspect of content validity.
	Content validity: Examines the extent to which a measurement method includes all major elements relevant to the construct being measured. For an instrument or scale, content evidence is obtained from the literature, representatives of the relevant population, and content experts (Bandalos, 2018).
	Construct validity: Focuses on determining whether the instrument actually measures the theoretical construct that it purports to measure, which involves examining the fit between the conceptual and operational definitions of a variable.
	Validity from factor analysis: An analysis technique conducted to determine the various dimensions or subconcepts of the construct being measured that are represented as subscales in a newly developed scale or instrument (Bandalos, 2018; DeVellis, 2017; Waltz et al., 2017).
	Convergent validity: The extent to which two measures that assess similar or related constructs are positively correlated with each other. For example, subjects completing two scales to measure depression should have positively correlated scores.
	Divergent validity: The extent to which two measures or instruments assess opposite concepts, such as hope and hopelessness. The instruments are administered to study participants at similar times, resulting in negatively correlated scores on the measures or scales.
	Validity from contrasting (or known) groups: An instrument or scale is given to two groups that are expected to have opposite or contrasting scores; one group scores high on the scale and the other scores low.
	Validity from discriminant analysis: An analysis technique conducted to determine the correlation between measures that are expected to assess dissimilar and unrelated constructs. The validity of the measures is suggested if the instruments show minimal correlation because they are not expected to be correlated (Kazdin, 2017).
	Successive verification of validity: Developed when an instrument is used over time in a variety of studies with different populations and settings.
	Criterion-related validity: Validity that is strengthened when a study participant's score on an instrument can be used to infer his or her performance on another variable or criterion (Waltz et al., 2017).
	Predictive validity: The extent to which an individual's score on a measure can be used to predict future performance or behavior on a criterion. The correlation of a measure with future performance on a criterion.
	Concurrent validity: Focuses on the extent to which an individual's score on an instrument or scale can be used to estimate his or her present or concurrent performance on another variable or criterion. The correlation of a measure with performance on a criterion at the same point in time.

obtain a reliable or precise measure of BP (Weber et al., 2014). The test-retest of a measurement method might involve a longer period of time between measurements if the variable being measured changes slowly. For example, the diagnosis of osteoporosis is made by a bone mineral density (BMD) study of the hip and spine. BMD scores are determined with a dual energy x-ray absorptiometry (DEXA) scan. Because the BMD does not change rapidly in people, even with treatment, test-retest over a period of 1 to 2 months could be used to show reliable or consistent DEXA scan scores for patients. After the study participants have been retested with the same instrument, such as the DEXA scan, researchers perform a correlational analysis on the scores from the two measurement times. This correlation is called the **coefficient of stability**, and the closer the coefficient is to 1.00 the more stable the instrument. Coefficients of stability for physiological measures should be at least 0.90 or preferably 0.95 to 0.99 (Bandalos, 2018; Ryan-Wenger, 2017).

For some tests or scales, test-retest reliability has not been as effective as originally anticipated. The procedure presents numerous problems. Participants may remember their responses from the first testing time, leading to overestimation of the reliability. In addition, they may be changed by the first testing and may respond to the second test differently, leading to underestimation of the reliability. Many of the phenomena studied in nursing, such as hope, pain, and anxiety, change over short intervals (Bandalos, 2018). Therefore the assumption that if the instrument is reliable, values will not change between the two measurement periods may not be justifiable. If the factor being measured does change, then the value obtained is a measure of change and not a measure of reliability (Polit & Yang, 2016). If the measures stay the same even though the factor being measured has changed, the instrument may lack reliability. If researchers are going to examine the reliability of an instrument with test-retest, they need to determine the optimum time between administrations of the instrument based on the variable being measured and the study participants (Cappelleri et al., 2014).

Stability of a measurement method needs to be examined as part of instrument development and discussed when the instrument is used in a study. When describing test-retest results, researchers need to discuss the process and the time period between administering an instrument and the rationale for this time frame. The values for the coefficients of stability for selected scales or educational tests should be at least 0.70 and preferably 0.80 (Bandalos, 2018). For example, Radloff (1977) developed the CES-D that was examined for stability using test-retest reliability in a general population of adults. The CES-D, when administered 1 week apart, was found to have stability reliability with coefficients greater than 0.70.

Equivalence Reliability

Equivalence reliability involves examining the consistency of scores between two forms of the same measure or instrument or two observers measuring the same event (see Table 16.2). Comparison of two forms of the same instrument to determine their equivalence in measuring a concept is referred to as **alternate-forms reliability** or **parallel-forms reliability**. **Interrater reliability** is the extent to which different observers, assessors, or raters agree on the scores they provide in assessing or rating subjects' performance in a study (Bandalos, 2018; Kazdin, 2017).

Alternate-form reliability. Alternate forms of a measurement method are complicated in the development of normative knowledge testing. However, when repeated measures are part of the design, alternative forms of measurement, although not commonly used, would improve the design. Demonstrating that one is testing the same content in both tests is extremely complex; thus the procedure is rarely used in clinical research (Barlett & Frost, 2008; Bialocerkowski et al., 2010).

The procedure for developing parallel forms involves using the same objectives and procedures for both forms to develop two similar instruments. These two instruments when completed by the same group of study participants on the same occasion, or on two different occasions, should have approximately equal means and standard deviations. In addition, these two instruments should correlate equally with a related variable. For example, if two instruments were developed to measure pain, the scores from these two scales should correlate equally with a perceived anxiety score. If both forms of the instrument are administered on the same occasion, a reliability coefficient can be calculated to determine equivalence. A coefficient of 0.80 or higher indicates strong equivalence (Bandalos, 2018; Waltz et al., 2017).

Interrater reliability. Determining interrater reliability is important when observational measurement is used in quantitative, mixed methods, and outcomes studies (Creswell & Creswell, 2018; Waltz et al., 2018). Interrater reliability values need to be reported when observational data are collected or when judgments are made by two or more data gatherers. Two techniques determine interrater reliability. Both techniques require that two or more raters independently observe and record the same event using the protocol developed for the study or that the same rater observes and records an event on two occasions. The latter ensures that a data collector consistently collects data from one time to another or has **intrarater reliability** (Bandalos, 2018).

To judge interrater reliability adequately, the raters need to observe at least 10 subjects or events. A digital recorder can be used to record the raters' observations to determine their consistency in recording essential study information. Every data collector used in the study must be tested for interrater reliability and trained until they are consistent in rating and recording information related to data collection. However, raters know when they are being watched, and their accuracy and consistency are usually better than when they believe they are not being watched. Interrater reliability declines (sometimes dramatically) when the raters are assessed covertly. You can develop strategies to monitor and reduce the decline in interrater reliability, but they may entail considerable time and expense (Bandalos, 2018).

One procedure for calculating interrater reliability requires a simple computation involving a comparison of the agreements obtained between raters on the coding form with the number of possible agreements. This calculation is performed using the following formula:

> Number of Agreements
> ÷ Number of Possible Agreements
> = Interrater Reliability

The interrater reliability value multiplied by 100% equals the percent of agreement. This formula tends to overestimate reliability, a particularly serious problem if the rating requires only a dichotomous judgment, such as present or absent. In this case, there is a 50% probability that the raters will agree on a particular item through chance alone. If more than two raters are involved, a statistical procedure to calculate coefficient alpha (discussed later in this chapter) may be used. ANOVA may also be used to test for differences among raters.

Determining the equivalence of scores in interrater reliability testing varies based on the measures used and might include percent agreement (previously discussed), Pearson correlations, or Cohen kappa (Bandalos, 2018; Kazdin, 2017). There is no absolute value below which interrater reliability is unacceptable. However, any value less than 0.80 (80%) raises concern about the reliability of the data because there is greater than 20% chance of error. (The formula for calculating this error is presented later in this chapter.) The more ideal interrater reliability value is 0.90, which means 90% reliability with reduced error. Researchers should include the process for determining interrater reliability and the value achieved in their research report. For longitudinal studies, it is important to test interrater reliability during the conduct of the study and retain data collectors as needed.

Internal Consistency

Internal consistency testing is conducted to determine the degree of homogeneity or consistency of items within a multi-item scale. The original approach to determining internal consistency was **split-half reliability**. This strategy was a way of obtaining test-retest reliability without administering the test twice. The instrument items were split in odd-even or first-last halves, and a correlational procedure was performed between the two halves. In the past, researchers generally reported the Spearman-Brown correlation coefficient in their studies (Nunnally & Bernstein, 1994). One of the problems with the procedure was that, although items were usually split into odd-even items, it was possible to split them in a variety of ways. Each approach to splitting the items would yield a different reliability coefficient. The researcher could continue to split the items in various ways until a satisfactorily high coefficient was obtained.

More recently, testing the internal consistency of all the items in the instrument has been developed, resulting in a better approach to determining reliability. Although the mathematics of the procedure are complex, the logic is simple. One way to view it is as though one conducted split-half reliabilities in all the ways possible and then averaged the scores to obtain one reliability score. Internal consistency testing examines the extent to which all the items in the instrument consistently measure a concept. **Cronbach alpha coefficient** is the statistical procedure used for calculating internal consistency for interval and ratio level data. This reliability coefficient is essentially the mean of the interitem correlations and can be calculated using most data analysis programs, such as the Statistical Program for the Social Sciences. If the data are dichotomous, such as a symptom list that has responses of "present" or "absent," the Kuder-Richardson (KR 20 or KR 21) formulas can be used to calculate the internal consistency of the instrument (Bandalos, 2018; Kazdin, 2017). The KR 21 assumes that all the items on a scale or test are equally difficult; the KR 20 is not based on this assumption. Waltz et al. (2017) includes the formulas for calculating both KR 20 and KR 21.

Cronbach alpha coefficients can range from 0.00, indicating no internal consistency or reliability, to 1.00, indicating perfect internal reliability with no measurement error. Alpha coefficients of 1.00 are not obtained in study results because all instruments have some measurement error. However, many respected psychosocial scales used for 15 to 30 years to measure study variables in a variety of populations have strong, 0.8 or greater, internal reliability coefficients. The coefficient of 0.80 (or 80%) is determined by calculating Cronbach alpha, and the percentage of error is calculated by (1 − coefficient squared) × 100%. Thus the error for this scale would be $(1 − 0.8^2) × 100\% = (1 − 0.64) × 100\% = 0.36 × 100\% = 36\%$ (Cappelleri et al., 2014). Scales with 20 or more items usually have stronger internal consistency coefficients than scales with 10 to 15 items or less. Often scales that measure complex constructs such as QoL have subscales that measure different aspects of QoL, such as health, mental health, physical functioning, and spirituality. Some of these complex scales with distinct subscales, such as the QoL scale, have somewhat lower Cronbach alpha coefficients because the scale is measuring different aspects of an overall concept. Subscales usually have lower Cronbach alpha coefficients than the total scale, but they must demonstrate internal consistency in measuring the identified subconcepts (Bandalos, 2018).

Newer instruments, such as those developed in the last 5 years, initially show limited to moderate internal reliability (0.70−0.79) when used to measure concepts in a variety of samples. The subscales of these new instruments may have internal reliability ranging from 0.60 to 0.69. However, when the authors of these scales continue to refine them based on available reliability and validity information, the reliability of both the total scale and the subscales usually improves. Reliability coefficients less than 0.60 are considered low and indicate limited instrument reliability or consistency in measurement with high random error (Bandalos, 2018). Higher levels of reliability or precision (0.90−0.99) are important for physiological measures, such as laboratory values, to guide treatment decisions (Stone & Frazier, 2017).

The quality of an instrument's reliability must be examined in terms of the type of study, measurement method, and population. Because the reliability of an instrument can vary from one population or sample to another, it is important that the reliability of the scale and subscales be determined and reported for the sample in each study (Bandalos, 2018; Kazdin, 2017).

Reliability plays an important role in the selection of measurement methods for use in a study. Reliable instruments or scales enhance the power of a study to detect significant differences or relationships occurring in the population under study (Bandalos, 2018). The strongest measure of reliability is obtained from heterogeneous samples versus homogeneous samples. Heterogeneous samples have more between-participant variability, and this is a stronger evaluation of reliability than homogeneous samples with limited between-participant variation (see Chapter 15 for types of samples). Researchers need to perform reliability testing for each instrument used in their study, before performing other statistical analyses, to ensure that the reliability is acceptable (≥ 0.70). In research reports, investigators need to identify the reliability coefficients for the scales and subscales from previous research and for the current study (Bandalos, 2018; Waltz et al., 2017).

Lynch and colleagues (2019) conducted a predictive correlational study to determine if selected psychological factors (psychological stress and depressive symptoms) and physiological factor (cortisol) are predictive of health outcomes (body mass index [BMI] and central adiposity) in children age 10 to 12 years. The following study excerpt includes reliability information for the scales used to measure psychological stress and depressive symptoms.

"Psychological Stress

Psychological stress was conceptualized as events or situations that the children perceived as stressful and was measured by the Feel Bad Scale (FBS) (Lewis, Siegel, & Lewis, 1984). The FBS has 20 items that originated from focus groups on fifth and sixth graders' interviews about situations that 'made them feel bad' (Lewis et al., 1984). Participants were asked to report how they would feel if the situation described happened to them and rate it on a Likert-type scale. Participants first rated the intensity of the item by using a 5-point scale with 1 representing *not bad* to 5 representing *terrible*. Next, participants were asked to indicate how often, if ever, the situation had occurred on a 5-point scale with 1 for *never* to 5 for *always*. Lewis et al. (1984) reported the ratings of internal consistency of coefficient alpha at 0.82 in a sample of ethnically diverse group of children, and factor analysis supported construct validity of the FBS. In this study, the Cronbach's alpha coefficient was 0.89.

Depressive Symptoms

Depressive symptoms were measured by the Children's Depression Inventory (CDI), a 27-item self-report questionnaire designed to measure depressive symptoms in children aged 7–17 years old (Kovacs, 1992). The instrument encompasses cognitive, affective, and behavioral functioning of depression. Each item describes a depressive symptom such as disturbance in mood, sleep, appetite, or interpersonal relationships. Scores range from 0 to 52 with higher scores indicating increasing depressive symptoms. A cutoff score of 13 has been suggested to indicate children with mild depressive symptoms and a cutoff of 19 to denote children with severe symptoms (Kovacs, 1992). In previous studies, the alpha coefficients for internal consistency ranged from 0.74 to 0.83 (Kovacs, 1992). The alpha coefficient for this sample was 0.90." (Lynch et al., 2019, p. 44)

Lynch and colleagues (2019) reported the FBS had a strong Cronbach alpha (0.82) from a previous study (Lewis et al., 1984); and the CDI had acceptable to strong Cronbach alphas (0.74−0.83) from previous research (Kovacs, 1992). In addition, the Cronbach alphas for the FBS and CDI were very strong in this study, reducing the potential for measurement error. Table 16.3 was developed to summarize essential information about the study variables psychological stress and depressive symptoms, the scales (FBS and CDI) used to measure these variables, Cronbach alphas for this study, and the description of the variables (means and ranges). The FBS and CDI appeared to be reliable measures for the study variables in this population of children aged 10 to 12 years old. Lynch et al. (2019) concluded, "In addition to regular screening for BMI and WC, nurses and other health care professionals need to consider psychological factors [psychological stress and depressive symptoms] that contribute to childhood obesity" (p. 42).

Instruments must be both reliable and valid for measuring a study variable in a selected population. If an instrument has low reliability values, it cannot be valid because its measurement is inconsistent, which increases measurement error (Bandalos, 2018; Waltz et al., 2017). You cannot assume that instruments with strong reliability, as in the Lynch et al. (2019) study, will be valid for a particular study or population. You need to examine the validity of the instruments in research reports and the ones you select for your own study.

VALIDITY

The **validity** of an instrument indicates the extent to which it actually reflects or is able to measure the construct being examined. The *Standards for Educational and Psychological Testing* were revised by the American

TABLE 16.3 Psychometric Properties of the Scales Used to Measure Psychological Stress and Depressive Symptoms in Children (N = 147)

Variable	Scales	Cronbach Alpha	Mean (*SD*)	Study Range	Scale Range
Psychological stress	FBS	0.89	12.44 (54.90)	200–500	20–500
Depressive symptoms	CDI	0.90	11.14 (8.98)	0–37	0–52

CDI, Children's Depression Inventory; *FBS*, Feel Bad Scale; *SD*, standard deviation.
Developed from content in the following research report: Lynch, T., Axuero, A., Lochman, J. E., Park, N., Turner-Henson, A., & Rice, M. (2019). The influence of psychological stress, depressive symptoms, cortisol on body mass and central adiposity in 10- to 12-year-old children. *Applied Nursing Research, 44*(1), 42−49.

Psychological Association (APA, 2014) to operationalize measurement validity in terms of five types of evidence. When investigating validity, the types of evidence examined include evidence based on (1) test or scale content, (2) response processes, (3) internal structure, (4) relations to other variables, and (5) consequences of testing. These types of evidence are often examined using several validity procedures. The validity procedures conducted to determine the accuracy of instruments or scales are usually reported in articles focused on instrument development. The development of an instrument's validity is complex, includes several validity procedures, and develops over years with the use of the instrument in studies. The multiple types of validity discussed in the literature are confusing, especially because the types are not discrete but are interrelated. In this text, three main categories of validity (content validity, construct validity, and criterion-related validity) are presented and linked to the five types of evidence previously identified (Bandalos, 2018). The readability of an instrument is also discussed because this affects the validity and reliability of an instrument in a study.

Validity, similar to reliability, is not an all-or-nothing phenomenon but a matter of degree. No instrument is completely valid. One determines the degree of validity of a measure rather than whether it has validity. Determining the validity of an instrument often requires years of work. Many authors equate the validity of the instrument with the rigorousness of the researcher. The assumption is that because the researcher develops the instrument, the researcher also establishes the validity. However, this is an erroneous assumption because validity is not a commodity that a single researcher can achieve.

Validity is an ideal state—to be pursued, but not to be attained. As the roots of the word imply, *validity* includes truth, strength, and value. Some authors might believe that validity is a tangible resource, which can be acquired by applying enough appropriate techniques. However, we reject this view and believe measurement validity is similar to integrity, character, or quality, to be assessed relative to purposes and circumstances and built over time by researchers conducting a variety of studies (Bandalos, 2018; Kazdin, 2017). Fig. 16.9 illustrates validity (the shaded area) by the extent to which the instrument A-1 reflects concept A. As measurement of the concept improves, validity improves. The extent

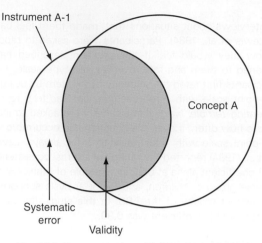

Fig. 16.9 Representation of instrument validity.

to which the instrument A-1 measures items other than the concept is referred to as systematic error (identified as the unshaded area of A-1 in Fig. 16.9). As systematic error decreases, validity increases.

Validity varies from one sample to another and from one situation to another; therefore validity testing affirms the appropriateness of an instrument for a specific group or purpose rather than establishing validity of the instrument itself (Bandalos, 2018; Waltz et al., 2017). An instrument may be valid in one situation but not valid in another. Instruments used in nursing studies that were developed for use in other disciplines need to be examined for validity in terms of nursing knowledge. An instrument developed to measure cognitive function in educational studies might not capture the cognitive function level of elderly adults measured in a nursing study. Nurse researchers are encouraged to reexamine their instruments' validity in each of their study situations. However, researchers often indicate that their measurement methods have good validity but do not describe the specific validity results from previous research or the current study. An enhanced discussion of the instruments' validity would improve the quality of such research reports. The following sections include the common types of content, construct, and criterion-related validity reported in nursing studies (see Table 16.2).

Content Validity

The discussion of content validity also includes face validity and the content validity index. In the 1960s and

1970s, the only type of validity that most studies addressed was referred to as **face validity**, which verified basically that the instrument looked as if it was valid or gave the appearance of measuring the construct it was supposed to measure. Face validity is a subjective assessment that might be made by researchers, expert clinicians, or even potential study participants. Because this is a subjective judgment with no clear guidelines for making the judgment, face validity is considered the weakest form of validity (Kazdin, 2017). However, it is still an important aspect of the usefulness of the instrument because the willingness of subjects to complete the instrument relates to their perception that the instrument measures the construct about which they agreed to provide information (Thomas, 1992). Face validity is often considered a precursor of or an aspect of content validity.

Content validity examines the extent to which a measurement method includes all major elements relevant to the construct being measured. For an instrument or scale, content evidence is obtained from the following three sources: the literature, representatives of the relevant population, and content experts (Bandalos, 2018; DeVon et al., 2007). Documentation of content validity begins with development of the instrument. The first step of instrument development is to identify what is to be measured; this is referred to as the universe or domain of the construct. You can determine the domain through a concept analysis or an extensive literature search (Cappelleri et al., 2014). Qualitative research methods can also be used for this purpose.

Jansson and colleagues (2015a) developed the Patient Advocacy Engagement Scale (Patient-AES) for health professionals working in acute care settings (hospitals). The health professionals included nurses, social workers, and medical residents who are required by accreditation guidelines and their codes of ethics to engage in patient advocacy in the course of their work. However, Jansson et al. (2015a) noted that no scale "had been developed to measure the extent to which specific health professionals engage in patient advocacy in the course of their work in acute care hospitals" (p. 162). Different types of validity for the Patient-AES are presented throughout this section, with the following study excerpt describing the initial development of the Patient-AES and its content validity.

"A definition of patient advocacy developed by Jansson (2011) was adapted for this project: ...An intervention to help patients obtain services and rights and benefits that would (likely) not otherwise be received by them and that would advance their well-being...

To identify appropriate patient problems, we began with Jansson's (2011) typology of 118 patient problems in seven categories. This list represented an array of problems beyond the biological or physiological, consonant with a biopsychosocial framework that considers the impact of the social and cultural environment as well as psychological factors upon individuals' well-being...

Jansson's (2011) seven categories of patient problems were: (1) ethical problems; (2) problems related to quality of care; (3) lack of culturally responsive care; (4) lack of preventive care; (5) lack of affordable or accessible care; (6) lack of care for mental health issues and distress; and (7) lack of care that addresses household and community barriers to care. A review of 800 sources confirmed that specific problems in these categories often adversely affect patient health outcomes." (Jansson et al., 2015a, pp. 163–164)

"The Patient Advocacy Engagement Scale (Patient-AES) was constructed using an applied mode of classical test theory (Nunnally & Bernstein, 1994). The stages...included instrument development and instrument validation. The instrument development stage included three steps: (1) preliminary planning; (2) generating an initial item pool; and (3) refining the scale. The instrument validation stage included four steps: (1) data collection; (2) estimation of content validity; (3) estimation of construct validity; and (4) estimation of reliability." (Jansson et al., 2015a, p. 164)

"Instrument Development

Step 1: Preliminary planning. We assembled a stakeholder panel in fall 2012 whose nine members had expertise in patient advocacy...

Step 2: Generating an item pool. We identified 44 specific patient problems from the list of 118 (Jansson, 2011) by excluding problems not likely to be seen by health professionals during a 2-month period. Items were developed and grouped in the seven categories developed by Jansson (2011).... Participants were asked, 'During the last 2 months, how often have you engaged in patient advocacy to address a patient's problem related to each of these numbered issues below?' After reading the definition of patient advocacy, respondents were asked to report on the five-point frequency [with the anchors

1 (never), 2 (seldom), 3 (sometimes), 4 (frequently), and 5 (always)] how often they engaged in advocacy with regard to each of the 44 problems during the prior 2 months." (Jansson et al., 2015a, pp. 165–166)

Jansson et al. (2015a) provided a detailed description of the development and selection of items for their Patient-AES. These researchers, building on Jansson's (2011) previous work, conducted an extensive review of the literature (800 sources) to determine potential items for their scale. A helpful strategy commonly used in determining items for a scale is to develop a blueprint or matrix, which was done by Jansson et al. (2015a) using the seven categories of patient problems. The blueprint specifications should be submitted to an expert panel to validate that they are appropriate, accurate, and representative. At least five experts are recommended, although a minimum of three experts is acceptable if you cannot locate additional individuals with expertise in the area. Researchers might seek out individuals with expertise in various fields—for example, one individual with knowledge of instrument development, a second with clinical expertise in an appropriate field of practice, and a third with expertise in another discipline relevant to the content area. Jansson et al. (2015a) assembled a stakeholder panel that included nine members with expertise in patient advocacy.

The experts need specific guidelines for judging the appropriateness, accuracy, and representativeness of the specifications. Berk (1990) recommended that the experts first make independent assessments and then meet for a group discussion of the specifications. The instrument specifications then can be revised and resubmitted to the experts for a final independent assessment. Davis (1992) recommended that researchers provide expert reviewers with theoretical definitions of concepts and a list of which instrument items are expected to measure each of the concepts, which was done by Jansson et al. (2015a).

The item format, item content, and procedures for generating items must be carefully described. Items are then constructed for each cell in the matrix, or observational methods are designated to gather data related to a specific cell. Researchers are expected to describe the specifications used in constructing items or selecting observations. Sources of content for items must be documented. Then researchers can assemble, refine, and arrange the items in a suitable order before submitting them to the content experts for evaluation. Specific instructions for evaluating each item and the total instrument must be given to the experts. Jansson et al. (2015a) described in detail their process for refining the scale. Table 16.4 includes the seven-patient advocacy dimensions and the items associate with each that were developed for the Patient-AES. (Table 16-4 was Table 3 from the Jansson et al. [2015a] article.)

"Step 3: Refining the scale. These 44 items were reduced to 33 by a panel of three experts, selected from among the project's stakeholders: the associate professor of social work who pioneered research on advocacy related to ethical issues in hospitals, the clinical associate professor with expertise in advocacy for senior citizens, and the professor of nursing who had done extensive research on advocacy for persons with HIV/AIDS [human immunodeficiency virus/acquired immunodeficiency syndrome]. These experts were asked to eliminate any items that they viewed as repetitive, poorly worded, confusing, or not essential. The experts also slightly reworded some items.... The 33 items in seven categories are listed in [Table 16.4]" in this study. (Jansson et al., 2015a, p. 166)

Content Validity Ratio and Index

In developing content validity for an instrument, researchers can calculate a **content validity ratio** (CVR) for each item on a scale by rating it 0 (not necessary), 1 (useful), or 3 (essential). A method for calculating the CVR was developed by Lawshe (1975) and is presented in Table 16.5. Minimum CVR scores for including items in an instrument can be based on a one-tailed test with a 0.05 level of significance.

The content validity score calculated for the complete instrument is called the **content validity index** (CVI). The CVI was developed to obtain a numerical value that reflects the level of content-related validity evidence for a measurement method. In calculating CVI, experts rate the content relevance of each item in an instrument using a four-point rating scale. Lynn (1986) recommended standardizing the options on this scale to read as follows: "1 = not relevant; 2 = unable to assess relevance without item revision or item is in need of such revision that it would no longer be relevant; 3 = relevant but needs minor alteration; 4 = very relevant and succinct" (p. 384) (see Table 16.5).

TABLE 16.4 **Item Content Validity Based on Proportion of Ratings of Relevant or Very Relevant by Seven Experts**

Dimension	Item	I-CVI
Patient advocacy for patient rights	1. Informed consent to a medical intervention	0.86
	2. Accurate medical information	0.86
	3. Confidential medical information	0.71
	4. Advanced directives	0.86
	5. Competence to make medical decisions	0.86
Patient advocacy for quality care	6. Lack of evidence-based health care	0.71
	7. Medical errors	1.00
	8. Whether to take specific diagnostic tests	1.00
	9. Fragmented care[a]	1.00
	10. Nonbeneficial treatment	1.00
Patient advocacy for culturally competent care	11. Information in patients' preferred language	1.00
	12. Communication with persons with limited literacy or health knowledge	1.00
	13. Religious, spiritual, and cultural practices[a]	0.86
	14. Use of complementary and alternative medicine[a]	0.57
Patient advocacy for preventive care	15. Wellness examinations	0.86
	16. At-risk factors[a]	1.00
	17. Chronic disease care	1.00
	18. Immunizations[a]	1.00
Patient advocacy for affordable care	19. Financing medications and healthcare needs	1.00
	20. Use of publicly funded programs	1.00
	21. Coverage from private insurance companies	0.71
Patient advocacy for mental health care	22. Screening for specific mental health conditions	1.00
	23. Treatment of mental health conditions while hospitalized	1.00
	24. Follow-up treatment for mental health conditions after discharge	1.00
	25. Medications for mental health conditions	1.00
	26. Mental distress stemming from health conditions	1.00
	27. Availability of individual counseling and or group therapy[a]	1.00
	28. Availability of support groups[a]	0.86
Patient advocacy for community-based care	29. Discharge planning	0.86
	30. Transitions between community-based levels of care	1.00
	31. Referrals to services in communities	1.00
	32. Reaching out to referral sources on behalf of the patient	0.71
	33. Assessment of home, community, and work environments	1.00

Note: I-CVI = item content validity index. The overall scale CVI (S-CVI) was 0.92.
[a]Item excluded from calculation of S-CVI and final scale based on I-CVI and confirmatory factor analysis.
From Jansson, B. S., Nyamathi, A., Duan, L., Kaplan, C., Heidemann, G., & Ananias, D. (2015a). Validation of the patient advocacy engagement scale for health professionals. *Research in Nursing & Health, 38*(2), 169.

In addition to evaluating existing items, the experts were asked to identify important areas not included in the Patient-AES. The calculations for the individual CVIs are reprinted in Table 16.5. The format for these calculations was developed by Lynn (1986) and is presented in the right side of Table 16-5.

Complete agreement needs to exist among the expert reviewers to retain an item, when there are seven or fewer reviewers. If few reviewers are used and many of the experts support most of the items on an instrument, this often results in an inflated CVI and inflation in the evidence for the instrument's content validity. Before sending the instrument to experts for evaluation, researchers need to decide how many experts must agree on each item and on the total instrument for the content to be considered valid. Items that do not achieve

TABLE 16.5   Two Methods of Calculating the Content Validity Ratio (CVR) and the Content Validity Index (CVI)

RATING SCALE	LAWSHE (1975)			LYNN (1986)			
	SCALE USED FOR RATING ITEMS			SCALE USED FOR RATING ITEMS			
	0	1	3	1	2	3	4
	Not Necessary	Useful	Essential	Irrelevant			Extremely Relevant
Calculations	To calculate CVR (a score for individual scale items)			CVI for each scale item is the proportion of experts who rate the item as a 3 or 4 on a four-point scale. *Example:* If 4 of 6 content experts rated an item as relevant (3 or 4), CVI would be 4/6 = 0.67.			
	$CVR = (n_e - N/2) \div (N/2)$			This item would not meet the 0.83 level of endorsement required to establish content validity using a panel of six experts at the 0.05 level of significance. Therefore it would be dropped.			
	Note: n_e = The number of experts who rated an item as "essential"			CVI for the entire scale is the proportion of the total number of items deemed content valid. *Example:* If 77 of 80 items were deemed content valid, CVI would be 77/80 = 0.96.			
	N = the total number of experts. *Example:* If 8 of 10 experts rated an item as essential, CVR would be $(8 - 5) \div 5 = 3 \div 5 = 0.60$						
Acceptable range	Depends on number of reviewers			Depends on number of reviewers			

Adapted from DeVon, H. A., Block, M. E., Moyle-Wright, P., Ernst, D. M., Hayden, S. J., Lazzara, D. J., et al. (2007). A psychometric toolbox for testing validity and reliability. Journal of Nursing Scholarship, 39(2), 158.

minimum agreement by the expert panel must be eliminated from the instrument, revised, or retained based on a clear rationale (Bandalos 2018; DeVon et al., 2007; Lynn, 1986). Jansson et al. (2015a) described their content validity testing process for the Patient-AES in the following excerpt.

"Estimation of content validity is a process in which the appropriateness, quality, and representativeness of each item is evaluated to determine the degree to which the items, taken together, constitute an adequate operational definition of a construct…. A panel of seven experts (five members of the project stakeholder group and two recruited from participating hospitals) who had not reviewed the instrument in the refinement stage were asked to rank the 33 items in the Patient-AES [see Table 3 (Table 16.4 in this text)] as: (1) not relevant, (2) somewhat relevant, (3) relevant, or (4) very relevant. Using these ratings, the item-level content validity index (I-CVI) and scale-level content validity (S-CVI) were determined. I-CVI was defined as the proportion of items that achieved a rating of 3 or 4 by the panel of expert reviewers. Polit, Beck, and Owen (2007) recommended that when there are seven experts, an I-CVI score above 0.71 can be considered good, and a score above 0.86 can be considered excellent. We follow this criterion of 0.71 as the minimally acceptable standard for I-CVI. As shown in Table 3 [Table 16.4] [in the far right column], the I-CVI of the Patient-AES items ranged from 0.57 to 1.00, with 28 items scoring 0.86 or higher, four items scoring between 0.71 and 0.86, and one item scoring 0.57. In general, these results showed good to excellent content validity, with the exception of the item measuring advocacy to address unresolved problems related to complementary and alternative medicine. This item was discussed in a subsequent meeting of the stakeholders and the research team and retained because it measures an aspect of patient care that they viewed as important and is often overlooked in traditional medical settings, and therefore one with a high need for advocacy. The overall S-CVI for patient advocacy, calculated using the average agreement approach (Polit et al., 2007), was 0.92, suggesting good overall content validity." (Jansson et al., 2015a, p. 168)

BOX 16.1 Readability Level of an Instrument

Readability level is the approximate level of educational mastery required to comprehend a given piece of text. Researchers need to evaluate and report the level of education participants need to read a study's instrument or the readability level of the instrument. The readability level must be appropriate to promote reliability and validity of an instrument (Bandalos, 2018; Waltz et al., 2017).

Jansson and colleagues (2015a) provided excellent detail about the development of the Patient-AES and the process for determining the scale's content validity. They also provided extensive information about the expert review panel for conducting the content validity testing. The strength of the review panel is their research and clinical expertise in determining patient advocacy needs. Table 16.4 (Table 3 from Jansson et al. [2015a] article) clearly presents the 33 items for the Patient-AES, the seven dimensions or subscales for the Patient-AES with their items, and the I-CVI for each item of the scale.

With some modifications, the content validity procedure previously described can be used with existing instruments, many of which have never been evaluated for content-related validity. With the permission of the author or researcher who developed the instrument, you could revise the instrument to improve its content-related validity (Lynn, 1986). In addition, the panel of experts or reviewers evaluating the items of the instrument for content validity might also examine it for readability and language acceptability from the perspective of possible study participants and data collectors (Bandalos, 2018; DeVon et al., 2007).

Readability Level of an Instrument

The **readability level** of a questionnaire, scale, educational test, or other documents is the approximate level of educational mastery that is required to comprehend the given piece of text (Box 16.1). The readability level of an instrument or scale used to measure study variables must be at an acceptable level for the population studied. If study participants cannot read and understand the items on a scale, the reliability and validity of the scale will be negatively affected resulting

in increased measurement error. Assessing the readability level of an instrument is simple and takes only seconds with the use of a computer. There are more than 30 readability formulas. These formulas count language elements in the document and use this information to estimate the degree of difficulty a reader may have in comprehending the text. Readability formulas are now a standard part of word-processing software.

Although readability has never been formally identified as a component of content validity, it is essential that subjects be able to comprehend the items of an instrument. Jansson et al. (2015a) could have strengthened the measurement section of their research report by including the readability level of the Patient-AES, even though the study participants were healthcare professionals.

Construct Validity

Construct validity focuses on determining whether the instrument measures the theoretical construct that it purports to measure, which involves examining the fit between the conceptual and operational definitions of a variable (see Chapter 6). Therefore construct validity testing attempts to validate the theory (concepts and relationships) supporting the instrument (Bandalos, 2018). The instrument's evidence based on content, response processes, and internal structure is examined to determine construct validity (APA, 2014; Kazdin, 2017). Construct validity is developed using a variety of techniques, and the ones included in this text are validity from factor analysis, convergent validity, divergent validity, validity from contrasting groups, and validity from discriminant analysis (see Table 16.2).

Validity From Factor Analysis

Factor analysis is a valuable approach for determining evidence of an instrument's construct validity. This analysis technique is conducted to determine the various dimensions or subcomponents of a phenomenon of interest. To conduct factor analysis, the instrument must be administered to a large, representative sample of participants at a specified time (Aberson, 2019). Usually the data are initially analyzed with **exploratory factor analysis** (EFA) to examine relationships among the various items of the instrument. Items that are closely related are clustered into a factor. The researcher needs to preset the minimum loading for an item to be included in a factor. The minimum loading is usually set at 0.30 but might be as high as 0.50 (Bandalos, 2018; Waltz et al., 2017). Determining and naming the factors identified through EFA require detailed work on the part of the researcher. In the Lynch et al. (2019) study, introduced earlier, they reported that factor analysis supported the construct validity of the FBS used to measure psychological stress in children aged 10 to 12 years old.

Researchers can validate the number of factors or subcomponents in the instrument and measurement equivalence among comparison groups through the use of **confirmatory factor analysis** (CFA). Items that do not fall into a factor (because they do not correlate with other items) may be deleted (Bandalos, 2018; Kazdin, 2017; Waltz et al., 2017). A more extensive discussion of EFA and CFA is presented in Chapter 23.

Jansson and colleagues (2015a) conducted a CFA to determine the factor structure for their Patient-AES. The initial 33 items of the Patient-AES were sorted into seven subscales: patient advocacy for patient rights, patient advocacy for quality care, patient advocacy for culturally competent care, patient advocacy for preventive care, patient advocacy for affordable care, patient advocacy for mental health care, and patient advocacy for community-based care (see Table 16.4). After CFA was conducted, the Patient-AES was reduced to 26 essential items. The CFA results and the reliability of the Patient-AES and seven subscales are presented in the following study excerpt.

Construct Validity

"Confirmatory factor analysis was conducted to verify the latent structure of the hypothesized seven-factor model. Seven cross loading items had factor loadings ≥ 0.32 and were removed...: items 9, 13, 14, 16, 18, 27, and 28 (Table 3) [see Table 16.4 in this text]. The final CFA model was composed of seven latent factors and 26 items.... There were no double-loading items or correlated errors in the final CFA.... Consistent with theory, the measure captured the seven aforementioned domains of patient advocacy, with five items loading on the latent factor of patients' ethical rights, four items loading on quality care, two items loading on culturally competent care, two items loading on preventive care, three items loading on affordable care, five items loading on mental health care, and five items loading on community-based care. The factor loadings from the CFA of all 26 items ranged from 0.53 to 0.96, and the interfactor correlations ranged from 0.2 to 0.8 (Table 4) [see Table 16.6].

Reliability

The test–retest Pearson correlation coefficients for seven subscales were all statistically significant and ranged from 0.57 to 0.83 [see Table 16.6]. The test–retest r for entire scale was 0.81, indicating adequate stability of the overall scale and its subscales.

Cronbach α for the seven subscales ranged from 0.55 to 0.94. The Patient Advocacy for Preventive Care subscale had the lowest α of 0.55 but contains only two items. Given the large impact of number of items on the Cronbach α value, we judged the relatively low value as an acceptable level of internal consistency. The Cronbach α value for overall scale was 0.94, supporting the internal consistency of the Patient-AES." (Jansson et al., 2015a, p. 169)

Jansson et al. (2015a) CFA results supported the conceptual structure of the Patient-AES and added to the construct validity of the scale (Bandalos, 2018). The final 26-item Patient-AES included seven subscales that were supported with the CFA. In addition, the Patient-AES and subscales had moderate to strong test-retest reliability, supporting the stability of the scale (see Table 16.6). The internal consistency reliability testing for the Patient-AES scale was very strong (Cronbach alpha = 0.94). The internal consistency alphas for the subscales were strong, ranging from 0.82 to 0.91, except for the patient advocacy for preventive care ($\alpha = 0.55$). The limited internal consistency for this subscale increases the potential for measurement

TABLE 16.6 Means, Standard Deviations, Test-Retest Stability, and Intercorrelations of Items in the Seven-Factor Final Patient Advocacy Engagement Scale ($N = 295$)

Dimension	Number of Items	Mean (*SD*)	Test–Retest Reliability (*r*)	Cronbach α	INTERFACTOR CORRELATION (*r*)					
					1	2	3	4	5	6
Patient advocacy for patient rights	5	14.8 (4.9)	0.62	0.82						
Patient advocacy for quality care	4	9.5 (3.7)	0.68	0.83	0.7					
Patient advocacy for culturally competent care	2	6.7 (2.2)	0.62	0.87	0.5	0.4				
Patient advocacy for preventive care	2	5.9 (2.1)	0.73	0.55	0.8	0.8	0.7			
Patient advocacy for affordable care	3	9.1 (3.5)	0.56	0.85	0.5	0.2	0.6	0.6		
Patient advocacy for mental health care	5	13.6 (5.7)	0.83	0.91	0.6	0.3	0.5	0.6	0.7	
Patient advocacy for community-based care	5	15.6 (5.6)	0.57	0.89	0.6	0.3	0.5	0.7	0.8	0.7

SD, Standard deviation.
Note: The 26-item scale as a whole had a mean score of 75.3 (*SD* 20.6), test–retest $r = 0.78$, and Cronbach α = 0.94.
From Jansson, B. S., Nyamathi, A., Duan, L., Kaplan, C., Heidemann, G., & Ananias, D. (2015a). Validation of the Patient Advocacy Engagement Scale for health professionals. *Research in Nursing & Health, 38*(2), 170.

error (Bandalos, 2018). Jansson et al. (2015a) provided a rationale for the low internal consistency value and judged it "acceptable for this study" (p. 169).

Convergent Validity

Convergent validity, a type of construct validity, is the extent to which two measures that assess similar or related constructs positively correlate with each other (see Table 16.2) (Kazdin, 2017). Convergent validity might be examined when researchers revise an instrument to measure a construct for their study. The values obtained from the revised scale are correlated with the values of another scale, which measures a similar construct. In another instance, an existing instrument takes 20 minutes to administer, and the researcher reduces the items on the scale so that it takes 10 minutes to complete. The instruments or scales are administered to a sample concurrently, and the values from the scales are evaluated with correlational analyses. If the values from the scales are moderately to

highly positively correlated, the construct validity of each instrument is strengthened (Bandalos, 2018).

Schiele, Emery, and Jackson (2019) conducted a correlational study to examine "the relationship of illness uncertainty and disease knowledge with emotional distress and health-related quality of life (HRQoL) among patients with CHD [congenital heart disease]" (p. 325). The sample include 169 individuals ranging in ages from 15 to 39. The researchers measured emotional distress by assessing the symptoms of depression and anxiety with the Adult Self-Report (ASR) and the Youth Self-Report (YSR) scales. Extensive convergent validity was reported for the ASR from previous studies in the following excerpt.

"Correlations of the depression/anxiety subscales [of the ASR] with other standard measures are generally high: correlations of 0.69 to 0.78 with the depression and anxiety dimensions of the Symptom Checklist-90-

Revised; correlations of 0.67 with structured diagnostic interviews; correlations of -0.65 with the Global Assessment of Functioning scale; and correlations of greater than 0.50 with the MMPI-2 [Minnesota Multiphasic Personality Inventory 2] depression, paranoia, psychasthenia, and schizophrenia scales… In the present study, the ASR demonstrated good internal consistency in both the depressive ($\alpha = 0.85$) and anxiety ($\alpha = 0.82$) subscales, in patients 18 years and older." (Schiele et al., 2019, p. 328)

Schiele et al. (2019) provided strong convergent validity values of 0.50 to 0.78 for the ASR with other scales. The ASR also had very strong internal consistency values for the depression and anxiety subscales with Cronbach alphas of 0.85 and 0.82, respectively. The ASR demonstrates strong reliability and validity in the study, which reduces the potential for measurement error.

Divergent Validity

Divergent validity is the extent to which measures or instruments assess opposite concepts, such as hope and hopelessness. The two measures are administered to subjects at similar times and should result in negatively correlated scores or values on the instruments (Kazdin, 2017). For example, if a scale measures hope, you could search for an instrument that measures hopelessness or despair. Ideally, the values obtained with the hope scale would negatively correlate with the values obtained with the despair scale, providing evidence of divergent validity. If possible, you should administer the scales to test for convergent validity and divergent validity at the same time (Waltz et al., 2017). This approach of combining convergent and divergent validity testing of instruments is called **multitrait-multimethod** (MT-MM).

The MT-MM approach can be used when researchers are examining two or more constructs being measured by two or more measurement methods (see Fig. 16.7) (Bandalos, 2018). Correlational procedures are conducted with the different scales and subscales. If the convergent measures positively correlate and the divergent measures negatively correlate with other measures, validity for each of the instruments is strengthened.

As discussed previously, Schiele et al. (2019) measured depression and anxiety of adults with CHD using the ASR scale. Extensive convergent validity was discussed earlier, but the researchers also provided evidence of divergent validity because the ASR was reported to

have a correlation of -0.65 with the Global Assessment of Functioning scale. These two scales were developed to measure opposite concepts, so this strong negative correlation value supports the divergent validity of the ASR and Global Assessment Functioning scales. Schiele et al. (2019) concluded, "When individuals with CHD feel uncertain about their disease course and outcomes, knowledge about the future cardiovascular risks may result in higher levels of distress" (p. 325). Therefore nurses need to be cautious about the disease knowledge they provide adolescents and adults with CHD.

Validity From Contrasting (or Known) Groups

To test the validity of an instrument, identify groups that are expected (or known) to have contrasting scores on the instrument and generate hypotheses about the expected response of each of these known groups to the construct (see Table 16.2). Next, select samples from at least two groups that are expected to have opposing responses to the items in the instrument. For example, individuals with depression and those without depression could be asked to complete the CES-D (Radloff, 1977). The scores for the CES-D range from 0 to 60; individuals with scores greater than 15 indicate significant symptomatology for depression and those with scores of 15 or less have limited depression symptomatology. Therefore the validity of the CES-D would be supported if the individuals with depression score higher (> 15) than those without depression (≤ 15).

Evidence of Validity From Discriminant Analysis

Validity from discriminant analysis is obtained by administering measures that are expected to assess dissimilar and unrelated constructs and analyzing the data for correlations. The validity of the measures is suggested if the instruments show little or no correlation because they are not expected to correlate (see Table 16.2) (Kazdin, 2017). For example, you would not expect an instrument to measure empathy to be correlated with measures of other constructs such as anxiety or depression. Testing of this discrimination involves administering the instruments simultaneously to a sample and performing a discriminant analysis (Kerlinger & Lee, 2000).

The Patient-AES that Jansson et al. (2015a) developed for healthcare professionals working in acute care hospitals might be analyzed for correlations with the values obtained from a nurse burnout scale. The two scales would be administered to the nurses in acute care hospitals at a similar time, and the values from the scales would be analyzed with discriminant analysis. Because the scales measure dissimilar or unrelated concepts, the instruments' scores should show minimal correlation (Kazdin, 2017).

Successive Verification of Validity

After the initial development of a scale, it is hoped that other researchers would use it in additional studies. When a scale is used in a variety of studies, the validity and reliability information of the scale is increased. An instrument's **successive verification of validity** develops over time when an instrument is used in multiple studies with different populations in various settings. For example, Jannson, Nyamathi, Heidemann, Duan, and Kaplan (2015b) conducted a predictive correlational study to determine if age, gender, race, and type of health professional (nurse, social worker, and medical residents) were predictive of patient advocacy engagement as measured by Patient-AES. The researchers found that younger age was significantly predictive of higher engagement in patient advocacy but not gender or race. Social workers had significantly higher levels of patient advocacy engagement than other health professionals (Jansson et al., 2015b).

Barrientos-Trigo, Gil-García, Romeo-Sánchez, Badanta-Romero, and Porcel-Gálvez (2019) conducted a systematic review (see Chapter 19) that evaluated the psychometric properties of instruments measuring nursing-sensitive outcomes (Moorhead, Swanson, Johnson, & Maas, 2018). They found that the Patient-AES and another scale had the "best psychometric properties and should be implemented in acute care settings to improve the quality of care, assess the effectiveness of nursing interventions, reduce health expenditures, and reduce the occurrence of adverse events" (Barrientos-Trigo et al., 2019, p. 209). This review reported that Patient-AES is valuable in measuring the nursing outcome patient advocacy in practice, which strengthens the validity of this scale.

Criterion-Related Validity

Criterion-related validity is strengthened when a study participant's score on an instrument can be used to infer his or her performance on another variable or criterion. The two types of criterion-related validity are predictive validity and concurrent validity. **Predictive validity** is the extent to which an individual's score on a scale or instrument can be used to predict future performance or behavior on a criterion (Bandalos, 2018; Waltz et al., 2017). For example, some nurse researchers want to determine the ability of scales developed to measure selected health behaviors to predict the future health status of individuals. One approach might be to examine reported stress levels of selected individuals in highly stressful careers, such as nursing, and see whether stress is linked to the nurses' future incidence of depression. French, Lenton, Walters, and Eyles (2000) completed an expanded evaluation of the reliability and validity of the Nursing Stress Scale (NSS) with a random sample of 2280 nurses working in a wide range of healthcare settings. They noted that, during construct validity assessment, the NSS included nine subscales, originally developed as factors through factor analysis: death and dying, conflict with physicians, inadequate preparation, problems with supervisors, workload, problems with peers, uncertainty concerning treatment, patients and their families, and discrimination. CFA supported the factor structure. Cronbach alpha coefficients of eight of the subscales were 0.70 or higher. Hypothetically, predictive validity could be examined if correlation analyses were calculated for the nurses' scores on the NSS and their depression scores (using the CES-D) at 1, 3, and 5 years. The predictive validity of the NSS would be strengthened if the nurses with high NSS scores had higher depression scores at the different time points. The accuracy of predictive validity is determined through regression analysis (Waltz et al., 2017).

Concurrent validity focuses on the extent to which an individual's score on an instrument or scale can be used to estimate his or her present or concurrent performance on another variable or criterion. Thus the difference between concurrent validity and predictive validity is the timing of the measurement of the other criterion. Concurrent validity is examined within a short period of time, and predictive validity is examined in the future, as previously discussed (Kazdin, 2017; Waltz et al., 2017). In the Lynch et al. (2019) study introduced earlier, the authors measured depressive symptoms in children 10 to 12 years old with the CDI. A score of 13 on the CDI indicates the children have mild depressive symptoms, and a score of 19 denotes severe depressive symptoms. The scores on the CDI can be used to determine current levels (mild or severe) of depression for children in clinical practice.

ACCURACY, PRECISION, AND ERROR OF PHYSIOLOGICAL MEASURES

Accuracy and precision of physiological and biochemical measures tend not to be reported in published studies. These routine physiological measures are assumed to be accurate and precise, an assumption that is not always correct. Some of the most common physiological measures used in nursing studies are BP, heart rate, temperature, height, and weight. These measures often are obtained from the patient's record with no consideration given to their accuracy. It is important to consider the possibility of differences between the obtained value and the true value of physiological measures (Ryan-Wenger, 2017).

The evaluation of physiological measures may require a slightly different perspective from that applied to behavioral measures, in that standards for most biophysical measures are defined by national and international organizations such as the Clinical and Laboratory Standards Institute (CLSI, 2019) and the International Organization for Standardization (ISO, 2019a). CLSI develops standards for laboratory and other healthcare-related biophysical measures. The ISO is the world's largest developer and publisher of international standards and includes a network of 160 countries (see ISO website for details at http://www.iso.org/iso/home.htm). The ISO standards were developed for a broad mission, but the goals specific to research include:

- Make the development, manufacturing, and supply of products and services more efficient, safer, and cleaner
- Share technological advances and good management practice
- Disseminate innovations

- Safeguard consumers and users in general of products and services
- Make life simpler by providing solutions to common problems (ISO, 2019b)

Another measurement resource is the Bureau International des Poids et Measures (BIPM, 2019). The unique role of the BIPM is to:

> "(1) Coordinate the realization and improvement of the world-wide measurement system to ensure it delivers accurate and comparable measurement results;
> (2) Undertake selected scientific and technical activities that are more efficiently carried out in its own laboratories on behalf of member states; and
> (3) Promote the importance of metrology to science, industry, and society, in particular through collaboration with other intergovernmental organizations and international bodies and in international forums" (BIPM, 2019; http://www.bipm.org/en/about-us/role.html).

Using these resources, you can locate the standards for different biophysical equipment, products, or services that you might use in a study or in clinical practice. When discussing a physiological measure in a study, researchers need to address the accuracy, precision, and error rate of the measurement method (Table 16.7).

Accuracy

Accuracy involves determining the closeness of the agreement between the measured value and the true value of the quantity being measured. Accuracy is similar to validity in which evidence of content-related validity addresses the extent to which the instrument measured the construct or domain defined in the study (see Table 16.7). New measurement devices are compared with existing

TABLE 16.7	**Determining the Quality of Physiological Measures**
Quality Indicator	**Description**
Accuracy	Addresses the extent to which the physiological instrument or equipment measures what it is supposed to in a study. The focus is on the agreement between the measured value and the true or actual value of a physiological variable (Ryan-Wenger, 2017).
Precision	Degree of consistency or reproducibility of the measurements made with physiological instruments or equipment on the same variables under specified conditions. The smaller the change sensed in the instrument, the greater the precision of the instrument (Polit & Yang, 2016; Ryan-Wenger, 2017).
Error	Sources of error in physiological measures can be grouped into the following five categories: (1) environment, (2) user, (3) study participant, (4) equipment, and (5) interpretation.

standardized methods of measuring a biophysical property or concept (Ryan-Wenger, 2017). For example, measures of oxygen saturation with a pulse oximeter were strongly correlated with arterial blood gas measures of oxygen saturation, which supports the accuracy of the pulse oximeter. Thus there should be a very strong, positive correlation (≥ 0.95) between pulse oximeter and blood gas measures of oxygen saturation to support the accuracy of the pulse oximeter.

Accuracy of physiological measures depends on (1) the quality of the measurement equipment or device, (2) the detail of the data collection plan or protocol, and (3) the expertise of the data collector (Ryan-Wenger, 2017). The data collector or person conducting the biophysical measures must conduct the measurements in a standardized way that is usually directed by a measurement protocol. For example, the measurement protocol for obtaining accurate and precise BP readings for a study or clinical practice are presented in Box 16.2.

The protocol in Box 16.2 was developed by the American Society of Hypertension and the International Society of Hypertension for their clinical practice guidelines for the management of hypertension in the community (Weber et al., 2014). Research continues to determine the best protocol and its implementation for measuring BP. For example, Tice, Cole, Ungvary, George, and Oliver (2019) questioned clinicians' accountability for providing a 5-minute rest before taking patients' blood pressure

measurements (BPMs). Thus they studied the effect of a 5-minute rest before BPMs were taken in a primary care clinic setting. Tice et al. (2019) found that the 5-minute rest significantly improved the accuracy of the BPMs and recommended nurses standardize their BPMs in everyday practice. Consistently implementing a standardized, detailed protocol greatly increases the accuracy and precision of physiological measures.

Some measurements, such as arterial pressure, can be obtained by the biomedical device producing the reading and automatically recorded in a computerized database. This type of data collection greatly reduces the potential for error and increases accuracy and precision.

The biomedical device or equipment used to measure a study variable must be examined for accuracy. Researchers should document the extent to which the biophysical measure is an accurate measurement of a study variable and the level of error expected. Reviewing the ISO (2019b) and CLSI (2019) standards could provide essential accuracy data and information about the company that developed the device or equipment. Contact the company that developed the physiological equipment to obtain recalibration and maintenance recommendations.

Selectivity, an element of accuracy, is "the ability to identify correctly the signal under study and to distinguish it from other signals" (Gift & Soeken, 1988, p. 129). Because body systems interact, the researcher must choose instruments that have selectivity for the dimension being studied. For example, electrocardiographic readings allow one to differentiate electrical signals coming from the myocardium from similar signals coming from skeletal muscles.

To determine the accuracy of biochemical measures, review the standards set by CLSI (2019) and determine whether the laboratory where the measures are going to be obtained is certified. Most laboratories are certified, so researchers could contact experts in the agency about the laboratory procedure and ask them to describe the process for data collection and analysis, and the typical values obtained for specimens. You might also ask these experts to judge the appropriateness of the biophysical device for the construct being measured in the study. Use contrasted groups' techniques by selecting a group of subjects known to have high values on the biochemical measures and comparing them with a group of subjects known to have low values on the same measure. In addition, to obtain concurrent validity, compare the results of the test with results from the use of a known

---

BOX 16.2 Protocol for Obtaining Blood Pressure (BP) Readings

1. Calibrate the BP equipment for accuracy according to equipment guidelines.
2. Have the individual empty his or her bladder.
3. Place the person in a chair with back support and allow 5 minutes of rest.
4. Remove restrictive clothing from the individual's arm.
5. Measure the person's upper arm and select the appropriate cuff size.
6. Instruct the person to place his or her feet flat on the floor.
7. Place the individual's arm on a table at heart level when taking the BP reading.
8. Take two to three BP readings each 5 minutes apart.
9. Calculate an average of BP readings.
10. Enter the averaged BP reading into a computer.
(Weber et al., 2014)

standard, such as the example of the comparison of pulse oximeter values with blood gas values for oxygen saturation.

Sensitivity, another aspect of the accuracy of physiological measures, relates to "the amount of change of a parameter that can be measured correctly" (Gift & Soeken, 1988, p. 130). If changes are expected to be small, the instrument must be very sensitive to detect the changes (Polit & Yang, 2016). For example, a glucometer that could detect incremental changes of five points in a patient's blood sugar would not be sensitive enough to use when adjusting regular insulin doses. Sensitivity is associated with effect size (see Chapter 15). With some instruments, sensitivity may vary at the ends of the spectrum, which is referred to as the frequency response. The stability of an instrument is also related to sensitivity, which may be judged in terms of the ability of the system to resume a steady state after a disturbance in input. For electrical systems, this feature is referred to as freedom from drift (see Chapter 17) (Gift & Soeken, 1988).

Precision

Precision is the degree of consistency or reproducibility of measurements made with physiological instruments or devices. There should be close agreement in the replicated measures of the same variable under specified conditions (Ryan-Wenger, 2017). Precision is similar to reliability. The precision of most physiological devices or equipment is determined by the manufacturer and is part of quality control testing done in the agency using the device. Similar to accuracy, precision depends on the collector of the biophysical measures and the consistency of the measurement equipment. The protocol for collecting the biophysical measures improves precision and accuracy (see the example in Box 16.2).

The data collectors need to be trained to ensure consistency, which is documented with intrarater (within a single data collector) and interrater (among data collectors) percentages of agreements (see the earlier discussion of interrater reliability). The kappa coefficient of agreement is one of the most common and simplest statistics conducted to determine intrarater and interrater accuracy and precision for nominal level data (Cohen, 1960; Ryan-Wenger, 2017). The equipment used to measure physiological variables needs to be maintained according to the standards set by ISO and the manufacturers of the devices. Many devices need to be recalibrated according to set criteria to ensure consistency in measurements. Because

of fluctuations in some physiological measures, test-retest reliability might be inappropriate.

Two procedures are commonly used to determine the precision of biochemical measures. One is the Levy-Jennings chart. For each analysis method, a control sample is analyzed daily for 20 to 30 days. The control sample contains a known amount of the substance being tested. The mean, standard deviation, and known value of the sample are used to prepare a graph of the daily test results. Only one value of 22 is expected to be greater than or less than two standard deviations from the mean. If two or more values are more than two standard deviations from the mean, the method is unreliable in that laboratory. Another method of determining the precision of biochemical measures is the duplicate measurement method. The same technician performs duplicate measures on randomly selected specimens for a specific number of days. The results are essentially the same each day if there is high precision. Results are plotted on a graph, and the standard deviation is calculated on the basis of difference scores. The use of correlation coefficients is not recommended (DeKeyser & Pugh, 1990).

Lynch and colleagues (2019) included physiological variables in their study of the "influence of psychological stress, depressive symptoms, and cortisol on body mass and central adiposity in 10- to 12-year-old children" (p. 42). This study was introduced earlier with the discussion of reliability and validity for the scales used to measure psychological stress and depressive symptoms (see Table 16.3). The variables of BMI, WC, and cortisol levels for this sample of 147 children are described in Table 16.8 to increase your understanding of the study results. The measurement of the BMI (including height and weight), WC, and cortisol levels are detailed in the following study excerpt.

"**Height and Weight**
Height was measured to the nearest ¼ inch using a portable stadiometer, and weight was measured to the nearest ¼ pound by use of a freestanding balance beam scale according to established recommendations by Heyward and Wagner (2004). Measurements were converted to metric units for analyses. BMI was calculated based on the following formula: weight in kilograms (kg) divided by the square of height in meters (m²), with overweight defined as a BMI in the 85th to 94th percentile and obesity defined as a BMI at or

TABLE 16.8 Means, Standard Deviations (*SDs*), and Ranges for Physiological Variables (*N* = 147)

Physiological Variables	Mean (*SD*)	Study Range
Waist circumference (cm)	76.65 (5.28)	51.18–114.30
Cortisol (nmol/l)[a]	6.75 (6.75)	1.97–46.08
Body mass index (kg/m^2)	21.93 (5.01)	13.42–36.54

[a]*n* = 144

Developed from content in the following research report: Lynch, T., Axuero, A., Lochman, J. E., Park, N., Turner-Henson, A., & Rice, M. (2019). The influence of psychological stress, depressive symptoms, cortisol on body mass and central adiposity in 10- to 12-year-old children. *Journal of Pediatric Nursing, 44*(1), 42−49.

above the 95th percentile (Centers for Disease Control and Prevention, 2015).

Waist Circumference

WC, an indicator of central adiposity, was measured according to protocol by Heyward and Wagner (2004). WC was measured twice to the nearest 1/16 in. and converted to centimeters. An average reading from the two measurements was calculated. Anthropometric reference data to include WC percentiles established from the NHANES (National Health and Nutrition Examination Surveys) studies based on age and sex were used in analysis (Fryar, Gu, Ogden, & Flegal, 2016).

Cortisol

Salivary specimens for cortisol were obtained using the passive drool method and collected at mid-morning (9:30 AM–11:00 AM), at least one hour after breakfast and prior to lunch, to potentially minimize circadian variability and standardize the collection time. Collection, transfer, and storage of saliva specimens were followed by the Parameter Cortisol Assay protocol (R & D Systems, 2012) and the literature (Hanneman, Cox, Green, & Kang, 2011). Cortisol level was determined by a standard two-step sandwich enzyme-linked immunosorbent assay (ELISA) using commercially prepared high-sensitivity kits (R & D Systems, MN, USA). To help ensure intra-assay accurateness, samples were assayed in duplicate. The assay sensitivity for salivary cortisol was 0.07 ng/ml and mean intra- and inter-assay coefficients of variation were 6.9% and 13.6%, respectively, indicating high sensitivity and precision." (Lynch et al., 2019, pp. 44−45)

Lynch and colleagues (2019) used nationally established protocols for the measurement of height, weight, and WC to ensure accuracy and precision of the data

collected. Extensive details were provided for the collection, transfer, and storage of saliva to ensure the accuracy and precision of these specimens. The cortisol levels were determined by implementing standard steps with commercial high-sensitivity kits. In addition, duplicate samples were assayed to ensure accuracy. These researchers clearly documented the accuracy, precision, and sensitivity of the cortisol values obtained in their study.

Lynch et al. (2019) reported, "No statistically significant relationships were found between psychological stress and cortisol or between depressive symptoms and cortisol…. Depressive symptoms were reported by normoweight, overweight, and obese children. Depressive symptoms accounted for variance in body mass and central adiposity…. In addition to regular screening of BMI and WC, nurses and other health professionals need to consider psychological factors that contribute childhood obesity" (p. 42).

Error

Sources of **error in physiological measures** can be grouped into the following five categories: (1) environment, (2) user, (3) study participant, (4) machine, and (5) interpretation. The environment affects both the machine and the subject. Environmental factors include temperature, barometric pressure, and static electricity. User errors are caused by the person using the instrument and may be associated with variations by the same user, different users, changes in supplies, or procedures used to operate the equipment. Study participant errors occur when either the person alters the machine or the machine alters the person. In some cases, the machine may not be used to its full capacity. Machine error may be related to calibration or to the stability of the machine. Signals transmitted from the machine are also a source of error and can cause misinterpretation (Ryan-Wenger, 2017).

Sources of error in biochemical measures are biological, preanalytical, analytical, and postanalytical. Biological variability in biochemical measures is due to factors such as age, gender, and body size. Variability in the same individual is due to factors such as diurnal rhythms, seasonal cycles, and aging. Preanalytical variability is due to errors in collecting and handling of specimens. These errors include sampling the wrong patients; using an incorrect container, preservative, or label; lysis of cells; and evaporation. Preanalytical variability may also be due to patient intake of food or drugs, exercise, or emotional stress. Analytical variability is associated with the method used for analysis and may be due to materials, equipment, procedures, and personnel used. The major source of postanalytical variability is transcription error. This source of error can be greatly reduced by data being directly and automatically entered into the computer (DeKeyser & Pugh, 1990; Stone & Frazier, 2017).

When the scores obtained in a study are at the interval or ratio level, a commonly used method of analyzing the agreement between two different measurement strategies is the Bland-Altman chart (Bland & Altman, 2010; King & Eckersley, 2019). This chart is a scatter plot of the differences between observed scores on the *y*-axis and the combined mean of the two methods on the *x*-axis. The distribution of the difference scores is examined in context of the limits of agreement that are drawn as a horizontal line across the chart or scatter plot (see Chapter 23). The limits are set by the researchers and might include one or two standard deviations from the mean or might be the clinical standards of the maximum amount of error that is safe. The data points are examined for level of agreement (congruence) and for level of bias (systematic error). Outliers are readily visible from the chart, and each outlier case should be examined to identify the cause of such a large discrepancy. Clinical laboratory standards indicate that "more than three outliers per 100 observations suggest there are major flaws in the measurement system" (Ryan-Wenger, 2017, p. 381).

SENSITIVITY, SPECIFICITY, AND LIKELIHOOD RATIOS

An important part of building evidence-based practice is the development, refinement, and use of quality diagnostic tests and measures in research and practice. Clinicians want to know which diagnostic test to order, such as a laboratory or imaging study, to help screen for and accurately determine the absence or presence of an illness (Straus, Glasziou, Richardson, Haynes, 2019). When you order a diagnostic test, how can you be sure that the results are valid or accurate? This question is best answered by current, quality research to determine the sensitivity and specificity of the test.

Sensitivity and Specificity

The **accuracy of a screening test** or a test used to confirm a diagnosis is evaluated in terms of its ability to assess correctly the presence or absence of a disease or condition as compared with a gold standard. The **gold standard** is the most accurate means of currently diagnosing a particular disease and serves as a basis for comparison with newly developed diagnostic or screening tests (Campo, Shiyko, & Lichtman, 2010). If the test is positive, what is the probability that the disease is present? If the test is negative, what is the probability that the disease is not present? When you talk to the patient about the results of his or her tests, how sure are you that the patient does or does not have the disease? **Sensitivity** and **specificity** are the terms used to describe the accuracy of a screening or diagnostic test (Table 16.9). There are four possible outcomes of a screening test for a disease or condition: (1) **true positive**, which accurately identifies the presence of a disease; (2) **false positive**, which indicates a disease is present when it is not; (3) **false negative**, which indicates that a disease is not present when it is; or (4) **true negative**, which indicates accurately that a disease is not present (Campo et al., 2010; Grove & Cipher, 2020; Melnyk & Fineout-Overholt, 2019). On the 2 × 2 contingency table shown in Table 16.9, look at the intersection of the columns and rows. For example, a false positive is at the intersection of the row positive result and the column disease not present or absent. False negative is at the intersection of the row negative result and the column disease present. Use this table

TABLE 16.9	**Results of Sensitivity and Specificity of Screening Tests**		
Diagnostic Test Result	**Disease Present**	**Disease Not Present or Absent**	**Total**
Positive test	a (True positive)	b (False positive)	a + b
Negative test	c (False negative)	d (True negative)	c + d
Total	a + c	b + d	a + b + c + d

a = The number of people who have the disease and the test is positive (true positive).
b = The number of people who do not have the disease and the test is positive (false positive).
c = The number of people who have the disease and the test is negative (false negative).
d = The number of people who do not have the disease and the test is negative (true negative).
From Grove, S. K., & Cipher, D. (2020). *Statistics for nursing research: A workbook for evidence-based practice* (3rd ed.). St. Louis, MO: Elsevier Saunders.

to help you visualize sensitivity and specificity and these four outcomes (Grove & Cipher, 2020; Straus et al., 2019).

Sensitivity and specificity can be calculated based on research findings and clinical practice outcomes to determine the most accurate diagnostic or screening tool to use in identifying the presence or absence of a disease for a population of patients. The calculations for sensitivity and specificity are provided as follows:

$$\text{Sensitivity Calculation} = \text{Probability of Patients With the Disease Who have a Positive Test Result}$$
$$= a/(a + c)$$
$$= \text{True Positive Rate}$$

Sensitivity is the ability of the diagnostic or screening test to correctly detect the presence of a disease. The ways the researcher or clinician might refer to the test sensitivity include the following:
- Highly sensitive test is very good at identifying the patient with a disease.
- If a test is highly sensitive, it has a low percentage of false negatives.
- Low sensitivity test is limited in identifying the patient with a disease.
- If a test has low sensitivity, it has a high percentage of false negatives.
- If a sensitive test has negative results, the patient is less likely to have the disease (Grove & Cipher, 2020; Straus et al., 2019)

$$\text{Specificity Calculation} = \text{Probability of Patients Without the Disease Who have a Negative Test Result}$$
$$= d/(b + d)$$
$$= \text{True Negative Rate}$$

Specificity is the ability of a diagnostic or screening test to correctly detect the absence of a disease. The ways the researcher or clinician might refer to the test specificity include the following:
- Highly specific test is very good at identifying patients without a disease.
- If a test is very specific, it has a low percentage of false positives.
- Low specificity test is limited in identifying patients without a disease.
- If a test has low specificity, it has a high percentage of false positives.
- If a specific test has positive results, the patient is more likely to have the disease (Grove & Cipher, 2020).

Clinicians and researchers also calculate the false positive and false negative rates using the following formulas.

$$\text{False positive Calculation} = \text{Probability of Patients Without a Disease Who have a Positive Test Result}$$
$$= b/(b + d)$$
$$= \text{False Positive Rate}$$

TABLE 16.10 Outcomes of the Ask Suicide Screening Questions (ASQ) for Repeat Emergency Department (ED) Visits by 6-Month Follow-Up

Diagnostic Test Result	Visit With Suicide Presenting Complaint	No Visit With Suicide Presenting Complaint	Total
ASQ Positive	28 (a)	250 (b)	278 (a + b)
ASQ Negative	2 (c)	194 (d)	196 (c + d)
Total	30 (a + c)	444 (b + d)	474 (a + b + c + d)

a = Number of individuals with repeat ED visit with suicide presenting complaint who had positive ASQ (true positive).
b = Number of individuals with no repeat ED visit with suicide presenting complaint who had a positive ASQ (false positive).
c = Number of individuals with repeat ED visit with suicide presenting compliant who had a negative ASQ (false negative).
d = Number of individuals with no repeat ED visit with suicide presenting compliant who had a negative ASQ (true negative).

False Negative Calculation = Probability of Patients With a Disease Who have a Negative Test Result

$$= c/(c + a)$$

$$= \text{False Negative Rate}$$

Calculations of Sensitivity and Specificity Based on Research Results

Ballard and colleagues (2017) conducted a study to determine the sensitivity and specificity of the Ask Suicide Screening Questions (ASQ) in a pediatric emergency department (ED). Suicide is now the second leading cause of death in children and adolescents ages 10 to 19 years. The following study excerpt describes the ASQ used in this study.

"The *Ask Suicide Screening Questions* (ASQ) is a four-item non-proprietary suicide screening instrument that can be administered to patients in the ED for psychiatric or non-psychiatric reasons, aged 10 to 21 years, by nurses regardless of psychiatric training (Horowitz et al., 2012). All questions are asked to the patient, and a *yes* response to any of the four items is considered a positive screen. The four items are the following: 'In the past few weeks, have you wished you were dead?', 'In the past few weeks, have you felt that you or your family would be better off if you were dead?', 'In the past week, have you been having thoughts about killing yourself', and 'Have you ever tried to kill yourself?' The ASQ was developed from a study of 524 patients across three pediatric EDs using the *Suicide Ideation Questionnaire* (SIQ) as the criterion standard…. In the initial development study, for psychiatric patients, the ASQ was found to have a sensitivity of 97.6%, a specificity of 65.6%, and a negative predictive value of 96.9% compared with the SIQ." (Ballard et al., 2017, pp. 175–176)

"The ASQ was implemented with a compliance rate of 79%. Fifty-three percent of the patients who screened positive (237/448) did not present to the ED with suicide-related complaints. These identified patients were more likely to be male, African American, and have externalizing behavior diagnoses. The ASQ demonstrated a sensitivity of 93% and specificity of 43% to predict return ED visits with suicide-related presenting complaints within 6 months of the index visit." (Ballard et al., 2017, p. 174)

The results of the Ballard et al. (2017) study are shown in Table 16.10, so you can understand the calculations of sensitivity, specificity, and the negative predictive value (NPV) for this study (Umberger, Hatfield, & Speck, 2017).

Sensitivity Calculation = Probability of Disease

$$= \frac{a}{(a + c)} \times 100\%$$

$$= \text{True Positive Rate}$$

Sensitivity = Probability of Suicidal Complaint

$$= \frac{28}{(28 + 2)} \times 100\%$$

$$= \frac{28}{30} \times 100\%$$

$$= 0.933 \times 100\%$$

$$= 93.3\%$$

Specificity Calculation = Probability of No Disease

$$= \frac{d}{(b+d)} \times 100\%$$

= True Negative Rate

Specificity = Probability of Suicidal Complaint

$$= \frac{194}{(250+194)} \times 100\%$$

$$= \frac{194}{444} \times 100\%$$

$$= 0.437 \times 100\%$$

$$= 43.7\%$$

NPV = Percentage of people who probably do not have the disease when the test is negative

$$= \frac{d}{(c+d)} \times 100\%$$

$$NPV = \frac{194}{(2+194)} \times 100\%$$

$$= 0.9898 \times 100\%$$

$$= 98.98\%$$

The sensitivity of 93.3% indicates the percentage of patients with a positive ASQ who presented to the ED with suicidal complaint (true positive rate) within 6 months. The specificity of 43.3% indicates the percentage of the patients with a negative ASQ who did not present to the ED with suicidal complaint (true negative rate) within 6 months. NPV was extremely strong (98.98%) in identifying children and adolescents who had a negative ASQ, who probably did not have suicidal complaints. These children and adolescents would not need additional assessment or treatment for suicidal intentions.

Ballard and colleagues (2017) described the process for developing the ASQ from the SIQ, which had been considered the criterion standard. The scoring for the ASQ was described and easily accomplished by nurses. The ASQ had strong sensitivity (97.6%), specificity (65.6%), and NPR (96.9%) when compared with the SIQ during development. In this study, the ASQ also presented strong sensitivity (93.3%) and specificity (43.7%) as presented in the calculations related to Table 16.10 data. The NPV was not noted in the study but was calculated to be 98.98%, which is very strong in determining children and adolescents who did not have suicidal intentions (Umberger et al., 2017). Ballard and colleagues (2017) encouraged nurses to incorporate the ASQ into the standard care of pediatric ED settings. This brief screening instrument "can identify patients who do not directly report suicide-related presenting complaints at triage and who may be at particular risk for future suicidal behaviors" (Ballard et al., 2017, p. 174).

Likelihood Ratios

Likelihood ratios (LRs) are additional calculations that can help researchers and clinicians determine the accuracy of diagnostic or screening tests, which are based on the sensitivity and specificity results. The LRs are calculated to determine the likelihood that a positive test result is a true positive and that a negative test result is a true negative. The ratio of the true positive results to false positive results is known as the **positive likelihood ratio** (Campo et al., 2010; Straus et al., 2019). The positive LR is calculated as follows, using the data from the Ballard et al. (2017) study:

Positive LR = sensitivity ÷ (100% − specificity)

Positive LR for suicide complaints

$$= 93.3\% \div (100\% - 43.7\%)$$

$$= 93.3\% \div 56.3\%$$

$$= 1.657 = 1.66$$

The negative LR is the ratio of true negative results to false negative results and is calculated as follows:

Negative LR = (100% − Sensitivity) ÷ Specificity

Negative LR suicide complaints

$$= (100\% - 93.3\%) \div 43.7\%$$

$$= 6.7\% \div 43.7\%$$

$$= 0.153 = 0.15$$

The very high LRs (or those that are > 10) rule in the disease or indicate that the patient has the disease or condition. The very low LRs (or those that are < 0.1) almost rule out the chance that the patient has the disease (Grove & Cipher, 2020; Straus et al., 2019). Understanding sensitivity, specificity, NPV, and LR increases your ability to read clinical studies and determine the most accurate diagnostic test to use in clinical practice (Melnyk & Fineout-Overholt, 2019).

KEY POINTS

- Measurement is the process of assigning numbers to objects, events, or situations in accord with some rule.
- Measurement theory and the rules within this theory have been developed to direct the measurement of abstract and concrete concepts.
- There are two types of measurement: direct and indirect.
- Healthcare technology has made researchers familiar with direct measures of concrete variables, such as height, weight, heart rate, temperature, and BP.
- Indirect measurement is used with abstract concepts when the concepts are not measured directly but when the indicators or attributes of the concepts are used to represent the abstractions. Common abstract concepts measured in nursing include pain, anxiety, depression, and QoL.
- Measurement error is the difference between what exists in reality and what is measured by a research instrument.
- Instrumentation is the application of specific rules to develop a measurement device or instrument.
- The levels of measurement, from lower to higher, are nominal, ordinal, interval, and ratio.
- Reliability refers to how consistently the measurement technique measures the concept of interest and includes stability reliability, equivalence reliability, and internal consistency.
- Stability reliability is concerned with the consistency of repeated measures of the same concept or attribute with an instrument or scale over time.
- Equivalence reliability includes interrater and alternate forms reliability.
- Internal consistency is the degree of homogeneity or consistency of items within a multi-item scale. Each item on a scale is correlated with all other items to determine the consistency of the scale in measuring a concept.
- The validity of an instrument is determined by the extent to which it actually reflects the abstract construct being examined or measured. Content, construct, and criterion-related validity are covered in this text.
- Content validity examines the extent to which the measurement method includes all major elements relevant to the construct being measured. Face validity is often considered part of content validity.

- Construct validity focuses on determining whether the instrument measures the theoretical construct it purports to measure, which involves examining the fit between the conceptual and operational definitions of a variable.
- Construct validity is developed using a variety of techniques such as validity from factor analysis, convergent validity, divergent validity, validity from contrasting groups, validity from discriminant analysis, and successive verification of validity.
- Criterion-related validity is strengthened when a study participant's score on an instrument can be used to infer his or her performance on another variable or criterion. The two types of criterion-related validity are predictive validity and concurrent validity.
- Understanding physiological measures used in research requires a different perspective from that of psychosocial measures and requires examination of the measures for accuracy, precision, and error.
- Accuracy involves determining the closeness of the agreement between the measured value and the true value of the variable being measured.
- Precision is the degree of consistency or reproducibility of measurements made with physiological instruments or devices.
- Sources of error in physiological measures can be grouped into the following five categories: (1) environment, (2) user, (3) study participant, (4) machine, and (5) interpretation.
- The accuracy of screening or diagnostic tests is determined by calculating the sensitivity, specificity, and LRs for the test.
- Sensitivity is the proportion of patients with the disease who have a positive test result or true positive rate.
- Specificity is the proportion of patients without the disease who have a negative test result or true negative rate.
- LRs are additional calculations that can help researchers and clinicians to determine the accuracy of diagnostic or screening tests, which are based on the sensitivity and specificity results. The ratio of the true positive results to false positive results is known as the positive LR. The negative LR is the ratio of true negative results to false negative results.

REFERENCES

Aberson, C. L. (2019). *Applied power analysis for the behavioral sciences* (2nd ed.). New York, NY: Routledge Taylor & Francis Group.

American Nurses Credentialing Center (ANCC). (2019). *Magnet Recognition Program® overview*. Retrieved from www.nursecredentialing.org/Magnet/ProgramOverview.

American Psychological Association (APA). (2014). *Standards for educational and psychological testing*. Washington, DC: APA.

Ballard, E. D., Cwik, M., Van Eck, K., Goldstein, M., Alfes, C., Wilson, M. E., … Horowitz, L. M. (2017). Identification of at-risk youth by suicide screening in a pediatric emergency department. *Prevention Science, 18*(2), 174–182. doi:10.1007/s11121-016-0717-5

Bandalos, D. L. (2018). *Measurement theory and applications for the social sciences*. New York, NY: Guilford Press.

Bannigan, K., & Watson, R. (2009). Reliability and validity in a nutshell. *Journal of Clinical Nursing, 18*(23), 3237–3243. doi:10.1111/j.1365-2702.2009.02939.x

Barrientos-Trigo, S., Gil-García, E., Romero-Sánchez, J. M., Badanta-Romero, B., & Porcel-Gálvez, A. M. (2019). Evaluation of psychometric properties of instruments measuring nursing-sensitive outcomes: A systematic review. *International Nursing Review, 66*(2), 209–223. doi:10.1111/inr.12495

Bartlett, J. W., & Frost, C. (2008). Reliability, repeatability and reproducibility: Analysis of measurement errors in continuous variables. *Ultrasound Obstetric Gynecology, 31*(4), 466–475. doi:10.1002/uog.5256

Berk, R. A. (1990). Importance of expert judgment in content-related validity evidence. *Western Journal of Nursing Research, 12*(5), 659–671. doi:10.1177/019394599001200507

Bialocerkowski, A., Klupp, N., & Bragge, P. (2010). Research methodology series: How to read and critically appraise a reliability article. *International Journal of Therapy & Rehabilitation, 17*(3), 114–120.

Bland, J. M., & Altman, D. M. (2010). Statistical methods for assessing agreement between two methods of clinical measurement. *International Journal of Nursing Studies, 47*(8), 931–936. doi:10.1016/j.ijnurstu.2009.10.001

Bureau International des Poids et Measures (BIPM). (2019). *About the BIPM*. Retrieved from http://www.bipm.org/en/about-us/

Campbell, D. T., & Fiske, D. W. (1959). Convergent and discriminant validation by the multitrait-multimethod matrix. *Psychological Bulletin, 56*(2), 81–105.

Campo, M., Shiyko, M. P., & Lichtman, S. W. (2010). Sensitivity and specificity: A review of related statistics and controversies in the context of physical therapist education. *Journal of Physical Therapy Education, 24*(3), 69–78.

Cappelleri, J. C., Lundy, J. J., & Hays, R. D. (2014). Overview of classical test theory and item response theory for the quantitative assessment of items in developing patient-reported outcomes measures. *Clinical Therapeutics, 36*(5), 648–662. doi:10.1016/j.clinthera.2014.04.006

Centers for Disease Control and Prevention. (2015). *Body mass index*. Retrieved from https://www.cdc.gov/healthyweight/assessing/bmi/index.html

Clinical and Laboratory Standards Institute (CLSI). (2019). *About CLSI: Committed to continually advancing laboratory practice*. Retrieved from http://clsi.org/about-clsi/

Cohen, J. A. (1960). A coefficient of agreement for nominal scales. *Education & Psychological Measurement, 20*(1), 37–46.

Creswell, J. W., & Clark, V. L. P. (2018). *Designing and conducting mixed methods research* (3rd ed.). Los Angeles, CA: Sage.

Creswell, J. W., & Creswell, J. D. (2018). *Research design: Qualitative, quantitative, and mixed methods approaches* (5th ed.). Los Angeles, CA: Sage.

Creswell, J. W., & Poth, C. N. (2018). *Qualitative inquiry & research design: Choosing among five approaches* (4th ed.). Los Angeles, CA: Sage.

Davis, L. L. (1992). Instrument review: Getting the most from a panel of experts. *Applied Nursing Research, 5*(4), 194–197.

DeKeyser, F. G., & Pugh, L. C. (1990). Assessment of the reliability and validity of biochemical measures. *Nursing Research, 39*(5), 314–317. doi:10.1016/j.hrtlng.2009.12.011

DeVellis, R. F. (2017). *Scale development: Theory and applications* (4th ed.). Los Angeles, CA: Sage.

DeVon, H. A., Block, M. E., Moyle-Wright, P., Ernst, D. M., Hayden, S. J., Lazzara, D. J., … Kostas-Polston, E. (2007). A psychometric toolbox for testing validity and reliability. *Journal of Nursing Scholarship, 39*(2), 155–164. doi:10.1111/j.1547-5069.2007.00161.x

French, S. E., Lenton, R., Walters, V., & Eyles, J. (2000). An empirical evaluation of an expanded nursing stress scale. *Journal of Nursing Measurement, 8*(2), 161–178.

Fryar, C. D., Gu, Q., Ogden, C. L., & Flegal, K. M. (2016). *Anthropometric reference data for children and adults: United States, 2011–2014*. Washington, DC: U.S. Government Printing Office.

Gift, A. G., & Soeken, K. L. (1988). Assessment of physiologic instruments. *Heart & Lung, 17*(2), 128–133.

Grove, S. K., & Cipher, D. J. (2020). *Statistics for nursing research: A workbook for evidence-based practice* (3rd ed.). St. Louis, MO: Elsevier.

Hanneman, S. K., Cox, C. D., Green, K. E., & Kang, D. (2011). Estimating intra- and interassay variability in salivary cortisol. *Biological Research for Nursing, 13*, 243–250. doi:10.1177/1099800411404061

Heyward, V., & Wagner, D. (2004). *Applied composition assessment* (2nd ed.). Champaign, IL: Human Kinetics.

Horowitz, L. M., Bridge, J. A., Teach, S. J., Ballard, E., Klima, J., Rosenstein, D. L. . . . Pao, M. (2012). Ask suicide-screening questions (ASK); A brief instrument for the pediatric emergency department. *Achieves of Pediatric and Adolescent Medicine, 166*(12), 1170–1176. doi:10.1001/archpediatrics.2012.1276

International Organization for Standardization (ISO). (2019a). *All about Iso*. Retrieved from http://www.iso.org/iso/home/about.htm

International Organization for Standardization (ISO). (2019b). *Benefits of ISO standards*. Retrieved from http://www.iso.org/iso/home/standards/benefitsofstandards.htm

Jansson, B. S. (2011). *Improving healthcare through advocacy: A guide for the health and helping professions*. Hoboken, NJ: John Wiley & Sons.

Jansson, B. S., Nyamathi, A., Duan, L., Kaplan, C., Heidemann, G., & Ananias, D. (2015a). Validation of the Patient Advocacy Engagement Scale for health professionals. *Research in Nursing & Health, 38*(2), 162–172. doi:10.1002/nur.21638

Jansson, B. S., Nyamathi, A., Heidemann, G., Duan, L., & Kaplan, C. (2015b). Predicting patient advocacy engagement: A multiple regression analysis using data from health professionals in acute-care hospitals. *Social Work in Health Care, 54*, 559–581. doi:10.1080/00981389.2015.1054059

Kaplan, A. (1963). *The conduct of inquiry: Methodology for behavioral science*. New York, NY: Harper & Row.

Kazdin, A. E. (2017). *Research design in clinical psychology* (5th ed.). Boston, MA: Pearson.

Kerlinger, F. N., & Lee, H. B. (2000). *Foundations of behavioral research* (4th ed.). Fort Worth, TX: Harcourt College Publishers.

King, A., & Eckersley, R. (2019). *Statistics for biomedical engineers and scientists: How to visualize and analyze data*. London, UK: Academic Press Elsevier.

Knapp, T. R. (1990). Treating ordinal scales as interval scales: An attempt to resolve the controversy. *Nursing Research, 39*(2), 121–123.

Knapp, T. R., & Brown, J. K. (2014). Ten statistics commandments that almost never should be broken. *Research in Nursing & Health, 37*(4), 347–351. doi:10.1002/nur.21605

Kovacs, M. (1992). *Children's depression inventory manual*. North Tonawanda, NY: MultiHealth Systems, Inc.

Lawshe, C. H. (1975). A quantitative approach to content validity. *Personnel Psychology, 28*(4), 563–575.

Leedy, P. D., & Ormrod, J. E. (2019). *Practical research: Planning and design* (12th ed.). New York, NY: Pearson.

Lewis, C. E., Siegel, J. M., & Lewis, M. A. (1984). Feeling bad: Exploring sources of distress among pre-adolescent children. *American Journal of Public Health, 74*, 117–122.

Lynch, T., Axuero, A., Lochman, J. E., Park, N., Turner-Henson, A., & Rice, M. (2019). The influence of psychological stress, depressive symptoms, cortisol on body mass and central adiposity in 10- to 12-year-old children. *Journal of Pediatric Nursing, 44*(1), 42–49. doi:10.1016/j.pedn.2018.10.007

Lynn, M. R. (1986). Determination and quantification of content validity. *Nursing Research, 35*(6), 382–385.

Melnyk, B. M., & Fineout-Overholt, E. (2019). *Evidence-based practice in nursing and healthcare: A guide to best practice* (4th ed.). Philadelphia, PA: Wolters Kluwer.

Moorhead, S., Swanson, E., Johnson, M., & Maas, M. L. (2018). *Nursing outcomes classification (NOC): Measurement of health outcomes* (6th ed.). St. Louis, MO: Elsevier.

Nunnally, J. C., & Bernstein, I. H. (1994). *Psychometric theory* (3rd ed.). New York, NY: McGraw-Hill.

Polit, D. F., Beck, C. T., & Owen, S. V. (2007). Is the CVI an acceptable indicator of content validity? Appraisal and recommendations. *Research in Nursing & Health, 30*(4), 459–467. doi:10.1002/nur.20199

Polit, D. F., & Yang, F. M. (2016). *Measurement and the measurement of change: A primer for the health professions*. Philadelphia, PA: Wolters Kluwer.

R & D Systems. (2012). *Parameter cortisol assay*. Retrieved from https://resources.rndsystems.com/pdf/datasheets/kge008.pdf

Radloff, L. S. (1977). The CES-D scale: A self-report depression scale for research in the general population. *Applied Psychological Measures, 1*(3), 385–394.

Ryan-Wenger, N. A. (2017). Precision, accuracy, and uncertainty of biophysical measurements for research and practice. In C. F. Waltz, O. L. Strickland, & E. R. Lenz (Eds.), *Measurement in nursing and health research* (5th ed., pp. 427–445). New York, NY: Springer.

Schiele, S. E., Emery, C. F., & Jackson, J. L. (2019). The role of illness uncertainty in the relationship between disease knowledge and patient-reported outcomes among adolescents and adults with congenital heart disease. *Heart & Lung, 48*(4), 325–330. doi:10.1016/j.hrtlng.2018.10.026

Spielberger, C. D., Gorsuch, R. L., & Lushene, P. R. (1970). *Manual for the State-Trait Anxiety Inventory (Form Y)*. Palo Alto, CA: Consulting Psychologists Press.

Stevens, S. S. (1946). On the theory of scales of measurement. *Science, 103*, 677–680.

Stone, K. S., & Frazier, S. K. (2017). Measurement of physiological variables using biomedical instrumentation. In C. F. Waltz, O. L. Strickland, & E. R. Lenz (Eds.), *Measurement in nursing and health research* (5th ed., pp. 379–424). New York, NY: Springer.

Straus, S. E., Glasziou, P., Richardson, W. S., & Haynes, R. B. (2019). *Evidence-based medicine: How to practice and teach EBM* (5th ed.). Edinburgh: Churchill Livingstone Elsevier.

Tice, J. R., Cole, L. G., Ungvary, S. M., George, S. D., & Oliver, J. S. (2019). Clinician accountability in primary care clinic time-interval blood pressure measurements study: Practice implications. *Applied Nursing Research, 45*(1), 69–72. doi:10.1016/j.apnr.2018.12.006.

Thomas, S. (1992). Face validity. *Western Journal of Nursing Research, 14*(1), 109–112.

Umberger, R. A., Hatfield, L. A., & Speck, P. M. (2017). Understanding negative predictive value of diagnostic tests used in clinical practice. *Dimensions of Critical Care Nursing, 36*(1), 22–29. doi:10.1097/DCC.0000000000000219

Waltz, C. F., Strickland, O. L., & Lenz, E. R. (2017). *Measurement in nursing and health research* (5th ed.). New York, NY: Springer.

Weber, M. A., Schiffrin, E. L., White, W. B., Mann, S., Lindholm, L. H., Kenerson, J. G., … Harrap, S. B. (2014). Clinical practice guidelines for the management of hypertension in the community: A statement by the American Society of Hypertension and the International Society of Hypertension. *Journal of Clinical Hypertension, 16*(1), 14–26.

Wong-Baker FACES Foundation. (2019). *Wong-Baker FACES® Pain Rating Scale.* Retrieved with permission from http://www.wongbakerfaces.org/.

Measurement Methods Used in Developing Evidence-Based Practice

Susan K. Grove

http://evolve.elsevier.com/Gray/practice/

Nursing research examines a wide variety of phenomena, requiring an extensive array of measurement methods. However, nurse researchers have sometimes found limited instruments available to measure phenomena central to the studies essential for generating evidence-based practice (Melnyk & Fineout-Overholt, 2019; Polit & Yang, 2016). Therefore nurse researchers have made it a priority over the last 30 years to develop valid and reliable instruments to measure phenomena of concern to nursing. As a result, the number and quality of measurement methods used in nursing research have expanded.

Knowledge of measurement methods is important to all aspects of nursing, including research, education, practice, and administration. For example, critical appraisal of a study requires nurses to grasp measurement theory and understand the state of the science for instrument development, relative to a phenomenon of interest. When evaluating someone else's research, you might want to know whether the researcher was using an older tool that has been surpassed by a more precise and accurate physiological measure. In measuring psychosocial variables, often an older scale might be more reliable and valid in measuring a concept of interest. It might help you to know that measuring a particular phenomenon has been a problem with which nurse researchers have struggled for many years. Your understanding of the successes and struggles in measuring nursing phenomena may stimulate your creative thinking and lead you to contribute your own research to developing measurement approaches.

This chapter describes common measurement approaches used in nursing research, including physiological

measures, observations, interviews, questionnaires, scales, and existing databases. Other measurement strategies discussed include Q-sort methodology, the Delphi technique, and diaries, which are used less often in nursing studies. This chapter also introduces you to the process for locating existing instruments, determining their reliability and validity, and assessing their readability for use in your own study. Directions are provided for describing an instrument in a research report. The chapter concludes with a brief description of the process of scale construction and issues related to translating an instrument into another language. You will probably use this chapter as a resource to read about selective measurement methods when critically appraising studies and selecting a measurement method for your own research.

PHYSIOLOGICAL MEASUREMENT

Much of nursing practice is oriented toward physiological dimensions of health. Therefore many of our research questions require us to be able to measure these dimensions. Of particular importance are studies linking physiological, psychological, and social variables. The need for physiological research reached national attention in 1993 when the National Institute of Nursing Research (NINR) recommended an increase in physiologically based nursing studies because 85% of NINR-funded studies involved nonphysiological variables (Cowan, Heinrich, Lucas, Sigmon, & Hinshaw, 1993). The NINR (2016) strategic plan reported: "For the past three decades, NINR has supported research on new and better ways to manage adverse symptoms and improve quality of life (QoL). Nursing science develops and applies new knowledge in biology and behavior, including genomics and biomarkers, to improve our understanding of symptoms, such as pain, fatigue, and sleep disturbance, as well as impaired cognition and disordered mood." The increased funding for adverse symptom research and the growing number of biophysical nurse researchers have expanded the quality and quantity of physiological measures used to study relevant physiological, pathological, and genetic variables (NINR, 2019a, b).

Physiological measures include two categories, biophysical and biochemical. **Biophysical measures** are devices, equipment, or methods used to measure physiological and pathological variables, such as the stethoscope and sphygmomanometer to measure blood pressure (BP). Biophysical measures can be acquired in a variety of ways from instruments within the body (in vivo), such as a reading from an arterial line, or from application of an instrument on the outside of a subject (in vitro), such as a BP cuff (Stone & Frazier, 2017). A **biochemical measure** determines microchemical values, such as laboratory values determining biological functions.

Physiological variables can be measured either directly or indirectly. **Direct measures** are measurements that count and quantify the variable itself. They are objective, and consequently not subjective to judgment issues. They are also specific to that particular variable being measured. **Indirect measures** are measurements that are obtained to represent count or quantity of a variable by measuring one or more characteristics or properties that are related to it. They are often more subjective than are direct measures and may be affected by judgment or experience in administration (Ryan-Wenger, 2017). For example, patients might be asked to report any irregular heartbeats during waking hours over a 24-hour period (an indirect measurement of heart rhythm), or each patient's heart could be monitored with a Holter monitor over the same 24-hour time frame (direct measure of heart rhythm). When possible, researchers usually select direct measures of study variables because of the accuracy and precision of these measurement methods. However, if a direct measurement method does not exist, an indirect measure could be used in the initial investigation of a physiological variable. Sometimes researchers use both direct and indirect measurement methods to expand the understanding of a physiological variable. The following sections describe how to obtain physiological measures by self-report, observation, laboratory tests, and electronic monitoring. The measurement of physiological variables across time is also addressed. This section concludes with a discussion of how to select physiological measures for a particular study and describe that method in the research report.

Obtaining Physiological Measures by Self-Report

Self-report has been used effectively in research to obtain biophysical information and may be particularly useful when subjects are not in closely monitored settings such as hospitals, clinics, or research facilities. Physiological variables that are often measured by self-report include elements of sleep, patterns of daily activities, eating patterns, patterns of joint stiffness, variations in degree of mobility, and exercise patterns. For some variables, self-report may be the only means of obtaining the information. Such may be the case when study participants experience a biophysical phenomenon that cannot be observed or measured by others. Nonobservable physiological concepts and variables include pain, nausea, dizziness, hot flashes, fatigue, and dyspnea (Stone & Frazier, 2017; Waltz, Strickland, & Lenz, 2017). These nonobservable physiological variables include adverse symptoms, an area needing further development to address the NINR's priority for symptom management.

Using self-report measures may enable nurses to study research questions that were not previously considered, which could be an important means to build knowledge in areas not yet explored. The insight gained could alter the way nurses manage patient situations that are now considered problematic and thereby improve patient outcomes (Moorhead, Swanson, Johnson, & Maas, 2018). However, self-report is an indirect, subjective way to measure physiological variables, and studies are strengthened by having both subjective and objective measurements of these variables, if possible (Leedy & Ormrod, 2019).

Joseph, Hanneman, and Bishop (2019) examined the relationships among the variables of physical activity, acculturation, and immigrant status of 262 Asian women living in Houston, Texas. The self-report instrument used to measure physical activity is described in the following study excerpt.

"Physical Activity

Physical activity was operationally defined as scores on the International Physical Activity Questionnaire (IPAQ-long form), a 27-item instrument for estimating frequency (days/week) and duration (hours/week) of physical activities of different intensities (e.g., walking, gardening, etc.) during the previous 7 days across the domains of occupational, housework/house maintenance, leisure time, transportation, physical activity, and sedentary behavior (Craig et al., 2003). The transportation scale, which includes walking and bicycling, had a mean of 1 and a median score of 0 in the sample…and, therefore, was deleted as a type of physical activity in the present analysis. Total physical activity score was computed as the sum of the occupational, household, and leisure time subscale scores. The IPAQ scoring protocol (IPAQ, 2005) was used, whereby metabolic equivalent of task (MET)—a unit for describing the energy expenditure of a specific activity (Office of Disease Prevention and Health Promotion, 2018)—was computed and multiplied by hours spent in a given activity to yield MET hours/week. Validity and reliability estimates of the IPAQ are comparable to other physical activity self-report measures, and the instrument is applicable to a broad range of cultures (Craig et al., 2003). Adequate (Nunnally & Bernstein, 1994) concurrent validity and test-retest reliability have been estimated (Craig et al., 2003)." (Joseph et al., 2019, p. 53)

Joseph and colleagues (2019) detailed the structure and scoring for the IPAQ, which was a *self-report measure of physical activity* developed by Craig et al. (2003). The IPAQ was reported to be applicable to a broad range of cultures and to have validity and reliability estimates that were comparable to other physical activity *self-report measures*. Sources were cited to support the reliability and validity of the IPAQ (Craig et al., 2003; IPAQ, 2005), but no specific information about validity and reliability was provided from previous research or this study.

The total physical activity score included the subscales of occupational, household, and leisure time, which supports construct validity by factor analysis for the IPAQ (see Chapter 16). The IPAQ scoring protocol was used to calculate the MET to determine the energy expenditure of each specific activity, providing a more objective measure of physical activity. The use of indirect and direct measures of physical activity in this study strengthens the understanding of these women's

physical activities (Bandalos 2018; Waltz et al., 2017). However, you do not have adequate information about the IPAQ in this study to critically appraise its quality.

Joseph et al. (2019) found that the physical activities of Asian Indian women living in Texas were associated with acculturation. These women had "different physical activity patterns according to their level of acculturation and immigrant status: low acculturation-immigrant women have high levels of occupational and total physical activity, and highly acculturated women, regardless of immigrant status, have high levels of leisure physical activity and sedentary behavior" (p. 56). The researchers recommended future studies include a national sample of Asian Indian women that were balanced for immigrant status and occupational role so the caloric expenditure of occupational and leisure physical activities might be examined.

Obtaining Physiological Measures by Observation

Researchers sometimes obtain data about physiological parameters by using observational data collection measures. These measures provide criteria for quantifying various levels or states of physiological functioning. In addition to collecting clinical data, this method provides a means to gather data from the observations of caregivers. This source of data has been particularly useful in studies involving critically ill patients in intensive care units and patients with Alzheimer disease, advanced cancer, and severe mental illness. Observation is also an effective way to gather data on frail elderly adults, infants, and young children. Studies involving home health agencies and hospices often use observation tools to record physiological dimensions of patient status (Bandalos, 2018; Leedy & Ormrod, 2019).

McLellan, Gauvreau, and Connor (2017) conducted a retrospective record review to validate the more recently developed Children's Hospital Early Warning Score (CHEWS) with the previously validated Brighton Pediatric Early Warning Score (PEWS). The PEWS was originally developed for early detection of critical deterioration of all noncardiac pediatric patients. The CHEWS was a modified version of the PEWS observational tool that was developed to identify pediatric cardiac patients at risk for critical deterioration, enabling clinicians to intervene early and prevent further deterioration. More details and a copy of the CHEWS observational tool are presented later in the observation measurement section of this chapter.

Obtaining Physiological Measures From Laboratory Tests

Laboratory tests are usually very precise and accurate and provide direct measures of many physiological variables. Biochemical measures, such as total cholesterol, triglycerides, hemoglobin, and hematocrit, must be obtained through invasive procedures (Stone & Frazier, 2017). Sometimes these invasive procedures are part of routine patient care, and researchers, with institutional review board (IRB) approval, can obtain the results from the patient's record. Although nurses perform some biochemical measures in the nursing unit, these measures often require laboratory analysis. When invasive procedures are not part of routine care but are instead performed specifically for a study, great care must be taken to protect the subjects and to follow guidelines for informed consent and IRB approval (see Chapter 9). Neither the patients nor their insurers can be billed for invasive procedures that are not part of routine care. Thus, to obtain data for the procedures performed strictly for research, investigators need to seek external funding or obtain support from the institution in which the patient is receiving care.

If you conduct a study that includes laboratory values, you must ensure the accuracy and precision of the laboratory measures and the methods for collecting and analyzing specimens for your study. The laboratory performing the analyses must be certified and in compliance with national standards developed by the Clinical and Laboratory Standards Institute (CLSI, 2019). Data collectors need to be trained to ensure that intrarater reliability and interrater reliability are maintained during the data collection process (see Chapter 16) (Waltz et al., 2017).

Guevara, Parra, and Rojas (2019) conducted a randomized controlled trial (RCT) to determine the effects of the *Teaching: Individual* intervention on the outcomes (glycosylated hemoglobin and systolic BP) of patients with diabetes and hypertension. This study included 200 patients (98 subjects in the intervention group and 102 in the control group) recruited from cardiovascular risk programs of 21 primary care centers. All the study participants were randomized to either the intervention group or the control group. The patients' glycosylated hemoglobin levels (HbA1c) were calculated by a

laboratory at three points in this study, and other laboratory values were obtained from the patients' records.

"The intervention group received, in addition to the usual care, the *Teaching: Individual* Intervention, defined as 'Implementation of the planning and evaluation of a teaching program designed to meet the particular needs of a patient.'... Control group participants continued receiving usual care in the health center they usually attended.... The usual care consisted of interdisciplinary management by the health team providing care, according to classification of the patient's cardiovascular risk...

Secondary outcomes: changes of mean score glycosylated hemoglobin levels from baseline (0 month) at 6 and 12 months, measured in peripheral venous blood, analyzed by immunoturbidimetry in whole blood by an accredited laboratory, and changes of mean systolic blood pressure levels in 24 h from baseline at 6 and 12 months, measured by ambulatory blood pressure monitoring (WatchBP 03-microlife).... Nurses applied questionnaires and took physical measurements, while laboratory assistant conducted blood testing" (Guevara et al., 2019, pp. 4–5)

"HDL [high density lipoprotein], LDL [low density lipoprotein], total plasma cholesterol levels, and plasma triglycerides levels were taken from medical records. Patients who did not wish to participate in the study were asked for consent to include their social characteristics, levels of adherence to treatment and reasons for not participating, to enable comparison with the participant group...[I]n order to guarantee data quality, the project's epidemiologist (LZR) conducted periodic recorded data audits, according to the operating manual of the study." (Guevara et al., 2019, p. 6)

Guevara and colleagues (2019) provided a limited discussion of the collection and analysis of the venous blood to determine the HbA1c values for the study participants. The blood was collected by a laboratory assistant, who has expertise in the collection and management of blood specimens. However, it is unclear if more than one assistant collected the blood specimens and whether they were trained according to the study protocol for collection and management of specimens. The researchers did specify that the analysis of blood was done by experts in a certified lab, supporting the precision and accuracy of the HgbA1c lab results (CLSI, 2019).

Obtaining the HgbA1c as part of the study protocol is a stronger measure of a physiological variable than obtaining the HDL, LDL, total plasma cholesterol levels, and plasma triglycerides levels from the patients' medical record. The measurement of the patients' HgbA1c values at three points in time was highly controlled because it was a key study outcome. The cholesterol and triglyceride values were collected from the medical record to describe the sample and determine if the intervention and control groups were different prior to implementing the study. There is greater potential for error in obtaining data from a medical record, but it was appropriate in this study to describe sample characteristics. In addition, Guevara et al. (2019) ensured that the data were audited for accuracy, reducing the potential for measurement error. The researchers found that the individualized teaching program was effective in significantly reducing the patients' HbA1c levels and systolic BP readings.

Obtaining Physiological Measures Through Electronic Monitoring

The availability of electronic monitoring equipment has greatly increased the possibilities for both the number and type of physiological measurements in nursing studies, particularly in critical care environments. Understanding the processes of electronic monitoring can make procedures less formidable to individuals critically appraising published studies and individuals considering using electronic monitoring methods for measurement.

To use electronic monitoring, usually sensors are placed on or within study participants. The sensors measure changes in body functions such as electrical energy. Fig. 17.1 shows the process of electronic measurement. Many sensors need an external stimulus to trigger the measurement process. Transducers convert an electrical signal to numerical data. Electrical signals often include interference signals as well as the desired signal, so you may choose to use an amplifier to decrease interference and amplify the desired signal. The electrical signal is digitized (converted to numerical digits or values) and stored in a computer. In addition, it is immediately displayed on a monitor. The display equipment may be visual or auditory, or both. One type of display equipment is an oscilloscope that displays the data as a waveform; it may provide information such as time, phase, voltage, or frequency of the target event or behavior. The final phase is the recording, data processing, and transmission that might be done through computer, camera, graphic recorder, or digital audio recorder. A graphic recorder provides a printed version of the data. Some electronic equipment simultaneously records multiple physiological measures that are displayed on a monitor. The equipment is often linked to a computer or might be wireless, which allows the researcher to store, review, and retrieve the data for analysis. Computers often contain complex software for detailed analysis of data and provide a printed report of the analysis results (Stone & Frazier, 2017).

The advantages of using electronic monitoring equipment are the collection of accurate and precise data, recording of data accurately within a computerized system, potential for collection of large amounts of data frequently over time, and transmission of data

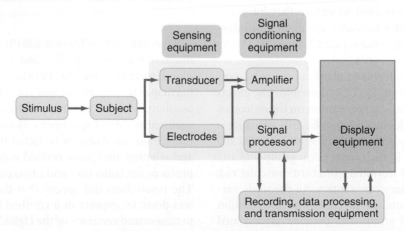

Fig. 17.1 Process of electronic measurement.

electronically for analysis. One disadvantage of using certain sensors to measure physiological variables is that the presence of a transducer within the body can alter the actual physiological value. For example, the presence of a flow transducer in a blood vessel can partially block the vessel and alter blood flow, resulting in an inaccurate reflection of the flow (Ryan-Wenger, 2017).

Ng, Wong, Lim, and Goh (2010) compared the Cadi ThermoSENSOR wireless skin-contact thermometer readings with ear and axillary temperatures in children on a general pediatric medical unit in a Singapore hospital. The ThermoSENSOR thermometer provides a continuous measurement of body temperature and transmits the readings wirelessly to a central server. The measurement with the ThermoSENSOR thermometer is described in the following excerpt.

"Developed by Cadi Scientific in Singapore as part of an integrated wireless system for temperature monitoring and location tracking, this system uses a reusable skin-contact thermometer or sensor called the *ThermoSENSOR*. This thermometer takes the form of a small disc that can be easily adhered to the patient's skin, and each disc is assigned a unique radio frequency identification (RFID) number (Figure 1 [Fig. 17.2 in this text]). The thermometer measures body temperature continuously and transmits a temperature reading and the RFID number approximately every 30 seconds to a computer or server through one or more signal receivers (nodes) installed in the vicinity of the patient." (Ng et al., 2010, pp. 176–177)

"Before the study, a ThermoSENSOR wireless temperature monitoring system was installed in the ward. A wireless signal receiver (node) was installed in the ceiling of each of the five-bedded rooms.... These receivers were connected to the hospital's local area network (LAN)... Web-based application software designed for use with the wireless system and installed on the computer was used to configure the computer to receive, store, and display the temperature and RFID data. A total of 32 sensors were used for the study (Figure 2 [Fig. 17.3 in this text]).

The ThermoSENSOR uses a thermistor as the sensing element. When in use, the sensor is attached to the patient using a two-layer dressing system that prevents the sensor from coming in direct contact with the skin (see Figure 1 [Fig. 17.2])…. The manufacturer provided the following specifications for the sensor: operating ambient temperature range, 10° C to 50° C; thermistor accuracy, ± 0.2° C for temperature range of 32.0° C to 42.0° C; data transmission rate, every 30 seconds on average; radio frequency, 868.4 MHz; typical transmission range, 10 m

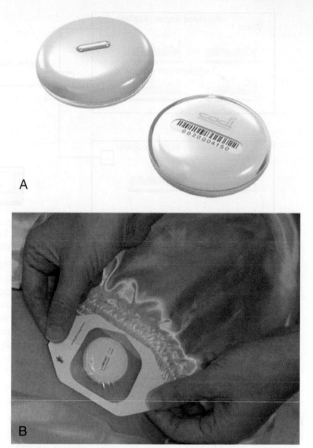

Fig. 17.2 (A) OR wireless thermometer. The disc has an elliptical cross section, and the sensing element consists of a metal strip located at the center of the skin-contact side. (B) ThermoSENSOR. The device has been placed over the first piece of hypoallergenic adhesive film dressing on the lower abdomen and is about to be secured to the lower abdomen by a second piece of the same dressing. (From Ng, K., Wong, S., Lim, S., & Goh, Z. [2010]. Evaluation of the Cadi ThermoSENSOR wireless skin-contact thermometer against ear and axillary temperatures in children. *Journal of Pediatric Nursing, 25*[3], 177.)

(unblocked); power source, internal 3-V lithium coin-cell battery; battery life, 12 months (continuous operation); dimensions, diameter of 36 mm, height of 11.6 mm; weight, 10 g without battery; applicable radio equipment standards, ETSI 300 220, ETSI EN 301 489." (Ng et al., 2010, pp. 177–178)

Ng et al. (2010) provided detailed descriptions and pictures of both the ThermoSENSOR thermometer and the wireless setup by which signals were captured

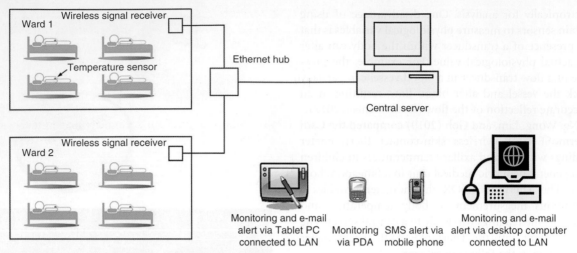

Fig. 17.3 Setup of the ThermoSENSOR wireless temperature monitoring system. Each sensor transmits data wirelessly to a signal receiver (node) that is within the prescribed transmission range. The signal receiver uploads the data to a central server through the local area network *(LAN)* through which the data can be accessed from computers and other devices that are connected, wirelessly or by wired means, to the LAN. The server can be configured to send out e-mail and short message service *(SMS)* alerts. (From Ng, K., Wong, S., Lim, S., & Goh, Z. [2010]. Evaluation of the Cadi ThermoSENSOR wireless skin-contact thermometer against ear and axillary temperatures in children. *Journal of Pediatric Nursing, 25*[3], 177.)

and transmitted. The thermometer was consistently applied to the abdomen of each child. The manufacturer specifications of the thermometer documented that it was an accurate device to measure temperature. The wireless system was described in detail with documentation of its precision and accuracy in obtaining and transferring the children's temperatures to a computer for recording, display, and analysis of the data. The findings of the study indicated that ThermoSENSOR wireless skin-contact thermometer readings were comparable to both ear and axillary temperature readings and would be an accurate way to measure temperature in research and clinical practice.

Genetic Advancements in Measuring Nucleic Acids

The Human Genome Project has greatly expanded the understanding of deoxyribonucleic acid (DNA) that contains the code for controlling human development. The US Human Genome Project was initiated in 1990 by the US Department of Energy (DOE) and the National Institutes of Health and completed in 2003. The genome is the entire DNA sequence in an organism, which includes the genes. The genes carry information

for making all the proteins required by the organism that are used to determine how the body looks, functions, and behaves. The DNA is a double-stranded helix and serves as the code for the production of the single-stranded messenger ribonucleic acid (RNA) (DOE Office of Science, 2019).

"Project goals were to:
- identify all the approximately 20,000–25,000 genes in human DNA.
- determine the sequences of the 3 billion chemical base pairs that make up human DNA.
- store this information in databases.
- improve tools for data analysis.
- transfer related technologies to the private sector.
- address the ethical, legal, and social issues that may arise from the project." (DOE, 2019)

Advancements in genetics have facilitated the development of new technologies that have permitted the analysis of normal and abnormal genes for the detection and diagnosis of genetic diseases. Through the use of molecular cloning, sufficient quantities of DNA and RNA have been produced to permit analysis in research. The Southern blotting technique is the standard way for analyzing the structure of DNA. The Northern blotting technique is used for RNA analysis. Analyses of both normal and mutant genes are of interest, and the Western blotting technique is used to examine mutant proteins in cells obtained from patients with diseases. In addition, polymerase chain reaction (PCR) can selectively amplify DNA and RNA molecules for study (Stone & Frazier, 2017). It is important that nurses be aware of the advances in technologies to measure nucleic acids and use them in their programs of research.

A major genetic resource is the National Human Genome Research Institute (NHGRI) located online at https://www.genome.gov/. The vision of the NHGRI (2019b) is "to improve the health of all humans through advances in genomics research. As a leading authority in the field of genomics, our mission is to accelerate scientific and medical breakthroughs that improve human health. We do this by driving cutting-edge research, developing new technologies, and studying the impact of genomics on society." NHGRI (2019a) details the funding for genomic research, research being conducted in this area, and noted genomic researchers. Both NIGRI (2019b) and NINR (2019a) provide educational opportunities to prepare future genetic researchers. Nurses are becoming more involved in the conduct of genetic research through doctoral and postdoctoral programs specialized in this area and through the NINR (2019a) Summer Genetics Institute.

Many expert nurse researchers and leaders have been working to identify the biomarkers that should be common data elements (CDEs) for symptom and self-management science. Page and colleagues (2018) developed a position paper to "(a) identify a 'minimum set' of biomarkers for consideration as CDEs in symptom and self-management science,…(b) evaluate the benefits and limitations of such a limited array of biomarkers with implications for symptom science, (c) propose a strategy for the collection of the endorsed minimum set of biologic samples to be employed as CDEs for symptom science, and (d) conceptualize this minimum set of biomarkers consistent with NINR symptoms of fatigue, depression, cognition, pain, and sleep disturbance" (p. 276). These 20 nursing experts recommended that the "minimum set of biomarker CDEs include pro- and anti-inflammatory cytokines, a hypothalamic-pituitary-adrenal axis marker, cortisol, the neuropeptide brain-derived neurotrophic factor, and DNA polymorphisms" (Page et al., 2018, p. 276). They believed the use of these

biomarker CDEs in biobehavioral research would promote generalization and reproducibility of research findings.

Kubik, Permenter, and Saremian (2015) conducted a comparative descriptive study to determine the stability of the human papillomavirus (HPV) DNA when retested 21 days after the collection date. The sample included 50 BD SurePath specimens that initially tested positive for high-risk HPV using the Roche Cobas 4800 assay. The BD SurePath liquid-based Papanicolaou (Pap) test is approved for only Pap testing by the US Food and Drug Administration, but these specimens are often used for HPV testing. In the Kubik et al. (2015) study, initial and repeat testing for HPV were performed per manufacturer instructions using 1 mL of SurePath specimen. When the specimens were retested 21 days after their collection date, eight tested negative (false negative rate of 16%). False negative occurs when the test results are negative for a disease but the individual has the disease (see Chapter 16). The genetic testing used for HPV DNA is discussed in the following study excerpt.

> "The Roche Cobas 4800 assay is a fully automated, in vitro test for detection of HPV that uses amplification of target DNA via PCR and nucleic acid hybridization for the detection of 14 HR-HPV types in a single analysis" (Kubik et al., 2015, p. 52).
> The PCR assay "provides specific genotyping for HPV types 16 and 18" (which account for approximately 70% of the cervical cancers worldwide) and pools the results of all the other high risk "HPV types (31, 33, 35, 39, 45, 51, 52, 56, 58, 59, 66, and 68). The system uses β-globin as an internal control to assess specimen quality and potential inhibitors of the amplification process." (Kubik et al., 2015, p. 52)

Kubik and colleagues (2015) described the accuracy and precision of the Roche Cobas 4800 assay for genotyping many types of high-risk HPV. The researchers also documented the accuracy and precision of the SurePath Pap specimens that were collected according to manufacturers' specifications. The steps taken to promote precision and accuracy in this genetic research greatly reduced the potential for error, supporting the credibility of the results.

Kubik et al. (2015) concluded: "Aged BD SurePath–preserved Pap test specimens older than 21 days from collection date may produce false-negative HPV DNA testing results when testing with assays such as Roche Cobas 4800, most likely due to degradation of DNA" (p. 51). The researchers recommended additional large sample studies to facilitate the development of guidelines "to limit the age of the specimen to less than two weeks to prevent false-negative test results and improve diagnostic accuracy and patient care" (Kubik et al., 2015, p. 51).

Obtaining Physiological Measures Across Time

Many nursing studies use physiological measures that focus on a single point in time. Thus there is insufficient information on normal variations in physiological measures across time and much less information on changes in physiological measures across time in individuals with abnormal physiological states. Circadian rhythms, activities, emotions, dietary intake, or posture can also affect physiological measures. Researchers need to determine to what extent these factors affect the ability to interpret measurement outcomes. An important question to ask is, "How labile is the measure?" Some measures vary within the individual from time to time, even when conditions are similar. When a clinician observes variation in a physiological value, it is important to know whether the variation is within the normal range or signals a change in the patient's condition. For example, you notice that a patient on telemetry has an increase in pulse to 105 beats per minute. You would interpret the pulse rate differently when the patient's typical heart rate is 60 compared to a patient with a typical heart rate of 100 beats per minute.

Some of the specimens collected from patients and research subjects can vary with the passage of time, and researchers need to determine when the analysis of the specimen is most accurate. The deterioration rate of a specimen also needs to be examined and a time limit set for discarding a specimen. As described in the previous section, Kubik et al. (2015) retested 50 SurePath Pap specimens 21 days after their initial collection. The Pap specimens that were 21 days or older had a 16% false negative result (indicating that eight women did not have HPV when they did). Kubik et al. (2015) determined the Pap specimens should be discarded after 2 weeks. However, additional research is needed to set national standards in this area.

Selecting a Physiological Measure

Researchers designing a physiological study have fewer printed resources for selecting methods of measurement than do researchers conducting studies using psychosocial variables. Multiple books and electronic sources are available that discuss various methods for measuring psychosocial variables. In addition, numerous articles in nursing journals describe the development of psychosocial scales. However, literature guiding the selection of physiological measures in nursing is still sparse. We recommend that you consider the factors in Box 17.1 when selecting a physiological measure for a study.

BOX 17-1   Factors Directing the Selection of a Physiological Measure for a Study

1. What physiological variables are relevant to the study?
2. Will the variables need to be measured continuously or at a particular point in time (Leedy & Ormrod, 2019)?
3. Will repeated measures be needed (Kazdin, 2017)?
4. Do certain characteristics of the population under study place limits on the measurement approaches that can be used?
5. How has the variable been measured in previous research?
6. Is more than one measurement method available to measure the physiological variable being studied (Stone & Frazier, 2017)?
7. Which measurement method is the most accurate and precise for the population you are studying (Ryan-Wenger, 2017)?
8. Could the study be designed to include more than one measurement method for the variable being studied (Kazdin, 2017; Leedy & Ormrod, 2019)?
9. Where can the measurement device or devices be obtained that will measure the physiological variable being studied?
10. Can the measurement device be obtained from the manufacturer for use in the study, or must it be purchased?
11. What are the national and international standards for the measurement device or equipment that has been designated (Bureau International des Poids et Measures [BIPM], 2019; Clinical and Laboratory Standards Institute [CLSI], 2019; International Organization for Standardization [ISO], 2019a, b)?

The sources most commonly used to identify physiological measurement methods are previous studies that have measured a particular physiological variable. Literature reviews or meta-analyses can provide reference lists of relevant studies. Because the measure you select might have been used in studies unrelated to the current research topic, it is usually important to examine the research literature broadly. Other disciplines, such as engineering and biomedical science, have technology and other devices for measuring physiological and pathological variables.

Each physiological variable measured in a study must be linked to an appropriate concept in the study framework that is explicitly presented in the research report. Operationalizing the concept in a particular way requires comparing different options and providing a logical rationale for your selection. It is often a good idea to use diverse physiological measures of a single concept, which reduces the impact of extraneous variables that might affect measurement. The operationalization of a physiological variable in a study should clearly indicate the physiological measure(s) to be used (see Chapter 6).

You also need to evaluate the accuracy and precision of physiological measures to be used in your study. Until recently, researchers commonly used information from the equipment manufacturer to describe a measurement method. This information is useful but may be biased. Additional sources (CLSI, 2019; ISO, 2019a, b; Ryan-Wenger, 2017; Stone & Frazier, 2017) and research articles should be reviewed for more information about physiological measures.

You need to consider problems you might encounter when using various approaches to physiological measurement. One factor of concern is the sensitivity of the measure. Will the measure detect differences finely enough to avoid a Type II error—known as a false negative—that occurs when the investigator claims there is no difference between groups or relationships among variables when one really exists (see Chapter 21). Physiological measures are usually norm referenced (see Chapter 16). Data obtained from a study participant are compared with a norm as well as with other participants. You need to determine whether the norm used for comparison is relevant for the population you are studying. Laboratories are certified ensuring the analyses conducted in them meet a national standard (CLSI, 2019). New physiological measures are compared with the **gold standard** or the current best measurement method for a physiological variable.

Many measurement strategies require the use of specialized equipment. Often the equipment is available in the patient care area and is part of routine patient care in that unit. Otherwise, the researcher may need to purchase, rent, or borrow the equipment specifically for the study. You need to be skilled in operating the equipment or obtain the assistance of someone who has these skills. You need to ensure that the equipment is operated in an optimal fashion and is used in a consistent manner. Sometimes equipment must be recalibrated, or reset, regularly to ensure consistent readings. For example, BP equipment needs to be recalibrated every 4 months to ensure the BP readings are accurate and precise in clinical practice, and the BP equipment should be recalibrated more often in research. The federal guidelines guiding the recalibration of healthcare equipment are presented in Box 17.2.

Reporting Physiological Measures in Studies

When the results of a physiological study are published, researchers must describe the measurement technique in considerable detail to allow an adequate critical appraisal of the study, enable others to replicate the study, and promote clinical application of the results. A detailed description of physiological measures in a research report includes the following:

1. Description of the equipment or device used in performing the measurement
2. Identification of the name of the equipment manufacturer

BOX 17-2 Federal Guidelines Guiding the Recalibration of Healthcare Equipment

- In accordance with the manufacturers' instructions
- In accordance with national and international standards (International Organization for Standardization [ISO], 2019b)
- In accordance with criteria set up by the laboratory (Clinical and Laboratory Standards Institute [CLSI], 2019)
- At least every 6 months
- After major preventive maintenance or replacement of a critical part
- When quality control indicates a need for recalibration (Bureau International des Poids et Measures [BIPM], 2019; CLSI, 2019; ISO, 2019b)

3. Account of the accuracy and precision of the equipment or device based on previous research, the manufacturers' specifications, and national and international standards

4. Explanation of the exact procedure followed to measure the physiological variable

5. Overview of the process used to collect, record, retrieve, and store data

The examples discussed in this section can provide direction for you to describe a physiological measure in a study and to detail the process used for collecting and managing physiological data to ensure quality outcomes.

OBSERVATIONAL MEASUREMENT

Observational measurement is the use of structured and unstructured inspection to gauge a study variable. This section focuses on structured observational measurement, which is more commonly used in quantitative research. Unstructured observation is frequently used in qualitative research and is presented in Chapter 12 (Creswell & Creswell, 2018; Leedy & Ormrod, 2019; Marshall & Rossman, 2016).

Structured Observation

Structured observation is the careful selection of specific behaviors, situations, or events that are to be inspected or examined in a study. The variable to be observed is identified and a detailed plan is developed to ensure that every aspect of the variable is observed in a similar manner for each study participant. Researchers determine how the observations are to be made, recorded, and coded. In most cases, the research team develops an observational checklist or category system to direct collecting, organizing, and sorting of the specific behaviors or events being observed. Extensive attention must be given to training data collectors, especially when the observations are complex and measured over time (Leedy & Ormrod, 2019; Waltz et al., 2017).

Category Systems

With observational category systems, the categories should be mutually exclusive. If categories overlap, the observer will be faced with making judgments regarding which category should contain each observed behavior, and data collection and recording may be inconsistent. In some category systems, only the behavior that is of interest is recorded. Most category systems require the

observer to make some inference from the observed event to the category. The greater the degree of inference required, the more difficult the category system is to use. Some systems are applicable in a wide variety of studies, whereas others are specific to the study for which they were designed. The number of categories used varies considerably with the study. An optimal number for ease of use, and therefore effectiveness of observation, is 10 to 15 categories.

Another type of category system used to direct the collection of observational data is a checklist. **Observational checklists** are techniques used to establish whether a behavior occurred. The observer places a tally mark on a data collection form each time he or she witnesses the behavior. Behavior other than that on the checklist is ignored. In some studies, the observer may place multiple tally marks in various categories while witnessing a particular event. However, in other studies, the observer is required to select a single category in which to place the tally mark. These data sometimes are stored electronically and are available to researchers for large database analysis. Measuring variables using observation requires a quality tool for data collection and consistent use of this tool by data collectors. If the observations in a study are being conducted using multiple data collectors, it is essential that the consistency or interrater reliability of the data collectors be determined at the start of the study and periodically during data collection (see Chapter 16) (Waltz et al., 2017).

Rating Scales

Rating scales (discussed in more detail later in this chapter) can be used for observation and for self-reporting. A rating scale allows the observer to rate the behavior or event on a scale. This method provides more information for analysis than the use of dichotomous data, which indicate only that the behavior either occurred or did not occur (see Table 16.1). The McLellan et al. (2017) study, introduced earlier in this chapter, was conducted to validate the CHEWS with the previously validated PEWS. The total sample for this study was $N = 1136$, and there was no significant difference between the pediatric patients included or excluded from data analysis. The CHEWS observational tool was developed to identify pediatric cardiac patients at risk for clinical deterioration. The CHEWS tool includes three physiological categories (behavior/neurological, cardiovascular, and respiratory) with a rating scale from 0 to 3 for each category in determining risk of deterioration. This observation tool is described in more detail in the following study excerpt.

"The final revised tool [Fig. 17.4], called the Cardiac Children's Hospital Earl Warning Score (C-CHEWS)... was successfully piloted, fully implemented and then formally validated (...sensitivity 95.3%, specificity 76.2%) in the pediatric cardiac population in a previous study (McLellan, Gauvreau, & Connor, 2013). In this study, the tool demonstrated excellent discrimination in identifying critical deterioration in children with cardiac disease and performed significantly better than the PEWS in identifying critical deterioration (McLellan et al., 2013). To optimize safety and to improve clarity, the hospital leadership decided to implement the cardiac tool throughout all inpatients area rather than having similar but different tools operating in the same institution. The C-CHEWS was renamed the Children's Hospital early Warning Score (CHEWS) and incorporated into the electronic health record [EHR]...

...Inter-rater reliability between staff nurses of all experience levels had previously been established for the CHEWS tool (100% score ≥ 3, kappa statistic 1.00) during the initial validation study and was not repeated (McLellan et al., 2013). The lead investigator trained all nurse data collectors in data extraction, data abstraction, and completion of study forms. A study nurse intermittently reviewed the collected records to identify, address, and reeducate data collection team members regarding any discrepancies in data abstraction to maintain inter-rater reliability of > 90% within the data collection team" [see Fig. 17.4]. (McLellan et al., 2017, pp. 53–54)

"Sensitivity for scores ≥ 3 was 91.4% for CHEWS and 73.6% for PEWS with specificity of 67.8% for CHEWS and 88.5% for PEWS. Sensitivity scores ≥ 5 was 75.6% for CHEWS and 38.9% for PEWS with specificity of 88.5% for CHEWS and 93.9% for PEWS. The early warning time from critical score (≥ 5) to critical deterioration was 3.8 h for CHEWS versus 0.6 h for PEWS (p < 0.001)." (McLellan et al., 2017, p. 52)

McLellan and colleagues (2017) provide extensive details regarding the behaviors to be observed, the scoring process, and the critical score indicating potential deterioration (see study narrative and Fig. 17.4). The validity and interrater reliability of the CHEWS from previous research (McLellan et al., 2013) were very strong. The same lead investigator, McLellan et al. (2017), in this study ensured the data collectors were trained, intermittently reviewed, and reeducated as needed. The interrater reliability was extremely strong in this study (> 90%). In addition, the sample ($N = 1136$) was reported to be representative of the study population, which increased the credibility of the study finding.

McLellan et al. (2017) found the CHEWS to be a significantly stronger observational tool for use in clinical practice than the PEWS for assessing the status of cardiac and noncardiac pediatric patients. The researchers concluded: "The CHEWS system demonstrated higher discrimination, higher sensitivity, and longer early warning time than the PEWS for identifying children at risk for critical deterioration" (McLellan et al., 2017, p. 52).

INTERVIEWS IN RESEARCH

Interviews involve verbal communication during which the subject provides information to the researcher. Although this data collection strategy is used most commonly in qualitative, mixed methods, and descriptive studies (Creswell & Clark, 2018; Creswell & Creswell, 2018), it is also used in other types of studies. The various approaches for conducting interviews range from unstructured interviews in which study participants are asked broad questions (see Chapter 12) to interviews in which the participants respond to a questionnaire, selecting from a set of specific responses. Although most interviews are conducted face to face or by telephone, computer-based interviews are also commonly used (Streiner, Norman, & Cairney, 2015).

Using the interview method for measurement requires detailed work with a scientific approach. Excellent books are available on the techniques of developing interview questions (Dillman, Smyth, & Christian, 2014; Streiner et al., 2015). If you plan to use this strategy, consult a text on interview methodology before designing your instrument. Because nurses frequently use interview techniques in nursing assessment, the dynamics of interviewing are familiar; however, using this technique for measurement in research requires greater sophistication (Waltz et al., 2017).

Structured Interviews

Structured interviews are verbal interactions with subjects that allow the researcher to exercise increasing

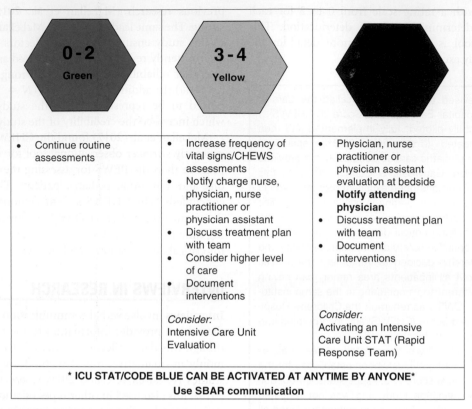

0 - 2 Green	3 - 4 Yellow	
• Continue routine assessments	• Increase frequency of vital signs/CHEWS assessments • Notify charge nurse, physician, nurse practitioner or physician assistant • Discuss treatment plan with team • Consider higher level of care • Document interventions *Consider:* Intensive Care Unit Evaluation	• Physician, nurse practitioner or physician assistant evaluation at bedside • **Notify attending physician** • Discuss treatment plan with team • Document interventions *Consider:* Activating an Intensive Care Unit STAT (Rapid Response Team)
* ICU STAT/CODE BLUE CAN BE ACTIVATED AT ANYTIME BY ANYONE* **Use SBAR communication**		

Fig. 17.4 The Children's Hospital Early Warning Score (CHEWS). (From McLellan, M. C., Gauvreau, K., & Connor, J. A. [2014]. Validation of the Cardiac Children's Hospital Early Warning Score: An early warning scoring tool to prevent cardiopulmonary arrests in children with heart disease. *Congenital Heart Disease, 9*[3], 54.)

amounts of control over the content of the interview for the purpose of obtaining essential data. The researcher designs the questions before data collection begins, and the order of the questions is specified. In some cases, the interviewer is allowed to explain the meaning of the question further or modify the way in which the question is asked so that the subject can understand it better. In more structured interviews, the interviewer is required to ask each question precisely as it has been designed (Waltz et al., 2017). If the study participant does not understand the question, the interviewer can only repeat it. The participant may be limited to a range of responses previously developed by the researcher, similar to those in a questionnaire (Dillman et al., 2014). For example, the interviewer may ask participants to select from the responses "weak," "average," or "strong" in describing their functional level. If the possible responses are lengthy or complex, they may be printed on a card so that study participants can review them visually before selecting a response.

Designing Interview Questions

The process for developing and sequencing interview questions progresses from broad and general to narrow and specific. Questions are grouped by topic, with fairly safe topics being addressed first and sensitive topics reserved until late in the interview process to make participants feel more comfortable in responding. Demographic information, such as age, ethnicity/race, and educational level, usually are collected last. These data are best obtained from other sources, such as the patients' EHRs to allow more time for the primary interview questions. The wording of questions in an interview is crafted toward the minimum expected educational level of the subjects, with the questions examined for readability level (see Chapter 16). Study participants may interpret the wording of certain questions in a variety of ways, and researchers must anticipate this possibility. After the interview protocol has been developed, it is wise to seek feedback from an expert on interview technique and from a content expert.

Interviewing children requires a special understanding of the art of asking them questions based on their age. The interviewer must use words that children tend to use to define situations and events. Interviewers also must be familiar with the language skills that exist at different stages of development. Children view topics differently than adults do, and their perception of time and the concepts of past and present are also different.

Pilot-Testing the Interview Protocol

After the research team has satisfactorily developed the interview protocol, team members need to pretest or pilot-test it on subjects similar to the individuals who will be included in their study. Pilot testing allows the research team to identify problems in the design of questions, sequencing of questions, and procedure for recording responses. The time required for the informed consent and interviewing processes also needs to be determined. Pilot testing provides an opportunity to assess the reliability and validity of the interview instrument (Waltz et al., 2017).

Training Interviewers

Skilled interviewing requires practice, and interviewers must be familiar with the content of the interview. They need to anticipate situations that might occur during the interview and develop strategies for dealing with them. One of the most effective methods of developing a polished approach is role playing. Playing the role of the subject can give the interviewer insight into the experience and facilitate an effective response to unscripted situations.

The interviewer should establish a permissive atmosphere in which the study participant is encouraged to respond to sensitive topics. He or she also must develop an unbiased verbal and nonverbal manner. The wording of a question, the tone of voice, a raised eyebrow, or a shifting body position can communicate a positive or negative reaction to the subject's responses—either of which can alter subsequent data (Dillman et al., 2014).

Interviews are conducted using specific protocol to ensure essential data are collected in a consistent way.

The interviewers must be trained to ensure consistency or interrater reliability among them in the implementation of the interview protocol. Strong interrater reliability values greater than 0.80 (80%) increase the consistency of the data collected (see Chapter 16) (Bandalos, 2018; Kazdin, 2017).

Preparing for an Interview

If you are serving as an interviewer in person, on the telephone, or by real-time computer communication, you need to make an appointment. For face-to-face interviews, choose a site for the interview that is quiet, private, and provides a pleasant environment. Before the appointment, carefully plan and develop a script for the instructions you will give the subject. For example, you might say, "I am going to ask you a series of questions about…. Before you answer each question you need to…. Select your answer from the following…, and then you may elaborate on your response. I will record your answer and then, if it is not clear, I may ask you to further explain some aspects."

Probing

Interviewers use probing to obtain more information in a specific area of the interview. In some cases, you may have to repeat a question. If your subject answers, "I don't know," you may have to press for a response. In other situations, you may have to explain the question further or ask the participant to explain statements that he or she has made. At a deeper level, you may pick up on a comment the participant made and begin asking questions to increase your understanding of what he or she meant. Probes should be neutral to avoid biasing participants' responses (Doody & Noonan, 2013).

Recording Interview Data

Data obtained from interviews are recorded, either during the interview or immediately afterward. The recording may be in the form of handwritten notes, video recordings, or audio recordings. With a structured interview, often an interview form is developed and then researchers can record responses directly on the form (Dillman et al., 2014). Data must be recorded without distracting the interviewee. Some interviewees have difficulty responding if it is obvious that the interviewer is taking notes or recording the conversation. In such a case, the interviewer may need to record data after completing the interview. If you wish to record the interview, you first must obtain IRB approval and then obtain the participant's permission.

Advantages and Disadvantages of Interviews

Interviewing is a flexible technique that can allow researchers to explore greater depth of meaning than they can obtain with other techniques. Interviewing allows you to use your interpersonal skills to encourage your participants' cooperation and elicit more information. The response rate to interviews is higher than the response rate to questionnaires, thus collecting data through interview instead of questionnaire yields a more representative sample. Interviews allow researchers to collect data from participants who are unable or unlikely to complete questionnaires, such as very ill subjects or those whose reading, writing, and ability to express their thoughts are marginal. Interviews are a form of self-report, and the researcher must assume that the information provided is accurate. Interviewing requires much more time than self-reports, questionnaires, and scales, and it is more costly. Because of time and cost, sample size usually is limited. Subject bias is always a threat to the validity of the findings, as is inconsistency in data collection from one participant to another (Dillman et al., 2014; Doody & Noonan, 2013; Waltz et al., 2017).

Rieder, Goshin, Sissoko, Kleshchova, and Weierich (2019) conducted semistructured interviews to examine if salivary biomarkers were predictive of "parenting stress in mothers under community criminal justice supervision" (p. 48). The sample included 23 women who were mothers to at least one minor child and were currently in contact with one or more of their children. The following excerpt describes the interviews conducted in this study.

"Procedure
All study procedures occurred during a single 60–90-minute session. This session took place in the participant's room or a private office at the residential treatment center or in the principal investigator's office. Participants were fully informed regarding all study procedures…. Following consent, the participants participated in a semi-structured interview and provided saliva samples at three timepoints, including before and immediately after discussing a stressful parenting event. At the end of the session, participants were

---

debriefed and compensated with a gift card to a local store ($20) and an age-appropriate children's book…

Interview We conducted a semi-structured interview to gather information on family structure, caregiving history for each of the women's children, child welfare history, and maternal criminal justice history (arrest, incarceration, community supervision), as well as how the women managed mothering under community supervision. The interview began with the following parenting stress reminder question: 'Sometimes things happen with our children that are extremely upsetting, things like when a child is hurt or sick, when a mother has to leave her child and live somewhere else, or when a child is taken away from his or her mother. Has anything like this happened with the child you have the most contact with right now?' This question also served as a stressor and allowed us to examine changes in stress system activity in response to a reminder of parenting stress. Interviews were audio recorded with consent." (Rieder et al., 2019, pp. 49–50)

Rieder and colleagues (2019) identified the questions used to initiate the interviews and the topics covered during their semistructured interview (family structure, child welfare history, and maternal criminal justice history). These seemed appropriate based on the purpose and design of the study (Kazdin, 2017). The interviews were conducted in private areas, such as the researcher's office or areas in the residential treatment center. Adequate time (60–90 minutes) was allowed for the interviews. However, the researchers did not identify who conducted the interviews. If more than one person was involved, what was their training and the interrater reliability value for the interviewing protocol? The study participants were treated with respect, as demonstrated by being fully informed about the study procedures, debriefed at the end of the study, and compensated with a gift card. Rieder et al. (2019) found that the biomarkers were predictors of parenting stress in mothers under criminal justice supervision. They recommended replication of their study with a larger sample.

QUESTIONNAIRES

A **questionnaire** is a written self-report form designed to elicit information that can be obtained from a subject's written responses. Information derived through questionnaires is similar to information obtained by interview, but the questions tend to have less depth. The subject is unable to elaborate on responses or ask for questions to be clarified, and the data collector cannot use probing strategies. However, questions are presented in a consistent manner, and there is less opportunity for bias than in an interview.

Questionnaires can be designed to determine facts about the study participants or persons known by the participants; facts about events or situations known by the participants; or beliefs, attitudes, opinions, levels of knowledge, or intentions of the participants. Questionnaires can be distributed to large samples directly, or indirectly through the mail or by computer. The design, development, and administration of questionnaires have been addressed in many excellent books that focus on survey techniques (Dillman et al., 2014; Harris, 2014; Saris & Gallhofer, 2014; Waltz et al., 2017).

Although items on a questionnaire appear easy to design, a well-designed item requires considerable effort. Similar to interviews, questionnaires can have varying degrees of structure. Some questionnaires ask open-ended questions that require written responses. Others ask closed-ended questions with options selected by the researcher. Data from open-ended questions are often difficult to interpret, and content analysis may be used to extract meaning (Miles, Huberman, & Saldaña, 2020). Open-ended questionnaire items are not advised if data are obtained from large samples or quantification of responses are needed.

Researchers frequently use computers to gather questionnaire data (Harris, 2014; McPeake, Bateson, & O'Neill, 2014). Computers are made available at the data collection site (such as a clinic or hospital), the questionnaire is presented on the screen, and subjects respond by using the keyboard or mouse. Data are stored in a computer file and are immediately available for analysis. Data entry errors are greatly reduced. Most researchers e-mail subjects and direct them to a website where they can complete the questionnaire online, allowing the data to be stored securely and analyzed immediately. Thus researchers can keep track of the number of subjects completing their questionnaire and the evolving results.

Using Questionnaires in Research

The first step in either selecting or developing a questionnaire is to identify the information desired. The research team develops a blueprint or table of specifications for the questionnaire. The blueprint identifies the essential content to be covered by the questionnaire; the content must be at the educational level of the potential subjects. It is difficult to stick to the blueprint when designing the questionnaire because it is tempting to add just one more question that seems to be a neat idea or a question that someone insists really should be included. However, as a questionnaire lengthens, fewer subjects are willing to respond, and more questions are left blank.

The second step is to search the literature for questionnaires or items in questionnaires that match the blueprint criteria. Sometimes published studies include questionnaires, but frequently you must contact the authors of a study to request a copy of their questionnaire and obtain their permission to use it. Researchers are encouraged to use questions in exactly the same form as questionnaires in previous studies to examine the questionnaire validity for new samples. However, questions that are poorly written need to be modified, even if rewriting makes it more difficult to compare the validity results of the questionnaire directly with those from previous studies (Harris, 2014).

In some cases, you may find a questionnaire in the literature that matches the questionnaire blueprint that you have developed for your study. However, you may have to add items to or delete items from the existing questionnaire to accommodate your blueprint. In some situations, items from two or more questionnaires are combined to develop an appropriate questionnaire. In all situations, you must obtain permission to use a questionnaire or the items from different questionnaires from the authors of these questionnaires (Saris & Gallhofer, 2014).

An item on a questionnaire has two parts: a question (or stem) and a response set. Each question must be carefully designed and clearly expressed (Dillman et al., 2014; Polit & Yang, 2016). Problems include ambiguous or vague language, leading questions that influence the response, questions that assume a preexistent state of affairs, and double questions.

In some cases, respondents interpret terms used in the question in one way when the researcher intended a different meaning. For example, the researcher might ask how heavy the traffic is in the neighborhood in which the family lives. The researcher might be asking about automobile traffic, but the respondent interprets the question in relation to drug traffic. The researcher might define neighborhood as a region composed of a three-block area, whereas the respondent considers a neighborhood to be a much larger area. Family could be defined as people living in one house or as all close blood relations. If a question includes a term that is unfamiliar to the respondent or for which several meanings are possible, the term must be defined (Harris, 2014; Waltz et al., 2017).

Leading questions suggest to the respondent the answer the researcher desires. These types of questions often include value-laden words and indicate the researcher's bias. For example, a researcher might ask, "Hospitals are stressful places to work, aren't they?" or "Is being placed on hospice care depressing?" These examples are extreme, and leading questions are usually constructed more subtly. The degree of formality and permissive tone with which the question is expressed, in many cases, are important for obtaining a true measure. A permissive tone suggests that any of the possible responses are acceptable. Questions implying a preexisting state of affairs often lead respondents to admit to a previous behavior regardless of how they answer. Examples are "How long has it been since you used drugs?" or, to an adolescent, "Do you use a condom when you have sex?"

Double questions ask for more than one bit of information: "Do you like critical care nursing and working closely with physicians?" It would be possible for the respondent to like working in critical care settings but dislike working closely with physicians. In this case, the question would be impossible to answer accurately. A similar question is, "Was the in-service program educational and interesting?" Questions with double negatives are often difficult for study participants to interpret. For example, one might ask, "Do you believe nurses should not question orders from other healthcare professionals? Yes or No." In this case, the wording of this question can be easily misinterpreted and the word *not* possibly overlooked. This situation can lead participants to respond in a way contrary to how they actually think or feel (Harris, 2014; Saris & Gallhofer, 2014).

Each item in a questionnaire has a **response set** that provides the parameters within which the respondent can answer. This response set can be open and flexible, as it is with open-ended questions, or it can be narrow and directive, as it is with closed-ended questions (Polit & Yang, 2016). For example, an open-ended question might have a response set of three blank lines (Creswell & Poth, 2018). With closed-ended questions, the response set includes a specific list of alternatives from which to select.

Response sets can be constructed in various ways. The cardinal rule is that every possible answer must have a response category. If the sample includes respondents who might not have an answer, a response category of "don't know" or "uncertain" should be included. If the information sought is factual, include "other" as one of the possible responses. However, recognize that the item "other" is essentially lost data. Even if the response is followed by a statement such as "Please explain," it is rarely possible to analyze the data meaningfully. If a large number of study participants ($> 10\%$) select the alternative "other," the alternatives included in the response set might not be appropriate for the population studied (Dillman et al., 2014; Harris, 2014).

The simplest response set is the dichotomous yes/no option. Arranging responses vertically preceded by a blank reduces errors. For example,

_____ Yes

_____ No

is better than

_____ Yes _____ No

because in the latter example, the respondent might not be sure whether to indicate yes by placing a response before or after the word.

Response sets must be mutually exclusive, which might not be the case in the following response set because a respondent might legitimately need to select two responses.

_____ Working full time

_____ Full-time graduate student

_____ Working part time

_____ Part-time graduate student

Mary Cazzell, a pediatric nurse practitioner at Cook Children's Medical Center in Fort Worth, Texas, developed the Self-Report College Student Risk Behavior Questionnaire, an eight-item questionnaire with a response set of yes and no possible answers. This questionnaire was developed and refined as part of her dissertation at The University of Texas at Arlington. Cazzell's (2010) questionnaire was developed based on the 87 risk behaviors identified in a national survey conducted by the US Centers for Disease Control and Prevention (CDC) on the *Youth Risk Behavior Surveillance System* (Brener et al., 2004). Cazzell included the most commonly identified adolescent risk behaviors from the CDC survey. Content validity of the questionnaire was developed by having a doctorally prepared social worker and a pediatric clinical nurse specialist, both risk behavior experts, evaluate the items. The content validity index calculated for the questionnaire was 0.88, supporting the inclusion of these eight items in the questionnaire. Cazzell (personal communication, 2015) presented her questionnaire at three national conferences and expanded question 2 on use of alcohol to target binge drinking (Fig. 17.5).

Questionnaire instructions should be pilot-tested on naïve subjects who are willing and able to express their reactions to the instructions. Each question should clearly instruct the subject how to respond (i.e., "Choose one," "Mark all that apply"), or instructions should be included at the beginning of the questionnaire. The subject must know whether to circle, underline, or fill in a circle as he or she responds to items. Clear instructions are difficult to construct and usually require several attempts. Cazzell (2010) provided clear directions and an

Self-Report College Student Risk Behavior Measure

Unique ID:

Shade Circles Like This --> ●
Not Like This --> ⊗   ☑

Answer YES or NO based on your participation in these behaviors over the past 30 days.

1. I smoked a cigarette (even a puff). ○ Yes   ○ No

2. I drank alcohol (even one drink). ○ Yes   ○ No
   If you answered YES to Question #2:

   a. If you are a female, did you have 4 or more drinks on one occasion? ○ Yes   ○ No

   b. If you are a male, did you have 5 or more drinks on one occasion? ○ Yes   ○ No

3. I used an illegal drug (even once). ○ Yes   ○ No

4. I had sexual intercourse without a condom. ○ Yes   ○ No

5. I rode in a car without wearing my seatbelt (even once). ○ Yes   ○ No

6. I drove a car without wearing my seatbelt (even once). ○ Yes   ○ No

7. I rode in a car with a person driving under the influence (even once). ○ Yes   ○ No

8. I drove a car while under the influence (even once). ○ Yes   ○ No

Fig. 17.5 Self-Report College Student Risk Behavior Questionnaire. (Adapted from Cazzell, M. [2010]. College student risk behavior: The implications of religiosity and impulsivity. Ph.D. dissertation, The University of Texas at Arlington. Proquest Dissertations & Theses. [Publication No. AAT 3391108.])

example of how to complete her questionnaire and directed the students to report their participation in these risk behaviors over the past 30 days (see Fig. 17.5).

After the questionnaire items have been developed, you need to plan carefully how they will be ordered. Questions related to a specific topic must be grouped together. General items are included first, with progression to more specific items. More important items might be included first, with subsequent progression to items of lesser importance. Questions of a sensitive nature or questions that might be threatening should appear near the end of the questionnaire. In some cases, the response to one item may influence the response to another. If so, the order of such items must be carefully considered. The general trend is to ask for demographic data about the subject at the end of the questionnaire (Dillman et al., 2014; Waltz et al., 2017).

An introductory page for computer-based questionnaires or a cover letter for a mailed questionnaire is needed to explain the purpose of the study and identify the researchers, the approximate amount of time required to complete the form, and organizations or institutions supporting the study. Because researchers indicate that completion of the questionnaire implies informed consent, researchers need to obtain a waiver of a signed consent from the IRB. Returning mailed questionnaires is much more complex. The instructions need to include an address to which the questionnaire can be returned. This address must be at the end of the questionnaire and on the cover letter and envelope. Respondents often discard both the envelope and the cover letter and do not know where to send the questionnaire after completing it. It is also wise to provide a stamped, addressed envelope for the subject to return the questionnaire. If possible, the best way to provide questionnaires to potential subjects is by e-mailing a Web address so that participants can easily complete the questionnaire at their leisure, and their responses are automatically submitted at the end of the questionnaire. Sending questionnaires by e-mail has many advantages, but one disadvantage is being able to access only individuals with e-mail. Researchers need to determine whether the population they are studying has e-mail access and, if they have e-mail, whether the addresses are available to the researchers. Another disadvantage for both mailed and e-mailed questionnaires is not being able to verify that the person who completes the questionnaire is the person to whom it was sent (Dillman et al., 2014).

Your questionnaire must be pilot-tested to determine clarity of questions, effectiveness of instructions, completeness of response sets, time required to complete the questionnaire, and success of data collection techniques. As with any pilot test, the subjects and techniques must be as similar as possible to those planned for the main study. In some cases, the open-ended questions are included in a pilot test to obtain information for the development of closed-ended response sets for the main study.

Questionnaire Validity

One of the greatest risks in developing response sets is leaving out an important alternative or response. For example, if the questionnaire item addressed the job position of nurses working in a hospital and the sample included nursing students, a category representing the student role would be necessary. When seeking opinions, there is a risk of obtaining a response from an individual who actually has no opinion on the research topic. When an item requests knowledge that the respondent does not possess, the subject's guessing interferes with obtaining a true measure of the study variable.

The response rate to questionnaires is generally lower than that with other forms of self-reporting, particularly if the questionnaires are sent out by mail. If the response rate is less than 40%, the representativeness of the sample is in question. However, the response rate for mailed questionnaires is usually small (25%–35%), so researchers are frequently unable to obtain a representative sample, even with randomization. There seems to be a stronger response rate for questionnaires that are sent by e-mail, but the response is still usually less than 40% (Saris & Gallhofer, 2014). Strategies that can increase the response rate for an e-mailed or mailed questionnaire are discussed in Chapter 20.

Study participants commonly fail to respond to all the questions on a questionnaire. This problem, especially with long questionnaires, can threaten the validity of the instrument. In some cases, study participants may write in an answer if they do not agree with the available choices, or they might write comments in the margin. Generally, these responses cannot be included in the analysis; however, you should keep a record of such responses. These responses might be used later to refine the questionnaire questions and responses.

Consistency in the way the questionnaire is administered is important to validity. Variability that could confound the interpretation of the data reported by the study participants is introduced by administering some questionnaires in a group setting, mailing some questionnaires, and e-mailing some questionnaires. There should not be a mix of mailing or e-mailing to business addresses and to home addresses. If questionnaires are administered in person, the administration needs to be consistent. Several problems in consistency can occur: (1) Some subjects may ask to take the form home to complete it and return it later, whereas others will complete it in the presence of the data collector; (2) some subjects may complete the form themselves, whereas others may ask a family member to write the responses that the respondent dictates; and (3) in some cases, a secretary or colleague may complete the form, rather than the individual whose response you are seeking. These situations may lead to biases in responses that are unknown to the researcher and can alter the true measure of the variables (Dillman et al., 2014; Harris, 2014).

Analysis of Questionnaire Data

Data from questionnaires are often at the nominal or ordinal level of measurement that limit analyses. Analysis may be limited to descriptive statistics, such as frequencies and percentages, and nonparametric inferential statistics, such as chi square, Spearman rank-order correlation, and Mann-Whitney U (see Chapters 22, 23, 24, and 25). However, in certain cases, ordinal data from questionnaires are treated as interval data, and t-tests and analysis of variance are used to test for differences between responses of various subsets of the sample (Grove & Cipher, 2020). Discriminant analysis may be used to determine the ability to predict membership in various groups from responses to particular questions.

SCALES

Scales, a form of self-report, are a more precise means of measuring phenomena than questionnaires. Most scales have been developed to measure psychosocial variables. However, self-reports can be obtained on physiological variables, such as pain, nausea, or functional capacity, by using scaling techniques, as discussed earlier in this chapter. Scaling is based on mathematical theory, and there is a branch of science whose primary concern is the development of measurement scales.

From the point of view of scaling theory, considerable measurement error, both random and systematic error, is expected in a single item (Bandalos, 2018; DeVellis, 2017; Waltz et al., 2017). Therefore, in most scales, the various items on the scale are summed to obtain a single score, and these scales are referred to as **summated scales**. Less random and systematic error exists when using the total score of a scale in conducting data analyses, although subscale comparisons are usually of interest and are conducted. Using several items in a scale to measure a concept is comparable to using several instruments to measure a concept (see Fig. 16.4). The various items in a scale increase the dimensions of the concept that are reflected in the instrument (DeVellis, 2017). The types of scales commonly used in nursing studies include rating scale, Likert scale, and visual analog scale (VAS).

Rating Scale

A **rating scale** lists an ordered series of categories of a variable that are assumed to be based on an underlying continuum. A numerical value is assigned to each category, and the fineness of the distinctions between categories varies with the scale, making this one of the crudest forms of scaling technique. The general public commonly uses rating scales. In conversations, one can hear statements such as "On a scale of 1 to 10, I would rank that…." Rating scales are easy to develop; however, one must be careful to avoid end statements that are so extreme that no subject would select them. A rating scale could be used to rate the medication adherence of a patient or the value placed by a patient on nurse-patient interactions. These types of rating scales are also used in observational measurement to guide data collection.

The Wong-Baker FACES® Pain Rating Scale is often used to assess the pain of children in clinical practice and in research. The FACES scale was developed over 30 years ago to measure children's pain, and research has supported the validity and reliability of this scale (Fig. 17.6) (Wong-Baker FACES Foundation, 2019). Pain in adults is often assessed with a numeric rating scale (NRS), such as the one presented in Fig. 17.7. McLellan et al. (2017) refined the CHEWS tool that was introduced earlier in this chapter (see Fig. 17.4). The CHEWS was an observational rating scale, with values 0 to 3, to identify children at risk for critical deterioration and to trigger nurses to intervene and prevent

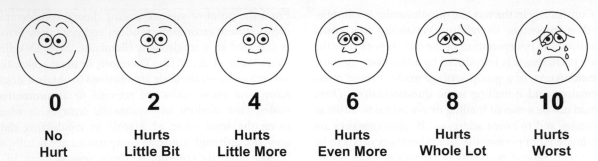

Fig. 17.6 Wong-Baker FACES® Pain Rating Scale. (From Wong-Baker FACES Foundation. [2015]. *Wong-Baker FACES® Pain Rating Scale*. Retrieved from http://www.wongbakerfaces.org/)

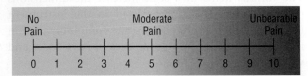

Fig. 17.7 Numeric rating scale (NRS).

further deterioration. These three rating scales are very different based on what is to be measured in a study. The FACES and NRS scales have a narrow focus on the concept of pain in children and adult populations, respectfully. The CHEWS scale has a broader focus of determining risk of critical deterioration by examining the children's behavioral/neurological, cardiovascular, and respiratory systems (Bandalos, 2018; DeVellis, 2017; McLellan et al., 2017).

Likert Scale

The **Likert scale** determines the opinion or attitude of a subject and contains a number of declarative statements with a scale after each statement. The Likert scale is the most commonly used of the scaling techniques in nursing and healthcare studies. The original version of the scale included five response categories. Each response category was assigned a value, with a value of 1 given to the most negative response and a value of 5 given to the most positive response (Bandalos, 2018; DeVellis, 2017; Nunnally & Bernstein, 1994).

Response choices in a Likert scale most commonly address agreement, evaluation, or frequency. Agreement options may include statements such as "strongly disagree," "disagree," "uncertain," "agree," and "strongly agree." Evaluation responses ask the respondent for an evaluative rating along a good/bad continuum, such as "very negative," "negative," "positive," and "very positive."

Frequency responses may include statements such as "never," "rarely," "sometimes," "frequently," and "all the time." The terms used are versatile and must be selected for their appropriateness to the stem. Likert scale responses often contain four to seven options. If the scale has an odd number of response options, then it includes a neutral or uncertain option. Use of the uncertain or neutral category is controversial because it allows the subject to avoid making a clear choice of positive or negative statements. Thus sometimes only four or six options are offered, with the uncertain category omitted. This type of scale is referred to as a **forced choice** version. Researchers who use the forced choice version consider an item that is left blank as a response of "uncertain" or "neutral." However, neutral responses are difficult to interpret, and if a large number of respondents select that option or leave the question blank, the data may be of little value (Bandalos, 2018). In addition, some computer-administered programs do not allow a subject to progress to the next item or section of another instrument if an item is left blank. In this instance, study participants either arbitrarily select an answer or close the program and never complete the instrument.

How the researcher phrases the stem of an item depends on the type of judgment the respondent is being asked to make. Agreement item stems are declarative statements, such as "Nurses should be held accountable for managing a patient's pain." Frequency item stems can be behaviors, events, or circumstances to which the respondent can indicate how often they occur. A frequency stem might be "You read research articles in nursing journals." An evaluation stem could be "The effectiveness of X drug for relief of nausea after chemotherapy." Items must be clear, concise, and concrete (DeVellis, 2017).

An instrument using a Likert scale usually consists of 15 to 30 items, each addressing an element of the concept being measured. Some scales have been reduced to 10 items to improve the response level of study participants. Response-set bias tends to occur when participants anticipate that either the positive or the negative ("agree" or "disagree") response is consistently provided either in the right or left column of the scale. Participants might note a pattern that agreeing with scale items consistently falls to the right and disagreeing to the left. Thus they might fail to read all questions carefully and just mark the right or left column based on whether they agree or disagree with scale items. Thus half the statements should be expressed positively and half should be expressed negatively, termed **counterbalancing**, to avoid inserting response-set bias into the participants' responses. Participants would need to mark some agreement items in the right column and others in the left column of the scale, based on the direction in which each item is written (DeVellis, 2017; Nunnally & Berstein, 1994).

Scale values of negatively worded items require reverse coding prior to analysis. For example, if a scale had a set of four responses ("1—strongly disagree," "2—disagree," "3—agree," and "4—strongly agree") and a study participant strongly disagreed with a negatively worded item, the score of 1 would be reverse-coded to a score of 4. Thus the scores for participants' agreement with certain positively worded items and, accordingly, their disagreement with negatively worded items (reverse coded) could be interpreted in a meaningful way. Usually the values obtained from each item in the instrument are summed to obtain a single score for each subject. Although the values of each item are technically ordinal-level data, the summed score is often analyzed as interval-level data, allowing more powerful parametric statistical analyses to be conducted (Grove & Cipher, 2020; Nunnally & Bernstein, 1994).

Salman and Lee (2019) conducted a predictive correlation study "to examine the effects of spiritual well-being on the relationship between depression and self-perceived health, and to describe the spiritual practices commonly used by Taiwanese elders" (p. 68). This study included a convenience sample ($N = 150$) of Taiwanese elders who were 65 years or older. The Center for Epidemiological Studies of Depression Scale (CES-D) was used to measure depression in this study (Fig. 17.8). The implementation of the CES-D is described by Salman and Lee (2019) in the following study excerpt.

> **"Depression**
> The Chinese version of the Center for Epidemiological Studies-Depression Scale (CES-D) was used to measure depression in this study. The CES-D scale (Radloff, 1977) was developed to assess depressive symptomatology in the general population, and it has been widely translated in multiple languages and used in diverse populations. Four dimensions of depressive symptoms, including depressed affect, positive affect, somatic and retarded activity, and interpersonal, are assessed in this scale (Radloff, 1977). The CES-D scale is a 4-point [Likert] rating scale with possible range of total scores between 0 and 60. It includes 20 items that ask the respondents to self-report the described symptoms that occurred in the past week [see Fig. 17.8]. A higher score on the CES-D scale indicates more depressive symptoms. Literature reported that the CES-D scale is a valid and reliable instrument. Excellent psychometric properties of the CES-D scale used in various populations and languages have been reported... Cronbach's alpha of 0.85 was found with the sample of this study. This study adapted the commonly used cutoff score of 16 on the CES-D scale to classify the participants into depressed or non-depressed groups." (Salman & Lee, 2019, p. 70)

Salman and Lee (2019) clearly described the CES-D used to measure depression in their study. The item response range (four-point Likert scale) and scoring of the scale (0 to 60) were discussed, with a commonly accepted score of 16+ indicating elevated depressive symptoms. This indicates the CES-D has criterion validity and has been used in many studies and in clinical practice to identify depression in various populations (Bandalos, 2018; Waltz et al., 2017). The four dimensions of the CES-D were identified supporting the construct validity of the scale. The reliability of the scale for this study was strong: $r = 0.85$. The discussion of the scale would have been strengthened by providing specific validity and reliability information from previous research.

Salman and Lee (2019) concluded, "Spiritual well-being has a mediating effect on the relationship between depression and self-perceived health status. The study provides support to the evidence that spiritual well-being plays a significant role that has positive impacts on health and may help elders who experience illness and health problems to deal with distress" (p. 73).

Center for Epidemiological Studies of Depression Scale DEPA					
THESE QUESTIONS ARE ABOUT HOW YOU HAVE BEEN FEELING LATELY. AS I READ THE FOLLOWING STATEMENTS, PLEASE TELL ME HOW OFTEN YOU FELT OR BEHAVED THIS WAY IN THE <u>LAST WEEK</u>. [*Hand card*]. FOR EACH STATEMENT, DID YOU FEEL THIS WAY: [Interviewer: You may help respondent focus on the whichever "style" answer is easier] 0 = **R**arely or none of the time (or less than 1 day)? 1 = **S**ome or a little of the time (or 1–2 days)? 2 = **O**ccasionally or a moderate amount of time (or 3–4 days)? 3 = **M**ost or all of the time (or 5–7 days)?					

	<u>R</u>	<u>S</u>	<u>O</u>	<u>M</u>	<u>NR</u>
1. I WAS BOTHERED BY THINGS THAT USUALLY DON'T BOTHER ME.	0	1	2	3	--
2. I DID NOT FEEL LIKE EATING; MY APPETITE WAS POOR.	0	1	2	3	--
3. I FELT THAT I COULD NOT SHAKE OFF THE BLUES EVEN WITH HELP FROM MY FAMILY AND FRIENDS.	0	1	2	3	--
4. I FELT THAT I WAS JUST AS GOOD AS OTHER PEOPLE.	0	1	2	3	--
5. I HAD TROUBLE KEEPING MY MIND ON WHAT I WAS DOING.	0	1	2	3	--
6. I FELT DEPRESSED.	0	1	2	3	--
7. I FELT THAT EVERYTHING I DID WAS AN EFFORT.	0	1	2	3	--
8. I FELT HOPEFUL ABOUT THE FUTURE.	0	1	2	3	--
9. I THOUGHT MY LIFE HAD BEEN A FAILURE.	0	1	2	3	--
10. I FELT FEARFUL.	0	1	2	3	--
11. MY SLEEP WAS RESTLESS.	0	1	2	3	--
12. I WAS HAPPY.	0	1	2	3	--
13. I TALKED LESS THAN USUAL.	0	1	2	3	--
14. I FELT LONELY.	0	1	2	3	--
15. PEOPLE WERE UNFRIENDLY.	0	1	2	3	--
16. I ENJOYED LIFE.	0	1	2	3	--
17. I HAD CRYING SPELLS.	0	1	2	3	--
18. I FELT SAD.	0	1	2	3	--
19. I FELT PEOPLE DISLIKED ME.	0	1	2	3	--
20. I COULD NOT GET GOING.	0	1	2	3	--

Fig. 17.8 Center for Epidemiological Studies of Depression Scale (CES-D). (Adapted from Radloff, L. S. [1977]. The CES-D scale: A self-report depression scale for research in the general population. *Applied Psychological Measurement, 1*[3], 385–394.)

The researchers recommended additional studies to test interventions for delivering culturally appropriate spiritual care to enhance the perceived health of elders.

Visual Analog Scale

One of the problems with scaling procedures is the difficulty of obtaining a fine discrimination of values. In an effort to resolve this problem, the **visual analog scale** was developed to measure magnitude, strength, and intensity of an individual's sensations or feelings (Wewers & Lowe, 1990). The VAS, as the term *analog* implies, is a continuous scale. Therefore this scale provides at least interval-level data, and some researchers argue that it provides ratio-level data (DeVellis, 2017). The VAS is particularly useful in scaling stimuli, such as measuring pain, mood, anxiety, alertness, craving for cigarettes, quality of sleep, attitudes toward environmental conditions, functional abilities, and severity of clinical symptoms (Bandalos, 2018; DeVellis, 2017; Waltz et al., 2017).

The stimuli must be defined in a way that the subject clearly understands. Only one major cue should appear for each scale. The VAS is a line 100 mm (or 10 cm) in length with right-angle stops at each end (Fig. 17.9). The line may be vertical or horizontal, and the bipolar anchors are placed beyond each end of the line. The anchors should not be placed above or below the line before the right-angle stop. These end anchors should include the entire range of sensations possible in the phenomenon being measured. Examples include "all" and "none," "best" and "worst," and "no pain" and "worst pain imaginable" (see Fig. 17.9).

The VAS is frequently used in healthcare research because it is easy to construct, administer, and score. The VAS can be administered using a drawn, printed, or computer-generated 100-mm line (DeVellis, 2017; Waltz et al., 2017). The research participant is asked to place a mark through the line to indicate the intensity of the sensation or stimulus. A ruler is used to measure the distance between the left end of the line and the mark placed by the subject. This measure is the value of the subject's sensation. With a computer-generated VAS, research participants can touch the VAS line on the computer screen to indicate the degree of their sensations, such as pain. The computer can determine the value of the sensation for each subject and store it in a database. The scale is designed to be used while the subject is seated. Whether use of the scale from the supine position influences the results by altering perception of the length of the line has yet to be determined. The VAS can be developed for children by using pictorial anchors at each end of the line rather than words (DeVellis, 2017).

Wewers and Lowe (1990) published an extensive evaluation of the reliability and validity of the VAS, although reliability is difficult to determine. Because the VAS is a single item that produces only one value for each subject, internal consistency cannot be calculated (DeVellis, 2017). Reliability of the VAS is most often determined with the test-retest method

(see Chapter 16), which is effective if the variable being measured is fairly stable, such as chronic pain. Because most of the variables measured with the VAS are labile, test-retest consistency might not be applicable. The VAS is more sensitive to small changes than are numerical and other rating scales and it can discriminate between two dimensions of pain. Validity of the VAS has most commonly been determined by comparing VAS scores with other measures of a concept.

Şentürk and Kartin (2018) conducted a RCT to determine the "effect of lavender oil application via inhalation pathway on hemodialysis [HD] patients' anxiety level and sleep quality" (p. 324). HD patients frequently experience sleep problems caused by their treatment, which leads to increased anxiety and daytime sleepiness. The daytime sleepiness reduces energy level, self-care abilities, and QoL. The researchers measured daytime sleepiness with a VAS that is described in the following study excerpt.

"Daytime Sleepiness Level (Visual Analog Scale)
The scale developed by Price et al. (1994) has been used in numerous studies to evaluate levels of pain and has been found to be valid and reliable. Visual Analog Scale has also been used in many studies to evaluate sleep level, which like pain is a subjective feeling.... The VAS sleepiness scale is a 10-cm scale evaluating daytime sleepiness within the previous week. The scale shows 'Very alert during the day' on the left side, and 'Very sleepy during the day' on the right side. The sleep value of the VAS is determined by measuring the distance between the marked point and the far left end of the scale. A 0 value indicates a good sleep level, while a value of 10 indicates a poor sleep level. The sleep level of an individual increases as the value falls. Because the duration of the application for the intervention group in the present study was 1 week, Daytime Sleepiness Level was evaluated by using VAS." (Şentürk & Kartin, 2018, p. 327)

Şentürk and Kartin (2018) clearly described the VAS used in their study and how the scale was administered and scored. These researchers found that the VAS was easy to use and an effective way to assess the daytime sleepiness of their subjects. The measurement discussion would have been strengthened by a discussion of specific reliability and validity information of the VAS based on previous research (DeVellis, 2017). The VAS

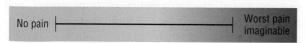

Fig. 17.9 Example of a visual analog scale to measure pain.

seemed to be an effective measure for daytime sleepiness in this study.

The researchers found that the intervention of inhaling lavender oil significantly reduced HD patients' daytime sleepiness as measured by the VAS. "Aromatherapy is a method that nurses can easily learn and use to relieve the sleep and anxiety problems of patients. Nurse practitioners need to receive basic training about the concepts and techniques of aromatherapy applications" (Şentürk & Kartin, 2018, p. 334).

Q-SORT METHODOLOGY

Q-sort methodology is a technique of comparative rating that preserves the subjective point of view of the individual. Cards are used to categorize the importance placed on various words or phrases in relation to the other words or phrases in the list. Each phrase is placed on a separate card. The number of cards should range from 40 to 100 (Tetting, 1988). The subject is instructed to sort the cards into a designated number of piles, usually 7 to 10 piles ranging from the most to the least important or from the most to least agreement (Tetting, 1988; van Hooft, Dwarswaard, Jedeloo, Bal, & van Staa, 2015). However, the subject is limited in the number of cards that may be placed in each pile. If the subject must sort 60 cards, Category One (of greatest importance) may allow only 2 cards; Category Two, 5 cards; Category Three, 10 cards; Category Four, 26 cards; Category Five, 10 cards; Category Six, 5 cards; and Category Seven (the least important), 2 cards. Placement of the cards fits the pattern of a normal curve. Study participants are usually advised to select first the cards they wish to place in the two extreme categories and then work toward the middle category, which contains the largest number of cards, rearranging the cards until they are satisfied with the results. When sorting the cards, subjects might be encouraged to make comments about the statements on the cards and provide a rationale for the categories into which they placed the cards (Akhtar-Danesh, Baumann, & Cordingley, 2008).

Q-sort methodology also can be used to determine the priority of items or the most important items to include in the development of a scale. In the previously mentioned example, the behaviors sorted into Categories One, Two, and Three might be organized into a 17-item scale. Correlational or factor analysis is used to analyze the data (Akhtar-Danesh et al., 2008; van Hooft et al., 2015). Simpson (1989) suggested using the Q-sort method for cross-cultural research, with pictures used rather than words for nonliterate groups.

van Hooft and colleagues (2015) used Q-sort methodology to examine nurses' perspectives on self-management support for people with chronic conditions. In this study, 49 registered nurses were asked to sort 37 statements into seven categories. Their use of Q-sort methodology is presented in the following study excerpt.

> "The first step of a Q-methodological study is the design of the collection of representative statements. These statements should cover all the relevant ground on a subject.... The purpose of a Q-methodological study is to identify different opinions on a topic, instead of generalization (Akhtar-Danesh et al., 2008). A limited sample is sufficient, therefore, as long as this sample holds a maximum variation of opinions...
>
> The statements are printed on separate cards with random numbers. The participants were asked to read the statements carefully and then sort them in three piles: agree, disagree, or neutral. Thereafter, they sorted the statements even more precisely on a Q-sort table with a forced-choice frequency distributions (Figure 7 [Fig. 17.10] on a range from '-3 least agree' to '+3 most agree.' This forced participants to make choices about which statement was more and which was less important to them. Next, participants in face-to-face interviews explained their motivations for the choice of the statements sorted on −3 and +3, and at random about other statements. The interviews lasted between 10 and 65 min and were recorded and transcribed ad verbatim." (van Hooft et al., 2015, p. 159)

van Hooft et al. (2015) conducted factor analysis on their data and identified "four distinct nurses' perspectives toward self-management support: the Coach, the Clinician, the Gatekeeper, and the Educator" (p. 165). Nurses in a Coach role focus on promoting patients' activities of daily living, and nurse Clinicians help patients adhere to their treatment regimes. Support from nurses in the Gatekeeper role helps reduce healthcare costs. Educator nurses focus on instructing patients and families in the management of the illness. Each perspective requires distinct competencies from nurses, and they need specific education to fulfill these roles of supporting patients in their management of chronic illnesses.

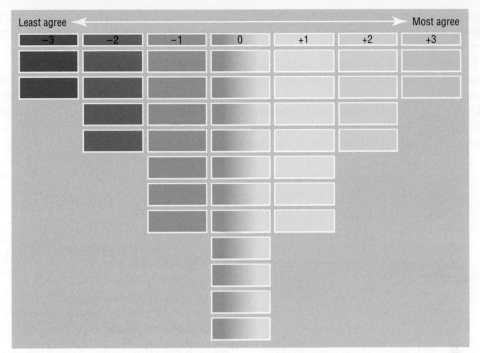

Fig. 17.10 Forced-choice frequency distribution in Q-sort. (Adapted from van Hooft, S. M., Dwarswaard, J., Jedeloo, S., Bal, R., & van Staa, A. [2015]. Four perspectives on self-management support by nurses for people with chronic conditions: A Q-methodological study. *International Journal of Nursing Studies, 52*[1], 161.)

DELPHI TECHNIQUE

The **Delphi technique** measures the judgments of a group of experts for the purpose of making decisions, assessing priorities, or making forecasts (Vernon, 2009). Using this technique allows a wide variety of experts to express opinions and provide feedback, nationally and internationally, without meeting together. When the Delphi technique is used, the opinions of individuals cannot be altered by the persuasive behavior of a few people at a meeting. Three types of Delphi techniques have been identified: classic or consensus Delphi, dialectic Delphi, and decision Delphi. In **classic Delphi**, the focus is on reaching consensus. **Dialectic Delphi** is sometimes called policy Delphi, and the aim is not consensus but identifying and understanding a variety of viewpoints and resolving disagreements. In **decision Delphi**, the panel consists of individuals in decision-making positions and the purpose is to come to a decision (Waltz et al., 2017).

To implement the Delphi technique, researchers identify a panel of experts who have a variety of

perceptions, personalities, interests, and demographics to reduce biases in the process. Members of the panel usually remain anonymous to one another. A questionnaire is developed that addresses the topics of concern. Although most questions call for closed-ended responses, the questionnaire usually contains opportunities for open-ended responses by each expert. Once they have completed the questionnaires, the respondents return them to the researcher, who then analyzes and summarizes the results. The statistical analyses usually include measures of central tendency and measures of dispersion. The role of the researcher is to maintain objectivity. The numerical outcomes of the most frequently selected items are returned to the panel of experts, along with a second questionnaire. Respondents with extreme responses to the first round of questions may be asked to justify their responses. The respondents return the second round of questionnaires to the researcher for analysis. This procedure is repeated until the data reflect consensus among the panel. Limiting the process to two or three rounds is not a good idea if consensus is the goal. In some studies, true consensus is reached, whereas in others, the majority rules. Some authors question whether the agreement reached is genuine (Vernon, 2009; Waltz et al., 2017). An adapted model of the Delphi technique is presented in Fig. 17.11 that might assist you in implementing this technique in a study (Couper, 1984).

Waltz et al. (2017) identified benefits and limitations of the Delphi technique. The benefits include increased access to experts and usually good response rates. The

Delphi design has simplicity and flexibility in its use; it is easily understood and implemented by researchers. Because the participants are anonymous, views can be expressed freely without direct persuasion from others.

There are also several potential problems that researchers could encounter when using the Delphi technique. There has been no documentation that the responses of experts are different from responses one would receive from a random sample of subjects. Because the panelists are anonymous, they have no accountability for their responses. Respondents could make hasty, ill-considered judgments because they know that no negative feedback would result. Feedback on the consensus of the group tends to centralize opinion, and traditional analysis with the use of means and medians may mask the responses of individuals who are resistant to the consensus sentiment. Therefore conclusions obtained with the Delphi technique could be misleading (Vernon, 2009; Waltz et al., 2017).

Roney and McKenna (2018) conducted a study using the Delphi technique to determine the education and research priorities related to nursing care of pediatric trauma patients. The study participants are members of the Society of Trauma Nurses (STN) and are recognized as experts in pediatric trauma care. The following study excerpt describes the Delphi technique they used.

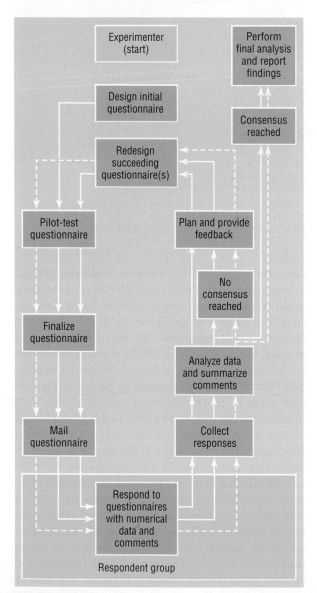

Fig. 17.11 Delphi technique sequence model. Multiple arrows indicate repeated cycles of review by experts.

"The Delphi technique is a hybrid research process that involves quantitative and qualitative approaches with multiple iterations designed to transform individual expert opinion to group consensus (Keeney, Hasson, & McKennon, 2011). The technique uses a group of experts in a specific field who anonymously reply to surveys and then receive feedback in the form of summarized group responses ('Delphi Method [RAND Corporation],' 2018). Consensus is reached as participants are required to first respond to a survey and then through subsequent survey rounds provide feedback based on group consensus from the previous round of surveying (Yeung, Woods, Dubrowski, Hodges, & Carnahan, 2015). The goal of using the Delphi technique is to narrow the range of responses and arrive at something closer to expert consensus ('Delphi Method [RAND Corporation],' 2018). There are many advantages to using this research method, which include the following: the ability to conduct a study in a geographically dispersed area without physically bringing participants together; discussion of broad and complex problems; and translation of scientific knowledge and professional experience into informed judgment to support effective decision making.... There is considerable variability in the number of participants in Delphi technique studies within healthcare publications as well as no standards established in any methodologically acceptable way related to sampling or sample size. Many published healthcare studies have as few as 10 participants.... Delphi studies with small numbers of participants from a defined field of study with similar training and knowledge of their field can yield [word missing] results (Boulkedid, Abdoul, Loustau, Sibony, & Alberti, 2011)... The Delphi technique has been used extensively in nursing research and specifically in trauma nursing research to develop a trauma care syllabus for intensive care unit nurses (Whiting & Cole, 2016), to establish regional standards in trauma nursing education (Haley et al., 2017), and to gain consensus for trauma nursing research priorities with adult patients.... Two of the members of the Pediatric Committee of STN (L.R., C.M.) approached the Pediatric Committee about the idea for this current study and received their support. After securing institutional review board approval, the researchers received permission from STN to complete this study with their members." (Roney & McKenna, 2018, p. 291)

"Round 1

Invitations to participate in this current study were sent to 1,440 STN members. Responses to Round 1 were received from 78 nurses representing trauma programs in 47 states, yielding a total of 373 education and 209 research items. The individual responses were cleaned, sorted, and organized into themes. Content analysis of Round 1 produced 22 educational and 26 research priorities. Education priorities...and research priorities... that received five or more responses were kept to move forward to Round 2 of surveying.

Round 2

A total of 25 members participated in both the first and second rounds of this study. The sum of all responses was calculated by the researchers. Ranked totals were calculated, and the lowest scores were the highest priorities for this study.... Participants were provided with the opportunity to comment on why they prioritized the education needs as they did in this round...

Round 3

A total of 25 participants participated in Round 1, Round 2, and Round 3 of this study, which reflects 100% retention of participants between Rounds 2 and 3. The

group of participants who completed all three rounds of the Delphi survey was very experienced, with a mean of 26.2 years as a registered nurse and 8.48 years in their current professional role." (Roney & McKenna, 2018, pp. 292–293)

Roney and McKenna (2018) provided a detailed description of the Delphi technique and how it was implemented in their study. The response rate for Round 1 was very low (5.42%) for the members of STN ($N = 1440$), decreasing the representativeness of the sample. A strength is that the responses represented 47 states. The response rate for Round 2 was stronger ($n = 25$ STN members; 28.74%) but still limited when compared to the original population. The response rate in Round 3 was $n = 25$ or 100% as compared to Round 2. The Delphi technique was appropriate for this study (identifying education and research priorities), and the steps were followed and reported in a quality way (Waltz et al., 2017). However, the sample size was very small ($n = 25$) based on the size of the population.

Roney and McKenna (2018) report: "Consensus on the education and research priorities was derived from a sample ($n = 25$) of trauma nursing experts. The pediatric trauma nursing education priorities identified were: (1) initial resuscitation; (2) assessment; and (3) evidence-based practice. The pediatric trauma nursing research priorities were: (1) impact of nursing care on outcomes; (2) initial resuscitation; and (3) critical care. Future efforts in educational program development and research should focus on these priorities" (p. 290).

DIARIES

A **diary** is a recording of events over time by an individual to document experiences, feelings, or behavior patterns. Diaries are also called logs or journals and have been used since the 1950s to collect data for research from various populations, including children, patients with acute and chronic illness, pregnant women, and elderly adults (Hyers, 2018; Nicholl, 2010). A diary, which allows recording shortly after an event, is thought to be more accurate than obtaining the information through recall during an interview. In addition, the reporting level of incidents is higher, and one tends to capture the participant's immediate perception of situations. Although diaries have been used primarily with adults, they are also an effective means of collecting data from school-age children.

The diary technique gives nurse researchers a means to obtain data on topics of particular interest within nursing that have not been accessible by other means. Some diaries include the collection of narrative data and are more common in qualitative studies (see Chapter 12) (Creswell & Poth, 2018; Hyers, 2018). However, diaries can take a variety of forms and might include filling in blanks, selecting the best response from a list of options, or checking a column, which are useful methods for collecting data in quantitative and mixed methods research. In experimental studies, diaries may be used to determine responses of subjects to experimental treatments. Some potential topics for diary data collection in quantitative research include expenses related to a healthcare event (particularly out-of-pocket expenses), self-care activities (frequency and time required), symptoms of disease, sexual activities, and care provided by family members at home. For example, Fig. 17.12 shows a page from a diary for patients to record their symptoms and how they were managed. This diary includes blanks to identify the symptoms and an option to check how the symptoms were managed, which produces numerical data.

Diaries can be paper, online, phone text-messaging formats, or apps on the iPad or smartphone. Some researchers are using blogs as a way to collect diary data (Lim, Sacks-Davis, Aitken, Hocking, & Hellard, 2010;

Nicholl, 2010). The format of the questions in diaries can vary based on the purpose of the study. As mentioned earlier, diaries with closed-ended questions are usually used in quantitative research, and participants are provided specific direction on the data to be recorded. The validity and reliability of diaries have been examined by comparing the results with data obtained through interviews and have been found to be acceptable. Participation in studies using health diaries has been good, and attrition rates are reported as low. Hyers (2018) and Nicholl (2010) provide some key points in Box 17.3 to consider when selecting a diary for collecting data in a study.

The use of diaries has some disadvantages. In some cases, keeping the diary may alter the behavior or events under study. For example, if a person were keeping a diary of the nursing care that he or she was providing to patients, the insight that the person gained from recording the information in the diary might lead to changes in care. In addition, patients can become more sensitive to items (e.g., symptoms or problems) reported in the diary, which could result in overreporting. Subjects may also become bored with keeping the diary and become less thorough in recording items, which could result in underreporting (Lim et al., 2010; Nicholl, 2010).

McCarthy, Matthews, Battaglia, and Meeks (2018) conducted a quasi-experimental study to determine the "feasibility of a telemedicine-delivered cognitive behavioral therapy for insomnia [CBTI] in rural breast cancer

Date	What symptom did you have?	Did you talk with a family member or friend about the symptom?		Did you talk with a health professional about it?		Did you take any pills or treatments for the symptom?	
		No	Yes	No	Yes	No	Yes, Specify

Fig. 17.12 Sample diary page.

BOX 17-3 **Key Points to Consider When Selecting a Diary for Data Collection in a Study**

1. Analyze the phenomenon of interest to determine whether it can be adequately captured using a diary.
2. Determine whether a diary is the best data collection approach when compared with interviews, questionnaires, and scales.
3. Decide whether the diary will be used alone or with other measurement methods.
4. Determine which format of the diary to use so that the most valid information can be obtained to address the study purpose without burdening the study participants.
5. Pilot-test any new or refined diary with the target population of interest to identify possible problems, determine whether the instructions and terminology are clear, ensure that the data can be recorded with this approach, and examine the ability of participants to complete diaries.
6. Determine the period of time that the diary will be completed to accomplish the purpose of the study, taking into consideration the burden on the participants. Typical diary periods are 2 to 8 weeks.

7. Provide clear instructions to participants on the use of a diary before the study begins to enhance the quality of data collected. Participants need to know how to use the diaries, what types of events are to be reported, and how to contact the researcher with questions.
8. Use follow-up procedures, such as phone calls or e-mails, during data collection to enhance completion rates.
9. Diaries might be e-mailed, mailed, or picked up by the researchers. Picking up the diary in person promotes a higher completion rate than mailing.
10. Plan data analysis procedures during diary development and refine these plans to ensure that the most appropriate analyses are used. Diary data are very dense and rich, and carefully prepared analysis plans can minimize problems (Alaszewski, 2006; Hyers, 2018; Lim et al., 2010; Nicholl, 2010).

---

survivors [BCSs]" (p. 607). This study included 18 women from the rural and frontier counties in Colorado who were "diagnosed and treated with surgery, radiation therapy, or chemotherapy for nonmetastatic breast cancer" (McCarthy et al., 2018, p. 608). The data for sleep were collected using a diary that is described in the following excerpt.

"Primary sleep-related outcomes were collected using daily sleep diaries that included the following parameters:
- Sleep efficiency (SE): ratio (%) of actual sleep time to time in bed multiplied by 100
- Sleep latency (SL): minutes to fall asleep after lights out
- Wake after sleep onset (WASO): sum of minutes awake after sleep onset
- Total sleep time (TST): sleep period minus SL and WASO
- Number of awakenings

The Consensus Sleep Diary (CSD) (Carney et al., 2012) is a subjective sleep assessment tool that standardizes instructions and core measures of sleep. It is a widely used clinical and research tool that monitors daily sleep characteristics and patterns (Carney et al., 2012). In this study, participants were instructed to fill

out the sleep diary every morning when they woke up. Items recorded included the estimated time they went to bed, time of lights out, time they fell asleep, time of last awakening, number of nighttime awakenings, and WASO. These data were used to calculate sleep parameters, including TST, SE, and SL. Reliability of sleep diaries has been supported with as few as three nights of data ($r = 0.8$).... Concurrent validity was previously supported in the comparison of duration of sleep between the CSD and an Actiwatch accelerometer (made by Philips Respironics) ($r = 0.49$) and the Pittsburgh Sleep Quality Index (PSQI) ($r = 0.75$) (Landry, Best, & Liu-Ambrose, 2015)." (McCarthy et al., 2018, pp. 609–611)

McCarthy et al. (2018) clearly described the five parameters of sleep that were measured using the CSD. The participants were provided instructions for when and how to use the CSD to promote consistency in the data collected. Strong reliability ($r = 0.80$) and concurrent validity from previous studies supported the use of the CSD in this study. The reliability of the CSD for this study was not noted. The sample size for this study was small ($N = 18$), which is not unusual for a feasibility study. A feasibility study is like a pilot study that is conducted to examine the flow of the study steps for possible problems. McCarthy et al. (2018) reported that the "nurse-led, telemedicine-delivered CBTI for rural BCSs is feasible and may be effective in managing insomnia" (p. 607). However, they recommended additional research with larger samples to determine the widespread effectiveness of this intervention for practice.

MEASUREMENT USING EXISTING DATABASES

Nurse researchers are increasing their use of existing databases to address the research problems they have identified in practice. The reasons for using these databases in studies are varied. With the EHR and computerization of other types of healthcare information, more large data sets have been developed internationally, nationally, regionally, and within clinical agencies. These databases include large amounts of information that have relevance in developing research evidence needed for practice (Melnyk & Fineout-Overholt, 2019). The costs and technology for secure storage of data have improved over the last 10 years, making these large data sets more reliable and accessible. Outcomes studies often are conducted using existing databases to expand understanding of patient, provider, and health agency outcomes (Moorhead et al., 2018). Another reason for the increased use of preexistent databases is that primary collection of data in a study is limited by the availability of participants and the expense of the data collection process. By using existing databases, researchers are able to have larger and more representative samples, conduct more longitudinal studies, experience lower costs during the data collection process, and limit the burdens placed on study participants (Johantgen, 2010).

There are also problems with using data from existing databases. The data in the database may not clearly address the researchers' study purpose. Most researchers identify a study problem and purpose and then develop a methodology to address these. The data collected are specific to the study and clearly focused on answering the research questions or testing the study hypotheses. However, with existing databases, researchers need to ensure that the data they require for their study are in the database that they are planning to use. Sometimes researchers must revise their study questions and variables based on what data exist in the database. The level of measurement of the study variables might limit the analysis techniques that can be conducted. There is also the question of the validity and reliability of the data in existing databases; unless these are specifically reported, researchers using these data files need to be cautious in their interpretation of findings.

Existing Healthcare Data

Existing healthcare data consist of two types: secondary and administrative. Data collected for a particular study are considered primary data. Data collected from previous research and stored in databases are considered secondary data when used by other researchers to address their study purposes. Because these data were collected as part of research, details can be obtained about the data collection and storage processes. Researchers should clearly indicate in the methodology section of a research report when secondary data analyses represent all or part of their total study data (Johantgen, 2010).

Data collected for reasons other than research are considered administrative data. Administrative data are collected within clinical agencies; obtained by national, state, and local professional organizations; and collected by federal, state, and local government agencies. The processes for collection and storage of administrative data are more complex and often more unclear than the data collection process for research (Johantgen, 2010). The data in administrative databases are collected by different people in different sites using different methods. However, the data elements collected for most administrative databases include demographics, organizational characteristics, clinical diagnosis and treatment, and geographical information. These database elements were standardized by the Health Insurance Portability and Accountability Act (HIPAA) of 1996 to improve the quality of databases. The HIPAA regulations can be viewed online at https://www.hhs.gov/hipaa/for-professionals/index.html (US Department of Health and Human Services [DHHS], 2017).

Sun, Sereika, Lingler, Tamres, and Erlen (2019) conducted a secondary analysis of primary research data to examine the association between caregivers' sleep quality and medication management when caring for community-dwelling persons with memory loss. The secondary analysis is described in the following study excerpt.

> "Methods
>
> This secondary analysis used baseline data from a 6-month randomized controlled trial (RCT) to examine the association between caregiver sleep quality and medication management. The purpose of the parent RCT was to test the efficacy of a problem-solving intervention to improve medication management provided by caregivers of community-dwelling persons with memory loss. Data from the 91 dyads were collect at four time points at 8-week intervals; only data at baseline from the caregivers and care recipients were used for the current study. Baseline data of the caregivers was collected through interviews by research staff at the care recipient's home. Also, caregivers were asked to complete an additional set of questionnaires during the following week and to return the questionnaire packet by postal mail to the research office. Details of the parent RCT protocol have been described previously (Erlen et al.; 2013; Lingler et al., 2016). The parent study was previously approved by the Institutional Review." (Sun et al., 2019, p. 16)

Sun and colleagues (2019) clearly indicated that a secondary analysis of data was conducted to address the purpose of their study. Erlen, Lingler, Sereika, and Tamres were researchers in the parent or primary studies and in this current secondary analysis. The PSQI was used to assess the caregivers' self-reported sleep quality. "For the current study, the internal consistency based on Cronbach's alpha was 0.72. Additionally, the PSQI yields the number of hours slept, a ratio level self-report" (Sun et al., 2019, p. 17). Details were also provided for the three self-report instruments that were used to measure medication management. Sun et al. (2019) found there was a significant association between sleep duration and PSQI hours slept and medication management. Nurses need to more frequently assess the sleep quality of caregivers, because poor sleep quality can contribute to errors in medication management for persons with memory loss.

SELECTION OF AN EXISTING INSTRUMENT

Selecting an instrument to measure a variable in a study is a critical process in research. The measurement method (the operational definition of the variable) selected must fit closely the conceptual definition of the variable (see Chapter 6). Researchers often conduct an extensive search of the literature to identify appropriate measurement methods for their studies. In many cases, they find instruments that measure some of the needed elements but not all, or the content may be related to but somehow different from what is needed for the planned study. Instruments found in the literature may have little or no documentation of their validity and reliability. Novice researchers often conclude that no appropriate method of measurement exists and that they must develop a tool. At the time, this solution seems to be the easiest because the researcher has a clear idea of what needs to be measured. This solution is not recommended unless all else fails. Instrument development is a complex, lengthy process that requires the expertise of sophisticated researchers. Using a new instrument in a study without first evaluating its validity and reliability is problematic and leads to questionable findings (Bandalos, 2018).

For novice researchers developing their first study, it is essential to identify existing instruments to measure their study variables. An adapted flow chart from Jones (2004) might help you to select an existing instrument for your study (Fig. 17.13). The major steps include (1) identifying an instrument from the literature; (2) determining whether the instrument is appropriate for measuring a study variable; and (3) examining the performance of the measurement method in research, such as identifying the reliability and validity of psychosocial instruments and the accuracy and precision of physiological measures (Waltz et al., 2017). These steps are detailed in the following sections.

Locating Existing Instruments

Locating existing measurement methods has become easier in recent years. A computer database, the Health and Psychosocial Instruments (HaPI), is available in many libraries and can be used to search for instruments that measure a particular concept or for information on a particular instrument. Sometimes a search on Medline or Cumulative Index to Nursing and Allied Health Literature might uncover an instrument that is useful. Many reference books have compiled published measurement tools, some of which are specific to instruments used in nursing research. Dissertations often contain measurement tools that have never been published, so a review of *Dissertation Abstracts* online might be helpful.

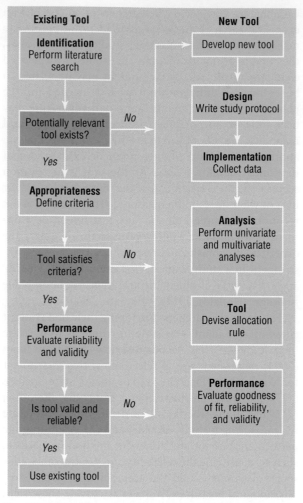

Existing Tool

Identification
Perform literature search

↓

Potentially relevant tool exists? →*No*→

Yes ↓

Appropriateness
Define criteria

↓

Tool satisfies criteria? →*No*→

Yes ↓

Performance
Evaluate reliability and validity

↓

Is tool valid and reliable? →*No*→

Yes ↓

Use existing tool

New Tool

Develop new tool

↓

Design
Write study protocol

↓

Implementation
Collect data

↓

Analysis
Perform univariate and multivariate analyses

↓

Tool
Devise allocation rule

↓

Performance
Evaluate goodness of fit, reliability, and validity

Fig. 17.13 Flow chart depicting the identification and assessment of an existing tool and development of a new tool.

Another important source of recently developed measurement instruments is word-of-mouth communication among researchers. Information on tools is often presented at research conferences years before publication. There are usually networks of researchers conducting studies on similar nursing phenomena. These researchers are frequently associated with nursing organizations and keep in touch through newsletters, correspondence, telephone, e-mail, computer discussion boards, and Web pages. Researchers are being encouraged to collect data on common elements across studies to advance the research needed for practice. Also the use of common measurement methods is thought to increase understanding of variables (Cohen, Thompson, Yates, Zimmerman, & Pullen, 2015).

Questioning available nurse investigators can lead to a previously unknown tool. These researchers can often be contacted by telephone, letter, or e-mail and are usually willing to share their tools in return for access to the data to facilitate work on developing validity and reliability information. You can also access health measures through the PROMIS® (Patient-Reported Outcomes Measurement Information System), which includes person-centered measures that evaluate and monitor physical, mental, and social health in adults and children (DHHS, 2019). Waltz et al. (2017) identified several strategies for locating existing instruments for studies (Box 17.4).

Evaluating Existing Instruments for Appropriateness and Performance

You may need to examine several instruments to find the one most appropriate for your study. When selecting an instrument for research, carefully consider how the instrument was developed, what the instrument measures, and how to administer it. Before you review existing instruments, be sure you have conceptually defined your study variable and are clear on what you desire to measure (see Chapter 6). You then need to address the following questions to determine the best instrument for measuring your study variable:

1. Does this instrument measure what you want to measure?
2. Does the instrument reflect your conceptual definition of the variable?
3. Is the instrument well constructed? (The process for constructing a scale is provided later in this chapter.)
4. Does your population resemble populations previously studied with the instrument (Waltz et al., 2017)?
5. Is the readability level of the instrument appropriate for your population?
6. How sensitive is the instrument in detecting small differences in the phenomenon you want to measure (i.e., what is the effect size)?
7. What is the process for obtaining, administering, and scoring the instrument? Are there costs associated with the instrument?
8. What skills are required to administer the instrument? Do you need training or a particular credential to administer the instrument?

(a) Search computerized databases by using the name of the instrument or keywords or phrases;

(b) generalize the search to the specific area of interest and related topics (research reports are particularly valuable);

(c) search for summary articles describing, comparing, contrasting, and evaluating the instruments used to measure a given concept;

(d) search journals, such as *Journal of Nursing Measurement,* that are devoted specifically to measurement;

(e) after identifying a publication in which relevant instruments are used, use citation indices to locate other publications that used them;

(f) examine computer-based and print indices, and compendia of instruments developed by nursing, medicine, and other disciplines; and

(g) examine copies of published proceedings and abstracts from relevant scientific meetings." (Waltz et al., 2017, p. 448)

9. How are the scores interpreted?

10. What is the time commitment of the study participants and researcher for administration of the instrument?

11. What evidence is available related to the reliability and validity of the instrument? Have multiple types of validity been examined (content validity; construct validity from factor analysis, convergence, and divergence validity; or evidence of criterion-related validity from prediction of concurrent and future events)? Chapter 16 provides a detailed discussion of instrument reliability and validity (also see Table 16.2) (Bandalos, 2018; DeVellis, 2017; Polit & Yang, 2016; Streiner et al., 2015; Waltz et al., 2017).

Assessing Readability Levels of Instruments

The readability level of an instrument is a critical factor when selecting an instrument for a study. Regardless of how valid and reliable the instrument is, it cannot be used effectively if study participants do not understand the items. Many word-processing programs and computerized grammar checkers report the readability level of written material (see Chapter 16). If the reading level of an instrument is beyond the reading level of the study population, you need to select another instrument for use in your study. Changing the items on an instrument to reduce the reading level can alter the validity and reliability of the instrument (Waltz et al., 2017).

INTRODUCTION TO SCALE CONSTRUCTION

Scale construction is a complex procedure that should not be undertaken lightly. There must be firm evidence of the need for developing another instrument to measure a particular phenomenon important to nursing practice. However, in many cases, measurement methods have not been developed for phenomena of concern to nurse researchers, or measurement tools that have been developed may be poorly constructed and have insufficient evidence of validity to be acceptable for use in studies. It is possible for researchers to carry out instrument development procedures on an existing scale with inadequate evidence of validity before using it in a study. Novice nurse researchers could assist experienced researchers in carrying out some of the field studies required to complete the development of scale validity and reliability.

The procedures for developing a scale have been well defined. The following discussion briefly describes this theory-based process and the mathematical logic underlying it. The theories on which scale construction is most frequently based include classical test theory, item response theory, and multidimensional scaling. Most existing instruments used in nursing research have been developed with classical test theory, which assumes a normal distribution of scores. The purpose of this section is to introduce you to scale construction, not provide the details for this complex, lengthy process. If you are considering constructing a scale, consult an expert researcher and the resources provided in this section (Bandalos, 2018; Borg & Groenen, 2010; Cappelleri, Lundy, & Hays, 2014; DeVellis, 2017; Nunnally & Bernstein, 1994; Polit & Yang, 2016; Streiner et al., 2015; Waltz et al., 2017).

Constructing a Scale Using Classical Test Theory

In classical test theory, the following process is used to construct a scale:

1. *Define the concept.* A scale cannot be constructed to measure a concept until the nature of the concept

has been delineated. The more clearly the concept is defined, the easier it is to write items to measure it (Bandalos, 2018; Spector, 1992). Concepts are defined through the process of concept analysis (see Chapter 8).

2. *Design the scale.* Items should be constructed to reflect the concept as fully as possible. The defining attributes identified by concept analysis may provide the subconcepts for which items will be developed. The process of construction differs depending on whether the scale is a rating scale, Likert scale, or VAS. Items previously included in other scales can be used if they have been shown empirically to be good indicators of the concept (Cappelleri et al., 2014; DeVellis, 2017). A blueprint may ensure that all elements of the concept are covered. Each item must be stated clearly and concisely and express only one idea. The reading level of items must be identified and considered in terms of potential respondents. The number of items constructed must be considerably larger than planned for the completed instrument because items are discarded during the item analysis step of scale construction. Nunnally and Bernstein (1994) suggested developing an item pool at least twice the size of that desired for the final scale.

3. *Review the items.* As items are constructed, it is advisable to ask qualified individuals to review them. Feedback is needed in relation to accuracy, appropriateness, or relevance to test specifications; technical flaws in item construction; grammar; offensiveness or appearance of bias; and level of readability. The items should be revised according to the critical appraisal. This is part of the development of content validity (see Chapter 16).

4. *Conduct preliminary item tryouts.* While items are still in draft form, it is helpful to test items on a limited number of subjects (15–30) who represent the target population. The reactions of respondents should be observed during testing to note behaviors such as long pauses, answer changing, or other indications of confusion about specific items. After testing, a debriefing session needs to be held during which respondents are invited to comment on items and offer suggestions for improvement. Descriptive and exploratory statistical analyses are performed on data from these tryouts while noting means, response distributions, items left blank, and outliers

(see Chapters 21, 22, and 23) (Grove & Cipher, 2020). Items need to be revised based on this analysis and on comments from respondents (Bandalos, 2018).

5. *Perform a field test.* All the items in their final draft form are administered to a large sample of subjects who represent the target population. Spector (1992) recommended a sample size of 100 to 200 subjects. However, the sample size needed for the subsequent statistical analyses depends on the number of items in the instrument. Some experts recommend including 10 subjects for each item being tested. If the final instrument was expected to have 20 items, and 40 items were constructed for the field test, 400 subjects would be required.

6. *Conduct item analyses.* The purpose of item analysis is to identify items that form an internally consistent or reliable scale and to eliminate items that do not meet this criterion. Internal consistency reliability implies that all items are consistently measuring a concept. Before these analyses are conducted, negatively worded items must be reverse-scored or given a score as though the item was stated positively. For example, the item might read, "I do not believe exercise is important to health," with the responses of 1 = strongly disagree, 2 = disagree, 3 = uncertain, 4 = agree, and 5 = strongly agree. If the subject marked a 1 for strongly disagree, this item would be reverse scored and given a 5, indicating the subject thinks exercise is very important to health. The analyses examine the extent of intercorrelation among the items. The statistical computer programs currently providing the set of statistical procedures needed to perform item analyses (as a package) are SPSS, SPSS/PC, and SYSTAT. These packages perform both item-to-item correlations and item-to-total score correlations. In some cases, the value of the item being examined is subtracted from the total score, and an item-remainder coefficient is calculated. This latter coefficient is most useful in evaluating items for retention in the scale.

7. *Select items to retain.* Depending on the number of items desired in the final scale, items with the highest coefficients are retained. Alternatively, a criterion value for the coefficient (e.g., 0.40) can be set, and all items greater than this value are retained. The greater the number of items retained, the smaller the item-remainder coefficients can be and still have an internally consistent scale. After this selection process, a

coefficient alpha is calculated for the shortened scale. This value is a direct function of the number of items and the magnitude of intercorrelations. Thus one can increase the value of a coefficient alpha by increasing the number of items or raising the intercorrelations through inclusion of more highly intercorrelated items. Values of coefficient alphas range from 0 to 1. The alpha value should be at least 0.70 to indicate sufficient internal consistency in a new tool (see Chapter 16) (Bandalos, 2018; Nunnally & Bernstein, 1994). An iterative process of removing or replacing items (or both), recalculating item-remainder coefficients, and recalculating the alpha coefficient is repeated until a satisfactory alpha coefficient is obtained. Deleting poorly correlated items raises the alpha coefficient, but decreasing the number of items lowers it. The initial attempt at scale development may not achieve a sufficiently high coefficient alpha. In this case, additional items need to be written, more data collected, and the item analysis redone.

8. *Conduct validity studies.* When scale development is judged to be satisfactory, studies must be performed to evaluate the validity of the scale (see Chapter 16 and Table 16.2). These studies require the researcher to collect additional data from large samples. As part of this process, scale scores must be correlated with scores on other variables proposed to be related to the concept being put into operation. Hypotheses must be generated regarding variations in mean values of the scale in different groups. Exploratory and confirmatory factor analysis (discussed in Chapters 16 and 23) is usually performed as part of establishing the validity of the instrument. Collect as many different types of validity evidence as possible (Bandalos, 2018; Cappelleri et al., 2014; DeVellis, 2017).

9. *Evaluate the reliability of the scale.* Various statistical procedures are performed to determine the reliability of the scale (see Chapter 16) (Waltz et al., 2017).

10. *Compile norms on the scale.* To determine norms, the scale must be administered to a large sample that is representative of the groups to which the scale is likely to be administered. Norms should be acquired for as many diverse groups as possible. Data acquired during validity and reliability studies can be included for this analysis. To obtain the large samples needed for this purpose, many researchers permit others to use their scale with the condition that data from these studies be provided for compiling norms.

11. *Publish the results of scale development.* Scales often are not published for many years after the initial development because of the length of time required to validate the instrument. Some researchers never publish the results of this work. Studies using the scale are published, but the instrument development process may not be available except by writing to the author. This information needs to be added to the body of knowledge, and colleagues should encourage instrument developers to complete the work and submit it for publication (Bandalos, 2018; Cappelleri et al., 2014).

Constructing a Scale Using Item Response Theory

Using item response theory to construct a scale proceeds initially in a fashion similar to that of classical test theory. There is an expectation of a well-defined concept to operationalize. Items are initially written in a manner similar to that previously described, and item tryouts and field testing are also similar. However, the process changes with the initiation of item analysis. The statistical procedures used are more sophisticated and complex than the procedures used in classical test theory. Using data from field testing, item characteristic curves are calculated by using logistic regression models (DeVellis, 2017; Nunnally & Bernstein, 1994). After selecting an appropriate model based on information obtained from the analysis, item parameters are estimated. These parameters are used to select items for the scale. This strategy is used to avoid problems encountered with classical test theory measures.

Scales developed by using classical test theory effectively measure the characteristics of subjects near the mean. The statistical procedures used assume a linear distribution of scale values. Items reflecting responses of respondents closer to the extremes tend to be discarded because of the assumption that scale values should approximate the normal curve. Scales developed in this manner often do not provide a clear understanding of study participants at the high or low end of values.

One purpose of item response theory is to choose items in such a way that estimates of characteristics at each level of the concept being measured are accurate. To accomplish this goal, researchers use maximal likelihood estimates. A curvilinear distribution of scale values is assumed. Rather than choosing items on the basis of the item remainder coefficient, the researcher specifies a test information curve. The scale can be tailored to have the desired measurement accuracy. By comparing a scale developed by classical test theory with one developed from the same items with item response theory, one would find differences in some of the items retained. Biserial correlations among items would be lower in the scale developed from item response theory than in the scale developed from classical test theory. Item bias is lower in scales developed by using item response theory because respondents from different subpopulations having the same amount of an underlying trait have different probabilities of responding to an item positively (DeVellis, 2017; Hambleton & Swaminathan, 2010).

Constructing a Scale Using Multidimensional Scaling

Multidimensional scaling is used when the concept being operationalized is actually an abstract construct believed to be represented most accurately by multiple dimensions. The scaling techniques used allow the researcher to uncover the hidden structure in the construct. The analysis techniques use proximities among the measures as input. The outcome of the analysis is a spatial representation, or a geometrical configuration of data points, that reveals the hidden structure. The procedure tends to be used to examine differences in stimuli rather than differences in people. A researcher might use this method to measure differences in perception of pain. This procedure is often used in the development of rating scales (Borg & Groenen, 2010).

TRANSLATING A SCALE TO ANOTHER LANGUAGE

Contrary to expectations, translating an instrument from the original language to a target language is a complex process. By translating a scale, researchers can compare concepts among respondents of different cultures. The goal of translation is achieving equivalence of the versions of a scale in different languages. Conceptual equivalence, semantic equivalence, and measurement equivalence are important to determine in translating a scale (Streiner et al., 2015; Waltz et al., 2017). **Conceptual equivalence** is focused on determining whether the people in the two cultures view the construct to be measured in the same way. The comparison requires that they first infer and then validate that the conceptual meaning about which the scale was developed is the same in both cultures. **Semantic equivalence** of the two scales refers to the meaning that is attached to each item on the scale by the different cultures. **Measurement equivalence** is conducted after the translation of a scale to establish the psychometric properties of the translated scale and to determine its correlation to the original.

Four types of translations can be performed: pragmatic translations, aesthetic-poetic translations, ethnographical translations, and linguistic translations. **Pragmatic translations** communicate the content from the source language accurately in the target language. The primary concern is the information conveyed. An example of this type of translation is the use of translated instructions for assembling a computer. **Aesthetic-poetic translations** evoke moods, feelings, and affect in the target language that are identical to those evoked by the original material. In **ethnographical translations**, the purpose is to maintain meaning and cultural content. In this case, translators must be familiar with both languages and cultures. **Linguistic translations** strive to present grammatical forms with equivalent meanings. Translating a scale is generally done in the ethnographical mode.

One strategy for translating a scale is called the **one-way translation**, which refers to the use of a bilingual translator who translates a questionnaire or scale from the source language into the target language. This method is simple and easy, but the disadvantage is that you are relying on the skills and knowledge of one translator. For example, an assessment of nurses' knowledge of human immunodeficiency virus was developed in English and translated by a Spanish-speaking nurse in the United States. When the assessment was used in the Dominican Republic (DR), the nurses had difficulty understanding some items due to the differences in Spanish as spoken in Mexico and in DR. This is the challenge of one-way translation. Another strategy for translating scales is called **forward and backward translation**, which involves translating the scale from the original language to the target language and then back-translate from the target language to the original language by using translators not involved in the original translation. Discrepancies are identified, and the procedure is repeated until troublesome problems are resolved. After this procedure, the two versions are administered to bilingual subjects and scored by standard procedures. The resulting sets of scores are examined to determine the extent to which the two versions yield similar information from the subjects. The forward and backward translation process provides a much stronger translation of an instrument. This procedure assumes that the subjects are equally skilled in both languages. One problem with this strategy is that bilingual subjects may interpret meanings of words differently from monolingual subjects. This difference in interpretation is a serious concern because the target subjects for most cross-cultural research are monolingual (Waltz et al., 2017).

Lee, Chinna, Abdulla, and Abidin (2019) investigated the "sematic equivalence between two translated versions of the heart quality of life (HeartQoL) questionnaire produced by the forward-backward (FB) and dual-panel (DP) methods" (p. 1). The English version of this questionnaire was translated to Malay or Bahasa Malaysia (BM), the national language of Malaysia. The translation process is briefly outlined in the following excerpt.

> "[T]he initial conceptual and item equivalence of the HeartQoL questionnaire was assessed prior to translation. This was done by affirming the relevance of HRQoL [health-related quality of life] concept in the Malaysian setting based on local literature...and confirmative feedback from two local cardiologists and five English-speaking patients." (Lee et al., 2019, p. 2)

> **"FB method**
> Four sequential processes were carried out as follows: (a) stage 1: forward translation of source version by two independent forward translators; (b) stage 2: synthesis of translated texts into a single version by the same team of forward translators; (c) stage 3: back-translation of the synthesized version by two independent back translators; and (d) stage 4: review of all versions by a committee of all forward and back translators in close correspondence with a methodologist and the developer of HeartQoL who played the role of adjudicator.... Each team of

forward and back translators consists of one certified translator and one medical personnel, who were native BM speakers and proficient English speakers.

> **DP method**
> A bilingual panel of members ($N = 5$), who were proficient in English and BM, performed independent translations, followed by synthesis of all versions in a panel meeting. The bilingual panel composed of two native BM-speaking Malay teachers and two non-native BM-speaking Chinese and Indian teachers. Their goal was to derive translated texts, which can be understood by the equivalent of a 12-year-old and non-native BM speakers. The fifth person on the panel was a non-medical university lecturer of Malay ethnicity who ensured that the English terms were correctly understood and correctly translated into BM words. The synthesized translation and alternative texts were reviewed by a monolingual lay panel ($N = 5$) in a focus group discussion. The panel members all spoke BM as their either first or second language, but two members spoke very little English." (Lee et al., 2019, pp. 3–4).

Lee and colleagues (2019) provided extensive details about the translation process and the analyses conducted to ensure that the two versions (English and BM) of the HeartQoL scale were semantically equivalent. Translation of a scale to another language is a very complex, time-consuming process, as indicated in this study, which is best managed by expert researchers, linguists, and clinicians. Lee et al. (2019) concluded that the FB and DP translation methods were effective in producing an equivalent version of the HeartQoL scale. They credited the quality of the translation to the skills of the translators on both sides (English and BM) and the fact that the HeartQoL scale was a relatively simple questionnaire with short sentences and no colloquial expressions.

▋ KEY POINTS

- Measurement approaches used in nursing research include physiological measures; observations; interviews; questionnaires; scales; and specialized measures such as Q-sort method, Delphi technique, diaries, and analyses using existing databases.

- Measurements of physiological variables can be either direct or indirect and sometimes require the use of specialized equipment or laboratory analyses.
- The Human Genome Project has increased the opportunities for nurses to be involved in genetic

- research and to include the measurement of nucleic acids in their studies.
- To measure observations, every variable is observed in a similar manner in each instance, with careful attention given to training data collectors.
- In structured observational studies, category systems are developed; checklists or rating scales are developed from the category systems and used to guide data collection.
- Interviews involve verbal communication between the researcher and the study participant, during which the researcher acquires information. Interviewers must be trained in the skills of interviewing, and the interview protocol must be pretested.
- A questionnaire is a printed or electronic self-report form designed to elicit information through the responses of a study participant. An item on a questionnaire usually has two parts: a stem or lead-in question and a response set.
- Scales, another form of self-reporting, are more precise in measuring phenomena than are questionnaires and have been developed to measure psychosocial and physiological variables. The types of scales included in this text are rating scale, Likert scale, and VAS.
- A rating scale is a crude form of measurement that includes a list of an ordered series of categories of a variable, which are assumed to be based on an underlying continuum. A numerical value is assigned to each category. A common example is asking patients to rate their pain on a scale from 0 to 10.
- The Likert scale contains declarative statements with a scale after each statement to determine the opinion or attitude of a study participant.
- The VAS is a 100-mm (10-cm) line with right-angle stops at each end with bipolar anchors placed beyond each end of the line. These end anchors must cover the entire range of sensations possible in the phenomenon being measured.

- Q-sort methodology is a technique of comparative rating that preserves the subjective point of view of the individual. Q-sort methodology might be used in research to determine the importance of selected concepts or variables in a study or to select items for scale development.
- The Delphi technique measures the judgments of a group of experts to assess priorities or make forecasts. It provides a means for researchers to obtain the opinions of a wide variety of experts across the United States without the need for the experts to meet.
- A diary, which allows a research participant to record an experience shortly after an event, is more accurate than obtaining the information through recall at an interview. In addition, the reporting level of incidents is higher, and one tends to capture the participant's immediate perception of situations.
- Nurse researchers are expanding their use of data from existing databases to answer their research questions and test their hypotheses. Health data are usually categorized into secondary data and administrative data.
- The choice of tools for use in a particular study is a critical decision that can have a major impact on the validity of the study. The researcher first must conduct an extensive search for existing tools. Once found, the tools must be carefully evaluated.
- Scale construction is a complex procedure that takes extensive expertise and time to complete. Theories on which scale construction is most frequently based include classical test theory, item response theory, and multidimensional scaling. Most existing instruments used in nursing research have been developed through the use of classical test theory.
- Translating a scale to another language is a complex process that allows concepts among respondents of different cultures to be compared if care is taken to ensure that concepts have the same or similar meanings across cultures.

REFERENCES

Akhtar-Danesh, N., Baumann, A., & Cordingley, L. (2008). Q-methodology in nursing research: A promising method for the study of subjectivity. *Western Journal of Nursing Research, 30*(6), 759–773. doi:10.1177/0193945907312979

Alaszewski, A. (2006). *Using diaries for social research*. London, UK: Sage.

Bandalos, D. L. (2018). *Measurement theory and applications for the social sciences*. New York, NY: Guilford Press.

Borg, J., & Groenen, P. J. (2010). *Modern multidimensional scaling: Theory and application* (2nd ed.). New York, NY: Springer.

Boulkedid, R., Abdoul, H., Loustau, M., Sibony, O., & Alberti, C. (2011). Using and reporting the Delphi method for selecting healthcare quality indicators: A systematic review. *Public Library of Science One, 6*(6), e20476. doi:10.137/journal.pone.0020476

Brener, N. D., Kann, L., Kinchen, S. A., Grunbaum, J. A., Whalen, L., Eaton, D., … Ross, J. G. (2004). Methodology of the Youth Risk Behavior Surveillance System. *Morbidity & Mortality Weekly Report, 53*(RR-12), 1–13.

Bureau International des Poids et Measures (BIPM). (2019). *About the BIPM*. Retrieved from http://www.bipm.org/en/about-us/

Cappelleri, J. C., Lundy, J. J., & Hays, R. D. (2014). Overview of classical test theory and item response theory for the quantitative assessment of items in developing patient-reported outcomes measures. *Clinical Therapeutics, 36*(5), 648–662. doi:10.1016/j.clinthera.2014.04.006

Carney, C. E., Buysse, D. J., Ancoli-Israel, S., Edinger, J. D., Krystal, A. D., Lichstein, K. L., & Morin, C. M. (2012). The consensus sleep diary: Standardizing prospective sleep self-monitoring. *Sleep, 35*, 287–302. doi:10.5665/sleep.1642

Cazzell, M. (2010). *College student risk behavior: The implications of religiosity and impulsivity*. Ph.D. dissertation, The University of Texas at Arlington. Proquest Dissertations & Theses. (Publication No. AAT 3391108).

Clinical and Laboratory Standards Institute (CLSI). (2019). *About CLSI: Committed to continually advancing laboratory practice*. Retrieved from https://clsi.org/about/about-clsi/.

Cohen, M. Z., Thompson, C. B., Yates, B., Zimmerman, L., & Pullen, C. H. (2015). Implementing common data elements across studies to advance research. *Nursing Outlook, 63*(2), 181–188. doi:10.1016/j.outlook.2014.11.006

Couper, M. R. (1984). The Delphi technique: Characteristics and sequence model. *Advances in Nursing Science, 7*(1), 72–77.

Cowan, M. J., Heinrich, J., Lucas, M., Sigmon, H., & Hinshaw, A. S. (1993). Integration of biological and nursing sciences: A 10-year plan to enhance research and training. *Research in Nursing & Health, 16*(1), 3–9.

Craig, C. L., Marshall, A. L., Sjostrom, M., Bauman, A. E., Booth, M. L., Ainsworth, B. E., … Oja, P. (2003). International physical activity questionnaire: 12-country reliability and validity. *Medicine & Science in Sports & Exercise, 35*(8), 1381–1395. doi::10.1249/01.Mss.0000078924.61453.Fb

Creswell, J. W., & Clark, V. L. P. (2018). *Designing and conducting mixed methods research* (3rd ed.). Los Angeles, CA: Sage.

Creswell, J. W., & Creswell, J. D. (2018). *Research design: Qualitative, quantitative, and mixed methods approaches* (5th ed.). Los Angeles, CA: Sage.

Creswell, J. W., & Poth, C. N. (2018). *Qualitative inquiry & research design: Choosing among five approaches* (4th ed.). Los Angeles, CA: Sage.

Department of Education Genomic Science. (2014). *Human Genome Project information Archive 1990–2003*. Retrieved from http://www.ornl.gov/sci/techresources/Human_Genome/home.shtml

DeVellis, R. F. (2017). *Scale development: Theory and applications* (4th ed.). Thousand Oaks, CA: Sage.

Dillman, D. A., Smyth, J. D., & Christian, L. M. (2014). *Internet, phone, mail, and mixed-mode surveys: The tailored design method*. Hoboken, NJ: John Wiley & Sons.

Doody, O., & Noonan, M. (2013). Preparing and conducting interviews to collect data. *Nurse Researcher, 20*(5), 28–32. doi:10.7748/nr2013.05.20.5.28

Erlen, A., Lingler, J., Sereika, S. M., Tamres, L. K., Happ, M. B., & Tang, F. (2013). Characterizing caregiver-mediated medication management in patients with memory loss. *Journal of Gerontological Nursing, 39*(4), 30–39. doi:10.3928/00989134-20130220-91

Grove, S. K., & Cipher, D. J. (2020). *Statistics for nursing research: A workbook for evidence-based practice* (3rd ed.). St. Louis, MO: Elsevier.

Guevara, S. L. R., Parra, D. I., & Rojas, L. Z. (2019). "Teaching: Individual" to increase adherence to therapeutic regimen in people with hypertension and type-2 diabetes: Protocol of the controlled clinical ENURSIN. *BMC Nursing, 18*, Article 22. doi:10.1186/s12912-019-0344-0

Haley, K., Martin, S., Kilgore, J., Lang, C., Rozzell, M., Coffey, C., … Deppe, S. (2017). Establishing standards for trauma nursing education: The Central Ohio trauma system's approach. *Journal of Trauma Nursing, 24*(1), 34–41. doi:10.1097/JTN.0000000000000260

Hambleton, R. K., & Swaminathan, H. (2010). *Item response theory: Principles and applications*. Boston, MA: Kluwer Academic.

Harris, D. F. (2014). *The complete guide to writing questionnaires: How to get better information for better decisions*. Durham, NC: BW&A.

Hyers, L. L. (2018). *Diary methods: Understanding qualitative research*. Oxford, UK: Oxford University Press.

International Organization for Standardization (ISO). (2019a). *All about ISO*. Retrieved from http://www.iso.org/iso/home/about.htm

International Organization for Standardization (ISO). (2019b). *Benefits of ISO standards*. Retrieved from http://www.iso.org/iso/home/standards/benefitsofstandards.htm

International Physical Activity Questionnaire. (2005). *Guidelines for data processing and analysis of the International Physical Activity Questionnaire (IPAQ)—Short and long forms*. Retrieved from https://sites.google.com/site/theipaq/

Johantgen, M. (2010). Using existing administrative and national databases. In C. F. Waltz, O. L. Strickland, & E. R. Lenz (Eds.), *Measurement in nursing and health research* (4th ed., pp. 241–250). New York, NY: Springer.

Jones, J. M. (2004). Nutritional methodology: Development of a nutritional screening or assessment tool using a multivariate technique. *Nutrition (Burbank, Los Angeles County, Calif.), 20*(3), 298–306. doi:10.1016/j.nut.2003.11.013

Joseph, N. M., Hanneman, S. K., & Bishop, S. L. (2019). Physical activity, acculturation, and immigrant status of Asian Indian women living in the United States. *Applied Nursing Research, 47*(1), 52–56. doi:10.1016/j.apnr.2019.04.007

Kazdin, A. E. (2017). *Research design in clinical psychology* (5th ed.). Boston, MA: Pearson.

Keeney, S., Hasson, F., & McKenna, H. (2011). *The Delphi technique in nursing and health research*. Oxford, UK: Wiley-Blackwell.

Kerlinger, F. N., & Lee, H. B. (2000). *Foundations of behavioral research* (4th ed.). Fort Worth, TX: Harcourt College Publishers.

King, A., & Eckersley, R. (2019). *Statistics for biomedical engineers and scientists: How to visualize and analyze data*. London, UK: Academic Press Elsevier.

Kubik, M. J., Permenter, T., & Saremian, J. (2015). Specimen age stability for human papilloma virus DNA testing using BD SurePath. *Lab Medicine, 46*(1), 51–54. doi:10.1309/LM87NED5LRSELUOQ

Landry, G. J., Best, J. R., & Liu-Ambrose, T. (2015). Measuring sleep quality in older adults: A comparison using subjective and objective methods. *Frontiers in Aging Neuroscience, 7*, 166. doi:10.3389/fnagi.2015.00166

Lee, W. L., Chinna, K., Abdulla, K. L., & Abidin, I. Z. (2019). The forward-backward and dual-panel translation methods are comparable in producing sematic equivalent versions of a heart quality of life questionnaire. *International Journal of Nursing Practice, 25*(1), e12715. doi:10.1111/ijn.12715

Leedy, P. D., & Ormrod, J. E. (2019). *Practical research: Planning and design* (12th ed.). New York, NY: Pearson.

Lim, M., Sacks-Davis, R., Aitken, C. K., Hocking, J. S., & Hellard, M. E. (2010). Randomized controlled trial of paper, online, and SMS diaries for collecting sexual behavior information from young people. *Journal of Epidemiology & Community Health, 64*(10), 885–889. doi:10.1136/jech.2008.085316

Lingler, J. H., Sereika, S. M., Amspaugh, C. M., Arida, J. A., Happ, M. E., Houze, M. P., … Erlen, J. A. (2016). An intervention to maximize medication management by caregivers of persons with memory loss: Intervention overview and two-month outcomes. *Geriatric Nursing, 37*(3), 186–191. doi:10.1016/j.gerinurse.2015.12.002

Marshall, C., & Rossman, G. B. (2016). *Designing qualitative research* (6th ed.). Thousand Oaks, CA: Sage.

McCarthy, M. S., Matthews, E. E., Battaglia, C., & Meek, P. M. (2018). Feasibility of a telemedicine-delivered cognitive behavioral therapy for insomnia in rural breast cancer survivors. *Oncology Nursing Forum, 45*(5). doi:10.1188/18.ONF.607-618

McLellan, M. C., & Connor, J. A. (2013). The cardiac children's hospital early warning score (C-CHEWS). *Journal of Pediatric Nursing, 28*(2), 171–178. doi:10.1016/j.pedn.2012.07.009

McLellan, M. C., Gauvreau, K., & Connor, J. A. (2013). Validation of the Cardiac Children's Hospital Early Warning Score: An early warning scoring tool to prevent cardiopulmonary arrests in children with heart disease. *Congenital Heart Disease, 9*(3), 194–202. doi:10.1111/chd.12132

McLellan, M. C., Gauvreau, K., & Connor, J. A. (2017). Validation of the Children's Hospital Early Warning System for critical deterioration recognition. *Journal of Pediatric Nursing, 32*(1), 52–58. doi:10.1016/j.pedn.2016.10.005

McPeake, J., Bateson, M., & O'Neill, A. (2014). Electronic surveys: How to maximize success. *Nurse Research, 21*(3), 24–26. doi:10.7748/nr2014.01.21.3.24

Melnyk, B. M., & Fineout-Overholt, E. (2019). *Evidence-based practice in nursing and healthcare: A guide to best practice* (4th ed.). Philadelphia, PA: Wolters Kluwer.

Miles, M. B., Huberman, A. M., & Saldaña, J. (2020). *Qualitative data analysis: A methods sourcebook* (4th ed.). Thousand Oaks: CA: Sage.

Moorhead, S., Swanson, E., Johnson, M., & Maas, M. L. (2018). *Nursing outcomes classification (NOC): Measurement of health outcomes* (6th ed.). St. Louis, MO: Elsevier.

National Human Genome Research Institute (NHGRI). (2019a). *Funding opportunities overview*. Retrieved from https://www.genome.gov/research-funding/Funding-Opportunities

National Human Genome Research Institute (NHGRI). (2019b). *NHGRI vision and mission*. Retrieved from https://www.genome.gov/about-nhgri/NHGRI-Vision-and-Mission

National Institute of Nursing Research (NINR). (2016). About NINR: Mission & strategic plan. Retrieved from http://www.ninr.nih.gov/aboutninr/ninr-mission-and-strategic-plan#.VabFp_lVhBc

National Institute of Nursing Research (NINR). (2019a). NINR: Summer Genetics Institute (SGI). Retrieved from http://www.ninr.nih.gov/training/trainingopportunities-intramural/summergeneticsinstitute#.Vumd5OIrKUk.

National Institute of Nursing Research (NINR). (2019b). *Spotlight on nursing research*. Retrieved from https://www.ninr.nih.gov/researchandfunding/spotlights-nursing-research-0#.

Ng, K., Wong, S., Lim, S., & Goh, Z. (2010). Evaluation of the Cadi ThermoSENSOR wireless skin-contact thermometer against ear and axillary temperatures in children. *Journal of Pediatric Nursing, 25*(3), 176–186. doi:10.1016/j.pedn.2008.12.002

Nicholl, H. (2010). Diaries as a method of data collection in research. *Pediatric Nursing, 22*(7), 16–20. doi:10.7748/paed2010.09.22.7.16.c7948

Nunnally, J. C., & Bernstein, I. H. (1994). *Psychometric theory* (3rd ed.). New York, NY: McGraw-Hill.

Office of Disease Prevention and Health Promotion. (2018). *Physical activity guidelines for Americans*. Retrieved from https://health.gov/paguidelines/2008/appendix1.aspx

Page, G. G., Corwin, E. J., Dorsey, S. G., Redeker, N. S., McCloskey, D. J., Austin, J. K., … Grady, P. (2018). Biomarkers as common data elements for symptom and self-management science. *Journal of Nursing Scholarship, 50*(3), 276–286. doi:10.1111/jnu.12378

Polit, D. R., & Yang, F. M. (2016). *Measurement and the measurement of change: A primer for the health professions*. Philadelphia, PA: Wolters Kluwer.

Price, D. D., Bush, F. M., Long, S., & Harkins, S. W. (1994). A comparison of pain measurement characteristics of mechanical visual analogue and simple numerical rating scales. *Pain, 56*, 217–226.

Radloff, L. S. (1977). The CES-D scale: A self-report depression scale for research in the general population. *Applied Psychological Measures, 1*(3), 385–394.

RAND Corporation. (2018). *Delphi method*. Retrieved from https://www.rand.org/topics/delphi-method.html

Rieder, J. K., Goshin, L. S., Sissoko, D. R. G., Kleshchova, O., & Weierich, M. R. (2019). Salivary biomarkers of parenting stress in mothers under community criminal justice supervision. *Nursing Research, 68*(1), 48–56. doi:10.1097/NNR.000000000000323

Roney, L., & McKenna, C. (2018). Determining the education and research priorities in pediatric trauma nursing: A Delphi study. *Journal of Trauma Nursing, 25*(5), 290–297. doi:10.1097/JTN.000000000000390

Ryan-Wenger, N. A. (2017). Precision, accuracy, and uncertainty of biophysical measurements for research and practice. In C. F. Waltz, O. L. Strickland, & E. R. Lenz (Eds.), *Measurement in nursing and health research* (5th ed., pp. 427–445). New York, NY: Springer.

Salman, A., & Lee, Y. (2019). Spiritual practices and effects of spiritual well-being and depression on elders' self-perceived health. *Applied Nursing Research, 48*(1), 68–74. doi:10.1016/j.apnr.2019.05.018

Saris, W. E., & Gallhofer, I. N. (2014). *Design, evaluation, and analysis of questionnaires for survey research* (2nd ed.). Hoboken, NJ: John Wiley & Son.

Şentürk, A., & Kartin, P. T. (2018). The effect of lavender oil application via inhalation pathway on hemodialysis patients' anxiety level and sleep quality. *Holistic Nursing Practice, 32*(6), 324–335. doi:10.1097/HNP.000000000000292

Simpson, S. H. (1989). Use of Q-sort methodology in cross-cultural nutrition and health research. *Nursing Research, 38*(5), 289–290.

Spector, P. E. (1992). *Summated rating scale construction: An introduction*. Newbury Park, CA: Sage.

Stone, K. S., & Frazier, S. K. (2017). Measurement of physiological variables using biomedical instrumentation. In C. F. Waltz, O. L. Strickland, & E. R. Lenz (Eds.), *Measurement in nursing and health research* (5th ed., pp. 379–425). New York, NY: Springer.

Streiner, D. L., Norman, G. R., & Cairney, J. (2015). *Health measurement scales: A practical guide to their development and use* (5th ed.). Oxford, UK: University Press.

Sun, R., Sereika, S. M., Lingler, J. H., Tamres, L. K., & Erlen, J. A. (2019). Sleep quality and medication management in family caregivers of community-dwelling persons with memory loss. *Applied Nursing Research, 46*(1), 16–19. doi:10.1016/j.apnr.2019.01.002

Tetting, D. W. (1988). Q-sort update. *Western Journal of Nursing Research, 10*(6), 757–765.

U.S. Department of Energy (DOE) Office of Science. (2019). *Human Genome Project information archive 1990-2003*. Retrieved from https://web.ornl.gov/sci/techresources/Human_Genome/project/

U.S. Department of Health and Human Services (DHHS). (2017). *Health information privacy: HIPAA for professionals*. Retrieved from https://www.hhs.gov/hipaa/for-professionals/index.html

U.S. Department of Health and Human Services (DHHS). (2019). *Health measures: PROMIS*. Retrieved from http://www.healthmeasures.net/explore-measurement-systems/promis#3

van Hooft, S. M., Dwarswaard, J., Jedeloo, S., Bal, R., & van Staa, A. (2015). Four perspectives on self-management support by nurses for people with chronic conditions: A Q-methodological study. *International Journal of Nursing Studies, 52*(1), 157–166. doi:10.1016/j.ijnurstu.2014.07.004

Vernon, W. (2009). The Delphi technique: A review. *International Journal of Therapy & Rehabilitation, 16*(2), 69–76. doi:10.12968/ijtr.2009.16.2.38892

Waltz, C. F., Strickland, O. L., & Lenz, E. R. (2017). *Measurement in nursing and health research* (5th ed.). New York, NY: Springer.

Wewers, M. E., & Lowe, N. K. (1990). A critical review of visual analogue scales in the measurement of clinical phenomena. *Research in Nursing & Health, 13*(4), 227–236.

Whiting, D., & Cole, E. (2016). Developing a trauma care syllabus for intensive care nurses in the United Kingdom: A Delphi study. *Intensive & Critical Care Nursing, 36*, 49–57. doi:10.1016/j.iccn.2016.03.006

Wong-Baker FACES Foundation. (2019). *Wong-Baker FACES® Pain Rating Scale*. Retrieved with permission from http://www.wongbakerfaces.org/.

Yeung, E., Woods, N., Dubrowski, A., Hodges, B., & Carnahan, H. (2015). Establishing assessment criteria for clinical reasoning in orthopedic manual physical therapy: A consensus-building study. *Journal of Manual & Manipulative Therapy, 23*(1), 27–36. doi:10.1179/20426186 13Y.0000000051

18

Critical Appraisal of Nursing Studies

Christy Bomer-Norton

http://evolve.elsevier.com/Gray/practice/

Professional nurses continually strive for evidence-based practice (EBP), which includes critically appraising studies, synthesizing research findings, and applying sound scientific evidence in practice. Nurse researchers also critically appraise studies in a selected area, develop a summary of current knowledge, and identify areas for subsequent study. The conclusion is that all nurses need skills in critically appraising research. The **critical appraisal of research** involves a systematic, unbiased, careful examination of all aspects of studies to judge their strengths, limitations, trustworthiness, meaning, and applicability to practice. This chapter provides a background for critically appraising studies in nursing and other healthcare disciplines. The expanding roles of nurses in conducting critical appraisals of research are addressed. Detailed guidelines are provided to direct you in critically appraising both quantitative and qualitative studies.

EVOLUTION OF CRITICAL APPRAISAL OF RESEARCH IN NURSING

EBP in nursing can be traced back to Florence Nightingale's use of statistics to understand patient outcomes in the 1800s (Mackey & Bassendowski, 2017). The process for critically appraising research has evolved gradually in nursing from a few to now many nurses who are prepared to conduct comprehensive, scholarly critiques.

Public research critiques, written or verbal, were rare before the 1970s, partially because of the harsh critiques that some nurse researchers endured in the 1940s and 1950s (Meleis, 2018). Nurses responding to research presentations in the 1960s and 1970s focused on the strengths of studies, and the weaknesses were minimized. Thus the effects of the study limitations and other weaknesses on the quality, credibility, and meaning of studies were often lost.

Incomplete critique or the absence of critique may have served to encourage budding nurse researchers as they gained basic research skills. However, now comprehensive critical appraisals of research are essential to evaluate and synthesize knowledge for nursing (Melnyk, Gallagher-Ford, & Fineout-Overholt, 2017). As a result of advances in the profession over the last 50 years, many nurses have the educational preparation and expertise to conduct critical appraisals of research. Nursing research textbooks, workshops, and conferences provide information on the critical appraisal process.

The critical appraisal of studies is essential for the development and refinement of nursing knowledge. Nurses examine the credibility and meaning of study findings by asking searching questions such as: Was the methodology of a study a valid choice for producing credible findings? Are the study findings trustworthy or an accurate reflection of reality (Cullen et al., 2018)? Do the findings increase our understanding of the nature of phenomena that are important in nursing? Are the findings from the present study consistent with those from previous studies? Are these studies' findings applicable to practice, theory, and/or knowledge development? The answers to these questions require careful examination of the research problem and purpose, the theoretical or philosophical basis of the study, the methodology, findings, and researcher's conclusions. Not only must the mechanics of conducting the study be evaluated, but also the abstract and logical reasoning the researchers used to plan and implement the study. If the reasoning process used to develop a study contains flaws, there are probably flaws in interpretation of the findings, decreasing the credibility of the study.

All studies have flaws; in fact, science itself is flawed. Science does not completely or perfectly describe, explain, predict, or control reality. However, improved understanding and an increased ability to predict and control phenomena depend on recognizing the weaknesses in studies and in science. In this chapter, **study weaknesses** are the errors or missteps that researchers consciously or unconsciously make in developing, implementing, and/or reporting studies. **Limitations** are specific types of study weaknesses that are reported by researchers; they can reduce the quality of study findings and, in quantitative studies, reduce the ability to generalize findings. Study limitations might be identified before, during, or after a study is conducted. They are identified in the research report and discussed in relationship to the study findings. All studies have limitations, and most include weaknesses that are not addressed by the researchers. You must decide whether a study is flawed to the extent that the evidence is not credible and is inappropriate to use in a systematic review of knowledge in an area (Aveyard, 2019). Although we recognize that knowledge is not absolute, we need to have confidence in the research evidence synthesized for practice.

All studies have strengths as well as weaknesses. Recognition of these strengths is essential to the generation of sound research evidence for practice. If only weaknesses are identified, nurses might discount the value of all studies and refuse to invest time in reading and examining research. The continued work of researchers also depends on recognizing the strengths of their studies. The strong points of a study added to the strong points from multiple other studies slowly builds solid research evidence for practice (Melnyk & Fineout-Overholt, 2019).

WHEN ARE CRITICAL APPRAISALS OF RESEARCH IMPLEMENTED IN NURSING?

In general, research is critically appraised to broaden understanding, summarize knowledge for practice, and provide a knowledge base for future studies. Critical appraisal allows the consumer of research to assess a study and determine its contribution to nursing. In addition, critical appraisals often are conducted after verbal presentations of studies, after publication of a research report, to select abstracts for a conference, to select articles for publication, and to evaluate research proposals for implementation and funding. In these instances, they underscore or rebut the research's observations, analyses, syntheses, and conclusions. Nursing students, practicing nurses, nurse educators, and nurse researchers all need to be involved in the critical appraisal of research.

Critical Appraisal of Studies by Students

In nursing education, conducting a critical appraisal of a study is often seen as a first step in learning the research process. Part of learning this process is being able to read and comprehend published research reports. However, conducting a critical appraisal of a study is not a basic skill, and a firm grasp of the content presented in previous chapters is essential for implementing this process. Students usually acquire basic knowledge of the research process and critical appraisal skills early in their baccalaureate nursing education. Advanced analysis skills usually are taught at the master's and doctoral levels (see Chapter 1).

By performing critical appraisals, students expand their analysis skills, strengthen their knowledge base, and increase their use of research evidence in practice. The *Essentials of Master's Education in Nursing* (American Association of Colleges of Nursing, 2011) identifies the competencies that nurses prepared at the master's level should accomplish. One of these competencies is the ability to translate evidence for use in practice. EBP requires critical appraisal and synthesis of study findings for practice (Aveyard, 2019). Therefore, critical appraisal of studies is an important part of your education and your practice as a nurse.

Critical Appraisal of Research by Practicing Nurses

Practicing nurses must appraise studies critically so that their practice is based on current research evidence and not merely tradition, supplemented by trial and error (Melnyk & Fineout-Overholt, 2019). Nursing actions must be updated in response to the current evidence generated through research. Practicing nurses need to formulate strategies for remaining current in their practice areas. Reading research journals, discussing study findings on a social media site, and posting or sharing current studies with peers can increase nurses' awareness of study findings, but these are insufficient for the purposes of critical appraisal. Nurses need to question the quality of studies and the credibility of findings and to share their concerns with other nurses. For example, nurses may form a research journal club in which studies are presented and critically appraised by members of the group (Dang & Dearholt, 2017). Skills in critical appraisal of research enable practicing nurses to synthesize the most credible, significant, and appropriate evidence for use in their practice. EBP is essential in healthcare agencies either seeking or maintaining Magnet status. The Magnet Recognition Program® was developed by the American Nurses Credentialing Center (2019) to recognize healthcare organizations that provide nursing excellence with care based on the most current research evidence.

Critical Appraisal of Research by Nurse Educators

Educators critically appraise research to expand their knowledge for practice and to develop and refine the educational process. The careful analysis of current nursing studies provides a basis for updating curriculum content for use in clinical and classroom settings. Educators influence students' perceptions of research and act as role models for their students by examining new studies, evaluating the information obtained from research, and indicating what research evidence to use in practice (Dang & Dearholt, 2017). In addition, educators may conduct or collaborate with others to conduct studies, which requires critical appraisal of previous relevant research.

Critical Appraisal of Studies by Nurse Researchers

Nurse researchers critically appraise previous research to plan and implement their next study (Adams & Lawrence, 2019). Many researchers have programs of research in selected areas (Beck, 2016), and they update their knowledge base by critiquing new studies in these areas. The outcomes of these appraisals influence the selection of research problems and purposes, the implementation of research methodologies, and the interpretations of study findings.

Critical Appraisal of Research Presentations and Publications

Critical appraisals following research presentations can assist researchers in identifying the strengths and weaknesses of their studies and generating ideas for further research. Experiencing the critical appraisal process can increase the ability of participants to evaluate studies and judge the usefulness of the research evidence for practice. Participants listening to study critiques might also gain insight into the conduct of research.

The nursing research journals *Scholarly Inquiry for Nursing Practice: An International Journal* and *Western Journal of Nursing Research* include commentaries after the research articles. In these journals, other researchers critically appraise the authors' studies, and the authors have a chance to respond to these comments. Published research critical appraisals often increase the reader's understanding of the study and the quality of the study findings (American Psychological Association [APA], 2020). Another, more informal critique of a published study might appear in a letter to the editor in which readers have the opportunity to comment on the strengths and weaknesses of published studies by writing to the journal editor.

Critical Appraisal of Abstracts for Conference Presentations

One of the most difficult types of critical appraisal is examining abstracts. The amount of information available usually is limited because many abstracts are restricted to 100 to 250 words. Nevertheless, reviewers must select the best-designed studies with the most significant outcomes for presentation at professional conferences. This process requires an experienced researcher who needs few cues to determine the quality of a study. Critical appraisal of an abstract usually addresses the following criteria: (1) appropriateness of the study for the conference program; (2) completeness of the research project; (3) overall quality of the study problem, purpose, methodology, results, and findings; (4) contribution of the study to the knowledge base of nursing; (5) contribution of the study to nursing theory; (6) originality of the work (not previously published); (7) implication of the study findings for practice; and (8) clarity, conciseness, and completeness of the abstract (APA, 2020).

Critical Appraisal of Research Articles for Publication

Nurse researchers who serve as peer reviewers for professional journals evaluate the quality of research articles submitted for publication. The role of these scientists is to ensure that the studies accepted for publication are well designed and contribute to the body of knowledge. Most of these reviews are conducted anonymously so that relationships or reputations do not interfere with the selection process. In most refereed journals, the experts who examine the research report have been selected from an established group of peer reviewers. Their comments or summaries of their comments are sent to the researcher. The editor also uses these comments to make selections for publication. The process for publishing a study is described in Chapter 27.

Critical Appraisal of Research Proposals

Critical appraisals of research proposals are conducted to approve student research projects, permit data collection in an institution, and select the best studies for funding by local, state, national, and international organizations and agencies. The process researchers use to seek the approval to conduct a study is presented in Chapter 28. The peer review process in federal funding agencies involves an extremely complex critical appraisal. Nurses are involved in this level of research review through the national funding agencies, such as the National Institute of Nursing Research (NINR, 2019), National Institutes of Health, and the Agency for Healthcare Research and Quality (2019). Some of the criteria used to evaluate the quality of a proposal for possible funding include (1) significance of the research problem and purpose for nursing, (2) appropriate use of methodology for the types of questions that the research is designed to answer, (3) appropriate use and interpretation of analysis procedures, (4) evaluation of clinical practice and forecasting of the need for nursing or other appropriate interventions, (5) construction of models to direct the research and interpret the findings, and (6) innovativeness of the study. The NINR (2019) website (https://www.ninr.nih.gov) provides details on grant development and research funding (see Chapter 29 on seeking funding for research).

> ### BOX 18.1 Critical Appraisal Guidelines for Quantitative and Qualitative Studies
>
> 1. Identifying the elements or processes of the study
> 2. Determining the study strengths and weaknesses
> 3. Evaluating the credibility, trustworthiness, and meaning of the study

NURSES' EXPERTISE IN CRITICAL APPRAISAL OF RESEARCH

Conducting a critical appraisal of a study is a complex mental process that is stimulated by raising questions. The three major steps for critical appraisal included in this text are (1) identifying the elements or processes of the study, (2) determining the study strengths and weaknesses, and (3) evaluating the credibility, trustworthiness, and meaning of the study (Box 18.1). The level of critique conducted is influenced by the education and experience of the individual appraising the study (Table 18.1). The initial critical appraisal of research by an undergraduate student often involves the identification of the elements or steps of the research process in a

TABLE 18.1 Educational Level With Associated Expertise in Critical Appraisal of Research

Educational Level	Expertise in Critical Appraisal of Research
Baccalaureate	Identify the steps of the quantitative research process in a study.
	Identify the elements of a qualitative study.
Master's	Determine study strengths and weaknesses in quantitative, qualitative, mixed methods, and outcomes studies.
	Evaluate the credibility, trustworthiness, and meaning of a study and its contribution to nursing knowledge and practice.
Doctorate or postdoctorate	Synthesize multiple studies in systematic reviews, meta-analyses, metasyntheses, and mixed methods research synthesis.

quantitative study. Some baccalaureate programs offer more in-depth research courses that also include critical appraisals of the processes of qualitative studies (Grove & Gray, 2019).

A critical appraisal of research conducted by a student at the master's level usually involves description of study strengths and weaknesses and evaluation of the credibility and meaning of the study findings for nursing knowledge and practice (see Table 18.1). Critical appraisals by master's level students and practicing nurses focus on a variety of studies, such as quantitative, qualitative, mixed methods, and outcomes studies.

At the doctoral level, students often critically appraise several studies in an area of interest and perform a complex synthesis of the research findings to determine the current empirical knowledge base for the phenomenon (see Table 18.1). These complex syntheses of quantitative, qualitative, mixed methods, and outcomes research include (1) systematic reviews, of research, (2) meta-analysis, (3) metasynthesis, and (4) mixed methods research synthesis (Aveyard, 2019; Whittemore, Chao, Jang, Minges, & Park, 2014). These summaries of current research evidence are essential for providing EBP and directing future research (Dang & Dearholt, 2017). Definitions of these types of complex syntheses are presented in Chapter 2, and Chapter 19 provides guidelines for critically appraising and conducting these research syntheses.

The major focus of this chapter is conducting critical appraisals of quantitative and qualitative studies using the steps previously discussed and outlined in Box 18.1. Critical appraisals of quantitative and qualitative studies involve implementing key principles that are outlined in Box 18.2. These principles stress the importance of examining the expertise of the authors; reviewing the entire study; addressing the strengths and weaknesses of the study; evaluating the credibility, trustworthiness, and meaning of the study findings; determining the usefulness or applicability of the findings for practice; and facilitating the conduct of future research (Creswell & Creswell, 2018; Creswell & Poth, 2018; Dane, 2018; Marshall & Rossman, 2016; Miles, Huberman, & Saldaña, 2020; Morse, 2018). These key principles provide a basis for the critical appraisal process for quantitative research that is discussed in the next section and the critical appraisal process for qualitative research that is discussed later in this chapter.

BOX 18.2 Key Principles for Critical Appraisal of Research

1. *Examine the research, clinical, and educational background of the authors.* The authors need a scientific and clinical background that is appropriate for the study conducted (Dane, 2018).
2. *Examine the organization and presentation of the research report.* The title of the research report needs to identify the focus of the study. The report usually includes an abstract, introduction, methods, results, discussion, and references. The abstract of the study needs to present the purpose of the study clearly and to highlight the methodology and major study results and findings (Adams & Lawrence, 2019). The body of the research report should be complete, concise, logically organized, and clearly presented. The references need to be complete and presented in a consistent format (APA, 2020).
3. *Read and critically appraise the entire study.* A research appraisal involves examining the quality of all aspects of the research report (see Box 18.1 and the critical appraisal guidelines provided throughout this chapter).
4. *Examine the significance of the problem studied for nursing practice and knowledge.* The foci of nursing studies need to be on the generation of quality knowledge to promote evidence-based practice.
5. *As you identify the strengths and weaknesses of the study, provide specific examples of and rationales for the identified study strengths and weaknesses.* Address the quality of the problem, purpose, theoretical or philosophical basis, methodology, results, and findings of quantitative and qualitative studies. Include examples and rationales for your critical appraisal and document your ideas with sources from the current literature. This strengthens the quality of your critical appraisal and documents the use of critical thinking skills.
6. *If you determine that the study resulted in valid and trustworthy findings, examine the usefulness or transferability of the findings to practice.* The findings for a study need to be linked with the findings from previous research and examined for use in practice.
7. *Suggest ideas and modifications for future studies.* Identify ideas and modifications for future studies to increase the strengths and decrease the limitations and other weaknesses of the current study.

CRITICAL APPRAISAL PROCESS FOR QUANTITATIVE RESEARCH

As you critically appraise studies, follow the steps of the critical appraisal process presented in Box 18.1. These steps occur in sequence, vary in depth, and presume accomplishment of the preceding steps. However, an individual with critical appraisal experience frequently performs multiple steps of this process simultaneously. This section includes the three steps of the research critical appraisal process applied to quantitative studies and provides relevant questions for each step. These questions are not comprehensive but have been selected as a means for stimulating the logical reasoning and analysis necessary for conducting a study review. Persons experienced in the critical appraisal process formulate additional questions as part of their reasoning processes. We cover the identification of the steps or elements of the research process separately because persons who are new to critical appraisal often only conduct this step. The questions for determining a study's strengths and weaknesses are covered together because this process occurs simultaneously in the mind of the person conducting the critical appraisal. Evaluation is covered separately because of the increased expertise needed to perform this final step.

Step I: Identifying the Steps of the Quantitative Research Process in Studies

Initial attempts to comprehend research articles are often frustrating because the terminology and stylized manner of the report are unfamiliar. Identification of the steps of the research process in a quantitative study is the first step in critical appraisal. It involves understanding the terms and concepts in the report; identifying study elements; and grasping the nature, significance, and meaning of the study elements. The following guidelines are presented to direct you in the initial critical appraisal of a quantitative study.

Guidelines for Identifying the Steps of the Quantitative Research Process

The first step involves reviewing the study title and abstract and reading the study from beginning to end (review the key principles in Box 18.2) (Adams & Lawrence, 2019). As you read, address the following questions about the research report: Was the writing style of the report clear and concise? Were the different parts of the research report plainly identified (APA, 2020)? Were relevant terms defined? You might underline the terms you do not understand and determine their meaning from the glossary at the end of this textbook. Read the article a second time and highlight or underline each step of the quantitative research process. An overview of these steps is presented in Chapter 3. To write a critical appraisal identifying the study steps, you need to identify each step concisely and respond briefly to the following guidelines and questions.

I. Introduction
   A. Describe the qualifications of the authors to conduct the study, such as research expertise, clinical experience, and educational preparation. Doctoral education, such as a PhD, and postdoctorate training provide experiences in conducting research. Have the researchers conducted previous studies, especially studies in this area? Are the authors involved in clinical practice or certified in their area of clinical expertise (Dane, 2018)?
   B. Discuss the clarity of the article title (variables and population identified). Does the title indicate the general type of study conducted—descriptive, correlational, quasi-experimental, or experimental (Kazdin, 2017)?
   C. Discuss the quality of the abstract. An abstract should include the study purpose, design, sample, intervention (if applicable), and results; highlight key findings (Adams & Lawrence, 2019; APA, 2020).

II. State the problem (see Chapter 5).
   A. Significance of the problem
   B. Background of the problem
   C. Problem statement

III. State the purpose (see Chapter 5).

IV. Examine the literature review (see Chapter 7).
   A. Were relevant previous studies and theories described?
   B. Were the references current? (Number and percentage of sources in the last 10 years and in the last 5 years?)
   C. Were the studies described, critically appraised, and synthesized (Melnyk & Fineout-Overholt, 2019)?
   D. Was a summary provided of the current knowledge (what is known and not known) about the research problem (Dale, Hallas, & Spratling, 2019)?

V. Examine the study framework or theoretical perspective (see Chapter 8).
  A. Was the framework explicitly expressed, or must the reviewer extract the framework from implicit statements in the introduction or literature review?
  B. Is the framework based on tentative, substantive, or scientific theory? Provide a rationale for your answer.
  C. Did the framework identify, define, and describe the relationships among the concepts of interest (Kazdin, 2017)? Provide examples of this.
  D. Is a model (diagram) of the framework provided for clarity? If a model is not presented, develop one that represents the framework of the study and describe it.
  E. Link the study variables to the relevant concepts in the model.
  F. How was the framework related to the body of knowledge of nursing (Smith & Liehr, 2018)?
VI. List any research objectives, questions, or hypotheses (see Chapter 6).
VII. Identify and define (conceptually and operationally) the study variables or concepts that were identified in the objectives, questions, or hypotheses. If objectives, questions, or hypotheses were not stated, identify and define the variables in the study purpose and the results section of the study. If conceptual definitions were not included, identify possible definitions for each major study variable. Indicate which of the following types of variables were included in the study. A study usually includes independent and dependent variables or research variables but not all three types of variables.
  A. Independent variables: Identify and define conceptually and operationally.
  B. Dependent variables: Identify and define conceptually and operationally.
  C. Research variables or concepts: Identify and define conceptually and operationally.
VIII. Identify demographic variables and other relevant terms.
IX. Identify the research design.
  A. Identify the specific design of the study. Draw a model of the design by using the sample design models presented in Chapters 10 and 11.
  B. Did the study include a treatment or intervention (see Chapter 11)? If so, is the treatment clearly described with a protocol and consistently implemented, which indicates intervention fidelity (Eymard & Altmiller, 2016)?
  C. If the study had more than one group, how were subjects assigned to groups (Kazdin, 2017)?
  D. Were extraneous variables identified and controlled for by the design or methods? Extraneous variables usually are discussed in research reports of quasi-experimental and experimental studies (Shadish, Cook, & Campbell, 2002).
  E. Were pilot study findings used to design this study? If yes, briefly discuss the pilot and the changes made in the study based on the pilot.
X. Describe the population, sample, and setting (see Chapter 15).
  A. Identify inclusion or exclusion sample or eligibility criteria that designate the target population.
  B. Identify the specific type of probability or nonprobability sampling method that was used to obtain the sample. Did the researchers identify the sampling frame for the study (Kazdin, 2017)?
  C. Identify the sample size. Discuss the refusal rate and include the rationale for refusal if presented in the article. Discuss the power analysis if this process was used to determine sample size (Aberson, 2019).
  D. Identify the sample attrition (number and percentage). Was a rationale provided for the study attrition?
  E. Identify the characteristics of the sample.
  F. Discuss the institutional review board approval. Describe the informed consent process used in the study (see Chapter 9).
  G. Identify the study setting and indicate whether it is appropriate for the study purpose.
XI. Identify and describe each measurement strategy used in the study (see Chapters 16 and 17). The following information should be provided for each measurement method included in a study. Identify each study variable that was measured and link it to a measurement method(s).
  A. Identify the name and author of each measurement strategy.
  B. Identify the type of each measurement strategy (e.g., Likert scale, visual analog scale, and physiological measure).
  C. Identify the level of measurement (nominal, ordinal, interval, or ratio) achieved by each

measurement method used in the study (Grove & Cipher, 2020).

D. Describe the reliability of each scale for previous studies, for this study, and for the pilot study if one was performed. Identify the precision of each physiological measure (Polit & Yang, 2016; Waltz, Strickland, & Lenz, 2017).

E. Identify the validity of each scale and the accuracy of physiological measures (Kazdin, 2017; Ryan-Wenger, 2017).

F. If data for the study were obtained from an existing database, did the researchers identify how, where, when, and by whom the original data were collected?

The following table includes the critical information about two measurement methods, the Beck Likert scale to measure depression and the physiological instrument to measure blood pressure. Completing this table allows you to identify essential measurement content for a study (Waltz et al., 2017).

Variable Measured	Name of Measurement Method/ Author	Type of Measurement Method	Level of Measurement	Reliability or Precision	Validity or Accuracy
Depression level	Beck Depression Inventory/ Beck	Likert scale	Interval	Cronbach alpha of 0.82–0.92 from previous studies and 0.84 for this study. Reading level at sixth grade.	Content validity from concept analysis, literature review, and reviews of experts. Construct validity: Convergent validity with Zung Depression Scale. Factor validity from previous research. Successive use validity with previous studies and this study. Criterion-related validity: Predictive validity of patients' future depressive episodes.
Blood pressure (BP)	Omron BP equipment: Healthcare Equipment Company	Physiological measurement method	Ratio	Test-retest values of BP measurement in previous studies. BP equipment new and recalibrated every 50 BP readings in this study. Average three BP readings to determine average BP.	Documented accuracy of systolic and diastolic BPs to 1 mm Hg by company developing Omron BP cuff. Designated protocol for taking BP. Average three BP readings to determine average BP.

XII. Describe the procedures for data collection and management (see Chapter 20).

XIII. Describe the statistical techniques performed to analyze study data (see Chapters 21, 22, 23, 24, and 25).

A. List the statistical procedures conducted to describe the sample.

B. Was the level of significance or alpha identified? If so, indicate what it was (0.05, 0.01, or 0.001).

C. Complete the following table with the analysis techniques conducted in the study: (1) identify the focus (description, relationships, predication, or differences) for each analysis technique, (2) list the statistical analysis technique performed, (3) list the statistic, (4) provide the specific results, and (5) identify the probability (p) of the statistical significance achieved by the result (Grove & Cipher, 2020; Hayat, Higgins, Schwartz, & Staggs, 2015).

Purpose of Analysis	Analysis Technique	Statistic	Results	Probability (p)
Description of Subjects' Pulse Rate	Mean	M	71.52	NA
	Standard deviation	SD	5.62	NA
	Range	Range	58–97	NA
Difference between men and women in systolic and diastolic blood pressures, respectively	t-Test	t	3.75	0.001
	t-Test	t	2.16	0.042
Differences of diet group, exercise group, and comparison group for pounds lost by adolescents	Analysis of variance	F	4.27	0.04
Relationship of depression and anxiety in elderly adults	Pearson correlation	r	0.46	0.03

XIV. Describe the researcher's interpretation of the study findings (see Chapter 26).

A. Are the findings related back to the study framework? If so, do the findings support the study framework?

B. Which findings are consistent with the expected findings?

C. Which findings were not expected?

D. Are the findings consistent with previous research findings (Astroth & Chung, 2018)?

XV. What study limitations did the researcher identify (Kazdin, 2017)?

XVI. How did the researcher generalize the findings?

XVII. What were the implications of the findings for nursing?

XVIII. What suggestions for further study were identified?

XIX. Was the researcher's description of the study design and methods sufficiently clear for replication?

Step II: Determining Study Strengths and Weaknesses

The next step in critically appraising a quantitative study requires determining the strengths and weaknesses of the study (see Box 18.1). To do this, you must have knowledge of what each step of the research process should be like. Use expert sources such as this textbook and other research sources (Aberson, 2019; Creswell & Creswell, 2018; Creswell & Poth, 2018; Grove & Cipher, 2020; Kazdin, 2017; Polit & Yang, 2016; Ryan-Wenger, 2017; Waltz et al., 2017). Another source for critical appraisal of research is the Critical Appraisal Skills Programme (CASP) that was developed in the United Kingdom with critical appraisal checklists provided online from CASP (2018). The ideal way to assess how well the research process was implemented is to compare the standards with the actual study steps. During this comparison, you examine the extent to which the researcher followed the rules for an ideal study and identify the study elements that are strengths or weaknesses. Your critical appraisal comments need to be supported with documentation from research references.

You also need to examine the logical links connecting one study element with another (Gravetter & Forzano, 2018). For example, the problem needs to provide background and direction for the statement of the purpose. In addition, you need to examine the logical reasoning in the study. The variables identified in the study purpose need to be consistent with the variables identified in the research objectives, questions, or hypotheses. The variables identified in the research objectives, questions, or hypotheses need to be conceptually defined in light of the study framework. The conceptual definitions provide the basis for the development of operational definitions (Dane, 2018). The study design and analyses need to be appropriate for the investigation of the study purpose and for the specific objectives, questions, or hypotheses (Astroth & Chung, 2018; Dale et al., 2019). Many study weaknesses result from breaks in logical reasoning. For example, biases caused by sampling, measurement methods, and the selected design impair the logical flow from design to interpretation of findings (Kazdin, 2017; Waltz et al., 2017). The previous level of critical appraisal addressed concrete aspects of the study. During analysis, the process moves to examining abstract dimensions of the study, which requires greater familiarity with the logic behind the research process and increased skill in critical thinking (Adams & Lawrence, 2019).

You also need to gain a sense of how clearly the researcher grasped the study situation and expressed it. The clarity of the researchers' explanation of study elements demonstrates their skill in using and expressing ideas that require abstract reasoning. With this examination of the study, you can determine which aspects of the study are strengths and which are weaknesses and provide rationale and documentation for your decisions.

Guidelines for Determining Study Strengths and Weaknesses

The following questions were developed to assist you in examining the different aspects of a study and determining whether they are strengths or weaknesses. The intent is not to answer each of these questions but to read the questions and make judgments about the elements or steps in the study. You need to provide a rationale for

your decisions and document from relevant research references such as those listed in the previous section and in the references at the end of this chapter. For example, you might decide the study purpose is a strength because it addresses the study problem, clarifies the focus of the study, and is feasible to investigate (Astroth & Chung, 2018; Kazdin, 2017).

I. Research problem and purpose
   A. Was the problem sufficiently delimited in scope so that it is researchable but not trivial?
   B. Is the problem significant to nursing (Brown, 2018)?
   C. Does the purpose narrow and clarify the focus of the study? Does the purpose clearly address the gap in nursing knowledge?
   D. Was this study feasible to conduct in terms of money commitment; the researchers' expertise; availability of subjects, facilities, and equipment; and ethical considerations?

II. Review of literature
   A. Was the literature review organized to show the progressive development of evidence from previous research (Brancati, 2018)?
   B. Was a theoretical knowledge base developed for the problem and purpose?
   C. Was a clear, concise summary presented of the current empirical and theoretical knowledge in the area of the study (CASP, 2018)?
   D. Did the literature review summary identify what was known and not known about the research problem, at the beginning of the study process (Brancati, 2018), and provide direction for the formation of the research purpose?

III. Study framework
   A. Is the framework presented with clarity? If a model or conceptual map of the framework is present, is it adequate for explaining the phenomenon of concern?
   B. Is the framework linked to the research purpose? If not, would another framework fit more logically with the study?
   C. Is the framework related to the body of knowledge in nursing and clinical practice at the time the study was conducted?
   D. If a proposition or relationship from a theory is to be tested, is the proposition clearly identified and linked to the study hypotheses (Smith & Liehr, 2018)?

IV. Research objectives, questions, or hypotheses
  A. Were the objectives, questions, or hypotheses expressed clearly?
  B. Were the objectives, questions, or hypotheses logically linked to the research purpose (Gravetter & Forzano, 2018)?
  C. Were hypotheses stated to direct the conduct of quasi-experimental and experimental research (Kazdin, 2017; Shadish et al., 2002)?
  D. Were the objectives, questions, or hypotheses logically linked to the concepts and relationships (propositions) in the framework (Smith & Liehr, 2018)?

V. Variables
  A. Were the variables reflective of the concepts identified in the framework?
  B. Were the variables clearly defined (conceptually and operationally) and based on previous research or theories (Smith & Liehr, 2018)?
  C. Is the conceptual definition of a variable consistent with the operational definition (construct validity)?
  D. Did the operational definitions capture both the concept and the breadth of its manifestations in the population of interest?

VI. Design
  A. Was the design used in the study the most appropriate design to obtain the needed data (Creswell & Creswell, 2018; Kazdin, 2017; Truluck & Leggett, 2016)?
  B. Did the design provide a means to examine all of the objectives, questions, or hypotheses?
  C. Was the treatment clearly described (Eymard & Altmiller, 2016)? Was the treatment appropriate for examining the study purpose and hypotheses? Did the study framework explain the links between the treatment (independent variable) and the proposed outcomes (dependent variables)?
  D. Was a protocol developed to promote consistent implementation of the treatment to ensure intervention fidelity? Did the researcher monitor implementation of the treatment to ensure consistency? If the treatment was not consistently implemented, what might be the impact on the findings?
  E. Did the researcher identify the threats to design validity (statistical conclusion validity, internal validity, construct validity, and external validity) and minimize them as much as possible? What threats to internal validity were actually controlled for in the design phase, and in what ways? (see Chapters 10 and 11) (Kazdin, 2017; Shadish et al., 2002)?
  F. Was the design logically linked to the sampling method and statistical analyses (Gray et al., 2017; Grove & Cipher, 2020; Kazdin, 2017)?
  G. If more than one group is included in the study, do the groups appear equivalent?
  H. If a treatment was implemented, were subjects randomly assigned to the treatment group, or were the treatment and comparison groups dependent? Were the treatment and comparison group assignments appropriate for the purpose of the study (Kazdin, 2017)?
  I. If a quasi-experimental design was implemented instead of an experimental one, was the decision justified by the researcher?

VII. Sample, population, and setting
  A. Was the sampling method adequate for producing a sample that was representative of the target population (Astroth & Chung, 2018)?
  B. If random sampling was used, was the type of sample actually obtained representative of the accessible population?
  C. What were the potential biases in the sampling method? Were any subjects excluded from the study because of age, socioeconomic status, or ethnicity without a sound rationale (Kazdin, 2017; Thompson, 2012)?
  D. Did the sample include an understudied or vulnerable population, such as young, elderly, pregnant, or minority subjects?
  E. Were the sampling criteria (inclusion and exclusion) appropriate for the type of study conducted?
  F. Was the sample size sufficient to avoid a Type II error? Was a power analysis conducted to determine sample size? If a power analysis was conducted, were the results of the analysis clearly described and used to determine the final sample size? Was the attrition rate projected in determining the final sample size (Aberson, 2019; Adams & Lawrence, 2019)?
  G. Were the rights of human subjects protected?
  H. Was the study setting appropriate for the study purpose?

I. What was the refusal rate for the study? If it was greater than 20%, how might this have affected the representativeness of the sample? Did the researchers provide rationale for the refusals?

J. What was the attrition rate for the study? Did the researchers provide a rationale for the attrition of study participants? How did attrition influence the final sample and the study results and findings (Adams & Lawrence, 2019)?

VIII. Measurements

A. Did the measurement methods selected for the study adequately measure the study variables (Polit & Yang, 2016; Waltz et al., 2017)?

B. Were the measurement methods sufficiently sensitive for detection of small differences between subjects? Should additional measurement methods have been used to improve the quality of the study outcomes (Waltz et al., 2017)?

C. Did the measurement methods used in the study have adequate validity and reliability? What additional reliability or validity testing might have improved the quality of the measurement methods (Kazdin, 2017; Waltz et al., 2017)?

D. Respond to the following questions, which are relevant to the measurement methods used in the study:

1. Scales and questionnaires
   (a) Were the instruments clearly described?
   (b) Were techniques for completion and scoring of the instruments provided?
   (c) Were validity and reliability of the instruments described (Kazdin, 2017)?
   (d) Did the researcher reexamine the validity and reliability of instruments for the present sample?
   (e) If an instrument was developed for the study, was the instrument development process described (Waltz et al., 2017)?

2. Observation
   (a) Were the entities that were to be observed clearly identified and defined?
   (b) Was interrater reliability described?
   (c) Were the techniques for recording observations described (Waltz et al., 2017)?

3. Interviews
   (a) Did the interview questions address concerns expressed in the research problem?
   (b) Were the interview questions relevant for the research purpose and objectives, questions, or hypotheses?
   (c) Did the design or sequence of the questions tend to bias subjects' responses (Waltz et al., 2017)?

4. Physiological measures
   (a) Were the physiological measures clearly described (Ryan-Wenger, 2017)? If appropriate, are the brand names, such as Hewlett-Packard, and models of instruments identified?
   (b) Were the accuracy, precision, and error of physiological instruments discussed (Ryan-Wenger, 2017)?
   (c) Were the physiological measures appropriate for the research purpose and objectives, questions, or hypotheses?
   (d) Were the methods for recording data from physiological measures clearly described? Was the recording of data consistent?

IX. Data collection

A. Was the data collection process clearly described?

B. Were the forms used to collect data organized to facilitate computerizing the data? Did the subjects enter their data into a computer?

C. Was the training of data collectors clearly described and adequate?

D. Was the data collection process conducted in a consistent manner (Dale et al., 2019)?

E. Were the data collection methods ethical?

F. Did the data collected address the research objectives, questions, or hypotheses?

G. Did any adverse events occur during data collection? If adverse events occurred, were these appropriately managed?

X. Data analysis

A. Were data analysis procedures appropriate for the type of data collected (Grove & Cipher, 2020)?

B. Were data analysis procedures clearly described? Did the researcher address any problems with missing data and how this problem was managed?

C. Did the data analysis techniques address the study purpose and the research objectives, questions, or hypotheses?

D. Were the results presented in an understandable way by narrative, tables, or figures, or a combination of methods (APA, 2020; Grove & Cipher, 2020)?

E. Were the statistical analyses logically linked to the design?

F. Is the sample size sufficient to detect significant differences if they are present (Astroth & Chung, 2018)?

G. Were the results interpreted appropriately?

XI. Interpretation of findings

A. Were findings discussed in relation to each objective, question, or hypothesis?

B. Were various explanations for significant and nonsignificant findings examined?

C. Were the findings clinically significant (Astroth & Chung, 2018)?

D. Were the findings linked to the study framework?

E. Were the study findings an accurate reflection of reality and valid for use in clinical practice?

F. Did the conclusions fit the results from the data analyses? Were the conclusions based on statistically significant and clinically important results?

G. Did the study have weaknesses not identified by the researcher?

H. Did the researcher generalize the findings appropriately?

I. Were the identified implications for practice appropriate, based on the study findings and the findings from previous research (Astroth & Chung, 2018)?

J. Were quality suggestions made for further research?

Step III: Evaluating a Study

Evaluation involves determining the credibility, trustworthiness, meaning, and usefulness of the study findings. This type of critical appraisal requires more advanced skills and might be performed by master's and doctoral level students in determining current nursing knowledge and its usefulness in practice (see Table 18.1). Evaluating research involves summarizing the quality of the research process and findings, determining the consistency of the findings with those from previous studies, and determining the usefulness of the findings for practice. The steps of the study are evaluated in light of previous studies, such as an evaluation of present hypotheses based on previous hypotheses, present design based on previous designs, and present methods of measuring variables based on previous methods of measurement. Evaluation builds on conclusions reached during the first two stages of the critical appraisal so that the credibility, meaning, trustworthiness, and usefulness of the study findings can be determined for nursing knowledge, theory, and practice.

Guidelines for Evaluating a Study

You need to reexamine the discussion section of the study focusing on the study findings, conclusions, implications for practice, and suggestions for further study. It is important for you to read previous studies conducted in the area to determine the quality, credibility, and meaning of the study based on previous research. Using the following questions as a guide, summarize your evaluation of the study and document your responses.

I. Did the study build on previous research problems, purposes, designs, samples, and measurement methods (Adams & Lawrence, 2019)? Provide examples to support your comments.

II. Could the weaknesses of the study have been corrected? How might that have been accomplished? Were recommendations for future study designs selected to remedy the weaknesses of the current study?

III. When the findings are examined in light of previous studies, do the findings build on previous findings?

IV. Do you believe the study findings are credible? How much confidence can be placed in the study findings?

V. Based on this study and the findings from previous research, what is now known and not known about the phenomenon under study?

VI. To what populations can the findings be generalized (Kazdin, 2017; Shadish et al., 2002)?

VII. Were the implications of the findings for practice discussed? Based on previous research, are the findings ready for use in practice (Melnyk & Fineout-Overholt, 2019; Melnyk et al., 2017)?

VIII. Were relevant studies suggested for future research?

CRITICAL APPRAISAL PROCESS FOR QUALITATIVE STUDIES

Critical appraisal of qualitative studies requires different detailed guidelines than those used when appraising a quantitative study (Marshall & Rossman, 2016; Sandelowski, 2008), because the different qualitative methodologies have different standards of quality than do quantitative research methods. However, appraisals of quantitative and qualitative studies follow the same three major steps in the appraisal process (see Box 18.1) and have a common purpose—determining the credibility and trustworthiness of the findings. The integrity of the design and methods affects the credibility and meaningfulness of qualitative findings and their usefulness in clinical practice (Melnyk & Fineout-Overholt, 2019). Burns (1989) first described the standards for rigorous qualitative research 30 years ago. Since that time, other criteria have been published (Melnyk & Fineout-Overholt, 2019; Morse, 2018), including one book on evaluating qualitative research (Roller & Lavrakas, 2015). The standards by which qualitative research should be appraised have been the source of considerable debate (Roller & Lavrakas, 2015). Nurses critically appraising qualitative studies need three prerequisite characteristics in applying rigorous appraisal standards. Without these prerequisites, nurses may miss potential valuable contributions qualitative studies might make to the knowledge base of nursing. These required prerequisite characteristics are addressed in the following section.

Prerequisites for Critical Appraisal of Qualitative Studies

The first prerequisite for appraising qualitative studies is an appreciation for the philosophical foundation of qualitative research (Melnyk & Fineout-Overholt, 2019) (Box 18.3). Qualitative researchers design their studies to be congruent with one of a wide range of philosophies,

such as phenomenology, symbolic interactionism, and hermeneutics, each of which espouses slightly different methods and approaches to gaining new knowledge (Corbin & Strauss, 2015; Marshall & Rossman, 2016). Without an appreciation for the philosophical perspective supporting the study being critically appraised, the appraiser may not appropriately apply standards of rigor that are congruent with that perspective (Melnyk & Fineout-Overholt, 2019). Although unique, the qualitative philosophies are similar in their views of the uniqueness of the individual and the value of the individual's perspective. Chapters 4 and 12 contain more information on the different philosophies that are foundational to qualitative research.

Guided by an appreciation of qualitative philosophical perspectives, nurses appraising a qualitative study can evaluate the methodology used to gather, analyze, and interpret the data (Miles et al., 2020). A basic knowledge of different qualitative methodologies is as essential for appraisal of qualitative studies as knowledge of quantitative research designs is for appraising quantitative studies (see Box 18.3) (Aveyard, 2019). Spending an extended time in the culture, organization, or setting that is the focus of the study is an expectation for ethnography studies but would not be expected for a phenomenological study (Creswell & Poth, 2018). A researcher using a grounded theory methodology is expected to analyze data to extract social processes and construct connections among emerging concepts (Bryant & Charmaz, 2019). Phenomenological researchers are expected to produce a rich, detailed description of a lived experience. Knowing these distinctions is a prerequisite to fair and objective critical appraisal of qualitative studies. What one expects to find in a qualitative research report may be the primary determinant of one's appraisal of the quality of that study (Morse, 2018).

Box 18.3 outlines the prerequisites of philosophical foundation, type of qualitative study, and openness to study participants that direct the implementation of the following guidelines for critically appraising qualitative studies. Appreciating philosophical perspectives and knowing qualitative methodologies are superficial, however, without respect for the participant's perspective. Qualitative philosophers are similar in their views of the uniqueness of the individual and the value of the individual's perspective. This basic value creates an openness to hearing a participant's story and perceiving the person's life, in context. This openness allows

> ### BOX 18.3 Prerequisites for Critically Appraising Qualitative Research
> - Appreciation for the philosophical foundation of qualitative research
> - Basic knowledge of different qualitative methodologies
> - Respect for the participant's perspective

qualitative researchers and nurses using the findings to perceive different truths and to acknowledge the depth, richness, and complexity inherent in the lives of all the patients we serve.

Step I: Identifying the Steps of the Qualitative Research Process in Studies

As with quantitative research, you will start by reviewing the title and abstract. Reading the article completely is essential when critically appraising a study, because you need to use all of the information that the researchers provided (Adams & Lawrence, 2019). If you are unfamiliar with the qualitative design that was used, this is a good time to look it up in Chapter 4 of this book or in other qualitative research sources listed in the references of this chapter.

Guidelines for Identifying the Steps of the Qualitative Research Process

The following questions are provided to help you identify the key elements of the study.
  I. Introduction
  A. Describe the researchers' qualifications. Take note of their employers, professions, levels of educational preparation, clinical expertise, and research experience. Have the researchers conducted previous studies on this topic or with this population? Some of the researchers' qualifications may be provided in the article, and additional information can be obtained through online searches.
  B. Does the title give you a clear indication of the concepts studied and the population? Can you determine from the title which qualitative design was used?
  C. Is the abstract inclusive of the purpose of the study, qualitative methodology, and sample (Adams & Lawrence, 2019)? The abstract should also contain key findings.
  II. Research problem
  A. Is the significance of the study established? In other words, why should you care about the problem that inspired the researcher to conduct this study (Creswell & Creswell, 2018)?
  B. Identify the problem statement. Is the research problem explicitly stated?
  C. Does the researcher identify a personal connection or motivation for selecting this topic to study? For example, the researcher may choose

to study the lived experience of men undergoing radiation for prostate cancer after the researcher's father underwent the same treatment. Acknowledging motives and potential biases is an expectation for qualitative researchers, but the researcher may not include this information in the article (Marshall & Rossman, 2016).
  III. Purpose and research questions
  A. Identify the purpose of the study. Is the purpose a logical approach to addressing the research problem of the study (Astroth & Chung, 2018)? Does the purpose have an intuitive fit with the problem?
  B. List research questions that the study was designed to answer.
  C. Are the research questions related to the problem and purpose?
  D. Are qualitative methods appropriate to answer the research questions?
  IV. Literature review
  A. Are quantitative and qualitative studies cited that are relevant to the focus of the study? What other types of literature are included?
  B. Were the references current at the time the research was published? For qualitative studies, the author may have included studies older than the 5-year limit typically used for quantitative studies. Findings of older qualitative studies may be relevant to a qualitative study that involves human processes, such as grieving or coping, that transcend time.
  C. Identify the disciplines of the authors of studies cited in the article. Does it appear that the researcher searched databases outside the Cumulative Index to Nursing and Allied Health Literature (CINAHL) for relevant studies? Research publications in other disciplines as well as literary works in the humanities may have relevance for some qualitative studies.
  D. Were the cited studies evaluated and their limitations noted?
  E. Did the literature review include adequate synthesized information to build a logical argument (Brancati, 2018; Gravetter & Forzano, 2018; Marshall & Rossman, 2016)? Another way to ask the question: Does the author provide enough evidence to support the assertion that the study was needed?

V. Philosophical foundation or theoretical perspective

The methods used by qualitative researchers are determined by the philosophical foundation of their work. The researcher may or may not state the philosophical stance on which the study is based. Despite this omission, you as a knowledgeable reader can recognize the philosophy through the description of the problem, formulation of the research questions, and selection of the methods to address the research questions.

A. Was a specific perspective (philosophy or theory) described from which the study was developed (Kazdin, 2017)? If so, what was that perspective?

B. If a broad philosophy, such as phenomenology, was identified, was the specific philosopher, such as Husserl or Heidegger, also identified?

C. Did the researcher cite a primary source for the philosophical foundation or theory (see Chapter 4)?

VI. Qualitative methodology

A. Identify the stated or implied research methodology used for the study.

B. Provide a paraphrased description of the research methodology used. In addition to reviewing Chapters 4 and 12, refer to Corbin and Strauss (2015), Creswell and Creswell (2018), and Creswell and Poth (2018) for descriptions of the different qualitative research perspectives or traditions.

VII. Sampling and sample

A. Identify how study participants were recruited.

B. Identify the types of sites where participants were recruited for the study.

C. Describe the inclusion and exclusion criteria of the sample.

D. Discuss the sample size. How was the sample size determined (theoretical saturation, no new themes generated, researcher understanding of the essences of the phenomenon, etc.)?

VIII. Data collection

A. Describe the data collection method.

B. Identify the period of time during which data collection occurred and the duration of any interviews.

C. Describe the sequence of data collection events for a participant. For example, were data collected from one interview or a series of interviews? Were focus group participants given an opportunity to provide additional data or review the preliminary conclusions of the researcher?

D. Describe any changes in the methods in response to the context and early data collection (Marshall & Rossman, 2016; Miles et al., 2020; Roller & Lavrakas, 2015).

IX. Protection of human study participants

A. Identify the benefits and risks of participation. Are there benefits or risks the researchers do not identify?

B. Are recruitment and consent techniques adjusted to accommodate the sensitivity of the subject matter and psychological distress of potential participants?

C. Describe the data collection and management techniques that acknowledge participant sensitivity and vulnerability. These might include how potential participants are identified or what resources are available if the participant becomes upset (Kazdin, 2017; Shadish et al., 2002).

X. Data management and analysis

A. Describe the data management and analysis methods used in the study by name, if possible (Marshall & Rossman, 2016; Miles et al., 2020).

B. Is an audit trail mentioned? An audit trail is a record of critical decisions that were made during the development and implementation of the study (Creswell & Poth, 2018). Chapter 12 provides information about audit trails.

C. Does the researcher describe other strategies used to minimize or allow for the effects of researcher bias (Miles et al., 2020; Patton, 2015)? For example, did two researchers analyze the data independently and compare their analyses?

XI. Findings

A. What are the findings of the study?

B. Does the researcher include participants' quotes to support themes or other processes identified as the findings (Corbin & Strauss, 2015; Patton, 2015)?

C. Do the findings ring true to the reader? The findings may seem true to you because of something you have experienced in your personal or professional life. When the findings resonate with the readers, the study's veracity is supported.

XII. Discussion
   A. Describe the limitations of the study.
   B. Identify whether the findings are compared to the findings of other studies or other relevant literature (Dale et al., 2019).
   C. Did the results offer new information about the phenomenon?
   D. What clinical, policy, theoretical, and other types of implications are identified?

Step II: Determining the Strengths and Weaknesses of the Study

Nurses prepared at the graduate level will compare each component of qualitative studies to the writings of qualitative experts, such as Corbin and Strauss (2015), Creswell and Creswell (2018), Creswell and Poth (2018), Miles et al. (2020), Morse (2018), and Roller and Lavrakas (2015). See also Chapters 4 and 12 in this text to review the processes considered appropriate for qualitative studies. By doing this comparison, you can determine the strengths and weaknesses of the study.

Guidelines for Determining the Strengths and Weaknesses of Qualitative Studies

I. Research report
   A. Are you able to identify easily the elements of the research report?
   B. Are readers able to hear the voice of the participants and gain an understanding of the phenomenon studied?
   C. Does the overall presentation of the study fit its purpose, method, and findings (Creswell & Creswell, 2018; Marshall & Rossman, 2016)?
II. Research problem, purpose, and questions
   A. Is the purpose a logical approach to addressing the research problem of the study (Creswell & Creswell, 2018)?
   B. Does the purpose have an intuitive fit with the problem?
   C. Are the research questions related to the problem and purpose?
III. Literature review
   A. Is the study based on a broad review of the literature? Does it appear that the author searched databases outside CINAHL for relevant studies?
   B. Is the review of the literature adequately synthesized and presented in a way that builds a logical argument (Brancati, 2018)? Another way to ask the question: Do the researchers provide enough evidence to support the conclusion that the study is needed?
IV. Methods
   A. Are the qualitative methods appropriate for the study purpose (Creswell & Poth, 2018)?
   B. Are the methods consistent with the philosophical tradition and qualitative methodology that was used? Determining whether there is consistency among the elements of the study termed *methodological congruence* is key to the quality of the study (Creswell & Poth, 2018; Hannes, 2011).
   C. Were the selected participants able to provide data relevant to the study purpose and research questions?
   D. Were the methods of data collection effective in obtaining data to address the study purpose?
   E. Were resources available to support participants who may have become upset? What resources did the researcher cite? Topics of qualitative studies may be sensitive topics that are difficult to mention (Creswell & Poth, 2018). Researchers concerned for their participants ensure that a mental health professional and other resources are available, should the participant become distressed (Shamoo & Resnik, 2015).
   F. Was the rationale provided for the selection of the particular data collection method used?
   G. Were the data collection procedures proscriptively applied or allowed to emerge with some flexibility? Flexibility within parameters of the method is considered appropriate for qualitative studies (Creswell & Poth, 2018).
   H. Did the data management and analysis methods fit the research purposes and data?
   I. Were the data analyzed sufficiently to allow new insights to occur?
   J. Were the methods used to ensure rigor adequate for eliciting the reader's confidence in the findings (Miles et al., 2020)? For example, were participants given the opportunity to validate their data after transcription and initial analysis? Did quotations support the themes or descriptions?

V. Findings

  A. Do the findings address the purpose of the study (Marshall & Rossman, 2016)?

  B. Are the findings of the study consistent with the qualitative methodology? For example, findings of a grounded theory study are presented as a description of concepts and social processes and the findings of an ethnography study are a description of a culture.

  C. Is there a coherent logic to the presentation of findings (Corbin & Strauss, 2015)?

  D. Are the interpretations of data congruent with data collected (Miles et al., 2020)?

  E. Did the researcher address variation in the findings by relevant sample characteristics, if applicable (Corbin & Strauss, 2015)?

VI. Discussion

  A. Did the researcher acknowledge the study limitations? Could any of these limitations been corrected before the end of the study?

  B. Did the researcher identify implications of the study that are consistent with the data and findings?

  C. What new insights or knowledge were gained from the study?

Step III: Evaluating a Study

"The sense of rightness and feeling of comfort readers experience reading the report of a study constitute the very judgments they make about the validity or trustworthiness of the study itself" (Sandelowski & Barroso, 2007, p. xix). Critical appraisal of research is not complete without making judgments about the validity of the study or, in the case of qualitative studies, making judgments about the trustworthiness. Balancing the strengths against the researcher-identified limitations and other weaknesses of the study, you determine the value or trustworthiness of study findings. Fig. 18.1 demonstrates that trustworthiness in qualitative research involves transparency, time, truth, and transformation, leading to transferability. Transparency, time, truth, and transformation are displayed as different aspects or facets of trustworthiness. Each of them plays a key role in whether the findings of a study are trustworthy. The arrow leading from trustworthiness indicates that trustworthy studies can potentially be transferable. Transferability of the findings to other populations is appropriate only if you determine that the findings are

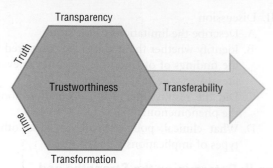

Fig. 18.1 Criteria for evaluating trustworthiness of qualitative findings.

trustworthy (Cullen et al., 2018). These characteristics of high-quality qualitative studies were synthesized from sets of criteria that included terms such as *credibility, reflexivity, confirmability,* and *dependability* (Hannes, 2011; Marshall & Rossman, 2016; Miles et al., 2020; Morse, 2018; Roller & Lavrakas, 2015). By examining transparency, truth, time, and transformation, you can make a judgment about the trustworthiness of the study findings. Although they will be described separately, the four characteristics overlap.

Guidelines for Evaluating a Qualitative Study

I. Transparency

  Transparency is the extent to which the researcher provided details about the study processes such as decisions made during data collection and analysis, ethical concerns that were noted, and personal perspectives that may bias the findings (Roller & Lavrakas, 2015). The researcher may indicate that field notes were written immediately after each interview. For example, such field notes may include thoughts on what worked or did not work in getting participants to talk freely as well as insights from the researcher's self-reflection of his or her response to the data. The openness of the researcher about how personal bias was managed increases your confidence in the findings. Terms used in assessing qualitative research that have similar meanings as transparency are *confirmability* and *dependability,* and rich or thick descriptions (Shamoo & Resnik, 2015). The questions are prompts to help you evaluate transparency.

  A. Were the researchers' assumptions made explicit about "sample population, data-gathering techniques, and expected outcomes" (Roller & Lavrakas, 2015, p. 93)?

B. Did the researcher describe how personal biases and preconceived ideas were identified and managed (Miles et al., 2020)?

C. Did the researcher indicate the use of journals, field notes, memos, and other forms of documentation written during the study?

D. Were any ethical issues discussed that arose during the study?

E. Were the characteristics of the participants described adequately for you to determine the relevance of the findings?

F. Was the rationale provided for any changes in the study methods?

G. Were the stages of data analysis from raw data to findings described (Miles et al, 2020)?

H. Were quotations or other participant data provided as exemplars of codes, themes, and patterns (Patton, 2015)?

II. Truth

Truth as a characteristic of qualitative studies is not absolute. Your evaluation is influenced by your confidence that the findings can be confirmed by reviewing the audit trail, field notes, or transcripts (note the overlap with transparency). Strategies implemented to increase rigor, such as comparing transcripts to audio recordings, sharing the findings with participants, and writing memos, also increase your confidence in the truth of the findings. Truth also includes the conceptual and experiential fit of the findings with your view of the phenomenon. Your view of the phenomenon also may expand as you empathize with the thoughts, feelings, and experiences of the participants. Some describe this as intuition or new insights that emerge as you read the article.

A. What strategies did the researcher use to confirm the accuracy and logic of the findings?

B. How do the findings fit with your previous views related to the phenomenon?

C. Are the findings believable?

III. Time

In qualitative research, the researcher is the instrument (Marshall & Rossman, 2016). Time must be spent in gathering data, developing relationships with participants and key informants, interviewing additional participants based on initial data analysis, and being immersed in the data during analysis and interpretation. These activities take time. Some

qualitative experts have described this study characteristic as "prolonged engagement" and "persistent observation" (Roller & Lavrakas, 2015, p. 21). As a researcher, you need time to reflect and analyze your own responses to the data as well as thoroughly analyze the data (Creswell & Poth, 2018). One indication of the amount of time spent engaged in the study is the depth and comprehensiveness of the descriptions (note the overlap with transparency).

A. How long did interviews last, how much time was spent in the field, and/or how much time was spent in observation (Miles et al., 2020)?

B. Does the time spent collecting and analyzing data seem adequate based on the size of the sample, complexity of the design, and scope of the phenomenon?

IV. Transformation

Data analysis and interpretation transform the words of participants, the observations of the ethnographer, and the text of a document into findings (Miles et al., 2020). Qualitative researchers who analyze the data at a superficial level will report the data as findings, without evidence of synthesis, comparison across participants, or creation of abstract themes or categories. To transform data, the researcher must organize, interpret, compare, and reorganize phrases and themes until the meaning of the data begins to emerge (Miles et al., 2020). Data analysis is "the heart of qualitative inquiry" (Streubert & Carpenter, 2011, p. 51). As you might expect, for transformation of the data to occur, the researcher must spend time to become focused and immersed in the data. Immersion requires persistent engagement with the data (note overlap with time).

A. Do the findings go beyond reporting facts and words to describing experiences with depth and insight?

B. Are there other possible interpretations of the data?

C. How do the meaning and interpretation of the data match or contrast with previous research findings?

D. What contributions do the findings of the study make to what is known about the phenomenon?

E. Has the researcher taken the time to hone the writing—to transform the stories of the participants to a narrative that exhibits both thoroughness and eloquence?

V. Transferability

Trustworthiness is a necessary but not sufficient condition for transferability. Transferability is the applicability of the findings to another population or phenomenon or, stated another way, the "ability to do something of value with the outcomes" (Roller & Lavrakas, 2015, p. 23). To be transferable, the findings must have meaning for similar groups or settings. The reader or user of the findings is the one who makes the determination of transferability (Creswell & Poth, 2018; Miles et al., 2020). If you have answered the previous questions and concluded the study is trustworthy, proceed with answering the following questions to determine the transferability of the findings to your practice.

A. How similar were the study participants to the persons or groups with whom you interact? Are there general truths that emerged from the research that might be used with similar populations or with people in similar circumstances?

B. What implications may the findings have for your practice?

C. What actions could be taken that are consistent with the findings?

D. How does the study move research, theory, knowledge, education, and practice forward?

KEY POINTS

- Critical appraisal of research involves carefully examining all aspects of a study to judge its strengths, weaknesses, meaning, credibility, and significance in light of previous research experience, knowledge of the topic, and clinical expertise.

- Critical appraisals of research are conducted to (1) summarize evidence for practice, (2) provide a basis for future research, (3) evaluate presentations and publications of studies, (4) select abstracts for a conference, (5) evaluate whether a manuscript should be published, and (6) evaluate research proposals for funding and implementation in clinical agencies.

- Nurses' levels of expertise in conducting critical appraisals depend on their educational preparation and experiences; nurses with baccalaureate, master's, doctoral, and postdoctoral preparation all have a role in examining the quality of research.

- The critical appraisal process for research includes the following steps: identifying the steps of the research process in a study; determining the study strengths and weaknesses; and evaluating the credibility, trustworthiness, and meaning of a study to nursing knowledge and practice (see Box 18.1).

- The identification step involves understanding the terms and concepts in the report and identifying the study steps.

- The second step of determining study strengths and weaknesses involves comparing what each step of the research process should be like with how the steps of the study were conducted. The logical development and implementation of the study steps also need to be examined for strengths and weaknesses.

- Study strengths and weaknesses need to be clearly identified, supported with a rationale, and documented with current research sources.

- The evaluation step involves examining the credibility, trustworthiness, and meaning of the study according to set criteria.

- Quantitative study design and analyses need to be appropriate for the investigation of the study purpose and for the specific objectives, questions, or hypotheses.

- In quantitative studies weaknesses often result from breaks in logical reasoning such as biases caused by sampling, measurement methods, and impairment of the logical flow from design to interpretation of findings by the selected design.

- Findings in a quantitative study need to be linked with the findings from previous research and examined for use in practice.

- To perform fair critical appraisals of qualitative studies, nurses need the prerequisites of an appreciation for the philosophical foundations of qualitative research, knowledge of different qualitative designs, and respect for the study participant's perspective (see Box 18.3).

- Each aspect of a qualitative study, such as problem, purpose, research questions, sample, data collection and analysis, and findings, needs to be examined for strengths and weaknesses.

- The trustworthiness of a qualitative study's findings is the extent to which the researcher demonstrated transparency, provided true findings, expended adequate time, and transformed the data into meaningful findings. Transparency, truth, time, and transformation are essential elements or aspects that determine whether a study's findings are trustworthy (see Fig. 18.1).

• Trustworthiness of a qualitative study is a necessary but not sufficient condition for transferability, the application of the findings to similar groups or settings. A study's findings may be trustworthy, but the sample, setting, or focus of the study may not be similar enough for transferring the findings to your population.

REFERENCES

Aberson, C. L. (2019). *Applied power analysis for the behavioral sciences* (2nd ed.). New York, NY: Routledge Taylor & Francis Group.

Adams, K., & Lawrence, E. (2019). *Research methods, statistics, and applications* (2nd ed.). Thousand Oaks, CA: Sage.

Agency for Healthcare Research and Quality (AHRQ). (2019). *Funding & grants.* Retrieved from https://www.ahrq.gov/funding/index.html./index.html

American Association of Colleges of Nursing (AACN). (2011). *Essentials of master's education in nursing.* Retrieved from https://www.aacnnursing.org/Education-Resources/AACN-Essentials

American Association of Colleges of Nursing (AACN). (2012). *QSEN Education Consortium. Graduate-level QSEN competencies: Knowledge, skills, and attitudes.* Retrieved from https://www.aacnnursing.org/Portals/42/AcademicNursing/CurriculumGuidelines/Graduate-QSEN-Competencies.pdf?ver=2017-07-15-135425-900

American Nurses Credentialing Center (ANCC). (2019). *ANCC Magnet Recognition Program*®. Retrieved from https://www.nursingworld.org/organizational-programs/magnet/

American Psychological Association (APA). (2020). *Publication manual of the American Psychological Association* (7th ed.). Washington, DC: Author.

Astroth, K. S., & Chung, S. Y. (2018). Focusing on the fundamentals: Reading quantitative research with a critical eye. *Nephrology Nursing Journal, 45*(3), 283–287.

Aveyard, H. (2019). *Doing a literature review in health and social care: A practical guide* (4th ed.). New York, NY: Open University Press.

Beck, C. (2016). *Developing a program of research in nursing.* New York, NY: Springer.

Brancati, D. (2018). *Social scientific research.* Thousand Oaks, CA: Sage.

Brown, S. J. (2018). *Evidence-based nursing: The research-practice connection* (4th ed.). Sudbury, MA: Jones & Bartlett.

Bryant, A., & Charmaz, K. (Eds.). (2019). *The Sage handbook of current developments in grounded theory.* Thousand Oaks, CA: Sage.

Burns, N. (1989). Standards for qualitative research. *Nursing Science Quarterly, 2*(1), 44–52. doi:10.1177/089431848900200112

Corbin, J., & Strauss, A. (2015). *Basics of qualitative research: Techniques and procedures for developing grounded theory* (4th ed.). Los Angeles, CA: Sage.

Creswell, J. W., & Creswell, J. D. (2018). *Research design: Qualitative, quantitative and mixed methods approaches* (5th ed.). Thousand Oaks, CA: Sage.

Creswell, J. W., & Poth, C. (2018). *Qualitative inquiry & research design: Choosing among five approaches* (4th ed.). Thousand Oaks, CA: Sage.

Critical Appraisal Skills Programme (CASP). (2018). *CASP checklists.* Retrieved from http://www.casp-uk.net/#!casp-tools-checklists/c18f8

Cullen, L., Hanrahan, K., Farrington, M., DeBerg, J., Tucker, S., & Kleiber, C. (2018). *Evidence-based practice in action: Comprehensive strategies, tools, and tips from the University of Iowa Hospitals and Clinics.* Indianapolis, IN: Sigma Theta Tau International.

Dale, J. C., Hallas, D., & Spratling, R. (2019). Critiquing research evidence for use in practice: Revisited. *Journal of Pediatric Health Care, 33*(3), 342–346. doi:10.1016/j.pedhc.2019.01.005

Dane, F. (2018). *Evaluating research: Methodology for people who need to read research* (2nd ed.). Thousand Oaks, CA: Sage.

Dang, D., & Dearholt, S. (2017). *Johns Hopkins nursing evidence-based practice: Model and guidelines* (3rd ed.). Indianapolis, IN: Sigma Theta Tau International.

Eymard, A. S., & Altmiller, G. (2016). Teaching nursing students the importance of treatment fidelity in intervention research: Students as interventionists. *Journal of Nursing Education, 55*(5), 288–291. doi:10.3928/01484834-20160414-09

Gravetter, F., & Forzano, L-A. (2018). *Research methods for the behavioral sciences* (6th ed.). Boston, MA: Cengage.

Grove, S. K., & Cipher, D. (2020). *Statistics for nursing research: A workbook for evidence-based practice* (3rd ed.). St. Louis, MO: Saunders.

Hannes, K. (2011). *Critical appraisal of qualitative research.* In J. Noyes, A. Booth, K. Hannes, J. Harris, S. Lewin, & C. Lockwood (Eds.), *Supplementary guidance for inclusion in qualitative research in Cochrane systematic reviews of interventions.* Retrieved from http://cqrmg.cochrane.org/supplemental-handbook-guidance

Hayat, M. J., Higgins, M., Schwartz, T. A., & Staggs, V. S. (2015). Statistical challenges in nursing education and research: An expert panel consensus. *Nursing Educator, 40*(1), 21–25. doi:10.1097/NNE.0000000000000080

Kazdin, A. (2017). *Research design in clinical psychology* (5th ed.). Boston, MA: Pearson.

Mackey, A., & Bassendowski, S. (2017). The history of evidence-based practice in nursing education and practice. *Journal of Professional Nursing, 33*(1), 51–55. doi:10.1016/j.profnurs.2016.05.009

Marshall, C., & Rossman, G. B. (2016). *Designing qualitative research* (6th ed.). Los Angeles, CA: Sage.

McCosker, H., Barnard, A., & Gerber, R. (2001). Undertaking sensitive research: Issues and strategies for meeting the safety needs of all participants. *Qualitative Social Research, 2*(1), 22. doi:10.17169/fqs-2.1.983

Meleis, A. I. (2018). *Theoretical nursing: Development and progress* (6th ed.). Philadelphia, PA: Lippincott.

Melnyk, B. M., & Fineout-Overholt, E. (2019). *Evidence-based practice in nursing & healthcare: A guide to best practice* (4th ed.). Philadelphia, PA: Lippincott Williams & Wilkins.

Melnyk, B. M., Gallagher-Ford, L., & Fineout-Overholt, E. (2017). *Implementing the EBP competencies in healthcare: A practical guide for improving quality, safety, & outcomes.* Indianapolis, IN: Sigma Theta Tau.

Miles, M. B., Huberman, A. M., & Saldaña, J. (2020). *Qualitative data analysis: A methods sourcebook* (4th ed.). Los Angeles, CA: Sage.

Morse, J. M. (2018). Reframing rigor in qualitative inquiry. In N. Denzin & Y. Lincoln (Eds.), *The Sage handbook of qualitative research* (5th ed., pp. 796–817). Thousand Oaks, CA: Sage.

National Institute of Nursing Research (NINR). (2019). *Building the scientific foundation for clinical practice.* Retrieved from https://www.ninr.nih.gov/

Patton, M. (2015). *Qualitative research & evaluation methods* (4th ed.). Los Angeles, CA: Sage.

Polit, D. F., & Yang, F. M. (2016). *Measurement and the measurement of change.* Philadelphia, PA: Wolters Kluwer.

Roller, M., & Lavrakas, P. (2015). *Applied qualitative research design: A total quality framework approach.* New York, NY: Guilford Press.

Ryan-Wenger, N. A. (2017). Evaluation of measurement precision, accuracy, and error in biophysical data for clinical research and practice. In C. F. Waltz, O. L. Strickland, & E. R. Lenz (Eds.), *Measurement in nursing and health research* (5th ed., pp. 371–383). New York, NY: Springer.

Sandelowski, M. (2008). Justifying qualitative research. *Research in Nursing and Health, 31*(3), 193–195. doi:10.1002/nur.20272

Sandelowski, M., & Barroso, J. (2007). *Handbook for synthesizing qualitative research.* New York, NY: Springer.

Shadish, W. R., Cook, T. D., & Campbell, D. T. (2002). *Experimental and quasi-experimental designs for generalized causal inference.* Chicago, IL: Rand McNally.

Shamoo, A., & Resnik, D. (2015). Responsible conduct of research (3rd ed.). Oxford, England: Oxford Univeristy Press.

Sherwood, G., & Barnsteiner, J. (2012). *Quality and safety in nursing: A competency approach to improving outcomes.* Ames, IA: Wiley-Blackwell.

Smith, M. J., & Liehr, P. R. (2018). *Middle range theory for nursing* (4th ed.). New York, NY: Springer.

Streubert, H., & Carpenter, D. (2011). *Qualitative research in nursing: Advancing the humanistic perspective* (5th ed.). Philadelphia, PA: Lippincott Williams & Wilkins.

Thompson, S. K. (2012). *Sampling* (3rd ed.). New York, NY: John Wiley & Sons.

Truluck, C. A., & Leggett, T. (2016). Critical appraisal of health professions research. *Radiologic Technology, 87*(3), 355–358.

Waltz, C. F., Strickland, O. L., & Lenz, E. R. (2017). *Measurement in nursing and health research* (5th ed.). New York, NY: Springer.

Whittemore, R., Chao, A., Jang, M., Minges, K. W., & Park, C. (2014). Methods of knowledge synthesis: An overview. *Heart and Lung: The Journal of Critical Care, 43*(5), 453–461. doi:10.1016/j.hrtlng.2014.05.014

19

Evidence Synthesis and Strategies for Implementing Evidence-Based Practice

Susan K. Grove

http://evolve.elsevier.com/Gray/practice/

Research evidence continues to expand at a rapid rate as numerous quality studies in nursing, medicine, and other healthcare disciplines are conducted and disseminated. These studies are commonly communicated via journal publications, the internet, books, conferences, and social media. The expectations of society and the goals of healthcare systems are the delivery of high-quality, safe, cost-effective health care to patients, families, and communities. The delivery of quality health care requires the use of the current best research evidence available. Healthcare systems are emphasizing the delivery of evidence-based care, and nurses and physicians are focused on developing evidence-based practice (EBP). Graduate nursing education programs emphasize achieving EBP competencies for the roles as advanced practice nurses (APNs) and administrators (Melnyk, Gallagher-Ford, & Fineout-Overholt, 2017). The emphasis on EBP in educational programs and clinical agencies has enhanced outcomes for students, patients, healthcare providers, and healthcare agencies (Hickman et al., 2018; Melnyk et al., 2018a).

Evidence-based practice is an important theme in this textbook and was defined earlier as the conscientious integration of best research evidence with clinical expertise and patient values and needs in the delivery of quality, cost-effective health care (see Chapter 1) (Cullen et al., 2018; Quality and Safety Education for Nurses [QSEN], 2012; Sherwood & Barnsteiner, 2017; Straus, Glasziou, Richardson, Rosenberg, & Haynes, 2011). **Best research evidence** is produced by the conduct and synthesis of numerous high-quality studies in a selected health-related area. Chapter 2

introduces the concept of best research evidence and the processes for synthesizing research. The research syntheses included in this text are systematic review, meta-analysis, metasynthesis, and mixed methods research synthesis (Higgins & Thomas, 2020; Paré, Trudel, Jaana, & Kitsiou, 2015; Whittemore, Chao, Jang, Minges, & Park, 2014).

This chapter builds on previous EBP discussions to provide you with strategies for implementing best research evidence in your practice and moving the profession of nursing toward EBP. Strengths, challenges, and current status of EBP in nursing are discussed. Guidelines are provided for synthesizing research to determine the best research evidence for a healthcare area. The Stetler and Iowa nursing models developed to facilitate EBP are described with examples provided. Expert researchers, clinicians, and consumers—through government agencies, professional organizations, and healthcare systems—have developed an extensive number of evidence-based guidelines. This chapter offers a framework for reviewing the quality of these evidence-based guidelines and for using them in practice. The chapter concludes with a discussion of nationally designated EBP centers and the role of translational research in promoting EBP.

STRENGTHS, CHALLENGES, AND CURRENT STATUS OF EVIDENCE-BASED PRACTICE IN NURSING

EBP is a goal for the nursing profession and each practicing nurse. At the present time, some nursing interventions are evidence based—that is, supported by the best research knowledge available from research syntheses. However, many nursing interventions require additional research to generate essential knowledge for making changes in practice (Hickman et al., 2018; Mackey & Bassendowski, 2017). Some healthcare agencies and administrators are supportive of EBP and provide resources to facilitate this process; however, other agencies and chief nurse executives (CNEs) place EBP as a low priority (Duncombe, 2018; Melnyk et al., 2016). Many nurses' knowledge of EBP is limited and requires expansion by educational programs and practice areas. The next two sections describe some of the strengths and challenges related to EBP to assist you in promoting EBP in your agency and delivering evidence-based care to your patients.

Strengths of Evidence-Based Practice in Nursing

The greatest strength of EBP is improved outcomes for patients, providers, and healthcare agencies (Hickman et al., 2018). Healthcare agencies nationally and internationally have promoted the synthesis of the best research evidence for thousands of healthcare topics by teams of expert researchers and clinicians. **Research synthesis** is a summary of relevant studies to determine the empirical knowledge in an area that is critical to the advancement of practice, research, and policy (Higgins & Thomas, 2020; Melnyk & Fineout-Overholt, 2019). Systematic reviews and meta-analyses are the most common research syntheses conducted to provide support for EBP guidelines. These guidelines identify the best treatment plan or **gold standard** for patient care in a selected health area for promotion of quality, safe, cost-effective healthcare outcomes. Healthcare providers have access to numerous evidence-based syntheses and guidelines to assist them in making the best clinical decisions for their patients.

Individual studies, research syntheses, and evidence-based guidelines assist students, educators, registered nurses (RNs), and APNs in promoting EBP. Expert APNs, including nurse practitioners (NPs), clinical nurse specialists, nurse anesthetists, and nurse midwives, are resources to other nurses and facilitate access to research evidence and the conduct of studies to ensure that patient care is based on the best research evidence available (Hickman et al., 2018).

Some healthcare agencies and CNEs are highly supportive of EBP as indicated by their attitudes and provision of resources to promote EBP. In a national study of CNEs, Melnyk et al. (2016) found that an organization with an EBP culture of conducting and using research evidence in practice had substantial improvements in several patient outcomes. An agency with an **EBP culture** includes setting EBP as an agency priority; developing organizational policies for EBP; training nurses in research methods and EBP strategies; designating mentors to promote EBP; improving access to research reports, syntheses, and guidelines; supporting and rewarding EBP activities; and providing official time to conduct research and evidence-based projects (Duncombe, 2018; Warren et al., 2016). Leaders in these clinical agencies recognize that EBP promotes quality patient outcomes, improves nurses' satisfaction, and facilitates achievement of accreditation requirements. The Joint Commission (2019) standards include accreditation criteria that emphasize patient care quality and safety achieved through EBP.

Many CNEs and healthcare systems are trying either to obtain or maintain Magnet recognition, which documents the excellence of nursing care in an agency. Magnet recognition is obtained through the American Nurses Credentialing Center (ANCC, 2019), and national and international healthcare agencies that currently have Magnet status can be viewed online at https://www.nursingworld.org/organizational-programs/magnet/find-a-magnet-organization/. The Magnet Recognition Program® recognizes EBP as a way to improve the quality of patient care and revitalize the nursing environment. Magnet recognition requires that healthcare agencies promote the following research activities: critically appraising and using research evidence in practice and policy development; budgeting for research activities; providing a research infrastructure with the help of consultants; supporting nurses as principle investigators with time and money; educating, training, and mentoring nursing staff in research activities and EBP; and tracking research and other scholarly outcomes (ANCC, 2019).

Challenges Related to Evidence-Based Practice In Nursing

The challenges to the EBP movement have been both practical and conceptual. Research evidence is strong in the medical management of diseases but limited regarding the effectiveness of many nursing interventions in managing diseases, preventing illnesses, and promoting health (Moore & Tierney, 2019). EBP requires synthesizing research evidence from RCTs and other types of interventional studies, but these types of studies are still limited in nursing (Duncombe, 2018; Leedy & Ormrod, 2019). A review of research evidence in high-impact nursing journals, including *Nursing Research, Research in Nursing & Health, Western Journal of Nursing Research, Journal of Nursing Scholarship,* and *Advances in Nursing Science,* indicate that studies are predominately nonexperimental and less than 30% are experimental and quasi-experimental. Quality RCTs, other experimental studies, and quasi-experimental studies are needed to generate evidence regarding nursing interventions for the management of disease, prevention of illness, and health promotion.

Systematic reviews and meta-analyses conducted in nursing have been limited compared with other disciplines. Bolton, Donaldson, Rutledge, Bennett, and Brown (2007) conducted a review of "systematic/integrative reviews and meta-analyses on nursing interventions and patient outcomes in acute care settings" (p. 123S). Their literature search covered 1999 to 2005 and identified 4000 systematic/integrative reviews and 500 meta-analyses covering the following seven topics selected by the authors: staffing, caregivers, incontinence, elder care, symptom management, pressure ulcer prevention and treatment, and developmental care of neonates and infants. The authors found a limited association between nursing interventions and processes and patient outcomes in acute care settings. They found the strongest evidence was for the use of patient risk-assessment tools and interventions by nurses to prevent patient harm (Bolton et al., 2007). To build evidence for practice, nurses need to be more active in conducting quality studies focused on nursing interventions and synthesizing research evidence (Friesen, Brady, Milligan, & Christensen, 2017; Hickman et al., 2018; Pintz, Zhou, McLaughlin, Kelly, & Guzzetta, 2018).

Another concern related to EBP is that the research evidence is generated based on population data and then applied in practice to individual patients. Sometimes it is difficult to transfer research knowledge to individual patients, who respond in unique ways or have unique needs (Weiss, Bobay, Johantgen, & Shirey, 2018). The National Institutes of Health (NIH, 2019a) are supporting translational research to improve the use of research evidence with different patient populations in various settings. Reed, Howe, Doyle, and Bell (2018) conducted a qualitative study to identify some simple rules for translating research evidence in complex healthcare systems. These rules "have potential to provide a common platform for academics, practitioners, patients, and policymakers to collaborate when intervening to achieve improvements in healthcare" (Reed et al., 2018, p. 92).

Some healthcare providers expressed concern that the development of evidence-based guidelines could lead to a controlled approach to health care with them having limited options for adapting care to their patients. However, the definition of EBP describes it as the conscientious integration of best research evidence with clinical expertise and patient values and needs. Nurse clinicians have a major role in determining how the best research evidence will be implemented to achieve quality outcomes. For example, APNs use the national evidence-based guidelines for the diagnosis and management of patients with hypertension (HTN). Two current guidelines exist for the management of HTN: (1) 2014 Evidence-Based Guideline for the Management of High Blood Pressure in Adults by the panel members of the Eighth Joint National Committee (JNC 8) (James et al., 2014) and (2) the Clinical Practice Guidelines for the Management of Hypertension in the Community by the American Society of Hypertension and the International Society of Hypertension (Weber et al., 2014). Evidence-based guidelines provide the gold standard for managing a particular health condition, but the healthcare provider and patient individualize the treatment plan.

A serious barrier to EBP is that some healthcare agencies and administrators do not provide the resources necessary for nurses to implement EBP. Their lack of support might include the following: (1) inadequate access to research journals and other sources of synthesized research findings and evidence-based guidelines, (2) inadequate knowledge on how to implement evidence-based changes in practice, (3) heavy workload with limited time to make research-based changes in practice, (4) limited authority or support to change patient care based on research findings, (5) limited funding to support research and EBP projects, and (6) minimal rewards for providing evidence-based care to patients and families (Alzayyat,

2014; Duncombe, 2018; Melnyk et al., 2016; Melnyk et al., 2018b; Spiva et al., 2017; Warren et al., 2016).

Current Status of Evidence-Based Practice

The success of EBP is determined by all involved, including nursing educational programs and faculty, healthcare agencies, administrators, RNs, APNs, physicians, and other healthcare professionals (Dang & Dearholt, 2018; Friesen et al., 2017; Kesten, White, Heitzler, Chaplin, & Bondmass, 2019). Educational programs have expanded their coverage of EBP. Many programs have adopted the American Association of Colleges of Nursing (AACN) Graduate QSEN Competencies, available online at http://qsen.org/competencies/graduate-ksas/. One of the competencies focused on EBP is defined as the integration of the "best current evidence with clinical expertise and patient/family preferences and values for delivery of optimal health care" (QSEN, 2012). The graduate QSEN EBP competencies were developed to assist faculty in preparing APNs and administrators for the delivery of EBP. Many graduate nursing programs include a separate course focused on EBP and additional content on EBP in clinical courses. In a recent study, Melnyk et al. (2018b) found "younger nurses and those with higher levels of education reported higher EBP competency" (p. 16). However, a recent systematic review of EBP in postgraduate nursing programs reported: "There is a paucity of empirical evidence supporting the best strategies to use in developing evidence-based practice skills and/ or research knowledge translation skills for master's nursing students" (Hickman et al., 2018, p. 69). Studies focused on developing and testing EBP strategies are essential if nurses are to become competent in providing EBP.

The QSEN EBP competencies also provided a basis for developing professional competencies in clinical practice (Sherwood & Barnsteiner, 2017). In 2014, Melnyk and colleagues developed EBP competencies for RNs and APNs to assist healthcare agencies in ensuring their clinicians were delivering the highest quality and safest evidence-based care. Melnyk et al. (2018b) conducted a national study of these 24 EBP competencies that included 2344 nurses from 19 healthcare systems. The EBP competencies and the nurses' reported EBP competency by educational level are presented in Fig. 19.1. Associate/diploma-prepared nurses demonstrate the weakest EBP competency and master-level

nurses had the strongest EBP competency. These researchers also found positive relationships between EBP competency scores and EBP beliefs, EBP mentorship, EBP knowledge, and EBP culture. However, the overall findings identified major deficits in achieving the EBP competencies that threaten healthcare quality, safety, and patient outcomes (see Fig. 19.1). Melnyk et al. (2018b) recommended, "Academic programs should ensure competency in EBP in students by the time of graduation and healthcare systems should set it as an expectation and standard for all clinicians" (p. 16). In summary, extensive work has been done to promote EBP in nursing, but additional studies and research syntheses must be conducted and innovative strategies implemented by nurses to achieve competency in EBP (Hickman et al., 2018; Melnyk et al., 2017; Melnyk et al., 2018a, 2018b; Spiva et al., 2017).

GUIDELINES FOR SYNTHESIZING RESEARCH EVIDENCE

Many nurses lack the expertise and confidence to critically appraise and synthesize research evidence in a selected nursing area. Master's and doctoral students often focus on clearly defined interventions when conducting research syntheses. A research synthesis is best done by more than one individual, including researchers and/or clinicians, and guided by specific guidelines or protocols (Higgins & Green, 2008, 2011; Higgins & Thomas, 2020; Pölkki, Kanste, Kääriäinen, Elo, & Kyngäs, 2013). Novice researchers should seek membership on these teams to increase their understanding of the research synthesis processes.

In this section, guidelines are provided for conducting systematic reviews, meta-analyses, metasyntheses, and mixed methods research syntheses to assist you in synthesizing research evidence for nursing practice. Numerous research syntheses have been conducted in nursing and medicine, so be sure to search for an existing synthesis or review of research in an area before undertaking such a project. MEDLINE (2019) has more than 25 million citations from journal articles in life sciences with a concentration of biomedicine. Approximately 2500 new systematic reviews are reported in English and indexed in MEDLINE each year. Table 19.1 identifies some common databases and EBP organizational websites that nurses can search for syntheses of healthcare research. The Cochrane Collaboration (2019)

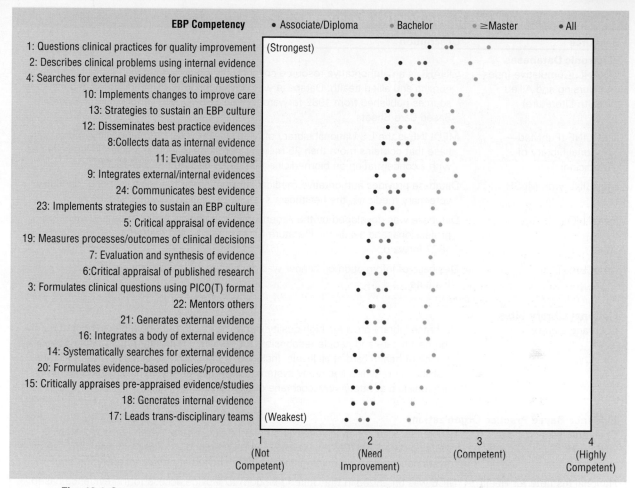

Fig. 19.1 Strongest to weakest items of nurses' reported evidence-based practice (*EBP*) competency by educational level. PICO(T), Patient population, intervention, comparison intervention or group, outcome, (time). (From Melnyk, B. M., Gallagher-Ford, L., Zellefrow, C., Tucker, S., Thomas, B., Sinnott, L. T., & Tan, A. [2018b]. The first US study on nurses' evidence-based practice competencies indicates major deficits that threaten healthcare quality, safety, and patient outcomes. *Worldviews on Evidence-Based Nursing, 15*[1], 21.)

library of systematic reviews is an excellent resource with more than 30,000 entries relevant to nursing and health care. The Cochrane Nursing Care Field was developed in 2009 to support the conduct and dissemination of research syntheses in nursing (Cochran Nursing, 2019). The Joanna Briggs Institute (2019) also provides resources for locating and conducting nursing research syntheses, if your facility subscribes to their services. If you can find no research synthesis for a selected nursing intervention or the review you find is outdated, you might use the following guidelines to conduct a systematic review of the relevant research.

Guidelines for Implementing and Evaluating Systematic Reviews

A **systematic review** is a structured, comprehensive synthesis of the research literature conducted to determine the best research evidence available for addressing a healthcare question. A systematic review involves identifying, locating, critically appraising, and synthesizing quality research evidence for expert clinicians to use to promote an EBP (Bettany-Saltikov, 2010a, 2010b; Dang & Dearholt, 2018). Systematic reviews must be conducted with rigorous research methodology to promote the accuracy of the findings and minimize

TABLE 19.1   Evidence-Based Practice Resources

Resource	Description
Electronic Databases	
CINAHL (Cumulative Index to Nursing and Allied Health Literature)	CINAHL is an authoritative resource covering the English-language journal literature for nursing and allied health. Database was developed in the United States and includes sources published from 1982 forward. Within EBSCO, you can search for Evidence-Based Care Sheets.
MEDLINE (PubMed—National Library of Medicine)	MEDLINE is the US National Library of Medicine® (NLM) premier bibliographical database that contains more than 25 million references to journal articles in life sciences with a concentration on biomedicine that dates back to the mid-1960s.
MEDLINE with MeSH	Database provides authoritative medical information on medicine, nursing, dentistry, veterinary medicine, the healthcare system, preclinical services, and more.
PsycINFO	Database was developed by the American Psychological Association and includes professional and academic literature for psychology and related disciplines from 1887 forward.
CANCERLIT	Database of information on cancer was developed by the US National Cancer Institute.
National Library Sites	
Cochrane Library	Cochrane Library provides high-quality evidence to inform people providing and receiving health care and people responsible for research, teaching, funding, and administration of health care at all levels. Included in the Cochrane Library is the Cochrane Collaboration, which has many systematic reviews of research. Cochrane Reviews are available at http://www.cochrane.org/reviews/.
Evidence-Based Practice Organizations	
Cochrane Nursing Care Network	Cochrane Collaboration includes 11 different fields, one of which is the Cochrane Nursing Care Field (CNCF), which supports the conduct, dissemination, and use of systematic reviews in nursing and can be searched at http://cncf.cochrane.org/.
National Institute for Health and Clinical Excellence (NICE)	NICE was organized in the United Kingdom to provide access to the evidence-based guidelines that have been developed. These guidelines can be accessed at http://nice.org.uk.
Joanna Briggs Institute	This international evidence-based organization, originating in Australia, has a search website that includes evidence summaries, systematic reviews, systematic review protocols, evidence-based recommendations for practice, critical appraisal tools, outcomes measures, and consumer information sheets. Search the Joanna Briggs Institute at http://joannabriggs.org/.
Registered Nurses Association of Ontario	Nurses, nurse practitioners, and nursing students are members of this organization that was formed to develop and implement evidence-based guidelines for this Canadian territory. These resources are available at https://rnao.ca/.
US Preventive Services Task Force	A panel of national experts was formed, as an independent organization, to develop evidence for preventive care with resources that can be accessed at https://www.uspreventiveservicestaskforce.org/.

reviewer bias. Pölkki et al. (2013) studied the quality of systematic reviews published in high-impact nursing journals and noted that the quality of the reviews varied considerably and that some reviews were conducted without guidelines or protocols to direct the process. Sun, Zhou, Zhang, and Liu (2019) examined the "reporting and methodological quality of systematic reviews and meta-analyses of nursing interventions in patients with Alzheimer's disease" (p. 308) and found these syntheses to be suboptimal without the consistent use of guidelines to direct them.

We recommend using the Preferred Reporting Items for Systematic Reviews and Meta-Analyses (PRISMA) Statement for reporting systematic reviews and meta-analyses (Liberati et al., 2009; Moher, Liberati, Tetzlaff, Altman, & PRISMA Group, 2009). The PRISMA Statement was developed by an international group of expert healthcare researchers and clinicians to improve the quality of reporting for systematic reviews and meta-analyses. The PRISMA guideline is still viewed as the gold standard for reporting systematic reviews and meta-analyses. Liu, Zhou, Yu, and Sun (2019) examined

"the effects of the PRISMA statement to improve the conduct and reporting of systematic reviews and meta-analyses of nursing interventions for patients with heart failure" (p. 1) and found a significant improvement since the PRISMA checklist was published. However, they recommended authors, reviewers, and editors adhere more strictly to the PRISMA and the Assessment of Multiple Systematic Reviews (AMSTAR) checklists in preparing systematic reviews and meta-analyses for publication. AMSTAR 2 is now available for critically appraising systematic reviews that include randomized and nonrandomized studies of healthcare interventions (Shea et al., 2017).

Kim and Park (2019) conducted a systematic review and meta-analysis to determine the "effects of smartphone-based mobile learning in nursing education for nurses and nursing students" (p. 21). Their systematic review and meta-analysis were conducted using the PRISMA Statement. Table 19.2 provides an adapted checklist of PRISMA items used in reporting systematic reviews and meta-analyses (Moher et al., 2009).

TABLE 19.2 Checklist of Items to Include in Reporting a Systematic Review or Meta-Analysis

Steps	Section/Topic	Checklist Item	Reported on Page Number
Step 1	**Title**	Identify the report as a systematic review, meta-analysis, or both in the study title.	
Step 2	**Abstract**	Provide a structured summary of the systematic review or meta-analysis, including purpose or questions directing the review, literature search process, study appraisal and synthesis methods, results, conclusions, and implications of key findings.	
Step 3	**Introduction**		
	Background and rationale	Describe the background and rationale for the review in the context of what is already known and not known.	
	Question(s) or objective(s)	Provide an explicit statement of questions being addressed with reference to PICOS (participants, intervention, comparative interventions, outcomes, and study design) format.	
	Guideline or protocol used	Indicate whether a specific guideline or protocol was used to direct the review. Most of the systematic reviews and meta-analyses are conducted using the Preferred Reporting Items for Systematic Reviews and Meta-Analyses (PRISMA) Statement.	

Continued

TABLE 19.2   Checklist of Items to Include in Reporting a Systematic Review or Meta-Analysis—cont'd

Steps	Section/Topic	Checklist Item	Reported on Page Number
	Methods		
Step 4	Eligibility criteria	Specify the study eligibility criteria such as type of participants in studies, intervention, measurement methods, and report characteristics (e.g., years considered, language, publication status). Provide a rationale for the eligibility criteria selected.	
Step 5	Information sources	Describe all information sources (e.g., databases with dates of coverage, contact with study authors to identify additional studies) in the search and date last searched. List and define all variables for which data were sought (e.g., PICOS, funding sources) and any assumptions and simplifications made.	
Step 6	Literature search	Present full electronic search strategy for at least one database, including any limits used, with enough detail so that it could be repeated by another researcher.	
	Results		
Step 7	Study selection	Describe the study selection process, including the number of studies screened, eligibility criteria assessment, and studies included in review, with reasons for excluding studies. This process is best presented in a flow diagram (see Fig. 19.2).	
Step 8	Critical appraisal of studies	Critical appraisal is best accomplished by constructing a table describing the characteristics of the included studies, such as the purpose, population, sampling method, sample size, sample acceptance and attrition rates, design, intervention (independent variable), outcomes (dependent variables), measurement methods for each outcome, and major results.	
Step 9	Results of the review	Results of the review include descriptions of the studies' participants, settings, interventions, measurement methods, and outcomes.	
	Population and setting	Describe the methods of handling data and combining results of studies. Describe the participants and settings for the different studies. Critically appraise the quality of the population for the review.	
	Interventions	If appropriate, identify the intervention(s) included in the studies. Critically appraise the similarities and differences of these interventions.	
	Measurement methods and outcomes	Describe and critically appraise the reliability and validity of measurement methods, such as scales and questionnaires, and the precision and accuracy of physiological measures included in the studies to measure key study variables or outcomes.	
Step 10	Meta-analysis	If a meta-analysis was included as part of the systematic review, describe the process for selecting the studies to be included in the analysis. Critically appraise the studies included in the meta-analysis and the results from this analysis.	
Step 11	**Discussion**	Develop a summary of the current best research evidence based on the review. Discuss the limitations and/or risks of bias in the review. Describe the implications of the evidence for practice, policy, and future research. State the conclusions obtained from the systematic review or meta-analysis.	

			Reported on Page Number
Steps	**Section/Topic**	**Checklist Item**	
Step 12	**Publication**	Develop the systematic review or meta-analysis for publication based on the PRISMA guidelines. Identify any sources of funding.	
Step 13	**Registration**	Register the review with the International Prospective Register of Systematic Reviews (PROSPERO).	

TABLE 19.2 Checklist of Items to Include in Reporting a Systematic Review or Meta-Analysis—cont'd

Adapted from Moher, D., Liberati, A., Tetzlaff, J., Altman, D. G., & PRISMA Group. (2009). Preferred reporting items for systematic reviews and meta-analyses: The PRISMA statement. Retrieved from http://www.prisma-statement.org.

Step 1: Title of the Literature Synthesis

The title of a literature synthesis needs to clearly reflect the type of synthesis conducted. The authors should identify if a systematic review, meta-analysis, or both were conducted. Having the type of synthesis in the title makes it easier to identify these sources when conducting a literature search. Kim and Park (2019) provided a precise title for their research synthesis: "Effects of smartphone-based mobile learning in nursing education: A systematic review and meta-analysis" (p. 20).

Step 2: Abstract

The report for a systematic review or meta-analysis should have an abstract that provides a concise summary of the focus, process, and outcomes of the synthesis. The abstract should include the clinical questions or purpose guiding the synthesis, literature search process, and data sources or types of studies included in the synthesis. The critical appraisal and synthesis methods should be highlighted as well as key results, conclusions, and implications of the findings for nursing. Kim and Park (2019) provided a quality abstract that included a purpose consistent with the report title, a brief discussion of the literature search process, assessment of the studies' quality using the Cochrane collaboration risk of bias (ROB) tool, key results, and conclusion. The conclusion was that the smartphone mobile learning intervention significantly improved students' knowledge, skill, confidence in performance, and learning attitude.

Step 3: Introduction (Including Rationale, Clinical Question, and Guidelines to Direct the Systematic Review)

A systematic review or meta-analysis includes an introduction that provides a background of what is known and not known in a selected area with a rationale for conducting the review. A purpose or clinical question is developed to focus the review process. As discussed earlier, systematic reviews and meta-analyses need to be conducted using a specified guideline, protocol, or checklist. The PRISMA Statement or guideline is often used because of its international acceptance for promoting consistency in reporting of systematic reviews and meta-analyses (Liberati et al, 2009; Moher et al., 2009).

Formulating a question involves identifying a relevant topic, developing a question of interest that is worth investigating, deciding whether the question will generate significant information for practice, and determining whether the question will clearly direct the review process and synthesis of findings. A well-stated question will define the nature and scope of the literature search, identify keywords for the search, determine the best search strategy, provide guidance in selecting articles for the review, and guide the synthesis of results (Bettany-Saltikov, 2010a, 2010b; Higgins & Thomas, 2020; Liberati et al., 2009; Liu et al., 2019; Moher et al., 2009).

The question developed might focus on a therapy or intervention, health promotion action, illness prevention strategy, diagnostic process, prognosis, causation, or experience (Bettany-Saltikov, 2010a). One of the most common formats used to develop a relevant clinical question to guide a systematic review is the participants, intervention, comparative interventions, outcomes (PICO) and study design (PICOS) format described in the *Cochrane Handbook for Systematic Reviews of Interventions* (Dang & Dearholt, 2018; Higgins & Thomas, 2020). PICOS format includes the elements identified in Box 19.1.

BOX 19.1   PICOS Format for Directing Literature Searches

P—**Population** or participants of interest (see Chapter 15)

I—**Intervention** needed for practice (see Chapter 11 for discussion of interventions)

C—**Comparisons** of the intervention with control, placebo, standard care, variations of the same intervention, or different therapies

O—**Outcomes** needed for practice (see Chapter 13 for discussion of outcomes research and Chapter 17 for discussion of measurement methods)

S—**Study design** (see Chapters 10 and 11 for discussion of study designs)

Kim and Park (2019) stated that "despite such advantages and the necessity of smartphone-based mobile learning, only a few studies on nursing education have identified and evaluated the effects of smartphone-based learning systematically" (p. 21). As mentioned earlier, they used the PRISMA criteria to direct their syntheses. Kim and Park (2019) stated the following specific purpose to guide their syntheses.

"The purpose of this study is to confirm the general characteristics (study design, setting, sample size, intervention, outcome variables, and so on) of the selected studies, by examining systematically the previous studies that evaluated the effects of smartphone-based mobile learning on nursing education and to analyze the effects of smartphone-based mobile learning by presenting the effect size of the intervention through a meta-analysis." (Kim & Park, 2019, p. 21)

Step 4: Eligibility Criteria for the Review

The Methods section of a systematic review includes eligibility criteria for the review, discussion of information sources, and the literature search process (see Table 19.2). Inclusion and exclusion criteria are developed to direct the literature search. These search criteria might focus on the following: (1) type of research methods, such as quantitative, qualitative, or outcomes research; (2) the population or type of study participants; (3) study designs, such as descriptive, correlational, quasi-experimental, experimental, qualitative, or mixed methods (Creswell & Creswell, 2018; Kazdin, 2017); (4) sampling

processes, such as probability or nonprobability sampling methods; (5) intervention and comparison of interventions; and (6) specific outcomes to be measured. The PICOS format is effective in identifying the key terms to be included in the search process. The search criteria also should indicate the years for the review, language, and publication status. The review might be narrowed by limiting the years reviewed, specifying the language as English, and the studies to those in print (Bettany-Saltikov, 2010b; Higgins & Thomas, 2020).

Kim and Park (2019) used inclusion and exclusion criteria and PICOS format to identify relevant studies to include in their systematic review and meta-analysis. They included only studies focused on the smartphone and excluded all other mobile devices. They excluded studies that were only in abstract, poster, monographs, or conference proceedings format. Only studies in English were included in the literature review and the years for the review were unlimited. The following describes their use of PICOS guidelines to direct their search of the literature.

"1) Population (P): nursing students
2) Intervention (I): mobile learning by using smartphones
3) Comparison (C): other group or placebo group that does not receive mobile learning by using smartphones
4) Outcome (O): cognitive load, confidence in performance, knowledge, learning attitude, learning satisfaction, skill, and self-efficacy
5) Design (S): Randomized controlled trials or quasi-experimental studies" (Kim & Park, 2019, p. 21)

Step 5: Information Sources

Once the eligibility criteria have been identified, relevant information sources are selected. Often searches have been limited to published sources in common databases, which excludes the grey literature from the research synthesis. **Grey literature** refers to studies that have limited distributions, such as theses and dissertations, unpublished research reports, articles in obscure journals, articles in some online journals, conference papers and abstracts, conference proceedings, research reports to funding agencies, and technical reports (Benzies, Premji, Hayden, & Serrett, 2006; Conn,

Valentine, Cooper, & Rantz, 2003; Higgins & Thomas, 2020). Most grey literature is difficult to access through database searches, is often not peer reviewed, and has limited referencing information. These are some of the main reasons for not including grey literature in searches for systematic reviews and meta-analyses. However, excluding grey literature from these searches might result in misleading, biased results (Higgins & Green, 2008; Higgins & Thomas, 2020). Studies with significant findings are more likely to be published than studies with nonsignificant findings and are usually published in more high-impact, widely distributed journals that are indexed in computerized databases. Studies with significant findings are more likely to have duplicate publications that need to be excluded when selecting studies to include in a research synthesis. Benzies et al. (2006) recommended considering the inclusion of grey literature in a systematic review or meta-analysis in the following situations:

- Interventions and outcomes are complex with multiple components.
- Lack of consensus is present concerning measurement of outcome.
- Context is important to implementing the intervention.
- Availability of research-based evidence is low volume and quality.

Authors of systematic reviews should identify the search strategies they used. Often it is best to construct a table that includes the search criteria so that they can be applied consistently throughout the search process (Liberati et al., 2009). Bagnasco and colleagues (2014) developed a protocol to guide them in conducting a systematic review of the factors influencing self-management by patients with type 2 diabetes. We think you would find this protocol helpful in planning a systematic review.

Many sources are identified through searches of electronic databases using the criteria previously discussed. However, publication bias might best be reduced by using the following rigorous search strategies.

1. Review the references of identified studies for additional studies. These are **ancestry searches** to use citations in relevant studies to identify additional studies.
2. Hand search certain journals for selected years, especially for older studies that were not identified in the electronic search.

3. Identify expert researchers in an area and search their names in the databases.
4. Contact the expert researchers regarding studies they have conducted that have not yet been published.
5. Search thesis and dissertation databases for relevant studies.
6. Review abstracts and conference reports of relevant professional organizations.
7. Search the websites of funding agencies for relevant research reports.
   (Bagnasco et al., 2014; Bettany-Saltikov, 2010b; Liberati et al., 2009)

Kim and Park (2019) detailed their literature search strategies that were guided by the PRISMA Statement (see Table 19.2). No date restriction was applied to the search, and only studies reported in English were included. The databases searched are discussed in step 6. The authors excluded most sources of grey literature, such as abstracts, conference proceedings, and dissertations, but did hand search the references of articles for additional studies.

Step 6: Comprehensive Search of the Research Literature

The next step for conducting a systematic review or meta-analysis requires an extensive search of the literature focused on the inclusion and exclusion criteria and strategies identified in steps 4 and 5. The different databases searched, date of the search, and search results are recorded for each database (see Chapter 7 for details on conducting and storing searches of databases). Table 19.1 identifies common databases that are searched by nurses in conducting syntheses of research and in searching for evidence-based guidelines. Key search terms usually are identified in the report (Cullen et al., 2018). Sometimes authors of systematic reviews provide a table that identifies search terms and criteria. The PRISMA Statement recommends presenting the full electronic search strategy used for at least one major database, such as Cumulative Index to Nursing and Allied Health Literature (CINAHL) or MEDLINE (Liberati et al., 2009). Search strategies used to identify grey literature and other unpublished studies should be described.

Kim and Park (2019) identified some of their key search terms, such as *nursing, students, education,* and *smartphone.* They received help from a professional librarian to conduct the search, and the specific search terms and search expressions were identified in the report. However, no search strategy was provided for any of the databases searched. The search process is briefly discussed in the following excerpt.

> "According to assessment of multiple systematic reviews [AMSTAR], a guideline for evaluating the quality of systematic reviews, at least two researchers should conduct the search for a systematic review (Shea et al., 2017). Therefore, the electronic database search of this review was performed independently by two researchers, and peer-reviewed journals published by July 2017 were included for literature search. In addition to PubMed, Cochrane Library, and Embase, the retrieved electronic databases include Cumulative Index to Nursing and Allied Health Literature (CINAHL), Educational Resource Information Center (ERIC), ProQuest Cental, and SCOPUS. To search for gray literature, all references were reviewed and handsearched, and the year was not limited." (Kim & Park, 2019, p. 22)

Step 7: Selection of Studies for Review

The results section of a systematic review includes the study selection process, critical appraisal of the selected studies, and results of the review (see Table 19.2). The following sections cover these areas in detail. The selection of studies for inclusion in the systematic review or meta-analysis is a complex process that initially involves review and removal of duplicate sources. Two or more authors and sometimes an external reviewer examine the remaining abstracts to ensure they meet the criteria identified in step 4. The abstracts might be excluded based on the study participants, interventions, outcomes, or design not meeting the search criteria. Sometimes the abstracts are not in English, are incomplete, or represent studies that are not obtainable. If contacting the authors of the abstracts cannot produce essential information, often the abstracts are excluded from the review (Bagnasco et al., 2014; Bettany-Saltikov, 2010b; Liberati et al., 2009; Pölkki et al., 2013).

After the abstracts that meet the designated criteria are identified, the next step is to retrieve the full-text citation for each study. It is best to enter these studies into a table and document how each study meets the eligibility criteria. If studies do not meet criteria, they should be removed and a rationale provided. Two or more authors of the review need to examine the studies

to ensure that eligibility or inclusion criteria are consistently implemented. Often the study selection process includes all members of the review team. This selection process is best demonstrated by the flow diagram in Fig. 19.2 that was developed by the PRISMA Group (Liberati et al., 2009). This flow diagram includes four phases: (1) identification of the sources, (2) screening of the sources based on set criteria, (3) determining whether the sources meet eligibility requirements, and (4) identifying the studies included in the review.

Kim and Park (2019) provided a detailed description of their search process, results, and final selection of sources for their systematic review and meta-analysis. The authors selected the search terms together, independently searched the literature, and screened the selected studies together. In the case of disagreement, the studies were reviewed and consensus was achieved. The stages for the selection of studies were summarized using a PRISMA flow diagram format.

> *"Selection process*
> A total of 3,419 articles were retrieved from the literature search. There were 469 articles from PubMed, 15 articles from Cochrane Library, 223 articles from Embase, 1,933 articles from CINAHL, 36 articles from ERIC, 82 articles from Web of Science, 333 articles from ProQuest Central, and 323 articles from SCOPUS. There were also five gray documents retrieved from other sources. Among the 3,419 articles, 678 duplicates were excluded, and 157 were identified based on the title and abstract review. A total of 94 articles were fully reviewed by the researchers except for 63 articles without full text among 157 articles. Among them, 35 were not mobile learning, 25 were not intervention studies, 17 were single group studies without a control group, and five did not report statistical results. A total of 11 articles were finally selected and among them, 10 articles were finally available for meta-analysis. The flow diagram of the study selection process is shown in Figure 1 [Fig. 19.3 in this textbook]." (Kim & Park, 2019, pp. 22–23)

Step 8: Critical Appraisal of the Studies Included in the Review

An initial critical appraisal of methodological quality occurs during the selection of studies to be included in the systematic review (Cullen et al., 2018). Kim and Park (2019) conducted an initial assessment independently using Cochran's ROB tool to select the 10 studies

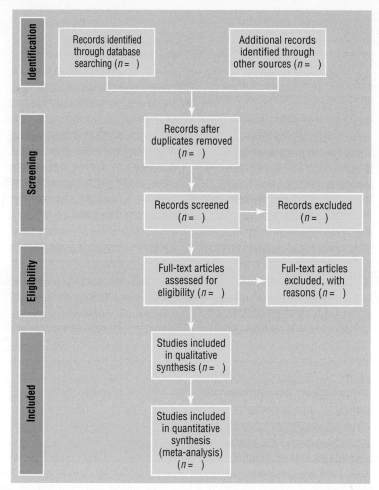

Fig. 19.2 PRISMA 2009 flow diagram. Identification, screening, eligibility, and inclusion of research sources in systematic reviews and meta-analyses. (Adapted from Moher, D., Liberati, A., Tetzlaff, J., Altman, D. G., & PRISMA Group. [2009]. *Preferred reporting items for systematic reviews and meta-analyses: The PRISMA statement*. Retrieved from http://www.prisma-statement.org.)

for the meta-analysis. Once the studies are selected, a more thorough critical appraisal takes place. This second appraisal is best accomplished by constructing a table describing the characteristics of the included studies, such as the purpose, population, sampling method, sample size, sample acceptance and attrition rates, design, intervention (independent variable), outcomes (dependent variables), measurement methods for each outcome, and major results (Higgins & Thomas, 2020; Liberati et al., 2009; Pölkki et al., 2013).

It is best if two or more experts independently review the studies and make judgments about their quality. The authors of the review contact the study investigators if it

is necessary to obtain important information about the study design or results not included in the publication. The critical appraisal of the studies reviewed is often difficult because of differences in types of participants, designs, sampling methods, intervention protocols, outcome variables and measurement methods, and presentation of results. Studies often are rank ordered based on their quality and contribution to the development of the review (Liberati et al., 2009).

Kim and Park (2019) summarized the characteristics of 11 studies that were presented in a table in the report. The critical appraisal process is briefly discussed in the following study excerpt.

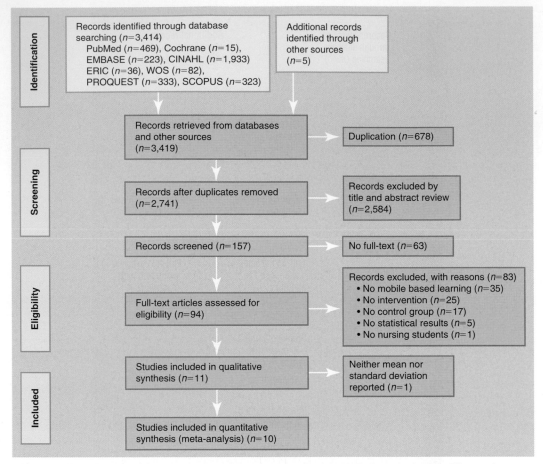

Fig. 19.3 Flow diagram of study selection. (Redrawn from Kim, J. H., & Park, H. [2019]. Effects of smartphone-based mobile learning in nursing education: A systematic review and meta-analysis. *Journal of Asian Nursing Research, 13*[1], 23.)

"Evaluation of quality of the literature
In this study, the quality of the selected studies was assessed using Cochrane's ROB tool. Evaluation items included random sequence generation, allocation concealment, blinding of study participants and personnel, blinding of outcome assessment, incomplete outcome data, selective outcome reporting, and other sources of bias. Other sources of bias were evaluated based on the provider's expertise and delivery time of smartphone-based mobile learning. Regarding the random sequence generation, 58.3% of the studies had low ROB, 33.4% had high ROB, and 8.3% had uncertain ROB due to a research method that was not presented in detail. In the allocation concealment, 41.7% had low ROB and 16.6%, uncertain ROB due to unclear

description. Regarding the blinding of study participants and personnel, 33.3% had low ROB. In the blinding of outcome assessment, 83.3% had low ROB. In the incomplete outcome data and selective outcome reporting, 66.7% had low ROB. Regarding the other sources of bias, 83.4% had low ROB." (Kim & Park, 2019, p. 23)

Step 9: Results of the Review

The results of a systematic review should include a description of the study participants, types of interventions, measurement methods, outcomes, and sometimes key study results. Kim and Park (2019) covered all these areas except measurement methods in their table of study characteristics. The results that focused on population, intervention, and outcomes are briefly presented in the following study excerpts.

Populations and settings. The participants, sample characteristics, and settings for each of the studies must be discussed and considered when synthesizing studies for systematic reviews and meta-analyses. The sample size and sampling methods are critically appraised for quality and consistency among the studies.

> "Table 1 shows characteristics of the 11 studies. All of them were published in 2011, and eight studies (72.7%) were published in the last 3 years, from 2014 to 2017. Countries of where the studies were conducted were South Korea, Taiwan, China, Spain, and Colombia. More than half of the studies (six studies) were performed in South Korea. Research participants were nursing students (11 studies)." (Kim & Park, 2019, p. 24)

Interventions in studies. Creating a table is a very efficient way to organize and summarize the results of different types of interventions. Liberati et al. (2009) recommended inclusion of the following in an intervention table summary: (1) study source; (2) structure of the intervention (stand-alone or multifaceted); (3) specific type of intervention, such as physiological treatment, education, counseling, or behavioral therapy; (4) delivery method such as demonstration and return demonstration, verbal, video, or self-administered; (5) statistical difference between the intervention and the control, standard care, placebo, or alternative intervention groups; and (6) the interventions' effect sizes.

Kim and Park's (2019) systematic review and meta-analysis focused on one intervention, the use of the smartphone as an educational delivery device. All the studies synthesized included a control or comparison groups that received traditional lecture or other conventional learning methods. "In general, smartphone-based learning was shown as a significant intervention in nursing education" (Kim & Park, 2019, p. 23).

Measurement methods and outcomes of the studies. Specific outcomes, including primary and secondary outcomes, of the studies are effectively summarized in a table. This table might include (1) the study source; (2) outcome or dependent variable, with an indication as to whether it was a primary or secondary outcome in the study; (3) measurement method used for each study

outcome; and (4) the quality of the measurement methods, such as the reliability and validity of a scale or the precision and accuracy of a physiological measure (see Chapter 16). Kim and Park (2019) identified the specific outcomes for each study included in their systematic review in a table. However, the researchers provided very limited information about the measurement methods used to assess the outcomes. Because the measurement methods were not described in this report, the quality of the outcomes cannot be appraised. The types of outcomes examined are summarized in the following excerpt.

> "The dependent variables [outcomes] that show effects of smartphone-based mobile learning were knowledge in six studies…, skills in seven studies…, confidence in performance in three studies…, learning attitude in two studies…, learning satisfaction in four studies…, cognitive load in two studies…, and self-efficacy in one study." (Kim & Park, 2019, p. 23)

Step 10: Conduct a Meta-Analysis If Appropriate

Some authors conduct a meta-analysis in the process of synthesizing sources for their systematic review (Cullen et al., 2018; Liberati et al., 2009). Because a meta-analysis involves the use of statistics to summarize the results of different studies, it usually provides strong, objective information about the effectiveness of an intervention or well-substantiated knowledge about a clinical problem. The authors of the review should provide a rationale for conducting the meta-analysis and detail the process they used. For example, the authors of a review might identify that a meta-analysis was conducted with a small group of similar studies to determine the effect of an intervention. Kim and Park (2019) conducted a meta-analysis as part of their systematic review, and the details of their meta-analysis are discussed later in this chapter.

Step 11: Discussion Section of the Review

In a systematic review or meta-analysis, discussion of the findings must include an overall evaluation of types of interventions implemented and outcomes measured in the reviewed studies. Methodological issues or limitations of the review also must be addressed. The discussion section requires a theoretical link back to the studies' frameworks to indicate the theoretical implications of the findings. Finally, the authors must present implications for research, practice, education, and policy development (see Table 19.2) (Bagnasco et al., 2014; Bettany-Saltikov, 2010b; Higgins & Thomas, 2020; Liberati et al., 2009). Kim and Park (2019) provided the following discussion of their findings, implications for research and practice, limitations, and conclusions.

"Findings

Most of the educational interventions included in this study contained relatively simpler and repetitive educational items such as exercising basic nursing skills, calculating medication dosage, and practicing communication.... By using mobile devices, users can be motivated to learn because they are familiar with the device and can learn anywhere at any time. Voluntary participation in learning has been proven to enhance the educational effect.... As a result of meta-analysis, there was an overall positive effect size for the outcome variables. They were observed to be significant in improving knowledge, skills, confidence in performance, and attitude toward learning but not in cognitive load and satisfaction with learning." (Kim & Park, 2019, pp. 26–27)

"Implications for Research and Practice

The reason that most studies were conducted on nursing students rather than on nurses is that university students are more familiar with and adept at using smartphone applications and use smartphones more effectively.... compared with nurses who work at hospitals. Nursing students also use smartphones relatively more freely and independently. However, as the number of nurses who can search for information through mobile phones and are familiar with mobile services is increasing; further research must be conducted to identify the effects of smartphone-based mobile learning on nurses...

Because the use of e-learning in nursing education had not been widely used, as a result, satisfaction with mobile learning was relatively lower than expected. Therefore, these issues must be considered in future research when planning and conducting an educational intervention that uses mobile devices." (Kim & Park, 2019, pp. 26–27)

"Limitations

The results of this study have the following limitations. It is likely that certain unpublished studies had been excluded as this study searched for and selected studies mostly in the eight databases for the systematic review

---

and meta-analysis. Therefore, the measured effect sizes might have been different from the actual number to some extent. Moreover, most of the articles included in the meta-analysis were quasi-experimental studies. As there was a lack of details regarding the period during which mobile learning was provided, there were limitations in conducting a meta-analysis of the differences in effect size depending on the intervention period. Therefore, future research must analyze the differences in effect size depending on the period of the studies, the standardization of a randomized experimental study, and the intervention period." (Kim & Park, 2019, p. 28)

"Conclusion

...The results of this study revealed that smartphone-based mobile learning was effective in improving nursing students' attitude toward learning and had a positive impact on the order of learning knowledge, skills, and confidence in learning. Considering that the ratio of smartphone-based mobile learning has been increasing and is expected to continue to rise, this study is significant in that it calculated effect sizes of mobile learning. However, certain limitations in generalizing the intervention effect must be recognized as most of the analyzed studies were quasi-experimental and not randomized trials. Therefore, future studies must conduct research pursuant to the randomized research guidelines." (Kim & Park, 2019, p. 28)

Step 12: Development of the Final Report for Publication and Step 13: Register the Research Synthesis

The final steps are the development of the systematic review and meta-analysis report for publication and the registration of the research synthesis. The report should include a title that identifies it as a systematic review and/or meta-analysis and an abstract that provides a concise summary of the review, as discussed earlier. The body of the report should include the content discussed in the previous steps and outlined in Table 19.2 (see Chapter 27 for details on publishing research reports). If the synthesis process is clearly detailed in the report, others can replicate the process and verify the findings (Higgins & Thomas, 2020; Pölkki et al., 2013). In addition, authors should register their systematic review; the most common registration system used is the International Prospective Register of Systematic Reviews (PROSPERO) (Sun et al., 2019).

The Kim and Park (2019) article indicated that a systematic review was conducted, but the major focus of this publication was the results from a meta-analysis. The publication provided extensive coverage of content consistent with the PRISMA checklist (Liberati et al., 2009), which is recognized as a quality guide for developing a systematic review or meta-analysis for publication (see http://www.prisma-statement.org).

Subsequently the PRISMA group published an additional guideline with a focus on conducting systematic reviews and meta-analyses of individual participant data (IPD) (Stewart et al. 2015). The PRISMA-IPD guideline involves collecting, checking, and reanalyzing individual-level data from studies to address a particular clinical question. The PRISMA-IPD might be considered a gold standard, since the specific participants' data from studies are reanalyzed to determine the results of a research synthesis. However, the difficulty occurs in obtaining the participants' actual data from studies while protecting their rights. More details on the PRISMA-IPD Statement can be found in the Stewart et al. (2015) article.

Critical Appraisal of a Published Systematic Review

Your critical appraisal of a systematic review focuses on whether each step of the PRISMA checklist was completed in a quality way and adhered to the questions presented in Table 19.3. You also will need to provide

TABLE 19.3 Checklist for Critically Appraising Published Systematic Reviews

Systematic Review Steps	Step Complete (Yes or No)	Comments: Quality and Rationale
1. Was the systematic review and/or meta-analysis conducted using the Preferred Reporting Items for Systematic Reviews and Meta-Analyses (PRISMA) Statement or another guideline?		
2. Were the title and abstract clearly presented?		
3. Was the clinical question clearly expressed and significant? Was the PICOS (participants, intervention, comparative interventions, outcomes, and study design) format used to develop the question and focus the review?		
4. Were the purpose and objectives or questions of the review clearly expressed and used to direct the review?		
5. Were the search criteria clearly identified? Was the PICOS format used to identify the search criteria and were the years covered and language and publication status of sources identified in the search criteria?		
6. Was a comprehensive, systematic search of the literature conducted using explicit criteria identified in step 4 of Table 19.2? Were the search strategies clearly reported with examples? Did the search include published studies, grey literature, and unpublished studies?		
7. Was the process for the selection of studies for the review clearly identified and consistently implemented? Was the selection process expressed in a flow diagram such as in Fig. 19.2?		
8. Were key elements (population, sampling process, design, intervention, outcomes, and results) of each study clearly identified and presented in a table?		
9. Was a quality critical appraisal of the studies conducted? Were the results related to participants, types of interventions, outcomes, outcome measurement methods, and risks of bias clearly discussed related to each study (i.e., in table and narrative format)?		

Continued

TABLE 19.3 **Checklist for Critically Appraising Published Systematic Reviews—cont'd**

Systematic Review Steps	Step Complete (Yes or No)	Comments: Quality and Rationale
10. Were the results of the review clearly described (i.e., in narrative and table format)? Were details of the study interventions compared and contrasted in a table? Were the outcome variables clearly identified and the quality of the measurement methods addressed?		
11. Was a meta-analysis conducted as part of the systematic review? Was a rationale provided for conducting the meta-analysis? Were the details of the meta-analysis process and results clearly described?		
12. Did the report conclude with a clear discussion section?		
a. Were the review findings summarized to identify the current best research evidence?		
b. Were the limitations of the review and how they might have affected the findings addressed?		
c. Were the implications for research, practice, education, and policy development addressed?		
13. Did the authors of the review develop a clear, concise, quality report for publication? Was the report inclusive of the items identified in the PRISMA Statement (Liberati et al., 2009)? Were sources of funding identified? Was the report registered with an appropriate organization?		

Adapted from Moher, D., Liberati, A., Tetzlaff, J., Altman, D. G., & PRISMA Group. (2009). *Preferred reporting items for systematic reviews and meta-analyses: The PRISMA statement*. Retrieved from http://www.prisma-statement.org

comments and rationale for the appraised strengths and limitations of the review. A brief critical appraisal of the Kim and Park (2019) systematic review was provided as the PRISMA steps were introduced earlier. In critically appraising systematic reviews and meta-analyses, you might use methodology articles (Bagnasco et al., 2014; Bettany-Saltikov, 2010a, 2010b; Pölkki et al., 2013; Sun et al., 2019); the Cochrane Collaboration handbook (Higgins & Thomas, 2020), the Cochrane Collaboration Library (2019), and Cochrane nursing (2019) websites; EBP texts (Dang & Dearholt, 2018; Melnyk & Fineout-Overholt, 2019) and other sources identified by your faculty advisors or experts in this area.

The critical appraisal of a systematic review or meta-analysis also includes an assessment of how current the literature synthesis is. This leads to the following question: How quickly do systematic reviews become outdated? Shojania et al. (2007) conducted a survival analysis of 100 quantitative systematic reviews published from 1995 to 2005 "to estimate the average time to changes in evidence that is sufficiently important

to warrant updating systematic reviews" (p. 224). The authors found that the average time before a systematic review should be updated was 5.5 years; however, 23% of the reviews needed updating within 2 years, and 15% in 1 year. Shojania et al. (2007) stressed that high-quality systematic reviews that were directly relevant to clinical practice require frequent updating to stay current. Numerous nursing and medical research syntheses have been conducted, so knowledge of the elements of systematic reviews and meta-analyses will assist you in critically appraising the quality of these reviews.

Conducting Meta-Analyses to Synthesize Research Evidence

A **meta-analysis** is a research synthesis strategy that involves statistically pooling the samples and results from previous studies with the same focus and research design (Kazdin, 2017). Meta-analyses provide one of the strongest levels of evidence about the effectiveness of an intervention (see Fig. 2.1) (Cooper, 2017; Higgins & Thomas, 2020). This approach has objectivity because it includes analysis techniques to determine the effect of an intervention while examining the influences of variations in the studies selected for the meta-analysis. The studies to be included in the analysis must be examined for variations or **heterogeneity** in such areas as sample characteristics, sample size, design, types of interventions, and outcomes variables and measurement methods. Meta-analysis is best conducted using studies that are more homogeneous in these areas. Heterogeneity in the studies to be included in a meta-analysis can lead to different types of biases, which are detailed in the following section (Cooper, 2017).

Statistically combining data from several studies results in a large sample size with increased power to determine the true effect of a specific intervention on a particular outcome (see Chapter 15 for discussion of power). The ultimate goal of a meta-analysis is to determine whether an intervention (1) significantly improves outcomes, (2) has minimal or no effect on outcomes, or (3) increases the risk of adverse events. Meta-analysis is also an effective way to resolve conflicting study findings and controversies that have arisen related to a selected intervention. As mentioned earlier, authors may conduct a meta-analysis as part of a systematic review that includes a group of similar studies to determine the effectiveness of an intervention.

Strong evidence for using an intervention in practice can be generated from a meta-analysis of multiple, quality studies such as RCTs and other experimental and quasi-experimental studies. However, the conduct of a meta-analysis depends on the accuracy, clarity, and completeness of information presented in individual study reports. Box 19.2 provides a list of information that should be included in intervention research reports to facilitate the conduct of a meta-analysis (Conn & Rantz, 2003; Cooper, 2017).

The steps for conducting a meta-analysis are similar to the steps for conducting a systematic review that were detailed in the previous section. The PRISMA Statement introduced earlier provides clear directions for developing a report for either a systematic review and/or a meta-analysis (see Table 19.2) (Moher et al., 2009). The following information is provided to increase your ability to appraise critically meta-analysis studies and to conduct a meta-analysis for a selected intervention (Andrel, Keith, & Leiby, 2009; Conn & Rantz, 2003; Cooper, 2017; Higgins & Thomas, 2020; Moore, 2012; Noordzij, Hooft, Dekker, Zoccali, & Jager, 2009; Turlik,

---

> **BOX 19.2 Recommended Reporting in Research Publications to Facilitate Meta-Analyses**
>
> **Demographic Variables Relevant to Population Studied**
> Age
> Gender
> Marital status
> Ethnicity
> Education
> Socioeconomic status
>
> **Methodological Characteristics**
> Sample size (experimental and control group sizes)
> Type of sampling method
> Sampling refusal rate and attrition rate
> Sample characteristics
> Research design
> Groups included in study—experimental, control, comparison, placebo groups
> Intervention protocol and fidelity discussion
> Data collection techniques
> Outcome measurements
> Reliability and validity of instruments
> Precision and accuracy of physiological measures
>
> **Data Analysis**
> Name of statistical tests
> Sample size for each statistical test
> Degrees of freedom for each statistical test
> Exact value of each statistical test
> Exact p value for each statistic test
> One-tailed or two-tailed statistical test
> Measures of central tendency (mean, median, and mode)
> Measures of dispersion (range, standard deviation)
> Post hoc test values for ANOVA (analysis of variance) test of three or more groups

2010) The meta-analysis by Kim and Park (2019), discussed earlier, focusing on the effects of smartphone-based mobile learning is presented again as an example.

Clinical Question for a Meta-Analysis

The clinical question developed for a meta-analysis is usually clearly focused as: "What is the effectiveness of a selected intervention?" The PICOS (see Box 19.1) format discussed earlier might be used to generate the clinical question (Moher et al., 2009). Kim and Park (2019) used a PICOS format to guide both their systematic review and meta-analysis.

Purpose and Questions to Direct a Meta-Analysis

Researchers must identify clearly the purpose of their meta-analysis and the questions or objectives that guide the analysis. The Cochrane Collaboration identified the following four basic questions to guide a meta-analysis to determine the effect of an intervention:

1. What is the direction of effect?
2. What is the size of effect?
3. Is the effect consistent across studies?
4. What is the strength of evidence for the effect? (Higgins & Thomas, 2020)

As discussed earlier, the meta-analysis by Kim and Park (2019) was guided by a specific research purpose that identified the foci of both the systematic review and the meta-analysis. "The purpose of this study is to confirm the general characteristics (study design, setting, sample size, intervention, outcome variables, and so on) of the selected studies, by examining systematically the previous studies that evaluated the effects of smartphone-based mobile learning on nursing education and to analyze the effects of smartphone-based mobile learning by presenting the effect size of the intervention through a meta-analysis" (Kim & Park, 2019, p. 21).

Search Criteria and Strategies for Meta-Analyses

The methods for identifying search criteria and selecting search strategies are similar for meta-analyses and systematic reviews. The search criteria usually are narrowly focused for a meta-analysis to identify selective studies examining the effect of a particular intervention. The search needs to be rigorous and include published sources identified through varied databases and unpublished studies and other grey literature identified through other types of searches (Melnyk & Fineout-Overholt, 2019).

The PICOS criteria were used by Kim and Park (2019) to guide the search for studies to include in the meta-analysis. The PICOS criteria and search strategies for the Kim and Park (2019) syntheses were presented in the previous section on systematic reviews. Eleven studies were critically appraised. (See Fig. 19.3 for details of the study selection process of the 10 studies for the meta-analysis, however, noting only 9 studies were included in the final analysis process.)

Possible Biases for Meta-Analyses and Systematic Reviews

Even with rigorous literature searches, authors of meta-analyses and systematic reviews are often limited primarily to published studies. The nature of the sources can lead to biases and flawed or inaccurate conclusions in the research syntheses. The common biases that can occur in conducting and reporting research syntheses include **publication bias**, such as time lag bias, location bias, duplicate publication bias, citation bias, and language bias; bias from poor study methodology; and outcome reporting bias. Publication bias occurs because studies with positive results are more likely to be published than studies with negative or inconclusive results. Higgins and Thomas (2020) reported that the odds were four times greater that positive study results would be published by researchers versus negative results. **Time-lag bias**, a type of publication bias, occurs because studies with negative results are usually published later, sometimes 2 to 3 years later, than studies with positive results. Sometimes studies with negative results are not published at all, whereas studies with positive results might be published more than once (**duplicate publication bias**). **Location bias** can occur if studies are published in lower impact journals and indexed in less-searched databases. A special case of location bias is dissertation research, which is often omitted from systematic reviews and meta-analyses because of the difficulty or cost involved in accessing them and the variations in the quality of the research. However, access to dissertations has improved with the full text of some being available online. Accessing dissertations is important because their findings may represent the most current research to date in an area. A **citation bias** occurs when certain studies are cited more often than others and are more likely to be identified in database searches. **Language bias** can occur if searches focus on studies in English, and important studies exist in other languages (Cooper, 2017).

Biases in studies' methodologies often are related to design and data analysis problems. The strengths and threats to design validity should be examined during critical appraisal of the studies for inclusion in a meta-analysis or systematic review (see Chapters 10 and 11 for discussion of design validity). The analyses conducted in studies need to be appropriate and complete (see Chapters 21, 22, 23, 24, and 25 on data analysis). **Outcome reporting bias** occurs when study results are not reported clearly and with complete accuracy. For example, reporting bias occurs when researchers selectively report positive results and not negative results;

or positive results might be addressed in detail with limited discussion of negative results. Higgins and Thomas (2020) provided a detailed discussion of potential biases in systematic reviews and meta-analyses.

An analysis method called the **funnel plot** can be used to assess for biases in a group of studies. Funnel plots provide graphic representations of possible effect sizes (*ESs*) or odds ratios for interventions in selected studies. To calculate the *ES* or strength of an intervention in a study, determine the difference between the experimental and control groups for the outcome measured. The mean difference between the experimental and control groups for several studies is easily determined if the outcome is measured by the same scale or instrument in each study (see Chapter 15 for calculation of *ES*). However, the **standardized mean difference** (SMD) must be calculated in a meta-analysis when the same outcome, such as learning satisfaction, is measured by different scales or methods.

Fig. 19.4 shows an example funnel plot of the SMDs from 13 individual studies. The SMDs from these particular studies are quite symmetrical and equally divided by the line through the middle of the funnel in the graph. A symmetrical funnel plot indicates little publication bias. Asymmetry of the funnel plot is widely thought to be the result of publication bias, but may also be the result of methodological bias, reporting bias, heterogeneity in individual studies' sample size or in research interventions, or chance (Cooper, 2017; Egger, Smith, Schneider, & Minder, 1997). In Fig. 19.4, studies with small sample sizes are toward the bottom of the graph, and studies with larger samples are toward the top. Kim and Park (2019) included a funnel plot of SMD and discussed the risk of publication bias in the following excerpt.

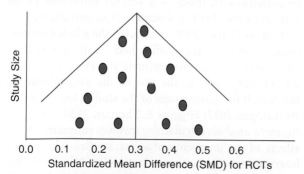

Fig. 19.4 Funnel plot of standardized mean differences (SMDs) for randomized controlled trials (RCTs) with limited bias.

> "*Publication bias*
> Figure 3 [Fig. 19.5 in this textbook] presents results of the publication bias analysis through the funnel plot, which showed a slight asymmetry. Egger's regression test was also used to evaluate publication bias and concluded that asymmetry existed in the funnel plot ($t = 3.08$, $df = 22$, $p = .005$). Therefore, trim-and-fill method was also assessed for checking publication bias. After filling five effect sizes to the left of the funnel plot, the corrected total mean effect size (*g*) was 0.63 (95% [confidence interval] CI: 0.17-1.09), which was still statistically significant. After conducting trim-and-fill method, Egger's regression test concluded that symmetry existed in the funnel plot ($t = -0.01$, $df = 27$, $p = .993$). The corrected total mean effect size was smaller than the overall mean effect size of 1.12 measured in 10 studies." (Kim & Park, 2019, p. 26)

Kim and Park's (2019) funnel plot showed asymmetry so a method called "trim and fill" was implemented. The asymmetry was thought to be due to limitations of the literature search and the researchers' removal of certain studies from the final meta-analysis. The trim-and-fill method provides ways to estimate the values of missing studies (see Fig. 19.5). With the addition of the missing effect sizes, the funnel plot was determined to be symmetrical, meaning there was no significant publication bias. This text just introduces funnel plots, so we encourage you to read additional sources to expand your understanding when conducting a meta-analysis (Cooper, 2017; Higgins & Thomas, 2020).

Results of Meta-Analysis for Continuous Outcomes

Many nursing studies examine continuous outcomes or outcomes that are measured by methods that produce interval or ratio level data (see Chapter 16). Physiological measures to examine blood pressure (BP) produce ratio level data. Likert scales, such as those to measure learning satisfaction, are considered to be interval level data (Grove & Cipher, 2020). The BP and learning satisfaction are considered continuous outcomes, and the data are analyzed with parametric statistics. Meta-analysis includes a two-step process: Step 1 is the calculation of a summary statistic for each study to describe the intervention effect, and step 2 is the summary (pooled) intervention effect that is the weighted average of the intervention effects, derived from the values of

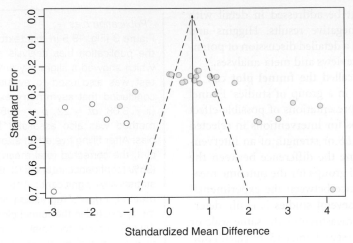

Fig. 19.5 Funnel plots of standard error by standardized mean difference with five effect size estimates added by the trim-and-fill analysis (open symbols). (Redrawn from Kim, J. H., & Park, H. [2019]. Effects of smartphone-based mobile learning in nursing education: A systematic review and meta-analysis. *Journal of Asian Nursing Research, 13*[1], 27.)

different studies. In step 1, to determine the effect of an intervention on continuous outcomes, the mean difference between two groups is calculated. The **mean difference** is a standard statistic that is calculated to determine the absolute difference between two groups. It is an estimate of the amount of change caused by the intervention (smartphone) on the outcomes (e.g., cognitive load, confidence in performance, knowledge, learning attitude, learning satisfaction, and skill) on average compared with the control groups, which included traditional lecture or other conventional learning methods. The mean difference can be calculated to determine the effect of an intervention only if the outcome is measured by the same scale in all of the studies (Higgins & Thomas, 2020).

SMD, or *d*, is used in studies as a summary statistic and is calculated in a meta-analysis when the same outcome is measured by different scales or methods across studies. The SMD is also sometimes referred to as the standardized mean effect size. Studies that have differences in means in the same proportion to the standard deviations have the same SMD *(d)* regardless of the scales used to measure the outcome variable. The differences in the means and standard deviations in the studies are assumed to be due to the measurement scales, not variability in the outcome (Higgins & Thomas,

2020). The SMD is calculated by meta-analysis software, and the formula is provided as follows:

$$SMD \ (d) = \frac{\text{difference in mean outcome between groups}}{\text{standard deviation of outcome among participants}}$$

Kim and Park (2019) did not provide information on the measurement methods of the studies included in their meta-analysis, so the quality of these methods cannot be assessed. The six outcomes were probably measured with Likert scales or other types of scales or questionnaires. Omitting the descriptions of the measurement methods is a serious limitation of the Kim and Park (2019) publication (Cooper, 2017).

Kim and Park (2019) conducted the *g* index formula because some of the studies had small sample sizes. The *d* index would overestimate the effect size of the intervention, such as the use of the smartphone for learning, if the sample sizes of the studies were less than 20 (Cooper, 2017; Higgins & Thomas, 2020). Step 2 of the meta-analysis calculations involves summarizing the effects of an intervention across studies. The pooled intervention effect estimate is calculated as a weighted average of the intervention effects estimated for the individual studies. A weighted average is defined by Higgins and Thomas (2020) as:

$$\text{Weighted average} = \frac{\text{sum of (estimate} \times \text{weight)}}{\text{sum of weights}}$$

In combining intervention effect estimates across studies, a random effects meta-analysis model or fixed effect meta-analysis model can be used. The assumption of using the **random effects model** is that all of the studies are not estimating the same intervention effect but rather related effects over studies that follow a distribution across studies. Kim and Park (2019) conducted the random effects model. When each study is estimating the exact same quality, a **fixed effects model** is used. Meta-analysis results can be obtained using software from SPSS and SAS statistical packages (see Chapter 21). Cochrane Collaboration Review Manager (RevMan) software can be used for conducting meta-analyses. This chapter provides a limited discussion of key ideas related to conducting meta-analyses, and you are encouraged to review Higgins and Thomas (2020) and other meta-analysis sources to increase your understanding of this process (Andrel et al., 2009; Cooper, 2017; Moore, 2012; Turlik, 2010). We also recommend the assistance of a statistician in conducting these analyses. The effects of the smartphone-based mobile learning intervention are presented in the following study excerpt using the *g* index for small samples.

"Figure 2 [Fig. 19.6 in this textbook] shows effects of smartphone-based mobile learning on nursing education. Forest plots were constructed for each outcome using the standardized mean effect size measured by the random effect model. Six outcomes were included in the meta-analysis: cognitive load, confidence in performance, knowledge, learning attitude, learning satisfaction, and skill. In general, smartphone-based mobile learning was shown as a significant intervention in nursing education; the total effect size of the intervention was *g* = 1.12 (95% CI: 0.72-1.52). The intervention lowered the cognitive load; however, group difference at postintervention was not statistically significant [*g* = −1.01 (95% CI: −2.32 ~ 0.31)]. At postintervention, there was a significant group difference in confidence in performance [*g* = 1.52 (95% CI: 0.46 ~ 2.58)]. There

were seven studies which examined that the effect intervention on knowledge and group difference was significant and large at postintervention [*g* = 1.47 (95% CI: 0.71 ~ 2.24)]. Regarding learning attitude, there was a significant group difference at postintervention [*g* = 1.69 (95% CI: 0.35 to 3.02)]. At postintervention, there was no significant group difference in learning satisfaction [*g* = 0.53 (95% CI: −0.38 ~ 1.44)]. There were seven studies which examined the effect intervention on skill and group difference was significant and large at postintervention [*g* = 1.41 (95% CI: 0.72 ~ 2.11)]." (Kim & Park, 2019, pp. 23, 25–26)

This meta-analysis supports the use of the smartphone-based mobile learning intervention in nursing education. Four of the six outcomes were statistically significant with the use of this intervention, but cognitive load and learning satisfaction were nonsignificant. Stronger studies, such as RCTs, are needed to examine the effect of this intervention in nursing education and in clinical practice. Additional findings from the Kim and Park (2019) synthesis was presented in the previous section focused on systematic review. The limitations, implications for research and practice, and conclusions were also presented earlier.

Results of a Meta-Analysis for Dichotomous Outcomes

When dichotomous outcome data are examined in a meta-analysis, risk ratios, odds ratio, and risk differences usually are calculated to determine the effect of the intervention on the measured outcome. These terms are introduced in this chapter, but more information is available in Cooper (2017), Higgins and Thomas (2020), and Straus et al. (2011). With dichotomous data, every participant will fit into one of two categories, such as clinical improvement versus no clinical improvement, effective versus ineffective screening device, or alive versus dead. **Risk ratio** *(RR)*, also called **relative risk**, is the ratio of the risk of subjects in the intervention group to the risk of subjects in the control group for having a particular health outcome. The intervention group might also be referred to as the exposed group and the control group as the unexposed group in some studies. The health outcome is usually adverse, such as the risk of a disease (e.g., cancer) or the risk of complications or

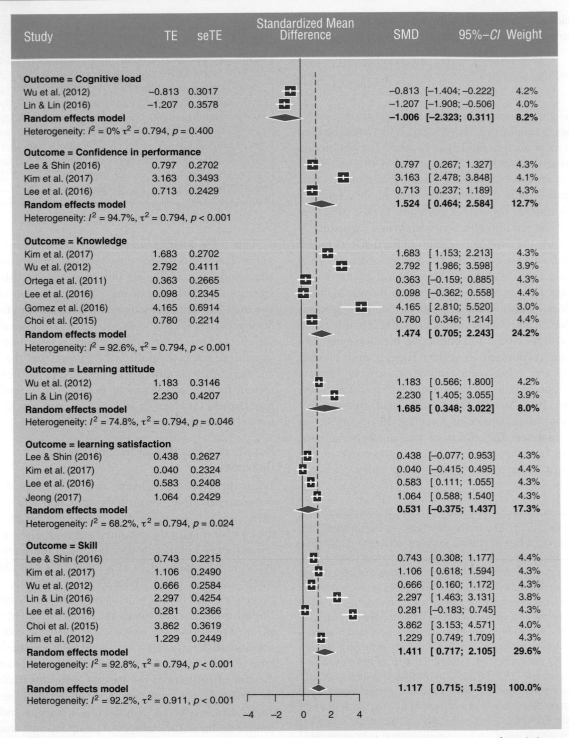

Fig. 19.6 Effects of smartphone-based mobile learning in nursing education. *CI,* Confidence interval; I^2, statistic for heterogeneity in studies included in meta-analysis; *SMD,* standardized mean difference. (Redrawn from Kim, J. H., & Park, H. [2019]. Effects of smartphone-based mobile learning in nursing education: A systematic review and meta-analysis. *Journal of Asian Nursing Research, 13*[1], 25.)

death (Grove & Cipher, 2020; Higgins & Thomas, 2020). The calculation for *RR* is:

$$\text{Relative risk } (RR) = \frac{\text{risk of event in experimental group}}{\text{risk of event in control group}}$$

The **odds ratio** *(OR)* is defined as the ratio of the odds of an event occurring in one group, such as the treatment group, to the odds of it occurring in another group, such as the standard care group (Grove & Cipher, 2020; King & Eckersley, 2019). The *OR* is a way of comparing whether two groups have the same odds of a certain event's occurrence (see Chapter 24). An example is the odds of medication adherence or nonadherence for an experimental group receiving an intervention of education and specialized medication packaging intervention versus a group receiving standard care. The calculation for *OR* is:

$$\text{Odds ratio } (OR) = \frac{\text{odds of event in experimental group}}{\text{odds of event in control or comparison group}}$$

The **risk difference** *(RD)*, also called the **absolute risk reduction**, is the risk of an event in the experimental group minus the risk of the event in the control or standard care group.

$$\text{Risk difference } (RD) = \text{risk for experimental group} - \text{risk for control group}$$

Funnel plots are used to examine publication bias in studies with dichotomous outcomes as well as continuous outcomes (see Fig. 19.5). Fig. 19.7 includes two example funnel plots for dichotomous outcomes, with the plot in Fig. 19.7A showing symmetry. An unbiased sample of studies should appear basically symmetrical in the funnel with the *OR*s of the studies fairly equally divided on either side of the line (see Chapter 24 for calculating *OR*). The funnel plot shown in Fig. 19.7B demonstrates asymmetry with possible publication bias in favor of larger studies with positive results when the studies having smaller effect and sample sizes are removed. This collection of studies in a meta-analysis could lead to the conclusion that a treatment was effective when it might not be when looking at a larger

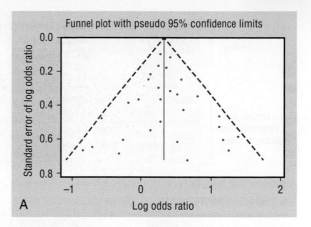

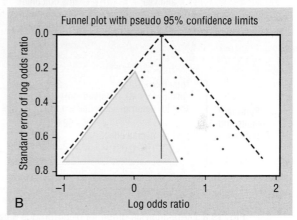

Fig. 19.7 A and B, Funnel plots examining publication bias. The green triangle in B emphasizes the asymmetry of this funnel plot. (Adapted from Androl, J. A., Keith, S. W., & Leiby, B. F. [2009]. Meta-analysis: A brief introduction. *Clinical & Translational Science, 2*[5], 376.)

collection of studies with negative and positive results as in the plot in Fig. 19.7A.

Meta-analysis results from studies with dichotomous data are often presented using a forest plot. Fig. 19.8 provides a format for presenting a forest plot in a meta-analysis study (Fernandez & Tran, 2009). A forest plot usually includes the following information: (1) author, year, and name of the study; (2) raw data from the intervention and control groups and total number in each group; (3) point estimate (*OR* or *RR*) and *CI*) for each study shown as a line and block on the graph; (4) numerical values for point estimate (*OR* or *RR*) and *CI* for each study; and (5) percent weights given to each study (Fernandez & Tran, 2009; Higgins & Thomas, 2020). In

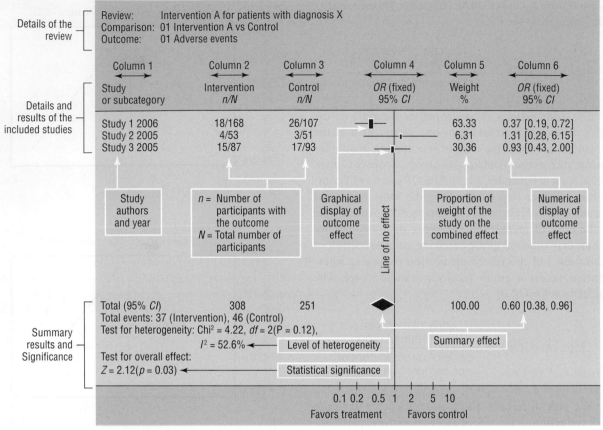

Fig. 19.8 Meta-analysis graph for dichotomous data. *CI,* Confidence interval; *OR,* odds ratio. (Adapted from Fernandez, R. S., & Tran, D. T. [2009]. The meta-analysis graph: Clearing the haze. *Clinical Nurse Specialist,* 23[2], 58.)

Fig. 19.8, column 1 identifies each of the studies using the clearest format for the studies being analyzed. Column 2 includes the number of participants with the outcome *(n)* and total number of participants in the intervention or experimental group *(N),* expressed as *n/N.* Column 3 includes the number of participants who displayed the outcome and the total number in the control group. Column 4 graphically presents the *OR* with a block and the 95% *CI* with a line. Column 5 displays the percent weights given to each of the three studies in this example. Column 6 shows the numerical values for the *OR* and 95% *CI.*

The bottom of the forest plot in Fig. 19.8 provides a summary of results and significance, including total events for intervention and control groups, a test for heterogeneity, and a test for overall effect. The unlabeled

line at the very bottom represents the *OR.* The scale of the line is logarithmic, not arithmetic. The large diamond in the plot is the summary of the effect of the studies included in the analysis. If the diamond is situated to the left of the line that is positioned at 1, the results favor the intervention or treatment. The *CI* does not include 1 if the results are statistically significant (Fernandez & Tran, 2009). The point estimates in Fig. 19.8 are consistently more on one side of the vertical line, which demonstrates homogeneity of the studies.

If the point estimates are fairly equally distributed on both the left and right sides of the vertical line, this shows heterogeneity of the studies included in the meta-analysis. Heterogeneity, introduced earlier, can exist in the sample size and characteristics, types of an intervention, designs, and outcomes of the studies. Heterogeneity statistics for random effects meta-analyses include chi-square tests (see Chapter 25), the I^2, and a test for differences across subgroups when it is appropriate (Higgins & Thomas, 2020). I^2 is a statistic that measures the inconsistency of studies that cannot be explained by chance. An I^2 of 25% indicates the studies are homogeneous and can be combined in a meta-analysis (Fernandez & Trans, 2009).

Magnus, Ping, Shen, Bourgeois, and Magnus (2011) conducted a meta-analysis of the effectiveness of mammography screening in reducing breast cancer mortality in women 39 to 49 years of age. Because mammography screening is significant in reducing breast cancer mortality of women older than 50 years and early detection of breast cancer increases survival, annual routine mammography screening has been recommended for all women age 40 to 47 years in the United States. Thus the "primary aim of the current study was, after a quality assessment of identified randomized controlled trials (RCTs), to conduct a meta-analysis of the effectiveness of mammography screening [intervention] in women ages 39–49 years [population] in reducing breast cancer mortality [dichotomous outcome]. The second aim was to compare and discuss the results of previously published meta-analyses" (Magnus et al., 2011, p. 845).

The following content briefly describes the methods and results of the meta-analysis conducted by Magnus et al. (2011). Several databases, such as PubMed/MEDLINE, OVID, COCHRANE, and Educational Resources Information Center (ERIC), were searched for relevant studies. To identify unpublished and ongoing research, dissertation and clinical trials databases were searched. The studies were assessed by two independent reviewers and nine RCTs met the eligibility criteria for inclusion in the meta-analysis. The studies were limited to English language and included data focused only on women 39–49 years of age. The studies also reported relative risk (RR)/odds ratio (OR) or frequency data. The RCTs were assessed for quality and essential data were extracted using predefined forms. "The seven RCTs with the highest quality score were combined, and a significant pooled RR estimate of 0.83 (95% confidence interval [CI] 0.72–0.97) was calculated" (Magnus et al., 2011, p. 845).

The results of the study were graphically represented using a forest plot (Fig. 19.9). The plot clearly identifies the names of the seven studies included in the meta-analysis on the left side of the figure. The RR and CI for each study are identified with a block and horizontal line. The numerical RR and 95% CI values are identified on the right side of the plot with the percent of weight given to each study. Most of the studies show homogeneity with ORs left of the vertical line except for the Stockholm study. The forest plot would have been strengthened by including the results from the test for heterogeneity and the test for overall effect. Magnus et al. (2011) concluded, "Mammography screenings were effective and generate a 17% reduction in breast cancer mortality in women 39–49 years of age. The quality of the trials varies, and providers should inform women in this age group about the positive and negative aspects of mammography screenings" (p. 845).

Conducting a Metasynthesis of Qualitative Research

Qualitative research synthesis is the process and product of systematically reviewing and formally interpreting and integrating the findings from qualitative studies (Bergdahl, 2019; France et al., 2019; Whittemore et al., 2014). Various synthesis methods for qualitative research have appeared in the literature, such as metasynthesis, metaethnography, qualitative metasummary, qualitative systematic review, and meta-aggregation (Barnett-Page & Thomas, 2009; Bergdahl, 2019; Butler, Hall, & Copnell, 2016; France et al., 2019; Sandelowski & Barroso, 2007; Walsh & Downe, 2005). Qualitative researchers disagree about the best method to use for synthesizing qualitative research or whether a single synthesis method would suffice. Although the methodology is not clearly developed for qualitative research synthesis, researchers recognize the importance of summarizing qualitative findings to generate important knowledge for practice and policy development (Beck, 2009; Bergdahl, 2019; Butler et al., 2016; France et al., 2019; Sandelowski & Barroso, 2007). Within the Cochrane Collaboration, the Cochrane Qualitative and Implementation Methods Group has been formed for the discussion and development of synthesis methodology in the area of qualitative research (Higgins & Thomas, 2020).

Currently most of the syntheses of qualitative research in the literature are identified as a metasynthesis. Methodological articles have been published to describe the process for conducting a metasynthesis, but this synthesis process is still evolving (Butler et al., 2016; France, Cunningham, et al., 2019). However, metaethnography has growing acceptance as a quality methodology for

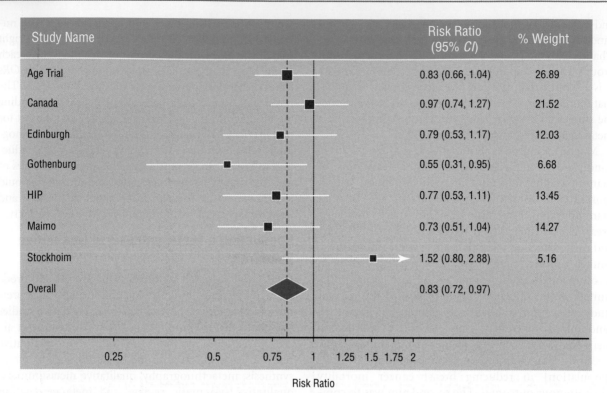

Fig. 19.9 Forest plot showing the individual randomized controlled trials and the overall pooled estimate from the seven original randomized controlled trials with a high-quality score addressing the impact of mammography screening on breast cancer mortality in women 39 to 49 years old. *CI*, Confidence interval. (Redrawn from Magnus, M. C., Ping, M., Shen, M. M., Bourgeois, J., & Magnus, J. H. [2011]. Effectiveness of mammography screening in reducing breast cancer mortality in women aged 39-49 years: A meta-analysis. *Journal of Women's Health, 20*[6], 848.)

promoting the completeness and clarity in the reporting of qualitative syntheses (France, Uny, et al., 2019). In this text, **metasynthesis** is defined as the systematic compilation, integration, and translation of qualitative study results using different conceptual views to consolidate knowledge of fundamental importance to nursing (Bergdahl, 2019). Therefore the focus is on interpretation rather than the combining of study results as with quantitative research synthesis. Metasynthesis involves the breaking down of findings from different studies to discover essential features and then the combining of these ideas into a unique, transformed whole. According to Sandelowski and Barroso (2007), a **metasummary** is a step in conducting metasynthesis that involves summarizing findings across qualitative reports to identify knowledge in a selected area. Metasummary is similar to meta-aggregation in summarizing

qualitative research findings and is not comprehensive enough to use in synthesizing knowledge to advance nursing science (Bergdahl, 2019).

A metasynthesis conducted by Luchsinger, Jones, McFarland, and Kissler (2019) to examine the nurse/patient relationships in care coordination is presented as an example. Metaethnography is the methodology used to develop and report this metasynthesis. Metaethnography was initially developed by Noblit and Hare (1988) for synthesizing qualitative studies. The seven phases for conducting a metaethnography are highlighted in Box 19.3. France, Cunningham, et al. (2019) provided detailed steps to conduct for each of the seven phases in Table 19.4. This table was developed to provide reporting guidance for researchers publishing a metaethnography of qualitative studies.

BOX 19.3 **Phases Guiding Metaethnography in Conducting a Metasynthesis**

Phase 1: Selecting metaethnography and getting started
Phase 2: Deciding what is relevant
Phase 3: Reading included studies
Phase 4: Determining how studies are related
Phase 5: Translating studies into one another
Phase 6: Synthesizing translations
Phase 7: Expressing the synthesis

Phase 1: Selecting Metaethnography and Getting Started

Initially, researchers identify the gap in nursing knowledge that needs to be filled. The focus, scope, and aims are then developed to address this gap in the knowledge base. The focus of the metasynthesis is usually an important area of interest for the individuals conducting it and is a topic with an adequate body of qualitative studies. The scope of a metasynthesis is an area of debate, with some qualitative researchers recommending a narrow, precise approach and others recommending a broader, more inclusive approach. Research questions or aims are formulated to guide the metasynthesis that is facilitated by the authors' research and clinical expertise, initial review of the relevant qualitative literature, and discussion with expert qualitative researchers (see Table 19.4) (Butler et al., 2016; France, Cunningham, et al., 2019).

Luchsinger et al. (2019) recognized the importance of nurses and nursing care to patient outcomes. Currently coordination of care research is heavily focused on quality outcomes. "For this meta-synthesis, the concepts of care coordination and nurse dose were combined into a construct called *coordinated nurse-patient relationships*" (Luchsinger et al., 2019, p. 42). Donabedian's (2005) systems theory approach to quality, including the three constructs of structure, process, and outcomes, was used to organize research findings.

TABLE 19.4 **The eMERG Meta-Ethnography Reporting Guidance**

No.	Criteria Headings	Reporting Criteria
Phase 1—Selecting Meta-ethnography and Getting Started		
Introduction		
1	Rationale and context for the meta-ethnography	Describe the gap in research or knowledge to be filled by the meta-ethnography and the wider context of the meta-ethnography
2	Aim(s) of the meta-ethnography	Describe the meta-ethnography aim(s)
3	Focus of the meta-ethnography	Describe the meta-ethnography review question(s) (or objectives)
4	Rationale for using meta-ethnography	Explain why meta-ethnography was considered the most appropriate qualitative synthesis methodology
Phase 2—Deciding What Is Relevant		
Methods		
5	Search strategy	Describe the rationale for the literature search strategy
6	Search processes	Describe how the literature searching was carried out and by whom
7	Selecting primary studies	Describe the process of study screening and selection and who was involved
Findings		
8	Outcome of study selection	Describe the results of study searches and screening
Phase 3—Reading Included Studies		
Methods		
9	Reading and data extraction approach	Describe the reading and data extraction method and processes

Continued

TABLE 19.4   The eMERG Meta-Ethnography Reporting Guidance—cont'd

No.	Criteria Headings	Reporting Criteria
Findings		
10	Presenting characteristics of included studies	Describe characteristics of the included studies
Phase 4—Determining How Studies Are Related		
Methods		
11	Process for determining how studies are related	Describe the methods and processes for determining how the included studies are related: • Which aspects of studies were compared AND • How the studies were compared
Findings		
12	Outcome of relating studies	Describe how studies relate to each other
Phase 5—Translating Studies Into One Another		
Methods		
13	Process of translating studies	Describe the methods of translation: • Describe steps taken to preserve the context and meaning of the relationships between concepts within and across studies • Describe how the reciprocal and refutational translations were conducted • Describe how potential alternative interpretations or explanations were considered in the translations
Findings		
14	Outcome of translation	Describe the interpretive findings of the translation
Phase 6—Synthesizing Translations		
Methods		
15	Synthesis process	Describe the methods used to develop overarching concepts ("synthesized translations") Describe how potential alternative interpretations or explanations were considered in the synthesis
Findings		
16	Outcome of synthesis process	Describe the new theory, conceptual framework, model, configuration, or interpretation of data developed from the synthesis
Phase 7—Expressing the Synthesis		
Discussion		
17	Summary of findings	Summarize the main interpretive findings of the translation and synthesis and compare them to existing literature
18	Strengths, limitations, and reflexivity	Reflect on and describe the strengths and limitations of the synthesis: • Methodological aspects—for example, describe how the synthesis findings were influenced by the nature of the included studies and how the meta-ethnography was conducted • Reflexivity—for example, the impact of the research team on the synthesis findings
19	Recommendations and conclusions	Describe the implications of the synthesis

From France, Cunningham, et al. (2019). Improving reporting of meta-ethnography: The eMERGe reporting guidance. *Psycho-Oncology, 28*, 452.

Luchsinger et al. (2019) identified the following purpose and research question to guide their synthesis of qualitative research.

> "Purpose
>
> The aim of the study was to synthesize the available qualitative literature on coordinated nurse patient relationships and explore the encounter from the perspective of nurses and patients in the care coordination experience.
>
> Research question
>
> Coordinated nurse patient relationships: What does a coordinated nurse patient relationship look like, using a systems theory approach from the perspective of nurses and patients in the care coordination experience? A systems theory approach (Donabedian, 2005) was used to synthesize the available qualitative literature on coordinated nurse/patient and caregiver relationships in the care coordination experience." (Luchsinger et al., 2019, p. 42)

Phases 2, 3, and 4: Designing a Multistage Literature Review Process

Most authors agree that a rigorous search of the literature needs to be conducted. Using metaethnography, the literature search includes phase 2, deciding what is relevant; phase 3, reading included studies; and phase 4, determining how studies are related (France, Cunningham, 2019; Noblit & Hare, 1988). The search should include databases, books, book chapters, and full reports of theses and dissertations. Special search strategies that were identified earlier must be engaged to identify grey literature because qualitative studies might be published in more obscure journals. The search criteria need to identify the years of the search, keywords to be searched, and language of sources. Metasyntheses usually are limited to qualitative studies only and do not include mixed method studies (Butler et al., 2016; Creswell & Creswell, 2018; France, Cunningham, et al., 2019; Walsh & Downe, 2005). Also, qualitative findings that have not been interpreted but are unanalyzed quotes, field notes, case histories, stories, or poems usually are excluded (Finfgeld-Connett, 2010). The search process is very fluid with the conduct of additional computerized and hand searches to identify more studies. However, it is important for researchers to document systematically the strategies that they used to search the literature and the sources found through these different search strategies.

The authors of a metasynthesis determine which studies are relevant based on the research questions or aims directing the synthesis. The studies are read, critically appraised, and data extracted during the review process (see Table 19.4). A flow diagram (similar to Fig. 19.2) is useful in identifying the process for selecting studies and determining how the studies' results are related to each other (France, Cunningham, et al., 2019). Luchsinger et al. (2019) provided the following description of their literature search, search criteria, and selection of studies for their metasynthesis. They used a PRISMA diagram to document their literature search process (see Fig. 19.2).

> "Databases were searched for qualitative studies published in English concerning nurse-patient relationships in care coordination and included CINAHL, Cochrane Library, Embase and PubMed. Key words searched included: (1) nurse patient relationships, and (2) transitions of care OR, nurse care coordination, and (3) qualitative. A ten-year limit was applied (2008–2018) to increase the sample size. After duplicates were removed, 159 articles were retrieved. Criteria for inclusion into the meta-synthesis were qualitative studies with content or applicability to adult patients, care coordination, care management, case management, and nursing care. The exclusion elements included content primarily focused on pediatrics, behavioral/mental health, oncology, and drug therapy. After inclusion and exclusion criteria were initially applied through title/abstract review, 67 publications remained. Two additional title/abstract reviews were conducted by the author on the literature for in-depth inclusion/exclusion criteria and an additional 56 publications were discarded from the sample, leaving 11 studies." (Luchsinger et al., 2019, p. 42)

Phase 5: Translating Studies Into One Another

Phase 5 of translating studies into one another includes a discussion of who is doing the translations and what steps are taken to "preserve the context and meaning of the relationships between concepts within and across studies" (France, Cunningham, et al., 2019, p. 452) (see Table 19.4). During this phase alternative interpretations or explanations are considered. Sometimes a table is developed as part of this comparison and translation of study findings, but this is also an area of debate. The table headings might include (1) author and year of source, (2) purpose or aim of the study, (3) design, (4), methodological orientation, (5) participants, (6) summary of findings, and (7) other key content relevant for comparison. This table provides a display of relevant study elements to facilitate the comparison and translation of study elements (Butler et al., 2016; France, Cunningham, et al., 2019; Sandelowski & Barroso, 2007; Walsh & Downe, 2005). The **comparative analysis** of studies involves examining methodology and findings across studies for similarities and differences. The frequency of similar findings might be recorded. The differences or contradictions in studies should be resolved or explained (or both). Varied analysis techniques often are used by the researchers to translate the findings of the different studies into a new or unique description (France, Cunningham, et al., 2019).

Luchsinger et al. (2019) detailed their steps for assessing, comparing, and translating qualitative study aspects as part of their synthesis process. They also developed a comparative analysis table of the studies included in their metasynthesis. The following excerpt briefly presents the data immersion and the findings from their translation of qualitative studies.

"The first step of a qualitative meta-synthesis is data immersion using a critical review tool. A team of four researchers independently completed a formal critical analysis of the eleven qualitative studies using a quality appraisal tool.... The research team utilized the tool to evaluate 17 domains of quality based on study design, qualitative methodology, sampling, data collection, data analysis, and credibility.... All research team members independently rated each study and then met via multiple video conferences to review the ratings and resolve any differences through group discussion until consensus was achieved. The full research team agreed that three studies did not provide enough data or did not provide enough detail to interpret and understand the qualitative study and were excluded from the final sample. A total of eight studies were included in the final sample." (Luchsinger et al., 2019, pp. 42–43)

Phases 6 and 7: Synthesizing Translations and Expressing the Synthesis

A metasynthesis report might include findings presented in different formats based on the knowledge developed and the perspective of the authors. A synthesis of qualitative studies in an area might result in the discovery of unique or more refined themes explaining the area of synthesis (see Table 19.4). The findings from a metasynthesis might be presented in narrative format or graphically presented in a conceptual map or model. The discussion of findings also needs to include identification of the limitations of the synthesis. The report often concludes with recommendations for further research and possibly implications for practice or policy development or both (Butler et al., 2016; France, Cunningham, et al., 2019).

Luchsinger and colleagues (2019) synthesized eight studies to identify themes and subthemes. The results of the metasynthesis were diagrammed using the constructs from Donabedian's (2005) theory, structure, process, and outcomes. The following excerpt summarizes the findings from this metasynthesis.

"The publications selected for the meta-synthesis were of varying quality and rigor. In addition, themes examining patients' perceptions about nurses as partners in chronic illness care..., examining the relationship between comorbidities and care processes within the context of care transitions..., factors influencing nurse care coordination in a patient-centered model..., and threats to safe discharge as exemplars of complex care transitions." (Luchsinger et al., 2019, p. 43)

"The associated derived subthemes were: (1) the patient and care giver happiness with the care coordination experience, (2) making an impact on cost, quality and need for care, (3) keeping the patient safe, (4) working with the patient to understand what they need to do to live with their disease, (5) being partners in care coordination, and (6) managing the transitions for patients...

The results of the meta-synthesis are diagramed [in Fig. 19.10] to illustrate that the structure of the coordinated nurse-patient relationship, the process of starting the coordinated nurse-patient relationship, and the outcomes of a coordinated nurse-patient relationship are interrelated and influenced by transitions theory. As the analysis unfolded, the process of starting and having a coordinated nurse-patient relationship was far more complex than originally perceived, the effects of transitions were higher than expected, and the applicability of transition theory to the results of these studies was identified. The integrated view, illustrated in the meta-synthesis, provides nursing leaders with additional insight into factors that promote an effective coordinated nurse-patient relationship....

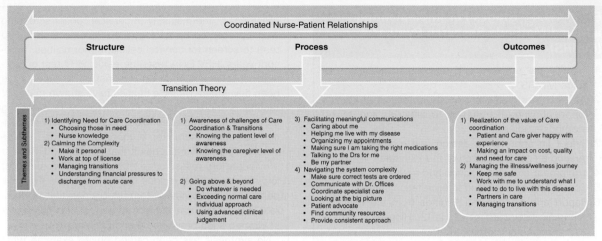

Fig. 19.10 The results of metasynthesis—influence of transition theory. (Redrawn from Luchsinger, J. S., Jones, J., McFarland, A. K., & Kissler, K. [2019]. Examining nurse/patient relationships in care coordination: A qualitative metasynthesis. *Applied Nursing Research, 49*[1], 48.)

Limitations in the studies were primarily related to sampling and relying on participant accounts of their experiences...

Conclusions: ... By examining the structure, process, and outcomes of the Coordinated Nurse-Patient relationship as perceived by nurses, patients, and caregivers, quality leaders can use this valuable information to evaluate program effectiveness. Careful considerations should be given to the outcomes and the importance of managing and navigating the complexity of transitions of care for patients living with chronic illnesses." (Luchsinger et al., 2019, p. 48)

Mixed Methods Research Synthesis

Currently nurse researchers are conducting more mixed methods studies that include both quantitative and qualitative research methods (Creswell & Clark, 2018; Creswell & Creswell, 2018) (see Chapter 14). Nurse researchers recognize the importance of synthesizing the findings of these studies to determine important knowledge for education, practice, and policy development. Harden and Thomas (2005) identified this process of combining findings from quantitative and qualitative studies as mixed methods synthesis. Higgins and Thomas (2020) referred to this synthesis of quantitative, qualitative, and mixed methods studies as a mixed methods systematic review. Sandelowski, Voils, Leeman, and Crandell (2012) identified this process as mixed methods–mixed research synthesis that they defined as a form of a systematic review in which the findings from qualitative and quantitative studies are integrated.

The synthesis of mixed methods studies involves aggregation and configuration. "**Research synthesis by aggregation** depends on both qualitative and quantitative findings being conceived as potentially addressing the same factors or aspects of a target phenomenon" (Sandelowski et al., 2012, p. 323). **Research synthesis by configuration** occurs when diverse individual findings or sets of aggregated findings are arranged into a coherent theoretical framework or model. Heyvaert, Maes, and Onghena (2013) termed the synthesis of qualitative, quantitative, and mixed methods studies **mixed methods research synthesis** (MMRS).

MMRS is the term used frequently in the literature and is included in this text. MMRS might include various study designs, such as a variety of types of qualitative research (see Chapter 4) and descriptive, correlational, and quasi-experimental quantitative studies (Creswell & Clark, 2018; Creswell & Poth, 2018; Heyvaert et al., 2013; Higgins & Thomas, 2020; Sandelowski et al., 2012). Conducting MMRS involves implementing a complex synthesis process that includes expertise in synthesizing knowledge from quantitative, qualitative, and mixed methods studies. There are different approaches to synthesizing the findings from studies using different methods, such as separate synthesis and integrated synthesis. **Separate synthesis** involves synthesizing the findings from quantitative studies separately from qualitative studies and integrating the findings from these two

---

BOX 19.4   Stages For Implementing a Mixed Methods Research Synthesis (MMRS)

1. Identify the problem and purpose or questions to guide MMRS.
2. Develop the review protocol with search strategies for identifying quantitative, qualitative, and mixed methods studies.
3. Select an appropriate design and method for conducting a rigorous search of the literature.
4. Implement a data extraction and evaluation stage.
5. Conduct an analysis and interpretation stage.
6. Report and discuss the findings from the research synthesis (Heyvaert et al., 2013; Higgins & Green, 2011; Higgins & Thomas, 2020).

---

syntheses in the final report. **Integrated synthesis** is used when quantitative and qualitative research findings are thought to extend, confirm, or refute each other and are synthesized concurrently (Heyvaert et al., 2013).

Further work is needed to develop the methodology for conducting MMRS. The steps seem to overlap with the systematic review process described previously. Some researchers use the PRISMA guideline when conducting their MMRS. The process might best be implemented by a team of researchers with expertise in conducting different types of studies and research syntheses. The basic framework for systematically synthesizing quantitative, qualitative, and mixed methods studies includes the stages presented in Box 19.4. The reader is encouraged to refer to the steps in systematic review and meta-analysis for conducting quantitative research syntheses (see Table 19.2) and to the metasynthesis discussion for synthesizing qualitative studies (see Table 19.4).

Identify the Problem and Purpose and/or Questions to Guide the Mixed Methods Research Synthesis

Tatar and colleagues (2018) determined the "factors associated with human papillomavirus (HPV) test acceptability in primary screening for cervical cancer by conducting a mixed methods research synthesis" (p. 40). The investigators thought it important to synthesize research in this area so healthcare providers and others might have the knowledge needed to encourage women to accept HPV testing for cervical cancer. The problem and purpose for this MMRS are presented in the following excerpt.

"Historically, the mainstay of cervical cancer screening was represented by cytology (i.e., Papanicolaou or Pap test) to screen for cervical cellular abnormalities. In recent years, HPV DNA tests (hereafter HPV test or testing) capable of identifying high-risk HPV types have been developed. Multiple studies have shown that HPV testing is more sensitive than cytology in detecting cervical intraepithelial neoplasia in primary cervical cancer screening (hereafter primary screening).... Overwhelming evidence suggests that a negative HPV test provides more reassurance to a woman that she is at low-risk for cervical lesions than a Pap test.... This evidence has led to new recommendations that incorporate HPV testing as a primary screen for cervical cancer in women aged between 30 and 65 years...

No synthesis has been carried out to examine what factors' impact (e.g. facilitators, barriers) on HPV test acceptability in primary screening. As new guidelines have been developed and are in the process of being implemented worldwide, we aimed to provide a comprehensive description of psychosocial factors related to HPV testing and to assess their influence on HPV testing acceptability in primary screening for cervical cancer with the ultimate goal to guide interventions to promote screening." (Tatar et al., 2018, p. 41)

Develop Search Protocol for Quantitative, Qualitative, and Mixed Methods Studies

Tatar et al. (2018) detailed their literature search strategies, which were guided by a PICOS format. The PICOS format is part of the PRISMA framework that was used to guide the conduct and reporting of this review (see Table 19.2) (Moher et al., 2009). The protocol for the review was registered through PROSPERO. The literature search strategy for this MMRS is briefly presented in the following excerpt.

"We searched Medline, Embase, PsycINFO, CINAHL, Global Health and Web of Science for journal articles between January 1, 1980 and October 31, 2017. The search strategy was developed for Medline by our team, validated by an experienced McGill librarian and then adapted for the other databases . . . . The following eligibility criteria were applied: 1) Population: women of all ages for whom primary cervical cancer screening is recommended, 2) Outcome: psychosocial factors related to acceptability of HPV testing in primary screening for cervical cancer, 3) Study design: empirical studies, without restrictions of study methodology, 4) Languages: English or French or German. The selection of references was performed by two researchers (OT and AN)." (Tatar et al., 2018, p. 41)

Select a Design and Method for Conducting a Rigorous Literature Search

Tatar et al. (2018) used the PRISMA guidelines for conducting their literature search (see Table 19.2 and the previous section on systematic reviews). The following excerpt briefly identifies the steps for their literature search.

"Records were first screened for eligibility based on titles and abstracts (phase one). Then, the full texts of retained records were retrieved and read; the final set of articles was identified based on eligibility criteria (phase two). Disagreements in phase one and two on whether or not an article should be included were mediated by the senior researcher (ZR). For this review, we did not retain studies related to self-sampling which represents a distinct strategy to increase screening uptake and merits separate consideration." (Tatar et al., 2019, p. 41)

Implement a Data Extraction and Evaluation Stage

Tatar et al. (2018) discussed their process for data extraction for quantitative and qualitative studies. Each individual study was assessed for bias separately by two of the researchers. The 16-item Quality Assessment Tool for Studies with Diverse Designs was used to evaluate the quality of each study (Sirriyeh, Lawton, Gardner, & Armitage, 2012). This tool was developed for the disciplines of nursing, psychology, and sociology with a total score of ≥ 60% and < 60% indicating high and low ROB, respectively. The following excerpt includes a brief discussion of data extraction and evaluation of studies included in Tatar and colleagues' (2018) MMRS.

"A data extraction sheet was developed in Excel and included author, title, publication date, country, objectives, study design, quantitative data collection and analysis methods, qualitative methodology, qualitative data collection methods and analysis, and number of participants. From qualitative studies, we extracted qualitative raw data without any interpretation

or analysis (e.g., quotes). From quantitative studies, we extracted outcomes of acceptability (e.g. proportions, means, odds ratios)...

We performed deductive-inductive qualitative thematic analysis to identify factors related to HPV testing. Deductively, we identified themes based on two frameworks widely used in health behavior research: The Health Belief Model (HBM) (Champion & Skinner, 2008) and the Theory of Planned Behavior (TPB).... Inductively, we developed new themes (i.e., not covered by HBM and TPB) through an iterative process, which consisted of reading the studies (and new themes) multiple times, allowing researchers to assure accurate interpretation of study results. Themes (hereinafter called factors) were further grouped into categories to enable a structured reporting of the results of the qualitative phase. The factors and categories were developed independently by two researchers (OT and ET) and then validated by the research team." (Tatar et al., 2018, p. 41

"The study selection flow diagram is presented [in a figure similar to Fig. 19.2]. We retained 22 primary studies: 5 of qualitative methodology..., 15 of quantitative methodology..., and 2 in which both methodologies were used.... Seventeen studies originate in high income countries (8-USA, 2-Canada, 5-Europe, and 2 in Australia) and five in low and middle income countries (1-Mexico, 1-El Salvador, 1-China, 1-India, and 1 in Nigeria). In 14 quantitative studies, statistical tests of significance to assess acceptability were reported; these studies were included in the integration phase...

Quality appraisal revealed low risk of bias in 18 studies and high risk of bias in 4 studies... In the high risk of bias studies, theoretical frameworks were not used, the validity and reliability of the measurement methods was not assessed, no sample size calculations were provided..., and few details were provided related to the recruitment procedure and research setting." (Tatar et al., 2018, p. 42)

Conduct an Analysis and Interpretation Stage

Tatar et al. (2018) provided a detailed description of their analysis and interpretation of the findings from 15 quantitative, 5 qualitative, and 2 mixed method studies used in their MMRS. We encourage you to access this review to gain an understanding of the complicated processes used to analyze and integrate the findings from the 22 studies included in this MMRS. The findings from this review were summarized in Fig. 19.11, which included a framework of the influencing factors on HPV test acceptability.

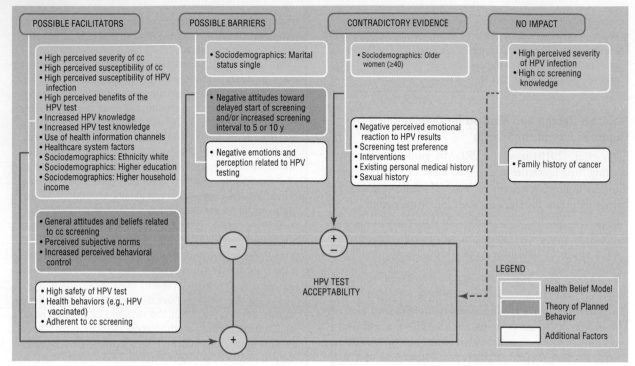

Fig. 19.11 Influence of factors on HPV test acceptability. *cc,* Cervical cancer; *HPV,* human papillomavirus. (Redrawn from Tatar, O., Thompson, E., Naz, A., Perez, S., Shapiro, G. K., Wade, K. ... Rosberger, Z. [2018]. Factors associated with human papillomavirus [HPV] test acceptability in primary screening for cervical cancer: A mixed methods research synthesis. *Preventative Medicine, 116*[1], 47.)

Report and Discuss the Findings From the Research Synthesis

Tatar et al. (2018) reported a quality discussion of their MMRS findings. They also identified the limitations of their review and the need for addition research in this area. They discussed their conclusions that included the implications for practice presented in the following excerpt.

> *"Conclusions*
> By synthesizing findings of both qualitative and quantitative studies, our review provides a wide perspective related to factors of HPV testing in primary cervical cancer screening. Our results can inform designing interventions to increase primary HPV-based cervical cancer screening uptake in high income countries, but even more so in low and middle income countries where the incidence of cervical cancer is highest and where, as suggested by previous research..., implementing a primary HPV testing program could be lifesaving." (Tatar et al., 2018, p. 49)

MODELS TO PROMOTE EVIDENCE-BASED PRACTICE IN NURSING

Two models developed to facilitate EBP in nursing are the Stetler Model of EBP (Stetler, 2001, 2010) and the Iowa Revised Model: Evidence-Based Practice to Promote Excellence in Healthcare (Cullen et al., 2018; Iowa Model Collaborative, 2017). This section introduces these two models, which might be used to implement evidence-based protocols, algorithms, and guidelines in clinical agencies.

Stetler Model of Evidence-Based Practice

An initial model for **research utilization** in nursing was developed by Stetler and Marram in 1976 and expanded and refined by Stetler in 1994, 2001, and 2010 to promote EBP for nursing. The **Stetler model** (2010), presented in Fig. 19.12, provides a comprehensive framework to enhance the use of research evidence by nurses to facilitate EBP. The research evidence can be

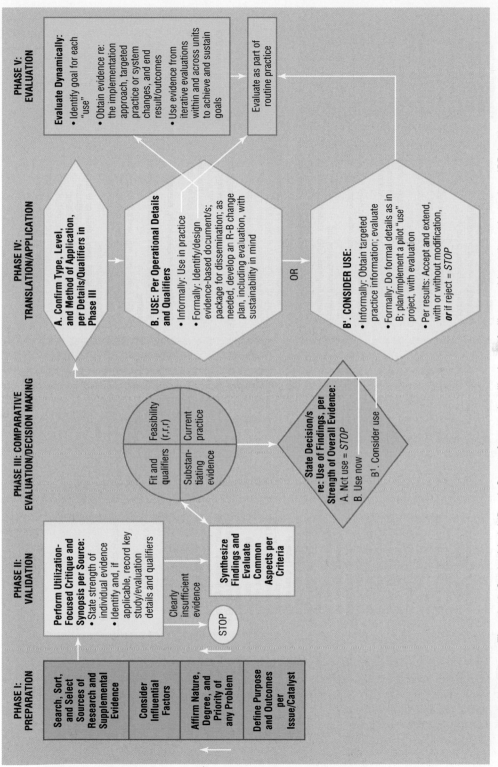

Fig. 19.12 Stetler Model, Part I: Steps of research utilization to facilitate evidence-based practice. *IRB*, Institutional Review Board; *R-B*, research-based; *RU*, Research Utilization. (From Stetler, C. B. [2010]. Stetler model. In J. Rycroft-Malone & T. Bucknall (Eds)., *Models and frameworks for implementing evidence-based practice: Linking evidence to action* (pp. 53–55). Oxford, England: Wiley-Blackwell.)

Continued

PHASE I: PREPARATION	PHASE II: VALIDATION	PHASE III: COMPARATIVE EVALUATION/DECISION MAKING	PHASE IV: TRANSLATION/APPLICATION	PHASE V: EVALUATION

PHASE I: PREPARATION

Purpose, Context, and Sources of Evidence:

- **Potential Issues/Catalysts:** = a problem, including unexplained variations; less-than-best practice; routine update of knowledge; validation/routine revision of procedures, etc; or innovative program goal [baseline]
- **Affirm/clarify perceived problem/s,** with internal evidence re: current practice
- Consider other influential internal and external factors, e.g., timelines
- Affirm and focus on high priority issues
- **Decide** if need to form a team, involve formal stakeholders, and/or assign project lead/facilitator
- Define desired, measurable outcome/s
- Seek out systematic reviews/guidelines first
- **Determine** need for an explicit type of research evidence, if relevant
- **Select** research sources with conceptual fit

PHASE II: VALIDATION

Credibility of Evidence and Potential for/Detailed Qualifiers of Application:

- **Critique and synopsize** essential components, operational details, and other qualifying factors, per source
  - See instructions for use of utilization-focused review tables, * with evaluative criteria, to facilitate this task; fill in the tables for group decision making or potential future synthesis
- Critique *systematic reviews and guidelines
- **Reassess fit** of individual sources
- **Rate** the level and quality of each individual evidence source per a "table of evidence"
- Differentiate statistical and clinical significance
- Eliminate noncredible sources
- **End the process** if there is clearly insufficient, credible external evidence that meets your need

*Stetler, Morsi, Rucki, et al. *Appl Nurs Res* 1998; 11(4):195–206 for noted tables, reviews, and synthesis process

PHASE III: COMPARATIVE EVALUATION/DECISION MAKING

Synthesis and Decisions/ Recommendations per Criteria of Applicability:

- **Synthesize the cumulative findings:**
  - Logically organize and display the similarities and differences across multiple findings, per common aspects or subelements of the topic under review
  - Evaluate degree of substantiation of each aspect/subelement; reference any qualifying conditions for application
- **Evaluate degree and nature of other criteria:** **feasibility (r,r,r = risk, resources, readiness);** pragmatic fit, including potential qualifying factors to application; and nature of **current practice, including the urgency/risk of current issues/needs
- **Make a decision whether/what to use:**
  - Can be a personal practitioner-level decision or a recommendation to others
  - Judge strength of decision; indicate if primarily "research-based" (R–B) or, per high use of supplemental info, "E–B"; note level of strength of recommendation/s per related* table; note any qualifying factors that may influence individualized variations
  - If decision = "Not use" research findings:
    - May conduct own research or delay use till additional research done by others
    - If still decide to act now, e.g., on evidence of consensus or another basis for practice, consider need for similar planned change and evaluation.
  - If decision = "Use/Consider Use," can mean a recommendation for or against a specific practice

PHASE IV: TRANSLATION/APPLICATION

Operational Definition of Use/Actions for Change:

- **Types** = cognitive/conceptual, symbolic and/or instrumental
- **Methods** = informal or formal; direct or indirect
- **Levels** = individual, group or department/organization
- **Direct instrumental use:** change individual behavior (e.g., via assessment tool or Rx intervention options); or change policy, procedure, protocol, algorithm, program, etc.
- **Cognitive use:** validate current practice; change personal way of thinking; increase awareness; better understand or appreciate condition/s or experience/s
- **Symbolic use:** develop position paper or proposal for change; or persuade others regarding a way of thinking
- **Formal dissemination and change/implementation strategies should be planned per relevant research and local barriers:**
  - Passive education is usually not effective as an isolated strategy. Use Dx analysis** and an ***implementation framework to develop a plan. Consider multiple strategies; e.g., opinion leaders, interactive education, reminders and audits.
  - Focus on context & to enhance sustainability of organization-related change
- **CAUTION: Assess whether translation/product or use goes beyond actual findings/evidence:**
  - Research evidence may or may not provide various details or a complete policy, procedure, etc.; indicate this fact to users, and note differential levels of evidence therein
- **Consider need for appropriate, reasoned variation**
- **WITH B*, where made a decision to use in the setting:**
  - With formal use, may need a dynamic evaluation to effectively implement and continuously improve/refine use of best available evidence across units and time
- **WITH B°, where made a decision to consider use and thus obtain additional, pragmatic information before a final decision:**
  - With formal consideration, do a pilot project
  - With a pilot, must assess if need IRB review, per relevant institutional criteria

PHASE V: EVALUATION

Alternative Evaluations:

- **Evaluation per type, method, level: e.g., consider conceptual use at individual level***
- **Consider cost-benefit** of change + various evaluation efforts
- **Use RU-as-a-process to enhance credibility of evaluation data**
- **For both dynamic and pilot evaluations, include:**
  - ***formative, regarding actual implementation and goal progress
  - ° summative, regarding identified end goal and end-point outcomes

NOTE: Model applies to all forms of practice, (i.e., educational, clinical, managerial, or other; to use effectively, read 2001 and 1994 model papers.

**E.g.: Rogers' re: implications of attributes of a change: Rycroft-Malone et al, §PARIHS (2002) and Green and Krueter's PRECEDE (1992) models re: implementation

§Stetler, 2003 on context §Stetler and Caramanica, 2007 on outcomes

Fig. 19.12, cont'd

used at the institutional or individual level. At the institutional level, synthesized research knowledge is used to develop or to update protocols, algorithms, policies, procedures, or other formal programs implemented in the institution. Individual nurses, including APNs, educators, administrators, and policymakers, use this model to summarize research and use the knowledge to influence educational programs, make practice decisions, and impact political decision making. The following sections briefly describe the five phases of the Stetler model: (1) preparation, (2) validation, (3) comparative evaluation and decision making, (4) translation and application, and (5) evaluation. Anderson and Jenson (2019) used the Stetler model to conduct an "integrative review of the literature to identify violence risk-assessment screening tools that could be used in acute care mental health settings" (p. 114). This review is used as an example in the discussion of the initial steps of the Stetler model.

Phase I: Preparation

The intent of Stetler's (2010) model is to ensure that a conscious, critical thinking process is initiated by nurses to use research evidence in practice. The first phase (preparation) involves selecting sources of research evidence; defining the issue, catalyst, or problem to be addressed; affirming the nature, degree, and priority of the problem; and defining the outcomes for the catalyst(s) (see Fig. 19.12). The agency's priorities and other external and internal factors that could be influenced by or could influence the proposed practice change must be examined. After the purpose of the evidence-based project has been identified and approved by the agency, a detailed search of the literature is conducted to determine the strength of the evidence available for use in practice. The research literature might be reviewed to solve a difficult clinical, managerial, or educational problem; to provide the basis for a policy, standard, algorithm, or protocol; or to prepare for an educational program or other type of professional presentation. The example of phase 1 from Anderson and Jenson's (2019) literature review to identify a violence risk-assessment screening tool is presented in the following excerpt.

"The method of inquiry was the Stetler model of evidence-based practice.... Phases 1 through 3 are discussed below. For the purpose of this article, phases 4

and 5 were not completed, because implementation was not within the scope of the present inquiry, which produced a recommendation.

Phase 1: preparation
Preparation consists of identifying the purpose, context, and sources of evidence (Grove, Burns, & Gray, 2013). A detailed search was conducted to determine the strength of the evidence, leading to the recommendation within this article." (Anderson & Jenson, 2019, p. 114)

Phase II: Validation

In the **validation phase**, research reports are critically appraised to determine their scientific soundness. If the studies are limited in number or are weak, or both, the findings and conclusions are usually considered inadequate or insufficient for use in practice, and the process stops. The quality of the research evidence is greatly strengthened if a systematic review or meta-analysis has been conducted in the area in which you want to make an evidence-based change. If the research knowledge base is strong in the selected area, a decision needs to be made regarding the priority of using the evidence in practice by the clinical agency (see Fig. 19.12). Phase 2 from the Anderson and Jenson (2019) article is briefly presented in the following excerpt.

"*Phase 2: Validation*
Validation outlines the need for a comprehensive literature search to determine the scientific soundness of current literature (Grove et al., 2013). The following section describes the primary literature review, which identified various violence risk–assessment screening tools used in acute care mental health settings.

Primary review. The aim of the primary literature review was to identify violence risk–assessment screening tools used in acute care mental health settings. A search of the EBSCOhost and CINAHL databases identified 60 articles. An additional search of PubMed, focusing on meta-analysis and systemic reviews, produced another 57 articles. Inclusion criteria for the literature search: written in English, peer-reviewed journals, and contained one or a combination of selected keywords (assessment; mental health; screening; tools; violence). Of the 117 articles identified, further review of the abstracts excluded studies within forensic mental health populations and publication dates before 2010.... Twenty articles were selected for further examination.

Fifteen violence risk–assessment screening tools were identified in the literature. Eight of the 15 tools were identified for evaluation.... Studies were excluded if they did not review validity and reliability of the tool and were published before 2010. Four of the 6 tools... warranted further exploration.

Secondary review. The aim of the secondary review was to further explore the literature identified as violence risk–assessment screening tools. Secondary review was conducted with searches in the CINAHL, PubMed, and PsycINFO databases, resulting in an additional 77 studies.... Of the 77 abstracts reviewed, 42 were selected for review and 32 were selected for further evaluation. Information from the primary and secondary searches [were provided in a figure]." (Anderson & Jenson, 2019, pp. 114–115)

Phase III: Comparative Evaluation and Decision Making

Comparative evaluation includes four parts: (1) fit and qualifiers of the evidence for the healthcare setting, (2) feasibility of using the research findings, (3) substantiation of the evidence, and (4) concerns with current practice (see Fig. 19.12). To determine the fit of the evidence in the clinical agency, the characteristics of the setting are examined to determine the forces that would facilitate or inhibit the evidence-based change. Stetler (2001, 2010) believed the feasibility of using research evidence for making changes in practice necessitated examination of the three *R*s: (1) potential risks, (2) resources needed, and (3) readiness of the people involved.

Substantiating evidence is produced by replication, in which consistent, credible findings are obtained from several studies in similar practice settings. The studies generating the strongest research evidence are RCTs, meta-analyses of RCTs, systematic reviews, and quasi-experimental studies. The final comparison involves determining whether the research information provides credible, empirical evidence for making changes in the current practice. The research evidence must document that an intervention increases the quality and safety in current practice by solving practice problems and improving patient outcomes. By conducting phase III, the overall benefits and risks of using the research evidence in a practice setting can be assessed. If the benefits (improved patient, provider, or agency outcomes) are much

greater than the risks (complications, morbidity, mortality, or increased costs) for the organization, the individual nurse, or both, then using the research-based intervention in practice is feasible.

Three types of decisions (decision making) are possible during this phase: (1) not to use the research evidence, (2) to use the research evidence now, and (3) to consider using the evidence (see Fig. 19.12). The decision not to make a change in practice is usually due to the poor quality of the research evidence, costs, and other potential problems. The decision to use research knowledge in practice now is determined mainly by the strength of the evidence. Depending on the research knowledge to be used in practice, the individual practitioner, hospital unit, or agency might make this decision. Another decision might be to consider using the available research evidence in practice, but not immediately. When a change is complex and involves multiple disciplines, the individuals involved often need additional time to determine how the evidence might be used and what measures will be taken to coordinate the involvement of different health professionals in the change. The application of phase 3 of Stetler's model from Anderson and Jenson's (2019) integrative review is presented in the following excerpt:

" *Phase 3: Comprehensive evaluation and decision making*
Phase 3 addresses evaluation of the literature and provides a recommendation for practice (Grove et al., 2013).... The recommendation for violence risk–assessment screening tools was based on predictive validity, calibration, discrimination, and reliability reported in the literature.

Comprehensive evaluation. Over past decades, several violence risk–assessment screening tools have been studied to establish predictive validity (based on calibration and discrimination) for assessing the likelihood of violence.... Calibration of an assessment is defined as the ability of the tool to predict risk with actual observed risk. Discrimination of an assessment is defined as the ability of the tool to assess tendency toward violence." (Anderson & Jenson, 2019, p. 115)

"The Brøset Violence Checklist and Violence Risk Screening-10 provided the best assessment for violence in the acute care mental health setting" (Anderson & Jenson, 2019, p. 112). These researchers concluded that a violence risk assessment tool is important to identify patients at risk for violence so interventions might be implemented to prevent violent episodes.

Phase IV: Translation and Application

The **translation and application phase** involves planning for and using the research evidence in practice. The translation phase involves determining exactly what knowledge will be used and how that knowledge will be applied to practice. The use of the research evidence can be informal or formal and direct or indirect (see Fig. 19.12) (Stetler, 2010). The application of research evidence includes direct instrumental use, cognitive use, and symbolic use. **Instrumental use** is the direct and formal application of research evidence to support the need for change in nursing interventions or practice protocols, algorithms, and guidelines. **Cognitive use** is a more informal, indirect use of the research knowledge to modify one's way of thinking or appreciation of an issue. Cognitive application may improve the nurse's understanding of a situation, allow analysis of practice dynamics, or improve problem-solving skills for clinical problems. **Symbolic use** occurs when position papers or proposals for change are developed to persuade others toward a new way of thinking (see Fig. 19.12).

The application phase includes the following steps for planned change: (1) Assess the situation to be changed, (2) develop a plan for change, and (3) implement the plan. During the application phase, educational programs, protocols, policies, procedures, or algorithms are developed based on research evidence and implemented in practice (Stetler, 2001, 2010). A pilot project on a single hospital unit or in a specific healthcare clinic might be conducted to implement the change in practice, and the results of this project could be evaluated to determine whether the change should be extended throughout the healthcare agency or system.

Phase V: Evaluation

The final phase of Stetler's model is evaluation of the effect of the evidence-based change on selected agency, providers, and patient outcomes. The **evaluation** process can include both formal and informal activities that are conducted by administrators, RNs, APNs, and other health professionals (see Fig. 19.12). Informal evaluations might include self-monitoring or discussions with

patients, families, peers, and other professionals. Formal evaluations can include case studies, medical records audits, quality improvement program, and outcomes research projects.

Sher (2018) implemented an "educational program for parents of neonates on nasal continuous positive airway pressure [NCPAP]" (p. 1) guided by the Stetler model. The practice problem focused on the stress of parents with preterm infants on NCPAP, who worried about holding their infant and the possible complications of NCPAP.

> "A review of the literature suggested family-centered educational programs are able to decrease stress and increase parental confidence. The purpose of this project was to develop a family-centered education program focused on the education of parents of infants on NCPAP in the NICU [neonatal intensive care unit].... Stetler's evidence-based practice model was used to guide this project.... Evidence was collected in a systematic review of published peer-reviewed journal articles. The Johns Hopkins Nursing evidence-based appraisal tool was used to evaluate relevant articles.... The curriculum, supporting handouts for participants, and implementation and evaluation plans were developed and were provided to the institution as a complete solution to the practice problem [phase 4 of Stetler's model]. The project may promote positive social change for caregivers, patients, and patients' families by enhancing outcomes such as improved infant behavior, increased parental emotional well-being, and increased caregiver satisfaction [phase 5 of Stetler's model]." (Sher, 2018, p. 1)

The goal of the Stetler (2001, 2010) model is to increase the use of research evidence in nursing to facilitate EBP. This model provides detailed steps to encourage nurses to become change agents and make the necessary improvements in practice based on the best current research evidence.

Sometimes only a snippet of evidence, such as a brief quotable passage, can lead to a change in nursing practice. For example, Dugan and Gabuya (2019) reported that sharing a research finding in their nursing research council led to the elimination of identification (ID) lanyards because of environmental contamination and spread of *Staphylococcus aureus* skin infections. Consensus was achieved to revise the hospital's ID badge policy to eliminate lanyards. This change was implemented throughout their hospital and later throughout all hospitals in the healthcare system (Dugan & Gabuya, 2019).

Iowa Model of Evidence-Based Practice

Nurses and other healthcare professionals can benefit from the direction provided by the Iowa Model of EBP. Titler and colleagues initially developed this EBP model in 1994 and revised it in 2001. The most current revision and validation of the Iowa model was published in 2017 by the Iowa Model Collaborative. "The Iowa Model-Revised remains an application-oriented guide for the EBP process. Intended users are point of care clinicians who ask questions and seek a systematic, EBP approach to promote excellence in health care" (Iowa Model Collaborative, 2017, p. 175) (Fig. 19.13). In a healthcare agency, triggers initiate the need for change, and the focus should always be to make changes based on best research evidence. These triggers can include clinical or patient identified issues; organization, state, or national initiative(s); new research evidence in a nursing area; accrediting agency requirements/regulations; and/or philosophy of care (Cullen et al., 2018). The triggers are evaluated and prioritized based on the needs of patients, nurse providers, and clinical agency. The next step is the statement of the question or purpose of the EBP project. Is the topic of this question a priority for nurses and the healthcare agency? If the answer is no, consider another issue/opportunity for an EBP project (see Fig. 19.13). If the topic is a priority, a team is formed to assemble, appraise, and synthesize the body of evidence available (Cullen et al., 2018; Iowa Model Collaborative, 2017).

In some situations, the research evidence is inadequate to make changes in practice, and additional studies are needed to strengthen the knowledge base. Sometimes the research evidence can be combined with other sources of knowledge (theories, scientific principles, expert opinion, and case reports) to provide fairly strong evidence for developing research-based protocols for practice. The strongest evidence is generated from meta-analyses of several RCTs, systematic reviews that usually include meta-analyses, and individual experimental studies (Cochrane Collaboration, 2019). If the evidence is sufficient, the team then designs and pilots the practice change. The next question the EBP team must address is, "Is the change appropriate for adoption in practice?" If the answer is no, then the practice change should be redesigned and pilot tested again (see Fig. 19.13).

If the outcomes of the pilot test are favorable, the next step is to integrate and sustain the practice change by identifying and engaging key personnel and hardwiring the change into the system (see Fig. 19.13). The indicators of the practice change are monitored over time by quality improvement to determine its impact on patients, nurses, and/or agency in terms of quality, safety, and costs. The team and other nurses involved in the EBP change should be reinfused as needed to sustain the practice change (Iowa Model Collaborative, 2017). The final step is to disseminate results of the evaluations of the practice change's efficacy (see Fig. 19.13).

Implementing the Iowa Model of Evidence-Based Practice

Lemus, McMullin, and Balinowski (2018) conducted an EBP project to develop and implement a guideline for patients identified as high risk for obstructive sleep apnea (OSA) to reduce the postoperative complications related to OSA. The Iowa model of EBP was used to guide the change in practice. This model includes three decision points that are briefly discussed in the following excerpt.

"The first decision point in the model was to determine if the topic is a priority for the organization [and healthcare professionals]. As previously stated, 27% of patients identified as high risk for OSA had adverse postoperative complications. Patient safety was a priority for the organization, and there was full support to proceed with the project. A multidisciplinary OSA team was formed consisting of perianesthesia nurses, APNs, a nurse manager, and ad hoc members including the Medical Director of Anesthesia, the Manager of the Respiratory Therapy Department, and the Medical Director of the Pulmonary/Sleep Lab departments.

More than 40 articles were critiqued and synthesized in the literature search phase.... Each article was critiqued by at least two members of the team. The evidence was then organized into a spreadsheet. Varying levels of evidence were found in the literature from literature reviews to meta-analysis...

The second decision point in the Iowa model was to question whether there was a sufficient research base to make a change in practice. Based on the synthesis of evidence, the OSA team determined that there was sufficient evidence to proceed. The team developed a guideline for the management of perioperative adult patients at high risk for OSA. An algorithm for practice was created for easy application of this guideline [Fig. 19.14]...

The Iowa Model Revised: Evidence-Based Practice to Promote Excellence in Health Care

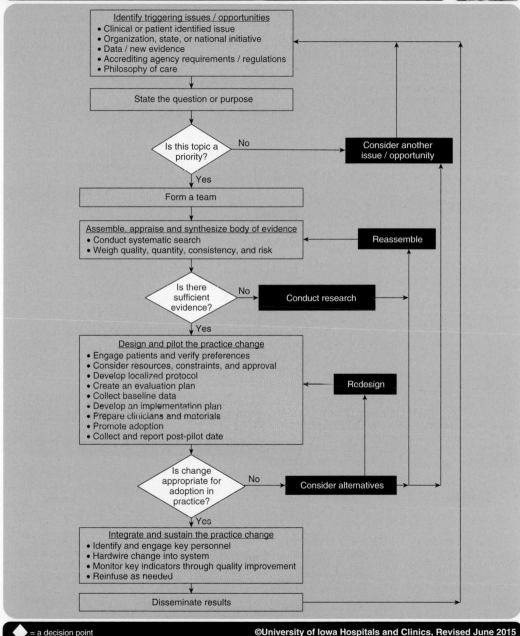

Fig. 19.13 The Iowa Model-Revised. (Used/reprinted with permission from the University of Iowa Hospitals and Clinics, Copyright 2015. For permission to use or reproduce the model, please contact the University of Iowa Hospitals and Clinics at 319-384-9098 or uihcnursingresearchandebp@uiowa.edu.)

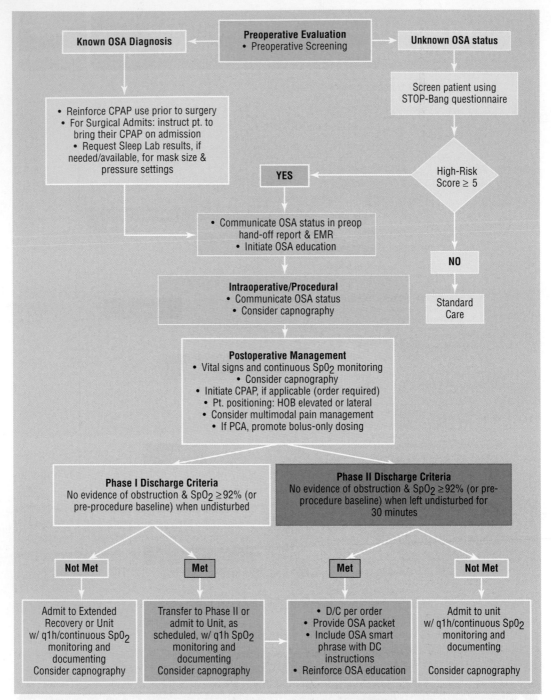

Fig. 19.14 OSA algorithm. *CPAP,* Continuous positive airway pressure; *D/C,* discharge; *DC,* discharge; *EMR,* electronic medical record; *HOB,* head of the patients' bed; *OSA,* obstructive sleep apnea; *PCA,* patient-controlled analgesia; *pt,* patient; *SpO₂,* peripheral capillary oxygen saturation. This figure is available in color online at www.jopan.org. (Redrawn from Lemus, L. P., McMullin, B., & Balinowski, H. [2018]. Don't ignore my snore: Reducing perioperative complications of obstructive sleep apnea. *Journal of PeriAnesthesia Nursing, 33*[3], 341.)

The guideline was piloted on outpatient orthopaedic patients admitted to the preoperative department of the main operating room. The postanesthesia care unit and a primarily orthopaedic unit were the two units in the pilot. Inpatient surgical patients were excluded from the pilot. The pilot unit nurses were educated on the OSA guideline through a self-learning module.... The written hand-off report for OSA was placed in the chart, and a for your information (FYI) label named FYI high-risk for OSA was entered by the preoperative registered nurse (RN) in the electronic medical record (EMR) for those patients screened high risk for OSA. These two methods were the initial communication for OSA status." (Lemus et al., 2018, p. 340)

"The third decision point in the Iowa model was to determine if the change was appropriate for adoption in practice. The practice change was instituted into practice, yet the process was revised because of unforeseen occurrences. The written hand-off report was underused or missing from the chart. The label FYI high-risk for OSA was eliminated from the EMR in response to risk management concerns. Auditing charts for guideline compliance was difficult. Therefore, the OSA team used the nursing diagnosis— Ineffective breathing pattern defined as inspiration/ expiration not adequate for ventilation. Because a nursing diagnosis was chosen, a nursing care plan based on practice recommendations in the OSA guideline was created... Communication of the nursing care plan in the EMR allowed for heightened awareness of patient OSA risk and a readily available resource for all nurses caring for this population, thereby promoting OSA guideline compliance and patient safety...

Results
A postguideline audit was conducted on all adult patients scheduled for elective surgery in the main operating room and screened high risk for OSA based on a STOP-Bang score ≥ 5 ($n = 164$) from September 2015 to February 2016. The charts were audited for oxygen desaturations, electrocardiographical changes, and respiratory treatments for 24 hours after anesthesia. The results of the postguideline audit revealed that 14.6% of patients at high risk for OSA experienced cardiopulmonary complications postoperatively. This was a decline from 27% of patients ($n = 136$) with a STOP-Bang score ≥ 3 experiencing complications at baseline." (Lemus et al., 2018, pp. 340–342)

Lemus and colleagues (2018) reported that the "step-by-step actions of the Iowa model facilitated the integration of an evidence-based guideline [see Fig. 19.14] into practice.... This patient safety initiative demonstrated that using an evidence-based guideline and nursing care plan specific to OSA was effective in improving patient outcomes in the perioperative setting" (p. 344).

IMPLEMENTING EVIDENCE-BASED GUIDELINES IN PRACTICE

Every day, research knowledge is generated and must be critically appraised and synthesized to determine the best evidence for use in practice (Melnyk & Fineout-Overholt, 2019; Whittemore et al., 2014). This section focuses on the development of EBP guidelines using the best research evidence and provides a model for using these guidelines in practice. The JNC 8 evidence-based guidelines for the management of high BP in adults is presented as an example (James et al., 2014).

Development of Evidence-Based Guidelines

Once a significant health topic or condition has been selected, guidelines are developed to promote effective assessment, diagnosis, and management of this health condition. Since the 1980s, the Agency for Healthcare Research and Quality (AHRQ) has had a major role in identifying health topics and developing evidence-based guidelines for practice. In the late 1980s and early 1990s, a panel of experts was charged with developing EBP guidelines. The AHRQ solicited the members of the panel, who usually included nationally recognized researchers in the topic area; expert clinicians, such as physicians, nurses, pharmacists, and social workers; healthcare administrators; policy developers; economists; government representatives; and consumers. The group designated the scope of the guidelines and conducted extensive reviews of the literature, including relevant systematic reviews, meta-analyses, metasyntheses, MMRSs, individual studies, and theories (Moriarity et al., 2019).

The best research evidence available was synthesized to develop recommendations for practice. Most of the evidence-based guidelines included systematic reviews, meta-analyses, and multiple individual studies. The guidelines were examined for their usefulness in clinical practice, their impact on health policy, and their cost effectiveness. Consultants, other researchers, and additional expert clinicians often were asked to review the guidelines and provide input (Moriarty et al., 2019). Based on the experts' critique, the AHRQ revised and packaged the guidelines for distribution to healthcare professionals. Some of the first guidelines focused on the following healthcare problems: (1) acute pain management in infants, children, and adolescents; (2) prediction and prevention of pressure ulcers in adults; (3) urinary incontinence in adults; (4) management of functional impairments with cataracts; (5) detection, diagnosis, and treatment of depression; (6) screening, diagnosis, management, and counseling about sickle cell disease; (7) management of cancer pain; (8) diagnosis and treatment of heart failure (HF); (9) low back problems; and (10) otitis media diagnosis and management in children.

The AHRQ initiated the National Guideline Clearinghouse (NGC) in 1998 to store EBP guidelines. The NGC included thousands of publicly available EBP guidelines and related documents. Regretfully this site was closed in July 2018 when the funding for this project was discontinued. Currently AHRQ is searching for organizations that might support the work of the NGC (2018). In addition, numerous government agencies, professional organizations, healthcare agencies, universities, and other groups provide evidence-based guidelines for practice. The websites in Box 19.5 are useful in identifying current evidence-based guidelines for nursing practice.

Another initiative of the AHRQ was the National Quality Measurement Center (NQMC) that was developed as a sister resource to the NGC and made available to the public in 2001. The NQMC mission was to provide practitioners, healthcare providers, health plans, integrated delivery systems, purchasers, and others an accessible mechanism for obtaining detailed information on quality measures. This website was also shut down in July 2018 with the NGC. However, other sources for measurement tools that can be used in research and practice are available through the Computerized Needs-Oriented Quality Measurement Evaluation System (CONQUEST), the Expansion of Quality of Care Measures (Q-SPAN) project, the Quality Measurement Network (QMNet) project, the Performance Measures Inventory (PMI), and the EvidenceNow tools and resources (AHRQ, 2019b; Moorhead, Swanson, Johnson, & Maas, 2018; NGC, 2018).

> **BOX 19.5 Websites for Identifying Evidence-Based Guidelines for Nursing Practice**
>
> - Academic Center for Evidence-Based Nursing: http://www.acestar.uthscsa.edu
> - Association of Women's Health, Obstetric, and Neonatal Nurses: http://awhonn.org
> - Centers for Disease Control Healthcare Providers: http://www.cdc.gov/CDCForYou/healthcare_providers.html
> - Centers for Health Evidence: http://www.cche.net
> - Guidelines Advisory Committee: http://www.gac-guidelines.ca
> - Guidelines International Network: http://www.g-i-n.net/
> - HerbMed: Evidence-Based Herbal Database, Alternative Medicine Foundation: http://www.herbmed.org/
> - National Association of Neonatal Nurses: http://www.nann.org/
> - National Institute for Clinical Excellence (NICE): http://www.nice.org.uk/
> - Oncology Nursing Society: http://www.ons.org/
> - PIER—the Physicians' Information and Education Resource (authoritative, evidence-based guidance to improve clinical care; ACP-ASIM members only): http://pier.acponline.org/index.html
> - Primary Care Clinical Practice Guidelines: http://www.medscape.com/pages/editorial/public/pguidelines/index-primarycare
> - US Preventive Services Task Force: http://www.uspreventiveservicestaskforce.org

Implementing the Eighth Joint National Committee Evidence-Based Guidelines for the Management of High Blood Pressure in Adults

Evidence-based guidelines have become the standards for providing care to patients in the United States and internationally. A few nurses have participated on committees that have developed these evidence-based guidelines, and many APNs are using them in their practices. The 2014 evidence-based guideline for the management of high BP in adults is presented as an example. This guideline was developed by the JNC 8 panel members who conducted a systematic review of RCTs to determine the best research evidence for management of HTN. The guideline includes nine revised recommendations for the management of HTN that are available in the James et al. (2014) article. The JNC 8 guideline also includes the 2014 Hypertension Guideline Management Algorithm. This algorithm provides clinicians with direction for (1) implementing lifestyle interventions, (2) setting BP goals, and (3) initiating BP-lowering medication based on age, diabetes, and chronic kidney disease (CKD) (James et al., 2014). Healthcare providers can use this algorithm to select the most appropriate treatment methods for each individual patient diagnosed with HTN.

APNs and RNs need to assess the usefulness and quality of each evidence-based guideline before they implement it in their practice. Fig. 19.15 presents the **Grove Model for Implementing Evidence-Based Guidelines in Practice**. In this model, nurses identify a practice problem, search for the best research evidence to manage the problem in their practice, and identify an evidence-based guideline. Assessing the quality and usefulness of the guideline involves examining the following: (1) the authors of the guideline, (2) the significance

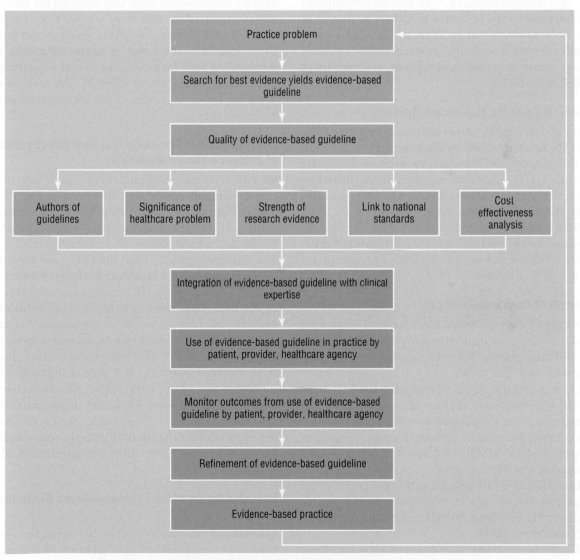

Fig. 19.15 Grove Model for Implementing Evidence-Based Guidelines in Practice.

of the healthcare problem, (3) the strength of the research evidence, (4) the link to national standards, and (5) the cost effectiveness of using the guideline in practice. The quality of the JNC 8 guideline is discussed using these five criteria.

Authors of the Guidelines

The panel members of the JNC 8 guideline were specifically selected from more than 400 nominees based on their "expertise in hypertension ($n = 14$), primary care ($n = 6$), ... pharmacology ($n = 2$), clinical trials ($n = 6$), evidence-based medicine ($n = 3$), epidemiology ($n = 1$), informatics ($n = 4$), and the development and implementation of clinical guidelines in systems of care ($n = 4$)" (James et al., 2014, p. 508). These panel members were specifically selected based on their strong, varied expertise to develop an evidence-based guideline for HTN.

Significance of the Healthcare Problem

James and colleagues (2014) addressed the significance of HTN in their article by identifying it as the most common condition managed by primary healthcare providers. HTN can lead to "myocardial infarction (MI), stroke, renal failure, and death if not detected early and treated appropriately" (James et al., 2014, p. 507). Therefore, providers want to use the best research evidence in managing HTN so patients will experience adequate control of their BP and reduce the burden of their disease.

Strength of Research Evidence

A modified Delphi technique (see Chapter 17) was used to identify the three highest-ranked questions related to high BP management. The systematic review was guided by questions to determine:

- Do hypertensive adults treated with anti-hypertensive pharmacologic therapy at selected BP levels experience improved healthoutcomes?
- Do adults treated with anti-hypertensive pharmacologic therapy to achieve a specified BP goal have improved health outcomes?
- Do adults receiving selected anti-hypertensive drugs or drug classes experience different benefits and/or sided effects related to selected health outcomes? (James et al., 2014).

The evidence review was focused on answering these three questions. The participants in the studies reviewed

were adults aged 18 and older with HTN. The studies with less than 100 participants or those with a follow-up period of less than 1 year were excluded. Only the studies with large sample sizes and follow-up that was adequate in yielding meaningful health-related outcomes were included in the systematic review. The panel also "limited its evidence review to only randomized controlled trials (RCTs) because they are less subject to bias than other study designs and represent the gold standard for determining efficacy and effectiveness" (James et al., 2014, p. 508).

The JNC 8 panel members had the services of an external methodology team that searched the literature and summarized the data from selected studies into an evidence table (James et al., 2014). Based on this review, panel members developed evidence statements that provided the basis for a guideline of nine recommendations for the management of HTN. The research evidence for the development of the JNC 8 guideline was extremely strong.

Link to National Standards and Cost Effectiveness of Evidence-Based Guideline

Quality evidence-based guidelines should link to national standards and be cost effective (see Fig. 19.15). The JNC 8 evidence-based guideline for the management of HTN built upon the JNC 7 national guideline for the assessment, diagnosis, and treatment of HTN. The recommendations from the JNC 7 are supported by the Department of Health and Human Services and disseminated through NIH publication 03-5231. Use of the JNC 8 guideline in practice is projected to be cost effective because the recommendations for management of HTN should lead to decreased incidences of MI, stroke, CKD, HF, and cardiovascular disease (CVD) related mortality and should improve health outcomes for adults with HTN. The Hypertension Guideline Management Algorithm in the James et al. (2014) article provides direction for the use of various antihypertensive drugs or drug classes to improve benefits and decrease harm in the management of adults with HTN.

Implementation of the Evidence-Based Guideline in Practice

Currently, APNs and physicians are using the JNC 8 evidence-based guideline or a variation of this guideline in their practice (Weber et al., 2014). Healthcare providers can assess the adequacy of the guideline for their practice and modify HTN treatments based on the individual health needs and values of their patients. The outcomes for patients, providers, and healthcare agencies are being examined using data from the electronic health record (EHR) and additional research. The outcomes examined usually include the following: (1) BP readings for patients; (2) incidence of diagnosis of HTN based on the JNC 8 guidelines; (3) appropriateness of the pharmacological therapies implemented to manage HTN; and (4) incidence of stroke, MI, HF, CKD, and CVD related mortality over 5, 10, 15, and 20 years. The healthcare agency outcomes include access to care by patients with HTN, patient satisfaction with care, and costs related to diagnosis and management of HTN, in addition to the HTN complications previously mentioned. This EBP guideline will be refined in the future based on clinical outcomes, outcome studies, and new RCTs. The use of this evidence-based guideline and additional guidelines promote an EBP for APNs and RNs (see Fig. 19.15).

EVIDENCE-BASED PRACTICE CENTERS

In 1997, the AHRQ launched its initiative to promote EBP by establishing 12 **Evidence-based Practice Centers** (EPCs) in the United States and Canada. The goals of the EPCs are described in the following excerpt.

"The EPCs develop evidence reports and technology assessments on topics relevant to clinical, social science/behavioral, economic, and other healthcare organization and delivery issues—specifically those that are common, expensive, and/or significant for the Medicare and Medicaid populations. With this program, AHRQ became a "science partner" with private and public organizations in their efforts to improve the quality, effectiveness, and appropriateness of health care by synthesizing the evidence and facilitating the translation of evidence-based research findings. Topics are nominated by non-federal partners such as professional societies, health plans, insurers, employers, and patient groups." (AHRQ, 2019a)

Under the EPC program, the AHRQ awards 5-year contracts to institutions to serve as EPCs. EPCs review all relevant scientific literature on clinical, behavioral, organizational, and financial topics to produce evidence reports and technology assessments. These reports are used to inform and develop coverage decisions, quality measures, educational materials, tools, guidelines, and research agendas. The AHRQ developed the following criteria as the basis for selecting a topic to be managed by an EPC.

- High incidence or prevalence in the general population and in special populations, including women, racial and ethnic minorities, pediatric and elderly populations, and those of low socioeconomic status.
- Significance for the needs of the Medicare, Medicaid, and other Federal health programs.
- High costs associated with a condition, procedure, treatment, or technology, whether due to the number of people needing care, high unit cost of care, or high indirect costs.
- Controversy or uncertainty about the effectiveness or relative effectiveness of available clinical strategies or technologies.
- Impact potential for informing and improving patient or provider decision making.
- Impact potential for reducing clinically significant variations in the prevention, diagnosis, or management of a disease or condition; in the use of a procedure or technology; or in the health outcomes achieved.
- Availability of scientific data to support the systematic review and analysis of the topic.
- Submission of the nominating organization's plan to incorporate the report into its managerial or policy decision making...
- Submission of the nominating organization's plan to disseminate derivative products to its members and plan to measure members' use of these products, and the resultant impact of such use on clinical practice. (AHRQ, 2019a)

The AHRQ (2019a) website provides names of the EPCs and the focus of each center. This site also provides a link to the evidence-based reports produced by these centers (https://www.ahrq.gov/research/findings/evidence-based-reports/index.html). These EPCs have had an important role in the development of evidence-based guidelines since the 1990s and will continue to make significant contributions to EBP in the future.

INTRODUCTION TO TRANSLATIONAL RESEARCH AND TRANSLATIONAL SCIENCE

Some of the barriers to EBP have resulted in the implementation of a type of research to promote the application of research knowledge to practice. This research strategy, translational research, was originally part of the National Center for Research Resources. However, in December 2011, the National Center for Advancing Translational Sciences (NCATS) was developed as part of the NIH Institutes and Centers (Chesla, 2008; NIH, 2019a). **Translational research** is an evolving strategy that is defined by the NIH as the translation of basic scientific discoveries into practical applications. It is the "process of turning observations in the laboratory, clinic and community into interventions that improve the health of individuals and the public—from diagnostics and therapeutics to medical procedures and behavioral changes" (NIH, 2019b).

Translation research is part of **translational science**, which is "the field of investigation focused on understanding the scientific and operational principles underlying each step of the translational process" (NCATS, 2019). Basic research discoveries from the laboratory setting should be tested in studies with humans before application is considered. In addition, the outcomes from human clinical trials should be adopted and maintained in clinical practice. Translational research is encouraged by both medicine and nursing to increase the use of evidence-based interventions in practice and to determine whether these interventions are effective in producing the outcomes desired (NCATS, 2019; Norris, Matsuda, & Sarik, 2019; Weiss et al., 2018).

NCATS (2019) developed a model of the **translational science spectrum**, which presents it focus and goals (Fig. 19.16). This model represents the concepts and their interaction in the translational science spectrum at each stage of research along the path from the biological basis of health and disease to interventions that improve the health of individuals and the public. The spectrum is not linear or unidirectional; each stage builds on and informs the others. At all stages of the spectrum, NCATS develops new approaches, demonstrates their usefulness, and disseminates the findings. Patient involvement is a critical feature of all stages in translation.

The NIH (2019b) wanted to encourage researchers to conduct translational research, so the Clinical and Translational Science Awards (CTSA) Consortium was implemented in October 2006. The consortium started with 12 centers located throughout the United States and expanded to 39 centers in April 2009. The program was fully implemented in 2012 with about 60 institutions involved in clinical and translational science. The details for the CTSA Program are available at the following website: https://ncats.nih.gov/ctsa.

Initially the CTSA Program was primarily focused on expanding the translation of medical research to practice. Therefore Westra and colleagues (2015) developed "a national action plan for sharable and comparable nursing data to support practice and translation research" (p. 600). This plan provides direction for the conduct and use of translation research to change nursing practice (Norris et al., 2019). Organizations such as the American Association of Critical Care Nurses have identified translational research as a priority (Deutschman et al., 2012). Weiss et al. (2018) aligned translational research with EBP in achieving and maintaining Magnet designation in hospitals. Dang and Dearholt (2018) detailed the importance of translation in facilitating evidence-based nursing practice at Johns Hopkins.

As you search the literature for relevant research syntheses and studies, you will note that translation studies are appearing more frequently. Wand and colleagues (2019) conducted a "multi-site translation research project to implement and evaluate an innovative model of mental health nursing care in three EDs [emergency departments] in Australia" (p. 10). The researchers reported the following results from their translational study.

> "There is incontrovertible evidence that the burden of mental health, drug health and behavioral problems in EDs is increasing. This necessitates the development of new models of care to meet mounting demands and support ED staff. However, implementing models of care that necessitate a significant change in workplace thinking and culture is complex and often messy. This multi-site pre-implementation study conducted as part of a larger translational research project illustrates how difficult transforming health care becomes when individuals place professional self-interest above improving service provision and the best interests of the public. Even with the weight of a solid evidence base, extensive consultation and significant high-level support, cooperation of key stakeholders is never guaranteed." (Wand et al., 2019, p. 15)

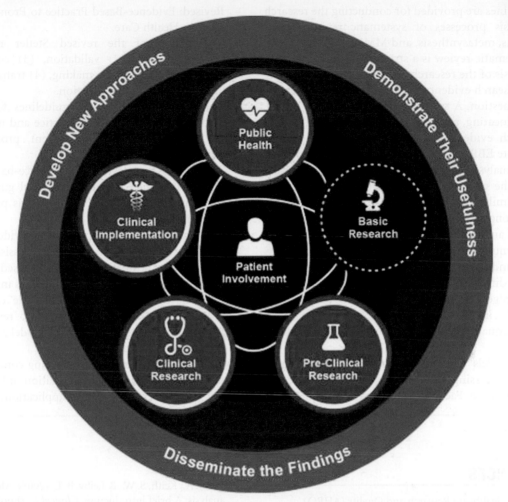

Fig. 19.16 National Science Spectrum. (From National Center for Advancing Translational Sciences. [NCATS, 2019]. *Translation science spectrum.* Retrieved from https://ncats.nih.gov/translation/spectrum.)

Additional translational studies are needed to translate research findings into practice and determining the outcomes of EBP on patients' health. However, national funding must be expanded to increase the conduct of translational research and other relevant outcomes studies in nursing (NIH, 2019a; Weiss et al., 2018).

KEY POINTS

- EBP is the conscientious integration of best research evidence with clinical expertise and patient values and needs in the delivery of quality, safe, cost-effective health care. Best research evidence is produced by the conduct and synthesis of numerous, high-quality studies in a health-related area.

- There are benefits and barriers associated with EBP. An important benefit is the delivery of care based on the most current research evidence. However, a barrier is the limited amount of interventional research, such as RCTs and quasi-experimental studies, that have been conducted in nursing.

- Guidelines are provided for conducting the research synthesis processes of systematic review, meta-analysis, metasynthesis, and MMRS.
- A systematic review is a structured, comprehensive synthesis of the research literature to determine the best research evidence available to address a healthcare question. A systematic review involves identifying, locating, appraising, and synthesizing quality research evidence for expert clinicians to use to promote EBP.
- Meta-analysis is a synthesis strategy that statistically pools the samples and results from previous studies with similar designs. Meta-analyses provide one of the strongest levels of evidence about the effectiveness of an intervention.
- Metasynthesis is the systematic compilation, integration, and translation of qualitative study results using different conceptual views to consolidate knowledge of fundamental importance to nursing.
- MMRSs involve the synthesis or integration of various quantitative, qualitative, and mixed methods studies.
- Two models have been developed to promote EBP in nursing: the Stetler Model of Research Utilization to Facilitate EBP and the Iowa Model

Revised: Evidence-Based Practice to Promote Excellence in Health Care.
- The phases of the revised Stetler model are (1) preparation, (2) validation, (3) comparative evaluation and decision making, (4) translation and application, and (5) evaluation.
- The Iowa model provides guidelines for making evidence-based changes in practice and monitoring the changes to determine patient, provider, and healthcare agency outcomes.
- The process for developing evidence-based guidelines is introduced, and the national guideline for the management of HTN in adults is provided as an example.
- The Grove Model for Implementing Evidence-Based Guidelines in Practice is provided to assist nurses in determining the quality of evidence-based guidelines and the steps for using these guidelines in practice.
- EPCs have an important role in the conduct of research, development of systematic reviews, and formulation of evidence-based guidelines for selected practice areas.
- Translational research is an evolving concept that is defined by the NIH as the translation of basic scientific discoveries into practical applications.

REFERENCES

Agency for Healthcare Research and Quality (AHRQ). (2019a). *Evidence-based practice centers (EPC): Program overview.* Retrieved from http://www.ahrq.gov/research/findings/evidence-based-reports/overview/index.html

Agency for Healthcare Research and Quality (AHRQ). (2019b). *The EvidenceNow key driver diagram.* Retrieved from https://www.ahrq.gov/evidencenow/tools/index.html

Alzayyat, A. S. (2014). Barriers to evidence-based practice utilization in psychiatric/mental health nursing. *Issues in Mental Health Nursing, 35*(2), 134–143. doi:10.3109/0161 2840.2013.848385

American Nurses Credentialing Center (ANCC). (2019). *ANCC Magnet Recognition Program® overview.* Retrieved from https://www.nursingworld.org/magnet

Anderson, K. K., & Jenson, C. E. (2019). Violence risk-assessment screening tools for acute care mental health settings: Literature review. *Archives of Psychiatric Nursing, 33*(1), 112–119. doi:10.1016/j.apnu.2018.08.012

Andrel, J. A., Keith, S. W., & Leiby, B. E. (2009). Meta-analysis: A brief introduction. *Clinical & Translational Science, 2*(5), 374–378. doi:10.1111/j.1752-8062.2009. 00152.x

Bagnasco, A., Di Giacomo, P., Mora, R., Catania, G., Turci, C., Rocco, G., et al. (2014). Factors influencing self-management in patients with type 2 diabetes: A quantitative systematic review protocol. *Journal of Advanced Nursing, 70*(1), 187–199. doi:10.1111/jan.12178

Barnett-Page, E., & Thomas, J. (2009). Methods for the synthesis of qualitative research: A critical review. *BMC Medical Research Methodology, 9*, 59. doi:10.1186/1471-2288-9-59

Beck, C. T. (2009). Metasynthesis: A goldmine for evidence-based practice. *AORN Journal, 90*(5), 701–710. doi:10.1111/jan.12178

Benzies, K. M., Premji, S., Hayden, K. A., & Serrett, K. (2006). State-of-the-evidence reviews: Advantages and challenges of including grey literature. *Worldview on Evidence-Based Nursing, 3*(2), 55–61. doi:10.1111/j.1741-6787.2006.00051.x

Bergdahl, E. (2019). Is meta-synthesis turning rich descriptions into thin reductions? A criticism of meta-aggregation as a form of qualitative synthesis. *Nursing Inquiry, 26*, e12273. doi:10.1111.nin.12273

Bettany-Saltikov, J. (2010a). Learning how to undertake a systematic review: Part 1. *Nursing Standard, 24*(50), 47–56. doi:10.7748/ns2010.08.24.50.47.c7939

Bettany-Saltikov, J. (2010b). Learning how to undertake a systematic review: Part 2. *Nursing Standard, 24*(51), 47–58. doi:10.7748/ns2010.08.24.51.47.c7943

Bolton, L. B., Donaldson, N. E., Rutledge, D. N., Bennett, C., & Brown, D. S. (2007). The impact of nursing interventions: Overview of effective interventions, outcomes, measures, and priorities for future research. *Medical Care Research & Review, 64*(2), S123–S143. doi:10.1177/1077558707299248

Butler, A., Hall, H., & Copnell, B. (2016). A guide to writing a qualitative systematic review protocol to enhance evidence-based practice in nursing and health care. *Worldviews on Evidence-Based Nursing, 13*(3), 241–249. doi:10.1111/wvn.12134

Champion, V. L., & Skinner, C. S. (2008). The health belief model. In K. Glanz, B. K Rimer, & K. Viswanath (Eds.), *Health behavior and health education: Theory, research and practice* (4th ed., pp. 45–62). San Francisco, CA: Jossey-Bass.

Chesla, C. A. (2008). Translational research: Essential contributions from interpretive nursing science. *Research in Nursing & Health, 31*(4), 381–390. doi:10.1002/nur.20267

Cochrane Collaboration. (2019). *Cochrane library.* Retrieved from https://www.cochranelibrary.com/

Cochrane Nursing. (2019). *About us.* Retrieved from https://nursing.cochrane.org/about-us

Conn, V. S., & Rantz, M. J. (2003). Research methods: Managing primary study quality in meta-analyses. *Research in Nursing & Health, 26*(4), 322–333. doi:10.1002/nur.10092

Conn, V. S., Valentine, J. C., Cooper, H. M., & Rantz, M. J. (2003). Methods: Grey literature in meta-analyses. *Nursing Research,* 52(4), 256–261.

Cooper, H. (2017). *Research synthesis and meta-analysis: A step-by-step approach* (5th ed.). Los Angeles, CA: Sage.

Creswell, J. W., & Clark, V. L. P. (2018). *Designing and conducting mixed methods research* (3rd ed.). Los Angeles, CA: Sage.

Creswell, J. W., & Creswell, J. D. (2018). *Research design. Qualitative, quantitative, and mixed methods approaches* (5th ed.). Los Angeles, CA: Sage.

Creswell, J. W., & Poth, C. N. (2018). *Qualitative inquiry & research design: Choosing among five approaches* (4th ed.). Los Angeles, CA: Sage.

Cullen, L., Hanrahan, K., Farrington, M., DeBerg, J., Tucker, S., & Kleiber, C. (2018). *Evidence-based practice in action: Comprehensive strategies, tools, and tips from the University of Iowa Hospitals and Clinics.* Indianapolis, IN: Sigma Theta Tau International.

Dang, D., & Dearholt, S. L. (2018). *John Hopkins nursing evidence-based practice: Model and guidelines* (3rd ed.). Indianapolis, IN: Sigma Theta Tau International.

Deutschman, C. S., Ahrens, T., Cairns, C. B., Sessler, C. N., Parsons, P. E., & Critical Care Societies Collaborative. Multisociety Task Force for Critical Care Research: Key issues and recommendations. (2012). *American Journal of Critical Care, 21*(1), 15–23. doi:10.4037/ajcc2012632

Donabedian, A. (2005). Evaluation the quality of medical care. *The Milbank Quarterly, 83*(4), 691–729. doi:10.1111/j.1468-0009.2005.00397.x

Dugan, K. A., & Gabuya, A. (2019). A "snippet" of evidence leads to practice change. *Nursing Management, 50*(6), 16–18. doi:10.1097/01.NUMA.0000558491.89888.f8

Duncombe, D. C. (2018). A multi-institutional study of the perceived barriers and facilitators to implementing evidence-based practice. *Journal of Clinical Nursing, 27*(5-6), 1216–1226. doi:10.1111/jocn.14168

Egger, M., Smith, G. D., Schneider, M., & Minder, C. (1997). Bias in meta-analysis detected by a simple graphical test. *British Medical Journal, 315*(7109), 629–634. doi:10.1136/bmj.315.7109.629

Fernandez, R. S., & Tran, D. T. (2009). The meta-analysis graph: Clearing the haze. *Clinical Nurse Specialist, 23*(2), 57–60. doi:10.1097/NUR.0b013e31819971fd

Finfgeld-Connett, D. (2010). Generalizability and transferability of meta-synthesis research findings. *Journal of Advanced Nursing, 66*(2), 246–254. doi:10.1111/j.1365-2648.2009.05250.x

France, E. F., Cunningham, M., Ring, N., Uny, I., Duncan, E. A. S., Jepson, R. G., et al. (2019). Improving reporting of meta-ethnography: The eMERGe reporting guidance. *Psycho-Oncology, 28*(3), 447–458. doi:10.1002/pon.4915

France, E. F., Uny, I., Ring, N., Turley, R., Maxwell, M., Duncan, E., et al. (2019). A methodological systematic review of meta-ethnography conduct to articulate the complex analytical phases. *BMC Medical Research Methodology, 19.* Article 35. doi:10.1186/s12874-019-0670-7

Friesen, M. A., Brady, J. M., Milligan, R., & Christensen, P. (2017). Findings from a pilot study: Bringing evidence-based practice to the bedside. *Worldviews on Evidence-Based Nursing, 14*(1), 22–34. doi:10.1111/Wvn.12195

Grove, S. K., & Cipher, D. J. (2020). *Statistics for nursing research: A workbook for evidence-based practice* (3rd ed.). St. Louis, MO: Elsevier.

Grove, S. K., Burns, N., & Gray, J. R. (2013). *The practice of nursing research: Appraisal, synthesis, and generation of evidence* (7th ed.). St. Louis, MO: Elsevier Saunders.

Harden, A., & Thomas, J. (2005). Methodological issues in combining diverse study types in systematic reviews.

International Journal of Social Research Methodology, 8(3), 257–271. doi:10.1080/13645570500155078

Heyvaert, M., Maes, B., & Onghena, P. (2013). Mixed methods research synthesis: Definition, framework, and potential. *Quality & Quantity, 47*(2), 659–676. doi:10.1007/s11135-011-9538-6

Hickman, L. D., DiGiacomo, M., Phillips, J., Rao, A., Newton, P. J., Jackson, D., et al. (2018). Improving evidence based practice in postgraduate nursing programs: A systematic review. Bridging the evidence practice gap (BRIDGE project). *Nurse Education Today, 63*(1), 69–75. doi:10.1016/j.nedt.2018.01.015

Higgins, J. P., & Green, S. (Eds.). (2011). *Cochrane handbook for systematic reviews of interventions* [Internet]. Version 5.1.0. London, England: The Cochrane Collaboration [Cited 2011 March 20]. Retrieved from http://handbook.cochrane.org/

Higgins, J. P. T., & Green, S. (2008). *Cochrane handbook for systematic reviews of interventions*. West Sussex, England: Wiley-Blackwell & The Cochrane Collaboration.

Higgins, J. P. T., & Thomas, J. (2020). *Cochrane handbook for systematic reviews of interventions* (2nd ed.). West Sussex, England: Wiley Cochrane Series.

Iowa Model Collaborative. (2017). Iowa model of evidence-based practice: Revisions and validation. *Worldviews on Evidence-Based Nursing, 14*(3), 175–182. doi:10.1111/wvn.12223

James, P. A., Oparil, S., Carter, B. L., Crushman, W. C., Denison-Himmelfarb, C., Handler, J., et al. (2014). 2014 Evidence-based guideline for the management of high blood pressure in adults: Report from the panel members appointed to the Eighth Joint National Committee (JNC 8). *Journal of American Medical Association, 311*(5), 507–520. doi:/10.1001/jama.2013.284427

Joanna Briggs Institute. (2019). *Joanna Briggs Institute: Evidence-based practice resources and publications*. Retrieved from https://joannabriggs.org/ebp

Kazdin, A. E. (2017). *Research design in clinical psychology* (5th ed.). Boston, MA: Pearson.

Kesten, K., White, K. A., Heitzler, E. T., Chaplin, L. T., & Bondmass, M. D. (2019). Perceived evidence-based practice competency acquisition in graduate nursing students: Impact of intentional course design. *Journal of Continuing Education in Nursing, 50*(2), 79–86. doi:10.3928/00220124-20190115-07

Kim, J. H., & Park, H. (2019). Effects of smartphone-based mobile learning in nursing education: A systematic review and meta-analysis. *Journal of Asian Nursing Research, 13*(1), 20–29. doi:10.1016/j.anr.2019.01.005

King, A., & Eckersley, R. (2019). *Statistics for biomedical engineers and scientists: How to visualize and analyze data*. London, England: Academic Press Elsevier.

Leedy, P. D., & Ormrod, J. E. (2019). *Practical research: Planning and design* (12th ed.). New York, NY: Pearson.

Lemus, L. P., McMullin, B., & Balinowski, H. (2018). Don't ignore my snore: Reducing perioperative complications of obstructive sleep apnea. *Journal of PeriAnesthesia Nursing, 33*(3), 338–345. doi:10.1016/j.jopN.2016.08.005

Liberati, A., Altman, D. G., Tetzlaff, J., Mulrow, C., Gotzsche, P. C., Ioannidis, J. P., et al. (2009). The PRISMA Statement for reporting systematic reviews and meta-analyses of studies that evaluate healthcare interventions: Explanation and elaboration. *Annals of Internal Medicine, 151*(4), W65–W94. doi:10.1371/journal.pmed.1000100

Liu, H., Zhou, X., Yu, G., & Sun, X. (2019). The effects of the PRISMA statement to improve the conduct and reporting of systematic reviews and meta-analyses of nursing interventions for patients with heart failure. *International Journal of Nursing Practice, 25*(3), e12729. doi:10.1111/ijn.12729

Luchsinger, J. S., Jones, J., McFarland, A. K., & Kissler, K. (2019). Examining nurse/patient relationships in care coordination: A qualitative metasynthesis. *Applied Nursing Research, 49*(1), 41–49. doi:10.1016/j.apnr.2019.07.006

Mackey, A., & Bassendowski, S. (2017). The history of evidence-based practice in nursing education and practice. *Journal of Professional Nursing, 33*(1), 51–55. doi:10.1016/profnurs.2016.05.Liberati009

Magnus, M. C., Ping, M., Shen, M. M., Bourgeois, J., & Magnus, J. H. (2011). Effectiveness of mammography screening in reducing breast cancer mortality in women aged 39–49 years: A meta-analysis. *Journal of Women's Health, 20*(6), 845–852. doi:10.1089/jwh.2010.2098

MEDLINE. (2019). *MEDLINE®: Description of the database*. Retrieved from https://www.nlm.nih.gov/bsd/medline.html

Melnyk, B. M. (2016). Editorial: Level of evidence plus critical appraisal of its quality yields confidence to implement evidence-based practice changes. *Worldviews on Evidence-Based Nursing, 13*(5), 337–339, doi:10.1111/Wvn.12181

Melnyk, B. M., & Fineout-Overholt, E. (2019). *Evidence-based practice in nursing and healthcare: A guide to best practice* (4th ed.). Philadelphia, PA: Wolters Kluwer.

Melnyk, B. M., Fineout-Overholt, E., Giggleman, M., & Choy, K. (2017). A test of the Advancing Research and Clinical practice through close Collaboration (ARCC©) model improves implementation of evidence-based practice, healthcare culture, and patient outcomes. *Worldviews on Evidence-Based Nursing, 14*(1), 5–9. doi:10.1111/wvn.12188

Melnyk, B. M., Gallagher-Ford, & Fineout-Overholt, E. (2017). *Implementing evidence-based practice competencies in healthcare: A practical guide for improving quality, safety, & outcomes*. Indianapolis, IN: Sigma Theta Tau International.

Melnyk, B. A., Gallagher-Ford, L., Thomas, B. K., Troseth, M., Wyngarden K., & Szalacha, L. (2016). A study of chief nurse executives indicates low prioritization of evidence-based practice and shortcomings in hospital performance metrics across the United States. *Worldview on Evidence-Based Nursing, 13*(1), 6–14. doi:10.1111/wvn.12133

Melnyk, B. M., Gallagher-Ford, L., Zellefrow, C., Tucker, S., Dromme, L. V., & Thomas, B. K. (2018a). Outcomes from the first Helene Fuld Health Trust National Institute for Evidence-Based Practice in Nursing and Healthcare Invitational Expert Forum. *Worldviews on Evidence-Based Nursing, 15*(1), 5–15. doi:10.1111/wvn.12272

Melnyk, B. M., Gallagher-Ford, L., Zellefrow, C., Tucker, S., Thomas, B., Sinnott, L. T., et al. (2018b). The first US study on nurses' evidence-based practice competencies indicates major deficits that threaten healthcare quality, safety, and patient outcomes. *Worldviews on Evidence-Based Nursing, 15*(1), 16–25. doi:10.1111/wvn.12269

Moher, D., Liberati, A., Tetzlaff, J., Altman, D. G., & PRISMA Group. (2009). *Preferred reporting items for systematic reviews and meta-analyses: The PRISMA statement.* Retrieved from http://www.prisma-statement.org

Moore, F., & Tierney, S. (2019). What and how but where does the why fit in? The disconnection between practice and research evidence from the perspective of UK nurses involved in a qualitative study. *Nurse Education in Practice, 34*(1), 90–96. doi:10.1016/j.nepr.2018.11.008

Moore, Z. (2012). Meta-analysis in context. *Journal of Clinical Nursing, 21*(19/20), 2798–2807. doi:10.1111/j.1365-2702.2012.04122.x

Moorhead, S., Swanson, E., Johnson, M., & Maas, M. L. (2018). *Nursing outcomes classification (NOC): Measurement of health outcomes* (6th ed.). St. Louis, MO: Elsevier.

Moriarty, F., Pottie, I. K., Dolovich, L., McCarthy, L., Rojas-Fernandez, C., & Farrell, B. (2019). Describing recommendations: An essential consideration for clinical guideline developers. *Research in Social and Administrative Pharmacy, 15*(1), 806–810. doi:10.1016/j.sapharm.2018.08.014

National Center for Advancing Translation Science (NCATS). (2019). *Translation science spectrum.* Retrieved from https://ncats.nih.gov/translation/spectrum

National Guideline Clearinghouse (NGC). (2018). *AHRQ: NGC to shut down July 16, 2018.* Retrieved from https://www.aafp.org/news/government-medicine/20180627guidelineclearinghouse.html

National Institutes of Health (NIH). (2019a). *About the National Center for Advancing Translational Sciences (NCATS).* Retrieved from https://ncats.nih.gov/about

National Institutes of Health (NIH). (2019b). *Clinical and translational research awards program.* Bethesda, MD: Author. Retrieved from https://ncats.nih.gov/ctsa

Noblit, G. W., & Hare, R. D. (1988). *Meta-ethnography: Synthesizing qualitative studies.* California, CA: Sage.

Noordzij, M., Hooft, L., Dekker, F. W., Zoccali, C., & Jager, K. J. (2009). Systematic reviews and meta-analyses: When they are useful and when to be careful. *Kidney International, 76*(11), 1130–1136. doi:10.1038/ki.2009.339

Norris, A. E., Matsuda, Y., & Sarik, D. A. (2019). Implementing quality: Implications for intervention and translational science. *Journal of Nursing Scholarship, 51*(2), 205–213. doi:10.1111/jnu.12449

Paré, G., Trudel, M., Jaana, M., & Kitsiou, S. (2015). Synthesizing information systems knowledge: A typology of literature reviews. *Information & Management, 52*(1), 183–199. doi:10.1016/j.im.2014.08.008

Pintz, C., Zhou, Q., McLaughlin, M. K., Kelly, K. P., & Guzzetta, C. E. (2018). National study of nursing research characteristics at Magnet®-designated hospital. *Journal of Nursing Administration, 48*(5), 247–258. doi:10.1097/NNA.000000000000609

Pölkki, T., Kanste, O., Kääriäinen, M., Elo, S., & Kyngäs, H. (2013). The methodological quality of systematic reviews published in high-impact nursing journals: A review of the literature. *Journal of Clinical Nursing, 23*(3-4), 315–332. doi:10.1111/jocn.12132

Quality and Safety Education for Nurses (QSEN). (2012). *Graduate QSEN competencies.* Retrieved from http://qsen.org/competencies/graduate-ksas/

Reed, J. E., Howe, C., Doyle, C., & Bell, D. (2018). Simple rules for evidence translation in complex systems: A qualitative study. *BMC Medicine, 16*(1), 92. doi:10.1186/s12916-018-1076-9

Sandelowski, M., & Barroso, J. (2007). *Handbook for synthesizing qualitative research.* New York, NY: Springer.

Sandelowski, M., Voils, C. I., Leeman, J., & Crandell, J. L. (2012). Mapping the mixed methods-mixed research synthesis terrain. *Journal of Mixed Methods Research, 6*(4), 317–331. doi:10.1177/1558689811427913

Shea, B. J., Reeves, B. C., Wells, G., Thuku, M. Hamel, C., Moran, J., et al. (2017). AMSTAR 2: A critical appraisal tool for systematic reviews that include randomised or non-randomised studies of healthcare interventions or both. *BMJ, 358*, j408. doi:10.1136/bmj.j4008

Sher, I. (2018). *Educational program for parents of neonates on nasal continuous positive airway pressure* [Doctoral dissertation, Walden University]. CINAHL.

Sherwood, G., & Barnsteiner, J. (2017). *Quality and safety in nursing: A competency approach to improving outcomes* (2nd ed.). Ames, IA: Wiley-Blackwell.

Shojania, K. G., Sampson, M., Ansari, M. T., Ji, J., Doucette, S., & Moher, D. (2007). How quickly do systematic reviews go out of date? Survival analysis. *Annals of Internal Medicine, 147*(4), 224–234. doi:10.7326/0003-4819-147-4-200708210-00179

Sirriyeh, R., Lawton, R., Gardner, P., & Armitage, G. (2012). Reviewing studies with diverse designs: The development and evaluation of a new tool. *Journal of Evaluation in Clinical Practice, 18*(4), 746–752. doi:10.1111/j.1365-2753.2011.01662.x

Spiva, L., Hart, P. L., Patrick, S., Waggoner, J., Jackson, C., & Threatt, J. L. (2017). Effectiveness of an evidence-based practice nurse mentor training program. *Worldviews on Evidence-Based Nursing, 14*(3), 183–191. doi:10.1111/Wvn.12219

Stetler, C. B. (1994). Refinement of the Stetler/Marram model for application of research findings to practice. *Nursing Outlook, 42*(1), 15–25. doi:10.1016/0029-6554(94)90067-1

Stetler, C. B. (2001). Updating the Stetler model of research utilization to facilitate evidence-based practice. *Nursing Outlook, 49*(6), 272–279. doi:10.1067/mno.2001.120517

Stetler, C. B. (2010) Stetler model. In J. Rycroft-Malone & T. Bucknall (Eds.), *Models and frameworks for implementing evidence-based practice: Linking evidence to action* (pp. 51–81). Oxford, England: Wiley-Blackwell.

Stetler, C. B., & Marram, G. (1976). Evaluating research findings for applicability in practice. *Nursing Outlook, 24*(9), 559–563.

Stewart, L. A., Clarke, M., Rovers, M., Riley, R. D., Simmonds, M., Stewart, G., et al. (2015). Preferred reporting for a systematic review and meta-analysis of individual participant data: The PRISMA-IPD statement. *Journal of the American Medical Association, 313*(6), 1657–1665. doi:10.1001/jama.2015.3656

Straus, S. E., Glasziou, P., Richardson, W. S., Rosenberg, W., & Haynes, R. B. (2011). *Evidence-based medicine: How to practice and teach EBM* (5th ed.). Edinburgh, Scotland: Churchill Livingstone Elsevier.

Sun, X., Zhou, X., Zhang, Y., & Liu, H. (2019). Reporting and methodological quality of systematic reviews and meta-analyses of nursing interventions in patients with Alzheimer's disease: General implications of the findings. *Journal of Nursing Scholarship, 51*(3), 308–316. doi:10.1111/jnu.12462

Tatar, O., Thompson, E., Naz, A., Perez, S., Shapiro, G. K., Wade, K., et al. (2018). Factors associated with human papillomavirus (HPV) test acceptability in primary screening for cervical cancer: A mixed methods research synthesis. *Preventative Medicine, 116*(1), 40–50. doi:10.1016/j.ypmed.2018.08.034

The Joint Commission. (2019). *About our standards*. Retrieved from http://www.jointcommission.org/standards_information/standards.aspx

Titler, M. G., Kleiber, C., Steelman, V. J., Rakel, B. A., Budreau, G., Everett, L. Q., et al. (1994). Infusing research into practice to promote quality care. *Nursing Research, 43*(5), 307–313.

Titler, M. G., Kleiber, C., Steelman, V. J., Rakel, B. A., Budreau, G., Everett, L. Q., et al. (2001). The Iowa model of evidence-based practice to promote quality care. *Critical Care Nursing Clinics of North America, 13*(4), 497–509. doi:10.1016/S0899-5885(18)30017-0

Turlik, M. (2010). Evaluating the results of a systematic review/meta-analysis. *Foot and Ankle Online Journal, 2*(7), 5. doi:10.3827/faoj.2009.0207.0005

Walsh, D., & Downe, S. (2005). Meta-synthesis method for qualitative research: A literature review. *Journal of Advanced Nursing, 50*(2), 204–211. doi:10.1111/j.1365-2648.2005.03380.x

Wand, T., Crawford, C., Bell, N., Murphy, M., White, K., & Wood, E. (2019). Documenting the pre-implementation phase for multi-site translational research project to test a new model emergency department-based mental health nursing care. *International Emergency Nursing, 45*(1), 10–15. doi:10.1016/j.ienj.2019.04.001

Warren, J. I., McLauglin, M., Bardsley, J., Eich, J., Esche, C. A., Kropkowski, L., et al. (2016). The strengths and challenges of implementing EBP in healthcare systems. *Worldviews on Evidence-Based Nursing, 13*(1), 15–24. doi:10.1111/wvn.12149

Weber, M. A., Schiffrin, E. L., White, W. B., Mann, S., Lindholm, L. H., Kenerson, J. G., et al. (2014). Clinical practice guidelines for the management of hypertension in the community: A statement by the American Society of Hypertension and the International Society of Hypertension. *Journal of Clinical Hypertension, 16*(1), 14–26. doi:10.1111/jch.12237

Weiss, M. E., Bobay, K. L., Johantgen, M., & Shirey, M. R. (2018). Aligning evidence-based practice with translational research. *Journal of Nursing Administration, 48*(9), 425–431. doi:10.1097/nna.0000000000000644

Westra, B. L., Latimer, G. E., Matney, S. A., Park, J. I., Sensmeier, J., Simpson, R. L., et al. (2015). A national action plan for sharable and comparable nursing data to support practice and translation research for transforming health care. *Journal of American Medical Informatics Association, 22*(3), 600–607. doi:10.1093/jamia/ocu011

Whittemore, R., Chao, A., Jang, M., Minges, K. E., & Park, C. (2014). Methods for knowledge synthesis: An overview. *Heart and Lung, 43*(5), 453–461. doi:10.1016/j.hrtlng.2014.05.014

20

Collecting and Managing Data

Daisha J. Cipher and Jennifer R. Gray

http://evolve.elsevier.com/Gray/practice/

Data collection is one of the most exciting parts of research. After all the planning, writing, and negotiating that precede it, the researcher is eager for this active part of research. However, before beginning, the researcher must spend time carefully preparing for this endeavor and double-checking each step. For quantitative research, preparation begins with clarifying exactly which data will be collected, how they will be collected, and how they will be recorded. The data to be collected are determined by the variables' operational definitions (see Chapter 6). Data collection strategies for qualitative studies are described in Chapter 12.

Data collection is the process of selecting subjects and gathering data from them. The actual steps of collecting data are specific to each study and depend on both the research design and measurement methods. Data may be collected from subjects by observing, testing, measuring, questioning, recording, or any combination of these methods, either conducted by the research team or retrieved from data sources. The primary investigator is actively involved in this process either by collecting data or by supervising data collectors.

This chapter describes practical aspects of quantitative data collection. Consistent with other phases of the

research process, decisions made later in the planning process may affect decisions made previously. Although presented in the chapter as a chronological series of steps, preparation for implementing a study, and specifically collecting the data, is actually a circular process that is refined through the planning and pilot study phases. The first section of the chapter is a brief discussion of the study protocol, which includes recruiting and consenting subjects, assigning subjects to groups if part of the study design, implementing an intervention, and collecting the data. Following that section, the focus of the chapter changes to the specific details of data collection, which begins with a description of factors that affect data collection decisions, such as cost and time. In the context of these factors, the researcher may need to develop or refine a demographic questionnaire, prepare for data entry, and revise a data collection plan.

Conducting a pilot test with a small group of subjects greatly strengthens the study. After necessary modifications of the study based on the pilot results, the researcher begins data collection, maintaining consistency among data collectors over time. Incoming data are coded and stored in ways that allow easy retrieval to answer the research question. Toward the end of the chapter, the common problems encountered during data collection and strategies for solving them are addressed. The chapter concludes with a discussion of the support and resources available to the researcher.

STUDY PROTOCOL

By the time you sketch plans for implementation of the study, the bulk of the methods have been finalized. How did you specify that subjects would be recruited? How many subjects are needed based on the power analysis? Were you planning on assigning your subjects randomly to groups? If so, at what point did you plan on making that assignment? It is optimal to assign subjects randomly to an intervention group or control group after baseline data are collected but before introducing the intervention. In this way, all subjects demonstrate the ability to complete questions and measures, but they have the opportunity to decline further participation before group assignment. For an interventional study, the way in which you will enact the research intervention was specified with your definition of the independent variable, but when did you envision that intervention as occurring, relative to baseline measurements?

You as the researcher will develop a flow diagram to illustrate the **study protocol** for implementing the study. A study protocol is the step-by-step plan for recruiting subjects, obtaining consent, collecting data, and implementing an intervention. The Consolidated Standards of Reporting Trials (CONSORT) 2010 Statement was developed from previous CONSORT guidelines for consistency and clarity in reporting randomized trials in publications (Schulz, Altman, & Moher, 2010). The flowchart for screening and enrollment of study participants recommended by the CONSORT 2010 guidelines should be followed. (Fig. 15.2 is the CONSORT figure from Lee and Park's [2019] study of the effects of auricular acupressure on pain and disability in adults with chronic neck pain.) To create such a flowchart, the researcher must keep excellent records of recruitment, enrollment, attrition, and reasons for attrition (see Chapter 15). Jull and Aye (2015) conducted a systematic review of five high-impact nursing journals and found improvement in the extent to which the CONSORT guidelines were followed, but they also identified areas for improvement.

FACTORS INFLUENCING DATA COLLECTION

When planning data collection, critical factors to consider are cost, number of researchers, time, availability of data collection tools, and methods of data collection. The researcher balances these with the need to maintain optimal reliability and validity of the study throughout data collection.

Cost Factors

Cost is a major consideration when planning a study. Box 20.1 provides a list of common costs associated with quantitative studies. Measurement tools, such as continuous electrocardiogram monitors, activity monitors, glucometers, or other devices used in physiological studies, may need to be rented, purchased, or borrowed from the manufacturer, a medical supply company, or a healthcare agency.

Researchers may be required to pay a fee to use instruments or questionnaires. Some of these instruments and questionnaires are available only if a copy is purchased for each participant or if a fee is paid for access of each participant to an electronic instrument. Data collection forms must be formatted or adapted to electronic use. Printing costs for materials such as teaching materials or questionnaires that will be used during the study must be considered. Providing subjects the required copy of the signed consent form doubles the expense of printing consent forms. Small payments to participants in the form of cash or gift cards should be considered as compensation for subjects' time and

---

BOX 20.1 Common Costs for Data Collection in Quantitative Studies

- Fee for use of instruments, data collection forms, and manual for scoring and coding
- Fee for use of survey software
- Duplication of questionnaires and consent forms
- Payment of nonvolunteer data collectors
- Equipment purchase or rental and maintenance costs
- Supplies related to physiological measures, such as glucometer test strips
- Laboratory analysis or test result analysis
- Fee for cloud storage to house data
- Compensation to subjects for time and travel
- Statistical or other consultation services

effort. Sometimes a researcher may choose to provide child care so that parents and other caregivers who would not otherwise be able to participate in the study can be included. In studies with mailed surveys, postage is a substantial expense. There may be costs involved in coding data for computer entry and for conducting data analysis. Consultation with a statistician early in the development of a research project and during data analysis must also be budgeted. The researcher may need to hire an assistant who can remain blinded for data entry or analysis or someone who can type the final report, develop graphics or presentations, or type and edit manuscripts for publication.

In addition to these direct costs of a research project, there are costs associated with the researcher's time and travel to and from the study site. The researcher may also identify the estimated expense of presenting the research findings at conferences and include those expenses in the budget, if allowable. To prevent unexpected expenses from delaying the study, estimated costs should be tabulated and totaled in a budget. This can be revised as needed. Seeking funding for at least part of the costs can facilitate the conduct of a study (see Chapter 29). Some proposals for funding require considerable time to write, so benefit versus cost should be pondered.

Size of Research Team

One researcher can implement a study as the primary investigator, but one-researcher studies require more time to complete. However, a master's thesis and doctoral dissertation are usually completed by an individual student supported by a faculty member. Having a research team of two or more people means having assistance in completing all of the tasks a study requires. The disadvantage of working with a team is that additional time is required for meetings and coordination of the members' activities. The larger, more complex the study, the less likely it is that the study will be implemented by one person. Funded studies are more likely to be implemented by a research team of two or more (see Chapter 29).

Time Factors

Researchers often underestimate the time required for participants to complete data collection forms and for the research team to recruit and enroll subjects for a study. The first aspect of time—the participant's time

commitment—must be determined early in the process because the time needed for participant involvement must be included in the informed consent process and document. While conducting the pilot study, make note of the time required to collect data from a subject and revise the consent form to reflect the expected time commitment accurately. The time needed for each individual subject is based on the average time pilot study subjects spent in completing data collection.

How long will it take to identify potential subjects, explain the study, and obtain consent? How much time will be needed for activities such as completing questionnaires or obtaining physiological measures? How long will it take to obtain approval of the institutional review board (IRB)? The number of days, weeks, or months required to obtain enough subjects for the research is a more difficult prediction, because unforeseen circumstances may make gaining IRB approval (see Chapter 9), securing access to subjects, obtaining consent, and collecting data a more extended processes than originally envisioned. Kelechi, Mueller, Madisetti, Prentice, and Dooley (2018) collected data for their three-site randomized trial for over 5 years. It took that long to accrue their sample of 276 persons with chronic venous disease. In some situations, researchers must obtain permission from administrators, managers, and even each subject's physician before they are permitted to collect data from the subject. Activities required for these stipulations, such as meeting the person in authority, explaining the study, and obtaining permission, require extensive time. In some cases, potential subjects are lost before the researcher can obtain permission, extending the time required to obtain the necessary number of subjects.

Novice researchers may have difficulty making reasonable estimates of time and costs related to a study. Validating those estimates with an academic advisor or on-site nurse researcher, after initial pilot study completion, is recommended. If cost and time factors are prohibitive, a trimmed-down study measuring fewer variables, using fewer measurement instruments, or consenting fewer subjects is a reasonable solution. The researcher, however, should thoroughly examine the consequences for design validity before making such revisions (Kazdin, 2017; Leedy & Ormrod, 2019).

Selection of Instruments

When several instruments or methods are available for measuring a variable, the researcher must select the best one for the specific study (Waltz, Strickland, & Lenz, 2017). Specifically, instruments and other measurements used in a study should fit, or be congruent with, the conceptual definitions for each study concept. In addition, practical considerations for instrument selection include item burden and reading level. Chapters 16 and 17 provide detailed information regarding the types and selection of quality measurement methods for a study.

Methods of Data Collection

Based on data needed to answer the research question and on instruments to be used in a study, the researcher must decide whether to present this instrument to subjects as a packet of pencil-paper instruments, a link to a website to access the instruments, or questions on an electronic tablet or other electronic interface. For some studies, the subject is equipped with an electronic sensor to automatically gather pertinent data. Some of the advantages and disadvantages of different approaches to data collection are presented in the following sections.

Researcher-Administered and Participant-Completed Instruments

If a subject's accurate blood pressure (BP), height, and weight are demographic variables, a self-report measure may be neither valid nor reliable for the purpose of the study. However, if the purpose of the study can be accomplished with a self-report survey method, you must decide whether the subject will complete the survey or whether the researcher will administer the survey. It may be best for the researcher to administer self-report pencil-paper instruments if the potential subjects have minimal language or literacy ability, whereas it may be best to consider electronic data collection or medical record extraction if the subjects are likely to have hearing impairments, transportation problems, or physical difficulties.

If the researcher is administering the survey, will this occur in person or by telephone? If self-administered, will the participant complete a pencil-paper copy or record their responses on an electronic device? The method you select for data collection may affect the cost of the study, response rate, and even the characteristics of your sample. Hobden, Bryant, Carey, Sanson-Fisher, and Oldmeadow (2017) conducted a study with patients at a drug and addiction clinic to compare collecting data by electronic tablet with collecting data by

telephone interview. Both methods were found to be acceptable to the participants, but the completion time was lower and the completion rate was higher with the tablet.

In a study conducted with American Indians in rural areas, researchers found a higher response rate with in-person data collection compared to telephone data collection (English, Espinoza, Pete, & Tjemsland, 2019). They also provided details about their methods.

> "The 2 administration modes necessitated distinct sampling strategies. For the telephone sample, a random-digit-dialing sample of landline telephone numbers was generated based upon the telephone prefix shared by all three participating Tribes. The cell phone random-digit-dialing sample was drawn using a systematic random sample stratified by county and service provider from a frame of blocks built from activated wireless phone numbers.... Samples for the in-person administration study phase were drawn at random from enrollment/census rosters in each tribe, inclusive of tribal members aged 18 years and older currently living on tribal lands.... Calls to a selected number were ceased if any of the following conditions occurred: (1) 15 attempts were made; (2) the selected phone number was disconnected; (3) the number was associated with a business; or (4) participant refusal." (English et al., 2019, p. S72)

Careful selection of the data collection method will consider the target population, accessibility to technology, and the type of data being collected.

If a mailed pencil-paper survey will be used, what will be done with undelivered or incomplete returns? Will the researcher search for correct mailing addresses and undertake a second mailing to contact subjects with forwarding addresses on record? Will reminders be sent if the survey is not received within a particular time frame, and, if so, what time frame will be given for respondents, and how many reminders will be sent (Dillman, Smyth, & Christian, 2014; Harwood, 2009)?

Scannable Forms

Some target populations may have limited access to technology, requiring use of more conventional types of data collection. Even with paper versions of data collection documents, there are ways to decrease the labor of data entry and improve the accuracy of data entry by preparing special data collection forms that can be scanned. These forms are developed and coded using optical character recognition (OCR). OCR requires exact placement on the page for each potential response. To maintain the precise location of each response on print copies of these instruments, careful attention must be given to printing or copying. The complete form is scanned and responses (data) are automatically recorded in a database. Additional features include data accuracy verification, selective data extraction and analysis, auditing and tracking, and flexible export interfaces.

Online and Electronic Device Data Collection

Computer software packages developed by a variety of companies (e.g., SurveyMonkey, Qualtrics, Google, and Research Electronic Data Capture [REDCap]) enable researchers to provide instruments and other data collection forms online to potential subjects. These software programs have unique features that allow the researcher to develop point-and-click automated forms that can be distributed electronically. The following questions should be considered with use of these programs:

- Are computers with online access and/or electronic devices available among the target population?
- For an online survey, what measures are in place to protect the confidentiality and anonymity of the data?
- Is the survey formatted so that it can be completed using other electronic devices such as smartphones and tablets?
- What strategies can be used to increase the likelihood that only eligible participants complete the survey?
- Will potential subjects receive a personalized e-mail message with a link to a website?
- How will e-mail addresses be obtained?
- Can the researcher or data collector offer help if subjects have questions about the study?

Online services can be easy to use for both researcher and study participants.

The International Business Machines (IBM) Corporation that owns Statistical Package for Social Sciences (SPSS) data analysis software also markets SPSS Data Collector. This product assists with survey development and includes the capacity to host online surveys (IBM, n.d.). In 2004, the National Institutes of Health (NIH) funded development of a secure internet environment for building online data surveys and data management packages (Harris et al., 2009). This free service is called REDCap (introduced earlier) and is used worldwide by research organizations and universities. McGinley et al. (2019) studied the perspectives of persons with multiple sclerosis related to stopping disease-modifying treatments. Using REDCap, the researchers collected data from 377 participants who were registered with the North American Research Committee on Multiple Sclerosis. The online service enhanced the feasibility of a national survey but only accessed patients who were motivated, had access to online services, and were listed on the registry.

An additional advantage of online data collection is that all postings are dated and timed. Ladores and Bray (2017) reviewed studies in which electronic diaries (EDs) were used for data collection. They found advantages and disadvantages for EDs compared to paper diaries (PDs). If subjects are instructed to complete a questionnaire before bedtime, time can be verified. If subjects are instructed to complete a daily diary, date of entry is automatically associated with each entry, discouraging subjects from posting all diary entries on the last day, just before returning the diary to the researcher (Fukuoka, Kamitani, Dracup, & Jong, 2011).

With the increased sophistication and capacity of laptops, tablet computers, and smartphones, data collectors can code data directly into an electronic file at the data collection site. There is increasing overlap between the functions of mobile phones and computers. Healthcare providers load applications to their smartphones that facilitate accurate assessment, diagnosis, and pharmacological and nonpharmacological management of patients. Some of these applications can be used to collect various data, and new apps are being developed for research purposes. When children and adolescents are the study subjects, using an iPad for data collection allows the use of a touchscreen interface on a device familiar to the target audience (Linder et al., 2013). Children and adults with disabilities may be able to use a touchscreen even if unable to manipulate a mouse or type in responses.

Researchers have reported that online or electronically delivered surveys may be more acceptable to subjects when responding to sensitive questions. Cárdenas and Stormshak (2019) recruited a sample of 274 emerging adults (adolescents) to test different delivery patterns of text messages to collect data about their risk behaviors and daily activities. Text messaging, also called short message service (SMS), was used to ask the participants questions about behaviors such as substance use, depressed mood, and interactions with parents. Their electronic responses were compared to their responses on a paper survey, with more alcohol use and time spent with friends reported by text message than the paper survey. The researchers concluded that measurement of some variables may vary across data collection method (Cárdenas & Stormshak, 2019).

Fig. 20.1 shows what a survey might look like on a mobile device. The screen displays two questions from a seven-item online survey created by the researchers using Qualtrics™. The respondents were students who were formerly enrolled in the Master of Science in Nursing program at The University of Texas at Arlington. They were e-mailed a survey link, and informed consent occurred when the students agreed to take the survey by reading a consent statement and selecting "I Accept." After the respondents accepted the consent statement, the survey items appeared. This IRB-approved study allowed for quick and convenient survey participation because the respondents could use either their mobile device, tablet, or computer to complete the survey (Cipher, Urban, & Mancini, 2019).

Another type of electronic device used in research is the Medication Event Monitoring System (MEMS), which uses pill bottle tops to record the times at which the bottle is opened. Because of the expense in a multiple medication regimen, the cap is placed on the pill bottle containing the most critical medication. Hartman, Lems, and Boers (2019) conducted a review of studies in which MEMS were used to determine adherence to the manner in which MEMS data were summarized. They concluded that most researchers calculated an adherence score based on the ratio of days of correct medication consumption to the total number of days.

Digital devices connected to a computer enable users to collect large amounts of data with few errors, data that can readily be analyzed with a variety of statistical software packages. An advantage of using digital devices for the acquisition and storage of physiological data is the increased accuracy and precision that can be achieved by reducing errors associated with manually recording or transcribing physiological data from a monitor (Ryan-Wenger, 2017). Ceyhan, Taşçı, Elmalı, and Doğan (2019) conducted a study to determine the efficacy of acupuncture in decreasing BP in adults with atrial fibrillation. A novel device was developed to systematically administer acupuncture at fixed specified intervals. The results revealed that the intervention group exhibited significantly lower heart rates, systolic BP, and diastolic BP over time, whereas the control group exhibited only lower diastolic BP.

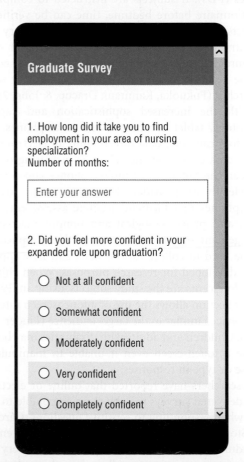

Fig. 20.1 Example of survey data collection on a mobile device.

"The acupressure device consisted of 2 control units. The first control unit had 4 apparatuses attached to arms and wrists and it was connected to [the] main unit with extension cables. After adjusting the pressure with the help of the apparatuses (tourniquets), the device applied constant pressure until tourniquets were removed. There were sensors on the apparatuses, sensor used can measure with precision of 0.1 kg/cm2, and the applied pressure can be viewed on the monitor simultaneously. The second control unit was designed to apply pressure to acupuncture point on chest and apply pressure by taking hold by hand in order to measure the stimulation level. It had only 1 pressure apparatus and sensor. Sensor and pressure head were [on] the device. The monitor of the device shows [the] level of pressure applied." (Ceyhan et al., 2019, p. 14)

Another advantage in electronic monitoring devices is that more data points can be recorded electronically than could be recorded manually. Computers linked to physiological monitoring systems can store multiple data values for multiple indicators, such as BPs, oxygen saturation levels, and sleep stages, as frequently as once per minute. Electronic sensors record signals that transducers translate into data. Because data can be electronically recorded, data collection is less labor intensive, and data are ready for analysis more quickly. The initial cost of equipment may be high but may be reasonable when compared to the cost of hiring and training human data collectors.

Some of the disadvantages of using electronic devices are the upfront expense, the need to support those unfamiliar with electronic devices, including nurses and subjects, and resistance from healthcare administrators because of concerns about security (Schick-Makaroff & Molzahn, 2015). In addition, using electronic devices requires more attention to data and device security and availability of wireless internet or a cellular network (Muigg, Kastner, Duftschmid, Modre-Osprian, & Haluza, 2019; Schick-Makaroff & Molzahn, 2015). An additional disadvantage of data collection with electronic devices is the potential for technical difficulty, resulting in loss of signal and resultant gaps in the data stream for seconds, minutes, or hours. If the malfunction occurs undetected in a repeated-measures study, some or all of the data for that particular subject may have to be discarded.

Physiological data typically require adequate electronic storage space on a computer or network of computers. Computer equipment interface machinery may require more space in an already crowded clinical setting; when possible, existing equipment should be used to collect data. Purchasing equipment, setting it up, and installing software can be time consuming and expensive at the beginning of a project. Thus initial studies usually require substantial funding. Another concern is

that the nurse researcher may focus on the machine and technology, decreasing time spent in observing and interacting with the subject (see Chapter 17 for more detail about physiological measures).

A serious concern with computerized data collection is the possibility of measurement error that can occur with equipment malfunctions and software errors. This threat can be reduced by regular maintenance and calibrations, reliability checks of the equipment and software, and frequent uploads of the data to cloud storage. **Cloud storage** is an increasingly popular means of storing data across computer servers and the internet that allows access to the data from anywhere with internet access.

Development of a Demographic Questionnaire

A few tested instruments contain demographic questions, but often researchers develop their own demographic questionnaires to capture the attributes of the sample as a whole, as well as differences that might be associated with the study variables. Data generated by subjects answering demographic questions are used to describe the sample. As you review the literature on your topic, make note of demographic variables other researchers have used to describe their samples. You may choose to ask other researchers for copies of their demographic questionnaires as a way of exploring options for composition and for different ways to measure demographics. Consider the importance of each piece of data and the subject's time required to collect it. The quantity of information provided should not be redundant. If the data can be obtained from patient records or any other written sources, researchers do not need to ask subjects to provide this information again.

Selecting Demographic Variables

Identifying data include variables such as patient record number, home address, and date of birth. Avoid collecting these data unless they are essential to answer the research question. For example, collecting a patient's age instead of date of birth is preferred because of the privacy regulations of the Health Insurance Portability and Accountability Act about the participant's health information (www.hhs.gov/ocr/hipaa) (see Chapter 9). Demographic variables are also defined and examples are provided in Chapter 6.

There are instances in which you do need to obtain subjects' contact information so they might be contacted for additional data collection. The subject's contact information, such as telephone number, e-mail address, and physical address, collected should be stored securely. Names and contact information of family members or friends may also be useful if subjects are likely to move or may be difficult to contact. This information can be obtained only with subjects' permission as part of their informed consent. To collect data from a patient's records, make sure to include permission to do this in the consent form, and ensure that the IRB has authorized the team to do this (see Chapter 9).

Common demographic descriptors are gender, race/ethnicity, and age. For gender, the answer responses may be male and female category. The researcher may also want to include an "other" category for participants who are bisexual, transgendered, or transsexual, when this is pertinent for the study focus. Human Rights Campaign (HRC) recommends dividing this question into "gender" and "gender identity," including the latter only if it yields information pertinent to data analysis. HRC recommends use of a self-identification fill-in blank for "gender" as the least-restrictive option (HRC, 2016).

At the writing of this book, federal guidelines regarding determinations of race and ethnicity for federally supported agencies require two questions, as shown in Box 20.2. How would a subject who is multiple races complete the form? Therefore researchers may ask for additional demographic information so as to clarify subjects' responses. The researcher may want to word the question to ask the participant's primary race or allow multiple responses. The current questions mandated by federal guidelines are overly simplistic and have resulted in confusing and inaccurate data (Cohn, 2015). The US Census Bureau is conducting pilot testing of different questions for the 2020 census. One option under consideration is the replacement of the current questions with a single question titled "Categories" that lists all current options plus Middle East and North Africa heritage. The instructions would be for the subject to select all that apply.

The National Ambulatory Medical Care Survey (NAMCS) is designed to collect data on ambulatory medical care services in the United States (Centers for Disease Control and Prevention [CDC], 2019). This survey uses cluster sampling of nonfederal medical clinics and health centers and collects data from office-based physicians who are primarily engaged in direct patient care. Fig. 20.2 displays an example of a NAMCS patient record form, which contains demographic variables and vital signs collected at the time of the office visit (CDC, 2019). The form collects data on age, sex, ethnicity, race, payment source, tobacco use, height, weight, temperature, systolic and diastolic BP, reason for visit, injury, continuity of care, diagnoses, prescriptions, and laboratory tests. This form can be an excellent template for researchers who are collecting similar information, because if assessed with the same coding, researchers can compare their study results with national results representing millions of medical clinic visits.

Developing Response Options for Demographic Questions

The response options for each single item on a questionnaire that allows only one response to be selected must be mutually exclusive but also exhaustive, which means that any given value for a specific variable must fit into only one category (see Chapter 16). For example, subjects are highly unlikely to recall or want to reveal exact income but would be more willing to indicate that the income is in a particular range. Box 20.3 lists income ranges that are both exclusive and exhaustive and would be appropriate for collecting demographic data from subjects. The researcher must decide how much detail is actually needed regarding income. Does the researcher seek to discover whether each participant's household income is below poverty level according to US federal poverty guidelines? To determine poverty level, the researcher must collect not only the household income,

---

BOX 20.2 Race and Ethnicity Questions for Demographic Questionnaires

Ethnicity
1. Hispanic or Latino
2. Non-Hispanic or Latino

Race
1. American Indian or Alaskan Native
2. Asian
3. Black or African American
4. Native Hawaiian or Other Pacific Islander
5. White

PATIENT INFORMATION

Patient medical record No.

Date of visit

Month	Day	Year
		2 0 2

ZIP Code Enter "1" if homeless.

Date of birth

Month	Day	Year

Age [____]
- 1 ☐ Years
- 2 ☐ Months
- 3 ☐ Days

Sex
- 1 ☐ Female - Is patient pregnant?
  - 1 ☐ Yes – Specify gestation week – Gestation week refers to the number of weeks plus 2 that the offspring has spent developing in the uterus → [____]
  - 2 ☐ No
- 2 ☐ Male

Ethnicity
- 1 ☐ Hispanic or Latino
- 2 ☐ Not Hispanic or Latino

Race - Mark (X) that apply.
- 1 ☐ White
- 2 ☐ Black or African American
- 3 ☐ Asian
- 4 ☐ Native Hawaiian or Other Pacific Islander
- 5 ☐ American Indian or Alaska Native

Expected source(s) of payment for THIS VISIT - Mark (X) all that apply.
- 1 ☐ Private insurance
- 2 ☐ Medicare
- 3 ☐ Medicaid or CHIP or other state-based program
- 4 ☐ Workers' compensation
- 5 ☐ Self-pay
- 6 ☐ No charge/Charity
- 7 ☐ Other
- 8 ☐ Unknown

Tobacco use
- 1 ☐ Not current
- 2 ☐ Current
- 3 ☐ Unknown

Prior tobacco use
- 1 ☐ Never
- 2 ☐ Former
- 3 ☐ Unknown

BIOMETRICS/VITAL SIGNS

Height [____] ft [____] in
OR
[____] cm

Weight [____] lb [____] oz
OR
[____] kg [____] gm

Temperature [____]
- 1 ☐ °C
- 2 ☐ °F

Blood pressure – If multiple measurements are taken, record the last measurement.

Systolic [____] / Diastolic [____]

REASON FOR VISIT

List the first 5 reasons for visit (i.e., symptoms, problems, issues, concerns of the patient) in the order in which they appear. Start with the chief complaint and then move to the patient history for additional reasons.

(1) Most important
(2) Other
(3) Other
(4) Other
(5) Other

Major reason for this visit
- 1 ☐ New problem (<3 mos. onset)
- 2 ☐ Chronic problem, routine
- 3 ☐ Chronic problem, flare up
- 4 ☐ Pre-surgery
- 5 ☐ Post-surgery
- 6 ☐ Preventive care (e.g., routine prenatal, well baby, screening, insurance, general exams)

Fig. 20.2 National Ambulatory Medical Care Survey patient record form.

BOX 20.3 An Example of Mutually Exclusive, Exhaustive Categories for Income

Income Range

Please check the range that most accurately reflects your family's income for a year, before taxes.

___ 1. Less than $30,000
___ 2. $30,000 to $49,999
___ 3. $50,000 to $69,999
___ 4. $70,000 or greater

---

but also how many people live in the household, which allows comparison with federal poverty guidelines (Department of Health and Human Services [DHHS], 2019) and classification of each subject as below or above poverty level.

Some researchers have used qualifying for the free or reduced lunch program as a proxy for low socioeconomic status (SES) in studies with children and families (Bohr, Brown, Laurson, Smith, & Bass, 2013). Bohr and colleagues compared the physical fitness of junior high students of higher and lower SES, using free or reduced lunch program as the indicator for lower SES. Boys of higher and lower SES were significantly different for only one type of fitness marker, performing "curl-ups," which was more likely to be a failed item for boys of higher SES than lower; in contrast, lower SES girls were significantly lower on all fitness measures than higher SES girls were. It is interesting that, for boys, differences in body mass index and percentage of body fat were also found to be statistically significant, with lower values found in boys of lower SES. It is not known whether this is a function of anthropometric variation, shortage of adequate calories, or more vigorous activity among boys of lower SES.

PREPARATION FOR DATA COLLECTION

When preparing for data collection, critical factors to consider are scheduling, entry methods, coding of the variables, and data retrieval (for any devices or online services used). Each of these factors impact the others in terms of resources and time required.

Creating a Data Collection Plan

Extensive planning increases accuracy of the data collected and validity of the study findings. Validity and strength of the findings from several carefully planned studies increase the quality of the research evidence that is then available for implementation in practice (Melnyk & Fineout-Overholt, 2019). Building on the preparations made for data collection and data entry, a data collection plan can now be developed. The **data collection plan** is a flowchart of interactions with subjects and decisions that should be made consistently. The plan for collecting data is specific to the study being conducted, beginning with recruitment. Fig. 20.3 is a flowchart of data collection steps that should be followed carefully, to maintain consistency.

A detailed plan ensures consistency of the data collection process. You as a researcher must first envision the overall activities that will occur during data collection. Write each step and develop the forms, training, and equipment needed for that step. Focus on who, what, when, where, why, and how. A data collection plan contains important details to ensure consistency of the data collected across subjects, which is critical to construct validity. Construct validity also is affected by the attention to details in planning and implementing the study (see Chapters 10 and 11). Some of these details include the timing of data collection, training data collectors, and identifying decision points.

Scheduling Data Collection

The specific days and hours of data collection may influence the consistency of the data collected and must be carefully considered. For example, the energy level and state of mind of subjects from whom data are gathered in the morning may differ from that of subjects from whom data are gathered in the evening. With hospitalized study participants, visitors are more likely to be present at certain times of day and may interfere with data collection or influence participant responses. Patient care routines vary with the time of day. Consultation with the nurses and other staff in the areas in which data collection will occur provides insight into the best times for data collection. In some studies, the care recently received or the care currently being provided may alter the data gathered. Subjects approached on Saturday to participate in the study may differ from subjects approached on weekday mornings. Subjects seeking care on Saturday may have full-time jobs, whereas subjects seeking care on weekday mornings may be either unemployed or too ill to work.

Will you collect data from more than one subject at a time, or do you think it would be simpler to focus attention on one subject at a time? How much time will be needed to collect data from each subject? If concurrent data collection is planned for several subjects, the length of time data collection will take per subject is determined by study design, setting, and available space. In addition, if the plan is for three subjects to complete data collection in the morning and three in the afternoon, what are the contingencies for subjects who arrive late or require additional time? Some subjects may be available only during lunch breaks or in the evening, after work hours.

What time of year will data be collected? For example, if the study is conducted during holiday seasons, data about sleeping, eating, or exercising may vary. Pediatric patients with asthma may experience more symptoms during the winter months than during the summer months. Planning data collection for a study of symptom management with this population would need to take this possibility into consideration.

Training Data Collectors

A high level of consistency in data collection, across subjects, is the goal. You may decide to collect all the data yourself for that reason. If you decide to use data collectors, they must be trained in responsible conduct of research and issues of informed consent, ethics, and confidentiality and anonymity (see Chapter 9). They must be informed about the research project, become familiar with the instruments to be used, and receive training in the data collection process. In addition to training, data collectors must have written guidelines or protocols that indicate which instruments to use, the order in which to introduce the instruments, how to administer the instruments, and a time frame for the data collection process (Harwood, 2009; Leedy & Ormrod, 2019). If nurses and other hospital staff collect the data for the study while performing day-to-day routines of patient care, observing their methods will identify the degree of consistency in both the collection and recording of data.

If more than one person is to collect data, consistency among data collectors (interrater reliability) must be ensured through testing (see Chapter 16). Additional training must continue until interrater reliability estimates are

ENROLLMENT AND SURVEY ADMINISTRATION PROCEDURES

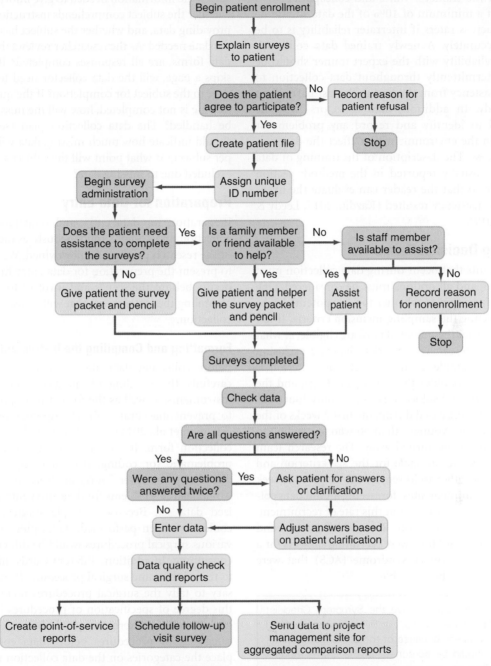

Fig. 20.3 Data collection flowchart.

at least 85% to 90% agreement between the expert trainer and the trainees. Waltz and colleagues (2017) suggest that a minimum of 10% of the data should be compared across raters if interrater reliability is to be reported accurately. A newly trained data collector's interrater reliability with the expert trainer should be assessed intermittently throughout data collection to ensure consistency from the first to the last participant in the study. In addition, data collectors must be encouraged to identify and record any problems or variations in the environment that affect the data collection process. The description of the training of data collectors is usually reported in the methods section of an article so that the reader can evaluate the likelihood that consistency resulted (Kazdin, 2017; Leedy & Ormrod, 2019).

Identifying Decision Points

Decision points that occur during data collection must be identified, and all options must be considered. One decision may pertain to whether too few potential subjects are meeting the sampling inclusion criteria. If too few subjects from the potential pool are eligible, at what point will the researcher consider changing exclusion criteria? For example, a study's inclusion criterion is first-time mothers older than 30 years of age, and the plan is to recruit 60 subjects. However, only four subjects have been consented during the first 2 weeks of the study, and persons younger than 30 who are willing to participate are being turned away. The research team may reconsider the rationale for the age criterion and perhaps decide either to lower the age range or to seek additional recruitment sites, foreseeing a total data collection period of 7.5 months at this rate of recruitment. In contrast, DeVon, Patmon, Rosenfeld, Fennessy, and Francis (2013) found they were recruiting subjects for a study on acute coronary syndrome (ACS) that were later determined to be ineligible.

"The initial plan was to have the Symptom Checklist completed by triage nurses, but this plan was modified early in the process because of the challenge of identifying who should be screened. In the first 6 months of data collection, we recruited many more patients who had ACS ruled out than was anticipated. To more accurately identify who was likely to be ruled in, we chose to delay the enrollment process until evidence of ischemia was available." (DeVon et al., 2013, p. 7)

Other decisions include whether the subject understands the information needed to give informed consent, whether the subject comprehends instructions related to providing data, and whether the subject has provided all the data needed. As the researcher reviews the completed data forms, are all responses completed? If the subject skips a page, will the data collector need to return that page to the subject for completion? If the question about income is not completed, how will the missing response be handled? The data collection plan (see Fig. 20.3) should indicate how much missing data will be allowed per subject. At what point will the subject's responses be excluded due to missing data?

Preparation for Data Entry

Preparation for data entry and preparation for data collection often occur simultaneously, as the two aspects of the research process are intertwined. We have chosen to present the preparation for data entry first because it occurs behind the scenes and involves formatting and compiling the instruments that will be used during data collection.

Formatting and Compiling the Instruments

Before collecting data, the researcher must consider carefully the wording of questions on surveys and instruments, as well as the format of response options, to prevent inaccurate subject responses or data entry (Dillman et al., 2014). Fig. 20.4 provides a sample data collection form. It includes four items that could be problematic for coding, data analysis, or both. The blank used to enter "Surgical Procedure Performed" would lead to problems for data entry into a computerized data set. Because multiple surgical procedures could have been performed, developing codes for the various surgical procedures would be difficult and time consuming. In addition, different words might be used to record the same surgical procedure. It may be necessary to tally the surgical procedures manually. Unless this degree of specification of procedures is important to the study, an alternative would be to develop larger categories of procedures before data collection and place the categories on the data collection form. A category "Other" might be useful for less frequently performed surgical procedures. This method would require the data collector to make a judgment regarding which category was appropriate for a particular surgical procedure. Another option would be to write in the category

DATA COLLECTION FORM

Demographics
____Subject Identification Number
____Age
____Gender
  1. Male
  2. Female
____Weight (in pounds)
____Height (in inches)
_____Surgical Procedure Performed
__/__/__Surgery Date (Month/Day/Year)
__/__/__Surgery Time (Hour/Minute/AM or PM)
Narcotics Ordered After Surgery_____
_____

Narcotic Administration
  Date   Time   Narcotic   Dose
1.
2.
3.
4.
5.
Instruction on Use of Pain Scale
__/__/__Date (Month/Day/Year)
__/__/__Time (Hour/Minute/AM or PM)
Comments:

    __Treatment Group
    1. TENS
    2. Placebo-TENS
    3. No-Treatment Control

Treatment Implemented
__/__/__Date (Month/Day/Year)
__/__/__Time (Hour/Minute/AM or PM)
Comments:

Dressing Change
__/__/__Date (Month/Day/Year)
__/__/__Time (Hour/Minute/AM or PM)
_____Hours since surgery
Comments:

Measurement of Pain
_____Score on Visual Analog Pain Scale
__/__/__Date Pain Measured
        (Month/Day/Year)
__/__/__Time Pain Measured
        (Hour/Minute/AM or PM)
_____Hours since surgery
Comments:

_____Data Collector Code
Comments:

Fig. 20.4 Example of a data collection form.

code number for a particular surgical procedure after the data collection form is completed but before data entry. If the specific surgical procedure is important to the study, recording the code the facility uses to bill for the procedure may be the best method.

Similar problems occur with the items "Narcotics Ordered After Surgery" and "Narcotic Administration." Unless these data are to be used in statistical analyses, it might be better to categorize this information manually for descriptive purposes. If these items are needed for planned statistical procedures, use care to develop appropriate coding. Detailed information may be needed to know the appropriateness of the narcotic doses given. The researcher might be interested in determining differences in the amount of narcotics administered in a given period in relation to weight and height. For blinded studies, do not record the treatment group assignments on the data collection form. Placing the treatment group code on the data collection form would be a mistake because the information would no longer be blinded and could influence data recorded by data collectors.

Data collection forms offer many response styles. The person completing the form (subject or data collector) might be asked to check a blank space before or after the words *male, female,* or *other* or to circle one of the words. Location of spaces for data on forms is important because careful placement makes it easier for subjects to complete the form without missing an item and for data entry staff to locate responses for computer entry. Locating responses on the left margin seems most efficient for data entry, but this layout may prove problematic for subject completion. The least effective arrangement is that in which data are positioned irregularly on a form, making it more likely that data will be missed during data collection and transcription.

You now have the individual instruments and data collection forms formatted consistently (Waltz et al., 2017). What is the best order for presenting the instruments? Should you ask subjects to complete the demographic questions first or last? Skilled researchers organize data collection forms and instruments so that the initial ones begin with less personal types of questions about age and education before asking more sensitive ones. Also, the researchers may choose not to leave the most important items for the last page of the questionnaire because of the risk of missing data if a participant becomes too fatigued or bored to complete all questions. Different types of questions require more or less time to answer, a factor that must be considered. Also, questions may ask for a response related to different time frames. For example, if one questionnaire asks about the past week and two other questionnaires ask about the past month, these should be organized so that the subject is not confused by going back and forth between time frames. If several instruments or forms are being used, putting them together in a booklet may minimize the likelihood that a questionnaire or form will be missed.

Developing a Codebook

All of the decisions the researcher makes about coding variables are documented in a codebook, either physical or virtual. A **codebook** identifies and defines each variable in the study and includes an abbreviated variable name ("income"), a descriptive variable label ("gross household annual income"), and the range of possible numerical values for every variable entered in a computer file ("0 = none; 1 = < $30,000; . . . 6 = > $100,000"). Prior to electronic files, the codebook was a binder or notebook available for the research team that contained all the information about variables, coding, and categories. Electronic versions of a codebook contain the same information as those in the past and can be shared easily with data collectors and other team members. Some codebooks also identify the source of each datum, linking the codebook with data collection forms and scales. The codebook is a useful repository of information, allowing not only a quick reference guide for decisions made during planning and analyses processes but a useful reference months or years later when data are analyzed for periodic reports to IRBs and funding agencies, retrieved for publication, reused for secondary analyses, shared anonymously with other researchers, or used for follow-up research on the same sample. Some computer programs, such as SPSS, allow researchers to print out data definitions after setting up a database. Fig. 20.5 is an example of data definitions from SPSS for Windows. The standard attributes are labels of characteristics of the variable. For example, the figure indicates that "motivation to migrate because of low pay" was measured at the ordinal level. The valid values are the response options for the item with the corresponding number. Fig. 20.6 is another example of codes for two variables. The codebook in Fig. 20.6 includes the source of the data for the variable of

Q1		Value
Standard Attributes	Position	2
	Label	I was motivated to migrate from my country because my pay was too low.
	Type	Numeric
	Format	F8
	Measurement	Ordinal
	Role	Input
Valid Values	1	Strongly Disagree
	2	Disagree
	3	Neutral
	4	Agree
	5	Strongly Agree
Missing Values	System	

Q 39		Value
Standard Attributes	Position	40
	Label	What is your gender?
	Type	Numeric
	Format	F8
	Measurement	Nominal
	Role	Input
Valid Values	1	Male
	2	Female
Missing Values	System	

Q50		Value
Standard Attributes	Position	54
	Label	Which of the following best describes your current employment situation?
	Type	Numeric
	Format	F8
	Measurement	Nominal
	Role	Input
Valid Values	1	Employed and working full time
	2	Employed and working part time
	3	Employed, currently on leave
	4	Self-Employed
	5	Unemployed
	6	Other
Missing Values	System	

Fig. 20.5 Example of data definitions from SPSS for Windows. (From the Nurse International Relocation Questionnaire 2 [Gray & Johnson, 2009].)

"mother's feeling, Day 3" as being the diary completed by the mother on Tuesday.

Developing a logical method of abbreviating variable names can be challenging. For example, the researcher might use a quality-of-life (QoL) questionnaire. It will

Variable Name	Variable Label	Source	Value Levels	Valid Range	Missing Data	Comments
A1 to A5	Family Apgar	Q2Family Apgar	1 = never 2 = hardly ever 3 = some of the time 4 = almost always 5 = always	1–5	9	Code as is (CAI)
MF3	Mother's feeling, Day 3	Tuesday diary, mother	1 = poor 2 = average 3 = good	1–3	9	Code 1 to 3 left to right

Fig. 20.6 Example of coding for hypothetical study.

be necessary to develop an abbreviated variable name for each item in the questionnaire. For example, the fourth item on a QoL questionnaire might be given the abbreviated variable name *QoL4*. A question asking the last time a home health nurse visited might be abbreviated *HHNLastvisit,* because variable names cannot have spaces. Although abbreviated variable names usually seem logical at the time the name is created, it is easy to confuse or forget these names unless they are clearly documented with a variable label. Again, the variable name is the abbreviation used to designate the variable, and the variable label is the phrase that describes the variable.

Determining the Logistics of Data Entry

If data are being collected on paper forms, the researcher must either scan a specially designed form for data entry or enter each individual datum into a computer program for analysis. When data are manually entered, the most accurate practice is to have two data collectors enter data separately and then compare the files for accuracy and to check entered data for out-of-range values (Kupzyk & Cohen, 2015). Kupzyk and Cohen also describe how to format spreadsheets such as those in Microsoft Excel so that out-of-range values cannot be entered. If data are collected electronically, data collection and entry are simultaneous. While setting up an online instrument to be completed by subjects, you will indicate the number or variable name and the code for each response for each variable (1 = Strongly disagree, 2 = Disagree, 3 = Neutral, 4 = Agree, 5 = Strongly agree).

Ensure that the question provides data at the level needed for the planned analysis. If you are planning inferential statistical analysis involving age, the question

needs to be open ended to elicit the number of years. However, if you ask the question with a list of options from which the subject selects (18–24 years, 25–32 years, etc.), the data will be ordinal and not suitable for parametric analyses (Grove & Cipher, 2020). Categorical data are assigned a number. For example, for gender, male would be coded "1," female "2," and other "3." The value of the number (lower or higher) does not mean a greater or smaller quantity in this case because measurement is at the nominal level: the number represents a name or category, not a numerical value (see Chapter 16 for more information about levels of measurement). The assigned number allows the data analysis program to count the frequency and percentage of each numbered category. Another common example is an item on a questionnaire about medical diagnoses or surgical procedures. Because multiple responses may need to be marked, each response is treated as a yes/no question and coded either "1" or "0." If physiological measures are to be included, decisions need to be made about how they will be entered as well. A BP may need to be entered as separate systolic and diastolic values. The variable name and the variable label, a short abbreviation, are recorded for each variable in the data analysis program.

With the first few pilot study subjects, it is good practice for the researcher to review the values obtained for all variables in terms of whether the data collected are interpretable and clear as stated. This practice encourages identification of items in questionnaires that might prove to be a problem during data entry because of overlapping or batched categories. For instance, the researcher may find that a single question contains not one but five variables: an item that asks whether the subject received support from her or his mother, father, sister, brother, or other relatives, followed by an item that asks the subject to indicate those who provided support, is unnecessarily tangled. It may, at first, seem logical to code mother as "1," father "2," sister "3," brother "4," and other "5." However, when a questionnaire allows an individual to select more than one source of support, each relative must be coded separately. Thus mother is one variable and would be a dichotomized value, coded "1" if circled and "0" if not circled. The father would be coded similarly as a second dichotomous variable, and so on. Identifying these items before data collection may allow items on the questionnaire or data collection form to be restructured to simplify computer entry (Dillman et al., 2014; Leedy & Ormrod, 2019).

Creating Rules for Data Entry

Rules for data entry may be finalized during pilot testing. For example, if a subject selects two responses for a single-response item, two decisions are possible: (1) the variable can be coded as missing, or (2) either the higher or the lower variable can become the default value. In the latter instance, a multiple-choice question indicating how many months have elapsed since a subject visited a dentist might be answered with both "6 to 11 months ago" and "12 to 17 months ago." The researcher, in this instance, would use "6 to 11 months ago" as the default value because the meaning of the question is not how long it's been since the responder saw a dentist but, rather, how long it's been since the responder *last* saw a dentist. If feasible, this particular question should then be reworded for the actual study as, "When was your last visit to a dentist?"

Even when items and responses are unambiguous, those entering the data will be faced with decisions. Therefore it is not sufficient to establish general rules for individuals entering data, such as "in this case always do X." This action still requires the person who is entering data to recognize a problem, refer to a general rule, and correct the data before entry. Correcting raw data is a judgment call and should be undertaken only when the person entering data is certain, beyond a doubt, of the actual value. The following provides suggestions for managing data entry problems to ensure accuracy and consistency in the entry and analysis of study data.

1. *Missing data.* Provide the data if possible or determine the impact of the missing data. In some cases, the subject must be excluded from at least some of the analyses, so the researcher must determine which

data are essential. Leave the variable blank when a datum is missing. Entering a zero will skew data analysis because the analysis program will include the value as a quantity.

2. *Items in which the subject provided two responses when only one was requested.* For example, if the question asked the subject to mark the most important item in a list of 10 items and the subject selected two of them, a decision must be made by the researcher as to how to resolve this problem, not left to a data entry person to decide. In the codebook and on the form itself, then, the researcher should indicate how that particular datum is to be coded and entered, so that the decision is documented and can be remade in the same manner when other subjects double-select a response.

3. *Items in which the subject has marked a response between two options.* This problem occurs frequently with Likert-type scales, particularly scales using forced-choice options. Given four options, the subject places a mark on the line between response 2 and response 3. In the codebook and on the form, indicate how the datum is to be coded. This is often best coded as a missing value, but coding rules should be consistent. A rationale can be constructed that supports using the highest value, lowest value, or a value halfway between the two. Removing the possibility of not clearly selecting an option is eliminated with electronic data collection, another advantage to that type of data collection.

4. *Items that ask the subject to write in some information such as occupation or diagnosis.* As noted earlier, such items are very time consuming to code and enter. The researcher should develop a list of codes for entering such data. Rather than leaving it up to the assistant to determine which code matches the subject's written response, the researcher should make decisions concerning coding and make a master list for any data entry assistants to use, so as to protect data integrity.

For paper instruments, after data have been checked and the necessary codes entered, it is prudent to make a copy of all completed forms rather than turning over the only set to an assistant for data entry. In addition, if someone other than the researcher is to enter the data, that person should receive the following information to facilitate setting up the database in advance:

• Dates for the beginning and ending of data collection

- Estimated number of subjects in the sample and how often batches of data will be entered
- Plan for documenting refusal rate, sample size, and attrition
- Copies of all scales, questionnaires, and data collection forms to be used
- Statistical package to be used for analysis of the data
- Statistical analyses to be conducted to describe the sample and to address the research purpose and the objectives, questions, or hypotheses
- Contact information for the statistician or project director with whom to consult for data entry or data analysis questions
- Computer directory location of the database in which the data will be entered and copied for backup
- Timeline for receiving the data—for example, will the data be delivered in batches, or will all the data be gathered and delivered at the same time

With this information, the assistant can develop the database in preparation for receiving data. The time needed to prepare the database varies depending on number of variables and complexity of response categories. Approximate dates for completion of data entry, analyses, or both must be negotiated before beginning data collection.

PILOT STUDY

Completing a pilot study is an essential step that saves difficulty later when the final steps of the research process are implemented. A pilot study may be conducted with several different aims, such as no prior research has been conducted on the topic, thereby making the power analysis difficult to perform. A pilot study will help to estimate the effect sizes needed for an accurate power analysis (Aberson, 2019; Grove & Cipher, 2020; Hayat, 2013). The aims of a pilot study may also assist with identifying problems that may interfere with study validity or challenges in using the instruments. Chapter 3 provides additional reasons to conduct a pilot study, but being clear about the aims will help you determine the appropriate sample size for the pilot study (Grove & Cipher, 2020). If the purpose is to try out the procedures, use the research plan to recruit three to five subjects who meet the eligibility criteria. Use the data collection methods that have been selected and prepared (see Fig. 20.3). Pay attention to how long it takes to recruit a subject, obtain informed consent, and

collect all data. At the conclusion of data collection, ask the participant to identify questions or aspects of the process that were unclear or confusing. Based on the pilot study and feedback of the first subjects, researchers may choose to modify data collection forms and methods of data collection to ensure the feasibility, validity, and reliability of the study. When the aim of the pilot study is to determine the effect size of an intervention or the internal consistency of an instrument, the necessary sample size to achieve the aim will be larger and can be determined by different statistical analyses (Aberson, 2019; Hertzog, 2008). If no changes are made in the procedures or instruments, pilot subjects are rolled over into the main study because they meet eligibility criteria.

ROLE OF THE RESEARCHER DURING DATA COLLECTION AND MANAGEMENT

The researcher applies ethical principles, people management strategies, and problem-solving skills constantly as data collection tasks are implemented. Even after pilot testing, whether related to the research plan or to situations external to the research, unforeseen events can occur, and support systems occasionally are needed for data collectors. For instance, a data collector in a subject's home may find that family members are neglecting a subject in the study who cannot get out of bed. The data collector will need assistance in reporting this to legal authorities. When multiple data collectors are involved, frequent interactions between data collectors and the team leader are essential for assessing any minor or major risks and reporting adverse effects to the IRB. In addition, the researcher's role includes maintaining control and managing the data.

Maintaining Controls and Consistency

Maintaining control and consistency of design and methods during subject selection and data collection protects the integrity or validity of the study. Researchers build controls into the design to minimize the influence of intervening forces on study findings. Maintenance of these controls is essential. For example, a study to describe changes in sleep stages during puberty may require controlling the environment of the bedroom to such an extent that a sleep laboratory is the only setting in which study integrity can be maintained. Control has stringent limitations in natural field settings. In some cases, these tenuous controls can fail without the researcher realizing that anything is amiss.

In addition to maintaining controls identified in the research plan, researchers continually watch for previously unidentified extraneous variables that might have an impact on the data being collected. An extraneous variable is any variable other than the independent variable that can affect the results of the study (McLeod, 2019). These variables are often study specific, becoming apparent during data collection. Some examples of an environmental extraneous variable are the lighting, temperature, or noise level of the data collection or experimental area. These conditions must be the same for all participants. Some examples of an extraneous variable particular to an individual are the participant's anxiety or emotional distress, intelligence, or reading level (McLeod, 2019). Extraneous variables identified at this time must be considered during data analysis and interpretation (see Chapter 26). These variables also must be noted in the research report to allow subsequent researchers to be aware of them.

Data Entry Period

Data must be carefully checked and problems corrected before the data entry phase, which should be essentially automatic and require no decisions regarding the data. Anything that alters the rhythm of data entry increases errors. For example, the subject's entry should be coded as it appears, and any reverse coding that may be needed should be done at a later time by computer manipulation in a consistent manner, rather than trying to have the data entry person recode during data entry. Follow the codebook that you have created very carefully.

If you enter your own data, develop a rhythm to the data entry process. Avoid distractions while entering data and limit your data entry periods to 2-hour intervals to reduce fatigue and error. Back up the database after each data entry period and store it on an encrypted flash drive, on a secure website, or in a fireproof safe. It is possible for the computer to crash and lose all of your precious data. If an assistant is entering the data, make yourself as available as possible to respond to questions and address problems. After entry, the data should be randomly checked for accuracy. Data checking is discussed in Chapter 21.

MANAGING DATA

Protecting the confidentiality of the data is a primary concern for the researcher. In general, the subject's name should not appear on data collection forms; only the subject's identification number should appear. The researcher may keep a master list of subjects and their code numbers, which is stored in a location separate from other data, and either encrypted in an electronic file or data repository, or locked in a file drawer, to ensure subjects' privacy. Often this master list of subjects and codes is kept with subjects' consent forms in a locked file drawer. This master list is required if contacting subjects again is necessary for additional data collection or if a subject contacts the researcher to withdraw from the study.

Once data collection begins, the researcher begins to accumulate large quantities of data. To avoid a state of total confusion, careful plans should be in place before data collection begins. Plans are needed to keep all data from a single subject together until analysis is initiated. The researcher must write the subject code number on each page of each form and check the forms for each subject to ensure that they all are present. Researchers have been known to sort their data by form, such as putting all the scales of one kind together, only to realize afterwards that they have failed to code the forms with subject identification numbers first. They then had no way to link each scale to the individual subject, and valuable data were lost.

Storage and Retrieval of Data

Space must be allotted for storing forms. File folders with a clear method of labeling allow easy access to data. Using different colors for forms is often useful. Large envelopes, approximately 8 by 11 inches, should be used to hold small pieces of paper or note cards that might fall out of a file folder. Plan to code data and enter them into the computer as soon as possible after data collection to reduce loss or disorganization of data. If data are recorded directly into a computer, data backup and storage in a separate location are imperative.

In this time of electronic storage devices and cloud storage, it is relatively easy to store data. The original data forms and database must be stored for a specified number of years dictated by the IRB, funding source, or journal publisher. There are several reasons to store data. The data can be used for secondary analyses. For example, researchers participating in a project related to a particular research focus may pool data from various studies for access by all members of the group. Data should be available to document the validity of the analyses and the published results of the study. Because of nationally publicized incidents of scientific misconduct (see Chapter 9) in which researchers fabricated data and published multiple manuscripts, researchers would be wise to preserve documentation supporting the appropriate and accurate collection of data. Issues that have been raised include how long data should be stored, the need for institutional policy regarding data storage, and access of team members to the data after the study is completed.

Some researchers store their data for 5 years after publication, whereas others store their data until they retire from a research career. Researchers should check with their funding sponsors and publishers for guidelines on how long to retain data. Most researchers store data in their offices or laboratories; others archive their data in central locations with storage fees or retrieval fees. Graduate students do have a responsibility to keep and securely store data collected in the course of their studies.

Wilson and Anteneise (2014), researchers at Johns Hopkins University, identified a flaw that threatened the security of cloud-stored data during file sharing. In cloud-based storage, privacy is reportedly protected because even the host company is not able to see the data. Encrypted electronic devices and neutral third-party agents are needed to protect the confidentiality of data during transmission. These electronic devices can be misplaced or stolen, threatening data confidentiality.

A serious concern with online data storage is the risk of some form of data breach. A **data breach** is a security incident in which confidential data are acquired, transmitted, or stolen by an unauthorized party or parties (University of California–Santa Cruz, 2015). Data breaches and their impact on health outcomes were examined by Choi, Johnson, and Lehmann (2019). Data breaches were categorized into hacking, improper disposal, loss, theft, unauthorized access, multiple forms of breach, and other. Collectively, these data breaches affected approximately 14 million individual patient records. Hospitals that experienced data breaches exhibited poorer health outcomes in the form of mortality and timeliness of care in the years following the breach. Thus data breaches had significant consequences for patients, providers, and payers.

Best practices for protecting patient and research subject data include locking up physical devices, data encryption, and stronger passwords (University of California–Santa Cruz, 2015). Single sign-on authentication may be used to improve password management. Do not use open or unencrypted wireless internet communications or e-mail to transmit sensitive data. Deletion of personal information from research files (either paper or electronic) is recommended if those data are unnecessary for study completion or no longer needed.

Policies are needed about the access that members of the team have following completion of the initial study (Sarpatwari, Kesselheim, Malin, Gagne, & Schneeweiss, 2014). Will graduate students who assist with a study receive a copy of the raw data, or will they have access to it after they leave the institution? The lack of policies related to access to data can have consequences. In the case of the Havasupai tribe versus Arizona State University (see Chapter 9), members of the research team continued to use data and samples after they moved to other universities without permission of the original subjects (McEwen, Boyer, & Sun, 2013).

Problem Solving

Little has been written about the problems encountered by nurse researchers. Research reports often read as though everything went smoothly. Research journals generally do not provide enough space for researchers to describe the problems encountered, and inexperienced researchers may receive a rosier impression than is realistic. Some problems are hinted at in a published paper in either the limitations section or in a discussion of areas for subsequent research. A more realistic sense of problems encountered by a researcher can be obtained through personal discussions with the primary author about the process of data collection for a particular sample or the use of a particular method or instrument.

"If anything can go wrong, it will, and at the worst possible time." This statement is often called **Murphy's law**, and it seems to prevail in research just as in other dimensions of life. For example, data collection frequently requires more time than was anticipated, and collecting data is often more difficult than expected. A problem can be perceived either as a frustration or as a challenge. The fact that the problem occurred is not as important as successfully resolving it. The final and perhaps most important task during the data collection period may be debriefing with the research team in weekly meetings to resolve problems that arise.

Despite conducting a pilot study, researchers may encounter challenges during the data collection process. Sometimes changes must be made in the way the data are collected, in the specific data collected, or in the timing of data collection. Potential subjects, as well as healthcare workers in a given area, react to a study in unpredictable ways. Institutional changes may force modifications in the research plan. Unusual or unexpected events may occur. Data collection processes must be as consistent as possible, but flexibility also is needed in dealing with unforeseen problems. Sometimes sticking with the original plan no matter what happens is a mistake. Skills in finding ways to resolve problems that protect the integrity of the study are critical.

In preparation for data collection, possible problems must be anticipated, and solutions for these problems must be explored. The following discussion describes some common problems and concerns and presents possible solutions. Problems that tend to occur with some regularity in studies have been categorized as people problems, researcher problems, institutional problems, and event problems.

People Problems

Nurses cannot place a subject in a laboratory test tube, instill one drop of the independent variable, and then measure the effect. Nursing studies often are conducted by examining subjects as they interact with their environments. In a laboratory setting, many aspects of the environment can be controlled, but other studies require a natural setting, to generate external validity. When research involves people, nothing is completely predictable. People, in their complexity and wholeness, have an impact on all aspects of nursing studies. Researchers, potential subjects, family members of subjects, healthcare professionals, institutional staff members, and others (i.e., innocent bystanders) interact within the study situation. As a researcher, you must be a keen observer and evaluate these interactions to determine their impact on your study.

Problems recruiting a sample. The first step in initiating data collection, recruiting a sample, may represent the tip of the people problem iceberg. Researchers may find that few people are available who fit the inclusion criteria or that many people refuse to participate in the study even though the request seems reasonable. Appropriate subjects, who were numerous a month earlier, seem to evaporate. Institutional procedures change, making many potential subjects ineligible for participation. At this juncture, inclusion and exclusion sampling criteria may need to be evaluated or additional sites for recruitment identified (see Chapter 15).

In research-rich institutions where studies are plentiful, patients paradoxically may be reluctant to participate in research. This lack of participation might arise because these patients are frequently exposed to studies, feel manipulated, or misunderstand what participation will involve. Patients may feel that they are being used as guinea pigs or fear that they will be harmed in some way that is external to the research. For example, recruiting Spanish-speaking women for a study of stress and acculturation may be met with high refusal rates if these women are worried about revealing their legal status in the United States. Fête, Aho, Benoit, Cloos, and Ridde (2019) conducted a study with a sample of migrants from multiple ethnocultural communities near Montreal, Canada. When recruitment of subjects was challenging, the researchers used certain sampling strategies, communication techniques, and an ethnically diverse research team to improve participation. Recruitment and retention of study participants is addressed in Chapter 15.

Subject attrition. After the sample is selected, certain problems might cause **subject attrition** (a loss of subjects from the study over time). For example, some subjects may agree to participate but then fail to follow through. Some may not complete needed forms and questionnaires or may fill them out incorrectly, and their data must be discarded.

To reduce these and related problems, a research team member can be available to subjects while they complete essential questions. Some subjects may not return for a second interview or may not be home for a scheduled visit. Although time has been invested to collect data from these subjects, if follow-up reveals that they do not want to continue as research subjects, their data may have to be excluded from analysis because of incompleteness. Generally, the more data collection time points there are in the study's design, the higher the risk for attrition. Attrition can occur because of subject burden accumulating over time, because healthy adults relocate for employment or family reasons, or because of death in a more critically ill population.

Sometimes subjects must be dropped from the study by the research team because of changes in health status. For example, a patient may be transferred out of the intensive care unit (ICU) in which the study is being conducted. Another possibility might be that the patient's condition may worsen and the patient no longer meets the inclusion criteria. The limits of third-party reimbursement may force the healthcare provider to discontinue the procedures or services being studied. The research team may drop a subject if it appears that participation is unusually burdensome. Other reasons for dropping a subject may be that the subject's better interests would be served outside the study, or if a subject initially determined to be mentally competent is reevaluated as someone with limited ability to consent.

Subject attrition occurs to some extent in all longitudinal studies. One way for you to deal with this problem is to anticipate the attrition rate and increase the planned number of subjects to ensure that a minimally desired number will complete the full study. A review of similar studies can allow you to anticipate your study's attrition rate. If subject attrition is higher than expected, it may be effective to offer a smaller token payment for the time and effort for initial data collection and increase the payment slightly for each data collection point. Attrition usually is higher in a placebo or control group, unless equalization of treatment is used. Sometimes in pretest-posttest or longitudinal studies, the sample size is smaller than expected by the end of the study due to attrition. If so, the effect of a smaller sample on the power of planned statistical analyses must be considered because this smaller sample may be inadequate to test the study's hypotheses (Grove & Cipher, 2020). If this is the case, a researcher may apply to the IRB for revision of the estimated size of the sample and then resume recruitment.

Researchers should report information about subjects' acceptance to participate in a study and attrition during the study to determine the degree to which the sample is representative of the study target population. Journal editors often require that manuscripts include a CONSORT or similar flowchart indicating the number of subjects meeting sample criteria, the numbers refusing to participate, and the reasons for refusal. If data are collected over time (repeated measures) or the study intervention is implemented over time, subjects often drop out of a study; and it is important to document when and how much attrition occurred. The flowchart

in Fig. 20.3 clearly identifies important aspects of the sampling process and reasons for attrition. This information enables researchers and clinicians to evaluate the representativeness of their sample for external validity and for any potential bias in interpreting the results.

Subject as an object. The quality of interactions between the researcher and subjects during the study is a critical dimension for maintaining subject participation. When researchers are under pressure to complete a study, people can be treated as objects rather than as subjects, particularly if electronic data collection is used. In addition to being unethical, such impersonal treatment alters interactions, diminishes subject satisfaction, and increases the likelihood for missing data and subject attrition. Subjects are scarce resources and must be treated with care. Treating the subject as an object can affect another researcher's ability to recruit from this population in the future.

Treating the subject as an object can be minimized by building strategies into the consent process, such as offering subjects a personal copy of their results, recognizing their valuable participation with small gifts as tokens of appreciation, or providing monetary reimbursement for their time and effort. Because of their sterling social skills, nurses are valuable members of interdisciplinary research teams: they establish relationships with subjects, aiding in retention.

External influences on subject responses. People external to the research who interact with the subject, the researcher, or both, can have an important impact on the data collection process. Family members may not agree to the subject's participation in the study or may not understand the study process. These individuals often influence the subject's decision to participate. Researchers benefit from taking time to explain the study and seeking the cooperation of family members.

Family members or other patients also may influence the subject's responses to scales or interview questions. In some cases, subjects may ask family members, friends, or other patients to complete study forms for them. The subject may discuss questions on the forms with other people who happen to be in the room. Therefore the data recorded may not reflect the subject's perceptions accurately. If interviews are conducted while others are in the room, the subject's responses may depend on his or her need to meet the expectations of the persons present. Sometimes a family member answers questions addressed verbally to the patient by the researcher. The setting in which a questionnaire is completed or an interview is conducted may determine the extent to which answers obtained are a true reflection of a subject's point of view. If the privacy afforded by the setting varies from one subject to another, subjects' responses may also vary and threaten the internal validity of the findings (Kazdin, 2017).

Usually, the most desirable setting for questionnaire completion is a private area away from distractions. If it is not possible to arrange for such a setting, the researcher can be present at the time the questionnaire is completed to decrease the influence of others. If the questionnaire is to be completed later or taken home and returned at a later time, the probability of influence by others increases, and return of questionnaire packet becomes less likely, even if the subject is provided with a stamped return envelope. The impact of the influence of others on the integrity of the data depends on the nature of the questionnaire items. For example, a marital relationship questionnaire may have different responses if the subject is allowed to complete it alone and return it immediately to the researcher, versus completing it aloud with the spouse in attendance.

Passive resistance. Healthcare professionals and institutional staff members working with study participants in clinical settings may affect the data collection process. DeVon and colleagues (2013) found that some nurses were initially enthusiastic about the study and later become less so, while another nurse indicated that research was not part of her job. Some professionals may verbalize strong support for the study and yet passively interfere with data collection. For example, nurses providing care may fail to follow guidelines agreed upon for providing specific care activities being studied, or they may forget to include information needed for the study in the patient records. The researcher may not be informed when a potential subject has been admitted, and a physician who has agreed that his or her patients can be participants may decide as each patient is admitted that this one is not quite right for the study. In addition, when the permission of the physician or nurse practitioner is required, the provider might be unavailable to the researcher.

Nonprofessional staff members may not realize the impact of the data collection process on their work patterns until the process begins. The data collection process may violate their beliefs about how care should be provided (or has been provided). If ignored, their resistance can completely undo a carefully designed study. For example, research on skin care may disrupt a bathing routine by nursing assistants so they may continue the normal routine regardless of the study protocol and thus invalidate the study findings. When there is funding to support subject recruitment and data collection, funds can be used to reimburse clinic or hospital staff members for their time, to create a raffle for one substantial gift, to offer a gift certificate to buy something needed for the clinic, or to send a nurse who assisted in data collection to a continuing education course. When funding is limited, staff members' enthusiasm for the study may be enhanced if they are able to participate in the research as authors or presenters in dissemination of the research findings.

Because of the potential impact of these people problems, the researcher must maintain open communication and nurture positive relationships with other professionals and staff members during data collection. Early recognition and acknowledgment of problems allow the researcher to resolve issues promptly, ideally with fewer serious consequences to the integrity of the study. However, not all problems can be resolved. Sometimes the researcher may need to seek creative ways to work around an individual or to counteract the harmful consequences of passive resistance.

What is cavalierly referred to as passive resistance on the part of staff members is sometimes related to lack of researcher presence. If a researcher, or an assistant, telephones the hospital unit's clerk daily to enquire about new admissions in the past 24 hours and to ask whether those patients are suitable for study inclusion, the unit clerk may wonder why the researcher is not putting in an appearance. The responsible researcher either goes to the research site daily and assesses potential subjects for recruitment, or delegates this daily responsibility to a member of the research team. In addition, being on-site for questions when interventions and documentation of information required by the research team are taking place and thanking them for their fine work are important ways to build goodwill and an effective quick-check of accuracy and quality.

Researcher Problems

Some problems are a consequence of a researcher's interaction with the study situation or lack of skill in data collection techniques. These problems are often difficult to identify because of the researcher's personal involvement. However, their effect on the study can be serious.

Researcher interactions. Researcher interactions can interfere with data collection in interview situations. To gain the cooperation of the subject, the researcher needs to develop rapport with the subject. One way to do this is to select data collectors who resemble the types of subjects being recruited as much as possible. Rapport may suffer if a young man collects data from female caregivers of elderly adults about their experience with end-of-life care. Similarly, a white middle-aged woman collecting data from young African American men or Hispanic teens is likely to be at more of an initial disadvantage, in terms of establishing immediate rapport, than would be a data collector who shares age or ethnic background with the subjects.

Lack of skill in data collection techniques. The researcher's skill in using a particular quantitative data collection technique can affect the quality of the data collected. A researcher who is unskilled at the beginning of data collection can practice the data collection techniques with the assistance of an experienced researcher. A pilot study to test data collection techniques is always helpful. If data collectors are being used, they also need opportunities to practice data collection techniques before the study is initiated. Sometimes a skill is developed during the course of a study; if this is the case, as one's skill increases, the data being collected may change and confound the study findings and threaten the validity of the study. If more than one data collector is used, the degree to which skills improve may vary across time and data collectors. The consistency of data collectors must be evaluated during the study to detect any changes in their data collection techniques.

Researcher role conflict. As a researcher, one is observing and recording events. Nurses who conduct clinical research often experience a conflict between their researcher role and their clinician role during data collection. In some cases, the researcher's involvement in the event, such as providing physical or emotional care to a patient during data collection, could alter the event and bias the results. It would be difficult to generalize study findings to other situations in which the researcher was not present to intervene. However, the needs of patients must take precedence over the needs of the study.

The dilemma is to determine when the needs of patients are great enough to warrant researcher intervention.

Some patient situations are life threatening, such as respiratory distress and changes in cardiac function, and require immediate action by anyone present, especially when that person is a nurse. Other patient needs are simple, can be addressed by any nurse available, and can be answered if the response is not likely to alter the results of the study. Examples of these interventions include giving the patient a bedpan, informing the nurse of the patient's need for pain medication, or helping the patient open food containers. These situations seldom cause a dilemma.

Solutions to other situations are not as easy. For example, suppose that the study involves examining the emotional responses of family members during and immediately after a patient's surgery. The study includes an experimental group that receives one 30-minute family support session before and during the patient's surgery and a control group that receives no support session. Both sets of families are being monitored for 1 week after surgery to measure level of anxiety and coping strategies. The researcher is currently collecting data from subjects in the control group. The data consist of demographic information and scales measuring anxiety and coping. After completing demographic information, one of the family members is experiencing great distress and verbally expresses her fears and the lack of support she has received from the nursing staff. Two other subjects from different families hear the expressed distress and concur; they move closer to the conversation and look to the researcher for information and support.

In this situation, a supportive response from the researcher is likely to modify the results of the study because these responses are part of the treatment to be provided to the experimental group only. This interaction is likely to narrow the difference between the two groups and decrease the possibility that the results will show a significant difference between the two groups. How should the researcher respond? Is it obligatory to provide support? To some extent, almost any response would be supportive. One alternative is to provide the needed support and not include these family members in the control group. Another alternative is to recruit the help of a nonprofessional to collect the data from the control group. However, most people would provide some degree of support in the described situation, even though their skills in supportive techniques may vary.

Other dilemmas include witnessing unethical behavior that interferes with patient care or witnessing subjects' unethical or illegal behavior (Humphreys et al., 2012). Consent forms are often required to stipulate that any member of the research team is legally required to report illegal behaviors that pose potential harm to the subject or others, such as neglect or abuse of children and elderly adults. Try to anticipate these dilemmas before data collection whenever possible and include this information in the consent form.

Pilot studies can help identify dilemmas likely to occur in a study and allow the research team to build strategies into the design to minimize or avoid them. However, some dilemmas cannot be anticipated and must be responded to spontaneously. There is no prescribed way to handle difficult dilemmas; each case must be dealt with individually. The wise researcher discusses any unethical and illegal behavior with members of the IRB, ethics committee members, or legal advisors. Situations related to potential harm must be reported to the IRB, and experts there can advise on the next step or course of action. After the dilemma is resolved, it is wise to reexamine the situation for its effect on study results and consider options in case the situation arises again.

Another type of conflict arises when a subject makes inaccurate statements or asks a question about health practices or treatment. Rather than offering professional advice or responding to the question, the research nurse should acknowledge that it is a good question but that the research protocol does not allow for a response during data collection. When data collection is complete, the research nurse can help the subject write down the question for the healthcare provider or provide patient-education materials for more information.

Institutional Problems

Institutions are in a constant state of change. They will not stop changing for the period of a study, and these changes often affect data collection. A nurse who has been most helpful in the study may be promoted or transferred. The unit on which the study is conducted may be reorganized, moved, or closed during data collection. An area used for subject interviews may be transformed into an office or a storeroom. Patient record forms may be revised, omitting data that you and your team are collecting. The medical record personnel may be reorganizing files and temporarily unable to provide needed records. Albrecht and Taylor's (2013) study of women with advanced ovarian cancer involved the pharmacy dispensing the study-related medications. Following IRB approval, it took 3 months for procedural issues with the pharmacy to be resolved.

These problems are, for the most part, completely outside your control in your role as researcher. Pay attention to the internal communication network of the institution for advanced warning of impending changes. Contacts within the institution's administrative decision makers could warn you about the impact of proposed changes on an ongoing study. In many cases, the IRB in the local hospital will have a nurse representative who can provide needed consultation. However, in many cases, data collection strategies might have to be modified to meet a newly emerging situation. Balancing flexibility with maintaining the integrity of the study may be the key to successful data collection. As a data collection site, the subject's home setting may be more desirable and convenient for a subject than a complex facility or institution, and response rates may improve. The disadvantage is that home visits are time intensive for the researcher, and the subject may not be home at the agreed-upon appointment time, despite confirmed appointments and reminder calls.

Event Problems

Unpredictable events can be a source of frustration during a study. Research tools ordered from a testing company can be lost in the mail. The printer may stop functioning just before 500 data collection forms are to be printed, or a machine to be used in data collection may break and require several weeks for repair. An internet connection could be lost or weak. Data collection forms can be misplaced, misfiled, or lost.

Local, national, or world events can also influence a subject's response to a questionnaire or the willingness to enroll in a study, as can changes in treatment protocols. Albrecht and Taylor (2013) noted that medical management of advanced ovarian cancer changed between seeking funding and implementing their study and, as a result, many of the women counted in the potential pool of subjects were no longer eligible. If data collection for the entire sample is planned for a single time, a snowstorm or a flood can require the researcher to cancel the session. Weather may decrease attendance far below the number expected at a support group or series of teaching sessions. A bus strike can disrupt transportation systems to such an extent that subjects who depend on public transportation can no longer reach the data collection site. A new health agency may open in the city, which may decrease demand for the care activities being studied. Conversely, an external event can also increase attendance at clinics to such an extent that existing resources are stretched and data collection is no longer possible. These events are also outside the researcher's control and are impossible to anticipate. In most cases, however, restructuring the data collection period can salvage the study. To do so, it is necessary to examine all possible alternatives for collecting the study data. In some cases, data collection can simply be rescheduled; in other situations, changes may need to be more complex. For example, recruiting women to participate in a study that requires an hour or longer of their time may necessitate that the researcher provide child care. Providing child care would be more costly and add complexity to the process, but it may be the best alternative for increasing participation.

RESEARCH/RESEARCHER SUPPORT

The researcher must have access to individuals or groups who can provide mentorship, support, and consultation during the data collection period. Support can usually be obtained from academic committees, IRB staff, and colleagues on the research team.

Support of Academic Committees

Although thesis and dissertation committees are basically seen as stern keepers of the sanctity of the research process, they also serve as support systems for novice researchers. Committee members must be selected from among faculty who are willing and able to provide the needed expertise and support. Experienced academic researchers are usually more knowledgeable about the types of support needed. Because they are involved directly in research, they tend to be sensitive to the needs of the novice researcher and more realistic about what can be accomplished within a given period of time.

Institutional Support

A support system within the institution in which the study is conducted is also important. Support might come from people serving on the institutional research committee or from nurses working on the unit in which the study is conducted. These people may have knowledge of how the institution functions, and their closeness to the study can increase their understanding of the problems experienced by the researcher and subjects. Do not overlook their ability to provide useful suggestions and assistance. The ability to resolve some of the problems encountered during data collection may depend on having someone within the power structure of the institution who can intervene.

Colleague Support

In addition to professional support, having at least one peer in your research world with whom to share the joys, frustrations, and current problems of data collection is important. This colleague can often serve as a mirror to allow you to see the situation clearly and perhaps more objectively. With this type of support, the researcher can share and release feelings and gain some distance from the data collection situation. Alternatives for resolving the problem can be discussed dispassionately.

Data Safety and Monitoring Board as Source of Support

If an intervention is being implemented that is deemed to be of low risk to the patient, such as a behavioral intervention to improve sleep quality, a data safety and monitoring plan will suffice. The plan includes monitoring consistent with the intervention's risks and benefits and the complexity of the study (NIH, 2017). In these situations, a plan is deemed adequate when it conforms to the IRB requirements for reporting any adverse event and includes annual progress reports. It requires that the researcher explicitly state the plan to review the data from each set number of subjects or from each 3-month or 6-month batch of recruited subjects, depending on the extent of the study.

If the study involves a population who may be susceptible to coercion or an intervention protocol posing higher than average risk to patient safety, a data safety and monitoring board (DSMB) is required. If the study is externally funded, the decision to involve a DSMB is usually made by the funding institution as a contingency for funding. A DSMB includes members who are not directly involved in the study and who can be objective about the findings. The DSMB will review the results of interim data analyses provided by the researcher and compare the results to the criteria for stopping the study, criteria that were determined prior to the beginning of the study. Because of the nature of the work, the DSMB should consist of very experienced researchers and clinical experts.

In a study conducted by Hocqueloux et al. (2019), the DSMB was involved in the decision to stop the study. The participants were persons living with human immunodeficiency virus (HIV) and receiving a combination therapy of three medications. They were randomized to continue on their three-drug therapy or to begin using a monotherapy. At 24 weeks, the DSMB reviewed the results and approved the study to continue to 48 weeks. When three participants experienced virologic failure in the monotherapy group, the DSMB and study sponsor decided to stop the study and return the treatment arm participants to the three-drug therapy.

SERENDIPITY

Serendipity is the accidental discovery of something useful or valuable that is not the primary focus of the inquiry. During the data collection phase of studies, researchers often become aware of elements or relationships that they had not identified previously. These aspects may be closely related to the study being conducted or have little connection with it. They come from increased awareness and close observation of the study situation. Serendipitous findings are important for the development of new insights in nursing theory. They can be important for understanding the totality of the phenomenon being examined. Additionally, they lead to areas of research that generate new knowledge. A relatively easy way to capture these insights as they occur is to maintain a research journal or make field notes. These events must be carefully recorded, even if their impact or meaning is not understood at the time, and they should be reported in the study findings.

KEY POINTS

- Careful planning is needed before collecting and managing data.
- A study protocol provides a plan for the implementation of the study.
- Factors such as cost, size of research team, and time affect decisions about data collection.
- The researcher has several decisions to make about measuring the study variables, including cost of the instrument, reading level, and method of data collection.
- Data may be collected with or without the assistance of the researcher. Data may be collected online, on scannable forms, or on printed surveys.
- Demographic questionnaires are developed to include the variables to describe the sample and are formatted to promote accuracy of the data.
- To prepare for data entry, the instruments are formatted and compiled prior to creating a codebook to promote consistent data entry.
- The logistics of data entry include who will enter the data and the rules for data entry, such as how missing data will be coded.

- A detailed data collection plan includes the chronology of recruiting and consenting subjects, scheduling data collection, training data collectors, and identifying decision points.
- When a pilot study is conducted, the lessons learned can refine the study protocol and data collection plan.
- During the study, the researcher maintains control and consistency, manages the data collection, and oversees the storage and retrieval of the data.
- Problems that tend to occur with some regularity in studies during data collection have been categorized as people problems, researcher problems, institutional problems, and event problems.
- Problems that arise during data collection involve recruitment and attrition issues, treatment of the subject as an object, external influences on subject responses, passive resistance from staff members or family, researcher interactions, lack of skill in data collection techniques, and researcher role conflicts.
- A successful study requires support that is often obtained from academic committees, healthcare agencies, work colleagues, and even data safety monitoring boards.

REFERENCES

Aberson, C. L. (2019). *Applied power analysis for the behavioral sciences* (2nd ed.). New York, NY: Routledge Taylor & Francis Group.

Albrecht, T., & Taylor, A. (2013). No stone left unturned: Challenges encountered during recruitment of women with advanced ovarian cancer for a phase I study. *Applied Nursing Research*, 26(4), 245–250. doi:10.1016/j.apnr.2013.05.003

Bohr, A., Brown, D., Laurson, K., Smith, P., & Bass, R. (2013). Relationship between socioeconomic status and physical fitness in junior high students. *Journal of School Health*, 83(8), 542–547. doi:10.1111/josh.12063

Cárdenas, L., & Stormshak, E. (2019). Measuring daily activities of emerging adults: Text messaging for assessing risk behaviors. *Journal of Child & Family Studies, 28*(2), 315–324. doi:10.1007/s10826-018-1267-1

Centers for Disease Control and Prevention (CDC). (2019). *National ambulatory medical care survey 2018 patient record*. Retrieved from https://www.cdc.gov/nchs/data/ahcd/2018_NAMCS_Patient_Record_Sample_Card.pdf

Ceyhan, Ö., Taşcı, S., Elmalı, F., & Doğan, A. (2019). The effect of acupressure on cardiac rhythm and heart rate among patients with atrial fibrillation: The relationship between heart rate and fatigue. *Alternative Therapies in Health and Medicine, 25*(1), 12–19.

Choi, S. J., Johnson, M. E., & Lehmann, C. U. (2019). Data breach remediation efforts and their implications for hospital quality. *Health Services Research*, 54, 971–980. doi:10.1111/1475-6773.13203

Cipher, D. J., Urban, R. W., & Mancini, M. E. (2019). Factors associated with student success in online and face-to-face delivery of master of science in nursing programs. *Teaching and Learning in Nursing, 14*(3), 203–207. doi:10.1016/j.teln.2019.03.007

Cohn, D. (2015). *Census considers new approach to asking about race-by not using the term at all.* Pew Research Center. Retrieved from http://www.pewresearch.org/fact-tank/2015/06/18/census-considers-new-approach-to-asking-about-race-by-not-using-the-term-at-all/

Department of Health and Human Services (DHHS). (2019). *U.S. poverty guidelines*. Retrieved from http://aspe.hhs.gov/poverty/19poverty.cfm

DeVon, H., Patmon, F., Rosenfeld, A., Fennessy, M., & Francis, D. (2013). Implementing clinical research in the high acuity setting of the emergency department. *Journal of Emergency Nursing, 39*(1), 6–12. doi:10.1016/j.jen.2012.08.012

Dillman, D. A., Smyth, J. D., & Christian, L. M. (2014). *Internet, phone, mail, and mixed-mode surveys: The tailored design method*. Hoboken, NJ: John Wiley & Sons.

English, K., Espinoza, J., Pete, D., & Tjemsland, A. (2019). A comparative analysis of telephone and in-person survey administration for public health surveillance in rural American Indian communities. *Journal of Public Health Management & Practice, 25*(5), S70–S76. doi:10.1097/PHH.0000000000001007

Fête, M., Aho, J., Benoit, M., Cloos, P., & Ridde, V. (2019). Barriers and recruitment strategies for precarious status migrants in Montreal, Canada. *BMC Medical Research Methodology, 19*(41), 1–14. doi:10.1186/s12874-019-0683-2

Fukuoka, Y., Kamitani, E., Dracup, K., & Jong, S. S. (2011). New insights into compliance with a mobile phone diary and pedometer use in sedentary women. *Journal of Physical Activity & Health, 8*(3), 398–403. doi:10.1123/jpah.8.3.398

Gray, J., & Johnson, L. (2009). *Nurse international relocation questionnaire 2*. Unpublished research tool. Retrieved from Jennifer.gray@oc.edu

Grove, S. K., & Cipher, D. J. (2020). *Statistics for nursing research: A workbook for evidence-based practice* (3rd ed.). St. Louis, MO: Saunders.

Harris, P. A., Taylor, R., Thielke, R., Payne, J., Gonzalez, N., & Conde, J. G. (2009). Research electronic data capture (REDCap)—A metadata-driven methodology and workflow process for providing translational research informatics support. *Journal of Biomedical Informatics, 42*(2), 377–381. doi:10.1016/j.jbi.2008.08.010

Hartman, L., Lems, W., & Boers, W. (2019). Outcome measures for adherence data from a medication event monitoring system: A literature review. *Journal of Clinical Pharmacy & Therapeutics, 44*(1), 1–5. doi:10.1111/jcpt.12757

Harwood, E. M. (2009). Data collection methods series: Part 3: Developing protocols for collecting data. *Journal of Wound Ostomy Continence Nursing, 36*(3), 246–250. doi:10.1097/WON.0b013e3181a1a4d3

Hayat, M. J. (2013). Understanding sample size determination in nursing research. *Western Journal of Nursing Research*, 35(7), 943–956. doi:10.1177/0193945913482052

Hertzog, M. (2008). Considerations for determining sample size for pilot studies. *Research in Nursing & Health, 31*(2), 180–191. doi:10.1002/nur.20247

Hobden, B., Bryant, J., Carey, M., Sanson-Fisher, R., & Oldmeadow, C. (2017). Computer tablet or telephone? A randomised controlled trial exploring two methods of collecting data from drug and alcohol outpatients. *Addictive Behaviors, 71*(1), 111–117. doi:10.1016/j.addbeh.2017.03.009

Hocqueloux, L., Raffi, F., Prazuck, T., Bernard, L., Sunder, S., Esnault, J. L., ... Valéry, A.(2019). Dolutegravir monotherapy versus dolutegravir/abacavir/lamivudine for virologically suppressed people living with chronic human immunodeficiency virus infection: The randomized noninferiority MONotherapy of tiviCAY trial. *Clinical Infectious Diseases, 69*(9), 1498–1505. doi:10.1093/cid/ciy1132

Human Rights Campaign (HRC). (2016). *Resources. Collecting transgender-inclusive gender data in workplace and other surveys.* Retrieved from http://www.hrc.org/resources/entry/collecting-transgender-inclusive-gender-data-in-workplace-and-other-surveys

Humphreys, J., Epel, E. S., Cooper, B. A., Lin, J., Blackburn, E. H., & Lee, K. A. (2012). Telomere shortening in formerly abused and never abused women. *Biological Research for Nursing, 14*(2), 115–123. doi:10.1177/1099800411398479

International Business Machines (IBM) Corporation. (n.d.). *IBM SPSS data collection.* Retrieved from https://www.ibm.com/support/home/product/K526560N53721Z75/spss/ibm_spss_data_collection

Jull, A., & Aye, P. (2015). Endorsement of the CONSORT guidelines, trial registration, and the quality of reporting randomised controlled trials in leading nursing journals: A cross-sectional analysis. *International Journal of Nursing Studies, 52*(6), 1071–1079. doi:10.1016/j.ijnurstu.2014.11.008

Kazdin, A. E. (2017). *Research design in clinical psychology* (5th ed.). Boston, MA: Pearson.

Kelechi, T., Mueller, M., Madisetti, M., Prentice, M., & Dooley, M. (2018). Effectiveness of cooling therapy (cryotherapy) on leg pain and self-efficacy in patients with chronic venous disease: A randomized controlled trial. *International Journal of Nursing Studies, 86*(1), 1–10. doi:10.1016/j.ijnurstu.2018.04.015

Kupzyk, K., & Cohen, M. (2015). Data validation and other strategies for data entry. *Western Journal of Nursing Research, 37*(4), 546–556. doi:10.1177/0193945914532550

Ladores, S., & Bray, L. (2017). Electronic diaries in healthcare: A review of literature. *Journal of Nursing Practice Applications & Reviews of Research, 7*(2), 13–21. doi:10.13178/jnparr.2017.0702.0705

Lee, S., & Park, H. (2019). Effects of auricular acupressure on pain and disability in adults with chronic neck pain. *Applied Nursing Research, 45*(1), 12–16. doi:10.1016/j.apnr.2018.11.005

Leedy, P. D., & Ormrod, J. E. (2019). *Practical research: Planning and design* (12th ed.). New York, NY: Pearson.

Linder, L., Ameringer, S., Erickson, J., Macpherson, C., Stegenga, K., & Linder, W. (2013). Using an iPad in research with children and adolescents. *Journal for Specialists in Pediatric Nursing, 18*(2), 158–164. doi:10.1111/jspn.12023

McEwen, J., Boyer, J., & Sun, K. (2013). Evolving approaches to the ethical management of genomic data. *Trends in Genetics, 29*(6), 375–382. doi:10.1016/j.tig.2013.02.001

McGinley, M., Cola, P., Fox, R., Cohen, J., Corboy, J., & Miller, D. (2019). Perspectives of individuals with multiple sclerosis on discontinuation of disease-modifying therapies. *Multiple Sclerosis Journal. Advance Online Publication.* doi:10.1177/1352458519867314

McLeod, S. A. (2019). *Extraneous variables.* Retrieved from https://www.simplypsychology.org/extraneous-variable.html

Melnyk, B. M., & Fineout-Overholt, E. (2019). *Evidence-based practice in nursing and healthcare: A guide to best practice* (4th ed.). Philadelphia, PA: Wolters-Kluwer.

Muigg, D., Kastner, P., Duftschmid, G., Modre-Osprian, R., & Haluza, D. (2019). Readiness to use telemonitoring in diabetes care: A cross-sectional study among Austrian practitioners. *BMC Medical Informatics and Decision Making, 19*(26), 1–10. doi:10.1186/s12911-019-0746-7

National Institutes of Health (NIH). (2017). *How to write a data and safety monitoring plan.* Retrieved from https://www.niams.nih.gov/grants-funding/conducting-clinical-trials/clinical-trial-policies-guidelines-and-templates/data-and

Ryan-Wenger, N. A. (2017). Precision, accuracy, and uncertainty of biophysical measurements for research and practice. In C. F. Waltz, O. L. Strickland, & E. R. Lenz (Eds.), *Measurement in nursing and health research* (5th ed., pp. 427–445). New York, NY: Springer.

Sarpatwari, A., Kesselheim, A., Malin, B., Gagne, J., & Schneeweiss, S. (2014). Ensuring patient privacy in data sharing for postapproval research. *New England Journal of Medicine, 137*(17), 1644–1649. doi:10.1056/NEJMsb1405487

Schick-Makaroff, K., & Molzahn, A. (2015). Strategies to use tablet computers for collection of electronic patient-reported outcomes. *Health and Quality of Life Outcomes, 13*, 2. doi:10.1186/s12955-014-0205-1

Schulz, K., Altman, D., & Moher, D. (2010). CONSORT 2010 statement: Updated guidelines for reporting parallel group randomized trials. *Annals of Internal Medicine, 152*(11), 1–8. doi:10.7326/0003-4819-152-11-201006010-00232

University of California–Santa Cruz. (2015). *Security breach examples and practices to avoid them.* Retrieved from https://its.ucsc.edu/security/breaches.html

Waltz, C. F., Strickland, O. L., & Lenz, E. R. (2017). *Measurement in nursing and health research* (5th ed.). New York, NY: Springer.

Wilson, D., & Anteneise, G. (2014). *"To share or not to share" in client-side encrypted clouds.* Preprinted by ArXiv.org. Retrieved from http://arxiv.org/pdf/1404.2697v1.pdf

21

Introduction to Statistical Analysis

Daisha J. Cipher

http://evolve.elsevier.com/Gray/practice/

Statistical analysis is often considered one of the most exciting steps of the research process. During this phase, you will finally obtain answers to the questions that led to the development of your study. Critical appraisal of the results section of a quantitative study requires you to be able to (1) identify the statistical procedures used; (2) judge whether these statistical procedures were appropriate for the hypotheses, questions, or objectives of the study and for the data available for analysis; (3) comprehend the discussion of statistical analysis results; (4) judge whether the author's interpretation of the results is appropriate; and (5) evaluate the clinical importance of the findings (see Chapter 18 for more details on critical appraisal).

As a neophyte researcher performing a quantitative study, you are confronted with many critical decisions related to statistical analysis that require statistical knowledge. To perform statistical analysis of data from a quantitative study, you need to be able to (1) determine the necessary sample size to power your study adequately; (2) prepare the data for analysis; (3) describe the sample; (4) test the reliability of the measurement methods used in the study; (5) perform exploratory analyses of the data; (6) perform analyses guided by the study objectives, questions, or hypotheses; and (7) interpret the results of statistical procedures. We recommend consulting with a statistician or expert researcher early in the research process to help you develop a plan for accomplishing these seven tasks. A statistician is also invaluable in conducting statistical analysis for a study and interpreting the results (Hayat, Higgins, Schwartz, & Staggs, 2015).

Critical appraisal of the results of studies and statistical analyses both require an understanding of the statistical theory underlying the process of analysis. This chapter and the following four chapters provide you with the information needed for critical appraisal of the results sections of published studies and for performance of statistical procedures to analyze data in studies and in clinical practice. This chapter introduces the concepts of statistical theory and discusses some of the more pragmatic aspects of quantitative statistical analysis: the purposes of statistical analysis, the process of performing statistical analysis, the method for choosing appropriate statistical analysis techniques for a study, and resources for conducting statistical analysis procedures. Chapter 22 explains the use of statistics for descriptive purposes, such as describing the study sample or variables. Chapter 23 focuses on the use of statistics to examine proposed relationships among study variables, such as the relationships among the variables dyspnea, fatigue, anxiety, and quality of life. Chapter 24 explores the use of statistics for prediction, such as using independent variables of age, gender, cholesterol values, and history of hypertension to predict the dependent variable of cardiac risk level. Chapter 25 guides you in using statistics to determine differences between groups, such as determining the difference in muscle strength and falls (dependent variables) between an experimental or intervention group receiving a strength training program (independent variable) and a comparison group receiving standard care.

CONCEPTS OF STATISTICAL THEORY

One reason nurses tend to avoid statistics is that many were taught the mathematical mechanics of calculating statistical formulas and were given little or no explanation of the logic behind the analysis procedure or the meaning of the results (Grove & Cipher, 2020). This mathematical process is usually performed by computer, and information about it offers little assistance to the individuals making statistical decisions or explaining results. We approach statistical analysis from the perspective of enhancing your understanding of the meaning underlying statistical analysis. You can use this understanding either for critical appraisal of studies or for conducting data analyses.

The ensuing discussion explains some of the concepts commonly used in statistical theory. The logic of statistical theory is embedded within the explanations of these concepts. The concepts presented in this chapter include probability theory, classical hypothesis testing, Type I and Type II errors, statistical power, statistical significance versus clinical importance, inference, samples and populations, descriptive and inferential statistical techniques, measures of central tendency, the normal curve, sampling distributions, symmetry, skewness, modality, kurtosis, variation, confidence intervals, and both parametric and nonparametric types of inferential statistical analyses.

Probability Theory

Probability theory addresses statistical analysis as the likelihood of accurately predicting an event or the extent of an effect. Nurse researchers are interested in the probability of a particular nursing outcome in a particular patient care situation. For example, what is the probability of patients older than 75 years of age with cardiac conditions falling when hospitalized? With probability theory, you could determine how much of the variation in your data could be explained by using a particular statistical analysis. In probability theory, the researcher interprets the meaning of statistical results in light of his or her knowledge of the field of study. A finding that would have little meaning in one field of study might be important in another (Good, 1983; Kerlinger & Lee, 2000). Probability is expressed as a lowercase p, with values expressed as a percentage or as a decimal value ranging from 0 to 1. For example, if the exact probability is known to be 0.23, it would be expressed as $p = 0.23$.

The p in statistics is defined as the probability of obtaining a statistical value as extreme or greater when the null hypothesis is true (Cohen, 1994). The p should be distinguished from Type I error (α) (discussed later in this chapter), which is the probability of rejecting the null hypothesis when the null is actually true. Nurse researchers typically consider a $p = 0.05$ value or less to indicate a real effect.

Classical Hypothesis Testing

Classical hypothesis testing refers to the process of testing a hypothesis to infer the reality of an effect. This process starts with the statement of a null hypothesis, which assumes no effect (e.g., no difference between groups, or no relationship between variables). The researcher sets the values of two theoretical probabilities: (1) the probability of rejecting the null hypothesis when it is in fact true (alpha [α], **Type I error**) and (2) the probability of retaining the null hypothesis when it is in fact false (beta [β], **Type II error**). In nursing research, alpha is usually set at 0.05, meaning that the researcher will allow a 5% or lower chance of making a Type I error. The beta is frequently set at 0.20, meaning that the researcher will allow for a 20% or lower chance of making a Type II error (Fisher, 1935, 1971).

After conducting the study, the researcher culminates the hypothesis testing process by making a rational decision either to reject or to retain the null hypothesis, based on the statistical results. The following steps outline each of the components of statistical hypothesis testing.

1. State your primary null hypothesis. (Chapter 6 discusses the development of the null hypothesis.)
2. Set your study alpha (Type I error); this is usually $\alpha = 0.05$.
3. Set your study beta (Type II error); this is usually $\beta = 0.20$.
4. Conduct power analyses (Cohen, 1988; Grove & Cipher, 2020).
5. Design and conduct your study.
6. Compute the appropriate statistic on your obtained data.
7. Compare your obtained statistic with its corresponding theoretical distribution in the tables provided in the appendices at the back of this book. For example, if you analyzed your data with a t-test, you would compare the t value from your study with the critical values of t in the table in Appendix B.

8. If your obtained statistic exceeds the critical value in the distribution table, you can reject your null hypothesis. If not, you must accept your null hypothesis. These ideas are discussed in more depth in Chapters 23, 24, and 25, in which the results of various statistical analyses are presented.

Significance testing addresses whether the data support the conclusion that there is a true effect in the direction of the apparent difference (Cox, 1958). This decision is a judgment and can be in error. The level of statistical significance attained indicates the degree of uncertainty in taking the position that the difference between groups (or the association between variables) is real. Classical hypothesis testing has been widely criticized for such errors in judgments (Cohen, 1994; Loftus 1993). Much emphasis has been placed on researchers providing indicators of effect rather than just relying on p values specifically, providing the magnitude of the obtained effect (e.g., a difference or relationship) as well as confidence intervals associated with the statistical findings. These additional statistics give consumers of research more information about the phenomenon being studied (Cohen, 1994; Gaskin & Happell, 2014).

Type I and Type II Errors

We choose the probability of making a Type I error when we set alpha, and if we decrease the probability of making a Type I error, we increase the probability of making a Type II error. The relationships between Type I and Type II errors are defined in Table 21.1. A Type II error occurs as a result of some degree of overlap between the values of different populations, so in some cases a value with a greater than 5% probability of being within one population may be within the dimensions of another population.

It is impossible to decrease both types of error simultaneously without a corresponding increase in sample size. The researcher must decide which risk poses the greatest threat within a specific study. In nursing research, many studies are conducted with small samples and physiological instruments that lack precision and accuracy or scales that lack reliability and validity in the measurement of study variables (see Chapter 16) (Waltz, Strickland, & Lenz, 2017). Many nursing situations include multiple variables that interact to lead to differences within populations. However, when one is examining only a few of the interacting variables, small differences can be overlooked and could lead to a false conclusion of no differences between the samples. In this case, the risk of a Type II error is a greater concern, and a more lenient level of significance is in order. Nurse researchers usually set the level of significance or $\alpha = 0.05$ for their studies versus a more stringent $\alpha = 0.01$ or 0.001. Setting $\alpha = 0.05$ reduces the risk of a Type II error of indicating study results are not significant when they are.

Statistical Power

Power is the probability that a statistical test will detect an effect when it actually exists. Power is the inverse of Type II error and is calculated as $1 - \beta$. Type II error is the probability of retaining the null hypothesis when it is in fact false. When the researcher sets Type II error at 0.20 before conducting a study, this means that the power of the planned statistic has been set to 0.80. In other words, the statistic will have an 80% chance of detecting an effect if it actually exists.

Reported studies failing to reject the null hypothesis (in which power is unlikely to have been examined) often have a low power level to detect an effect if one exists. Until more recently, the researcher's primary interest was in preventing a Type I error. Therefore great emphasis was placed on the selection of a level of significance, but little emphasis was placed on power. However, this point of view is changing as the seriousness of a Type II error is increasingly recognized in nursing studies (Taylor & Spurlock, 2018).

As stated in the steps of classical hypothesis testing previously, step 4 is "conducting a power analysis." Power analysis involves determining the required sample size needed to conduct your study after performing steps 1, 2, and 3. Power analysis can address the number of participants required for a study, or conversely the

TABLE 21.1	**Type I and Type II Errors**		
		DECISION	
		Reject Null	**Accept Null**
True Population Status	**Null is True.**	Type I error α	Correct decision $1 - \alpha$
	Null is False.	Correct decision $1 - \beta$	Type II error β

extent of the power of a statistical test. A researcher conducts a power analysis prior to the study beginning to determine the required number of participants needed to identify an effect. This process is called a **priori power analysis**. A power analysis performed after the study ends to determine the power of the statistical result is termed a **post hoc power analysis**. Optimally, the power analysis is performed prior to the study's beginning so that the researcher can plan to include an adequate number of participants. Otherwise, the researcher risks conducting a study with an inadequate number of participants and putting the study at risk for Type II error (Grove & Cipher, 2020).

Cohen (1988) identified four parameters of power: (1) significance level, (2) sample size, (3) effect size, and (4) power (standard of 0.80). If three of the four are known, the fourth can be calculated by using power analysis formulas. Significance level and sample size are straightforward. Chapter 15 provides a detailed discussion of determining sample size in quantitative studies that includes power analysis. **Effect size** is "the degree to which the phenomenon is present in the population or the degree to which the null hypothesis is false" (Cohen, 1988, pp. 9–10). For example, suppose you were measuring changes in anxiety levels, measured first when the patient is at home and then just before surgery. The effect size would be large if you expected a great change in anxiety. If you expected only a small change in the level of anxiety, the effect size would be small.

Small effect sizes require larger samples to detect these small differences (see Chapter 15 for a detailed discussion of effect size). If the power is too low, it may not be worthwhile to conduct the study unless a large sample can be obtained, because statistical tests are unlikely to detect differences or relationships that exist. Deciding to conduct a study in these circumstances is costly in time and money, frequently does not add to the body of nursing knowledge, and can lead to false conclusions. Power analysis can be conducted with hand calculations, computer software, or online calculators and should be performed to determine the sample size necessary for a particular study (Cohen, 1988). Power analysis can be calculated by using the free power analysis software G*Power (Faul, Erdfelder, Lang, & Buchner, 2007) or statistical software such as NCSS, SAS, and SPSS (see Table 21.2). In addition, many free sample size calculators are available online that are easy to use and understand. The workbook by Grove and Cipher (2020)

TABLE 21.2 Software Applications for Statistical Analysis

Software Application	Website
SPSS (Statistical Packages for the Social Sciences)	www.ibm.com/software/analytics/spss/
SAS (Statistical Analysis System)	www.sas.com
NCSS (Number Cruncher Statistical System)	www.ncss.com
Stata	www.stata.com
JMP	www.jmp.com

provides step-by-step instructions for six common power analyses using the software G*Power 3.1 (Faul, Erdfelder, Buchner, & Lang, 2009).

The power achieved should be reported with the results of the studies, especially studies that fail to reject the null hypothesis (have nonsignificant results). If power is high, it strengthens the meaning of the findings. If power is low, researchers need to address this issue in the discussion of limitations and implications of the study findings. Modifications in the research methodology that resulted from the use of power analysis also need to be reported.

Statistical Significance Versus Clinical Importance

The findings of a study can be statistically significant but may not be clinically important. For example, one group of patients might have a body temperature 0.1° F higher than that of another group. Statistical analysis might indicate that the temperatures of two groups are significantly different. However, the findings have little or no clinical importance because of the small difference in temperatures between groups. It is often important to know the magnitude of the difference between groups in studies. However, a statistical test that indicates significant differences between groups (e.g., a *t*-test) provides no information on the magnitude of the difference. The extent of the level of significance (0.01 or 0.0001) tells you nothing about the magnitude of the difference between the groups or the relationship between two variables. The magnitude of group differences can best be determined through calculating effect sizes and confidence intervals (see Chapters 22, 23, 24, and 25).

Inference

Statisticians use the terms **inference** and **infer** in a way that is similar to the researcher's use of the term *generalize*. Inference requires the use of inductive reasoning. One infers from a specific case to a general truth, from a part to the whole, from the concrete to the abstract, from the known to the unknown. When using inferential reasoning, you can never prove things; you can never be certain. However, one of the reasons for the rules that have been established with regard to statistical procedures is to increase the probability that inferences are accurate. Inferences are made cautiously and with great care. Researchers use inferences to generalize the findings from the sample in their study to the larger population.

Samples and Populations

Use of the terms *statistic* and *parameter* can be confusing because of the various populations referred to in statistical theory. A **statistic**, such as a mean ($\overline{X}$), is a numerical value obtained from a sample. A **parameter** is a true (but unknown) numerical characteristic of a population. For example, μ is the population mean or arithmetic average. The mean of the sampling distribution (mean of samples' means) can also be shown to be equal to μ. A numerical value that is the mean ($\overline{X}$) of the sample is a statistic; a numerical value that is the mean of the population (μ) is a parameter (Barnett, 1982; Grove & Cipher, 2020).

Relating a statistic to a parameter requires an inference as one moves from the sample to the sampling distribution and then from the sampling distribution to the population. The population referred to is in one sense real (concrete) and in another sense abstract. These ideas are illustrated as follows:

For example, perhaps you are interested in the cholesterol levels of women in the United States. Your population is women in the United States. You cannot measure the cholesterol level of every woman in the United States; therefore you select a sample of women from this population. Because you wish your sample to be as representative of the population as possible, you obtain your sample by using random sampling techniques (see Chapter 15). To determine whether the cholesterol levels in your sample are similar to those in the population, you must compare the sample with the population. One strategy would be to compare the mean of your sample with the mean of the entire population. However, it is highly unlikely that you know the mean of the entire population; you must make an estimate of the mean of that population. You need to know how good your sample statistics are as estimators of the parameters of the population. First, you make some assumptions. You assume that the mean scores of cholesterol levels from multiple, randomly selected samples of this population would be normally distributed. This assumption implies another assumption: that the cholesterol levels of the population will be distributed according to the theoretical normal curve—that is, that difference scores and standard deviations can be equated to those in the normal curve. The normal curve is discussed later in this chapter and in Chapter 22.

If you assume that the population in your study is normally distributed, you can also assume that this population can be represented by a normal sampling distribution. You infer from your sample to the sampling distribution, the mathematically developed theoretical population made up of parameters such as the mean of means and the standard error. The parameters of this theoretical population are the measures of the dimensions identified in the sampling distribution. You can infer from the sampling distribution to the population. As illustrated earlier, there is both a concrete population and an abstract population. The concrete population consists of all the individuals who meet your study sample criteria; the abstract population consists of individuals who will meet your sample criteria in the future or the groups addressed theoretically by your framework (see Chapter 8).

TYPES OF STATISTICS

There are two major classes of statistics: descriptive statistics and inferential statistics. **Descriptive statistics** are computed to reveal characteristics of the sample and to describe study variables. **Inferential statistics** are computed to draw conclusions and make inferences about the population, based on the sample data set (Plichta & Kelvin, 2013). The following sections define the concepts and rationale associated with descriptive and inferential statistics.

Descriptive Statistics

A basic yet important way to begin describing a sample is to create a frequency distribution of the variable(s) being studied. A frequency distribution is a plot of one variable, whereby the x-axis consists of the possible values of that variable and the y-axis is the tally of each value. For example, if you assessed a sample for a variable such as pain using a visual analog scale and your subjects reported particular values for pain, you could create a frequency distribution as illustrated in Fig. 21.1.

Measures of Central Tendency

The measures of central tendency are descriptive statistics. The statistics that represent **measures of central tendency** are the mean, median, and mode. All of these statistics are representations or descriptions of the center or middle of a frequency distribution. The **mean** is the arithmetic average of all of the values of a variable. The **median** is the exact middle value (or the average of the middle two values if there is an even number of observations). The **mode** is the most commonly occurring value in a data set (Grove & Cipher, 2020; Zar, 2010). It is possible to have more than one mode in a sample, which is discussed in Chapter 22. In a normal curve, the mean, median, and mode are equal or approximately equal (Fig. 21.2).

Normal Curve

The theoretical **normal curve** is an expression of statistical theory. It is a theoretical frequency distribution of all possible scores (see Fig. 21.2). However, no real distribution fits the normal curve exactly. The idea of the normal curve was developed by an 18-year-old mathematician, Gauss, in 1795, who found that data measured repeatedly in many samples from the same population by using scales based on an underlying continuum can be combined into one large sample (Gauss, 1809). From this large sample, one can develop a more accurate representation of the pattern of the curve in that population than is possible with only one sample. In most cases, the curve is similar, regardless of the specific data that have been examined or the population being studied. This theoretical normal curve is symmetrical and unimodal and has continuous values. The mean, median, and mode are equal. The distribution is completely defined by the mean and standard deviation, which are calculated and discussed further in Chapter 22.

Sampling Distributions

The shape of the distribution provides important information about the data. The outline of the distribution shape is obtained by using a histogram. Within this

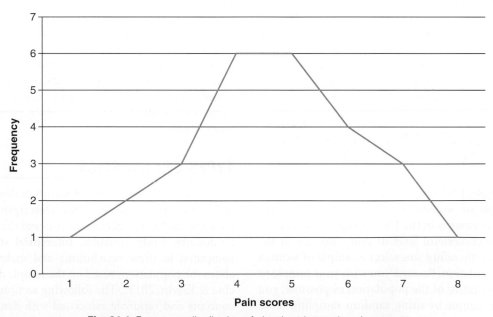

Fig. 21.1 Frequency distribution of visual analog scale pain scores.

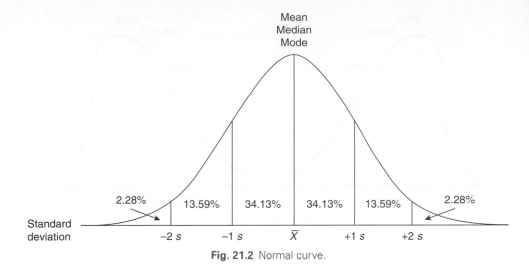

Fig. 21.2 Normal curve.

outline, the mean, median, mode, and standard deviation can be graphically illustrated (see Fig. 21.2). This visual presentation of combined summary statistics provides insight into the nature of the distribution. As the sample size becomes larger, the shape of the distribution more accurately reflects the shape of the population from which the sample was taken. Even when statistics, such as means, come from a population with a skewed (asymmetrical) distribution, the sampling distribution developed from multiple means obtained from that skewed population tends to fit the pattern of the normal curve. This phenomenon is referred to as the **central limit theorem.**

Symmetry

Several terms are used to describe the shape of the curve (and the nature of a particular distribution). The shape of a curve is usually discussed in terms of symmetry, skewness, modality, and kurtosis. A **symmetrical curve** is one in which the left side is a mirror image of the right side (Fig. 21.3). In these curves, the mean, median, and mode are equal and are the dividing point between the left and right sides of the curve.

Skewness

Any curve that is not symmetrical is referred to as **skewed** or **asymmetrical.** Skewness may be exhibited in the curve in various ways. A curve may be **positively skewed,** which means that the largest portion of data is

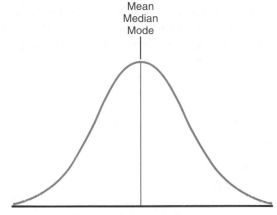

Fig. 21.3 Symmetrical curve.

below the mean. For example, data on length of enrollment in hospice are positively skewed. Most people die within the first 3 weeks of enrollment, whereas increasingly smaller numbers survive as time increases. A curve can also be **negatively skewed,** which means that the largest portion of data is above the mean. For example, data on the occurrence of chronic illness by age in a population are negatively skewed, with most chronic illnesses occurring in older age groups. Fig. 21.4 includes both a positively skewed distribution and a negatively skewed distribution.

In a **skewed distribution,** the mean, median, and mode are not equal. Skewness interferes with the validity

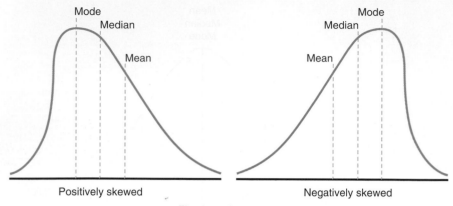

Fig. 21.4 Skewness.

of many statistical analyses; therefore statistical procedures have been developed to measure the skewness of the distribution of the sample being studied. Few samples are perfectly symmetrical; however, as the deviation from symmetry increases, the seriousness of the impact on statistical analysis increases (Plichta & Kelvin, 2013). In a positively skewed distribution, the mean is greater than the median, which is greater than the mode. In a negatively skewed distribution, the mean is less than the median, which is less than the mode (see Fig. 21.4). Grove and Cipher (2020) provide direction for determining the normality of a distribution in a study.

Modality

Another characteristic of distributions is their modality. Most curves found in practice are unimodal, which means that they have one mode, and frequencies progressively decline as they move away from the mode. Symmetrical distributions are usually unimodal. However, curves can also be bimodal (Fig. 21.5) or multimodal. When a bimodal sample is revealed, it may mean that the researcher has not applied an adequate sampling approach. An example of this may be when a researcher surveys a small sample of patients and presents them with

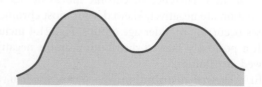

Fig. 21.5 Bimodal distribution.

a continuous response scale. For reasons particular (or idiosyncratic) to the survey sample, the responses obtained are primarily two distinct values. The frequency distribution will lack variability and appear as bimodal, when in fact the researcher should include a larger sample, thereby allowing for a greater variability in response values.

Kurtosis

Another term used to describe the shape of the distribution curve is kurtosis. **Kurtosis** explains the degree of peakedness of the curve, which is related to the spread or variance of scores. An extremely peaked curve is referred to as **leptokurtic**, an intermediate degree of kurtosis is referred to as **mesokurtic**, and a relatively flat curve is referred to as **platykurtic** (Fig. 21.6). Extreme kurtosis can affect the validity of statistical analysis because the scores have little variation in a leptokurtic curve. Many computer programs analyze kurtosis before conducting statistical analyses. A kurtosis of zero indicates that the curve is mesokurtic. Kurtosis values above zero indicate that the curve is leptokurtic, and values below zero that are negative indicate a platykurtic curve (Box, Hunter, & Hunter, 1978; Grove & Cipher, 2020).

Tests of Normality

Statistics are computed to obtain an indication of the skewness and kurtosis of a given frequency distribution. The **Shapiro-Wilk *W* test** is a formal test of normality that assesses whether the distribution of a variable is skewed, kurtotic, or both. This test has the ability to calculate both skewness and kurtosis for a study variable, such as pain measured with a visual analog scale.

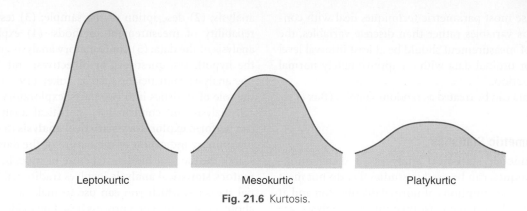

Leptokurtic   Mesokurtic   Platykurtic

Fig. 21.6 Kurtosis.

For large samples ($n > 2000$), the **Kolmogorov-Smirnov D test** is an alternative test of normality for large samples (Grove & Cipher, 2020).

Variation

The range, standard deviation, and variance are statistics that describe the extent to which the values in the sample vary from one another. The most common of these statistics to be reported in the literature is the standard deviation because of its direct association with the normal curve. If the frequency distribution of any given variable is approximately normal, knowing the standard deviation of that variable allows us to know what percentages of subjects' values on that variable fall between +1 and −1 standard deviation. Referring back to the hypothetical frequency distribution of pain in Fig. 21.1, when we calculate a standard deviation, we know that 34.13% of the subjects' pain scores were between the mean pain score and 1 standard deviation above the mean pain score. We also know that 34.13% of the subjects' pain scores were between the mean pain score and 1 standard deviation below the mean. The middle 95.44% of the subjects' scores were between −2 standard deviations and +2 standard deviations.

Confidence Intervals

When the probability of including the value of the parameter within the interval estimate is known, this is referred to as a **confidence interval**. Calculating a confidence interval involves the use of two formulas to identify the upper and lower ends of the interval (see Chapter 22 for calculations). Confidence intervals are usually expressed as "(38.6, 41.4)," with 38.6 being the lower end and 41.4

being the upper end of the interval. Theoretically, we can produce a confidence interval for any parameter of a distribution. It is a generic statistical procedure. Confidence intervals can also be developed around correlation coefficients (Glass & Stanley, 1970). Estimation can be used for a single population or for multiple populations. In **estimation**, we are inferring the value of a parameter from sample data and have no preconceived notion of the value of the parameter. In contrast, in **hypothesis testing**, we have an a priori theory about the value of the parameter(s) or some combination of parameters. A formula is provided for calculating confidence intervals, and example confidence intervals are provided for different analysis results in Chapters 22, 23, 24, and 25.

Inferential Statistics

Inferential statistics are computed to draw conclusions and make inferences about the greater population, based on the sample data set. There are two classes of inferential statistics: parametric and nonparametric statistics.

Parametric Statistics

The most commonly used type of statistical analysis is parametric statistics. The analysis is referred to as **parametric statistical analysis** because the findings are inferred to the parameters of a normally distributed population. These approaches to analysis emerged from the work of Fisher (1935) and require meeting the following three assumptions before they can justifiably be used.

1. The sample was drawn from a population for which the variance can be calculated. The distribution is usually expected to be normal or approximately normal (Conover, 1971; Zar, 2010).

2. Because most parametric techniques deal with continuous variables rather than discrete variables, the level of measurement should be at least interval level data or ordinal data with an approximately normal distribution.

3. The data can be treated as random samples (Box et al., 1978).

Nonparametric Statistics

Nonparametric statistical analyses, or distribution-free techniques, can be used in studies that do not meet the first two assumptions of normal distribution and at least interval-level data. Nonparametric analyses are conducted to analyze nominal and ordinal levels of data and interval-level data that are skewed. Most nonparametric techniques are not as powerful as their parametric counterparts (Tanizaki, 1997). In other words, nonparametric techniques are less able to detect differences and have a greater risk of a Type II error if the data meet the assumptions of parametric procedures; this is generally because nonparametric statistics are actually performed on ranks of the original data. When data have been converted into ranks, they inevitably lose accuracy. Because nonparametric statistics have lower statistical power, many researchers choose to submit ordinal data to parametric statistical procedures. If the instrument or measurement procedure yielding ordinal data has been rigorously evaluated, parametric statistics are justified (de Winter & Dodou, 2010). For example, researchers often analyze data from a Likert scale with strong reliability and validity as though they are interval-level data (see Chapter 17 for a description of Likert scales).

PRACTICAL ASPECTS OF STATISTICAL ANALYSIS

Statistics can be conducted for a variety of purposes, such as to (1) summarize, (2) explore the meaning of deviations in the data, (3) compare or contrast descriptively, (4) test the proposed relationships in a theoretical model, (5) infer that the findings from the sample are indicative of the entire population, (6) examine causality, (7) predict, or (8) infer from the sample to a theoretical model. These different purposes for statistical analysis are addressed in Chapters 22, 23, 24, and 25.

The process of quantitative statistical analysis consists of several stages: (1) preparation of the data for analysis; (2) description of the sample; (3) testing the reliability of measurement methods; (4) exploratory analysis of the data; (5) confirmatory analysis guided by the hypotheses, questions, or objectives; and (6) post hoc analysis. Statisticians such as Tukey (1977) divided the role of statistics into two parts: exploratory statistical analysis and confirmatory statistical analysis. You can perform **exploratory statistical analysis** to obtain a preliminary indication of the nature of the data and to search the data for hidden structure or models. **Confirmatory statistical analysis** involves traditional inferential statistics, which you can use to make an inference about a population or a process based on evidence from the study sample.

Although not all of these six stages are reflected in the final published report of the study, they all contribute to the insight you can gain from analyzing the data. Many novice researchers do not plan the details of statistical analysis until the data are collected and they are confronted with the analysis task. This research technique is poor and often leads to the collection of unusable data or the failure to collect the data needed to answer the research questions. Plans for statistical analysis need to be made during development of the study methodology. The following section covers the six stages of quantitative statistical analysis.

Preparing the Data for Analysis

Except in very small studies, computers are almost universally used for statistical analysis. When computers are used for analysis, the first step of the process is entering the data into a software package designed for data and/or statistical analyses. Table 21.2 lists examples of common statistical packages used for nursing research.

Before entering data, a codebook should be created that describes the measurement, coding, and scoring information for each variable as described in Chapter 20. Each variable must be labeled in the statistical software so that the variables involved in a particular analysis are clearly designated in the output. Develop a systematic plan for data entry that is designed to reduce errors during the entry phase and enter data during periods when you have few interruptions. In some studies, the data are already in a database and no data entry is needed. Examples of existing databases are electronic medical records and online surveys for which the responses are collected electronically.

In some cases, data must be reverse-scored before initiating statistical analysis. Items in scales are often arranged so that sometimes a higher numbered response indicates more of the construct being studied. For example, on a scale of 1 to 5, the highest number (5) designates higher levels of coping. Sometimes a higher numbered response indicates less of the construct being studied. In the example of the coping scale, resilience might be measured 1 to 5, with 1 representing higher levels of resilience and 5 representing lower levels of resilience. This arrangement prevents the subject from giving a global response to all items in the scale. To reduce errors, the values on these items need to be entered into the statistical software exactly as they appear on the data collection form. Values on the items are reversed by software commands.

Cleaning the Data

To examine the data carefully for errors, begin by printing a paper copy of the data file. When the size of the data file allows, you need to cross-check every datum on the printout with the original datum for accuracy. Otherwise, randomly check the accuracy of data points. Correct all errors found in the computer file. Perform an analysis of the frequencies of each value of every variable as a second check of the accuracy of the data. Search for values outside the appropriate range of values for that variable. Data that have been scanned into a computer program are less likely to have errors but should still be checked.

Identifying Missing Data

Identify all missing data points. Determine whether the missing information can be obtained and entered into the data file. If a large number of subjects have missing data on specific variables, you need to make a judgment regarding the availability of sufficient data to perform analysis with those variables. In some cases, subjects must be excluded from the analysis because of missing essential data. Missing data can also be imputed (estimated) via missing data statistical procedures. The rules involving the appropriateness of missing data imputations are complex, and there are many choices of statistical applications. The seminal publication on the topic of missing data imputation was written by Rubin (1976). You might seek the help of a statistician in making choices regarding the missing data in your study.

Data Transformations

Skewed or non-normally distributed data that do not meet the assumptions of parametric analysis can sometimes be transformed in such a way that the values are distributed closer to the normal curve. Various mathematical operations are used for this purpose. Examples of these operations include squaring each value, calculating the square root of each value, or calculating the logarithm of each value (Kim & Mallory, 2017). These operations can allow the researcher to yield a frequency distribution that more closely approximates normality, freeing the researcher to compute parametric statistics.

Data Calculations and Scoring

Sometimes a variable used in the analysis is not collected but calculated from other variables and is referred to as a **calculated variable**. For example, if data are collected on the number of patients on a nursing unit and on the number of nurses on a shift, one might calculate a ratio of nurse to patient for a particular shift. The data are more accurate if this calculation is performed with statistical software rather than manually. The results can be stored in the data file as a variable rather than being recalculated each time the variable is used in an analysis (Shortliffe & Cimino, 2006).

Data Storage and Documentation

When the data-cleaning process is complete, backups need to be made again; labeled as the complete, cleaned dataset; and carefully stored. Data cleaning is a time-consuming process that you will not wish to repeat unnecessarily. Be sure to back up the information each time you enter more data. It is wise to keep a second copy of the data filed at a separate, carefully protected site. If your data are being stored on a network, ensure that the network drive is being backed up at least once a day. After data entry, you need to store the original data in secure files for safekeeping. The data files need to be secured as designated by institutional review board policies. This usually includes password-protecting data files, storing data on encrypted flash drives, or storing on a network that requires two-factor authentication to access.

Rather than keep paper printouts of statistical output, it is recommended that you make portable document format (pdf) files of each output file and store these files in the same folder as your data sets and reports. Most word-processing software and statistical software packages can save data and output to pdf files. Converting output files into pdf files allows the researcher to transport those files and read them on any computer, even a computer that does not house the statistical software that created the original output file.

All files, including datasets and output files, need to be systematically named to allow easy access later when theses or dissertations are being written or research papers are being prepared for publication. We recommend naming files by time sequence. Name the file by its contents, and at the end of the file name, identify the date (month, day, and year) that the file was created or the analysis was performed. For example, the files named "Outcomes Data 020321" and "Means and Standard Deviations of Subscales 062321" represent a data file saved on February 3, 2021, and a statistical output file containing means and standard deviations of subscale scores saved on June 23, 2021, respectively.

Description of the Sample

After the data have been successfully entered into the software, saved, and stored, researchers start conducting the essential analysis techniques for their studies. The first step is to obtain as complete a picture as possible of the sample. The demographic variables such as age, gender, education, race, and ethnicity are analyzed with the appropriate analysis techniques and used to develop the characteristics of the sample. The analysis techniques used in describing the sample are covered in Chapter 22.

Testing the Reliability of Measurement Methods

Examine the reliability of the methods of measurement used in the study. The reliability of observational measures and multi-item scales and the precision of physiological measures may have been obtained during the data collection phase, but they also need to be noted at this point. Additional examination of the reliability of measurement methods, such as a Likert scale, is possible at this point. If you used an instrument that contained self-report items, such as true-false or Likert scale responses, internal consistency coefficients need to be calculated (see Chapter 16) (Waltz et al., 2017). The value of the coefficient needs to be compared with values obtained for the instrument in previous studies. If the coefficient is unacceptably low (< 0.6), you need to determine whether you are justified in performing

analysis on data from the instrument (see Chapter 16) (Grove & Cipher, 2020).

Exploratory Analysis of the Data

Examine all the data descriptively, with the intent of becoming as familiar as possible with the nature of the data. You might explore the data by conducting measures of central tendency and dispersion and examining outliers of the data. Neophyte researchers often omit this step and jump immediately into the analyses that were designed to test their hypotheses, questions, or objectives. However, they omit this step at the risk of missing important information in the data and performing analyses that are inappropriate for the data. The researcher needs to examine data on each variable by using measures of central tendency and dispersion. Are the data skewed or normally distributed? What is the nature of the variation in the data? Are there **outliers** with extreme values that appear different from the rest of the sample that cause the distribution to be skewed? The most valuable insights from a study sometimes come from careful examination of outliers (Tukey, 1977).

In many cases, as a part of exploratory analysis, inferential statistical procedures are used to examine differences and associations within the sample. From an exploratory perspective, these analyses are relevant only to the sample under study. There should be no intent to infer to a population. If group comparisons are made, effect sizes need to be determined for the variables involved in the analyses.

In some nursing studies, the purpose of the study is exploratory. In such studies, it is often found that sample sizes are small, power is low, measurement methods have limited reliability and validity, and the field of study is relatively new. If treatments are tested, the procedure might be approached as a pilot study. The most immediate need is tentative exploration of the phenomena under study. Confirming the findings of these studies requires more rigorously designed studies with much larger samples. Many of these exploratory studies are reported in the literature as confirmatory studies, and attempts are made to infer to larger populations. Because of the unacceptably high risk of a Type II error in these studies, negative findings should be viewed with caution.

Using Tables and Graphs for Exploratory Analysis

Although tables and graphs are commonly thought of as a way of presenting the findings of a study, these tools may be even more useful in helping the researcher to become familiar with the data (see Fig. 21.1 of the frequency distribution of visual analog scale pain scores). Tables and graphs need to illustrate the descriptive analyses being performed, even though they will probably not be included in a research report. These tables and figures are prepared for the sole purpose of helping researchers to identify patterns in their data and interpret exploratory findings, but they are sometimes useful in reporting study results to selected groups (Tukey, 1977). Visualizing the data in various ways can greatly increase insight regarding the nature of the data (see Chapter 22).

Confirmatory Analysis

As the name implies, **confirmatory analysis** is performed to confirm expectations regarding the data that are expressed as hypotheses, questions, or objectives. The findings are inferred from the sample to the population. Thus inferential statistical procedures are used. The design of the study, the methods of measurement, and the sample size must be sufficient for this confirmatory process to be justified. A written analysis plan needs to describe clearly the confirmatory analyses that will be performed to examine each hypothesis, question, or objective.

1. Identify the level of measurement of the data available for analysis with regard to the research objective, question, or hypothesis (see Chapter 16).
2. Select a statistical procedure or procedures appropriate for the level of measurement that will respond to the objective, answer the question, or test the hypothesis (Grove & Cipher, 2020; Plichta & Kelvin, 2013).
3. Select the level of significance that you will use to interpret the results, which is usually $\alpha = 0.05$.
4. Choose a one-tailed or two-tailed test if appropriate to your analysis. The extremes of the normal curve are referred to as **tails**. In a **one-tailed test of significance**, the hypothesis is directional and the extreme statistical values that occur in a single tail of the curve are of interest. In a **two-tailed test of significance**, the hypothesis is nondirectional or null and the extreme statistical values in both ends of the curve are of interest. Tailedness is discussed in more detail in Chapter 25.
5. Determine the risk of a Type II error in the analysis by performing a power analysis.

6. Determine the sample size available for the analysis. If several groups will be used in the analysis, identify the size of each group (Cohen, 1988; Grove & Cipher, 2020).
7. Evaluate the representativeness of the sample (see Chapter 15).
8. Develop dummy tables and graphics to illustrate the methods that you will use to display your results in relation to your hypotheses, questions, or objectives.
9. Perform the statistical analyses.
10. Most analyses are conducted by statistical software, and the output includes the statistical value obtained by analyzing the data, *p* value, and degrees of freedom *(df)* for each inferential analysis technique.
11. Reexamine the analysis to ensure that the procedure was performed with the appropriate variables and that the statistical procedure was correctly specified in the software program.
12. Interpret the results of the analysis in terms of the hypothesis, question, or objective.
13. Interpret the results in terms of the framework.

Post Hoc Analysis

Post hoc analyses are commonly performed in studies with more than two groups when the analysis indicates that the groups are significantly different but does not indicate which groups are different. For example, an analysis of variance (ANOVA) is conducted to examine the differences among three groups—experimental group, control group, and placebo group—and the groups are found to be significantly different. A post hoc analysis must be performed to determine which of the three groups are significantly different. Post hoc analysis is discussed in more detail in Chapter 25. In other studies, the insights obtained through the planned analyses generate further questions that can be examined with the available data.

CHOOSING APPROPRIATE STATISTICAL PROCEDURES FOR A STUDY

Multiple factors are involved in determining the suitability of a statistical procedure for a particular study. These factors can be related to the nature of the study, the nature of the researcher, and the nature of statistical theory. Specific factors include (1) the purpose of the study; (2) hypotheses, questions, or objectives; (3) research design;

(4) level of measurement; (5) previous experience in statistical analysis; (6) statistical knowledge level; (7) availability of statistical consultation; (8) financial resources; and (9) access to statistical software. Use items 1 through 4 to identify statistical procedures that meet the requirements of the study, and narrow your options further through the process of elimination based on items 5 through 9.

The most important factor to examine when choosing a statistical procedure is the study hypothesis. The hypothesis that is clearly stated indicates the statistics needed to test it. An example of a clearly developed hypothesis is, "There is a difference in employment rates between veterans who receive vocational rehabilitation and veterans who are on a waitlist control." This statement tells the researcher that a statistic to determine differences between two groups is appropriate for addressing this hypothesis.

One approach to selecting an appropriate statistical procedure or judging the appropriateness of an analysis technique is to use a decision tree. A decision tree directs your choices by gradually narrowing your options through the decisions you make. A decision tree that has been helpful in selecting statistical procedures is presented in Fig. 21.7.

One disadvantage of decision trees is that if you make an incorrect or uninformed decision (guess), you can be led down a path where you might select an inappropriate statistical procedure for your study. Decision trees are often constrained by space and do not include all of the information needed to make an appropriate selection. Detailed explanations and examples of how to use a statistical decision tree can be found in *Statistics for Nursing Research: A Workbook for Evidence-Based Practice* by Grove and Cipher (2020). The following examples of questions designed to guide the selection of analysis techniques for a study or the evaluation of statistical procedures in published research reports were extracted from selected sources (Andrews et al., 1981; Grove & Cipher, 2020).

1. How many variables does the problem involve?
2. How do you want to treat the variables with respect to the scale of measurement (nominal, ordinal, interval, or ratio)?
3. What do you want to know about the distribution of the variable?
4. Do you want to treat outlying cases differently from others?

5. How will you handle missing data?
6. What is the form of the distribution of data?
7. Is a distinction made between a dependent and an independent variable?
8. Do you want to test whether the means of the two variables are equal?
9. Do you want to treat the relationship between variables as linear?
10. How many of the variables are dichotomous?
11. Do you want to treat the ranks of ordered categories as interval scales?
12. Do the variables have the same distribution?
13. Do you want to treat the ordinal variable as though it were based on an underlying normally distributed interval variable?
14. Is the dependent variable at least at the interval level of measurement?
15. Do you want a measure of the strength of the relationship between the variables or a test of the statistical significance of differences between groups?
16. Are you willing to assume that an interval-scaled variable is normally distributed in the population?
17. Is there more than one dependent variable?
18. Do you want to statistically remove the linear effects of one or more covariates from the dependent variable?
19. Do you want to treat the relationships among the variables as additive?
20. Do you want to analyze patterns existing among variables or among individual cases?
21. Do you want to find clusters of variables that are more strongly related to one another than to the remaining variables? (Andrews et al, 1981; Grove & Cipher, 2020)

Each question confronts you with a decision. The decision you make narrows the field of available statistical procedures (see Fig. 21.7). Decisions must be made regarding the following:
1. Research design (see Chapters 10 and 11)
2. Number of variables (one, two, or more than two)
3. Level of measurement (nominal, ordinal, or interval)
4. Type of variable (independent, dependent, or research)
5. Distribution of variable (normal or non-normal)
6. Type of relationship (linear or nonlinear)
7. What you want to measure (strength of relationship or difference between groups)
8. Nature of the groups (equal or unequal in size, matched or unmatched, dependent [paired] or independent)

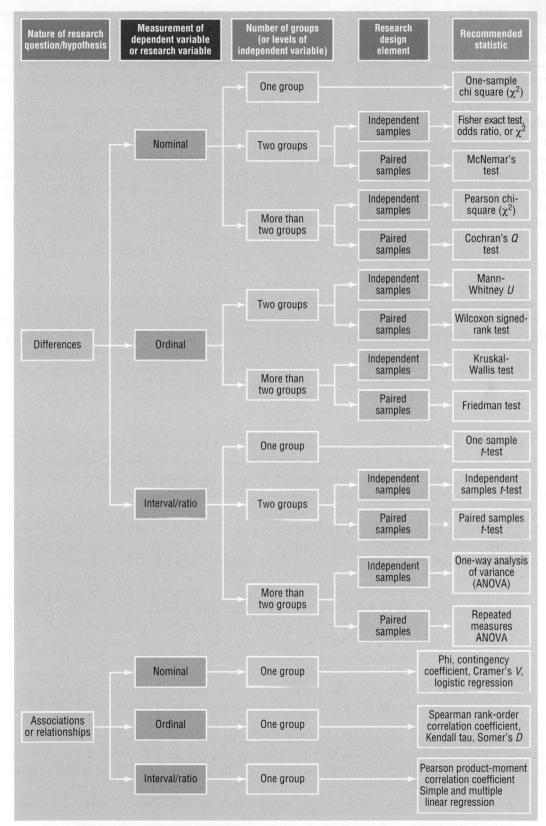

Fig. 21.7 Statistical decision tree for selecting an appropriate analysis technique.

9. Type of analysis (descriptive, classification, method-ological, relational, comparison, predicting outcomes, intervention testing, causal modeling, examining changes across time)

Examples

The following are some examples of using the questions listed previously, along with Fig. 21.7, to select the appropriate statistic.
1. A researcher has an associational study design and a research question that involves the linear association between two normally distributed variables both that are measured on an interval scale. The appropriate statistic would be the Pearson r correlation.
2. A researcher has an experimental study design with a comparative research question involving the difference between two groups on a dichotomous dependent variable. The Pearson chi-square test would be the appropriate statistic to test the difference between two groups on a dichotomous variable.
3. A researcher has an experimental study design with a comparative research question involving the difference

between three independent groups on a normally distributed dependent variable measured on an interval scale. The appropriate statistic would be a one-way ANOVA.
4. A researcher has an associational study design and a predictive research question that involves the linear association between a set of predictors and one normally distributed dependent variable that is measured on an interval scale. Multiple linear regression is the appropriate statistical procedure that tests the extent to which a set of variables predicts a normally distributed dependent variable.

In summary, selecting and evaluating statistical procedures requires that you make many judgments regarding the nature of the data and what you want to know. Knowledge of the statistical procedures and their assumptions is necessary for selecting appropriate procedures. You must weigh the advantages and disadvantages of various statistical options. Access to a statistician can be invaluable in selecting the appropriate procedures.

KEY POINTS

- This chapter introduces you to the concepts of statistical theory and discusses some of the more pragmatic aspects of quantitative statistical analysis, including the purposes of statistical analysis, the process of performing statistical analysis, the choice of the appropriate statistical procedures for a study, and resources for statistical analysis.
- Two types of errors can occur when making decisions about the meaning of a value obtained from a statistical test: Type I errors and Type II errors.
- A Type I error occurs when the researcher concludes a significant effect when no significant effect actually exists.
- A Type II error occurs when the researcher concludes no significant effect when an effect actually exists.
- The formal definition of the level of significance, or alpha (α), is the probability of making a Type I error when the null hypothesis is true.
- The p value is the exact value that can be calculated during a statistical computation to indicate the probability of obtaining a statistical value as extreme or greater when the null hypothesis is true.

- Power is the probability that a statistical test will detect a significant effect when it exists.
- Statistics can be used for various purposes, such as to (1) summarize, (2) explore the meaning of deviations in the data, (3) compare or contrast descriptively, (4) test the proposed relationships in a theoretical model, (5) infer that the findings from the sample are indicative of the entire population, (6) examine causality, (7) predict, or (8) infer from the sample to a theoretical model.
- The quantitative statistical analysis process consists of several stages: (1) preparation of the data for analysis; (2) description of the sample; (3) testing the reliability of measurement; (4) exploratory analysis of the data; (5) confirmatory analysis guided by hypotheses, questions, or objectives; and (6) post hoc analysis.
- A decision tree is provided to assist you in selecting appropriate analysis techniques to use in analyzing study or clinical data or in critically apprising the results section of published studies.

REFERENCES

Andrews, F. M., Klem, L., Davidson, T. N., O'Malley, P. M., & Rodgers, W. L. (1981). *A guide for selecting statistical techniques for analyzing social science data* (2nd ed.). Ann Arbor, MI: Survey Research Center, Institute for Social Research, University of Michigan.

Barnett, V. (1982). *Comparative statistical inference*. New York, NY: Wiley.

Box, G. E. P., Hunter, W. G., & Hunter, J. S. (1978). *Statistics for experimenters*. New York, NY: Wiley.

Cohen, J. (1988). *Statistical power analysis for the behavioral sciences* (2nd ed.). New York, NY: Academic Press.

Cohen, J. (1994). The earth is round ($p < .05$). *American Psychologist, 49*(12), 997–1003.

Conover, W. J. (1971). *Practical nonparametric statistics*. New York, NY: Wiley.

Cox, D. R. (1958). *Planning of experiments*. New York, NY: Wiley.

de Winter, J. C. F., & Dodou, D. (2010). Five-point Likert items: *t*-test versus Mann-Whitney-Wilcoxon. *Practical Assessment, Research, and Evaluation, 15*(11), 1–16.

Faul, F., Erdfelder, E., Buchner, A., & Lang, A. (2009). Statistical power analyses using G*Power 3.1: Tests for correlation and regression analyses. *Behavior Research Methods, 41*(4), 1149–1160. doi:10.3758/BRM.41.4.1149

Faul, F., Erdfelder, E., Lang, A.-G., & Buchner, A. (2007). G*Power 3: A flexible statistical power analysis program for the social, behavioral, and biomedical sciences. *Behavior Research Methods, 39*(2), 175–191. doi:10.3758/BRM.41.4.1149

Fisher, R. A. (1935). *The design of experiments*. New York, NY: Hafner.

Fisher, R. A. (1971). *The design of experiments* (9th ed.). New York, NY: MacMillan.

Gaskin, C. J., & Happell, B. (2014). Power, effects, confidence, and significance: An investigation of statistical practices in nursing research. *International Journal of Nursing Studies, 51*(5), 795–806. doi:10.1016/j.ijnurstu.2013.09.014

Gauss, C. F. (1809). *Theoria motus corporum coelestium in sectionibus conicis solem ambientium*. Hamburg: Friedrich Perthes and I. H. Besser.

Glass, G. V., & Stanley, J. C. (1970). *Statistical methods in education and psychology*. Englewood Cliffs, NJ: Prentice-Hall.

Good, I. J. (1983). *Good thinking: The foundations of probability and its applications*. Minneapolis, MN: University of Minnesota Press.

Grove, S. K., & Cipher, D. J. (2020). *Statistics for nursing research: A workbook for evidence-based practice* (3rd ed.). St. Louis, MO: Saunders.

Hayat, M. J., Higgins, M., Schwartz, T. A., & Staggs, V. S. (2015). Statistical challenges in nursing education and research: An expert panel consensus. *Nurse Educator, 40*(1), 21–25. doi:10.1097/NNE.0000000000000080

Kerlinger, F. N., & Lee, H. B. (2000). *Foundations of behavioral research* (4th ed.). New York, NY: Harcourt Brace.

Kim, M., & Mallory, C. (2017). *Statistics for evidence-based practice in nursing*. Burlington, MA: Jones & Bartlett Learning.

Loftus, G. R. (1993). A picture is worth a thousand *p* values: On the irrelevance of hypothesis testing in the microcomputer age. *Behavior Research Methods, Instrumentation, & Computers, 25*(2), 250–256.

Plichta, S. B., & Kelvin, E. A. (2013). *Munro's statistical methods for health care research*. Philadelphia, PA: Wolters Kluwer/ Lippincott Williams & Wilkins.

Rubin, D. B. (1976). Inference and missing data. *Biometrika, 63*(3), 581–592. doi:10.1093/biomet/63.3.581

Shortliffe, E. H., & Cimino, J. J. (2006). *Biomedical informatics: Computer applications in health care and biomedicine*. New York, NY: Springer Science.

Tanizaki, H. (1997). Power comparison of non-parametric tests: Small-sample properties from Monte Carlo experiments. *Journal of Applied Statistics, 24*(5), 603–632. doi:1080/02664769723576

Taylor, J., & Spurlock, D. (2018). Methodology corner: Statistical power in nursing education research. *Journal of Nursing Education, 57*(5), 262–264. doi:10.3928/01484834-20180420-02

Tukey, J. W. (1977). *Exploratory data analysis*. Reading, MA: Addison-Wesley.

Waltz, C. F., Strickland, O. L., & Lenz, E. R. (2017). *Measurement in nursing and health research* (5th ed.). New York, NY: Springer.

Zar, J. H. (2010). *Biostatistical analysis* (5th ed.). Upper Saddle River, NJ: Pearson Prentice-Hall.

22

Using Statistics to Describe Variables

Daisha J. Cipher

http://evolve.elsevier.com/Gray/practice/

There are two major classes of statistics: descriptive statistics and inferential statistics. Descriptive statistics are computed to reveal characteristics of the sample data set. Inferential statistics are computed to gain information about effects in the population being studied. For some types of studies, descriptive statistics are the only approach to analysis of the data. For other studies, descriptive statistics are the first step in the statistical analysis process, to be followed by inferential statistics. For all studies that involve numerical data, descriptive statistics are crucial to understanding the fundamental properties of the variables being studied. This chapter focuses on descriptive statistics and includes the most common descriptive statistics conducted in nursing research with examples from clinical studies.

USING STATISTICS TO SUMMARIZE DATA

Frequency Distributions

A basic yet important way to begin describing a sample is to create a **frequency distribution** of the variable(s) being studied. A frequency distribution can be displayed in a table or figure. A line graph figure can be used to plot one variable, whereby the x-axis consists of the possible values of that variable, and the y-axis is the tally of each value. The frequency distributions presented in this chapter include values of continuous variables. With a **continuous variable**, the higher numbers represent more of that variable, and the lower numbers represent less of that variable. Continuous variables may be interval or ratio scales of measurement. Common examples of continuous variables are age, income, blood pressure, weight, height, and temperature.

The frequency distribution of a variable can be presented in a **frequency table**, which is a way of organizing the data by listing every possible value in the first column of numbers and the frequency (tally) of each value in the second column of numbers. For example, consider the following hypothetical age data for patients from a primary care clinic. The ages of 20 patients were:

45, 26, 59, 51, 42, 28, 26, 32, 31, 55, 43, 47, 67, 39, 52, 48, 36, 42, 61, 57

First, we must sort the patients' ages from lowest to highest values:

26
26
28
31
32
36
39
42
42
43
45
47
48
51
52
55
57
59
61
67

Next, each age value is tallied to create the frequency. This is an example of an ungrouped frequency distribution. In an **ungrouped frequency distribution**, researchers list all categories of the variable for which they have data and tally each observation (Grove & Cipher, 2020). In this example, all the different ages of the 20 patients are listed and then tallied for each age.

Age	Frequency
26	2
28	1
31	1
32	1
36	1
39	1
42	2
43	1
45	1
47	1
48	1
51	1
52	1
55	1
57	1
59	1
61	1
67	1

Because most of the ages in this data set have frequencies of 1, it is better to group the ages into ranges of values. These ranges must be mutually exclusive. A patient's age can be classified into only one of the ranges. In addition, the ranges must be exhaustive, meaning that each patient's age fits into at least one of the categories (Plichta & Kelvin, 2013). For example, one may choose to have ranges of 10, so that the age ranges are 20 to 29, 30 to 39, 40 to 49, 50 to 59, and 60 to 69. A researcher may choose to have ranges of 5, so that the age ranges are 20 to 24, 25 to 29, 30 to 34, and so on. The grouping should be devised to provide the greatest possible meaning to the purpose of the study. If the data are to be compared with data in other studies, groupings should be similar to groupings of other studies in this field of research. Classifying data into groups results in the development of a **grouped frequency distribution** (Grove & Cipher, 2020). Table 22.1 presents a grouped frequency distribution of patient ages classified by ranges of 10 years. The range starts at 20 because there are no patient ages lower than 20; also, there are no ages higher than 69.

TABLE 22.1 Grouped Frequency Distribution of Patient Ages With Percentages

Adult Age Range	Frequency (f)	Percentage	Cumulative Percentage
20–29	3	15%	15%
30–39	4	20%	35%
40–49	6	30%	65%
50–59	5	25%	90%
60–69	2	10%	100%
Total	**20**	**100%**	

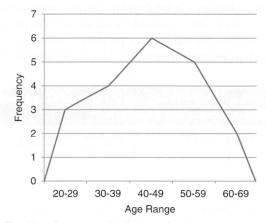

Fig. 22.1 Frequency distribution of patient age ranges.

Table 22.1 also includes percentages of patients with an age in each range and the cumulative percentages for the sample, which should add to 100%. This table provides an example of a **percentage distribution** that indicates the percentage of the sample with scores falling in a specific group or range (Grove & Cipher, 2020). Percentage distributions are particularly useful in comparing the data of the present study with results from other studies.

As discussed earlier, frequency distributions can be presented in figures. Frequencies are commonly presented in graphs, charts, histograms, and frequency polygons. Fig. 22.1 is the frequency distribution for age ranges, where the x-axis (horizontal line) represents the different age ranges, and the y-axis (vertical line) represents the frequencies of patients with ages in each of the ranges.

A frequency table is also an important method to represent nominal data (Grove & Cipher, 2020; Tukey,

1977). Common nominal variables include gender, race, ethnicity, and marital status. Table 22.2 presents an example of how the nominal variable "nursing graduate program enrollment" can be reported. The frequency and percentage distributions are presented for nominal data extracted from a sample of survey respondents of former nursing graduate students (Cipher, Urban, & Mancini, 2019).

As shown in Table 22.2, the frequencies indicate that of 125 survey respondents, 22 (17.6%) were enrolled in a Master of Science in Nursing (MSN) education program, 27 (21.6%) were enrolled in an MSN administration program, and 76 (60.8%) were enrolled in a nurse practitioner program. For nominal variables such as this, tables are a helpful method to inform researchers and others about the variable being studied. Graphically representing the values in a frequency table can yield visually important trends. Fig. 22.2 is a histogram that

was developed to represent the graduate program data visually.

Measures of Central Tendency

A **measure of central tendency** is a statistic that represents the center or middle of a frequency distribution (Kim & Mallory, 2017; Zar, 2010). The three measures of central tendency commonly reported in nursing studies include mode, median (MD), and mean ($\bar{X}$). The mode, median, and mean are defined and calculated in this section using a simulated subset of data collected from veterans with inflammatory bowel disease (Flores, Burstein, Cipher, & Feagins, 2015). Table 22.3 contains the body mass index (BMI) data collected from a subset of 10 veterans with inflammatory bowel disease. The BMI, a measure of body fat based on height and weight that applies to adult men and women, is considered an indicator of obesity when 30 or greater (National Heart, Lung, and Blood Institute, 2019). Because the number of study subjects represented is 10, the correct statistical notation to reflect that number is:

$$n = 10$$

The letter n is lowercase because it refers to a sample of veterans and italicized because it represents a statistic. If the data being presented represented the entire population of veterans, the correct notation would be an uppercase N (Zar, 2010). Because most nursing research is conducted using samples, not populations, all formulas in this chapter and in Chapters 23, 24, and 25 incorporate the sample notation, n.

Mode

The **mode** is the numerical value or score that occurs with the greatest frequency in a data set. It does not indicate the center of the data set. The data in Table 22.3

TABLE 22.2 Frequency Table of Graduate Nursing Program Enrollment

Smoking Status	Frequency	Percentage (%)
MSN Education Program	22	17.6%
MSN Administration Program	27	21.6%
Nurse Practitioner Program	76	60.8%
Total	**125**	**100.0%**

MSN, Master of Science in Nursing.

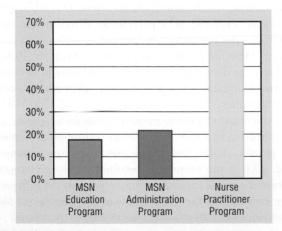

Fig. 22.2 Histogram of graduate nursing program enrollment. *MSN*, Master of Science in Nursing.

TABLE 22.3 Body Mass Index (BMI) Values in 10 Veterans With Inflammatory Bowel Disease

BMI	BMI
20.1	31.0
24.4	31.7
28.1	34.2
28.1	36.8
28.7	36.9

contain one mode: 28.1. The BMI value of 28.1 occurred twice in the data set. When two modes exist, the data set is referred to as **bimodal** (see Chapter 21). A data set that contains more than two modes is referred to as **multimodal** (Zar, 2010).

Median

The **median** is the score at the exact center of the ungrouped frequency distribution. It is the 50th percentile. To obtain the *MD,* sort the values from lowest to highest. If the number of values is an uneven number, the *MD* is the exact middle number in the data set. If the number of values is an even number, the *MD* is the average of the two middle values; thus the *MD* may not be an actual value in the data set (Zar, 2010). For example, the data in Table 22.3 consist of 10 observations, and the *MD* is calculated as the average of the two middle values.

$$MD = \frac{(28.7 + 31)}{2} = 29.85$$

Mean

The **mean** is the arithmetic average of all the values of a variable in a study and is the most commonly reported measure of central tendency. The mean is the sum of the scores divided by the number of scores being summed. Similar to the *MD,* the mean may not be a member of the data set. The formula for calculating the mean is as follows:

$$\bar{X} = \frac{\Sigma X}{n}$$

where
$\bar{X}$ = mean
Σ = sigma, the statistical symbol for summation
X = a single value in the sample
n = total number of values in the sample

The mean BMI for the veterans with inflammatory bowel disease is calculated as follows:

$$\bar{X} = \frac{\begin{array}{c}(20.1 + 24.4 + 28.1 + 28.1 + 28.7 + 31.0 + 31.7 \\ + 34.2 + 36.8 + 36.9)\end{array}}{10}$$

$$\bar{X} = \frac{300}{10} = 30.0$$

The mean is an appropriate measure of central tendency to calculate for approximately normally distributed populations with variables measured at the interval or ratio levels. It is also appropriate for ordinal-level data such as Likert scale or rating scale values (as described in Chapter 17), where higher numbers represent more of the construct being measured and lower numbers represent less of the construct, such as a 5-point rating scale, on which 1 represents "not at all confident" and 5 represents "completely confident" (Cipher et al., 2019; Waltz, Strickland, & Lenz, 2017).

The mean is sensitive to extreme scores such as outliers. An **outlier** is a value in a sample data set that is unusually low or unusually high in the context of the rest of the sample data (Zar, 2010). An example of an outlier in the data presented in Table 22.3 might be a value such as a BMI of 55. The existing values range from 20.1 to 36.9, indicating that no veteran had a BMI value greater than 36.9. If an additional veteran was added to the sample, and that person had a BMI of 55, the mean would be larger: 32.27 (mean = 355 ÷ 11 = 32.27). The outlier would also change the frequency distribution. Without the outlier, the frequency distribution is approximately normal, as shown in Fig. 22.3. The inclusion of the outlier changes the shape from an approximately normal distribution to a positively skewed distribution (see Fig. 22.3) (Plichta & Kelvin, 2013; Zar, 2010). The median is a better measure of central tendency than the mean for data that are positively skewed by an outlier (see Chapter 21 for discussion of skewness).

USING STATISTICS TO EXPLORE DEVIATIONS IN THE DATA

Although the use of summary statistics has been the traditional approach to describing data or describing the characteristics of the sample before inferential statistical analysis, the ability of summary statistics to clarify the nature of data is limited. For example, using measures of central tendency, particularly the mean, to describe the nature of the data obscures the impact of extreme values or deviations in the data. Significant features in the data may be concealed or misrepresented. Measures of dispersion, such as the range, difference scores, variance, and standard deviation, provide important insight into the nature of the data.

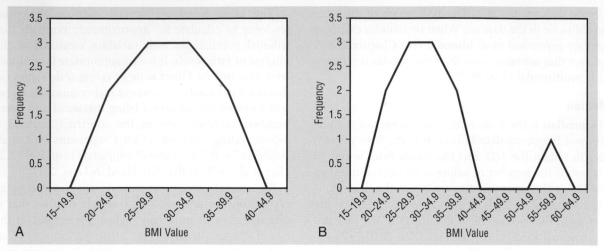

Fig. 22.3 Frequency distribution of body mass index (*BMI*) values (A) without outlier and (B) with outlier.

Measures of Dispersion

Measures of dispersion or variability are measures of individual differences of the members of the population and sample (Zar, 2010). They indicate how values in a sample are dispersed around the mean. These measures provide information about the data that is not available from measures of central tendency. They indicate how different the scores are—the extent to which individual values deviate from one another. If the individual values are similar, measures of variability are small, and the sample is relatively **homogeneous** in terms of those values. When there are wide variations or differences in the scores, the sample is considered **heterogeneous**. The **heterogeneity** of sample scores or values is determined by measures of dispersion or variability (Grove & Cipher, 2020). The measures of dispersion most commonly reported in nursing research are range, difference scores, variance, and standard deviation.

Range

The simplest measure of dispersion is the **range**. In published studies, range is presented in two ways: (1) the range is the lowest and highest scores, or (2) the range is calculated by subtracting the lowest score from the highest score. The range for the scores in Table 22.3 is 20.1 to 36.9 or can be calculated as follows: 36.9 − 20.1 = 16.8. In this form, the range is a difference score that uses only the two extreme scores for the comparison. The range is generally reported in published studies but is not used in further analyses.

Difference Scores

Difference scores are obtained by subtracting the mean from each score. Sometimes a difference score is referred to as a **deviation score** because it indicates the extent to which a score deviates from the mean. Most variables in nursing research are not "scores"; however, the term *difference score* is used to represent the deviation of a value from the mean. The difference score is positive when the score is above the mean, and it is negative when the score is below the mean. The difference scores (both positive and negative) add to zero or approximately zero based on rounding. Difference scores are the basis for many statistical analyses and can be found within many statistical equations. The formula for difference scores is:

$$X - \bar{X}$$

The **mean deviation** is the average difference score, using the absolute values. The formula for the mean deviation is:

$$\bar{X}_{deviation} = \frac{\Sigma |X - \bar{X}|}{n}$$

$$\bar{X}_{deviation} = \frac{9.9 + 5.6 + 1.9 + 1.9 + 1.3 + 1 + 1.7 + 4.2 + 6.8 + 6.9}{10}$$

$$\bar{X}_{deviation} = \frac{41.2}{10}$$

$$\bar{X}_{deviation} = 4.12$$

TABLE 22.4 Difference Scores of Body Mass Index			
X	$-\bar{X}$	$X - \bar{X}$	$\lvert X - \bar{X}\rvert$
20.1	−30	−9.9	9.9
24.4	−30	−5.6	5.6
28.1	−30	−1.9	1.9
28.1	−30	−1.9	1.9
28.7	−30	−1.3	1.3
31.0	−30	1.0	1.0
31.7	−30	1.7	1.7
34.2	−30	4.2	4.2
36.8	−30	6.8	6.8
36.9	−30	6.9	6.9
		Σ of absolute values = 41.2	

TABLE 22.5 Calculation of Variance for Body Mass Index			
X	$-\bar{X}$	$X - \bar{X}$	$(X - \bar{X})^2$
20.1	−30	−9.9	98.01
24.4	−30	−5.6	31.36
28.1	−30	−1.9	3.61
28.1	−30	−1.9	3.61
28.7	−30	−1.3	1.69
31.0	−30	1.0	1.00
31.7	−30	1.7	2.89
34.2	−30	4.2	17.64
36.8	−30	6.8	46.24
36.9	−30	6.9	47.61
		Σ	253.66

In this example using the data from Table 22.4, the mean deviation is 4.12. The result indicates that, on average, veterans' BMI values deviated from the mean by 4.12.

Variance

Variance is another measure of dispersion commonly used in statistical analysis. The equation for a sample variance (s^2) is provided. The lowercase letter s^2 is used to represent a sample variance. The lowercase Greek sigma (σ^2) is used to represent a population variance, in which the denominator is N instead of $n - 1$. Because most nursing research is conducted using samples, not populations, all formulas in the next several chapters that contain a variance or standard deviation incorporate the sample notation and use $n - 1$ as the denominator. Statistical software packages compute the variance and standard deviation using the sample formulas, not the population formulas.

$$s^2 = \frac{\Sigma\left(X - \bar{X}\right)^2}{n-1}$$

The variance is always a positive value and has no upper limit. In general, the larger the calculated variance for a study variable is, the larger the dispersion or spread of scores is for the variable. Table 22.4 displays how you might compute a variance by hand, using the BMI data. Table 22.5 shows calculation of the variance for BMI.

$$s^2 = \frac{253.66}{9}$$

$$s^2 = 28.18$$

Standard Deviation

Standard deviation (s) is a measure of dispersion that is the square root of the variance. The equation for obtaining a standard deviation is:

$$s = \sqrt{\frac{\Sigma\left(X - \bar{X}\right)^2}{n-1}}$$

Table 22.5 displays the computations for the variance. To compute the standard deviation, simply take the square root of the variance. You know that the variance of BMI values is $s^2 = 28.18$. Therefore the standard deviation of BMI values is $s = 5.31$. In published studies, sometimes the statistic reported by researchers for standard deviation is *SD*. Either *SD* or *s* might be used in a research report to indicate the standard deviation for a study variable.

The standard deviation is an important statistic, both for understanding dispersion within a distribution and for interpreting the relationship of a particular value to the distribution. The statistical workbook by Grove and Cipher (2020) provides you with a resource for calculating and interpreting the measures of central tendency and measures of dispersion in published studies, as well as computing those measures with statistical software. The following section summarizes the properties of the standard deviation as it relates to a normal distribution.

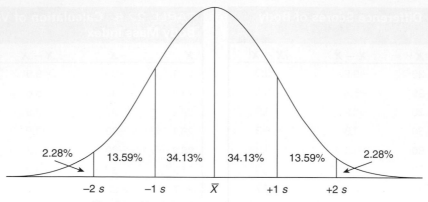

Fig. 22.4 Normal curve. *s*, Standard deviation (*SD*).

Normal Curve

The standard deviation of a variable tells researchers much about the entire sample of values. A frequency distribution of a variable that is *perfectly normally distributed* is shown in Fig. 22.4, otherwise known as the **normal curve**.

The normal curve is a perfectly symmetrical frequency distribution. The value at the exact center of a normal curve is the mean of the values. Note the vertical lines to the left and to the right of the mean. Those lines are drawn at +1 standard deviation (which indicates 1 *s* above the mean) and −1 standard deviation (which indicates 1 *s* below the mean), +2 standard deviations above the mean, −2 standard deviations below the mean, and so forth. When a frequency distribution is shaped like the normal curve, we know that 34.13% of the subjects scored between the mean and 1 standard deviation above the mean, and 34.13% of the subjects scored between the mean and 1 standard deviation below the mean. Because the normal curve is perfectly symmetrical, we also know that 50% of the subjects scored above the mean, and 50% of the subjects scored below the mean.

We can also say that 68.26% of the subjects scored between −1 and +1 standard deviation. This number is obtained by adding 34.13% and 34.13%. Furthermore, we can say that 95.44% of the subjects scored between −2 and +2 standard deviations. If we are given a mean and a standard deviation value for any variable that is normally distributed, we know certain facts about those data. For example, consider a score obtained on a subscale of the Short Form (36) Health Survey (SF-36). The SF-36 is a widely used health survey that yields eight subscales that each represent a domain of subjective health status (Ware & Sherbourne, 1992). The subscales have been normed on populations of respondents as having a mean of 50 and standard deviation of 10. The frequency distribution of responses for the subscale "physical functioning" can be drawn as seen in Fig. 22.5.

The mean is marked as 50 in the middle, and the standard deviations are marked at the lines. Therefore you know that 34.13% of the population scores fall between a 50 and a 60 on the "physical functioning" subscale. You also know that 95.44% of the population scores fall between 30 and 70 on the "physical functioning" subscale. Fig. 22.5 shows that only 2.28% of the population scores fall above the value of 70 (this is computed by subtracting 34.13% and 13.59% from 50%). Likewise, only 2.28% of the population scores fall below the value of 30.

When using examples such as these, researchers often use the statistic *z* instead of the term *standard deviation*. A *z* value is synonymous with a standard deviation unit. A *z* value of 1.0 represents 1 standard deviation unit above the mean. A *z* value of −1.0 represents 1 standard deviation unit below the mean (see Appendix A: *z* Values Table). Although a standard deviation value cannot have a negative value, a *z* value can be negative or positive. A *z* of 0 represents exactly the mean value. Any value in a data set can be converted to a *z* by using the following formula:

$$z = \frac{(X - \bar{X})}{s}$$

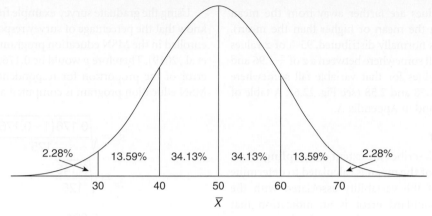

Fig. 22.5 Frequency distribution of SF-36 "physical functioning" scale values.

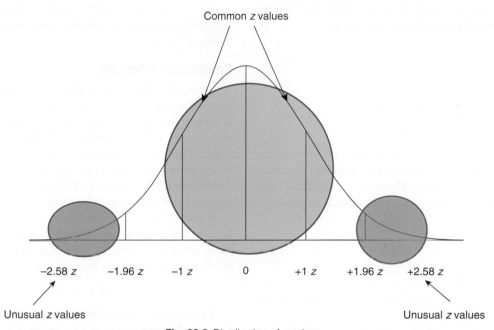

Fig. 22.6 Distribution of z values.

For example, a person scoring a 61 on the SF-36 "physical functioning" scale would have a z value of 1.1:

$$z = \frac{(61-50)}{10}$$

$$z = 1.1$$

It is important to note how z values represent standard deviations on the normal curve because this knowledge becomes necessary when performing significance testing in inferential statistics. For example, observe how a z value of 1.0 or −1.0 is much more common than a z value of 3.0 or −3.0. The farther the z value is from the mean, the more uncommon, unusual, and unlikely that value is to occur. This principle is revisited in Chapters 23, 24, and 25.

The distribution of the normal curve is drawn once more in Fig. 22.6 but this time with the z statistic, where z represents 1 standard deviation unit. Common values of z are smaller values and closer to the mean. Uncommon and unusual z values are farther away from the mean (either lower than the mean or higher than the mean). When a variable is normally distributed, 95% of z values for that variable fall somewhere between a z of -1.96 and 1.96; 99% of z values for that variable fall somewhere between a z of -2.58 and 2.58 (see Fig. 22.6). A table of z values can be found in Appendix A.

Sampling Error

A standard error describes the extent of **sampling error**. A **standard error of the mean** is calculated to determine the magnitude of the variability associated with the mean. A small standard error is an indication that the sample mean is close to the population mean. A large standard error yields less certainty that the sample mean approximates the population mean. The formula for the standard error of the mean ($s_{\bar{X}}$) is:

$$s_{\bar{X}} = \frac{s}{\sqrt{n}}$$

where
$s_{\bar{X}}$ = standard error of the mean
s = standard deviation
n = sample size

Using the BMI data for the veterans with inflammatory bowel disease, we know that the standard deviation of BMI values is $s = 5.31$. Therefore the standard error of the mean for BMI values is computed as follows:

$$s_{\bar{X}} = \frac{5.31}{\sqrt{10}}$$
$$s_{\bar{X}} = 1.68$$

The standard error of the mean for BMI data in this sample of veterans is 1.68.

A **standard error of the proportion** is calculated to determine the magnitude of the variability associated with a proportion, also expressed as a percentage. A small standard error of proportion is an indication that the sample proportion is close to the population proportion. The formula for the standard error of the proportion (s_p) is:

$$s_p = \sqrt{\frac{p(1-p)}{n}}$$

where
s_p = standard error of the proportion
p = proportion observed
n = sample size

Using the graduate survey example from Table 22.2, we know that the percentage of survey respondents who were enrolled in the MSN education program is 17.6% (Cipher et al., 2019). Therefore p would be 0.176, and the standard error of the proportion for respondents enrolled in the MSN education program is computed as follows:

$$s_p = \sqrt{\frac{0.176(1-0.176)}{125}}$$
$$s_p = \sqrt{\frac{0.145}{125}}$$
$$s_p = 0.034$$

The standard error of the proportion for the survey respondents enrolled in the MSN education program is 0.034, or 3.4%.

Confidence Intervals

To determine how closely the sample mean approximates the population mean or the sample proportion approximates the population proportion, the standard error is used to build a **confidence interval**. A confidence interval can be created for many statistics, such as a mean, proportion, odds ratio, and correlation. To build a confidence interval around a statistic, you must have the standard error value and the t value to adjust the standard error. The t is a statistic for the t-test that is calculated to determine group differences and is discussed in more detail in Chapter 25. The degrees of freedom calculation for a confidence interval is as follows:

$$df = n - 1$$

To compute the confidence interval for a mean, the lower and upper limits of that interval are created by multiplying the standard error by the t statistic, where $df = n - 1$. For a 95% confidence interval, the t value should be selected at $\alpha = 0.05$. For a 99% confidence interval, the t value should be selected at $\alpha = 0.01$.

Using the BMI data, we know that the standard error of the mean for BMI values is $s_{\bar{X}} = 1.68$. The mean BMI is 30.0. The 95% confidence interval for the mean BMI is computed as follows:

$$\bar{X} \pm s_{\bar{X}} t$$
$$30.0 \pm (1.68)(2.26)$$
$$30.0 \pm 3.80$$

As referenced in Appendix B, the *t* value required for the 95% confidence interval with *df* = 9 for a two-tailed test is 2.26. The previous computation results in a lower limit of 26.2 and an upper limit of 33.8.

This means that our confidence interval of 26.2 to 33.8 estimates the population mean BMI among veterans with inflammatory bowel disease with 95% confidence (Kline, 2004). Technically and mathematically, it means that if we computed the mean BMI on an infinite number of groups of veterans, and a confidence interval for each of those means, exactly 95% of the confidence intervals would contain the true population mean and 5% would not contain the population mean (Gliner, Morgan, & Leech, 2009).

If we were to compute a 99% confidence interval, we would require the *t* value that is referenced at α = 0.01 for a two-tailed test. The 99% confidence interval for BMI is computed as follows:

$$30.0 \pm (1.68)(3.25)$$
$$30.0 \pm 5.46$$

As referenced in Appendix B, the *t* value required for the 99% confidence interval with *df* = 9 for a two-tailed test is 3.25. The previous computation results in a lower limit of 24.54 and an upper limit of 35.46. Thus our confidence interval of 24.54 to 35.46 estimates the population mean BMI among veterans with inflammatory bowel disease with 99% confidence.

Using the graduate survey data, we know that the percentage of former MSN education program enrollees is 17.6%, and the standard error of the proportion is

s_p = 3.4%. The 95% confidence interval for the percentage of MSN education program enrollees is computed as follows:

$$p \pm s_p t$$
$$17.6\% \pm (3.4\%)(1.984)$$
$$17.6\% \pm 6.75\%$$

As referenced in Appendix B, the *t* value required for the 95% confidence interval with *df* = 124 for a two-tailed test is 1.984. As can be observed from the table, any *df* larger than *df* = 100 but smaller than *df* = 200 would require a *t* of 1.984 for a 95% confidence interval. The previous computation results in a lower limit of 10.85% and an upper limit of 24.35%. This means that our confidence interval of 10.85% to 24.35% estimates the population percentage of graduate nursing students who are enrolled in an MSN education program with 95% confidence.

Degrees of Freedom

The concept of degrees of freedom was used in reference to computing a confidence interval. For any statistical computation, **degrees of freedom** is the number of independent pieces of information that are free to vary to estimate another piece of information (Zar, 2010). In the case of the confidence interval, the *df* is *n* − 1. This means that there are *n* − 1 independent observations in the sample that are free to vary (to be any value) to estimate the lower and upper limits of the confidence interval.

KEY POINTS

- Data analysis begins with descriptive statistics in any study in which the data are numerical, including demographic variables for samples in quantitative and qualitative studies.
- Descriptive statistics allow the researcher to organize the data in ways that facilitate meaning and insight.
- Three measures of central tendency are the mode, median, and mean.
- The measures of dispersion most commonly reported in nursing studies are range, difference scores, variance, and standard deviation.

- The standard deviation and *z* represent certain properties of the normal curve that are used in significance testing.
- Standard error indicates the extent of sampling error.
- To determine how closely the sample mean approximates the population mean, the standard error of the mean is used to build a confidence interval.
- For any statistical computation, degrees of freedom are the number of independent pieces of information that are free to vary to estimate another piece of information.

REFERENCES

Cipher, D. J., Urban, R. W., & Mancini, M. E. (2019). Factors associated with student success in online and face-to-face delivery of master of science in nursing programs. *Teaching and Learning in Nursing, 14*(3), 203–207. doi:10.1016/j.teln.2019.03.007

Flores, A., Burstein, E., Cipher, D. J., & Feagins, L. A. (2015). Obesity in inflammatory bowel disease: A marker of less severe disease. *Digestive Diseases and Sciences, 60*(8), 2436–2445. doi:10.1007/s10620-015-3629-5

Gliner, J. A., Morgan, G. A., & Leech, N. L. (2009). *Research methods in applied settings* (2nd ed.). New York, NY: Routledge.

Grove, S. K., & Cipher, D. J. (2020). *Statistics for nursing research: A workbook for evidence-based practice* (3rd ed.). St. Louis, MO: Elsevier.

Kim, M., & Mallory, C. (2017). *Statistics for evidence-based practice in nursing*. Burlington, MA: Jones & Bartlett Learning.

Kline, R. B. (2004). *Beyond significance testing*. Washington, DC: American Psychological Association.

National Heart, Lung, and Blood Institute. (2019). *Classification of overweight and obesity by BMI, waist circumference, and associated disease risks*. Retrieved from https://www.nhlbi.nih.gov/health/educational/lose_wt/BMI/bmi_dis.htm

Plichta, S. B., & Kelvin, E. A. (2013). *Munro's statistical methods for health care research*. Philadelphia, PA: Wolters Kluwer/Lippincott Williams & Wilkins.

Tukey, J. W. (1977). *Exploratory data analysis*. Reading, MA: Addison-Wesley.

Waltz, C. F., Strickland, O. L., & Lenz, E. R. (2017). *Measurement in nursing and health research* (5th ed.). New York, NY: Springer.

Ware, J. E., & Sherbourne, C. D. (1992). The MOS 36-item short-form health survey (SF-36®): Conceptual framework and item selection. *Medical Care, 30*(6), 473–483.

Zar, J. H. (2010). *Biostatistical analysis* (5th ed.). Upper Saddle River, NJ: Prentice-Hall.

23

Using Statistics to Examine Relationships

Daisha J. Cipher

http://evolve.elsevier.com/Gray/practice/

Correlational analyses identify relationships or associations among variables. There are many different kinds of statistics that yield a measure of correlation. All of these statistics address a research question or hypothesis that involves an association or a relationship. Examples of research questions that are answered with correlation statistics are as follows: Is there an association between weight loss and depression? Is there a relationship between patient satisfaction and health status? A hypothesis is developed to identify the nature (positive or negative) of the relationship between the variables being studied. For example, a researcher may hypothesize that the frequency of home care visits are associated with improved health status among persons with spinal cord injuries (see Chapter 6 for question and hypothesis development) (Sippel et al., 2019).

This chapter presents the common analysis techniques used to examine relationships in studies. The analysis techniques discussed include the use of scatter diagrams before correlational analysis, bivariate correlational analysis, testing the significance of a correlational coefficient, spurious correlations, correlations between two raters or measurements, the role of correlation in understanding causality, and the multivariate correlational procedure of factor analysis.

SCATTER DIAGRAMS

Scatter plots or **scatter diagrams** provide useful preliminary information about the nature of the relationship between variables (Plichta & Kelvin, 2013). The researcher should develop and examine scatter diagrams before performing a correlational analysis. Scatter plots may be useful for selecting appropriate correlational procedures, but most correlational procedures are useful for examining linear relationships only. A scatter plot can be used to identify nonlinear relationships; if the data are nonlinear, the researcher should select statistical alternatives such as nonlinear regression analysis (Zar, 2010). A scatter plot is created by plotting the values of two variables on an *x*-axis and *y*-axis. As shown in Fig. 23.1, the ages at which veterans received a diagnosis of ulcerative colitis were plotted against their body mass indices (BMIs) (Flores, Burstein, Cipher, & Feagins, 2015). Specifically, each veteran's pair of values (age at diagnosis, BMI) was plotted on the diagram. The resulting scatter plot reveals a linear trend whereby older diagnostic ages tend to correspond with higher BMI values. The line drawn in Fig. 23.1 is a regression line that represents the concept of least squares. A **least-squares regression line** is a line drawn through a scatter plot that represents the smallest distance between each value and the regression line (Cohen & Cohen, 1983). Regression analysis is discussed in detail in Chapter 24.

BIVARIATE CORRELATIONAL ANALYSIS

Bivariate correlational analysis measures the magnitude of a linear relationship between two variables and is performed on data collected from a single sample (Kim & Mallory, 2017; Zar, 2010). The particular correlation statistic that is computed depends on the scale of measurement of each variable. Correlational techniques are available for all levels of data: nominal

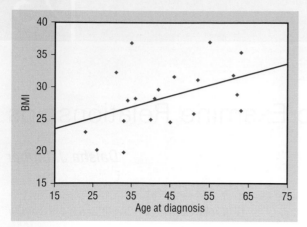

Fig. 23.1 Scatter plot of body mass index *(BMI)* and age at diagnosis among veterans with ulcerative colitis.

(phi, contingency coefficient, Cramer's V, and lambda), ordinal (Spearman rank-order correlation coefficient, gamma, Kendall's tau, and Somers's D), or interval and ratio (Pearson product-moment correlation coefficient). Fig. 21.7 illustrates the level of measurement for which each of these statistics is appropriate. Many of the correlational techniques (Kendall's tau, contingency coefficient, phi, and Cramer's V) are used in conjunction with contingency tables, which illustrate how values of one variable vary with values for a second variable. Contingency tables are explained further in Chapter 25.

Correlational analysis provides two pieces of information about the data: (1) the nature or direction of the linear relationship (positive or negative) between the two variables and (2) the magnitude (or strength) of the linear relationship. Correlation statistics are not an indication of causality, no matter how strong the statistical result.

In a **positive linear relationship**, the values being correlated vary together (in the same direction). When one value is high, the other value tends to be high; when one value is low, the other value tends to be low. The relationship between weight and blood pressure is considered positive because the more a patient weighs, the higher his or her blood pressure tends to be. In a **negative linear relationship**, when one value is high, the other value tends to be low. There is a negative linear relationship between level of pain and functional capacity because the more pain a person is experiencing, the lower is his or her ability to function. A negative linear relationship is sometimes referred to as an **inverse**

linear relationship—the terms *negative* and *inverse* are synonymous in correlation statistics (see Chapter 6 for diagrams of positive and negative relationships).

Sometimes the relationship between two variables is **curvilinear**, which reflects a relationship between the variables that change over the range of both variables. For example, one of the most famous curvilinear relationships is that of stress and test performance. Test performance tends to be better as test-takers have more stress but only up to a point. When students experience very high stress levels, test performance deteriorates (Lupien, Maheu, Tu, Fiocco, & Schramek, 2007; Yerkes & Dodson, 1908). Analyses designed to test for linear relationships or associations between two variables, such as Pearson correlation, cannot detect a curvilinear relationship.

Pearson Product-Moment Correlation Coefficient

The Pearson product-moment correlation was one of the first of the correlation measures developed and is the most commonly used (Plichta & Kelvin, 2013; Zar, 2010). This coefficient (statistic) is represented by the letter *r*, and the value of *r* is always between −1.00 and +1.00. A value of zero indicates no relationship between the two variables. A positive correlation indicates that higher values of *x* are associated with higher values of *y*, and lower values of *x* are associated with lower values of *y*. A negative or inverse correlation indicates that higher values of *x* are associated with lower values of *y*. The *r* value is indicative of the slope of the line (called a regression line) that can be drawn through a standard scatter plot of the values of two paired variables. The strengths of different associations are identified in Table 23.1 (Cohen, 1988; Grove & Cipher, 2020). Fig. 23.2 represents an *r* value approximately equal to zero, indicating no relationship or association between the two variables. An *r* value is rarely, if ever, exactly equal to zero. Fig. 23.3 shows an *r* value equal to 0.50,

TABLE 23.1	Strength of Association for Pearson *r*	
Strength of Association	**Positive Association**	**Negative Association**
Weak	0.00 to 0.29	0.00 to −0.29
Moderate	0.30 to 0.49	−0.49 to −0.30
Strong/large	0.50 to 1.00	−1.00 to −0.50

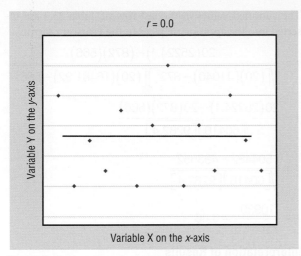

Fig. 23.2 Scatter plot of r equal to approximately 0.00, representing no relationship between two variables.

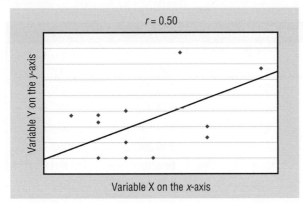

Fig. 23.3 Scatter plot of variables where r is 0.50, representing a strong positive correlation.

which is a strong positive relationship. Fig. 23.4 shows an r value equal to -0.50, which is a strong negative or inverse relationship.

As discussed earlier, the **Pearson product-moment correlation coefficient** is used to determine the relationship between two variables measured at least at the interval level of measurement. The formula for the Pearson correlation coefficient is based on the following assumptions:

1. Interval or ratio measurement of both variables (e.g., age, income, blood pressure, cholesterol levels). However, if the variables are measured with a Likert scale, and the frequency distribution is approximately normally distributed, these data are usually considered

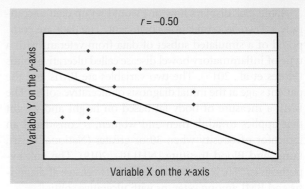

Fig. 23.4 Scatter plot of variables where r is -0.50, representing a strong inverse correlation.

interval level measurement and are appropriate for the Pearson r (de Winter & Dodou, 2010; Rasmussen, 1989; Waltz, Strickland, & Lenz, 2017).
2. Normal distribution of at least one variable
3. Independence of observational pairs
4. Homoscedasticity

Data that are **homoscedastic** are evenly dispersed both above and below the regression line, which indicates a linear relationship on a scatter plot (see Chapter 24 for more information on heteroscedasticity). Homoscedasticity reflects equal variance of both variables. In other words, for every value of x, the distribution of y values should have equal variability with respect to the regression line. If the data for the two variables being correlated are not homoscedastic, inferences made during significance testing could be invalid (Cohen & Cohen, 1983).

Calculation

The Pearson product-moment correlation coefficient is computed using one of several formulas; the following formula is considered the computational formula because it makes computation by hand easier (Zar, 2010).

$$r = \frac{n\sum xy - \sum x \sum y}{\sqrt{\left[n\sum x^2 - \left(\sum x\right)^2\right]\left[n\sum y^2 - \left(\sum y\right)^2\right]}}$$

where
r = Pearson product-moment correlation coefficient
n = total number of subjects
x = value of the first variable
y = value of the second variable
xy = x multiplied by y

Table 23.2 displays how one would set up data to compute a Pearson correlation coefficient. The data are composed of a simulated subset of data from veterans with a type of inflammatory bowel disease called ulcerative colitis (Flores et al., 2015). The two variables are BMIs and the patient's age at the initial diagnosis of ulcerative colitis. The BMI, a measure of body fat based on height and weight that applies to adult men and women, is considered an indicator of obesity when 30 or greater (National Heart, Lung, and Blood Institute [NHLBI], 2019). The null hypothesis is, "There is no correlation between age at diagnosis and BMI among veterans with ulcerative colitis."

A simulated subset of 20 veterans was randomly selected for this example so that the computations would be small and manageable. In actuality, studies involving Pearson correlations need to be adequately powered (Cohen, 1988). Observe that the data in Table 23.2 are arranged in columns, which correspond to the elements of the formula.

The summed values in the last row of Table 23.2 are inserted into the appropriate place in the Pearson r formula.

$$r = \frac{20(25224.1) - (872)(566)}{\sqrt{[(20)(41040) - 872^2][(20)(16481.92) - 566^2]}}$$

$$r = \frac{20(25224.1) - 20(872)(566)}{\sqrt{[60416][9282.4]}}$$

$$r = \frac{504482 - 493552}{\sqrt{[60416][9282.4]}}$$

$$r = \frac{10930}{23681.3} = 0.46$$

Interpretation of Results

The r is 0.46, indicating a moderate positive correlation between BMI and age at diagnosis among veterans with

TABLE 23.2	Computation of Pearson r Correlation Coefficient				
Participant Number	x (Age at Diagnosis)	y (BMI)	x^2	y^2	xy
1	33	19.7	1089	388.09	650.1
2	26	20.1	676	404.01	522.6
3	23	22.9	529	524.41	526.7
4	45	24.4	2025	595.36	1098
5	33	24.6	1089	605.16	811.8
6	40	24.8	1600	615.04	992
7	51	25.7	2601	660.49	1310.7
8	63	26.2	3969	686.44	1650.6
9	34	27.8	1156	772.84	945.2
10	41	28.1	1681	789.61	1152.1
11	36	28.1	1296	789.61	1011.6
12	62	28.7	3844	823.69	1779.4
13	42	29.5	1764	870.25	1239
14	46	31.5	2116	992.25	1449
15	52	31	2704	961	1612
16	61	31.7	3721	1004.89	1933.7
17	31	32.2	961	1036.84	998.2
18	63	35.3	3969	1246.09	2223.9
19	35	36.8	1225	1354.24	1288
20	55	36.9	3025	1361.61	2029.5
sum Σ	872	566.0	41,040	16,481.92	25,224.10

BMI, Body Mass Index.

ulcerative colitis. To determine whether this relationship is improbable to have been caused by chance alone, we consult the *r* probability distribution table in Appendix C. The formula for **degrees of freedom** *(df)* for a Pearson *r* is *n* − 2. Recall from Chapter 22 that every inferential statistic has its own formula for degrees of freedom (numbers of values that are free to vary). In our analysis, the *df* is 20 − 2 = 18. With *r* of 0.46 and *df* = 18, you need to consult the table in Appendix C to identify the critical value of *r* for a two-tailed test. The critical *r* value at alpha (α) = 0.05, *df* = 18 is 0.4438 that was rounded to 0.444 for this discussion. Our obtained *r* was 0.46, which exceeds the critical value in the table. It should be noted that if the obtained *r* was −0.46, it would also be considered statistically significant because the absolute value of the obtained *r* is compared to the critical *r* value. The sign of the *r* is only used to indicate whether the association is positive or negative.

Another way to determine the statistical significance of a statistic is to compute the exact *p* value, which is facilitated with statistical software. When this particular Pearson *r* was computed using statistical software, the exact *p* value associated with the *r* of 0.46 was *p* = 0.041. This indicates that the exact likelihood of obtaining this *t* value or larger when the null hypothesis is true is 4.1 in 100, or 4.1%. When reporting statistical interpretations for journal articles that use formatting from the American Psychological Association (APA, 2020), the exact *p* value is required.

The following interpretation is written as it might appear in a research article, formatted according to APA (2020) guidelines:

There was a significant correlation between BMI and age at diagnosis among veterans with ulcerative colitis, r(18) = 0.46, p = 0.041. Higher BMI values were associated with older ages at which the diagnosis occurred. (Grove & Cipher, 2020)

Every inferential statistic can be reflected by a **probability distribution** of that statistic. The table to which we referred in Appendix C to determine the significance of our obtained *r* was actually drawn from the probability distribution of *r* values. Chapter 22 illustrated the probability distribution of *z*, which appears identical to the normal curve. The Pearson *r* can be reflected by a theoretical distribution of *r* values. The shape of this distribution changes, depending on the size of the sample. When a Pearson correlation is computed using a large number of values (*n* > 120), the corresponding distribution of *r* values appears similar to the normal curve. The smaller the sample size, the flatter the *r* distribution; the larger the sample size, the more the *r* distribution approximates the normal curve, reflecting the range of paired values obtained. Sample size matters because the shape of the probability distribution determines whether our obtained statistic is statistically significant (Plichta & Kelvin, 2013; Zar, 2010).

For example, consider our obtained *r* of 0.46, previously calculated. At 18 *df*, the *r* probability distribution looks like that of Fig. 23.5. With a sample size of 20 (and 18 *df*), the middle 95% of the *r* probability distribution is delimited by −0.444 and 0.444. The mean *r*, theoretically, is *r* = 0. That is, most correlation coefficients computed between two variables equal zero, reflecting no relationships between the two variables. Therefore, an *r* value of zero is the most common and probable *r* value. It is much more improbable to obtain a high *r* value. At 18 *df*, *r* values within the limits of −0.444 and 0.444 are considered common and likely; values outside these limits are uncommon, unlikely, and improbable to have occurred by chance. The values outside these limits constitute 5% of the *r* distribution, which is where the concept of alpha (Type I error) originates. We obtained an *r* of 0.46 and rejected the null hypothesis that there was no association between age at diagnosis and BMI. Thus there is an association between age at diagnosis and BMI among veterans with

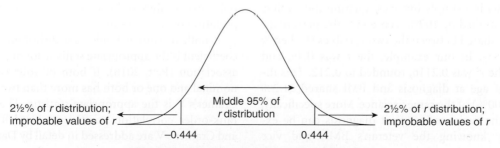

Fig. 23.5 Probability distribution of *r* at *df* = 18.

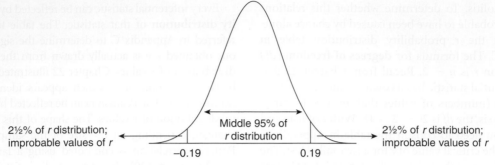

2½% of *r* distribution;
improbable values of *r*

Middle 95% of
r distribution

2½% of *r* distribution;
improbable values of *r*

−0.19   0.19

Fig. 23.6 Probability distribution of *r* at *df* = 100.

ulcerative colitis. In rejecting the null hypothesis, there is less than a 5% chance that we are making a Type I error (Cohen, 1988).

Compare Fig. 23.5 with Fig. 23.6, in which the probability distribution of *r* at *df* = 100 is displayed. Appendix C indicates that the critical *r* value at α = 0.05, *df* = 100 (and a sample size of 102) for a two-tailed test is *r* = 0.1946, rounded to 0.19. This means that the middle 95% of the *r* probability distribution at *df* = 100 is delimited by −0.19 and 0.19. Furthermore, *r* values within the limits of −0.19 and 0.19 are considered common and likely, and values outside these limits are uncommon, unlikely, and improbable to have occurred by chance. Observe the difference that the larger sample size makes in the critical *r* value needed to achieve significance. The larger the sample size, the smaller the *r* value needed to demonstrate statistical significance.

Effect Size

After establishing the statistical significance of *r*, the relationship subsequently must be examined for clinical importance. There are ranges for strength of association suggested by Cohen (1988), as displayed in Table 23.1. One can also assess the magnitude of association by obtaining the **coefficient of determination** for the Pearson correlation. Computing the coefficient of determination simply involves squaring the *r* value. The r^2 (multiplied by 100%) represents the percentage of variance shared between the two variables (Cohen & Cohen, 1983). In our example, the *r* was 0.46, and therefore the r^2 was 0.2116, rounded to 0.212. This indicates that age at diagnosis and BMI shared 21.2% (0.212 × 100%) of the same variance. More specifically, 21.2% of the variance in age at diagnosis can be explained by knowing the veteran's BMI, and vice

versa—21.2% of the variance in BMI can be explained by knowing the veteran's age at diagnosis. Statistical textbooks and online resources provide more direction in interpreting the Pearson correlation coefficient (*r*) and explaining its calculations (Grove & Cipher, 2020; Plichta & Kelvin, 2013).

Nonparametric Alternatives

If one or both of your variables do not meet the assumptions for a Pearson correlation, both **Spearman rank-order correlation coefficient** and **Kendall's tau** are more appropriate statistics. The Spearman rank-order correlation coefficient and Kendall's tau calculations involve converting the data to ranks, discarding any variance or normality issues associated with the original values (Pett, 2016).

If your data meet the assumptions for the Pearson correlation coefficient, it is the preferred analysis procedure. You would calculate a nonparametric alternative only if your data violate those assumptions. Because the Spearman correlation and Kendall's tau are based on ranks of the data, the properties of the original data are lost when they are converted to ranks. Because of this fact, most nonparametric statistics of association yield lower statistical power (Daniel, 2000; Pett, 2016). The statistical workbook by Grove and Cipher (2020) provides examples of the Spearman rank-order correlation coefficient from published studies and provides guidance in the interpretation of these results.

If both of your variables are dichotomous, the phi coefficient is the appropriate statistic for determining an association (Pett, 2016). If both of your variables are nominal and one or both has more than two categories, Cramer's V is the appropriate statistic. The Spearman rank-order correlation coefficient, Kendall's tau, phi, and Cramer's V are addressed in detail by Daniel (2000).

Role of Correlation in Understanding Causality

In any situation involving causality, a relationship exists between the factors involved in the causal process. Therefore the first clue to the possibility of a causal link is the existence of a relationship; however, a relationship does not mean causality. For example, blood glucose level may be related to or correlated with body temperature, but this does not mean that one causes the other. Two variables can be highly correlated but have no causal relationship. However, as the strength of a relationship increases, the possibility of a causal link increases. The absence of a relationship precludes the possibility of a causal connection between the two variables being examined, given adequate measurement of the variables (Waltz et al., 2017) and absence of other variables that might mask the relationship (Cohen & Cohen, 1983). A correlational study can be the first step in determining the connections among variables important to nursing practice within a particular population. Determining these dynamics can allow us to increase our ability to predict and control the situation studied. However, *correlations cannot be used to show causality.*

Spurious Correlations

Spurious correlations are relationships between variables that are not true. In some cases, these significant relationships are a consequence of chance and have no meaning. When you choose a level of significance of $\alpha = 0.05$, 1 in 20 correlations that you compute will be statistically significant by chance alone. There is really no true relationship between the two variables under study in the population; you just happened to draw a sample that showed a relationship where there typically is none. Other pairs of variables may be correlated because of the influence of other unrelated or confounding variables. For example, you might find a positive correlation between the number of deaths on a nursing unit and the number of nurses working on the unit. The number of deaths cannot be explained as occurring because of increases in the number of nurses. It is more likely that a third variable (units having patients with more critical conditions) explains both the increased number of nurses and the increased number of deaths. In many cases, the "other" variable remains unknown, although the researcher can use reasoning to identify and exclude most of these spurious correlations.

BLAND AND ALTMAN PLOTS

Bland and Altman plots are used to examine the extent of agreement between two measurement techniques (Bland & Altman, 1986, 2010). In nursing research, Bland and Altman plots are used to display visually the extent of interrater agreement and test-retest agreement (see Chapter 16 for discussion of reliability). For both instances, pairs of data are collected from each subject (from rater 1 and rater 2 or administration 1 and administration 2), and each subject's two values are subtracted from one another. The differences are plotted on a graph, displaying a scatter diagram of the differences plotted against the averages. Limits of agreement are defined as twice the standard deviation above and below the mean. Bland and Altman plots are primarily used to see how many of the values are outside these limits. Acceptable interrater or test-retest agreement is considered to be reflected when at least 95% of the values are within the limits of agreement on the plot (Altman, 1991).

Example

Table 23.3 displays a simulated subset of test-retest data from veterans with inflammatory bowel disease. These values are BMIs collected from 20 veterans, 1 month apart. Each veteran's BMI value at Assessment 1 and Assessment 2 is displayed in Table 23.3, along with the difference between each pair of scores.

A Bland and Altman plot of these data is illustrated in Fig. 23.7. The line of perfect agreement is drawn as a red line in the exact horizontal middle of the graph. The mean difference of the sample data is represented by the dotted middle line, and the limits of agreement are the two outside dotted lines. Observe that there are no values outside of the limits of agreement. Therefore all 20 pairs of data were within the limits of agreement. Incidentally, the r between the first and second assessments of the BMI was 0.97. However, the Bland and Altman plot does not always corroborate a Pearson correlation coefficient, and vice versa, because they are distinctly different methods (Bland & Altman, 1986).

Bland and Altman (1986) created the coefficient of repeatability *(CR)* as an indication of the repeatability of a single method of measurement. Because the same method is being measured repeatedly, the mean difference should be zero. Use the following formula to calculate a *CR*, where $S_{x_1-x_2}$ is the standard deviation of the difference scores.

$$CR = 1.96\left(S_{x_1-x_2}\right)$$

TABLE 23.3 Test-Retest Data for Body Mass Index Values Among Veterans With Inflammatory Bowel Disease

Assessment 1	Assessment 2	Difference
19.7	20.9	−1.2
20.1	20.7	−0.6
22.9	22.2	0.7
24.4	26.6	−2.2
24.6	24.4	0.2
24.8	25.3	−0.5
25.7	27.5	−1.8
26.2	25.2	1
27.8	29.2	−1.4
28.1	30.1	−2
28.1	27.3	0.8
28.7	28.4	0.3
29.5	31.3	−1.8
31.5	32.4	−0.9
31	29.8	1.2
31.7	30.7	1
32.2	32.5	−0.3
35.3	36.0	−0.7
36.8	35.3	1.5
36.9	36.5	0.4
		$\bar{X}: -0.315$

Table 23.3 displays each difference score, of which the mean is −0.315. The standard deviation of the difference scores is $s_{x_1 - x_2} = 1.17$. Therefore the CR is calculated as:

$$CR = 1.96(1.17)$$
$$CR = 2.29$$

Interpretation of Results

The mean difference between the two assessments of BMI was −0.315 (see Table 23.3). In other words, the average difference between the first and second assessments of BMI values was −0.315. A perfect average agreement would be 0, meaning that, on average, the two sets of values were exactly the same. The CR value, 2.29, is added to and subtracted from the mean difference to create lower and upper limits of acceptable agreement: −0.315 ± 2.29. Differences within −0.315 ± 2.29 (−2.61, 1.98) would not be deemed clinically important, according to Bland and Altman (2010). Differences between the two administrations that are less than −2.61 and greater than 1.98 are "unacceptable for clinical purposes" (Bland & Altman, 2010, p. 933). The CR is not an inferential statistic, and values of lower and upper limits of agreement are not interpreted the way one would interpret a confidence interval. Rather, they are formulas invented by Bland and Altman for heuristic purposes to make decisions on the extent of agreement between two measurements.

FACTOR ANALYSIS

Factor analysis refers to a collection of statistical techniques designed to examine interrelationships among large numbers of variables to reduce them to a smaller set of variables and to identify clusters of variables that are most closely linked together (i.e., **factors**). Factors are hypothetical constructs created from the original variables. The term *factor analysis* may apply to the statistical applications of exploratory factor analysis (EFA) (sometimes called principal components analysis) and confirmatory factor analysis (Tabachnick & Fidell, 2013). EFA is the procedure of choice for a researcher who is primarily interested in reducing a large number of variables down to a smaller number of components.

A common reason for performing EFA is to assist with validity investigations of a new measurement method or scale, particularly subjective assessments or instruments that pertain to attitudes, beliefs, values, or opinions. When researchers develop a new instrument, EFA can serve to

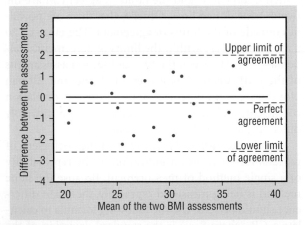

Fig. 23.7 Bland and Altman plot of test-retest data for body mass index (*BMI*) values for veterans with inflammatory bowel disease.

assist the researcher in investigating its content and construct validity, as described in Chapter 16 (Waltz et al., 2017). The results of EFA assist researchers in understanding which questions are redundant (or assess the same concept), which questions represent subsets of variables, and which items stand alone and reflect unique concepts.

Mathematically, EFA extracts maximum variance (explanatory power to predict one variable's value from another's value) from the data set with each factor. The first factor is the linear combination of the variables (or instrument items) that maximizes the variance of their factor scores. The second component is formed from residual correlations. Subsequent factors are formed from the residual correlations that have not yet been created.

Once the factors have been identified mathematically, the researcher attempts to explain why the variables are grouped as they are. Factor analysis aids in the identification of theoretical constructs and is also used to confirm the accuracy of a theoretically developed construct.

Example

The following example describes how EFA was used to investigate content and construct validity for the Maslach Burnout Inventory (MBI) (Poghosyan, Aiken, & Sloane, 2009). The MBI was developed in 1981 to assess burnout experienced by nurses (Maslach & Jackson, 1981). The MBI has been reported in many factor analytic studies since its original publication (Worley, Vassar, Wheeler, & Barnes, 2008). These sources are older because it takes years to develop a valid scale to measure concepts important to nursing practice (Waltz et al., 2017). Poghosyan and colleagues (2009) investigated the factor structure of the MBI in 54,738 nurses living in one of eight countries. The 22 items were answered on a 7-point Likert scale, ranging from never having those feelings to having those feelings a few times a week. Of the 22 items, all loaded on at least one of the subscales (with a factor loading of > 0.30). Using EFA, three factors were identified, confirming prior factor analytic reports. The factor loadings from the US nurses (the other countries were excluded for this example) are listed in Table 23.4.

The first factor, emotional exhaustion, accounted for the majority of the variance extracted from the EFA solution, followed by smaller percentages of variance explained by the second and third factors. Table 23.4 lists the factor loadings of each item. **Factor loadings** are the correlations between the item and the new factor. The MBI items that were not highly correlated with

TABLE 23.4 Item Factor Loadings on Three MBI Subscales

Factor Loading[a]	MBI Item
EMOTIONAL EXHAUSTION SUBSCALE	
0.93	Feel emotionally drained from work
0.94	Feel used up at the end of the workday
0.86	Feel fatigued when getting up in the morning
0.58	Feel like at the end of the rope
0.77	Feel burned out from work
0.75	Feel frustrated by job
0.72	Feel working too hard on the job
0.59	Working with people puts too much stress
0.60	Working with patients is a strain
PERSONAL ACCOMPLISHMENT SUBSCALE	
0.40	Can easily understand patients' feelings
0.50	Deal effectively with patients' problems
0.64	Feel positively influencing people's lives
0.46	Feel very energetic
0.62	Can easily create a relaxed atmosphere
0.63	Feel exhilarated after working with patients
0.73	Have accomplished worthwhile things in job
0.52	Deal with emotional problems calmly
DEPERSONALIZATION SUBSCALE	
0.61	Treat patients as impersonal "objects"
0.79	Become more callous toward people
0.71	Worry that job is hardening emotionally
0.64	Don't really care what happens to patients
0.41	Feel patients are to blame for their problems

[a]From US sample.
MBI, Maslach Burnout Inventory.
Adapted from Poghosyan, L., Aiken, L.H., & Sloane, D.M. (2009). Factor structure of the Maslach Burnout Inventory: An analysis of data from large scale cross-sectional surveys of nurses from eight countries. *International Journal of Nursing Studies, 46*(7), 894–902.

a factor (the factor loadings that were < 0.30) are not listed with that factor in Table 23.4. The first factor, named emotional exhaustion by the researchers, represented feelings of being exhausted and overextended by work. This factor was correlated with nine of the MBI items, and the factor loadings ranged from 0.58 to 0.94.

The second factor, personal accomplishment, was correlated with eight of the MBI items, all of which pertained to feelings of successful achievement and competence in the workplace. The factor loadings ranged from 0.40 to 0.73. The third factor, depersonalization, was correlated with five of the MBI items, all of which pertained to the respondent feeling impersonal and/or emotionless when delivering care to the patient. The factor loadings ranged from 0.41 to 0.79.

Naming the Factor

The three factors generated from the EFA were named according to the nature of the items that loaded on those factors. When naming the factor, the researcher must examine the items that cluster together in a factor and seem to explain that clustering. Variables with high loadings on the factor must be included, even if they do not fit the researcher's preconceived theoretical notions of which items fit together because they reflect a similar concept. The purpose is to identify the broad construct of meaning that has caused these particular variables to be so strongly intercorrelated. Naming this construct is an important part of the procedure because naming of the factor provides theoretical meaning (Tabachnick & Fidell, 2013).

Factor Scores

After the initial factor analysis, additional studies are conducted to examine changes in the phenomenon in various situations and to determine the relationships of the factors with other concepts. Factor scores are used during statistical analysis in these additional studies (Stevens, 2009; Tabachnick & Fidell, 2013). To obtain **factor scores,** the variables included in the factor are identified, and the scores on these variables are summed

for each study participant. Thus each participant has a score for each factor in the instrument. There are several methods of computing factor scores. One of the most common methods involves simply adding the participant's scores on the items that load on a factor. Using the MBI results as an example, to obtain a factor score for depersonalization, a respondent's score on the items that loaded on the depersonalizations subscale would be summed. For example, if a participant scored a 4 on "Treat patients as impersonal objects," a 2 on "Become more callous toward people," a 5 on "Worry that job is hardening emotionally," a 2 on "Don't really care what happens to patients," and a 3 on "Feel patients are to blame for their problems," that individual's factor score for depersonalization would be:

$$4+2+5+2+3=16$$

Another common method of computing a factor score is using the factor loadings to weight each study participant's score. Applying the same hypothetical scores as before, the factor loadings are multiplied by the item scores to create the factor score:

$$(0.61)4+(0.79)2+(0.71)5+(0.64)2+(0.41)3$$
$$=2.44+1.58+3.55+1.28+1.23=10.08$$

In the first method, each item is weighted equally in the equation because the weight is essentially 1. In the second method, each item is adjusted for the extent to which that item loads on that factor. The advantages and disadvantages of these factor score methods, in addition to descriptions of other methods for obtaining factor scores, are reviewed by DiStefano, Zhu, and Mîndrilă (2009).

KEY POINTS

- Correlational analyses identify relationships or associations between or among variables.
- The purpose of correlational analysis is also to clarify relationships among theoretical concepts or help identify potentially causal relationships, which can be tested by inferential analysis.
- All data for the analysis should have been obtained from a single population from which values are available for all variables to be examined.

- Correlational analysis provides two pieces of information about the data: the nature of a linear relationship (positive or negative) between the two variables and the magnitude (or strength) of the linear relationship.
- The Pearson product-moment correlation coefficient is the preferred computation when investigating the association among two variables measured at the interval or ratio level and when the variables meet the other required statistical assumptions.

- Spearman rank-order correlation coefficient and Kendall's tau are both nonparametric statistics that are calculated when the assumptions of a Pearson correlation cannot be met, such as variables that are non-normally distributed or are measured at the ordinal level.
- The first clue to the possibility of a causal link is the existence of a relationship, but a relationship does not mean causality.
- Bland and Altman plots are a graphical display of agreement between two administrations of an instrument or assessment, or two raters of a clinician-rated instrument.

- The *CR* is a value that is used to determine acceptable lower and upper limits of interrater agreement and test-retest agreement.
- EFA is a procedure that reduces a large number of variables down to a smaller number of components and is most often used during the construction of a new measurement method or scale.
- The results of EFA assist the researcher in understanding which questions assess the same concept and are redundant, which questions represent subsets of variables, and which items stand alone.

REFERENCES

Altman, D. G. (1991). *Practical statistics for medical research*. London, UK: Chapman & Hall.

American Psychological Association (APA) (2020). *Publication manual of the American Psychological Association* (7th ed.). Washington, DC: American Psychological Association.

Bland, J. M., & Altman, D. M. (1986). Statistical methods for assessing agreement between two methods of clinical measurement. *Lancet, 1*(8476), 307–310.

Bland, J. M., & Altman, D. M. (2010). Statistical methods for assessing agreement between two methods of clinical measurement. *International Journal of Nursing Studies, 47*(8), 931–936. doi:10.1016/j.ijnurstu.2009.10.001

Cohen, J. (1988). *Statistical power analysis for the behavioral sciences* (2nd ed.). Hillsdale, NJ: Lawrence Erlbaum Associates.

Cohen, J., & Cohen, P. (1983). *Applied multiple regression/correlation analysis for the behavioral sciences* (2nd ed.). Hillsdale, NJ: Erlbaum.

Daniel, W. W. (2000). *Applied nonparametric statistics* (2nd ed.). Pacific Grove, CA: Duxbury Press.

de Winter, J. C. F., & Dodou, D. (2010). Five-point Likert items: *t*-test versus Mann-Whitney-Wilcoxon. *Practical Assessment, Research, and Evaluation, 15* Article 11. doi:10.7275/bj1p-ts64

DiStefano, C., Zhu, M., & Mîndrilă, D. (2009). Understanding and using factor scores: Considerations for the applied researcher. *Practical Assessment, Research Evaluation, 14* Article 20. doi:10.7275/da8t-4g52

Flores, A., Burstein, E., Cipher, D. J., & Feagins, L. A. (2015). Obesity in inflammatory bowel disease: A marker of less severe disease. *Digestive Diseases and Sciences, 60*(8), 2436–2445. doi:10.1007/s10620-015-3629-5

Grove, S. K., & Cipher, D. J. (2020). *Statistics for nursing research: A workbook for evidence-based practice* (3rd ed.). St. Louis, MO: Saunders.

Kim, M., & Mallory, C. (2017). *Statistics for evidence-based practice in nursing*. Burlington, MA: Jones & Bartlett Learning.

Lupien, S. J., Maheu, F., Tu, M., Fiocco, A., & Schramek, T. E. (2007). The effects of stress and stress hormones on human cognition: Implications for the field of brain and cognition. *Brain & Cognition, 65*(3), 209–237. doi:10.1016/j.bandc.2007.02.007

Maslach, C., & Jackson, S. E. (1981). The measurement of experienced burnout. *Journal of Occupational Behaviour, 2*(2), 99–113. doi:1002/job.4030020205

National Heart, Lung, and Blood Institute (NHLBI). (2019). *Classification of overweight and obesity by BMI, waist circumference, and associated disease risks*. Retrieved from https://www.nhlbi.nih.gov/health/educational/lose_wt/BMI/bmi_dis.htm

Pett, M. A. (2016). *Nonparametric statistics for health care research: Statistics for small samples and unusual distributions* (2nd ed.). Thousand Oaks, CA: Sage.

Plichta, S. B., & Kelvin, E. (2013). *Munro's statistical methods for health care research* (6th ed.). Philadelphia, PA: Wolters Kluwer/Lippincott Williams & Wilkins.

Poghosyan, L., Aiken, L. H., & Sloane, D. M. (2009). Factor structure of the Maslach Burnout Inventory: An analysis of data from large scale cross-sectional surveys of nurses from eight countries. *International Journal of Nursing Studies, 46*(7), 894–902. doi:10.1016/j.ijnurstu.2009.03.004

Rasmussen, J. L. (1989). Analysis of Likert-scale data: A reinterpretation of Gregoire and Driver. *Psychological Bulletin, 105*(1), 167–170. doi:10.1037/0033-2909.105.1.167

Sippel, J. L., Bozeman, S. M., Bradshaw, L., Cipher, D. J., McCarthy, M., & Wickremasinghe, I. M. (2019). Implementation and initial outcomes of a spinal cord injury home care program at a large veterans affairs medical center. *Journal of Spinal Cord Medicine, 42*(2), 155–162. doi:10.1080/10790268.2018.1485311

Stevens, J. P. (2009). *Applied multivariate statistics for the social sciences* (5th ed.). London, England: Psychology Press.

Tabachnick, B. G., & Fidell, L. S. (2013). *Using multivariate statistics* (6th ed.). Needham Heights, MA: Allyn and Bacon.

Waltz, C. F., Strickland, O. L., & Lenz, E. R. (2017). *Measurement in nursing and health research* (5th ed.). New York, NY: Springer.

Worley, J. A., Vassar, M., Wheeler, D. L., & Barnes, L. B. (2008). Factor structure of scores from the Maslach Burnout Inventory: A review and meta-analysis of 45 exploratory and confirmatory factor-analytic studies. *Educational and Psychological Measurement, 68*(5), 797–823. doi:10.1177/0013164408315268

Yerkes, R. M., & Dodson, J. D. (1908). The relation of strength of stimulus to rapidity of habit-formation. *Journal of Comparative Neurology & Psychology, 18*(5), 459–482.

Zar, J. H. (2010). *Biostatistical analysis* (5th ed.). Upper Saddle River, NJ: Prentice-Hall.

24

Using Statistics to Predict

Daisha J. Cipher

http://evolve.elsevier.com/Gray/practice/

In nursing practice, the ability to predict future events is crucial. Clinical researchers might investigate whether hospital length of stay can be predicted by severity of illness. Health outcome researchers want to know what factors play an important role in patients' responses to health promotion, illness prevention, and rehabilitation interventions. Educators may be interested in knowing which variables are most effective in predicting scores of undergraduate nurses on the National Council Licensure Examination (NCLEX). Advanced practice nurses may be interested in what variables predict favorable treatment outcomes in their specialty clinics.

The statistical procedure most commonly used for prediction is regression analysis. The purpose of a regression analysis is to identify which factor or factors predict or explain the value of a dependent (outcome) variable. In some cases, the analysis is exploratory, and the focus is prediction. In others, selection of variables is based on a theoretical proposition, and the purpose is to develop an explanation that confirms the theoretical proposition (Cohen & Cohen, 1983).

In **regression analysis**, the independent (predictor) variable or variables influence variation or change in the value of the dependent variable. The goal is to determine how accurately one can predict the value of an outcome (or dependent) variable based on the value or values of one or more predictor (or independent) variables. This chapter describes some common statistical procedures used for prediction. These procedures include simple linear regression, multiple regression, logistic regression, and Cox proportional hazards regression.

SIMPLE LINEAR REGRESSION

Simple linear regression is a procedure that estimates the value of an outcome (dependent) variable based on the value of a predictor (independent) variable. Simple linear regression is an effort to explain the dynamics within a scatter plot by drawing a straight line (the **line of best fit**) through the plotted scores. This line is drawn to best explain the **linear relationship** or association between two variables. Knowing that linear relationship, we can, with some degree of accuracy, use regression analysis to predict the value of an outcome if we know the value of the predictor (Cohen & Cohen, 1983). Fig. 24.1 illustrates the linear relationship between gestational age and birthweight. As shown in the scatter plot, there is a strong positive association in preterm births between the two variables. In premature infants, more advanced gestational ages predict higher birthweights.

Use of simple linear regression involves the following assumptions (Zar, 2010):
1. Normal distribution of the dependent (y) variable
2. Linear relationship between x and y
3. Independent observations
4. No (or little) multicollinearity
5. Homoscedasticity

Data that are **homoscedastic** are symmetrically dispersed both above and below the line of prediction throughout the range of values, which indicates a linear relationship on a scatter plot. Homoscedasticity reflects equal variance of both variables. In other words, for all values of x, the distribution of y values

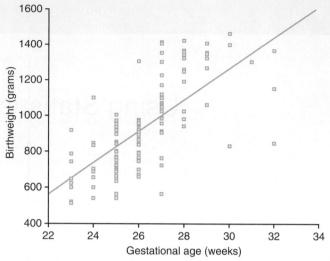

Fig. 24.1 Linear relationship between gestational age and birthweight.

should have equal variability (see Fig. 24.1). If the data for the predictor and dependent variables are not homoscedastic, inferences made during significance testing could be invalid (Cohen & Cohen, 1983; Grove & Cipher, 2020).

The homoscedasticity assumption can be checked by visual examination of a plot of the standardized residuals (the errors) by the regression standardized predicted value. Ideally, residuals are randomly scattered around zero (where zero represents perfect prediction) providing a relatively even distribution. **Heteroscedasticity** is indicated when the residuals are not evenly scattered around the line of prediction. Heteroscedasticity manifests itself in all kinds of uneven shapes. When the plot of residuals appears to deviate substantially from normal, more formal tests for heteroscedasticity should be performed. Formal tests for heteroscedasticity include the Breusch-Pagan test (Breusch & Pagan, 1979) and White test (White, 1980).

Formulas

In simple linear regression, the dependent variable is continuous, and the predictor can be any scale of measurement. However, if the predictor is nominal, it must be correctly coded prior to analysis with statistical software. Examples of coding nominal variables are presented later in this chapter. Once the data are ready, the parameters a and b are computed to obtain a regression equation. To understand the mathematical process, recall the algebraic equation for a straight line:

$$y = bx + a$$

where

y = dependent variable (outcome)

x = independent variable (predictor)

b = **slope of the line** (beta, or what the increase in value is along the x-axis for every unit of increase in the y value)

a = **y-intercept** (the point where the regression line intersects the y-axis)

A regression equation can be generated with a data set containing participants' x and y values. When this equation is generated, it can be used to predict y values of other participants, given only their x values. In simple or bivariate regression, predictions are made in cases with two variables. The score on variable y (dependent variable) is predicted from the same individual's known score on variable x (predictor).

No single regression line can be used to predict with complete accuracy every y value from every x value. You could draw an infinite number of lines through the scattered paired values. However, the purpose of the regression equation is to develop the line that allows the highest degree of prediction possible—the **line of best fit**. The procedure for developing the line of best fit is the **method of least squares**. The formulas for the beta (b) and y-intercept (a) of the regression equation are computed as follows. Note that when the b is calculated, that value is inserted into the formula for a.

$$b = \frac{n\sum xy - \sum x \sum y}{n\sum x^2 - \left(\sum x\right)^2} \qquad a = \frac{n\sum y - b\sum x}{n}$$

where
b = beta
a = y-intercept
n = total number of subjects
x = value of the predictor
y = value of the dependent variable
xy = x multiplied by y

Calculation of Simple Linear Regression

Table 24.1 displays how one would arrange data to perform linear regression by hand. Regression analysis is conducted with a computer for most studies, but this calculation is provided to increase your understanding of the aspects of regression analysis and how to interpret the results. This example uses data collected from a study of students enrolled in a registered nurse to bachelor of science in nursing (RN-to-BSN) program

(Mancini, Ashwill, & Cipher, 2015). The predictor in this example is number of academic degrees obtained by the student prior to enrollment, and the dependent variable is number of months it took for the student to complete the RN-to-BSN program. A student entering the program with only a certificate would have a predictor value of zero. The null hypothesis is "Number of degrees does not predict the number of months until completion of an RN-to-BSN program."

The data are presented in Table 24.1. A simulated subset of 20 students was selected for this example so that the computations would be small and manageable. In actuality, studies involving linear regression must be adequately powered (Aberson, 2019; Cohen, 1988; Grove & Cipher, 2020). Observe that the data in Table 24.1 are arranged in columns, which correspond to the elements of the formula. The summed values in the last row of the table are inserted into the appropriate place in the formula for b.

TABLE 24.1 Computation of Linear Regression Equation

Student ID	x (Number of Degrees)	y (Months to Completion)	x^2	xy
1	1	17	1	17
2	2	9	4	18
3	0	17	0	0
4	1	9	1	9
5	0	16	0	0
6	1	11	1	11
7	0	15	0	0
8	0	12	0	0
9	1	15	1	15
10	1	12	1	12
11	1	14	1	14
12	1	10	1	10
13	1	17	1	17
14	0	20	0	0
15	2	9	4	18
16	2	12	4	24
17	1	14	1	14
18	2	10	4	20
19	1	17	1	17
20	2	11	4	22
sum Σ	20	267	30	238

Calculation Steps

Step 1: Calculate b.

From the values in Table 24.1, we know that $n = 20$, $\Sigma x = 20$, $\Sigma y = 267$, $\Sigma x^2 = 30$, and $\Sigma xy = 238$. These values are inserted into the formula for b, as follows:

$$b = \frac{20(238) - (20)(267)}{20(30) - 20^2}$$

$$b = \frac{4760 - 5340}{600 - 400}$$

$$b = \frac{-580}{200}$$

$$b = -2.9$$

Step 2: Calculate a.

From step 1, we now know that $b = -2.9$, and we insert this value into the formula for a.

$$a = \frac{267 - (-2.9)(20)}{20}$$

$$a = \frac{325}{20}$$

$$a = 16.25$$

Step 3: Write the new regression equation.

$$y = -2.9x + 16.25$$

Step 4: Calculate R.

We can use our new regression equation from step 3 to compute predicted program completion for each student, using their number of degrees. The extent to which predicted program completion is the same as actual program completion is determined by the multiple R. The **multiple R** is defined as the correlation between the actual y values and the predicted y values using the new regression equation. The predicted y value using the new equation is represented by the symbol $\hat{y}$ to differentiate from y, which represents the actual y values in the data set. For example, Student 1 had earned one academic degree prior to enrollment, and the predicted months to completion for Student 1 is calculated as:

$$\hat{y} = -2.9(1) + 16.25$$
$$\hat{y} = 13.35$$

Thus the predicted $\hat{y}$ for Student 1 is 13.35 months for RN-to-BSN program completion. This procedure would be continued for the rest of the students, and the Pearson correlation between the actual months to completion (y) and the predicted months to completion ($\hat{y}$) would yield the multiple R value. In this example, the $R = 0.638$. The higher the R, the more likely that the new regression equation accurately predicts y because the higher the correlation, the closer the actual y values are to the predicted $\hat{y}$ values. Fig. 24.2 displays the regression line for which the x-axis represents possible numbers of degrees, and the y-axis represents the predicted months to program completion ($\hat{y}$ values).

Step 5: Determine whether the predictor significantly predicts y.

To know whether the predictor significantly predicts y, the beta must be tested against zero. In simple regression, this is most easily accomplished by using the R value from step 4:

$$t = R\sqrt{\frac{n-2}{1-R^2}}$$

$$t = 0.638\sqrt{\frac{20-2}{1-0.407}}$$

$$t = 3.52$$

The t value is then compared to the t probability distribution table (see Appendix B). The df for this t statistic is $n - 2$. The critical t value for a two-tailed test at alpha (α) = 0.05, $df = 18$ is 2.101, rounded to 2.10. Our obtained t was 3.52, which exceeds the critical value in the table, thereby indicating a significant association between the predictor x and y (outcome).

Another way to determine the statistical significance of a statistic is to compute the exact p value, which is facilitated with statistical software. When this particular regression example was computed using statistical software, the exact p value associated with the t statistic of 3.52 was $p = 0.002$. This indicates that the exact likelihood of obtaining this t value or larger when the null hypothesis is true is 2 in 1000, or 0.2%. When reporting statistical interpretations for journal articles that use formatting from the American Psychological Association (APA, 2020), the exact p value is required.

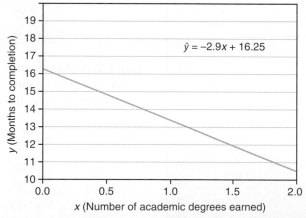

Fig. 24.2 Regression line represented by regression equation of months of program completion predicted by number of academic degrees earned. (From Grove, S. K., & Cipher, D. J. [2020]. *Statistics for nursing research: A workbook for evidence-based practice* [2nd ed.]. St. Louis, MO: Elsevier.)

Step 6: Calculate R^2.

After establishing the statistical significance of the R value, it must subsequently be examined for actual importance. This is accomplished by obtaining the **coefficient of determination** for regression—which simply involves squaring the R value. The R^2 represents the percentage of variance explained in y by the predictor. Cohen describes R^2 values of 0.02 as small, 0.13 as moderate, and 0.26 or higher as large effect sizes (Cohen, 1988). In our example, the R was 0.638, and therefore the R^2 was 0.407. Multiplying 0.407 × 100% indicates that 40.7% of the variance in months to program completion can be explained by knowing the student's number of earned academic degrees at admission (Cohen & Cohen, 1983).

The R^2 can be very helpful in testing more than one predictor in a regression model. Unlike R, the R^2 for one regression model can be compared with another regression model that contains additional predictors (Cohen & Cohen, 1983). For example, a researcher could add another predictor, such as student's admission grade point average (GPA), to the regression model of months to completion. The R^2 values of both models would be compared, the first with number of academic degrees as the sole predictor and the second with number of academic degrees and enrollment GPA as predictors. The R^2 values of the two models would be statistically compared to indicate whether the proportion of variance in $\hat{y}$ was significantly increased by including the second predictor, enrollment GPA, in the model.

The standardized beta (β) is another statistic that represents the magnitude of the association between x and y. β has the same limits as a Pearson r, meaning that the standardized β cannot be lower than -1.00 or higher than 1.00. This value can be calculated by hand but is best computed with statistical software. The standardized β is calculated by converting the x and y values to z scores, then correlating the x and y values using the Pearson r formula. The standardized β is often reported in the literature instead of the unstandardized b, and that is because b does not have lower or upper limits and therefore the magnitude of b cannot be judged. β, on the other hand, is interpreted as a Pearson r and the descriptions of the magnitude of β (as recommended by Cohen [1988]) can be applied to β. As presented in Chapter 23, Pearson r values of 0.10 = weak effect, 0.30 = moderate effect, and 0.50 or above = large effect. In this example, the standardized β is -0.638. Thus the magnitude of the association between x and y in this example is considered a large predictive association (Cohen, 1988).

Interpretation of Results

The following summative statements are written in APA (2020) format, as one might read the results in an article.

> Simple linear regression was performed with the number of earned academic degrees prior to enrollment as the predictor and months to program completion as the dependent variable. The student's number of degrees significantly predicted months to completion among students in an RN-to-BSN program, $\beta = -0.638$, $p = 0.002$, $R^2 = 40.7\%$. Higher numbers of earned academic degrees significantly predicted shorter program completion time.

MULTIPLE REGRESSION

Multiple linear regression analysis is an extension of simple linear regression in which more than one predictor is entered into the analysis (Grove & Cipher, 2020; Stevens, 2009). Because the relationships between multiple predictors and y are tested simultaneously, the calculations involved in multiple regression analysis are very complex. Multiple regression is best conducted using a statistical software package such as those presented in Table 21.2. However, full explanations and examples of the matrix algebraic computations of multiple regression are presented by Stevens (2009) and Tabachnick and Fidell (2019).

Interpretations of multiple regression findings are the same as with simple regression. The beta (b) values of each predictor are tested for significance, and a multiple R and R^2 are computed. The only difference is that in multiple regression, when all predictors are tested simultaneously, each b has been adjusted for every other predictor in the regression model. The b represents the independent relationship between that predictor and y, even after controlling for (or accounting for) the presence of every other predictor in the model.

Mancuso (2010) conducted a study of 102 subjects with diabetes to develop a predictive model of glycemic control, as measured by glycosylated hemoglobin (HbA1c). The five predictors for HbA1c were health literacy, patient trust, knowledge of diabetes, performance of self-care activities, and depression. The five predictors of glycemic control were tested with multiple regression

TABLE 24.2   Predictors of Glycosylated Hemoglobin (HbA1c) in Patients With Diabetes

Independent Variable	UNSTANDARDIZED COEFFICIENTS		STANDARDIZED COEFFICIENT		
	B	SE	β	t	Significance (p)
Health literacy	−0.063	0.080	−0.070	−0.782	0.436
Patient trust	−0.873	0.165	−0.459	−5.288	0.000[a]
Diabetes knowledge	0.012	0.011	0.100	1.116	0.267
Performance of self-care activities	0.005	0.135	0.003	0.040	0.968
Depression	0.036	0.014	0.226	2.589	0.011[a]

[a]$p < 0.05$, significant.
Data from Mancuso, J. M. (2010). Impact of health literacy and patient trust on glycemic control in an urban USA populations. *Nursing & Health Sciences, 12*(1), 94–104.

analysis. The analysis yielded five *b* and β values, each with a corresponding *p* value. As shown in Table 24.2, patient trust and depression were significant predictors of glycemic control (HbA1c), even after adjusting for the presence or contribution of every other predictor in the model. The *p* values for these two predictors were less than 0.05. Health literacy, diabetes knowledge, and performance of self-care activities did not significantly predict HbA1c levels ($p > 0.05$). R^2 was 0.285, indicating that patient trust and depression accounted for 28.5% of the variance in HbA1c (the measure of glycemic control).

The findings from this study have potential implications for the management of patients with diabetes. Because lower levels of patient trust were associated with higher HbA1c values, fostering communication and trusting collaboration between the patient and the healthcare provider could directly or indirectly improve glycemic control. Higher levels of depression were also associated with higher HbA1c values, and early interventions or referrals aimed at addressing depressive symptoms could be important in improving glycemic control. However, it is important to note that regression analysis is not an indication of cause and effect. Rather, these results can serve as a basis for further research aimed at investigating the influence of patient factors such as trust and depression on glycemic control.

Multicollinearity

Multicollinearity occurs when the independent variables in a multiple regression equation are strongly correlated with one another. The presence of multicollinearity does not affect predictive power (the capacity of the independent variables to predict values of the dependent variable in a specific sample); rather, it causes problems related to generalizability and to the stability of the findings. If multicollinearity is present, the equation lacks **predictive validity**, and the amount of variance explained by each variable in the equation is inflated. Additionally, when cross-validation is performed, the *b* values do not remain consistent across samples (Cohen & Cohen, 1983). Multicollinearity is minimized by carefully selecting the independent variables and thoroughly determining their correlation before the regression analysis. If high correlations among predictors are identified, the correlated predictors might be combined into one score or value yielding one predictor, or only one of the measures (scores) might be included in the regression equation.

The first step in identifying multicollinearity is to examine the correlations among the independent variables. Therefore you would perform multiple correlation analyses before conducting the regression analyses. The correlation matrix is carefully examined for evidence of multicollinearity. Many statistical software packages, such as SPSS, provide two statistics—tolerance and variance inflation factor (VIF)—that describe the extent to which your model has a multicollinearity problem. A tolerance of less than 0.20 and/or a VIF of 10 and above indicates a multicollinearity problem (Allison, 1999).

Types of Predictor Variables Used in Regression Analyses

Variables in a regression equation can take many forms. Traditionally, as with most multivariate analyses, variables are measured at the interval or ratio level. However, researchers also use nominal variables (referred to as **dummy variables**), multiplicative terms, and transformed terms. A mixture of types of variables may be used in a single regression equation. The following discussion describes the treatment of dummy variables in regression equations.

Dummy Variables

To use categorical variables in regression analysis, a coding system is developed to represent group membership. Categorical variables of interest in nursing that might be used in regression analysis include gender, income, ethnicity, social status, level of education, and diagnosis. If the variable is dichotomous, such as gender, members of one category are assigned the number 1, and all others are assigned the number 0. In this case, for gender the coding could be the following:

1 = female
0 = male

If the categorical variable has three values, two dummy variables are used (e.g., social class could be classified as lower class, middle class, or upper class). The first dummy variable (X_1) would be classified as follows:

1 = lower class
0 = not lower class

The second dummy variable (X_2) would be classified as follows:

1 = middle class
0 = not middle class

The three social classes would be represented in the data set in the following manner:

Lower class: $X_1 = 1$, $X_2 = 0$
Middle class: $X_1 = 0$, $X_2 = 1$
Upper class: $X_1 = 0$, $X_2 = 0$

The variables lower class and middle class would be entered as predictors in the regression equation in which both are tested against the reference category (i.e., upper class). Specifically, the b values for these two variables would represent whether y differs by lower class versus upper class and middle class versus upper class. When more than three categories define the values of the variable, increased numbers of dummy variables are used. The number of dummy variables is always one less than the number of categories (Aiken & West, 1991). An example of how one might analyze dichotomous dummy variables is presented in the next section.

ODDS RATIO

When both the predictor and the dependent variable are dichotomous (having only two values), the **odds ratio** *(OR)* is a statistic commonly used to obtain an indication of association and is defined as the ratio of the odds of an event occurring in one group to the odds of it occurring in another group (Gordis, 2014). Put simply, the *OR* is a way of comparing whether the odds of a certain event are the same for two groups. For example, the use of angiotensin-converting enzyme (ACE) inhibitors in a sample of veterans was examined in relation to having advanced adenomatous colon polyps (Kedika et al., 2011). The *OR* was 0.63, indicating that ACE inhibitor use was associated with a lower likelihood of developing adenomatous colon polyps in veterans.

Statistical Formula and Assumptions

Use of the *OR* involves the following assumptions (Gordis, 2014):

1. Only one datum entry is made for each subject in the sample. Therefore if repeated measures from the same subject are being used for analysis, such as pretests and posttests, the *OR* is not an appropriate test.
2. The variables must be dichotomous, either inherently or transformed to nominal values from quantitative values (ordinal, interval, or ratio).

The formula for the *OR* is:

$$OR = \frac{ad}{bc}$$

The formula for the *OR* designates the odds of occurrence in the numerator when the predictor is present and the odds of occurrence in the denominator when the predictor is absent. Note that the values must be coded accordingly. Table 24.3 displays the following notation to assist you in calculating the *OR* by noting which cells represent *a*, *b*, *c*, and *d*. For example, *a* represents the number of homeless veterans who had one or more emergency department (ED) visits.

Calculation of Odds Ratio

A retrospective corelational study examined the medical utilization by homeless veterans receiving treatment in a veterans affairs healthcare system (LePage, Bradshaw, Cipher, Crawford, & Hooshyar, 2014). A sample of veterans

TABLE 24.3 Notation in Cells of the Odds Ratio Table

	≥ 1 ED Visit	No ED Visits
Homeless	a	b
Not Homeless	c	d

ED, Emergency department.
a: Number of homeless veterans with ≥ 1 ED visit.
b: Number of homeless veterans with no ED visits.
c: Number of non-homeless veterans with ≥ 1 ED visit.
d: Number of non-homeless veterans with no ED visits.

TABLE 24.4 Homelessness and Emergency Department Visits Among Veterans

	≥ 1 ED Visit	No ED Visits
Homeless	807	1398
Not Homeless	15,198	84,631

ED, Emergency department.

seen in the VA North Texas Health Care System in 2010 ($N = 102{,}034$) was evaluated for homelessness at any point during the year, as well as chronic medical and psychiatric diseases, and medical utilization. The two variables in this example are dichotomous: homelessness in 2010 (yes/no) and having made at least one visit to the ED in 2010 (yes/no). The data are presented in Table 24.4. The null hypothesis is, "There is no association between homelessness and emergency department visits among veterans."

Calculation Steps

The computations for the OR are as follows:
Step 1: Fit the cell values into the OR formula.

$$OR = \frac{ad}{bc} = \frac{(807)(84631)}{(1398)(15198)} = \frac{68297217}{21246804} = 3.21$$

$$OR = 3.21$$

Step 2: Compute the 95% confidence interval (CI) for the OR.

OR values are often accompanied by a CI, which consists of a lower and upper limit value. An OR of 1.0 is an indication of no association between the variables (null hypothesis). In this example, the calculated OR of 3.21 will possibly allow rejection of that null hypothesis if the CI around 3.21 does not include the

value 1.00. As demonstrated in Chapter 22, the CI for any statistic is composed of three components: (computed statistic) $\pm SE(t)$. To compute a 95% CI for the OR, you must first convert the OR into the natural logarithm (ln) of the OR. The natural logarithm of a number X is the power to which e would have to be raised to equal X (where e is approximately 2.718288, a mathematical constant). For example, the natural logarithm of e itself would be 1, because $e^1 = 2.718288$.

Convert the OR to the $ln(OR)$
$$ln(3.21) = 1.17$$

Step 3: Compute the standard error of $ln(OR)$.

$$SE_{ln(OR)} = \sqrt{\frac{1}{a} + \frac{1}{b} + \frac{1}{c} + \frac{1}{d}}$$

$$SE_{ln(OR)} = \sqrt{\frac{1}{807} + \frac{1}{1398} + \frac{1}{15198} + \frac{1}{84631}}$$

$$SE_{ln(OR)} = \sqrt{\begin{array}{l}.001239 + .000715 \\ + .0000658 + .0000118\end{array}}$$

$$SE_{ln(OR)} = 0.045$$

Step 4: Create the CI still using the $ln(OR)$, with a t of 1.96.

$$95\%\ CI = ln(OR) \pm SE(t)$$
$$95\%\ CI = 1.17 \pm 0.045(1.96)$$
$$[1.082, 1.258]$$

Step 5: Convert the lower and upper limits of the CI back to the original OR unit.

Place the lower limit, 1.082, as the exponent of e: $e^{1.082} = \mathbf{2.95}$

Place the upper limit, 1.258, as the exponent of e: $e^{1.258} = \mathbf{3.52}$

This means that the interval of 2.95 to 3.52 estimates the population OR with 95% confidence (Grove & Cipher, 2020; Kline, 2004). Moreover, because the CI does not include the number 1.0, the OR indicates a significant association between homelessness and ED visits.
Step 6: Interpret the directionality of the OR.

An OR of $\cong 1.0$ indicates that exposure (to homelessness) does not affect the odds of the outcome (ED visit).

An *OR* of > 1.0 indicates that exposure (to homelessness) is associated with a higher odds of the outcome (ED visit).

An *OR* of < 1.0 indicates that exposure (to homelessness) is associated with a lower odds of the outcome (ED visit).

The *OR* for the study was 3.21, indicating that the odds of having made an ED visit among veterans who were homeless was higher than those who were not homeless. We can further note that homeless veterans were over three times (or 221%) more likely to have made an ED visit (LePage et al., 2014). This value was computed by subtracting 1.00 from the *OR* (3.21 − 1.00) = 2.21 × 100% = 221%. The difference between the obtained *OR* and 1.00 represents the extent of the lesser or greater likelihood of the event occurring.

Interpretation of Results

The following summative statements are written in APA (2020) format, as one might read the results in an article.

> An odds ratio was computed to assess the association between homelessness and emergency department visits. Homeless veterans were significantly more likely to have made an emergency department visit in 2010 than the non-homeless veterans (36.6% versus 15.2%, respectively; OR = 3.21, 95% CI [2.95, 3.52]).

LOGISTIC REGRESSION

Logistic regression replaces linear regression when the researcher wants to test a predictor or predictors of a dichotomous dependent variable. The output yields an adjusted *OR* for each predictor, meaning that each predictor's *OR* represents the relationship between that predictor and *Y*, after adjusting for the presence of the other predictors in the model (Tabachnick & Fidell, 2019). As is the case with multiple linear regression, each predictor serves as a covariate to every other predictor in the model. In other words, when all predictors are tested simultaneously, each *b* has been adjusted for every other predictor in the regression model. Logistic regression is best conducted using a statistical software package. Full explanations and examples of the mathematical computations of logistic regression are presented in Tabachnick and Fidell (2019). A brief overview is provided in this

chapter, with an example of simple logistic regression using actual clinical data.

Some common examples of dependent variables that are analyzed with logistic regression are patient lived or died, responded or did not respond to treatment, and employed or unemployed. The logistic regression model can be considered more flexible than linear regression in the following ways:

1. Logistic regression can have continuous predictors, nominal predictors, or a combination of the two, with no assumptions regarding normality of the distribution.
2. Logistic regression can test predictors with a non-linear relationship between the predictor (independent) variable and the outcome (dependent) variable.
3. With a logistic regression model, you can compute the odds of a person's outcome. Each predictor is associated with an *OR* that represents the independent association between that predictor and the outcome (*y*) (Tabachnick & Fidell, 2019).

Because the dependent variable is either 1 or 0, logistic regression analysis produces a regression equation that yields probabilities of the outcome occurring for each person. If the predictor is continuous, we can determine the probability of the outcome occurring with a predictor score of some value *x*. If the predictor is dichotomous, we can determine the probability of the outcome occurring with a predictor value of 1 and a predictor value of 0.

Calculation of Logistic Regression

Because the dependent variable in logistic regression is dichotomous, the predicted $\hat{y}$ is always in the range of 0 to 1, which is interpreted as a probability. Similar to linear regression, the predicted $\hat{y}$ values are calculated from a *b* (or more than one *b* in the case of multiple predictors) and a *y*-intercept. In contrast to linear regression, the *b* and *y*-intercept are the exponents of the number *e* (2.718). An exponent of *e* is commonly referred to as the natural logarithm. In other words, the natural logarithm of a given number is the power to which *e* would have to be raised to equal that number. When the *b* and *y*-intercept serve as natural logarithms, it allows the result to yield a probability (a value between 0 and 1).

Recall the example from the homelessness and ED visits data (LePage et al., 2014). If a veteran was homeless, the probability of that veteran making at least one ED visit is calculated as follows:

Given: For these data, $b = 1.17$ and the y-intercept (a) is -1.72.

$$\hat{y} = \frac{e^{1.17(1)+-1.72}}{1+e^{1.17(1)+-1.72}}$$

$$\hat{y} = \frac{e^{-0.55}}{1+e^{-0.55}} \quad so \quad \hat{y} = \frac{0.577}{1.577} = 0.37$$

The probability of making an ED visit if the veteran was homeless is $0.37 \times 100\%$, or 37%. The probability of making an ED visit if the veteran was *not* homeless is 15%, as shown in the next calculation. The risk of making an ED visit was greater if the veteran was homeless.

$$\hat{y} = \frac{e^{1.17(0)+-1.72}}{1+e^{1.17(0)+-1.72}}$$

$$\hat{y} = \frac{e^{-1.72}}{1+e^{-1.72}} \quad so \quad \hat{y} = \frac{0.18}{1.18} = 0.15$$

Odds Ratio in Logistic Regression

Each predictor is associated with an *OR* in a logistic regression model. If the predictor is dichotomous, the *OR* is interpreted as, "With an *x* value of 'yes,' the odds of the outcome occurring is [*OR* value] times as likely." The homelessness and ED visits example yielded an *OR* of 3.21. As stated previously, this *OR* indicates that homeless veterans were 3.21 times as likely to make an ED visit.

If the predictor is continuous, the *OR* is interpreted as, "For every 1-unit increase in *x*, the odds of the outcome occurring are either more or less likely, depending on the *OR* value." For example, the association between years of education and obtaining employment among persons with a spinal cord injury was investigated (Ottomanelli, Sippel, Cipher, & Goetz, 2011). The predictor was years of education, and the dependent variable was employment (yes/no). The *OR* was 1.10, indicating that for every additional year of education, the patient was 1.10 times as likely (or 10% more likely) to have obtained employment.

In the same study, the association between being male and obtaining employment among persons with spinal cord injury was investigated (Ottomanelli et al., 2011). The predictor was being male (yes/no), and the dependent variable was employment (yes/no). The *OR* was 1.00, indicating that patients who were male were 1.00 times as likely (or just as likely) as females to have

obtained employment. In other words, the likelihood of employment was equal among males and females.

COX PROPORTIONAL HAZARDS REGRESSION

When testing predictors of a dependent variable that is time related, the appropriate statistical procedure is Cox proportional hazards regression (or Cox regression) (Hosmer, Lemeshow, & May, 2008). The dependent variable in Cox regression is called the **hazard**, a neutral word intended to describe the risk of event occurrence (e.g., risk of obtaining an illness, risk of complications from medications, or risk of relapse). The primary output in a Cox regression analysis represents the relationship between each predictor variable and the hazard, or rate of event occurrence.

Cox regression is a type of survival analysis that can answer questions pertaining to the amount of time that elapses until an event occurs. Examples of the types of questions that can be answered using Cox regression follow. A group of nurse practitioners begins a doctoral program. What variables predict how long it will take the students to graduate? A group of depressed adults completes a cognitive therapy program. What variables predict the time elapsed from the end of treatment until a patient's first relapse?

The major difference between using Cox regression as opposed to linear regression is the ability of survival analysis to handle cases where survival time is unknown. For example, in the study of treatment for streptococcal pharyngitis (strep throat), perhaps only 20% of cases relapse. The other 80% do not relapse by the end of the researcher's study. Thus it is unknown how long it will be until the remainder of the patients relapse. Survival times that are known only to exceed a certain value are called **censored data**. Censored data can also occur when a participant drops out of the study. Cox regression calculations take into account censored data when estimating the relationships between predictors and *y*—in contrast to linear regression analyses, which would delete or exclude those cases from analysis (Hosmer et al., 2008).

Logistic regression yields an *OR* for each predictor that represents the association between each predictor and *y*, whereas Cox regression yields a **hazard ratio** *(HR)*. An *HR* is interpreted almost identically to an *OR* with the exception that the *HR* represents the risk of the event occurring sooner.

TABLE 24.5   Cox Proportional Hazards Regression Results of Stroke Recurrence

Predictor	Hazard Ratio (Adjusted)[a]	p Value	95% Confidence Interval
Treatment with fluoxetine	0.594	0.025	0.376–0.938
Carotid or intracranial arterial stenosis>50%	2.013	0.015	1.145–3.540
Low-density lipoprotein (LDL) cholesterol at baseline	1.170	0.045	1.004–1.364
Systolic blood pressure at baseline	1.010	0.034	1.001–1.019

Note: Full explanations and examples of the computations of Cox regression are presented in Hosmer et al. (2008).
[a]Adjusted for all other model predictors.
Data from He, Y., Cai, Z., Zeng, S., Chen, S., Tang, B., Liang, Y., ... Guo, Y. (2018). Effect of fluoxetine on three-year recurrence in acute ischemic stroke: A randomized controlled clinical study. *Clinical Neurology and Neurosurgery, 168*, 6; Hosmer, D. W., Lemeshow, S., & May, S. (2008). *Applied survival analysis: Regression modeling of time to event data* (2nd ed.). Hoboken, NJ: John Wiley & Sons.

An example of Cox regression used in clinical research is presented in Table 24.5. Predictors of ischemic stroke recurrence in a sample of 404 persons with a history of stroke were tested with Cox regression (He et al., 2018). This study specifically focused on the effectiveness of fluoxetine, a selective serotonin reuptake inhibitor (SSRI), in preventing a recurrence of stroke. Patients with a history of ischemic stroke were randomized to a fluoxetine treatment condition (20 mg daily for 90 days plus conventional secondary preventive treatment for stroke) or a control (conventional secondary preventive treatment for stroke) and followed for 3 years. Among those predictors of stroke recurrence tested, Cox regression analysis yielded four significant predictors. Table 24.5 lists the predictors and *HR*s, each with a corresponding *p* value and 95% *CI*. These four predictors were tested simultaneously, and therefore the *HR*s are called **adjusted hazard ratios**, which means that each *HR* has been adjusted for every other predictor in the regression model. The results of the adjusted *HR* values indicated that treatment with fluoxetine, having a carotid or intracranial arterial stenosis of greater than 50%, baseline low-density lipoprotein (LDL) cholesterol, and baseline systolic blood pressure all were significant predictors of a stroke recurrence, even after controlling for the presence of every other predictor in the model. Full explanations and examples of the computations of Cox regression are presented by Hosmer and colleagues (2008).

The findings from this study could have indications for the treatment of stroke recurrence in clinical practice. Fluoxetine appeared to reduce the risk of stroke recurrence by 40.6%, even after controlling for stenosis, LDL cholesterol, and systolic blood pressure. Although this study did not test the effect of varying doses and durations of fluoxetine, 20 mg daily for 90 days plus conventional secondary preventive treatment appeared to have a substantial impact on the risk of stroke recurrence. The researchers suggested that fluoxetine works to prevent stroke recurrence by improving negative emotions, inhibiting platelet aggregation, and optimizing the control of traditional risk factors of stroke.

KEY POINTS

- The purpose of a regression analysis is to predict or explain as much of the variance in the value of the dependent variable as possible.
- The independent (predictor) variable or variables cause variation in the value of the dependent (outcome) variable.
- Simple linear regression provides a means to estimate the value of a dependent variable based on the value of an independent variable.
- Multiple regression analysis is an extension of simple linear regression in which more than one independent variable is entered into the analysis to predict a dependent variable.
- Multicollinearity occurs when the predictors in a multiple regression equation are strongly intercorrelated and result in unstable findings.
- The *OR* is a way of comparing whether the odds of a certain event are the same for two groups.

- Logistic regression replaces linear regression when the intent is to test a predictor or predictors of a dichotomous dependent variable.
- When testing predictors of a dependent variable that is time related, the appropriate statistical procedure is Cox proportional hazards regression (or Cox regression).
- The HR represents the risk of the event occurring sooner than the end time specified in the study.

REFERENCES

Aberson, C. L. (2019). *Applied power analysis for the behavioral sciences* (2nd ed.). New York, NY: Routledge Taylor & Francis Group.

Aiken, L. S., & West, S. G. (1991). *Multiple regression: Testing and interpreting interactions.* Newbury Park, UK: Sage.

Allison, P. D. (1999). *Multiple regression: A primer.* Thousand Oaks, CA: Pine Forge Press.

American Psychological Association (APA). (2020). *Publication manual of the American Psychological Association* (7th ed.). Washington, DC: APA.

Breusch, T. S., & Pagan, A. R. (1979). A simple test for heteroscedasticity and random coefficient variation. *Econometrica: Journal of the Econometric Society, 47*(5), 1287–1294. doi:10.2307/1911963

Cohen, J. (1988). *Statistical power analysis for the behavioral sciences* (2nd ed.). New York, NY: Academic Press.

Cohen, J., & Cohen, P. (1983). *Applied multiple regression/correlation analysis for the behavioral sciences* (2nd ed.). Hillsdale, NJ: Erlbaum.

Gordis, L. (2014). *Epidemiology* (5th ed.). Philadelphia, PA: Saunders.

Grove, S. K., & Cipher, D. J. (2020). *Statistics for nursing research: A workbook for evidence-based practice* (3rd ed.). St. Louis, MO: Saunders.

He, Y., Cai, Z., Zeng, S., Chen, S., Tang, B., Liang, Y., … Guo, Y. (2018). Effect of fluoxetine on three-year recurrence in acute ischemic stroke: A randomized controlled clinical study. *Clinical Neurology and Neurosurgery, 168*, 1–6. doi:10.1016/j.clineuro.2018.02.029

Hosmer, D. W., Lemeshow, S., & May, S. (2008). *Applied survival analysis: Regression modeling of time to event data* (2nd ed.). Hoboken, NJ: John Wiley & Sons.

Kedika, R., Patel, M., Pena Sahdala, H. N., Mahgoub, A., Cipher, D. J., & Siddiqui, A. A. (2011). Long-term use of angiotensin converting enzyme inhibitors is associated with decreased incidence of advanced adenomatous colon polyps. *Journal of Clinical Gastroenterology, 45*(2), e12–e16. doi:10.1097/MCG.0b013e3181ea1044

Kline, R. B. (2004). *Beyond significance testing: Reforming data analysis methods in behavioral research.* Washington, DC: American Psychological Association.

LePage, J. P., Bradshaw, L. D., Cipher, D. J., Crawford, A. M., & Hooshyar, D. (2014). The effects of homelessness on veterans' healthcare service use: An evaluation of independence from comorbidities. *Public Health, 128*(11), 985–992. doi:10.1016/j.puhe.2014.07.004

Mancini, M. E., Ashwill, J., & Cipher, D. J. (2015). A comparative analysis of demographic and academic success characteristics of on-line and on-campus RN-to-BSN students. *Journal of Professional Nursing, 31*(1), 71–76. doi:10.1016/j.profnurs.2014.05.008

Mancuso, J. M. (2010). Impact of health literacy and patient trust on glycemic control in an urban USA populations. *Nursing & Health Sciences, 12*(1), 94–104. doi:10.1111/j.1442-2018.2009.00506.x.

Ottomanelli, L., Sippel, J., Cipher, D. J., & Goetz, L. (2011). Factors associated with employment among veterans with spinal cord injury. *Journal of Vocational Rehabilitation, 34*(1), 141–150. doi:10.3233/JVR-2011-0542

Stevens, J. P. (2009). *Applied multivariate statistics for the social sciences* (5th ed.). London, UK: Psychology Press.

Tabachnick, B. G., & Fidell, L. S. (2019). *Using multivariate statistics* (7th ed.). Needham, NY: Pearson.

White, H. (1980). A heteroskedasticity-consistent covariance matrix estimator and a direct test for heteroskedasticity. *Econometrica: Journal of the Econometric Society, 48*(4), 817–838. doi:10.2307/1912934

Zar, J. H. (2010). *Biostatistical analysis* (5th ed.). Upper Saddle River, NJ: Prentice Hall.

25

Using Statistics to Determine Differences

Daisha J. Cipher

http://evolve.elsevier.com/Gray/practice/

The statistical procedures in this chapter examine differences between or among groups. There are statistical procedures available for examining differences with nominal, ordinal, and interval/ratio level data. The procedures vary considerably in their power to detect differences and in their complexity. How one interprets the results of these statistics depends on the design of the study. If the design is quasi-experimental or experimental and the study is well designed and has no major issues in regard to threats to internal and external validity, causality can be considered and the results can be inferred or generalized to the target population (Kazdin, 2017). If the design is comparative descriptive, differences identified are associated only with the sample under study. The parametric statistics used to determine differences that are discussed in this chapter are the independent samples *t*-test, paired or dependent samples *t*-test, and analysis of variance (ANOVA). If the assumptions for parametric analyses are not achieved or if study data are at the ordinal level, the nonparametric analyses of Mann-Whitney *U*, Wilcoxon signed-rank test, and Kruskal-Wallis *H* are appropriate techniques to use to test the researchers hypotheses. This chapter concludes with a discussion of the Pearson chi-square test, which is a nonparametric technique for analyzing nominal-level data.

CHOOSING PARAMETRIC VERSUS NONPARAMETRIC STATISTICS TO DETERMINE DIFFERENCES

Parametric statistics are always associated with a certain set of assumptions that the data must meet; this is because the formulas of parametric statistics yield valid results only when the properties of the data are within the confines of these assumptions (Grove & Cipher, 2020; Zar, 2010). If the data do not meet the parametric assumptions, there are nonparametric alternatives that do not require those assumptions to be met, usually because nonparametric statistical procedures convert the original data to rank-ordered data (Pett, 2016).

Many statistical tests can assist researchers in determining whether their data meet the assumptions for a given parametric test. The most common assumption (which accompanies all parametric tests) is that the data are normally distributed. The K^2 test and the Shapiro-Wilk test are formal tests of normality that assess whether distribution of a variable is non-normal—that is, skewed or kurtotic (see Chapter 21) (D'Agostino, Belanger, & D'Agostino, 1990; Grove & Cipher, 2020). The Shapiro-Wilk test is used with samples of less than 1000 subjects. When the sample is larger, the Kolmogorov-Smirnov D test is more appropriate. All of these statistics are found in mainstream statistical software packages and are accompanied by a *p* value. Significant normality tests with $p \leq 0.05$ indicate that the distribution being tested is significantly different from the normal curve, violating the normality assumption. The nonparametric statistical alternative is listed in each section in the event that the data do not meet the assumptions of each parametric test illustrated in this chapter.

t-TESTS

One of the most common parametric analyses used to test for significant differences between group means of two samples is the *t*-test. The **independent samples *t*-test** was developed to examine differences between two independent groups; the **paired samples** or **dependent *t*-test** was developed to examine differences between two paired or matched groups, or a comparison of two measurements in the same group. The details of the independent and paired samples *t*-tests are described in this section.

t-Test for Independent Samples

The most common parametric analysis technique used in nursing studies to test for significant differences between two independent samples is the independent samples *t*-test. The samples are independent if the study participants in one group are unrelated to or different from the participants in the second group. Use of the *t*-test for independent samples involves the following assumptions (Zar, 2010):

1. Sample means from the population are normally distributed.
2. The dependent or outcome variable is measured at the interval/ratio level.
3. The two samples have equal variance.
4. All observations within each sample are independent.

The *t*-test is robust to moderate violation of its assumptions. **Robustness** means that the results of analysis can still be relied on to be accurate when an assumption has been violated. If the dependent variable is measured with a Likert scale, and the frequency distribution is approximately normally distributed, these data are usually considered interval-level measurement and are appropriate for an independent samples *t*-test (see Chapter 16) (de Winter & Dodou, 2010; Rasmussen, 1989). The *t*-test is not robust with respect to the between-samples or within-samples independence assumptions, and it is not robust with respect to an extreme violation of the normality assumption unless the sample sizes are extremely large. Sample groups do not have to be equal for this analysis—instead, the concern is for equal variance (Grove & Cipher, 2020). A variety of *t*-tests have been developed for various types of samples. The formula and calculation of the independent samples *t*-test is presented next.

Calculation

The formula for the *t*-test is:

$$t = \frac{\bar{X}_1 - \bar{X}_2}{s_{\bar{X}_1 - \bar{X}_2}}$$

where

$\bar{X}_1$ = mean of group 1

$\bar{X}_2$ = mean of group 2

$s_{\bar{X}_1 - \bar{X}_2}$ = the standard error of the difference between the two groups

To compute the *t*-test, one must compute the denominator in the formula, which is the standard error of the difference between the means. If the two groups have different sample sizes, one must use this formula:

$$s_{\bar{X}_1 - \bar{X}_2} = \sqrt{\frac{(n_1 - 1)s_1^2 + (n_2 - 1)s_2^2}{n_1 + n_2 - 2}\left(\frac{1}{n_1} + \frac{1}{n_2}\right)}$$

where

n_1 = group 1 sample size

n_2 = group 2 sample size

s_1 = group 1 variance

s_2 = group 2 variance

If the two groups have the same number of subjects in each group, one can use this simplified formula:

$$s_{\bar{X}_1 - \bar{X}_2} = \sqrt{\frac{s_1^2 + s_2^2}{n}}$$

where

n = sample size in each group, because this short formula is based on equal *n* per group.

A retrospective associational or correlational study was conducted to examine the medical utilization of homeless veterans receiving treatment in a veterans affairs healthcare system (LePage, Bradshaw, Cipher, Crawford, & Hooshyar, 2014). A sample of veterans seen in the Veterans Affairs healthcare system in 2010 ($N = 102,034$) was evaluated for homelessness at any point during the year, as well as chronic medical and psychiatric diseases, and medical utilization.

A simulated subset of data for these patients was selected for this example so that the computation would be small and manageable (Table 25.1). In actuality, studies involving *t*-tests need to be adequately powered to identify significant differences between groups accurately (Aberson, 2019; Cohen, 1988; Grove & Cipher, 2020). The independent variable in this example is homelessness in 2010 (yes/no, nominal scale of measurement), and the dependent variable is the total number of outpatient visits in 2010 (ratio scale of measurement). The null hypothesis is, "There is no difference between homeless and not homeless veterans for the number of outpatient visits."

TABLE 25.1   Outpatient Visits by Veteran Homelessness Status

Patient Number	Homeless Veterans' Number of Outpatient Visits	Patient Number	Non-Homeless Veterans' Number of Outpatient Visits
1	36	11	28
2	18	12	33
3	23	13	3
4	15	14	9
5	28	15	13
6	40	16	16
7	18	17	22
8	38	18	10
9	15	19	12
10	16	20	8
Σ	**247**		**154**

The computations for the *t*-test are as follows:

Step 1: Compute means for both groups, which involves the sum of scores for each group divided by the number in the group.
   The mean for Group 1, Homeless: $\bar{X}_1 = 24.7$
   The mean for Group 2, Not Homeless: $\bar{X}_2 = 15.4$

Step 2: Compute the numerator of the *t*-test.

$$24.7 - 15.4 = 9.3$$

It does not matter which group is designated as Group 1 or Group 2. Another possible correct method for step 2 is to subtract Group 1's mean from Group 2's mean, such as:

$$\bar{X}_2 - \bar{X}_1 = 15.4 - 24.7 = -9.3$$

This will result in the exact same *t*-test results and interpretation for a two-tailed test, although the *t*-test value will be negative instead of positive. The sign of the *t*-test does not matter in the interpretation of the results—only the *magnitude* of the *t*-test (Grove & Cipher, 2020).

Step 3: Compute the standard error of the difference.
a. Compute the variances for each group.
   s^2 for Group 1 = 100.68
   s^2 for Group 2 = 89.82

b. Insert into the standard error of the difference formula.

$$s_{\bar{X}_1 - \bar{X}_2} = \sqrt{\frac{s_1^2 + s_2^2}{n}}$$

$$s_{\bar{X}_1 - \bar{X}_2} = \sqrt{\frac{100.68 + 89.82}{10}}$$

$$s_{\bar{X}_1 - \bar{X}_2} = \sqrt{19.05}$$

$$s_{\bar{X}_1 - \bar{X}_2} = 4.36$$

Step 4: Compute *t* value.

$$t = \frac{\bar{X}_1 - \bar{X}_2}{s_{\bar{X}_1 - \bar{X}_2}}$$

$$t = \frac{9.3}{4.36}$$

$$t = 2.13$$

Step 5: Compute the degrees of freedom *(df)*.

$$df = n_1 + n_2 - 2$$
$$df = 10 + 10 - 2$$
$$df = 18$$

Step 6: Locate the critical *t* value in the *t* distribution table (Appendix B) and compare it to the obtained *t* value.
   The critical *t* value for a two-tailed test with 18 *df* at alpha (α) = 0.05 is 2.101, which is rounded to 2.10. This means that if we viewed the *t* distribution for $df = 18$, the middle 95% of the distribution would be delimited by -2.10 and 2.10, as shown in Fig. 25.1.
   Another way to determine the statistical significance of a statistic is to compute the exact *p* value, which is facilitated with statistical software. When this particular *t*-test example was computed using statistical software, the exact *p* value associated with the *t* statistic of 2.13 was $p = 0.047$. This indicates that the exact likelihood of obtaining this *t* value or larger when the null hypothesis is true is 4.7 in 100, or 4.7%. When reporting statistical interpretations for journal articles that use formatting from the American Psychological Association (APA, 2020), the exact *p* value is required.

Interpretation of Results

Our obtained *t* is 2.13, exceeding the critical value, which means that the *t*-test is *significant* and represents a real difference between the two groups. The following

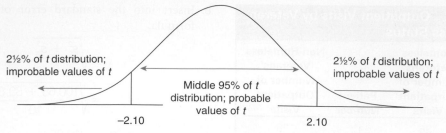

Fig. 25.1 Probability distribution of *t* at *df* = 18.

summative statement is written in the APA (2020) format, as one might read the results in an article.

An independent samples t-test computed on number of outpatient visits revealed that homeless veterans had significantly higher numbers of outpatient visits in 2010 than non-homeless veterans, t(18) = 2.13, p = 0.047; $\overline{X}$ = 24.7 versus 15.4.

With additional research in this area, knowledge of housing status might assist healthcare professionals to improve the healthcare needs of homeless veterans. This knowledge could lead to the more frequent implementation of preventive and health maintenance programs for the homeless veteran population (LePage et al., 2014).

Nonparametric Alternative

If the data do not meet the assumptions involving normality or equal variances for an independent samples *t*-test, the nonparametric alternative is the **Mann-Whitney *U* test**. Mann-Whitney *U* calculations involve converting the data to ranks, discarding any variance or normality issues associated with the original values. In some studies, the data collected are ordinal level, and the Mann-Whitney *U* test is appropriate for analysis of the data. The Mann-Whitney *U* test is 95% as powerful as the *t*-test in determining differences between two groups. For a more detailed description of the Mann-Whitney *U* test, see the statistical textbooks by Daniel (2000), Pett (2016), and Plichta and Kelvin (2013). The statistical workbook by Grove and Cipher (2020) has exercises for expanding your understanding of *t*-tests and Mann-Whitney *U* results from published studies.

t-Tests for Paired Samples

When samples are related, the formula used to calculate the *t* statistic is different from the formula previously described for independent groups. One type of **paired samples** refers to a research design that assesses the same group of people two or more times, a design commonly referred to as a **repeated measures design**. Another research design for which a paired samples *t*-test is appropriate is the case control research design (Kazdin, 2017). **Case control designs** involve a matching procedure whereby a control subject is matched to each case, in which the cases and controls are different people but matched demographically (Gordis, 2014). Paired or dependent samples *t*-tests can also be applied to a **crossover** study design, in which subjects receive one kind of treatment and subsequently receive a comparison treatment (Gliner, Morgan, & Leech, 2009; Gordis, 2014). However, similar to the independent samples *t*-test, this *t*-test requires that differences between the paired scores be independent and normally or approximately normally distributed.

Calculation

The formula for the paired samples *t*-test is:

$$t = \frac{\overline{D}}{s_{\overline{D}}}$$

where

$s_{\overline{D}}$ = mean difference of the paired data

$\overline{D}$ = standard error of the difference

To compute the *t*-test, one must compute the denominator in the formula, the standard error of the difference:

$$s_{\overline{D}} = \frac{s_D}{\sqrt{n}}$$

where

s_D = standard deviation of the differences between the paired data

n = number of subjects in the sample

TABLE 25.2 Esophageal Impedance Values at Baseline and Two-Week Follow-Up

Participant #	Esophageal Impedance, Baseline	Esophageal Impedance, Two-Week Follow-Up	Difference Scores
1	2249	773	1476
2	3993	1329	2664
3	1422	1113	309
4	3676	1670	2006
5	2004	1231	773
6	3271	2660	611
7	2130	1784	346
8	2947	2000	947
9	2000	850	1150
10	3021	1674	1347
Σ	26,713	15,084	11,629

Using an example from a study of adults with gastroesophageal reflux disease (GERD), symptoms of gastroesophageal reflux were examined over time (Dunbar et al., 2016). Twelve adults with GERD were followed over a period of 2 weeks while being required to be free of all proton-pump inhibitor medications (i.e., the intervention). A subset of these data ($n = 10$) is presented in Table 25.2.

The independent variable in this example was treatment over time, meaning that the whole sample received the intervention for 2 weeks. The dependent variable was esophageal impedance, which is an index of mucosal integrity, where higher numbers are more desirable and indicative of healthy esophageal functioning. Impedance was measured with a pH electrode positioned 5 cm above the lower esophageal sphincter. For this example, the null hypothesis is, "There is no change in esophageal impedance from baseline to follow-up for patients with GERD."

The computations for the *t*-test are as follows:

Step 1: Compute the difference between each subject's pair of data (see last column of Table 25.2).

Step 2: Compute the mean of the difference scores, which becomes the numerator of the *t*-test.

$$\bar{D} = 11629.00 \div 10$$

$$\bar{D} = 1162.90$$

Step 3: Compute the standard error of the difference.
a. Compute the standard deviation of the difference scores:

$$s = \sqrt{\frac{\Sigma(x - \bar{x})^2}{n - 1}}$$

$$s = \sqrt{\frac{4995908.90}{10 - 1}}$$

$$s = 745.05$$

b. Insert into the standard error of the difference formula:

$$s_{\bar{D}} = \frac{s_D}{\sqrt{n}}$$

$$s_{\bar{D}} = \frac{745.05}{\sqrt{10}}$$

$$s_D = \frac{745.05}{3.16}$$

$$s_{\bar{D}} = 235.78$$

Step 4: Compute *t* value.

$$t = \frac{\bar{D}}{s_{\bar{D}}}$$

$$t = \frac{1162.90}{235.78}$$

$$t = 4.93$$

Step 5: Compute degrees of freedom.

$$df = n - 1$$
$$df = 10 \quad 1$$
$$df = 9$$

Step 6: Locate the critical *t* value on the *t* distribution table in Appendix B and compare it with the obtained *t* value.

The critical *t* value for 9 *df* for a two-tailed test at $\alpha = 0.05$ is 2.262 rounded to 2.26. Our obtained *t* is 4.93, exceeding the critical value (see *t* table in Appendix B). This means that if we viewed the *t* distribution for $df = 9$, the middle 95% of the distribution would be delimited by -2.26 and 2.26.

Another way to determine the statistical significance of a statistic is to compute the exact *p* value, which is facilitated with statistical software. When this particular *t*-test example was computed using statistical software, the exact *p* value associated with the *t* statistic of 4.93 was $p = 0.001$. This indicates that the exact likelihood of obtaining this *t* value or larger when the null hypothesis is true is 1 in 1000, or 0.1%. When reporting statistical interpretations for journal articles that use formatting from the APA (2020), the exact *p* value is required.

Interpretation of Results

Our obtained $t = 4.93$ exceeds the critical *t* value in the table, which means that the *t*-test is statistically significant and represents a real difference between participants' baseline and post−esophageal impedance levels. The following summative statement is written in APA (2020) format, as one might read the results in an article.

> *A paired samples t-test computed on esophageal impedance levels revealed that the patients who were free of all proton-pump inhibitor medications for 2 weeks had significantly decreased esophageal impedance levels from baseline to follow-up, t(9) = 4.93, p = 0.001; $\overline{X}$ = 2671.3 versus 1508.4.*

During the 2-week observation period, patients experienced a decrease in esophageal impedance (an undesirable trend for persons with GERD). Thus the removal of proton-pump inhibiting medications appeared to play a role in the deterioration of the esophageal mucosal integrity (Dunbar et al., 2016).

Nonparametric Alternative

If the interval/ratio level data do not meet the normality assumptions for a paired samples *t*-test, the nonparametric alternative is the **Wilcoxon signed-rank test**. The Wilcoxon signed-rank test calculations involve converting the data to ranks, discarding any variance or normality issues associated with the original values. This analysis technique is also appropriate when the study data are ordinal level, such as self-care abilities

identified as low, moderate, and high based on the Orem Self-Care Model (Orem, 2001). This test is thoroughly addressed by Daniel (2000), Pett (2016), and Plichta and Kelvin (2013) in their statistical textbooks. The statistical workbook for nursing research by Grove and Cipher (2020) has an exercise for expanding your understanding of the Wilcoxon signed-rank results from published studies.

ONE-WAY ANALYSIS OF VARIANCE

ANOVA is a statistical procedure that compares data between two or more groups or conditions to investigate the presence of differences between those groups on some continuous dependent variable. In this chapter, we focus on the one-way ANOVA, which involves testing one independent variable and one dependent variable (as opposed to other types of ANOVAs such as factorial ANOVAs that incorporate multiple independent variables).

Why ANOVA and not a *t*-test? Remember that a *t*-test is formulated to compare two sets of data or two groups at one time. Thus data generated from a clinical trial that involves four experimental groups, Treatment 1, Treatment 2, Treatment 1 and 2 combined, and a Control, would require six *t*-tests. Consequently, the chance of making a Type I error (α error) increases substantially (or is inflated) because so many computations are being performed. Specifically, the chance of making a Type I error is the number of comparisons multiplied by the α level. Thus ANOVA is the recommended statistical technique for examining differences between more than two groups (Zar, 2010).

ANOVA is a procedure that culminates in a statistic called the **F statistic**. This value is compared against an *F* distribution (see Appendix D) to determine whether the groups significantly differ from one another on the dependent variable studied. The basic formula for the *F* is:

$$F = \frac{\text{Mean square between groups}}{\text{Mean square within groups}}$$

The term *mean square* (MS) is used interchangeably with the word *variance*. The formulas for ANOVA compute two estimates of variance: the between-groups variance and the within-groups variance. The **between-groups variance** represents differences between the groups or conditions being compared, and the **within-groups variance** represents differences among (within) each group's data.

Calculation

A descriptive comparative study was conducted with a cross-sectional survey of former nursing graduate students (Cipher, Urban, & Mancini, 2019). The survey respondents were asked a number of questions about their graduate program experience. One survey item queried the extent to which they were confident in their expanded career role after graduation, where 1 = not at all confident, 2 = somewhat confident, 3 = moderately confident, 4 = very confident, and 5 = completely confident.

The independent variable in this example is type of graduate program from which the respondent graduated (master of science in nursing [MSN] administration program, MSN education program, or nurse practitioner [NP] program), and the dependent variable is self-reported confidence in the expanded career role at graduation. The null hypothesis is, "There is no difference between the three program groups in level of confidence in expanded role after graduation." A simulated subset was selected for this example so that the computations would be small and manageable (Table 25.3). In actuality, studies involving ANOVA must be adequately powered to detect differences accurately among study groups (Aberson, 2019; Cohen, 1988; Grove & Cipher, 2020).

The steps to perform an ANOVA are as follows:

Step 1: Compute correction term, C.

$$C = \frac{G^2}{N}$$

Square the grand sum (G), and divide by total N:

$$C = \frac{78^2}{24} = 253.50$$

Step 2: Compute total sum of squares (SS).

$$\left(\sum X^2\right) - C$$

Square every value in data set, sum, and subtract C:

$$(3^2 + 3^2 + 2^2 + 4^2 + 5^2 + 4^2 + 3^2 \ldots + 4^2)$$
$$-253.5 = 286 - 253.5 = 32.5$$

Step 3: Compute between groups sum of squares.

$$\sum \frac{\left(\sum X_{group}\right)}{n} - C$$

Square the sum of each column and divide by N. Add each, and then subtract C.

$$\frac{28^2}{8} + \frac{31^2}{8} + \frac{19^2}{8} - 253.5$$
$$(98.00 + 120.13 + 45.13) - 253.50 = 9.76$$

TABLE 25.3 Confidence in Expanded Role at Graduation by Type of Graduate Nursing Program

Respondent Number	MSN Administration	Respondent Number	MSN Education	Respondent Number	Nurse Practitioner
1	3	9	3	17	3
2	3	10	4	18	4
3	2	11	3	19	1
4	4	12	5	20	2
5	5	13	3	21	1
6	4	14	3	22	2
7	3	15	5	23	2
8	4	16	5	24	4
Σ	28		31		19
Grand total (G)					78

MSN, Master of science in nursing.

TABLE 25.4   Analysis of Variance Summary Table

Source of Variation	SS	df	MS	F
Between groups	9.76	2	4.88	4.52
Within groups	22.74	21	1.08	
Total	32.50	23		

df, Degrees of freedom; F, F statistic; MS, mean square; SS, sum of squares.

Step 4: Compute within groups sum of squares.

$$SS_{within} = SS_{total} - SS_{between}$$

Subtract the between groups sum of squares (step 3) from total sum of squares (step 2).

$$32.50 - 9.76 = 22.74$$

Step 5: Create an ANOVA summary table similar to Table 25.4.

a. Insert the sum of squares values in the first column.

b. The degrees of freedom are in the second column. Because the F is a ratio of two separate statistics (mean square between groups and mean square within groups) both have different df formulas—one for the numerator and one for the denominator:

Mean square between groups df = number of groups – 1

Mean square within groups $df = N$ − number of groups

For this example, the df for the numerator is $3 - 1 = 2$.

The df for the denominator is $24 - 3 = 21$.

c. The mean square between groups and mean square within groups are in the third column in Table 25.4. These values are computed by dividing the SS by the df. Therefore the MS between = $9.76 \div 2 = 4.88$. The MS within = $22.74 \div 21 = 1.0828$, rounded to 1.08.

d. The F is the final column and is computed by dividing the MS between by the MS within. Therefore $F = 4.88 \div 1.08 = 4.5185$, rounded to 4.52.

Step 6: Locate the critical F value on the F distribution table (see Appendix D) and compare the obtained F value with it. The critical F value for 2 and 21 df at $\alpha = 0.05$ is 3.47. Our obtained F is 4.52, which exceeds the critical value.

Another way to determine the statistical significance of a statistic is to compute the exact p value, which is facilitated with statistical software. When this particular ANOVA example was computed using statistical software, the exact p value associated with the F statistic of 4.52 was $p = 0.024$. This indicates that the exact likelihood of obtaining this F value or larger when the null hypothesis is true is 2.4 in 100, or 2.4%. When reporting statistical interpretations for journal articles that use formatting from the APA (2020), the exact p value is required.

Interpretation of Results

The obtained $F = 4.52$ exceeds the critical value in the table, which means that the F is statistically significant and that the population means are not equal. We can reject our null hypothesis that the three groups have the same level of confidence in their expanded career roles after graduation. However, the F does not tell us which groups differ from one another. Further testing, termed *multiple comparison tests* or *post hoc tests,* are required to complete the ANOVA process and determine all of the significant differences among the study groups.

Post hoc tests have been developed specifically to determine the location of group differences after ANOVA is performed on data from more than two groups (e.g., Is the significant difference between the MSN administration and MSN education groups, between MSN administration and NP, or between MSN education and NP?) These tests were developed to reduce the incidence of a Type I error. Frequently used post hoc tests are the Tukey Honestly Significant Difference (HSD) test, the Newman-Keuls test, the Scheffé test, and the Dunnett test (Plichta & Kelvin, 2013). When these tests are calculated, the alpha level is reduced in proportion to the number of additional tests required to locate statistically significant differences. For example, for several of the aforementioned post hoc tests, if many groups' mean values are being compared, the magnitude of the difference is set higher than if only two groups are being compared. Post hoc tests are tedious to perform by hand and are best handled with statistical computer software programs. The statistical workbook for nursing research by Grove and Cipher (2020) has exercises for expanding your interpretation and understanding of ANOVA and post hoc procedure results from published studies.

The following summative statements are written in APA (2020) format, as one might read the results in an article. The Tukey Honestly Significant post hoc test is reported here as an example of how to write the results of a post hoc test.

Analysis of variance performed on confidence ratings revealed significant differences between the three program groups, F(2, 21) = 4.52, p = 0.024. Post hoc comparisons using the Tukey HSD comparison test indicated that the graduates of the NP program had significantly lower confidence ratings of their expanded career role than both the graduates of the MSN administration program and the MSN education program ($\overline{X}$= 2.38 vs 3.50 and 3.88, respectively). There were no significant differences in confidence scores between the MSN administration students and the MSN education students.

Nonparametric Alternative

If the data do not meet the normality assumptions for an ANOVA, the nonparametric alternative is the Kruskal-Wallis test. Calculations for the Kruskal-Wallis test involve converting the data to ranks, discarding any variance or normality issues associated with the original values. Similar to the ANOVA, the **Kruskal-Wallis test** is a nonparametric analysis technique that can accommodate the comparisons of more than two groups. This test is thoroughly addressed in textbooks by Daniel (2000) and Plichta and Kelvin (2013).

Other ANOVA Procedures

There are other kinds of ANOVA that accommodate other research designs involving various numbers of independent and dependent variables, such as factorial ANOVA, repeated measures ANOVA, and mixed factorial ANOVA. These ANOVA procedures are presented and explained in comprehensive statistics textbooks such as King and Eckersley (2019) and Zar (2010).

PEARSON CHI-SQUARE TEST

The chi-square (χ^2) test compares differences in proportions of nominal-level variables. When a study requires that researchers compare proportions (percentages) in one category versus another category, the χ^2 is a statistic that reveals whether the difference in proportion is statistically improbable. The χ^2 has its own theoretical distribution and associated χ^2 table (see Appendix E).

A **one-way chi-square** is a statistic that compares different levels of one variable only. For example, a researcher may collect information on gender and compare the proportions of males to females. If the one-way chi-square is statistically significant, it would indicate that the difference in gender proportions was significantly greater than what would be expected by chance (Daniel, 2000; Pett, 2016).

A **two-way chi-square** is a statistic that tests whether proportions in levels of one variable are significantly different from proportions of the second variable. For example, the presence of advanced colon polyps was studied in three groups of patients: patients having a normal body mass index (BMI), patients who were overweight, and patients who were obese (Siddiqui et al., 2009). The research question tested was, "Is there a significant difference between the three groups (normal, overweight, and obese) in the presence of advanced colon polyps?" The results of the chi-square analysis indicated that a larger proportion of obese patients fell into the category of having advanced colon polyps compared with normal-weight and overweight patients, suggesting that obesity may be a risk factor for developing advanced colon polyps.

Assumptions

The use of the Pearson chi-square test involves the following assumptions (Daniel, 2000):

1. Only one datum entry is made for each subject in the sample. Therefore if repeated measures from the same subject are being used for analysis, such as pretests and posttests, a chi-square is not an appropriate test (the **McNemar's test** is the appropriate test) (Daniel, 2000).
2. The variables must be categorical (nominal), either inherently or transformed to categorical from ordinal, interval, or ratio values. For example, BMI values might be categorized into normal and overweight.
3. For each variable, the categories are mutually exclusive and exhaustive. No cells may have an "expected" frequency of zero. In the actual data, the "observed" cell frequency may be zero. However, the Pearson chi-square test is not sensitive to small sample sizes, and other tests such as the Fisher's exact test are more appropriate when testing very small samples (Daniel, 2000; Pett, 2016; Yates, 1934).

The test is distribution free, or nonparametric, which means that no assumption has been made for a normal distribution of values in the population from which the sample was taken (Daniel, 2000; Pett, 2016).

The formula for a two-way chi-square is:

$$\chi^2 = \frac{n[(A)(D) - (B)(C)]^2}{(A + B)(C + D)(A + C)(B + D)}$$

A **contingency table** displays the relationship between two or more categorical variables (Daniel, 2000; Pett, 2016). The contingency table is labeled as follows:

A	B
C	D

With any chi-square analysis, the degrees of freedom must be calculated to determine the significance of the value of the statistic. The following formula is used for the *df* calculation:

$$df = (R - 1)(C - 1)$$

where

R = number of rows
C = number of columns

Calculation

A retrospective comparative study examined whether longer antibiotic treatment courses were associated with increased antimicrobial resistance in patients with spinal cord injury (Lee et al., 2014). Using urine cultures from a sample of spinal cord–injured veterans, two groups were created: those with evidence of antibiotic resistance and those with no evidence of antibiotic resistance. All veterans were divided into two groups based on having had a history of recent (in the last 6 months) antibiotic use for more than 2 weeks, or no history of recent antibiotic use for more than 2 weeks.

The data are presented in Table 25.5. The null hypothesis is, "There is no difference between antibiotic users and nonusers on the presence of antibiotic resistance."

The computations for the Pearson chi-square test are as follows:

Step 1: Create a contingency table of the two nominal variables (see Table 25.5).

TABLE 25.5 Antibiotic Use and Antibiotic Resistance in Veterans With Spinal Cord Injuries

	Antibiotic Use	No Recent Antibiotic Use	Total
Antibiotic Resistance	8	7	15
No Antibiotic Resistance	6	21	27
Total	14	28	Grand total = 42

Step 2: Fit the cells into the formula:

$$\chi^2 = \frac{n[(A)(D) - (B)(C)]^2}{(A + B)(C + D)(A + C)(B + D)}$$

$$\chi^2 = \frac{42[(8)(21) - (7)(6)]^2}{(8 + 7)(6 + 21)(8 + 6)(7 + 28)}$$

$$\chi^2 = \frac{42[126]^2}{(15)(27)(14)(28)}$$

$$\chi^2 = \frac{666792}{158760}$$

$$\chi^2 = 4.20$$

Step 3: Compute the degrees of freedom.

$$df = (2 - 1)(2 - 1) = 1$$

Step 4: Locate the critical χ^2 value in the χ^2 distribution table in Appendix E and compare it to the obtained χ^2 value.

The chi-square table in Appendix E includes the critical values of chi-square for specific degrees of freedom at selected levels of significance. The obtained χ^2 value is compared with the table's χ^2 values. If the value of the statistic is equal to or greater than the value identified in the chi-square table, the difference between the two variables is statistically significant. The critical χ^2 for $df = 1$ and $\alpha = 0.05$ is 3.842, rounded to 3.84. Our obtained χ^2 is 4.20, thereby exceeding the critical value and indicating a significant difference between antibiotic users and nonusers on the presence of antibiotic resistance.

Another way to determine the statistical significance of a statistic is to compute the exact *p* value, which is facilitated with statistical software. When this particular chi-square example was computed using statistical software, the exact p value associated with the χ^2 of 4.20 was $p = 0.04$. This indicates that the exact likelihood of obtaining this χ^2 value or larger when the null hypothesis is true is 4 in 100, or 4.0%. When reporting statistical interpretations for journal articles that use formatting from the APA (2020), the exact p value is required.

Furthermore, we can compute the rates of antibiotic resistance among antibiotic users and nonusers by using the numbers in the contingency table (see Table 25.5) from step 1. The antibiotic resistance rate among the antibiotic users can be calculated as $8 \div 14 = 0.571 \times 100\% = 57.1\%$. The antibiotic resistance rate among the nonantibiotic users can be calculated as $7 \div 28 = 0.25 \times 100\% = 25\%$.

Interpretation of Results

The following summative statement is written in APA (2020) format, as one might read the results in an article.

> *A Pearson chi-square analysis indicated that 2-week antibiotic users had significantly higher rates of antibiotic resistance than those who had not recently used antibiotics, $\chi^2(1) = 4.20$, $p = 0.04$ (57.1% vs 25%, respectively).*

This finding suggests that extended antibiotic use may be a risk factor for developing resistance in spinal cord–injured patients and further research is needed to investigate resistance as a direct effect of antibiotics.

◾ KEY POINTS

- Parametric statistics conducted to determine differences are accompanied by certain assumptions, and the data must be tested for whether they meet those assumptions before computing the statistic.
- Many tests of normality can assist the researcher in determining the suitability of the data for the use of parametric statistics.
- In the event that the data do not meet the assumptions of the parametric statistic, there are nonparametric alternatives that do not adhere to the assumptions of the parametric test.
- The t-test is one of the most commonly used parametric analyses to test for significant differences between statistical measures of two samples or groups.
- The independent samples t-test indicates a difference between two unrelated groups of subjects, whereas the paired samples t-test indicates a difference in two assessments of the same subjects or two groups matched on selected variables.
- The Mann-Whitney U test is the nonparametric alternative to the independent samples t-test when the study data violate one or more of the independent samples t-test assumptions.

- The Wilcoxon signed-rank test is the nonparametric alternative to the paired or dependent samples t-test when the study data violate one or more of the paired samples t-test assumptions.
- A one way ANOVA can be used to examine data from two or more groups and compares the variance within each group with the variance between groups.
- A one-way ANOVA conducted on three or more groups that yields a significant result requires the use of post hoc analysis procedures for determining the location of group differences.
- The Kruskal-Wallis test is the nonparametric alternative to the ANOVA when the study data violate one or more of the ANOVA assumptions.
- The chi-square test compares proportions (percentages) in one category of a variable of interest with proportions in another category.
- The McNemar test is the appropriate statistical test to conduct when analyzing nominal level data obtained from repeated measures from the same subject, such as pretests and posttests.

REFERENCES

Aberson, C. L. (2019). *Applied power analysis for the behavioral sciences* (2nd ed.). New York, NY: Routledge.

American Psychological Association (APA). (2020). *Publication manual of the American Psychological Association* (7th ed.). Washington, DC: APA.

Cipher, D. J., Urban, R. W., & Mancini, M. E. (2019). Factors associated with student success in online and face-to-face delivery of master of science in nursing programs. *Teaching and Learning in Nursing, 14*(3), 203–207. doi:10.1016/j.teln.2019.03.007

Cohen, J. (1988). *Statistical power analysis for the behavioral sciences* (2nd ed.). New York: Academic Press.

D'Agostino, R. B., Belanger, A., & D'Agostino Jr., R. B. (1990). A suggestion for using powerful and informative tests of normality. *The American Statistician, 44*(4), 316–321. doi:10.2307/2684359

Daniel, W. W. (2000). *Applied nonparametric statistics* (2nd ed.). Pacific Grove, CA: Duxbury Press.

de Winter, J. C. F., & Dodou, D. (2010). Five-point Likert items: *t*-test versus Mann-Whitney-Wilcoxon. *Practical Assessment, Research, and Evaluation, 15*(11), 1–16.

Dunbar, K. B., Agoston, A. T., Odze, R. D., Huo, X., Pham, T. H., Cipher, D. J., … Spechler, S. J. (2016). Association of acute gastroesophageal reflux disease with esophageal histologic changes. *Journal of the American Medical Association, 315*(19), 2104–2112. doi:10.1001/jama.2016.5657

Gliner, J. A., Morgan, G. A., & Leech, N. L. (2009). *Research methods in applied settings* (2nd ed.). New York, NY: Routledge.

Gordis, L. (2014). *Epidemiology* (5th ed.). Philadelphia, PA: Saunders.

Grove, S. K., & Cipher, D. J. (2020). *Statistics for nursing research: A workbook for evidence-based practice* (3rd ed.). St. Louis, MO: Saunders.

Kazdin, A. E. (2017). *Research design in clinical psychology* (5th ed.). Boston, MA: Pearson.

King, A., & Eckersley, R. (2019). *Statistics for biomedical engineers and scientists: How to visualize and analyze data.* London, UK: Academic Press Elsevier.

Lee, Y. R., Tashjian, C. A., Brouse, S. D., Bedimo, R. J., Goetz, L. L., Cipher, D. J., et al. (2014). Antibiotic therapy and bacterial resistance in patients with spinal cord injury. *Federal Practitioner, 31*(3), 13–17.

LePage, J. P., Bradshaw, L. D., Cipher, D. J., Crawford, A. M., & Hooshyar, D. (2014). The effects of homelessness on veterans' healthcare service use: An evaluation of independence from comorbidities. *Public Health, 128*(11), 985–992. doi:10.1016/j.puhe.2014.07.004

Orem, D. E. (2001). *Nursing: Concepts of practice* (6th ed.). St. Louis, MO: Mosby.

Pett, M. A. (2016). *Nonparametric statistics for health care research: Statistics for small samples and unusual distributions* (2nd ed.). Los Angeles, CA: Sage

Plichta, S. B., & Kelvin, E. (2013). *Munro's statistical methods for health care research* (6th ed.). Philadelphia, PA: Wolters Kluwer/Lippincott Williams & Wilkins.

Rasmussen, J. L. (1989). Analysis of Likert-scale data: A reinterpretation of Gregoire and Driver. *Psychological Bulletin, 105*(1), 167–170.

Siddiqui, A. A., Nazario, H., Mahgoub, A., Pandove, S., Cipher, D. J., & Spechler, S. J. (2009). Obesity is associated with an increased prevalence of advanced adenomatous colon polyps in a male veteran population. *Digestive Disease & Sciences, 54*(7), 1560–1564. doi:10.1007/s10620-009-0811-7

Yates, F. (1934). Contingency tables involving small numbers and the χ^2 test. *Journal of Royal Statistical Society, 1*(2), 217–235.

Zar, J. H. (2010). *Biostatistical analysis* (5th ed.). Upper Saddle River, NJ: Prentice-Hall.

Interpreting Research Outcomes

Susan K. Grove

http://evolve.elsevier.com/Gray/practice/

When data analysis is complete, there is a feeling that the answers are known and the study is finished. However, there remains the need to finish the research process by interpreting the results of the statistical and qualitative analyses. Even a first-time researcher amasses considerable knowledge of the problem area, related literature, potential applications, and needs of the discipline. They also have a beginning understanding of what the study signifies and the extent to which the findings can be generalized. Because of all the preparation that went into the study, the researcher is very knowledgeable in this particular area of inquiry. For masters and doctoral students, aside from the thesis or dissertation committee members, hardly anyone understands all that the researcher understands. Healthcare professionals, in general, represent the primary audience for the results of the research, either through presentation or publication. So before dissemination, the results must be explained so that others will understand their significance. This detailed examination and an explanation of study results are called **interpretation of research outcomes**.

Interpretation of research outcomes requires reflection upon three general aspects of the study and their interactions: the primary findings, validity issues, and the resultant body of knowledge in the area of investigation. These issues will determine how the researcher writes the Discussion section of the research report, which presents the study findings, limitations, conclusions, generalizations, implications of the findings for practice, and the recommendations for subsequent inquiry in the area. The order of information included in the Discussion section varies based on researcher preference and the study content covered.

There is a tendency to rush the interpretation of the findings, but it is not a step to be minimized or hurried. This interpretation process takes time for reflection, and researchers need to step back from the details of the study and reexamine the big picture. Researchers should consider their findings dispassionately, as if another person had conducted the study, because possessive ownership does not assist the process. Discussion with others in the field such as fellow healthcare workers, and with peers and other academically based persons and mentors, is helpful as well. How do they view the study in relation to the area of inquiry? What do they envision for application potential, either now or with subsequent research that builds upon this and other studies?

This chapter focuses primarily on the interpretation of findings from quantitative and outcomes research (Creswell & Creswell, 2018; Kazdin, 2017; Kleinpell, 2017; Leedy & Ormrod, 2019). Interpretations of results and findings for qualitative research are presented in Chapter 12 and for mixed methods research in Chapter 14. The process of interpreting quantitative research findings includes several steps that are identified in Box 26.1. Incorporated into the explanation of each of these steps are examples from a quantitative correlational study conducted by Lynch and colleagues (2019).

EXAMPLE STUDY

Lynch et al. (2019) supported the need for their study by reporting that body mass index (BMI) and central

"Given the gaps in knowledge related to psychological stress, depressive symptoms, cortisol, body mass, and central adiposity in children, the purpose of this study was to examine the influence of psychological stress and depressive symptoms on body mass and central adiposity in 10-to-12-year-old children and to determine the mediating role of cortisol in the relationships among psychological stress, depressive symptoms, body mass, or central adiposity. Specifically, we sought to address the following research questions in 10-to-12-year-old children: 1) What is the relationship between psychological stress and depressive symptoms? 2) How much of the variance in body mass and central adiposity is explained by psychological stress and depressive symptoms after controlling for sex, puberty, race/ethnicity, and SES [socioeconomic status]? and 3) Does cortisol mediate the relationships between psychological stress, depressive symptoms, and body mass or central adiposity after controlling for sex, puberty, race/ethnicity, and SES?" (Lynch et al., 2019, p. 43)

adiposity increased in US children aged 6 to 11 years from 2013 to 2016 (Centers for Disease Control and Prevention [CDC], 2018). In addition, the increased BMI and central adiposity have resulted in health problems of high blood pressure (BP) and type 2 diabetes in these children that continue into adulthood. Currently, direct healthcare costs associated with childhood obesity are estimated at $14 billion annually.

The conceptual framework developed to guide this study included the concepts of psychosocial factors, physiological factors, and health outcomes that are linked to the study variables in Fig. 26.1. The review of literature identified a strong association between psychological stress and depressive symptoms and between depression and increased percentage of body fat in adults. However, very few studies have been conducted with children, linking depressive symptoms, psychological stress, and BMI or central adiposity in children. In the following excerpt, Lynch et al. (2019) identified the gap in knowledge in this area and the purpose and research questions developed to guide this study.

Lynch and colleagues (2019) conducted a correlational study with a convenience sample of 147 children ages 10 to 12 years. These study participants were recruited from one middle school and three elementary schools in a rural, southeastern US city. The key study variables (psychological stress, depressive symptoms, cortisol, height and weight, and waist circumference [WC]) were measured with a variety of psychological and physiological methods that are summarized in Table 26.1. Example quotes from the Lynch et al. (2019) study are presented in the following sections, focusing on identification of study findings, limitations, generalizations, implications for nursing,

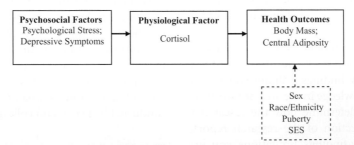

Fig. 26.1 Conceptual framework. (From Lynch, T., Azuero, A., Lochman, J. E., Park, N., Turner-Henson, A., & Rice, M. [2019]. The influence of psychological stress, depressive symptoms, and cortisol on body mass and central adiposity in 10- to 12-year-old children. *Journal of Pediatric Nursing, 44*[1], 43.) *SES*, Socioeconomic status.

TABLE 26.1 Summary of Study Psychological and Physiological Measures

Variable	Measure	Type of Measure
Psychological stress	The 20-item Feel Bad Scale (FBS) was used to measure children's perceived stress. FBS was developed from focus groups with fifth and sixth graders (Lewis, Siegel, & Lewis, 1984).	Likert scale of five points ranging from 1 for never to 5 for always with scores ranging from 20 to 100
Depressive symptoms	The 27-item Children's Depression Inventory (CDI) was used to measure depressive symptoms. CDI was designed to measure depression in children ages 7 to 17 years with each item measuring a depressive symptom that disturbs mood, sleep, appetite, or interpersonal relationships (Kovacs, 1992).	Self-report questionnaire with scores ranging from 0 to 52. Score of 13 indicates mild depression and score of 19 denotes severe depression
Cortisol	"Cortisol level was determined by a standard two-step sandwich enzyme-linked immunosorbent assay (ELISA) using commercially prepared high-sensitivity kits (R & D Systems, MN, USA)" (Lynch et al., 2019, p. 45).	Biomedical instrument (Stone & Frazier, 2017)
Height and weight	"Height was measured to the nearest ¼ inch using a portable stadiometer, and weight was measured to the nearest ¼ pound by use of a freestanding balance beam scale according to established recommendations by Heyward and Wagner (2004)" (Lynch et al., 2019, p. 44).	Physiological measure (Ryan-Wenger, 2017)
Waist circumference (WC)	"WC, an indicator of central adiposity, was measured according to protocol by Heyward and Wagner (2004). WC was measured twice to the nearest 1/16 in. and converted to centimeters" (Lynch et al., 2019, p. 44).	Physiological measure (Ryan-Wenger, 2017)

Content abstracted from Lynch, T., Azuero, A., Lochman, J. E., Park, N., Turner-Henson, A., & Rice, M. (2019). The influence of psychological stress, depressive symptoms, and cortisol on body mass and central adiposity in 10- to 12-year-old children. *Journal of Pediatric Nursing, 44*(1), 44–45.

recommendations for further study, and final conclusions (see Box 26.1).

Identification of Study Findings

The first step the researcher makes in interpretation is examination of the results of the study, and then phrasing those results as language instead of statistical analysis printouts (Grove & Cipher, 2020). Evaluating evidence, translating the study results, and interpreting them provide the basis for developing the **findings**. Although much of the process of developing findings from results occurs in the mind of the researcher, evidence of such thinking can be found in published research reports (Kazdin, 2017; Leedy & Ormrod, 2019). As noted earlier, it is important during this process to talk with colleagues or mentors to clarify meanings or expand implications of the research findings. Key results and findings are presented as an example from the study conducted by Lynch et al. (2019). As is a common practice, these researchers

began the results section by describing the participants of the study in the narrative and using a table.

"The final sample included 147 completed data sets. Of the 147 children, 84 were female and 63 male (60 ten-year-olds [35 female, 25 male]; 64 eleven-year-olds [36 female, 28 male]; and 23 twelve-year-olds [13 female, 10 male]). The mean age was 10.75 years (*SD* 0.71). Demographic data including age, sex, race/ethnicity, pubertal status, and socioeconomic status are presented in a table.... The majority of children (57.8%) were overweight (17.7%) or obese (40.1%) based on BMI percentiles for age and sex (Centers for Disease Control and Prevention, 2015). Using anthropometric percentiles for WC, the mean WC for the sample was at the 75th percentile (Fryar, Carroll, & Ogden, 2016), with 38% (*n* = 56) of children with WC values at or above this percentile." (Lynch et al., 2019, p. 45)

In the results section, Lynch et al. (2019) also provided the results of the descriptive statistics used to summarize the data for the primary variables. Table 26.2 contains these results, including a mean, standard deviation (*SD*), and range for each variable. The researchers also provided some interpretation of whether the scores were low or high and possible reasons.

"The majority of children (57.8%) were overweight (17.7%) or obese (40.1%) based on BMI percentiles for age and sex (Centers for Disease Control and Prevention, 2015). Using anthropometric percentiles for WC, the mean WC for the sample was at the 75th percentile (Fryar et al., 2016), with 38% ($n = 56$) of children with WC values at or above this percentile...

Twenty-four (16.3%) of the participants reported mild to moderate depressive symptoms, while 23.1% ($n = 34$) indicated severe levels of depressive symptoms.... Children in the overweight ($n = 26$) category reported depressive symptoms with 15.4% ($n = 4$) reporting mild to moderate symptoms and 34.6% ($n = 9$) indicating severe levels of depressive symptoms. Finally, of the 59 children in the obese category 49.1% ($n = 29$) reported depressive symptoms of which 16.9% ($n = 10$) were mild to moderate and 32.2% ($n = 19$) severe levels.

Of the 147 children, 46.3% ($n = 68$) had FBS [Feel Bad Scale] scores higher than the mean value of 124.44 for the group. Of the 68 students who scored higher than the mean, 4.4% ($n = 3$) had BMI values between the 85th and 94th percentile, and 58.8% ($n = 40$) had BMI values at or above the 95th percentile." (Lynch et al., 2019, p. 45)

TABLE 26.2 Means, Standard Deviations, and Ranges for Study Variables ($N = 147$)

Variable	Mean (*SD*)	Range
Body mass index (kg/m^2)	21.93 (5.01)	13.42–36.54
Waist circumference (cm)	76.65 (5.28)	51.18–114.30
Cortisol (nmol/l)[a]	6.75 (6.75)	1.97–46.08
Depressive symptoms	11.14 (8.98)	0–37
Psychological stress	12.44 (54.90)	200–500

[a]$n = 144$.

From Lynch, T., Azuero, A., Lochman, J. E., Park, N., Turner-Henson, A., & Rice, M. (2019). The influence of psychological stress, depressive symptoms, and cortisol on body mass and central adiposity in 10- to 12-year-old children. *Journal of Pediatric Nursing, 44*(1), 45.

After describing the sample and the primary variables, researchers consider the statistical output relative to the hypotheses or research questions.

Interpretation of Inferential Data Analysis Results

Interpretation of results for each research hypothesis or question yields five possible results: (1) significant results that are in keeping with the results predicted by the researcher; (2) nonsignificant results; (3) significant results that oppose the results predicted by the researcher, sometimes referred to as unexpected results; (4) mixed results; and (5) serendipitous results (Kazdin, 2017; Shadish, Cook, & Campbell, 2002). Table 26.3 provides a list of possible results with examples from the Lynch et al. (2019) study.

Significant and Predicted Results

Significant results that coincide with the researcher's predictions validate the proposed logical links among the elements of a study. These results support the logical links developed by the researcher among the purpose, framework, questions or hypotheses, variables, and measurement methods (Kazdin, 2017; Shadish et al., 2002; Waltz, Strickland, & Lenz, 2017). Although this outcome is very gratifying, the researcher needs to consider alternative explanations for the positive findings. What other elements could possibly have led to the significant results? Are the statistically significant results meaningful? Sometimes with very large sample sizes, a result will be statistically significant but the effect size may be very small, or the result may lack clinical or practical importance of the changes. Kazdin (2017) recommends using the following to judge clinical importance of findings: (1) magnitude or strength of the change in the participants from pretreatment to posttreatment; (2) posttreatment participants fall within normative levels of functioning; (3) posttreatment participants no longer meet diagnostic criteria, no longer have the clinical problem, or are considered recovered; (4) researchers' subjective evaluation of the study participants indicates improvement; or (5) study participants demonstrate improved quality of life and/or social functioning. Any of these conditions indicate the clinical importance of the study findings.

Nonsignificant Results

Unpredicted **nonsignificant** or inconclusive **results** are often referred to as **negative results**. The negative

TABLE 26.3 Interpretation of Results for Lynch et al. (2019) Study

Result	Example
Significant, predicted results	"A positive relationship between psychological stress and depressive symptoms was found ($r = 0.559$, $p < .001$)" (Lynch et al., 2019, p. 45).
Nonsignificant results	"The lack of relationships between psychological stress and cortisol, and between depressive symptoms and cortisol precluded the testing of cortisol for mediation among the study variables" (Lynch et al., 2019, p. 46).
Mixed results	"Depressive symptoms were significantly related to Body Mass Index (BMI) ($\beta = 0.37$, $p < .001$); however, psychological stress did not relate to BMI" (Lynch et al., 2019, p. 45). "Depressive symptoms were found to contribute significantly to central adiposity ($\beta = 0.40$, $p < .001$), while psychological stress did not contribute significantly to the model" (Lynch et al., 2019, p. 46).
Significant results opposite of predictions (unexpected)	No unexpected significant results were noted in this study.

Content abstracted from Lynch, T., Azuero, A., Lochman, J. E., Park, N., Turner-Henson, A., & Rice, M. (2019). The influence of psychological stress, depressive symptoms, and cortisol on body mass and central adiposity in 10- to 12-year-old children. *Journal of Pediatric Nursing, 44*(1), 44–45.

results could be a true reflection of reality (Kazdin, 2017; Teixeira da Silva, 2015). In this case, the reasoning of the researcher or the theory used by the researcher to develop the hypothesis is in error, but the study was scientifically sound. If so, the negative findings are an important addition to the body of knowledge. Negative results could help refine the hypotheses for a subsequent study.

With nonsignificant results, it is important to determine whether adequate power of 0.8 or higher was achieved for the data analysis. The researcher needs to conduct a power analysis to determine whether the sample size was adequate to prevent the risk of a Type II error (Aberson, 2019; Grove & Cipher, 2020; Kazdin, 2017). A Type II error means that in reality the findings were significant, but because the sample size was inadequate the statistical tests failed to show significance.

Negative results could also be due to poor operationalization of variables. For example, the independent variable or intervention was not implemented in an optimal way, or the dependent variables were measured with methods that lacked reliability and validity (see Chapter 16) (Waltz et al., 2017). Negative results might also be due to the following: a sample that was inexplicably nonrepresentative of the study population (see Chapter 15), uncontrolled-for and unmeasured extraneous variables (see Chapter 6), use of inappropriate

statistical techniques, or faulty data analysis (Grove & Cipher, 2020). Unless these weak links are detected, the reported results could lead to faulty information in the body of knowledge (Kazdin, 2017). Negative results, to reiterate, do not mean that there are no relationships among the study variables or differences between groups; they indicate that the study failed to find any relationships or group differences.

Significant and Not Predicted Results

Significant results that are the opposite of those predicted, if the results are valid, are an important addition to the body of knowledge. These are sometimes referred to as *unexpected results.* An example would be a study in which the researchers proposed that social support and ego strength were positively related. If the study showed that high social support was related to low ego strength, the result would be the opposite of that predicted. Such results, when verified by other studies, indicate that the theory being tested needs modification and refinement. These types of studies can provide important information that might affect nursing practice.

Mixed Results

Mixed results are probably the most common outcome of studies that examine more than one relationship. In a study, one variable may uphold the characteristics predicted, whereas another does not. In the Lynch et al.

(2019) study, depressive symptoms were significantly related to the outcome BMI, as predicted in the study framework, but psychological stress was not significantly related to BMI (see Table 26.3). Mixed results might also occur when two dependent measures of the same variable show opposite results. For example, the FACES scale might indicate a child is in pain but the vital signs of heart rate and respiration are normal. Each result should be considered individually for interpretation.

Serendipitous Results

Serendipitous results are discoveries or researcher observations that were not the focus of the study. Most researchers examine as many elements of data as possible in addition to the elements directed by the research objectives, questions, or hypotheses. In doing so, they sometimes discover a relationship or variable distribution heretofore unearthed. Serendipitous results should be reported because they are legitimate discoveries of the study.

Example Study Results

Lynch et al. (2019) presented their study results in the usual order with the description of the sample (as previously discussed) and the description of the primary variables (see Table 26.2). The discussion for a descriptive study includes only descriptive results, but with other designs, both descriptive and inferential results are discussed for significant and nonsignificant findings (Grove & Cipher, 2020; Kazdin, 2017). Lynch et al. (2019) conducted a cross-sectional, predictive correlational design so descriptive statistics (frequencies, percentages, means, standard deviations, and ranges) and inferential statistics (Pearson correlation and simple and multiple regression) were conducted. The study results were presented in tables and the narrative of the report. The inferential statistical results were organized by the three research questions introduced earlier. Lynch et al. (2019) identified significant, nonsignificant, and mixed results, which are briefly presented in Table 26.3.

The Pearson correlation coefficients were discussed in the study narrative, indicating those that were significant and what the relationship meant. The following results address this research question: "1) What is the relationship between psychological stress and depressive symptoms?" (Lynch et al., 2019, p. 43).

> "A positive relationship between psychological stress and depressive symptoms was found ($r = 0.559$, $p < .001$), with those reporting higher psychological stress also having higher depressive symptoms…. Depressive symptoms were significantly related to BMI ($\beta = 0.37$, $p < .001$); however, psychological stress did not relate to BMI." (Lynch et al., 2019, p. 45)

Multiple regression was conducted to address an additional research question: "2) How much of the variance in body mass and central adiposity is explained by psychological stress and depressive symptoms?" (Lynch et al., 2019, p. 43). The following excerpt indicates that depressive symptoms were significant predictors of both BMI and central adiposity. However, psychological stress was not significantly related to or a significant predictor of BMI or central adiposity.

> "After controlling for puberty, sex, race/ethnicity, and SES, the independent variables depressive symptoms and psychological stress explained a significant amount of the variance in BMI scores $F (7, 139) = 4.49$, $p < .001$, ΔR^2 0.14… the study variables (psychological stress and depressive symptoms) were added to the model to test for significant variance in central adiposity. The full model including the control variables, depressive symptoms, and psychological stress revealed a significant contribution of 24.9% to the amount of variance explained in central adiposity, $F (7, 139) = 7.93$, $p < .001$, ΔR^2 0.25. Depressive symptoms were found to contribute significantly to central adiposity ($\beta = 0.40$, $p < .001$), while psychological stress did not contribute significantly in the model." (Lynch et al., 2019, p. 46)

The third research question focused on the following: "Does cortisol mediate the relationships between psychological stress, depressive symptoms, and body mass or central adiposity after controlling for sex, puberty, race/ethnicity, and SES?" (Lynch et al., 2019, p. 43). The study framework (see Fig. 26.1) identified cortisol as a possible mediator between selected psychosocial factors (psychological stress and depressive symptoms) and health outcomes (body mass and central adiposity), but this proposition was not supported by the study results as indicated by the following excerpt.

"To address the third research question, simple linear regression models were used to determine whether, after puberty, sex, race/ethnicity, and SES were controlled, cortisol mediated the relationships between psychological stress and body mass and/or between depressive symptoms and body mass. The lack of relationships between psychological stress and cortisol, and between depressive symptoms and cortisol precluded the testing of cortisol for mediation among the study variables." (Lynch et al., 2019, pp. 45–46)

Comparison With the Literature

The results of a study should be examined in light of previous findings. In the Discussion portion of a research report, selected individual results are discussed, both those related to demographics and those examining study variables. The results are not presented again in their entirety because that would be redundant with the Results section. Here the results are discussed in relation to whether the major results were expected or unexpected and whether they were consistent or inconsistent with similar findings in the literature. Consistency in findings across studies is important for developing theories and refining scientific knowledge for the nursing profession. Therefore, any inconsistencies must be explored to determine reasons for the differences. Replication of studies (Kazdin, 2017) and synthesis of findings from existing studies using meta-analyses and systematic reviews are critical for the development of empirical knowledge for an evidence-based practice (EBP) (Higgins & Thomas, 2020; Melnyk & Fineout-Overholt, 2019).

Lynch et al. (2019) provided a detailed discussion of their findings and compared them with the findings of other researchers. The following study excerpt highlights some of these comparisons. As expected, some of the findings were consistent with previous research and others were not. The researchers addressed the inconsistent findings and provided possible reasons for these findings. Because several findings from the Lynch et al. (2019) study were inconsistent with previous study finding, this area requires further study.

"The majority of the participants in this study were overweight or obese with more being obese than overweight. Children in the obese category in this study exceed that of those reported in the national NHANES [National Health and Nutritional Examination Survey] study (18.4%) (Hales et al., 2018) but are similar to the estimated 50% in the southern region of states (Singh, Kogan, & van Dyck, 2010). The prevalence of overweight and obesity in children aged 10 to 17 years in the state where data were collected is estimated to be 35.5% (National Survey of Children's Health, 2016), which is lower than the percentage of 57.8% in our sample of children...

The WC mean in this group of children was above the national average. This finding differs from Xi and colleagues' report from national data that found children aged 6 to 11 years had an average WC of 65 cm (Xi et al., 2014)...

A majority of children had cortisol values within normal range; however, 8.3% had cortisol values above the norm. In this sample, the cortisol values were not associated with elevated body mass or central adiposity. This finding contrasts with that of Chu et al. (2017), who found a positive relationship between cortisol and body composition in children. Because few studies exist with children, it is difficult to draw any conclusions about the relationships between cortisol and body mass or between cortisol and central adiposity...

A positive relationship was found between psychological stress and depressive symptoms, and this finding is in line with those of other studies of adolescents (Braet, Vlierberghe, Vandevivere, Theuwis, & Bosmans, 2012; Mazurka, Wynne-Edwards, & Harkness, 2016)...

Whereas depressive symptoms were significant in explaining both body mass and central adiposity, psychological stress was not significant. This, despite the fact that psychological stress was related to both BMI and WC. This finding differs from other investigations (Brumby, Kennedy, & Chandrasekara, 2013; Roberts, Troop, Connan, Treasure, & Campbell, 2007) that noted the significant contribution of psychological stress between body weight and central adiposity in adults...

Last, there were no significant relationships found between psychological stress and cortisol and between depressive symptoms and cortisol. This finding is inconsistent with other studies (Dockray, Susman, & Dorn, 2009; Francis, Granger, & Susman, 2013) who found that depressive symptoms were associated with increased cortisol and psychological stress linked to cortisol elevations in children." (Lynch et al., 2019, pp. 46–47)

IDENTIFICATION OF LIMITATIONS THROUGH EXAMINATION OF DESIGN VALIDITY

Limitations of a study may include the scope and its methodology but are essentially validity-based limitations to generalizations of the findings. It is critical for the development of science and EBP that limitations are acknowledged (Kazdin, 2017; Ioannidis, 2007; Shadish et al., 2002). The suggested language in research reports and critical appraisals is "limitation," not "weakness" or "shortcoming," because limitations address usefulness instead of impaired worth. There are four elements of design validity: construct validity, internal validity, external validity, and statistical conclusion validity (see Chapters 10 and 11). These types of design validity should be examined for a study before writing the Discussion section of the research report. Table 26.4 identifies some common types of limitations or threats to these types of design validity. In the following sections, each type of design validity is reviewed and applied to the Lynch et al. (2019) study.

Construct Validity Limitations

Construct validity issues involve whether or not a central study concept was operationalized, or made measurable, in the way that best represented the concept's presence or range of values (Kazdin, 2017; Shadish et al., 2002). Threats to construct validity may be due to faulty reasoning that occurs when the

researcher selects measurements for study variables (see Table 26.4). However, measurement options for some concepts and constructs are limited, and the researcher must make trade-offs and select the most feasible instrument or method to measure a study variable from the available options.

For purposes of writing the Discussion section, instrument validity is considered a subtype of construct validity, because it reflects operationalization of variables. If the validity of an instrument is poor, this is a construct validity limitation because the instrument did not measure what it was intended to measure (see Chapter 16) (Waltz et al., 2017). If the reliability of an instrument is poor, a different problem is present: The instrument's exact values cannot be trusted. However, when the range of error of an instrument with poor reliability can be determined, meaningful statistical analysis based on broad categories of value instead of exact values is still possible.

Lynch et al. (2019) provided a detailed description of the FBS and Children's Depression Inventory (CDI) that were used in their study, which were introduced in Table 26.1. Consent was obtained from the participants' parents and assent from the participants. Following the consent process, demographic information was collected from the parents. Validity and reliability for the scales used to measure psychological stress and depressive symptoms are addressed in the following study excerpt. The different types of validity and reliability are italicized or identified in brackets.

TABLE 26.4	The Four Elements of Design Validity—Their Impact on Limitations	
Element of Design Validity	**General Underlying Flaw or Threat**	**Relationship to Limitations**
Construct validity	Inaccurate operationalization; measurement irregularities	Results and findings related to the poorly operationalized or poorly measured construct are flawed and may be invalid.
Internal validity	Failure to measure the effect of, or control for, extraneous variables' effects	Hypothesis-testing results may be inapplicable to the concepts studied. Descriptive tests may be valid.
External validity	Population not well represented by the sample	Results pertain to a subset of the population similar in geographical location, language, gender, age, race, underlying health system, and sometimes all of these.
Statistical conclusion validity	Inappropriate statistical test (rarely identified); inadequate sample size	Sample size, because if statistically significant results were not achieved, the research generates no empirical evidence.

"Psychological Stress

Psychological stress was conceptualized as events or situations that the children perceived as stressful [content validity] and was measured by the Feel Bad Scale (FBS) (Lewis, Siegel, & Lewis, 1984).... Lewis et al. (1984) reported the ratings of internal consistency of coefficient alpha at 0.82 in a sample of ethnically diverse group of children, and factor analysis supported construct validity of the FBS. In this study, the Cronbach's alpha coefficient was 0.89 [internal consistency].

Depressive Symptoms

Depressive symptoms were measured by The Children's Depression Inventory (CDI).... The instrument encompasses cognitive, affective, and behavioral functioning of depression. Each item describes a depressive symptom such as disturbance in mood, sleep, appetite, or interpersonal relationships [content validity]. Scores range from 0 to 52 with higher scores indicating increasing depressive symptoms. A cutoff score of 13 has been suggested to indicate children with mild depressive symptoms [predictive validity] and a cutoff of 19 to denote children with severe symptoms [predictive validity] (Kovacs, 1992). In previous studies, the alpha coefficients for *internal consistency* ranged from 0.74 to 0.83 (Kovacs, 1992). The alpha coefficient for this sample was 0.90 [internal consistency]." (Lynch et al., 2019, p. 44)

Lynch et al. (2019) reported that the internal consistency reliability of both scales was adequate based on previous research and very strong in this study with a Cronbach's alpha of 0.89 for the FBS and 0.90 for the CDI. A limitation of the study is the lack of construct validity evidence for the FBS and CDI scales from previous studies. A construct validity strength is that both scales were developed to measure psychological stress and depressive symptoms in children.

The variables height, weight, waist circumference, and cortisol were measured using physiological methods and biophysical instruments (Stone & Frazier, 2017). The precision and accuracy of these measures (Ryan-Wenger, 2017) are presented in the following study excerpt.

"Height and Weight

Height was measured to the nearest ¼ inch using a portable stadiometer, and weight was measured to the nearest ¼ pound by use of a freestanding balance beam scale according to established recommendations by Heyward and Wagner (2004). Measurements were converted to metric units for analyses. BMI was calculated based on the following formula: weight in kilograms (kg) divided by the square of height in meters (m²), with overweight defined as a BMI in the 85th to 94th percentile and obesity defined as a BMI at or above the 95th percentile (Centers for Disease Control and Prevention, 2015).

Waist Circumference

WC, an indicator of central adiposity, was measured according to protocol by Heyward and Wagner (2004). WC was measured twice to the nearest 1/16 in. and converted to centimeters. An average reading from the two measurements was calculated. Anthropometric reference data to include WC percentiles established from the NHANES (National Health and Nutrition Examination Survey) studies based on age and sex were used in analysis (Fryar, Gu, Ogden, & Flegal, 2016).

Cortisol

Salivary specimens for cortisol were obtained using the passive drool method and collected at mid-morning (9:30 AM–11:00 AM), at least one hour after breakfast and prior to lunch, to potentially minimize circadian variability and standardize the collection time. The collection, transfer, and storage of saliva specimens followed the Parameter Cortisol Assay protocol (R & D Systems, 2012) and the literature (Hanneman, Cox, Green, & Kang, 2011). Cortisol level was determined by a standard two-step sandwich enzyme-linked immunosorbent assay (ELISA) using commercially prepared high-sensitivity kits (R & D Systems, MN, USA). To help ensure intra-assay accurateness, samples were assayed in duplicate. The assay sensitivity for salivary cortisol was 0.07 ng/ml and mean intra- and inter-assay coefficients of variation were 6.9% and 13.6%, respectively, indicating high sensitivity and precision." (Lynch et al., 2019, pp. 44–45)

Height and weight were measured with quality equipment according to established recommendations to promote precision and accuracy (Ryan-Wenger, 2017). For example, height was measured to the nearest 0.25 inch and weight to the nearest 0.25 pound to ensure precision and accuracy of the measures. WC was measured twice according to the study protocol to the nearest 0.0625 inch, ensuring accuracy and precision of this measurement. National standards were used to establish the WC percentiles for the participants.

Cortisol levels were determined using precisely collected salivary specimens, and the specimens were collected, transferred, and stored according to national protocol. The cortisol levels were determined according to a standardized process with high-sensitivity kits. Lynch et al. (2019) detailed the steps taken to ensure sensitivity and precision of the cortisol levels. In summary, the quality measurement methods that were consistently implemented in this study provided strength to the construct validity of the study findings.

Construct Validity Problems With Study Implementation

In studies with an intervention, problems with implementation can cause validity issues. Intervention fidelity is one of these. Did the research team implement the intervention the same way every time, thereby achieving intervention fidelity (Kazdin, 2017; Melnyk & Fineout-Overholt, 2019)? If not, construct validity related to the intervention might be a limitation. The intervention is defined in a certain way at the beginning of the study (see Chapter 6) and establishes the way the independent variable should be enacted throughout the study (see Chapter 11).

Sometimes data collection does not proceed as planned, and unforeseen situations alter the collection of data (see Chapter 20). This is a problem of construct validity when the variables are not measured as planned for all study subjects. What is the effect if one subject completes the instruments at home and another completes them at the community center before a support group? What is the effect if one day during the study, the BP is measured using a different machine than is used the other days of the study? Lynch et al. (2019) stressed that data were collected in a consistent way from parents and their children using established recommendations and protocols to ensure accuracy and precision of the physiological measures and reliability of the scales. The detailed, structured collection of data in this study reduced the potential for construct validity limitations.

Internal Validity Limitations

Internal validity is the extent to which the researcher controls for the effect of extraneous variables in the design or methods of a study. Extraneous variables are those that might affect the value of dependent or outcome variables and are neither controlled for nor measured in the study design (see Table 26.4). Internal validity influences the confidence researchers can have that the intervention caused the difference in the

outcome variable, as opposed to some other factor (Kazdin, 2017; Leedy & Ormrod, 2919). Sample selection, method of subject assignment to group if applicable, and timing of measurements, among other decisions, can also introduce extraneous variables in both interventional and noninterventional studies. Depending on design, the researcher may control for the most powerful of the apparent extraneous variables before the study begins (see Chapter 6). However, there are dozens of potentially extraneous variables, and the researcher can control only for a small number of them in the design phase (Kazdin, 2017). Because internal validity issues occur most often in intervention research, every attempt is made to control extraneous variables related to the study intervention, measurement methods, sampling process, and setting (Leedy & Ormrod, 2019). Lynch et al. (2019) conducted a noninterventional correlational study that did not include a discussion of extraneous variables. However, the researchers did identify the limitation of collecting a saliva specimen only once from each study participant at a designated time. They recommended that repeated saliva specimens be collected at different times in future studies to expand the understanding of the children's cortisol levels.

External Validity Limitations

External validity is the extent to which study results are generalizable to the target population. The way a sample is selected is the largest determinant of the research's eventual external validity (Kazdin, 2017; Shadish et al., 2002). External validity is strongest for studies with large, randomly selected samples, and it is still stronger when that sample is drawn from many different sites (see Table 26.4). Is the sample representative of the target population for the variable of interest? When a researcher reports the results of a study conducted with a nonrandomly obtained sample, it strengthens the external validity of the results when the researcher can provide population demographics and demonstrate that the sample demographics are markedly similar to those of the entire population.

Lynch and colleagues (2019) selected their study participants using a sample of convenience. All students aged 10 to 12 years from three schools in a rural setting were invited to participate in the study. Attrition is nonapplicable because the study included a one-time data collection; however, the refusal rate should have been addressed but was not (see Chapter 15). Participants were recruited from one middle school and three elementary schools in a rural southeastern city. The sample was predominately Caucasian (67.3%) with a limited percentage of African Americans (11.6%) and Hispanics (17.7%). Therefore the nonrandom sampling process, single rural setting, and race/ethnicity distribution decreased the external validity of the study and limited the generalizability of the findings. Key study limitations are presented in the following study excerpt.

> *"Limitations*
> Several limitations must be considered. The study was conducted in one school system in the southeastern U.S. Although African American and Hispanic children were represented in the study, the sample included a majority of Caucasian children, and the study was not powered to examine differences based on race/ethnicity or sex. Studies in other geographic locations may generate different results, which limits generalizability…
>
> Because the study design was cross-sectional, and data were collected at one point in time, no causal relationships among the variables can be concluded. Thus, it is possible that the directions of psychological stress and depressive symptoms with body mass and central adiposity are reversed. Similar studies with larger, more diverse samples conducted over time may help to inform what underlying mechanism contribute to the development of increased body mass and central adiposity." (Lynch et al., 2019, p. 47)

Statistical Conclusion Validity Limitations

Statistical conclusion validity involves examining the adequacy of the sample size and the researchers' decisions regarding the statistical analyses conducted in a study (see Table 26.4). Lynch et al. (2019) conducted a prior power analysis that indicated a sample size of 136 participants was adequate to address the research questions but not to examine subgroups created by gender or ethnicity. The sample size of the study was small ($n = 147$) for a predictive correlational study design and limited the analyses that could be performed (Aberson, 2019; Grove & Cipher, 2020). In addition, the nonsignificant or negative results, such as those for the relationships between psychological stress and BMI, WC, and cortisol levels and between depression symptoms and cortisol levels, might have resulted from the limited sample size. When negative results are obtained, the researcher needs to conduct a post hoc power analysis to determine whether the study had sufficient power to detect relationships or differences that were present. If the power of the study was .80 or greater, the reader could have increased confidence that the nonsignificant results were accurate (Aberson, 2019). Lynch et al. (2019) did not report a post hoc power analysis for the nonsignificant results; thus the limited sample size might have resulted in a Type II error (Grove & Cipher, 2020).

Error intrudes in all measurement (Kazdin, 2017; Waltz et al., 2017) and, subsequently, additional errors occur during the processes of data management and analysis. Choosing the correct statistical test is critical during the planning of the study, and consultation with a biostatistician is recommended. Continuing consultation with the biostatistician during data analysis is also recommended to ensure that the data meet the assumptions of the selected tests and missing data are handled appropriately. The Grove and Cipher (2020) text provides an algorithm with detailed explanations and examples to assist you in selecting appropriate statistical techniques when conducting data analyses. In their text, George and Mallery (2019) provide the steps for conducting analyses using the IBM Statistical Package for Social Sciences (SPSS) program. Lynch et al. (2019) did not provide information about how missing data were handled, but their structured process for collecting physiological data and data from self-report questionnaires implied that few, if any, data were missing. However, three of the saliva specimens were inadequate for analysis, so cortisol levels for 144 participants were included in the analysis of cortisol data.

Before submitting a study for publication, each analysis reported in the paper should be double-checked, and the interpretations of the statistical analyses closely examined. Documentation for each statistical value or analysis statement reported in the paper is filed with a copy of the article. The documentation includes the date of the analyses, the page number of the computer printout showing the results or the electronic file containing the output of the statistical analyses, the sample size for each analysis, and the number of missing values (see Chapters 20 and 21) (Grove & Cipher, 2020). The following excerpt from Lynch et al. (2019) describes their data analyses.

"Analysis
To address the research questions, SPSS (Statistical Package for Social Sciences) 23.0 (IBM Corp., Armonk, NY) was used to calculate descriptive statistics including means, standard deviations, and ranges. Bivariate correlation using Pearson's product-moment correlation was used to address the first research question, and hierarchical multiple regression analyses were used to address the second research question. For research question three, based on the principles of the mediation model proposed by Baron and Kenny (1986), simple linear regression and multiple regression analyses were planned. Cortisol is deemed to function as a mediator a) if there is a significant relationship between the independent variables and the hypothesized mediator; b) if there is a significant relationship between the independent variables and the dependent variables and; c) if there is a significant relationship between the hypothesized mediator and the independent variables." (Lynch et al., 2019, p. 45)

The data analysis section clearly identified the analysis software package used and types of analyses conducted to address each of the research questions. Because the relationships between cortisol levels and the independent and dependent variables were not significant, cortisol was not considered a mediator between these variables. The Results section was strengthened by including the specific significant results and the significance level (p) for the Pearson correlation and regression analyses results.

GENERALIZING THE FINDINGS

Generalization extends the implications of the findings from the sample studied to a larger population or from the situation studied to similar situations, within the limitations imposed by design validity issues (see Chapters 10 and 11). It is important to note that some generalization may be possible in the presence of limitations to both internal and external validity. However, in the presence of multiple limitations, generalizability is limited to the sample and accessible population (Kazdin, 2017; Leedy & Ormrod, 2019).

Table 26.5 summarizes the links of the design validity flaws or limitations to the generalization of study findings. When the measurement of a construct is flawed, the study findings related to the construct also are flawed. As a result, no generalizations of findings related to the flawed construct or constructs should be made (Shadish et al., 2002). An internal validity limitation must be considered in terms of both variables and study outcome. The design selected or the implementation of the study did not control for extraneous factors adequately. For example, members of a control group are inadvertently provided the study intervention, or the setting for the study undergoes a change in ownership during a study of nurse satisfaction. These threats to internal validity should be noted in the limitations section of the research report, and they directly affect the extent to which the findings can be generalized. When external validity is limited, generalization can always be

TABLE 26.5	**The Four Elements of Design Validity—Generalization**	
Element of Design Validity	**Underlying Threat to Design Validity**	**Relationship to Generalization**
Construct validity	Inaccurate operationalization; measurement irregularities	No generalizations using the poorly operationalized or poorly measured construct(s) can be made.
Internal validity	Failure to measure the effect of, or control for, extraneous variables' effects	Generalization must be made conditionally, so as to include possible effects of the extraneous variable.
External validity	Population not well represented by the sample	Cautious generalization to other samples or groups who have similar demographic characteristics.
Statistical conclusion validity	Inappropriate statistical test (rarely identified); inadequate sample size	No empirical evidence was generated, but if the results show "trends," they can inform the reader.

made back to the sample itself and possibly to other groups at the same or similar sites, with similar demographic characteristics (see Table 26.5). For limitations to statistical conclusion validity that involve inadequate sample size, no generalizations related to the research question can be made.

Generalizations apply to the current study findings, in conjunction with previous studies in the same area. For instance, an interventional study comparing toothbrushing and plaque-removal focused toothbrushing in intubated patients in the intensive care unit builds upon recent literature comparing various styles of oral hygiene for their effectiveness in reducing bacterial overgrowth. Because there is extensive evidence already in this problem area, cautious generalization of findings could be made based on the study results and the evidence provided by other studies. Generalizations like these, based on accumulated evidence from many studies, are called **empirical generalizations**. These generalizations are important for verifying hypotheses and theoretical statements and can contribute to development of new theories. Empirical generalizations are foundational to scientific discovery and, within nursing, provide a basis for generating evidence-based guidelines to manage specific practice problems (Melnyk & Fineout-Overholt, 2019). Chapter 19 provides a detailed discussion of research synthesis processes and strategies for promoting evidence-based nursing practice.

How far can generalizations be made? The answer to this question is debatable. From a narrow perspective, one cannot really generalize from the sample with which the study was conducted because samples differ from the population. The conservative position, represented by Kerlinger and Lee (2000), recommends caution in considering the extent of generalization. Conservatives consider generalization particularly risky if the sample was small, homogeneous, and not randomly selected (Kandola, Banner, O'Keefe-McCarthy, & Jassal, 2014; Kazdin, 2017).

The less conservative view allows generalization from the sample to the accessible population (the population from which the sample was drawn) if the population demographics are essentially the same as those of the sample. If an intervention is effective in an outpatient clinic that sees only three or four subjects with a certain disorder each week, it will most likely continue to be effective in the same clinic with subsequent outpatients. In practice, this is exactly what occurs. If an intervention

seems to work, it is continued at the same site. If the researchers publish their findings, by the time the study is published, other outpatients will have been treated as well, producing more results that may contradict or strengthen the findings.

The least conservative view also considers what will be generalized and the implications of false generalization. For example, single-site small-sample study is conducted to test the intervention of having a 1-minute strategic planning session with the patient early in the shift, so that the patient is aware of the nurse's plans for tasks to be completed, and the nurse is aware of the patient's planned activities for the shift. The dependent variables are complaints, amount of sleep, and morning glucose values. If the research demonstrates that, for this sample, the intervention resulted in fewer complaints, more sleep, and more in-range morning glucose values, what would be the generalization potential of the research?

This intervention is benign, cost-free, and takes very little of the nurse's time. The intervention is also consistent with nursing theories and can be classified as a socially appropriate step toward involving the patient in care. If a Type I error occurred in the research and the intervention was in actuality ineffective, what would be the implications of false generalization? The least conservative view might recommend this intervention in a research report based on related literature on patient involvement in care and on the low risk of making a false generalization relate to the intervention.

Lynch et al. (2019) conducted a predictive correlational study in a relatively new area focused on examining the relationships of psychosocial factors (psychological stress and depressive symptoms) to health outcomes (BMI and central adiposity) with mediation by the physiological factor, cortisol (see Fig. 26.1). This conceptual framework was not supported by the study findings. The researchers did not recommend generalization of their findings for a variety of reasons. As discussed earlier, the nonrandom sampling method, predominately Caucasian sample, and relatively small sample size limited the generalizability of the findings (Lynch et al., 2019). The researchers recommended additional studies with a larger sample size to determine the potential for generalization of the findings. In addition, the collection of saliva specimens was a limitation, and additional research is needed to determine the relationships between psychological stress and depressive symptoms and cortisol levels.

Therefore the researchers' conservative approach to generalization is appropriate.

CONSIDERING IMPLICATIONS FOR PRACTICE, THEORY, AND KNOWLEDGE

Implications of research findings for nursing are the meanings of the results for the body of nursing knowledge and practice. As with generalizations, implications for practice can be summative, including both the current study and related literature in the same area of evidence. Implications for practices are often based, in part, on whether treatment decisions or outcomes would be different in view of the study findings (Kazdin, 2017; Melnyk & Fineout-Overholt, 2019).

In terms of practice, implications can be drawn from any part of the study findings, descriptive or inferential, but they must arise from those findings, not merely from general principles of nursing practice. The researcher must be cautious and base the implications on the findings. This legitimate identification of implications includes generalizations for teaching or early intervention when description of subjects includes knowledge deficits or potential for harm. Such is the case for Lynch et al.'s (2019) identified implications for practice, which focused on the expanding problems of depression and childhood obesity. To address these problems, Lynch et al. (2019) recommended regular screening for depressive symptoms and assessment of children's BMI and WC to identify overweight and obese children. The following study excerpt presents the practice implications identified in this study.

"Practice Implications
Given that the participants in this study reported psychological stress and depressive symptoms regardless of elevations in BMI and WC, it would be important to address such psychological issues in children beginning early in childhood. It is important to promote regular screening for depressive symptoms and psychological stress in children within primary prevention assessments by healthcare professionals. Although it may be beneficial to assign school nurses to assess depressive symptoms in the school setting, it may not be feasible to expect that every school will employ a full-time nurse to screen children or that the nurses would have time to perform screenings. Should evidence

emerge that psychological stress or depressive symptoms lead to obesity in children, this may open new strategical approaches in reducing overweight and obesity. In addition, nurses can play an essential role in educating clinicians that both BMI and WC need to be included at child well visits. Incorporating body composition measurements such as BMI and WC may provide valuable monitoring of children over time and provides opportunities for early intervention in overweight and obese prevention." (Lynch et al., 2019, p. 47)

Implications for knowledge development exist in practically all research that generates valid findings. Each study, even if its findings are all negative ones, contributes to the body of knowledge in the discipline.

SUGGESTING FURTHER RESEARCH

Examining a study's implications and generalizations should culminate in **recommendations for further research** that emerge from the present study and from previous studies in the same area of interest. In every study, the researcher gains knowledge and experience that can be used to design a better study next time. Formulating recommendations for future studies will stimulate you to define more clearly how your study might have been improved.

These recommendations must also take into consideration the design validity-related limitations identified in the current study. For instance, if construct validity was seriously flawed, further research recommendations might include redesigning the research and conducting it again, not replicating it, because a replication would include the same flawed operational definition (Kazdin, 2017). If negative findings and low power indicate the possibility of a Type II error, recommending repeating the study with a larger sample may be appropriate (Aberson, 2019; Kazdin, 2017). However, if other factors contributed to statistical conclusion validity, the study should be redesigned and these limitations corrected prior to repeating the study.

Recommendations for further research related to internal validity limitations might include a different type of design that eliminates subjects with the extraneous variable of concern, matches subjects in intervention and control groups with respect to the variable, or measures the effects of extraneous variables (see Chapters 10 and 11). The researcher is in the best position to make suggestions as to how an important extraneous variable might be controlled for in the design process (Kazdin, 2017; Leedy & Ormrod, 2019).

Recommendations for further research related to external validity limitations are specific to sample selection and number of sites used in the research. Recommendations for future studies should reverse those limitations, making the study stronger, larger, and more representative. When nonrandom sampling has been used, subsequent research with random sampling allows improved external validity. When a small, single-site sample has been used, further research with a larger sample, using two or more sites, improves external validity (see Chapter 15). Lynch et al. (2019) provided the following suggestions for further research, which were identified with the discussion of limitations.

> "Future studies need to include larger numbers of African American and Hispanic children to determine consistency of findings.... Because a diurnal rhythm exists in healthy individuals, dysregulation in cortisol secretion could not be established with one sample. Therefore, measurement of cortisol at different times will need to be considered for future studies. In addition, psychological stress and depressive symptoms need to be studied over time to determine whether blunted cortisol effects or some dysregulation of the HPA [hypothalamic-pituitary-adrenal] axis is occurring." (Lynch et al., 2019, p. 47)

FORMING FINAL CONCLUSIONS

Conclusions are derived from the study findings and are a synthesis of what the researcher deems the most important findings. Preliminary conclusions are formed when the output of data analyses is reviewed, but they are refined during the process of interpretation. Most researchers provide a summary of their conclusions at the end of the research report. As the researchers' last word on the topic, it is the most likely aspect of the paper to be remembered by the reader.

One of the risks in developing conclusions in research is going beyond the data—specifically, forming conclusions that the data do not warrant, as noted related to causality. Going beyond the data may be due to faulty logic or preconceived ideas and allowing personal biases to influence the conclusions. When forming conclusions, it is important to remember that research never proves anything; rather, research offers support for a position when the study design and statistical analyses were appropriate. A common flaw in logic occurs when the researcher finds statistically significant relationships between A and B by correlational analysis and then concludes that A causes B. This conclusion is inaccurate because a correlational study does not examine causality (Grove & Cipher, 2020). Another example of a flawed conclusion occurs when the researcher tests the causal statement that *A causes B* and finds statistical support for the statement under the study's conditions. It is inappropriate to state that, absolutely, in all situations, a causal relationship exists between A and B. This conclusion cannot be scientifically proven. A more credible conclusion is to state the conditional probabilities of a causal relationship. For example, stating that if A occurs, then B occurs under conditions x, y, and z is more appropriate (Kazdin, 2017; Kerlinger & Lee, 2000; Shadish et al., 2002). Another way to appropriately state the conclusion is that if A occurs, then B has an 80% probability of occurring.

The conclusions developed by Lynch and colleagues (2019) were appropriate based on the study findings, limitations, and implications for practice. These conclusions focused on screening children for depressive symptoms and monitoring them for overweight and obesity.

> **"Conclusions**
> Overweight and obesity as measured by BMI and WC were evident in the majority of children in this sample. This is of concern as obesity and overweight in children track to adulthood and are associated with chronic diseases such as diabetes, cardiovascular disease, and cancer. Further, more than one-third of children in this sample, no matter weight status, reported depressive symptoms, something not reported previously in the literature (Benson, Williams, & Novick, 2012). Depressive symptoms can impact academic achievement, interpersonal relationships, and potentially result in thoughts of self-harm or suicide and is a factor in the development of chronic diseases, such as cardiovascular disease. It is essential then to assess not only depressive symptoms but also overweight and obesity during this crucial developmental period. If depressive symptoms are noted, school nurses need to make referrals for further assessment and possible treatment." (Lynch et al., 2019, p. 47)

Going beyond the data occurs more frequently in published studies than one would like to believe. Be sure to check the validity of your logic related to the conclusions before disseminating your findings.

KEY POINTS

- Interpretation of research outcomes requires reflection upon three general aspects of the research and their interactions: the primary findings, validity issues, and the resultant body of knowledge in the area of investigation.
- Interpretation includes several intellectual activities, such as examining evidence, forming conclusions, identifying study limitations, generalizing the findings, considering implications, and suggesting further research.
- The first step in interpretation is examining all of the evidence available that supports or contradicts the validity of the results. Evidence is obtained from various sources, including the research plan, measurement reliability and validity (or physiological measures' precision and accuracy), data collection process, data analysis process, data analysis results, and previous studies.
- The outcomes of data analysis are the most direct evidence available of the results related to the research purpose and the objectives, questions, or hypotheses.
- Five possible results are (1) significant results that are in keeping with those predicted by the researcher, (2) nonsignificant results, (3) significant results that are opposite those predicted by the researcher, (4) mixed results, and (5) serendipitous results.

- Findings are a consequence of evaluating evidence, which includes the findings from previous studies.
- Conclusions are derived from the findings and are a synthesis of the findings.
- Limitations may be related to threats to construct validity, internal validity, external validity, and statistical conclusion validity. Each aspect of validity should be clearly identified and discussed in relation to the conclusions of the study.
- The limitations of a study decrease the generalizability of the findings.
- Generalization extends the implications of the findings from the sample studied to a larger target population.
- Implications of the study for nursing are the meanings of study conclusions for the body of nursing knowledge, theory, and practice.
- Completion of a study and examination of implications should culminate in recommending further studies that emerge from the present study and previous studies.
- The conclusions are a summary of your most important study findings. Use caution to not go beyond what you found; however, emphasize one or two main findings you want the reader to remember.

REFERENCES

Aberson, C. L. (2019). *Applied power analysis for the behavioral sciences* (2nd ed.). New York, NY: Routledge Taylor & Francis Group.

Baron, R., & Kenny, D. (1986). The moderator-mediator variable distinction in social psychological research: Conceptual, strategic, and statistical considerations. *Journal of Personality and Social Psychology, 51*, 1173–1182. doi:10.1037/0022-3514.51.6.1173

Benson, L., Williams, R., & Novick, M. (2012). Pediatric obesity and depression: A cross-sectional analysis of absolute BMI as it relates to children's depression index scores in obese 7- to 17-year-old children. *Clinical Pediatrics, 52*(1), 24–29. doi:10.1177/0009922812459949

Braet, C., Vlierberghe, L. V., Vandevivere, E., Theuwis, L., & Bosmans, G. (2012). Depression in early, middle, and late adolescence: Differential evidence for the cognitive diathesis-stress model. *Clinical Psychology & Psychotherapy, 25*(5), 369–383. doi:10.1002/cpp.1789

Brumby, S., Kennedy, A., & Chandrasekara, A. (2013). Alcohol consumption, obesity, and psychological distress in farming communities—an Australian study. *Journal of Rural Health, 29*, 311–319. doi:10.1111/jrh.1201

Centers for Disease Control and Prevention. (2015). *Body mass index*. Retrieved from https://www.cdc.gov/healthyweight/assessing/bmi/index.html

Centers for Disease Control and Prevention. (2018). Childhood obesity facts. Retrieved from https://www.cdc.gov/healthyschools/obesity/facts.htm

Chu, L., Sheng, K., Liu, P., Ye, K., Wang, Y., Li, C., et al. (2017). Increased cortisol levels and cortisone levels in overweight children. *Medical Science Monitor Basic Research, 23*, 25–30. doi:10.12659/msmbr.902707

Creswell, J., & Creswell, J. D. (2018). *Research design: Qualitative, quantitative, and mixed methods approaches* (5th ed.). Los Angeles, CA: Sage.

Dockray, S., Susman, E. J., & Dorn, L. D. (2009). Depression, cortisol reactivity, and obesity in childhood and adolescence. *Journal of Adolescent Health, 45*(4), 344–350. doi:10.1016/j.jadohealth.2009.06.014

Francis, L. A., Granger, D. A., & Susman, E. J. (2013). Adreno-cortical regulation, eating in the absence of hunger and BMI in young children. *Appetite, 64*(1), 32–38. doi:10.1016/j.appwt.2012.11.008

Fryar, C. D., Carroll, M. D., & Ogden, C. L. (2016). *Prevalence of overweight and obesity among children and adolescents aged 2–19 years: United States, 1963–1965 through 2013–2014.* Retrieved from https://www.cdc.gov/nchs/data/hestat/obesity_child_13_14/obesity_child_13_14.pdf

Fryar, C. D., Gu, Q., Ogden, C. L., & Flegal, K. M. (2016). *Anthropometric reference data for children and adults: United States, 2011–2014.* Washington, DC: US Government Printing Office.

George, D., & Mallery, P. (2019). *IBM SPSS statistics 25 step by step: A simple guide and reference* (15th ed.). New York, NY: Taylor & Francis.

Grove, S. K., & Cipher, D. J. (2020). *Statistics for nursing research: A workbook for evidence-based practice* (3rd ed.). St. Louis, MO: Elsevier.

Hales, C. M., Fryar, C. D., Carroll, M. D., Freedman, D. S., & Ogden, C. L. (2018). Trends in obesity prevalence in US youth and adults by sex and age, 2007-2008 to 2015-2016. *Journal of the American Medical Association, 319*(16), 1723–1725. doi:10.1001/jama.2018.3060

Hanneman, S. K., Cox, C. D., Green, K. E., & Kang, D. (2011). Estimating intra- and interassay variability in salivary cortisol. *Biological Research for Nursing, 13*, 243–250. doi:10.1177/1099800411404061

Heyward, V., & Wagner, D. (2004). *Applied composition assessment* (2nd ed.). Champaign, IL: Human Kinetics.

Higgins, J. P. T., & Thomas, J. (2020). *Cochrane handbook for systematic reviews of interventions* (2nd ed.). West Sussex, England: Wiley Cochrane Series.

Ioannidis, J. (2007). Limitations are not properly acknowledged in the scientific literature. *Journal of Clinical Epidemiology, 60*(4), 324–329. doi:10.1016/j.jclinepi.2006.09011

Kandola, D., Banner, D., O'Keefe-McCarthy, S., & Jassal, D. (2014). Sampling methods in cardiovascular nursing research: An overview. *Canadian Journal of Cardiovascular Nursing, 24*(3), 15–18.

Kazdin, A. E. (2017). *Research design in clinical psychology* (5th ed.). Boston, MA: Pearson.

Kerlinger, F. N., & Lee, H. P. (2000). *Foundations of behavioral research* (4th ed.). Fort Worth, TX: Harcourt College.

Kleinpell, R. M. (2017). *Outcome assessment in advanced practice nursing* (4th ed.). New York, NY: Springer.

Kovacs, M. (1992). *Children's depression inventory manual.* North Tonawanda, NY: Multi-Health Systems, Inc.

Leedy, P. D., & Ormrod, J. E. (2019). *Practical research: Planning and design* (12th ed.). New York, NY: Pearson.

Lewis, C. E., Siegel, J. M., & Lewis, M. A. (1984). Feeling bad: Exploring sources of distress among pre-adolescent children. *American Journal of Public Health, 74*, 117–122. doi:10.2105/ajph.74.2.117

Lynch, T., Azuero, A., Lochman, J. E., Park, N., Turner-Henson, A., & Rice, M. (2019). The influence of psychological stress, depressive symptoms, and cortisol on body mass and central adiposity in 10-to-12-year-old children. *Journal of Pediatric Nursing, 44*(1), 42–49. doi:10.1016/j.pedn.2018.10.007

Mazurka, R., Wynne-Edwards, K. E., & Harkness, K. L. (2016). Stressful life events prior to depression onset and cortisol response to stress in youth with first onset versus recurrent depression. *Journal of Abnormal Child Psychology, 44*(6), 1173–1184. doi:10.1007/s10802-015-0103-y

Melnyk, B. M., & Fineout-Overholt, E. (2019). *Evidence-based practice in nursing and healthcare: A guide to best practice* (4th ed.). Philadelphia, PA: Wolters Kluwer.

National Survey of Children's Health (NSCH). (2016). *Child and adolescent health measurement initiative.* Data Resource Center for Child and Adolescent Health. Retrieved from www.childhealthdata.org

R & D Systems. (2012). *Parameter cortisol assay.* Retrieved from https://resources.rndsystems.com/pdfs/datasheets/kge008.pdf

Roberts, C., Troop, N., Connan, F., Treasure, J., & Campbell, I. C. (2007). The effects of stress on body weight: Biological and psychological predictors of change in BMI. *Obesity, 15*(12), 3045–3055. doi:10.1038/oby.2007.363

Ryan-Wenger, N. A. (2017). Precision, accuracy, and uncertainty of biophysical measurements for research and practice. In C. F. Waltz, O. L. Strickland, & E. R. Lenz (Eds.), *Measurement in nursing and health research* (5th ed., pp. 427–445). New York, NY: Springer.

Shadish, W. R., Cook, T. D., & Campbell, D. T. (2002). *Experimental and quasi-experimental designs for generalization causal inference.* Chicago, IL: Rand McNally.

Singh, G. K., Kogan, M. D., & van Dyck, P. C. (2010). Changes in state-specific childhood obesity and overweight prevalence in the United States from 2003 to 2007. *Archives of Pediatrics and Adolescent Medicine, 164*(7), 598–607. doi:10.1001/archpediatrics.2010.84

Stone, K. S., & Frazier, S. K. (2017). Measurement of physiological variables using biomedical instrumentation.

In C. F. Waltz, O. L. Strickland, & E. R. Lenz (Eds.), *Measurement in nursing and health research* (5th ed., pp. 379–424). New York, NY: Springer.

Teixeira da Silva, J. (2015). Negative results: Negative perceptions limit their potential for increasing reproducibility. *Journal of Negative Results in Biomedicine, 14*, 12. doi:1186/s12952-015-0033-9

Waltz, C. F., Strickland, O. L., & Lenz, E. R. (2017). *Measurement in nursing and health research* (5th ed.). New York, NY: Springer.

Xi, B., Mi, J., Zhao, M., Zhang, T., Jia, C., Li, J., ... Steffen, L. (2014). Trends in abdominal obesity among US children and adolescents. *Pediatrics, 134*(2), e334–e339. doi:10.1542/peds.2014-0970

27

Disseminating Research Findings

Suzanne Sutherland

http://evolve.elsevier.com/Gray/practice/

The study is now complete, and the researcher breathes a sigh of relief. After completing a study, the researcher may feel unskilled in presenting the information and overwhelmed by the idea of publishing. Or perhaps the graduate student is so exhausted by the labor-intensive process of completing a thesis or dissertation that dissemination of the findings beyond the academic requirements is delayed. The study documents are placed in a drawer with the intent to communicate the findings later. Someday, when there's more time to tackle the writing needed to submit the results for conference presentation or to create a whole article. Then time passes, and dissemination becomes less and less a priority.

Whether caused by lack of knowledge, feelings of inadequacy, fatigue, or competing priorities, findings of valuable nursing studies often are not communicated outside the research team, and the benefit of the knowledge gained is lost to the world. Failure to communicate research findings may be considered a failure to fulfill the promise to subjects that their input would be used to increase knowledge and benefit others with the same condition. After involving members of an institutional review board (IRB) committee to approve your study and after subjects consented and participated in your study, you have an ethical obligation to complete the process. When researchers do not disseminate, the valuable resources of time, funding, and data are wasted. And you owe it to yourself to publish the results of your hard work.

Communicating research findings, the final step in the research process, involves developing a research report and disseminating study findings through presentations and publications to audiences of nurses, healthcare professionals, policymakers, and healthcare consumers. The most usual methods of dissemination are presentations at conferences and professional meetings, and publication of findings in professional research journals (Hanneke & Link, 2019).

Disseminating findings provides many advantages for the researcher, the nursing profession, and the consumer of nursing services. By presenting and publishing findings, researchers advance the knowledge particular to a given discipline, which is essential for providing evidence-based practice (EBP). For individual researchers, communicating study findings often leads to professional advancement and recognition as a researcher in one's field of specialization. By communicating findings, the researcher also promotes critical analysis of previous studies, encourages research replication, and identifies additional research problems. Over time, findings from many studies are synthesized with the ultimate goal of providing evidence-based health care to patients, families, and communities (Craig & Dowding, 2020; Melnyk & Fineout-Overholt, 2019).

To facilitate communication of research findings for nurse clinicians and researchers, this chapter describes the basic content of a written research report common to quantitative and qualitative studies. Differences in report content relative to the type of study will be identified. You will also learn about the different sections of a research report, how to select a journal in which to publish, and when and how to use tables and figures. Other types of dissemination will be described as well, such as presentations.

COMPONENTS OF A RESEARCH REPORT

A **research report** is the written description of a completed study designed to communicate study findings efficiently and effectively to nurses and other healthcare professionals. The information included in the report depends on the study, the intended audience, and the mechanisms chosen for dissemination. Usually, research reports include four major sections or content areas: (1) introduction that usually includes a literature review, (2) methods, (3) results, and (4) discussion of the findings (Pyrczak & Bruce, 2017). Box 27.1 contains a general outline for the content in each section.

Specific journals may require other sections, or your university might include other sections in the final thesis or dissertation report. Some journals limit the Introduction section to a brief review of the literature that identifies the gap in knowledge, a statement about the underlying theoretical framework, and the clear purpose of the study. Other journals may require a free-standing background section that includes the significance of the study and a review of literature. The Methods section describes how the study was implemented, including sampling, measurement methods, data collection, and data analysis. When preparing to publish the results of your thesis or dissertation in a professional journal, recognize the need to drastically reduce the content and revise the paper to fit the format and tone of the journal. The Results sections of reports for qualitative studies are usually longer than those of quantitative studies because of the inclusion of quotes from participants, but may include fewer tables than quantitative studies do. The Discussion section briefly identifies the limitations of the study, presents the findings in relation to other literature, and discusses the implications of the findings for the intended journal audience.

Title

The title of your research report must indicate what you have studied so as to attract the attention of interested readers. The title should be concise and consistent with the study purpose and the research objectives, questions, or hypotheses. A title may include the major study variables and population and the type of study conducted, but should not include the findings of a study (Pyrczak & Bruce, 2017). Some journals limit the length of manuscript titles; others discourage use of colons. The Public Library of Science ([PLOS], 2019) publishes several open-access, online scientific journals.

BOX 27.1   Outline for a Research Report

Introduction
- Background and significance of the problem
- Purpose of study
- Brief review of relevant literature (may include theoretical framework and conceptual definitions for quantitative studies and philosophical perspective for qualitative studies)
- Gap in knowledge the study will address
- Research objectives, questions, or hypotheses

Methods
- Research design
  Quantitative study: include intervention if applicable
  Qualitative study: approach to the study such as phenomenology, grounded theory, ethnography, or exploratory-descriptive qualitative research
- Setting
- Sampling method, consent process
- Human subject protections, including institutional review board (IRB) approval
- Data collection methods
  Quantitative studies: measurement with instrument descriptions and scoring
  Qualitative studies: interviews, observation, document analysis, focus groups
- Data collection process
- Data analysis

Results
- Description of sample (may use tables or figures)
- Presentation of results of data analysis
  Quantitative studies results: Organized by objectives, questions, or hypotheses
  Qualitative studies results: Organized by themes, cultural characteristics, or format specific to the methods
- Use narrative, tables, and figures to present results

Discussion
- Major findings compared with previous research
- Limitations of study
- Conclusions
- Implications for practice, education, or administration
- Future studies that are indicated, based on the remaining research gap

References
- Include references cited in paper, using format specified by journal

Their submission guidelines request that authors submit a long title of 250 characters or less and a short title of 100 characters or less. The *International Journal of Nursing Studies* (IJNS) website (IJNS, 2019) provides a specific format for manuscript titles. The title begins with the topic or question of the study. Following a colon, the subtitle includes the study method design or type of paper.

An example of a title for a mixed methods study is "Nursing teamwork in the care of older people: A mixed-methods study" (Anderson et al., 2019). The title identifies the design (mixed methods), the central concept (nursing teamwork), and the population (older people). This title might have been stronger, had it indicated that the researchers focused upon quality of care and the experience of teamwork. Adebiyi, Mosaku, Irinoye, and Oyelade's (2018) quantitative study was entitled "Socio-demographic and clinical factors associated with relapse in mental illness." The title for their report strongly implies the design (correlational) because of use of the word *associated*. The authors specified the primary outcome variable, relapse in mental illness, as it was predicted by sociodemographic and clinical factors, without revealing findings in the title, as recommended by Pyrczak & Bruce (2017). The authors did not specify multiple logistic regression in their title. Although the term is more specific for the type of correlational analysis performed, it may be quite off-putting for readers unfamiliar with statistical analyses. The aim is to interest potential readers without daunting them.

Abstract

The abstract of a study summarizes the key aspects of the study in 100 to 300 words and is the first component of a research report. Often scholars decide whether to read the full report on the basis of the abstract. In addition, submission to present a poster or oral presentation at a conference usually requires an abstract, written in keeping with the specifications of that particular conference. More information about preparing an abstract for conferences is included later in this chapter.

Structured abstracts have specific headings such as problem, methods, and results (Pyrczak & Bruce, 2017), as well as conclusions and sometimes other key study components. Al-Ghareeb, McKenna, and Cooper (2019) provided a structured abstract for their mixed methods study of the influence of anxiety on student nurses' performance in a simulated clinical setting.

Abstract

"Background
Anxiety has a powerful impact on learning due to activation of anxiety hormones, which target related receptors in the working memory. Experiential learning requires some degree of challenge and anxiety. Patient simulation, as a form of experiential learning, has been an integrated component of health professional education internationally over the last two decades, especially in undergraduate nursing education. Little information is available to determine if and how anxiety impacts nursing students' clinical performance during simulation.

Objectives
To investigate physiological and psychological anxiety during emergency scenarios in high-fidelity simulation and understand the effect of anxiety on clinical performance.

Design
First Act was the model for the simulation intervention. Second and third year undergraduate nursing students attended a two-hour simulation session and completed a demographic questionnaire plus pre-simulation self-reported psychological anxiety scale. A heart rate variability monitor was attached to each student's chest to measure heart rate variability (as a sign of anxiety) before engaging in two video-recorded simulated emergency scenarios (cardiac and respiratory) with a professional actor playing the patient. Performance was rated by a clinician followed by video-assisted debriefing. Finally, heart monitors were removed and students repeated self-reports of psychological anxiety.

Results
Students' psychological anxiety was high pre-simulation and remained high post-simulation. With regard to physiological anxiety, students were anxious at the start of the simulation but became more relaxed toward the end as they gained familiarly with the simulation environment ($p < .007$). Clinical performance increased significantly in the second scenario ($p < .001$). Factors found to positively affect clinical performance were length of enrolment in the nursing degree ($p = .001$), current employment in a nursing or allied healthcare field ($p = .030$), and previous emergency experience ($p = .047$). The relationship between physiological anxiety and clinical performance was statistically not significant, although there was an indication that low level anxiety led to optimal performance.

Conclusion
High-fidelity patient simulation has the capacity to arouse novice nurses psychologically and physiologically while

managing emergency situations. Indicative outcomes suggest that optimal performance was apparent when anxiety levels were low, indicating that they had received insufficient training to deal with situations that induced moderate to high anxiety levels." (Al-Ghareeb et al., 2019, p. 57)

Al Ghareeb et al. (2019) used the journal's headings to write their structured abstract. Unstructured abstracts include the same elements but are written in narrative format. Anderson et al. (2019) provided an unstructured abstract, containing the elements introduction/problem, methods, results, and conclusion, in their study's report.

"Healthcare is increasingly complex and requires the ability to adapt to changing demands. Teamwork is essential to delivering high quality care and is central to nursing. The aims of this study were to identify the processes that underpin nursing teamwork and how these affect the care of older people, identify the relationship between perceived teamwork and perceived quality of care, and explore in depth the experience of working in nursing teams. The study was carried out in three older people's wards in a London teaching hospital. Nurses and healthcare assistants completed questionnaires ($n=65$) on known dynamics of teamwork (using the Nursing Teamwork Survey) together with ratings of organisational quality (using an adapted AHRQ HSPS [Agency for Healthcare Research and Quality Hospital Survey on Patient Safety Culture] scale). A sample ($n=22$; 34%) was then interviewed about their perceptions of care, teamwork and how good outcomes are delivered in everyday work. Results showed that many care difficulties were routinely encountered, and confirmed the importance of teamwork (e.g. shared mental models of tasks and team roles and responsibilities, supported by leadership) in adapting to challenges. Perceived quality of teamwork was positively related to perceived quality of care. Work system variability and the external environment influenced teamwork, and confirmed the importance of team adaptive capacity. The CARE [Concepts for Applying Resilience Engineering] model shows the centrality of teamwork in adapting to variable demand and capacity to deliver care processes, and the influence of broader system factors on teamworking." (Anderson et al., 2019, p. 119)

Following the abstract are the four major sections of a research report: Introduction, Methods, Results, and Discussion.

Introduction

The Introduction section of a research report discusses the background and significance of the problem, so as to inform the reader of the reason the study was conducted (see Box 27.1). Statements are supported with citations from the literature. The introduction may also describe the study framework or philosophical perspective and identify the research purpose (aims, objectives, questions, or hypotheses, if applicable). The study aims or purpose and specific research questions emanate from the phenomenon or research problem, clarify the study focus, and identify expected outcomes of the investigation (see Chapters 5 and 6). You developed this content for the research proposal, and now you summarize it in the final report. Depending on the type of research report, the review of literature and framework might be separate sections or separate chapters as in a thesis or dissertation.

Review of Literature

The review of literature section of a research report documents the current knowledge of the problem investigated. The sources included in the literature review are the sources that you used to develop your study and interpret the findings. A review of literature can be two or three paragraphs or several pages long. In journal articles, the review of literature is concise and usually includes a maximum of 15 to 20 sources. Theses, and especially dissertations, include an extensive literature review, for the purpose of demonstrating the student's thorough grasp of the research problem. The summary of the literature review clearly identifies what is known, what is not known (knowledge gap), and the contribution of this study to the current knowledge base. The objectives, questions, or hypotheses that were used to direct the study often are stated at the end of the literature review. See Chapter 7 for more information on writing a review of the literature.

Framework

A research report includes the study framework. In this section, you identify and define the major concepts in the framework and describe the relationships among the concepts (see Chapter 8). You can develop a schematic map or model to clarify logical interweaves of principal concepts within the framework. If a particular proposition or relationship is being tested in a quantitative study, that proposition should be stated clearly. Developing a framework and identifying the proposition(s) examined in a study serve to connect the framework and research purpose to the objectives, questions, or hypotheses. The concepts in the framework must be linked to the study variables and are used to define the variables conceptually (see Chapters 6 and 8 for examples). The philosophical perspective for a qualitative study may provide a theoretical context for the concepts and possibly structure for the data collection, such as interview questions.

Methods

The Methods section of a research report describes how the researcher conducted the study. This section must be concise, yet provide sufficient detail for nurses to appraise critically or replicate the study procedures. In this section, you will describe the study design, sample, setting, data collection tools and process, and plan for data analysis. If your research project included a pilot study, you will describe the reason for the pilot, its implementation, and its results succinctly. You will also describe any changes made in the research project based on the pilot study (Pyrczak & Bruce, 2017), and mention whether pilot data were or were not included in the analysis of results.

Design

The study design should be explicitly stated. Review Chapters 10 and 11 for information on quantitative study designs and Chapters 4 and 12 for qualitative study methods. Al-Ghareeb et al. (2019) were explicit in stating the following:

> "The larger study, of which this research was a part, employed mixed methods, in particular an embedded design that involved measuring psychological and physiological anxiety, and clinical performance. This paper focuses on findings of students' performance and anxiety levels arising from heart rate variability monitoring." (Al-Ghareeb et al., 2019, p. 58)

Even when a research report provides only part of the result of a larger study, the design for the entire study is identified in the report. Al-Ghareeb et al. (2019) presented their quantitative results related to student performance, anxiety levels, and heart rate, but they appropriately identified the design of the entire study.

Sample and Setting

This section of the research report should describe the sampling method, criteria for selecting the sample,

sample size, and sample characteristics (see Chapter 15). Specifics of subject recruitment, including refusal or acceptance rates, should be reported. In the Methods section, Chan et al. (2018) described subject recruitment and the inclusion/exclusion criteria for their longitudinal study of an advance care planning program for elders and their families. The authors included both anticipated refusal and acceptance rates in their introductory paragraphs and included actual refusal rates in the description of the sample.

In the section about the sample and subjects, researchers are expected to include information about how subjects' rights were protected and informed consent was obtained. In a published study, the setting is often described in one or two sentences, and agencies are not identified by name unless permission has been obtained.

Data Collection Process and Procedures

This section of the report describes methods used to collect data. The description of the data collection process in the research report includes details such as who collected the data, the types of data collected, whether data were collected through measurement or a qualitative method, and the procedure for collecting data, including frequency and timing.

In the Methods section of a quantitative study, instruments and their reliability and validity are described. The description of each instrument includes the concepts or variables measured by the instrument, the number of items, the type of response set (i.e., Likert scale), and the possible range of scores. If an instrument has subscales, they are described in detail. The reliability and validity results from previous studies are included with the type of participants who completed the instruments.

For qualitative studies, the author includes how and where the interviews, focus groups, or observations occurred. Qualitative researchers will include in this section of the report the details about recording and transcribing the interviews or focus groups. Steps taken to enhance study credibility are also included such as one person conducting all the interviews or having an observer make field notes during a focus group.

Because of different approaches to research problems, data collection is an area of the report that varies greatly depending on the type of study.

Analysis Plan

Data must be transformed into results through analysis. For quantitative reports, the analysis plan consists of statistical analyses for each research aim, question, or hypothesis. For qualitative study reports, this section highlights the name and process of the method of analysis. The researchers will also include how they documented the decisions they made during data analysis. For mixed methods studies, the analysis plan includes analyses for both quantitative and qualitative data but, more important, the processes the researcher used to integrate the two types of data into a comprehensive answer to the research questions (see Chapter 14).

Results

The Results section usually begins with a description of the sample and subgroups, if applicable, followed by what was learned through implementation of the study methods. Researchers can present the demographic characteristics of their sample in narrative format; however, most quantitative researchers present the characteristics of their sample in a table. Guidelines for preparing tables will be discussed later in the chapter.

For each research objective, question, or hypothesis in quantitative and outcomes research, the author provides the results. Statistical results are reported in a narrative description accompanied by tables (Grove & Cipher, 2020) (see Chapters 21, 22, 23, 24, and 25). Themes that emerge from qualitative analysis often are supported by direct quotes of the participants. The report of a grounded theory study will include the description of the emergent theory, often accompanied by a model or diagram of the concepts and relationships identified (see Chapter 12).

Discussion

The Discussion section ties the other sections of your research report together by connecting parts of the report with one another. For instance, the introduction plus the methods give rise to the results, and then the review of the literature plus the results form the basis for the conclusions. Discussion includes your major findings, limitations of the study, conclusions drawn from the findings, implications of the findings for nursing, and recommendations for further research. Your major findings are actually an interpretation of the results and should be discussed in relation to the study framework or philosophical perspective. You should compare your findings with those from previous research and describe how what you found extends existing knowledge.

Discussion of the findings also includes the limitations that were identified while conducting the study.

The limitations are threats to validity and should be noted as such. For example, limitations related to measurement, such as self-report for unhealthy behaviors, are threats to construct validity. A study might have other limitations related to the sample (e.g., size, response rate, attrition) that threaten external validity or are related to the design (e.g., convenience sample, only one clinical site, lack of random assignment) that threaten internal validity. These limitations influence the generalizability of the findings from quantitative and outcomes research and the transferability of the findings from qualitative research (Pyrczak & Bruce, 2017). Refer to Chapter 26 for more information on how to interpret study findings of quantitative and outcomes studies and Chapter 12 for more information on interpreting findings of qualitative studies.

The research report includes the conclusions or the knowledge generated from the findings. Frequently, conclusions are stated in tentative or speculative terms, because one modest study does not produce conclusive findings that can be generalized to the larger population. If your quantitative study is valid and the findings are consistent with previous studies, you will make a statement related to generalization. If your study is qualitative, you will discuss the transferability of the findings. You might provide a brief rationale for accepting certain conclusions and rejecting others. The conclusions should be discussed in light of their implications for knowledge, theory, and practice. If there is enough evidence for application, you will describe how the findings and conclusions might be implemented in specific practice areas.

Conclude your research report with recommendations for further research. Based on the limitations, identify how revising the methods for future studies on the same topic may produce findings with greater validity. For example, are the findings sufficient for application? If not, what designs might result in a more rigorous study? If several descriptive studies have been reported, should a correlational study be the next step? If sufficient correlational evidence has been reported, is it time to develop a model or test for causation using an interventional design? If a model was developed during a grounded theory study, is it time to use the model as the framework for a quantitative study? The Discussion section of the report identifies the value of your study by describing its contribution to knowledge. By the time the study is published, career researchers are designing and conducting a subsequent study to address their own recommendations for future research.

Reference Citations

The final section of the research report is the reference list, which includes all sources that were cited in the report. Most of the sources in the reference list are relevant studies that provided a knowledge base for conducting the study or reference books supporting the methods. The editors of many nursing and psychology journals use the format described in detail in the *Publication Manual of the American Psychological Association* (American Psychological Association [APA], 2020). Sources must be cited in the text of the report using a consistent format as specified by the journal. The formatting guidelines for the journal to which you plan to submit your manuscript for publication must be followed exactly. Some journals request that the references include only citations published in the past 5 years, except for landmark studies. Other journals may limit the number of references to less than 50 (e.g., the journal *Nursing Research* limits the number of references to "approximately 40").

TYPES OF RESEARCH REPORTS

The sections of a research report provide an outline for you to follow when writing a manuscript for publication. As a reader, the headings provide clues about where to find the specific content about the study. Especially in the Methods section, the content varies, depending on whether the study's methodology was quantitative or qualitative.

Quantitative Research Reports

In reports of quantitative studies, you would expect to see numerical and statistical information that you would not find in qualitative research reports. For example, when a clinical trial or experiment has been conducted, the report must address the statistical power analysis used to determine how many subjects per group were needed to find a statistically significant difference for a given alpha level, such as $\alpha \leq 0.05$. If fewer subjects enroll or complete the study than the number indicated in the original power analysis, statistically significant findings may be absent, even if the group difference appears to be clinically relevant. Lack of statistically significant findings due to a sample that is too small is known as Type II statistical error (see Chapters 15 and 21).

The number of subjects who completed the study should be identified in the report. If your subjects were divided into groups (experimental, comparison, or control groups), identify the method for assigning subjects to groups and the number of subjects in each. For randomized clinical trials (RCTs), the expectation is that you will follow the Consolidated Standards of Reporting Trials (CONSORT, 2010). The guidelines recommend a flow diagram of the enrollment, recruitment, response rate, size of groups, and attrition rate (Schulz, Altman, & Moher, 2010). Following the guidelines facilitates systematic reviews by providing the information reviewers need to determine the quality of a study. See Chapter 11, specifically Figs. 11.23 and 11.34 for examples of CONSORT flow diagrams.

Details about measures or instruments used in the data collection process are crucial if nurses are to critically appraise and replicate a study. The details include each measure's scaling and range of scores and how often each was used. These details about scaling, subscales, range of scores, and scoring can be provided most concisely in a table. Table 27.1 is an example. Reliability and validity information previously published for each instrument should be provided. In addition, the report includes the instrument's reliability in the current study and any further support of validity obtained from the current study. If you have used physiological measures, be sure to identify their manufacturers and address their accuracy, precision, selectivity, sensitivity, and sources of error (Pyrczak & Bruce, 2017) (see Chapter 16).

The presentation of results depends on the end product of the data analysis, your own preference, and any journal instructions. Generally, what is presented in a table is not restated in the text of the narrative. When reporting results in a narrative format, the value of the calculated statistic (t, F, r, or χ^2), the degrees of freedom *(df)*, and probability (*p*-value) should be included (Grove & Cipher, 2020). Word-processing programs include the Greek-letter statistics in the collection of symbols that the user can insert into a manuscript. When reporting any nonsignificant results, it is important to include the effect size and power level for that analysis so that readers could evaluate the risk of Type II error (Grove & Cipher, 2020).

Students often have difficulty putting all these Greek-letter statistical findings back into words for the text of the Results section. The APA *Publication Manual* (APA, 2020) provides direction for how to present various statistical results in a research report. Statistical values should be reported with two decimal digits of accuracy. Although computer output of data may include results reported to several decimal places, this is unnecessary

TABLE 27.1 Variables, Instruments, and Scoring Used to Test a Pain Management Program		
Variable	**Instrument Description**	**Instrument Scoring**
Pain intensity	Pain severity subscale of Brief Pain Inventory (Cleeland, 2009), four items with 11-point numerical rating scale (0 = no pain; 10 = pain as bad as you can imagine)	Mean score on the four items; the higher the score, the greater the pain intensity
Functional interference	Pain interference subscale of Brief Pain Inventory (Cleeland, 2009), seven items with 11-point numerical rating scale (0 = no pain; 10 = pain as bad as you can imagine)	Mean score on the seven items; the higher the score, the greater the functional interference
Depression	Short version Personal Health Questionnaire Depression Scale (PHQ-8) (Kroenke, Spitzer, Williams, & Löwe, 2010), eight items with 4-point rating scale (0 = not at all to 3 = nearly every day)	Sum score on the eight items; the higher the score, the greater the depression
Pain self-efficacy	Pain Self-Efficacy Questionnaire (PSEQ) (Tonkin, 2008); 10 items with 7-point Likert scale (0 = not at all confident to 6 = completely confident)	Sum score on the 10 items; the higher the score, the greater the self-efficacy
Opioid misuse	Current Opioid Misuse Measure (COMM) (Inflexxion, 2010); 17-item self-assessment of pain-related symptoms and behaviors with 5-point Likert scale (0 = never to 4 = very often)	Sum score on the 17 items; the higher the score, the greater the opioid misuse

Adapted from Wilson, M., Roll, J., Corbett, C., Barbosa-Leiker, C. (2015). Empowering patients with persistent pain using an internet-based self-management program. *Pain Management Nursing*, 16(4), 503-14. doi:10.1016/j.pmn.2014.09.009

for the report. For example, reporting the χ^2 value as 11.14 is sufficient, even if the computed value is 11.13965 (APA, 2020). The *p*-value, on the other hand, should be reported as the exact value. The exception is that if the computer output reads $p = 0.0000$, it should be reported as $p < 0.001$ because the computer rounds the value to zero, whereas *p* cannot actually assume that value (Grove & Cipher, 2020).

Presentation of Results in Figures and Tables

Figures and tables are used to present a large amount of detailed information concisely and clearly. Researchers use figures and tables to demonstrate relationship and to document change over time, so as to reduce the number of words in the text of the report (APA, 2020; American Society of Agronomy, Crop Science Society of America, & Soil Science Society of America [ASA-CSSA-SSSA], 2019; Saver, 2006). However, figures and tables are useful only if they are appropriate for the results you have generated and if they are well constructed (Saver, 2006). Box 27.2 provides guidelines for developing accurate and clear figures and tables for a research report. More extensive guidelines and examples for developing tables and figures for research reports can be found in the APA *Publication Manual* (APA, 2020).

BOX 27.2   Guidelines for Developing Tables and Figures in Research Reports

- Select the results to include in the report.
- Identify a few key tables and figures that explain or support the major points.
- Develop simple tables and figures.
- Consider a table or figure for each research question or objective.
- Ensure that tables and figures are complete and clear without reference to the narrative.
- Give each table or figure a brief title.
- Number tables and figures separately in the report (e.g., Table 1, 2; Figure 1, 2).
- Review figures and tables in the journal to which you plan to submit your manuscript for formats acceptable to the journal.
- Use descriptive headings, labels, and symbols—remember to provide a key for abbreviations or symbols used in tables and figures.
- Include actual probability values or indicate whether statistically significant by asterisks.
- Refer to each table and figure in the narrative (e.g., Table 1 presents . . .).
- Use the narrative to summarize main ideas without repeating the specifics of figures and tables.

Compiled from APA (2020); Pyrczak and Bruce (2017); ASA-CSSA-SSSA (2019).

Figures. Figures are diagrams or pictures that illustrate either a conceptual framework or the study results. Researchers often use computer programs to generate sophisticated black-and-white or color figures. Conceptual frameworks are described both in the text and graphically (see examples in Chapter 8). Other common figures included in nursing research reports are bar graphs and line graphs. Journals often require high-resolution images for reproduction. The APA *Publication Manual* (APA, 2020, p. 225) has a figure checklist for you to review when deciding whether to include a figure. Generally, figures require specific formatting and may have less detail than readers want, so potential authors should carefully check with journal guidelines (Saver, 2006).

Bar graphs typically have horizontal or vertical bars that represent the size or amount of the group or variable studied. The bar graph is also a means of comparing one group with another. Henderson, Ossenberg, and Tyler (2015) conducted a mixed methods study of novice nurses' perceptions of the learning environment in a

structured program to facilitate the assimilation of new graduates. The quantitative data they collected included the nurses' responses to a survey that measured recognition, affiliation, accomplishment, influence, and dissatisfaction. They added items to the influence subscale to address influence up and influence down and included an engagement subscale from another instrument. Henderson et al. (2015) reported the means on the subscales using a bar graph (Fig. 27.1), on which the higher bar displayed a higher mean. The researchers placed the mean for each subscale in a table below the bar. Providing the numerical results effectively supplemented the graph, but it could have been improved by including the standard deviation as well.

A **line graph** is developed by joining a series of points with a line. It displays the values of a variable in comparison with a second variable, usually time. In this type of graph, the vertical scale (*y*-axis) is used to display the values of the first variable, and the horizontal scale (*x*-axis) is used to display the values of the second variable. A line graph figure requires at least three data

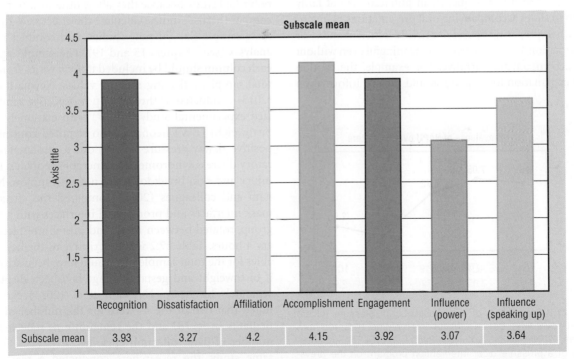

Subscale mean	Recognition	Dissatisfaction	Affiliation	Accomplishment	Engagement	Influence (power)	Influence (speaking up)
Subscale mean	3.93	3.27	4.2	4.15	3.92	3.07	3.64

Fig. 27.1 Novice nurses' (*n* = 78) perceptions of the clinical learning organizational culture: Bar graph of subscale means. (Adapted from Henderson, A., Ossenberg, C., & Tyler, S. [2015]. "What matters to graduates": An evaluation of a structured clinical support program for newly graduated nurses. *Nurse Education in Practice, 15*[3], 228.)

points on the horizontal axis to show a trend or pattern. However, complexity does not enhance the ability to convey the data in a meaningful way, so it is recommended that no more than 10 time points should be included on a single line graph, and there should be no more than four lines or groups per graph, except when physiological data for intervals of seconds or minutes are presented.

Fig. 27.2 is a simple line graph developed by Mallah, Nassar, and Kurdahi Badr (2015) to depict the change in the prevalence of hospital-acquired pressure ulcers (HAPU) after interventions in a clinical facility. Fig. 27.2 is easy to interpret because it includes five data points along the *x*-axis (quarters of the year), and the *y*-axis represents percentage prevalence. The figure clearly shows the effect of a group of interventions that were implemented in the third quarter of 2012. The researchers found that there was a statistically significant difference in prevalence rates from the first quarter of 2012 to the first quarter of 2013 ($\chi^2 = 7.64$, $p < 0.01$).

Researchers may use other types of figures to display sample characteristics. A pie chart is an example of a figure that is seen less frequently in publications but fairly often in slides accompanying oral presentations. Remember when preparing figures to provide sufficient and clear information so that the figure is meaningful even without the accompanying narrative. For example, the caption and explanation for a figure should include information about the study, such as key concepts, type and size of the sample, and abbreviations used in the figure.

For meta-analysis reports that synthesize the results of many studies, figures called forest plots are used for presentation of results. A forest plot has been described as "a graphical display of one common statistical conclusion from a number of studies directing the same problem" (Seth, 2019, p. 108). As is the case with pooled analyses, in general, it combines the inferences of a number of previously performed studies, so as to produce a conclusion that is statistically powerful. Refer to Chapter 19 for more information on forest plots and other figures that may be used in reporting meta-analyses.

Tables. **Tables** are used more frequently in research reports than figures and can be developed to present results from numerous statistical analyses in a small amount of space. Tabular results are presented in columns and rows so that the reader can review them easily. Table 27.2 is an example that presents descriptive statistics for the sample and variables, using means *(Ms)*, ranges, and standard deviations *(SDs)*. *Ms* and *SDs* of the study variables should be included in the published study because they allow other researchers to compare across studies, calculate the effect sizes to estimate sample size for new studies, and conduct meta-analyses (see Chapters 15 and 19). The sample size for each column should be included if the *n* varies from the total sample, reflecting missing values. Newnam et al. (2015) conducted a "three group prospective randomized experimental study" (p. 37) with extremely low-birthweight (BW) neonates who required continuous positive airway pressure (CPAP) due to neonatal respiratory distress syndrome. In vulnerable neonates, nasal injury and skin breakdown are not uncommon. Newnam and colleagues (2015) compared the effects of mask interfaces and prong nasal interfaces with a third group, rotated between mask and prong interfaces every 4 hours. Table 27.2 was descriptive of the key variables for the total sample but would have been stronger if birthweight and gestational age had been displayed separately by group. Newnam et al. (2015) carefully noted that two of the *n*s were for the number of participants ($n = 78$) and the remaining *n*s reflected the number of data collection episodes ($n = 730$). In the same study, the researchers conducted a regression analysis (see Chapter 24). Table 27.3 is an example of the results of the regression analysis. Newnam et al. (2015) provided a summary of the table in the text of the article as well.

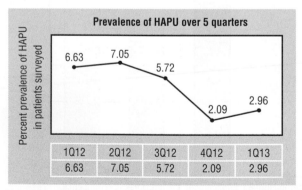

Fig. 27.2 Prevalence of hospital-acquired pressure ulcers (HAPU) over time: Before and after intervention. (Adapted from Mallah, Z., Nassar, N., & Kurdahi Badr, L. [2015]. The effectiveness of a pressure ulcer intervention program on the prevalence of hospital acquired pressure ulcers: Controlled before and after study. *Applied Nursing Research, 28*[2], 110.) *1Q12,* First quarter of 2012; *2Q12,* second quarter of 2012; *3Q12,* third quarter of 2012; *4Q12,* fourth quarter of 2012; *1Q13,* first quarter of 2013.

TABLE 27.2 Sample Description Demographic Variables for Total Sample

Variable	N	Mean	Minimum	Maximum	SD
Birthweight (g)	78[a]	873.36	500.00	1460.00	220.70
Birth gestational age (weeks)	78[a]	26.77	23.00	32.00	1.90
Current weight (g)	730[b]	1065.24	720.00	3170.00	373.99
Current age (weeks)	730[b]	3.87	0.14	14.43	3.23
Time to CPAP initiation (weeks)	730[b]	3.87	0.14	14.43	3.23
Number of CPAP days	730[b]	4.32	1.00	16.00	3.22
CPAP flow rate (lpm)	730[b]	5.35	4.00	7.00	0.66
Oxygen supplementation (%)	730[b]	0.25	0.21	0.60	0.60

CPAP, Continuous positive airway pressure; *lpm*, liter per minute.
[a]Total number of participants in the study.
[b]Number of data collection episodes.
From Newnam, K., McGrath, J., Salyer, J., Estes, J., Jallo, N., & Bass, W. (2015). A comparative effectiveness study of continuous positive airway pressure-related skin breakdown when using different nasal interfaces in the extremely low birth weight neonate. *Applied Nursing Research*, 28(1), 39.

TABLE 27.3 Regression Model: Identified Predictors of Skin Breakdown Risk Factors During Nasal CPAP Use in the Neonate Less Than 1500 g

Model	R	R^2	Standard Error	Df1	Df2	F	p-Value
Model 1: mean postmenstrual age at time of nasal CPAP (constant)	0.399	0.159	0.48	1	73	13.82	< 0.001
Model 2: mean postmenstrual age at time of nasal CPAP; number of CPAP days (constant)	0.492	0.221	0.46	1	72	11.51	0.006

Note: Dependent variable: mean NSCS sum score.
CPAP, Continuous positive airway pressure.
From Newnam, K., McGrath, J., Salyer, J., Estes, J., Jallo, N., & Bass, W. (2015). A comparative effectiveness study of continuous positive airway pressure-related skin breakdown when using different nasal interfaces in the extremely low birth weight neonate. *Applied Nursing Research*, 28(1), 40.

"To best evaluate the effect of additional risk factors and their influence on the incidence and frequency of skin breakdown, a regression model was developed, guided by factors identified in the literature. Factors included in the model were BW, length of therapy, PMA [postmenstrual age] at the time of CPAP, environmental temperature, amount of CPAP flow administered and nursing interventions that include positioning techniques, nasal suctioning type (oral/nasal), suctioning interval and the use of nasal saline during suctioning [see Table 27.3]. The mean PMA made the largest unique contribution (16% variance explained; $\beta = 0.46$; $p < 0.001$) although the number of CPAP days also made a statistically significant contribution (25% variance explained; $\beta = 0.31$; $p = 0.006$). The model accounted for 22% of total variance of skin breakdown ($R^2 = 0.22$; $F = 11.51$, $p = 0.006$)." (Newnam et al., 2015, p. 39)

Tables also are used to identify correlations among variables, and often the table presents a correlation matrix generated from the data analysis. The correlation matrix indicates the correlation values (coefficients) obtained when examining relationships between pairs of variables (bivariate correlations). When a statistical program, such as the Statistical Package for Social Sciences ([SPSS], IBM, n.d.), SPSS, displays a correlation table as the result of a multivariate analysis, the values from all pairs of data are displayed twice. In a research report, usually only the left lower diagonal half of the entire table is presented, to eliminate redundancy (Table 27.4). In the table, the correlations in parentheses are the duplicate correlations: These values would not appear in the research report. None of the correlational values of this study were found to be statistically significant. If some had been, however, the table would have identified them

TABLE 27.4 Correlation Matrix for Major Study Variables: Patient Volume, Waiting Time, Ophthalmologist Quality, Overall Hospital Quality

	Patient Volume	Waiting Time	Ophthalmologist Quality	Overall Hospital Quality
Patient volume	1.0000	(−0.1778)	(0.4748)	(0.1518)
Waiting time	−0.1778	1.0000	(−0.1434)	(−0.1144)
Ophthalmologist quality	0.4748	−0.1434	1.0000	(0.1176)
Overall hospital quality	0.1518	−0.1144	0.1176	1.0000

From Ruwaard, S., & Douven, R. (2018). Hospital choice for cataract treatments: The winner takes most. *International Journal of Health Policy and Management, 7*(12), 1120–1129.

by placing one or more asterisks (*, **, ***) next to each significant *p*-value. The reader must carefully interpret the significance (*p*-value) of each correlation coefficient because significance is dependent upon sample size.

In addition to the other elements of the Discussion section that are common to all research reports, reports of quantitative and outcomes studies usually address the generalizability of the findings to other samples and populations. Demographic and health characteristics of the sample are compared to the same characteristics of the population to examine the extent to which the sample is representative of the target population. Convenience samples are less representative of the target population than are randomly selected samples.

Qualitative Research Report

Reports for qualitative research are as diverse as the different types of qualitative studies. The types of qualitative research are presented in Chapter 4, and methods for specific types of qualitative studies are presented in Chapter 12. The intent of a qualitative research report is to describe the dynamic implementation of the project and the unique, creative findings obtained (Creswell & Creswell, 2018; Marshall & Rossman, 2016). Similar to a quantitative report, a qualitative research report needs a clear, concise title that identifies the focus of the study.

The abstract for a qualitative research report briefly summarizes the key parts of the study and usually includes the following: (1) aim of the study, (2) qualitative approach (e.g., phenomenology), (3) methods (including sample, setting, and process of data collection), (4) brief synopsis of findings, and (5) implications of the findings (Miles, Huberman, & Saldaña, 2020; Munhall, 2012). The example of an unstructured abstract provided earlier in the chapter was developed for a

mixed methods study, in which the qualitative aspect of the study was to explore the in-depth dimensions of teamwork (Anderson et al., 2019). The abstract contains all five of the requisite elements for a qualitative research report.

Tong, Sainsbury, and Craig (2007) developed a checklist that included three domains to be included in qualitative research reports: "(i) research team and reflexivity, (ii) study design, and (iii) data analysis and reporting" (p. 349). The Consolidated Criteria for Reporting Qualitative Research (COREQ) is their 32-item checklist for studies in which the data are collected through interviews and focus groups (Tong et al., 2007). COREQ has not had the widespread acceptance of the CONSORT Statement, but provides a standard by which qualitative researchers can evaluate the thoroughness of their research report.

The Methods section for a qualitative study includes the specific qualitative design, such as phenomenology or ethnography; a detailed description of the data collection method, such as interview or observation; and the data management and analysis plan. In the presentation of the qualitative approach, the researcher provides the philosophical basis for and the assumptions of the qualitative method with citations from primary sources rather than from current textbooks. In addition, a rationale for selecting this type of qualitative study should be specified (Creswell & Creswell, 2018; Marshall & Rossman, 2016).

Unique to qualitative research, the researchers may be expected to describe their relevant educational and clinical background for conducting the study. This documentation helps the reader evaluate the worth of the study because the researcher serves as the primary data-gathering instrument and also analyzes and interprets data to produce the results (Creswell & Creswell, 2018;

Munhall, 2012). The researcher provides detail about all data collection processes, including training of project staff, entry into the setting, selection of participants, and ethical considerations extended to the participants throughout the study. When data collection tools are used, such as observation guides, initial questions for open-ended interviews, or forms to record facts extracted from documents, they are described in the report and also displayed as an inset or an appendix. The flexible, dynamic way in which a researcher collects data is described, including the range of time the researcher used for conducting each interview and the amount of time the researcher spent collecting observational data. In addition, the researcher describes how data were recorded and the amount of data collected. For example, if your data collection involved participant observation, you should describe the number, length, structure, and focus of the observation and participation periods. In addition, you should identify the tools (e.g., digital devices) for recording the data from these periods of observation and participation. What processes were used to transcribe audio recordings for analysis? How was the accuracy of transcription confirmed? The plan described in the methods section for analyzing data includes the person(s) who coded the data, how they were trained, and the software product used, if any.

Data analysis procedures are performed during or after the data collection process, depending on method, and this timing should be specified (Marshall & Rossman, 2016; Miles et al., 2020; Munhall, 2012). Present your results in a manner that clarifies for the reader the phenomenon under investigation. These results include descriptions, themes, social processes, and theories that emerged from the study of life experiences, cultures, behaviors, or healthcare problems. Sometimes, these theoretical ideas are organized into conceptual maps, models, or tables. Researchers often gather additional data or reexamine existing data to verify their theoretical conclusions, and this process is described in the report (Marshall & Rossman, 2016; Miles et al., 2020). Some qualitative study findings lack clarity and quality, which makes it difficult for practitioners to understand and apply them. Some of the problems with qualitative study results are mismatching of quotes with theoretical concepts, lack of clarity in identifying patterns and themes in the data, and misrepresentation of data and data analysis procedures in the report (Sandelowski & Barroso, 2002).

Researchers must clearly and accurately develop their findings and present them in a way that a diverse audience of practitioners and researchers can understand. Sandelowski and Leeman (2012) recommended writing sentences that reflect the identified themes. Clearly, writing themes will take practice, because you want to preserve "the complexity of the phenomena these ideas were meant to represent" and yet summarize key ideas (Sandelowski & Leeman, 2012, p. 1407).

The Discussion section includes conclusions, study limitations, implications for nursing, and recommendations for further research in the same manner that quantitative research reports do. Conclusions are a synthesis of the study findings in relation to relevant theoretical and empirical literature. Limitations are identified, and their influence on the formulation of the conclusions is addressed. Small sample size in qualitative research is not a limitation; failure to explain the phenomenon of interest fully due to inadequate data collection and analysis is.

Theses and Dissertations

Theses and **dissertations** are research reports that students develop in depth as part of the requirements for a degree. The university, nursing school or college, and members of the student's research committee provide specific requirements for the final thesis or dissertation. Traditionally, theses and dissertations are organized by chapters, the content of which are specified by the college or university. The content of a thesis follows the general outline of reports (see Box 27.1). Chapter 28 also provides guidelines for the content of thesis and dissertation proposals. Graves et al. (2018) surveyed various doctoral programs regarding the formatting of dissertations, focusing on the option of publishable papers as chapters for a dissertation. The authors identified multiple issues regarding this option, centering on intellectual property rights and faculty burden related to editing student manuscripts but were, overall, supportive of the option as being helpful for the careers of new researchers. Morse (2005) raised additional issues for qualitative dissertations that are comprised of publishable articles, considering these a move away from the holism that a qualitative inquiry must possess. In addition, splitting the study into three to five 15-page articles robs the reports of the richness and depth that characterize the complete and well-reflected-upon nature of qualitative excellence. The advantages for graduates are the experience of writing for publication, the presence of publications on their curriculum vitae (resumé) when they apply for academic positions, and the time advantage of not having to write a five-chapter tome.

AUDIENCES FOR COMMUNICATION OF RESEARCH FINDINGS

Before developing a research report, you will first determine who will benefit from knowing the findings. The greatest impact on nursing practice can be achieved by communicating nursing research findings to a variety of audiences, including nurses, other health professionals, healthcare consumers, and policymakers.

Nurses and Other Healthcare Professionals

Nurses, including administrators, educators, practitioners, and researchers, must be aware of research findings for use in practice and as a basis for conducting additional studies. Nurse researchers communicate their research broadly by presenting at conferences sponsored by non-nursing specialty organizations such as the American Heart Association, American Public Health Association, American Cancer Society, American Lung Association, National Hospice Organization, and National Rural Health Association, at which attendees have an active interest in application of findings. Other health professionals should make themselves aware of knowledge newly generated by nurse researchers and facilitate the use of that knowledge in the healthcare system as part of the delivery of evidence-based care (Craig & Dowding, 2020). Nurse researchers and other health professionals conducting research on the same problem might collaborate to publish an article, a series of articles, a book chapter, or a book. This type of interdisciplinary collaboration increases communication of research findings and facilitates synthesis of research knowledge to promote EBP.

Policymakers

Policymakers at the local, state, and federal levels use research findings to generate health policy that has an impact on consumers, individual practitioners, and the healthcare system. Susan Chapman's work is unusual, in that it utilizes quantitative, qualitative, and mixed methods approaches to amass evidence that can impact

policy changes. Rather than the more common research with individuals as the source of data, Chapman, Wides, and Spetz (2010) provided an excellent example of communicating policy-related quantitative descriptive research findings using the *Medicare Claims Processing Manual,* reports from the National Council of State Boards of Nursing, and congressional reports as their sources of data. They tabulated their data and concluded that more data are needed in these documents about the type of care provided. They also concluded from their analysis that the payment system for advanced practice nurses needed to be remodeled (Chapman et al., 2010).

Building upon this, Chapman and Blash (2017) described new roles for the medical assistant (MA) in the face of the physician shortage and strategies to meet care needs with nonphysician providers using thematic qualitative analysis of the findings of studies on the topic. Themes identified included factors driving MA role innovation, role description, training required, and wage gains. Outcomes were categorized as patient and staff satisfaction, quality of care, and efficiency. More recently, in a mixed methods study, Chapman, Phoenix, Hahn, and Strod (2018) examined the contribution of psychiatric mental health nurse practitioners within public behavioral health services in terms of utilization and economic contribution. In these three papers, Chapman and colleagues synthesized findings from multiple studies to develop policy recommendations.

Consumers

Nurse researchers frequently neglect healthcare consumers as an audience for research reports. Consumers are interested in research findings about illnesses that they or their family members currently face. There is a need to provide consumers with evidence-based guidelines and educational materials to assist them in making quality healthcare decisions.

The findings from nursing studies can be communicated rapidly to the public through a variety of means (Hanneke & Link, 2019). Some universities prepare and disseminate press releases about research findings. The researcher may write a summary of the study for a local newspaper. Even local articles have the potential of being picked up by a national wire service and published in other papers across the nation. Findings also can be communicated to consumers by being published in news magazines, such as *Time* and

Newsweek, or popular health magazines, such as *American Baby* and *Health.* Television and radio are other valuable media for communicating research findings to consumers and other healthcare providers.

Freelance journalists often contact authors of scientific articles, and these writers have the skills to translate research findings into language for consumers. Ot'Alora et al. (2018) conducted randomized Phase II trials of the efficacy of the psychedelic 3,4-methylenedioxymethamphetamine (MDA)–assisted psychotherapy for severe, chronic posttraumatic stress disorder (PTSD). Smith (2018), in an article for *WebMD Magazine,* subsequently was able to catch consumers' attention with the title "Psychedelic Drugs to Treat Depression, PTSD?" to disseminate excerpted data from the research publication, with a human-interest focus, for a targeted public audience. Paraphrased results reported in lay publications are not considered duplicate publications, so they do not represent scientific misconduct.

In addition to print media, the increase of digital media allows the nurse researcher wide dissemination of study findings. Health articles published for consumer magazines and online distribution reach millions of readers at a time (e.g., webmd.com or *WebMD Magazine*). One caution of digital media is that the report must be clear about study limitations and additional confirmatory studies that must be conducted before generalization is appropriate. There is a tendency by the writers of lay publications to reword a correlational relationship in a study as a causative one, implying that everything from lack of adequate rest through nutritional practices to an array of risk-taking activities definitively causes serious diseases and conditions, whereas the study itself produced only correlational evidence.

STRATEGIES FOR PRESENTATION OF RESEARCH FINDINGS

Nurses communicate research findings to their peers through presentations at conferences and meetings. **Presentations** are structured, formal reports of a completed research study that are communicated orally or through a poster. The formal research report must be edited for dissemination. The specifics of conference presentation require judicious selection of the most relevant parts of the total study. Sigma, the international honor society for nursing, sponsors international, national, regional, and local research conferences.

Specialty organizations, such as the American Association of Critical Care Nurses, Oncology Nurses' Society, and Association of Women's Health, Obstetrics, and Neonatal Nursing, sponsor research conferences. Many universities and some healthcare agencies provide financial support (sponsorship) for research conferences. For various reasons, nurses are not always able to attend these research conferences. To increase the communication of research findings and disseminate the new knowledge more widely, conference sponsors may provide websites with electronic posters and recordings of the research presentations. Some sponsors publish abstracts of studies with the conference proceedings, publish the abstracts in a research journal supplement, or provide materials electronically on their websites. To be selected to present at a conference, the researcher must submit an abstract describing the study.

The Abstract Submission Process

The sponsors of a research conference circulate a call for abstracts months, sometimes as much as a year, before the conference. Many research journals and newsletters publish these requests for abstracts, and they are available electronically. In addition, conference sponsors e-mail requests for abstracts to universities, major healthcare agencies, and nurse researcher listservs.

Acceptance as a presenter is based on the quality of the submitted abstract. The abstract should be reflective of the theme of the conference and the organizers' criteria for reviewing the abstract. As noted earlier, an **abstract** is a clear, concise summary of a study. The abstract submitted for a verbal presentation has a word limit. It is usually based on results from a completed study that has not as yet been published.

Before submitting an abstract for a conference, pay attention to the description of the conference, which includes its overview, goal, and expected attendees. How well does your study fit with the goals of the conference? Especially if your paper or poster will be presented concurrently with other research presentations, will attendees be interested enough in your study to attend your presentation? The call for abstracts stipulates the format for the abstract. Frequently, abstracts are limited to one page, single-spaced, and include the content outlined in Box 27.3. Use the abstract guidelines for the conference to ensure that all required elements are included. When abstracts are submitted online, you may be limited to a set number of characters instead of words. For electronic

---

BOX 27.3   Outline for an Abstract Submitted for a Conference

I. **Title of the Study**
II. **Introduction**
   Statement of the problem and purpose
   Identification of the framework
III. **Methodology**
   Design
   Sample size
   Identification of data analysis methods
IV. **Results**
   Major findings
   Conclusions
   Implications for nursing
   Recommendations for further research

Note: The title and authors with affiliations, a conflict-of-interest statement, a brief reference list of one or two key citations, and the acknowledgment of funding source are not usually considered in the word limitations for the abstract.

---

submissions, write and revise the abstract in a separate document. Depending on the instructions, you may copy and paste the text into a box on the web page or attach the file. Some conference planning committees require that you submit two versions of your abstract: one with names and affiliations that would appear in their program or published abstracts, and another that removes all names and affiliations so that the abstract is anonymous and reviewers are blinded.

The title of your abstract must create interest, and the body of your abstract sells the study to the reviewers. Writing an abstract requires practice; frequently, a researcher rewrites an abstract many times until it meets all the criteria, including the word limit, outlined by the conference sponsors. Careful attention to the criteria of the sponsoring agency should increase the chances of having your abstract accepted. There is a helpful online tutorial called "Writing a WINning Abstract" (Lentz, 2011).

Some conference organizers ask that you specify whether you want to be considered for an oral podium or a poster presentation, whereas others decide on a poster versus oral podium presentation based on their own criteria or scoring system. Generally, abstracts that utilize smaller sample sizes and describe preliminary findings or pilot studies are less likely to be accepted for an oral podium presentation. Read the instructions

carefully because they may stipulate that the abstract content has not been published or presented elsewhere. Instructions also indicate whether accepted abstracts are to be published, usually as a supplemental issue of the sponsor's affiliated professional journal.

Podium Presentation of Research Findings

Through podium presentations, researchers have an opportunity to share their findings with many persons at one time, answer a limited number of questions about their studies, interact formally with other interested professionals, and receive a small amount of immediate feedback on their study, concisely provided. Research project findings frequently are presented at conferences as preliminary findings of completed studies. The researchers may not have completely finalized the implications and conclusions, but the interaction with other researchers may facilitate that process and expand their thinking. When research findings are published, the data must not be published elsewhere, and any presentation of these data at a conference should be acknowledged in ensuing presentations and publications. In addition to having your abstract accepted, presenting findings at a conference verbally also involves developing a research report, delivering the report, and responding to questions.

Developing an Oral Research Presentation

You will develop your presentation to fit the audience and the time designated for each presentation. The interests and size of the audience vary, depending on whether you were accepted for a concurrent session with an audience that selects your presentation to attend based on the title and their interest, or for a plenary session with the entire audience of conference participants. If you are unsure of the composition of your conference audience, ask others who have attended the conference or ask the contact person for the conference.

Time is probably the most important factor in developing a presentation because many presenters are limited to 10 or 15 minutes, with an additional 5 minutes for questions. If you choose to accompany your presentation with slides, as a general guideline you should include about one slide per presentation minute. Your title slide, acknowledgment slide, and final slide of references or slide calling for questions from the audience should be included in the timing because other factors may encroach on your total allotted time. For example, the moderator will introduce you and may give other instructions to the attendees, tasks that may last a few minutes.

Your presentation should be paced so as to fit your allocated time exactly. The audience is there to hear what is new in your area of research, not to hear the entire background and review of literature that brought you to this current research. Although it is important to address the major sections of a research report, which are Introduction (including background and literature review), Methods, Results, and Discussion, in your presentation, most attendees are more interested in the study results and findings than a review of the literature or history of a tool's development. For guidance, in a 10-minute presentation you should spend 20% (2 minutes or two slides) of your total time on the title and introduction/background/literature review, 20% on the methodology, 40% on the results, and 20% on the discussion and implications for practice and research. In planning the allotted time for your presentation, it is helpful to know whether questions from the audience will be allowed during your presentation, allowed at the end of your presentation, or held until the end of the entire session, at which time participants direct their questions to one or more of the presenters in the session.

Your title slide should provide the audience with the gap in knowledge that you addressed in your study. Your introduction should acknowledge funding sources and collaborators, if applicable, as well as any conflict of interest. A very brief review of key background literature and a simple diagram of the conceptual framework should lead directly into the research questions or hypotheses that address the knowledge gap. The methodology content includes a brief identification of the design, sampling method, measurement techniques, and analysis plan. The content covered in the results section should start with a simple table of the sample characteristics followed by a slide of results for each question or hypothesis. The presentation should conclude with a brief discussion of findings, implications of findings for clinical practice, and recommendations for subsequent research. Most presenters find that the shorter the presentation time, the greater the preparation time needed. If you are limited to 10 minutes, you must be very selective about which one or two research questions or hypotheses will be your focus. If you have 15 or 20 minutes, you may still choose to limit your

presentation to three research questions or hypotheses but allow more time to discuss the details regarding the contributions and limitations of your research. Start developing your presentation early because some conferences require that you submit your slides up to 6 weeks prior to the conference. Ahead of time, the conference organizers download all computerized slide presentations that are to be given in a specific room within a given session onto one laptop computer or tablet, to save time on the day of the presentation. It is wise to bring a duplicate presentation with you on a thumb drive or disc, or to e-mail it to yourself as an attachment, just in case yours fails to be properly downloaded. For longer presentations, consider using figures, pictures, or possibly a little animation, to emphasize key points and maintain the audience's attention. Bear in mind, however, that your abstract was accepted for its content, not its cuteness.

PowerPoint slides provide an excellent format for presenting an oral research report; they include easy-to-read fonts, color, creative backgrounds, visuals or pictures to clarify points, and animation options. Although you can construct your own PowerPoint presentation, consulting an audiovisual expert will ensure that your materials are clear and properly constructed, with the print large enough and dark enough for the audience to read. When the PowerPoint slides have been developed, view them from the same vantage point as the audience to ensure that each slide is clear and can be visualized without darkening the room.

The information presented on each slide should be limited to eight lines or fewer, with six or fewer words per line. A single slide should contain information that can be easily read and examined in 30 seconds to 1 minute. Use a standard font such as Times Roman or Ariel. Unusual fonts may not be available on the laptop being used by the conference and not display correctly. All words in both title and body of a slide should be bolded, so that they will be visible throughout the audience. Only major points are presented on visuals, so use single words, short phrases, or bulleted points to convey ideas, not complete sentences. Do not read your slides aloud; rather, trust the audience to be able to read. Use the slide as a cue or reminder of what you planned to say. Figures such as bar graphs and line graphs may convey ideas more clearly than tables.

Tables and figures that are included should contain only the most important information and must be in a font that can be seen clearly by the audience. If a large table is required, provide it to attendees as a handout and focus on the key points from the table on your slide. Pictures of the research setting and equipment and photographs of the research team help the audience visualize the research project. A laser pointer may be useful to guide the audience to your key point on the slide, but the deliberate and careful use of color is more appealing to the audience, can increase the clarity of the information presented, and can call attention to a particular important statistical test and *p*-value without the need for a laser pointer. When using color, avoid using particular shades of red for bulleted points or highlighted wording, particularly if you have a dark background; red may display correctly on a computer monitor, but it becomes difficult to see when projected to a large audience.

Preparing the script and visuals for a presentation is difficult, so enlist the assistance of an experienced researcher and audiovisual expert. Rehearse your presentation in a large room with experienced researchers so as to confirm readability, and use their comments to refine your script, slides, and presentation style. If your presentation is too long, synthesize parts of your script into handouts for important content. You may want to prepare handouts for the participants, even if your presentation is shorter. Be sure that the handouts include your name, your contact information, the name of your employer, and an acknowledgment of any funding you received to conduct the study.

Delivering a Research Report and Responding to Questions

A novice researcher may benefit from attending conferences and examining the presentation styles of other researchers before preparing an oral report. Even though each researcher develops his or her own presentation style, observing others can allow you to identify approaches that communicate succinctly and engage the audience. An effective presentation requires practice. You will, of course, rehearse your presentation several times, with the script, until you are comfortable with the timing, the content, and your presentation style. When practicing, advance the slides and use the other presentation modalities so that you are comfortable with the equipment.

The first thing the audience hears from you should not be, "(tap-tap) Is this thing on?" Rehearse with special attention to verbal mannerisms such as, "Umm," "you know," "like," and tongue clicks, and to visual mannerisms and body language. Stand up straight. Enunciate. SLOW DOWN. Take a deep breath and slow down even more. If the audience cannot understand what you say, your presentation is wasted. The rules "Never alibi, never complain" are good to remember. It is always advantageous to check out the room in which you will be presenting to see how chairs are arranged and how the podium and screen are situated. Before your turn to present, check to make sure that your slides are available on the computer, practice opening the file, and ensure that you know how to advance from one slide to the next.

Most conferences organize their oral presentations by topic into a session moderated by an expert in the field. The session usually includes a presentation by the researcher, a comment by the session's moderator, and a question period before moving to the next speaker. If your presentation is too long for the allotted time, the moderator may stop your presentation to ensure that there will be an opportunity for questions from the audience before proceeding to the next speaker. When preparing for a presentation, try to anticipate the questions that members of the audience might ask and rehearse your answers (Box 27.4). As you practice your presentation with colleagues, ask them to raise questions. Frequently, the questions they pose will be the same ones the audience will raise. If you practice making clear, concise responses to specific questions, you will be less anxious during your presentation. When giving a presentation, have someone make notes of the audience's questions, suggestions, or comments, because often this input is useful when preparing a manuscript for publication or developing the next study.

At the end of the presentation, remember to say thank you into the microphone, and to thank the moderator of the session, either then or later. Walking by the technology table at the end of the session and thanking the computer technician is also good form.

Poster Presentation of Research Findings

Your research abstract may be accepted at a conference as a poster presentation rather than a podium presentation. A **poster session** is a collection of all the posters being displayed in one central location at a conference. A poster is a visual presentation of your study, all on one surface. Through poster presentation, researchers have

BOX 27.4 Specific Answers to Several Sample Presentation Questions With Rationale

Question	Answer	Action and Rationale
Why did you not control for the extraneous variable of (_____)?	Good question. This is the first study on the topic and little was known about the problem area, so I merely performed the intervention and measured its effects. I controlled for the variable in post hoc fashion by comparing the group with the variable with the other group. Now that I know the strength of that extraneous variable, in subsequent research I would certainly advise controlling for the effects of it in the design phase.	Acknowledgment that questioner is correct: such a tactic would be interesting for a subsequent study. The "why" was answered honestly.
Why did you use a single site with a preponderance of one racial group rather than multiple sites?	Thank you for that question. I am familiar with the clinic site and wanted to do my first study in a place in which I was sure of the details of the workplace. In subsequent research, I agree that multiple sites would improve the external validity of the study.	Acknowledgment of a sound suggestion and provision of an answer to the "why" question. The effect of multiple sites on design validity was identified, as well.
I had some trouble reading your slides in this big room. What were the notations at the bottom of the fourth, fifth, and tenth slides?	If you would leave me your e-mail address after this session, I would be happy to send you my PowerPoint. Anyone with the same problem, please feel free to request this.	"Never alibi, never complain." No excuse was provided, and no criticism of the technology was made. A solution was provided. Also, the presenter was not derailed into the act of clicking backward through the slides to read the notations aloud.
Why did you study this? It all seems so obvious that this intervention would work.	As a clinician, I will admit that I felt confident that the intervention would be effective. You are correct. However, there is no published research on this problem, so I wanted to measure effectiveness and generate some hard evidence for nursing practice.	Did not respond in the same tone, nor to the implied devaluing of your study. Instead, addressed the value of the research to the profession.
What was the refusal rate for the study subjects? And if it was low, why was it so low?	The refusal rate was 0%. This was probably because of the benign type of intervention and the small amount of time required for participation. I already have a rapport with the clinic patients, too, having worked there for many years.	An honest admission that the research subjects might have participated because it was not difficult to do so and because of the person requesting participation.
Do you plan a second study and what will be its design?	At this time, no subsequent research is planned. However, I am interested in a qualitative study, asking the clients why they thought the intervention was effective.	Answered the question. Also offered an opinion of a direction that subsequent research could legitimately take.
You don't seem very familiar with the statistical analyses of your research. I notice that you mispronounced one test, the Scheffé comparison.	Thank you for pronouncing that correctly for me. I need to study up on how to say the names of the statistical tests, in the future.	Didn't rise to the bait of this ridiculously contentious question. Instead, defused by thanking.

an opportunity to share their findings with a handful of persons at one time, answer unlimited questions, interact informally with other interested professionals, and receive thoughtful feedback, gently offered. Having the opportunity to present a poster should not be minimized. In nursing, a poster presentation is a legitimate means of communicating findings—in fact, it is as legitimate as a podium presentation.

Before developing a poster, read the directions. Follow the conference sponsor's specifications for (1) the size limitations or format restrictions for the poster, (2) the size of the poster display area, and (3) the background and potential number of conference participants. Your institution may have a template with the logo that you are required to use, so that the audience can identify your affiliation more easily. A poster usually includes the following content: the title of the study; investigator and institution names; purpose; research objectives, questions, or hypotheses (if applicable); framework; design; sample; essential data collection procedures and instruments; results; conclusions; implications for nursing; recommendations for further research; a few key references; and acknowledgments. Box 27.5 provides suggestions for developing a poster.

A quality poster presents a study completely, yet can be comprehended in 5 minutes or less. For clarity and visual appeal, a poster often uses pictures, tables, or figures to communicate the study. In fact, recent research examined a pharmacy conference audience's preference for informatic items on a poster versus text. The nurses

attending the conference expressed a preference for the infographic-type presentation: minimum text, many illustrations, diagrams, and visual displays (Young, Bridgeman, & Hermes-DeSantis, 2018). High-quality posters have a polished, professional look and present the key aspects of the study using a balance of text, figures, and color. Bold headings are used for the different parts of the research report, followed by concise narratives or bulleted phrases. Summary and implications sections are placed prominently and at eye level, given the limited time for viewing many posters during a session and your desire to make the findings known. Use of an eye-catching diagram or brightly colored photograph illustrating the content is useful for attracting conference attendees who are interested in what is portrayed while discouraging attendees whose interests lie elsewhere from approaching. Because rich narrative text is so meaningful in qualitative studies, authors are advised to bold and enlarge the font for a few particularly meaningful quotes, and use artwork or photos that conceptualize the quote in a visual way. The size of the text on a poster must be large enough to be read at 3 feet (approximately 20-point font), but the title or banner should be readable at 20 feet. Matte finish is preferable to glossy finish because in less favorable lighting, glossy finishes predispose to glare. Lamination protects the poster from damage and lends to the finished product a slight shine that does not produce glare.

Posters take a range of 10 to 20 hours to develop, depending on the complexity of the study and the experience of the researcher. Novice researchers usually need more than 20 hours to develop a poster. Important points in poster development include planning ahead, seeking the assistance of others, and limiting the information on the poster, one of the most difficult things to do. Many universities provide detailed online information about poster presentation (New York University [NYU] Libraries, 2019). There are several modalities for creation of a visually engaging and well-organized poster, including PowerPoint, with which most new researchers are familiar. Many universities have digital laboratories and personnel available to assist in poster development for a study that was completed to meet academic requirements.

Conference organizers often provide boards for displaying posters. The poster can be rolled to prevent creases and easily transported to the conference in a

---

BOX 27.5 Principles for Developing a Poster

1. Start planning early with a clear focus.
2. Follow conference guidelines carefully.
   a. Poster size
   b. Hanging or freestanding
3. Use bullet points or abbreviated wording.
4. Include pictures and graphics that add to the content.
5. Balance text and pictures with white space.
6. Use a large font size for viewing from a distance.
7. Place the eye-catching materials of the poster in the upper right or upper center.
8. A photograph that contains emotional content appeals to creativity or surprises viewers can draw them to your poster.

protective tube. Office supply stores and shipping companies provide online services such as designing, printing, and shipping the poster to the conference venue. Posters can also be printed on fabric and easily packed in a suitcase, which is especially practical for an international conference. Because accidents can occur, it is wise to email oneself the poster; then if the actual poster is lost or damaged in transit, it can be reprinted onsite.

Poster sessions usually last 1 to 2 hours; you should remain by your poster during this time and offer to answer any questions when a viewer is present. Most researchers provide conference participants with a copy of the accepted abstract. You may choose to prepare a single-page handout of the poster with your contact information, particularly if you cannot stand by the poster for the full allotted time. Some conferences require posters to be displayed for the entire run of the conference. Leaving contact information on or near the poster will be appreciated by interested attendees who want to communicate with you.

One major advantage of a poster session is the opportunity for one-to-one interaction between the researcher and the viewer. Frequently, at the end of the poster session individuals interested in a study stay to speak with the researcher. Have a notepad on hand to record comments and contact information for individuals conducting similar research. Exchanging business cards and writing key information on the back of the card is a useful practice. Poster sessions provide an excellent opportunity to begin networking with other researchers involved in the same area of research. Conference participants occasionally request your study instruments or other items, so it is essential that you keep a record of their contact information and specific requests.

STRATEGIES FOR PUBLICATION OF RESEARCH FINDINGS

Podium and poster presentations are valuable means of communicating findings rapidly, but their impact is limited and findings should not have been published previously. Even if the accepted abstract is published in a supplemental volume of a journal associated with the conference sponsors, you should be planning publication of the full findings in a research journal as you prepare for the oral podium or poster presentation. **Published research** findings are permanently recorded

in a journal or book and usually reach a larger audience than do presentations. Because journals are the most common venue used by nurses to disseminate findings in print, we will focus on that type of publication. Following the description of those factors, the process of developing a manuscript will be discussed.

Factors to Consider Before Publication

This section will explain factors to consider when preparing to submit a manuscript, such as previous presentation of findings and negative findings. Another potentially challenging decision is who will be authors on the manuscript and the order in which their names will be listed.

Previous Presentation of Findings

When study findings have been presented prior to publication, there should be an acknowledgment in the published report that the contents of the paper were presented at a particular research conference. The presentation and comments from the audience can provide a basis for finalizing your article for publication. Many journal editors are conference attendees and may request your paper for an article when they hear your oral presentation or see your poster. Many researchers present their findings at a conference or two and never submit the paper for publication.

Negative Findings

Studies with negative findings (no significant difference or relationship) frequently are not submitted for publication (Mlinarić, Horvat, & Šupak Smolčić, 2017), which can contribute to scientific bias. The bias is apparent in scientists' unawareness of the negative findings, as well as in eventual meta-analysis publications, which report stronger evidence than is actually the case (Mlinarić et al., 2017). When statistical power is sufficient and measures are reliable, negative findings may be an accurate reflection of reality. Negative findings can be as important to the development of knowledge as positive findings are because they inform other researchers of what did not work, preventing subsequent waste of research resources. Eliminating rival hypotheses advances science (Mlinarić et al., 2017). Many authors strategize placing nonsignificant findings within a journal that has previously published an article describing positive findings on the same topic.

Authorship

While you are developing your study and writing the proposal, outline your plans for dissemination of the findings. At the outset of the endeavor, which is the planning phase, you and other members of your research team should discuss and determine authorship credit. This discussion can become a complex issue when the research is a collaborative project among individuals from different disciplines with varied degrees of research education and experience.

There are several terms related to authorship credit that are important to understand. **Honorary authorship** refers to listing a senior researcher's name on an article with that person making no contribution to the manuscript (Shamoo & Resnik, 2015). **Ghost authorship** is the situation in which an individual or company, such as the manufacturer of a medication used in a research intervention, was involved in a study and the ensuing manuscript but is not listed as an author to avoid the appearance of a conflict of interest (Shamoo & Resnik, 2015). Both types of authorship are unethical. To avoid such situations, the International Committee of Medical Journal Editors (ICMJE) developed authorship guidelines that have become the standard for most professional journals. Journal editors require authors to specify their contributions to a study and to the manuscript, including signing a form that documents the contributions. Box 27.6 lists the four criteria on which authorship should be based (ICMJE, 2019). Shamoo and Resnik (2015) provide additional discussion related to authorship that may be helpful for specific situations, such as nonresearch manuscripts and faculty-student relationships.

Developing the Manuscript

Developing a manuscript for publication includes the following steps: (1) selecting a journal, (2) developing a query letter, (3) preparing a manuscript, (4) submitting the manuscript for review, and (5) revising the manuscript. In this section, this process will be described.

Selecting a Journal

Selecting a journal for publication of your study requires knowledge of the basic requirements of the journal, the journal's review process, and recent articles published in the journal. A **refereed journal** is peer reviewed and uses referees or expert reviewers to determine whether a manuscript is acceptable for publication. In nonrefereed

> **BOX 27.6   Authorship Criteria of the International Committee of Medical Journal Editors: Requirements to Be an Author**
>
> - Substantial contributions to the conception or design of the work or the acquisition, analysis, or interpretation of data for the work; AND
> - Drafting the work or revising it critically for important intellectual content; AND
> - Final approval of the version to be published; AND
> - Agreement to be accountable for all aspects of the work in ensuring that questions related to the accuracy or integrity of any part of the work are appropriately investigated and resolved.
>
> In addition to being accountable for the parts of the work she or he has done, an author should be able to identify which coauthors are responsible for specific other parts of the work. In addition, authors should have confidence in the integrity of the contributions of their coauthors.
>
> All those designated as authors should meet all four criteria. All who meet the four criteria should be identified as authors.

From International Committee of Medical Journal Editors (ICMJE). (2019). *Defining the role of authors and contributors.* Retrieved from http://www.icmje.org/recommendations/browse/roles-and-responsibilities/defining-the-role-of-authors-and-contributors.html

journals, the editor makes the decision to accept or reject a manuscript, but this decision usually is made after consultation with a nursing expert.

Some journals are published only online. Of these, some charge a fee for open access. It is important to establish that your target journal is not a predatory journal. A **predatory journal** is involved in solicitation of manuscripts and requires authors to pay an article processing charge of hundreds or thousands of dollars to have a manuscript published. It may be difficult to differentiate legitimate open-access journals from predatory ones. Ensure that the journal you select is a reputable journal that is indexed in databases such as the Cumulative Index to Nursing and Allied Health Literature (CINAHL). In addition, the librarian at your institution can be extremely helpful in assisting you in this determination. For publication in a reputable open-access journal, a faculty author may have the fee paid by the university. Occasionally, fees may be waived by the journal. Some of these journals require peer review of submitted manuscripts, similar to non-predatory journals.

Most refereed journals require manuscripts to be reviewed anonymously, or blinded, by two or three reviewers. Expertise and objectivity are characteristics of ideal reviewers (Shamoo & Resnik, 2015) who can evaluate the quality of a manuscript and its potential contribution to knowledge. Reviewers are asked to determine the strengths and weaknesses of a manuscript, and their comments are sent anonymously from the journal editor to the contact author. Most academic institutions support the refereed system and may credit only publications that appear in peer-reviewed journals in support of faculty members seeking tenure and promotion.

Opportunities to publish research have grown as research journals have become more plentiful. Publishing opportunities in nursing continue to increase. The *Journal Citation Reports* (Web of Science Group, 2019) includes more than 260 journals with *nursing* or *nurse* in their titles. The Nursing and Allied Health Resources Section (NAHRS) of the Medical Library Association created a report of 512 nursing journals in 2016. The report incorporates the type of review that manuscripts receive, the percentage of submitted manuscripts accepted for publication, and the types of articles published (NAHRS, 2016). When deciding on a potential journal for a study, the NAHRS report, the *Journal Citations Report,* and other similar reports can provide invaluable information about four criteria to consider when selecting a journal: (1) the intended readers who would benefit from reading the findings, (2) the fit of the study's topic to the journal's focus, (3) the journal's reported elapsed time between acceptance of a manuscript and its publication, and (4) the impact factor for the journal.

Intended audience. The content for a study may be most suitable for a small specialty group audience, or perhaps a broader spectrum of nurses would think the research interesting and pertinent to their practice. Nurse researchers should not limit their options to nursing journals if a wider audience of health professionals is the proper target for findings of the study. Additional clues about possible audiences can be found in the references cited in the research report. For example, if your reference list includes several articles from genomics journals, one of those journals may be an appropriate choice for your article. If it is important

for the findings to be reported as soon as possible, consider an online journal or a journal that has monthly issues rather than quarterly issues.

Fit of the topic to the journal's focus. Having a manuscript accepted for publication depends not only on the quality of the manuscript but also on how closely the manuscript matches the goals of the journal and its subscribers or audience (MedSurg Nursing, 2019). Reviewing articles recently published in the journal being considered can be helpful in assessing this match. A detailed review of this sort lets you know whether a research topic has been addressed recently and whether the research findings would be of interest to that journal's readers. This process enables you to identify and prioritize a few journals that would be appropriate for publishing your findings. Reviewing the journal's impact factor, the timeline for their review process, and the waiting period from acceptance to publication date also can impact your decision on submission targets for your manuscript.

Time between acceptance and publication. The editors of journals that are considered to be highly reputable and well established receive more manuscripts than their journals can ever publish. Journals that have a broad focus, such as *Nursing Research* and *Journal of Nursing Scholarship,* receive many submissions and may have a backlog of accepted manuscripts. Authors may wait over a year for a manuscript to be published. Newer and specialty journals receive fewer manuscripts. Online journals may publish a manuscript as soon as it is accepted, revised, and checked for format. As a result, the time from acceptance to publication may be shorter, which is especially desirable if you are seeking promotion or trying to complete a requirement for your doctoral program.

Journal impact factor. *Journal Citation Reports* (Web of Science Group, 2019) provides quantitative measures for evaluating scientific journals, including data on journal impact factors. Garfield (2006), the originator of the **impact factor**, defined it to be a measure of the frequency with which the "average article" in a journal has been cited in a given period of time. The impact factor for a journal is calculated based on a 3-year period and can be considered to be the average number of times published papers are cited in the first 2 years after publication. The impact factor cannot be calculated until the publication of a year's worth of issues; for that reason, the most current impact factor available may reflect data from 1 to 2 years earlier. The impact factor for a journal usually can be found on the journal's website. The higher the number, the better. In general, specialty journals in nursing have lower impact factors than broad-based medical journals such as *Journal of the American Medical Association* or *New England Journal of Medicine.*

Developing a Query Letter

A **query letter** is a letter an author sends to an editor, to ask about the editor's interest in reviewing a manuscript. This letter should be no more than one page in length and usually includes the abstract and the researcher's qualifications for writing the article. The length of the manuscript and the numbers of tables or figures may be useful information to include, and the editor may be interested to know when, if ever, something on this topic was last published in that journal. Some editors appreciate a list of potential reviewers that you might suggest. Address your query letter in an e-mail to the current editor of a journal. Indicate in the letter the title of the manuscript you would like to submit, why publishing the manuscript is important, and why the readers of the journal would be interested in reading the manuscript. Even if a query letter is not required by a journal, some researchers send one because the response (positive or negative) enables them to make the final selection for submitting their manuscript to a journal. Often an editor responds that the journal is planning a special issue on a particular topic and provides the due dates so that you can prepare well in advance. Other journals, such as *Advances in Nursing Science,* publish only special topic issues. You can select an appropriate issue for your submission by reviewing their websites with due dates by topic.

Preparing a Manuscript

A manuscript is written according to the format outlined by each different journal. Guidelines for developing a manuscript usually are published in the individual issues of the journal or on journal websites. Oermann et al. (2018) conducted research concerning the author guidelines provided by 245 nursing journals. The authors found that, overall, guidelines were accurate and of assistance to authors. Following the journal recommendations for specific reporting guidelines improved the accuracy and completeness of submitted manuscripts. Many journals will not review a manuscript

until it is written and formatted according to the author guidelines. Author guidelines are comprised of directions for manuscript preparation, a discussion of copyright and conflict of interest, and guidelines for submission of the manuscript. Most journals accept only online submissions of electronic files.

Writing research reports for publication requires technical writing skills that are not used in other types of publications. Technical writing condenses information and is stylistic. The *Publication Manual of the American Psychological Association* (APA, 2020); *A Manual for Writers of Research Papers, Theses, and Dissertations* (Booth et al., 2018); and the *Chicago Manual of Style* (Colbert-Lewis, 2018) are considered useful sources for quality technical writing. Most journals stipulate the format style required for their journal. In a review of 245 nursing journals, Oermann et al. (2018) noted that about half (51%) required APA format. If a journal requires a format different from that of your original manuscript, there are format translators available through most universities that will convert one format to another. Computer programs are available with bibliography systems that enable you to compile a consistent reference list formatted in any commonly accepted journal style. With these programs, researchers can maintain a permanent file of reference citations. When a reference list is needed for a manuscript, the researchers can select the appropriate references from the collection and use the program to reformat for the requirements of a particular journal.

A quality research report has no errors in punctuation, spelling, or sentence structure. It is also important to avoid confusing words, clichés, jargon, and excessive wordiness and abbreviations. Word processing programs have tools with the capacity to proofread manuscripts for errors. However, as the author, you still must respond to the software's prompts and correct the sentences that the program has identified as problematic. These program tools also perform a word count, to ensure that your manuscript adheres to the limitations specified in the journal guidelines.

Knowledge about the author guidelines provided by the journal and a background in technical writing will help you develop an outline for a proposed manuscript. You can use the outline to develop a rough draft of your article, which you will revise numerous times. Present the content of your article logically and concisely under clear headings, and select a title that creates interest and reflects the content. The *Publication Manual* (APA, 2020) provides detailed directions regarding appropriate terms to use in describing study results and manuscript preparation. Consider using an article from the journal as a guide or template; this can help inform you as to the general length of the Introduction and Discussion sections, the presentation format for tables, the reference citation format, and the wording of acknowledgments. For a journal with an international focus, it is important to specify that your sample is from a particular geographic area such as the United States. If the journal is British, appropriate spelling is important (e.g., *hospitalization* would be spelled *hospitalisation*); software spellcheck tools have options for American English, British English, and other languages.

Developing a well-written manuscript is difficult. Often universities and other agencies offer writing seminars to assist students and faculty members in preparing a publication. Graduate students might consider working with a faculty member to publish a manuscript. Some faculty members who chair thesis and dissertation committees assist their students in developing an article for publication in exchange for second authorship. The *Publication Manual* (APA, 2020) has a section on how to reduce the content of a thesis or dissertation so as to create a manuscript of suitable size for publication.

When you are satisfied with your manuscript, ask one or two colleagues to review it for accuracy, organization, completeness of content, and writing style. If you are writing the article with a research team, your coauthors are the colleagues whom you would ask to review the manuscript. Ask a friend or family member who is not a health professional to read the article, as well. Although friends and family members may not understand the topic or statistical results, they should be able to read the paper and understand the primary messages being communicated. If they don't understand and can explain where they lost the thread of the argument, what an opportunity for you, as a writer! Gennaro (2018), the editor of a major nursing journal, stated, "When other people don't understand my thoughts, their confusion helps me gain clarity" (p. 239).

The reference list for the manuscript must be complete and in the correct format. To double-check all references doesn't mean that you should read each one twice. It means that you will, first, read each item in the entire reference list to confirm that all requisite parts of

the reference are present. Then you will recheck for proper spelling, italicization, and capitalization of all required elements. Next, you must check all in-text citations to be sure that they appear in the reference list and check all entries in the reference list to make sure that they appear as in-text citations. Finally, website addresses for all electronic sources are selected just prior to submission, to confirm that they still access the required information.

Submitting a Manuscript for Review

Guidelines in each journal indicate the name of the editor and the address for manuscript submission. Submit your manuscript to one journal at a time; only when you confirm that your manuscript is not accepted should you submit to a different journal. Most journals now accept only manuscripts submitted electronically, and the editor provides a portable document format (PDF) version to reviewers when they accept the offer to review the manuscript. When submitting the manuscript, include your complete mailing address, phone number, fax number, and e-mail address. The corresponding author who submits the manuscript usually receives notification of receipt of the manuscript within 24 to 48 hours if submitted electronically, and in many cases the notification is sent to all authors listed on the title page of the manuscript.

Scholarly journals use a peer review process to evaluate the quality of manuscripts submitted for publication. As noted previously in the chapter, peer reviewers who do not know the identity of the authors evaluate the quality and acceptability of the manuscript. For reviewers to remain blinded, journal instructions will indicate that any materials in the manuscript that identify the authors or institutions should be omitted and replaced with brackets to indicate that something was intentionally removed from the text—[removed for blind review].

For research papers, reviewers are asked to evaluate the validity of the study. Reviewers consider whether the methodology was adequate for addressing the research question or hypotheses and whether the findings are trustworthy and correctly interpreted. For example, if results were not statistically significant, was a power analysis performed? Reviewers also evaluate whether the discussion was appropriate, given the findings, and whether the author adequately discussed clinical implications of the findings without going beyond the actual data. Reviewers also are asked to comment on the relevance of the reference citations, the usefulness of any tables or figures, and the consistency among title, abstract, and text. Reviewers also look for the strengths and limitations of the study, which the authors should convey in their discussion. Every study has its limitations, and a limitation is not a reason for rejecting the manuscript. However, reviewers want to see that the authors have accurately identified and addressed limitations for the readers. The author's failure to identify limitations of the study implies that the author does not understand what a limitation is.

Responding to Requests to Revise a Manuscript

After reviewing a manuscript, the journal editor gathers the evaluations of all reviewers and reaches one of four possible decisions: (1) acceptance of the manuscript as submitted; (2) acceptance of the manuscript, pending minor revisions; (3) tentative acceptance of the manuscript pending major revisions; or (4) rejection of the manuscript. Acceptance of a manuscript as submitted is extremely rare. When this occurs, the editor sends a letter that indicates acceptance and the likely date of publication.

Most manuscripts are accepted pending revisions or accepted tentatively and returned to the author for minor or major revisions, before publication. Unfortunately, too many of these returned manuscripts are never revised. If you perceive the review to be negative, you would do well to set aside the review for a few days to allow the emotional response to subside. An author may incorrectly interpret the request for revision as a rejection and assume that a revised manuscript would also be rejected. This assumption usually is not true because revising a manuscript based on reviewers' comments improves the quality of the manuscript. When editors return a manuscript for revision, they include reviewers' actual comments or a summary of the comments to direct the revision. These reviewers and the editor have devoted time to reviewing your manuscript, and you should make the necessary revisions or respond with your rationale for not making a specific change requested by a reviewer and return the revised manuscript to the same journal for reconsideration.

On a practical note, create a two-column table in a new document, number all the reviewers' comments, and list them in separate rows in the first column. Review each comment carefully and decide whether the recommendation or modification will improve the quality of the research report without making inaccurate statements about the study. When appropriate, revise accordingly and note the page number where the changes can be found in the second column on the row corresponding to the comment. In some cases, you may disagree with a reviewer's recommendation. If so, provide a rationale for your disagreement with literature support in the second column, but do not ignore any comment or recommendation. If two reviewers provided conflicting comments, consult the journal editor, who will provide guidance about how to respond to the suggestions. When you have revised your manuscript based on the reviewers' comments, it should be resubmitted with a cover letter and the table of reviewers' comments and your responses. Sometimes the revised manuscript and your cover letter are returned to the reviewers, and still further modification is requested in the paper before it is published. Some published manuscripts have been revised three times before being accepted by the first journal to which they were submitted. Although these experiences are frustrating, they provide the opportunity to improve your writing skills and logical development of ideas.

In the case that the manuscript is rejected, realize that manuscripts are rejected for various reasons. The most common reason for manuscript rejection is that the writer did not follow the author guidelines (Suhonen, 2016). Other reasons cited are lack of clarity and writing that is not up to expectations (Suhonen, 2016). Sometimes the topic of the article has been well covered in the literature recently, and so the study is no longer of interest (Gennaro, 2018). The editor or reviewers may determine that the topic is not relevant to the journal's audience. Most rejection notices include the reason for the rejection. When a manuscript is rejected, make changes as appropriate, correct any writing concerns the reviewers identified, and send the manuscript to another journal.

Formats for Publication

As you consider where to publish your research findings, there are formats other than print journals. In this section, we will describe the unique aspects of publishing in online journals and books.

Online Journals

Many print journals have converted to online formats. These journals continue to provide their traditional print version but also maintain a website with access to some or all of the articles in the printed journal. The number of nursing journals being published only online is growing.

Not all online journals are refereed or provide peer review, however. The author should investigate potential online journals by determining whether submissions are peer reviewed and whether the journal has an editorial board (see earlier comments about predatory journals). Peer review is essential to scholars in the university tenure track system and to the development of nursing science. Because online journals do not have advertisers to offset their operating costs, some journals require a processing fee for submitting and publishing an article in the journal. Carefully review the information provided on the journal's website for specific information on fees and other charges. A way to establish the legitimacy of an online journal is to determine whether the journal, and subsequently each article, has a Digital Object Identifier (DOI). The International DOI Foundation assigns permanent DOIs to all types of digital work. The DOI will never change, even if the location for that work changes. The use of DOIs is expected to increase and become accepted as the permanent identifier for scientific and scholarly publications (International DOI Foundation, 2018).

Online publication has several advantages, including continuous publication. There is no wait for approved articles to be published because the editor does not have to wait until the next issue is scheduled for publication. The notion of an issue is becoming antiquated as a result of electronic publishing. Approved articles are placed online almost immediately. Rapid availability of research findings can facilitate the development of science and promote EBP. The constraint on length of the manuscript, imposed because of the cost of print publishing, usually does not exist. Multiple tables, figures, graphics, and even streaming audio and video are possibilities with online journals. Animations can be created to assist the reader to visualize ideas. Links may be established with full-text versions of citations from other online sources. It is possible to track the number of times the article has been accessed to assess its impact on the scientific community. Electronic listservs and chat rooms may be available to discuss the paper. All of these capabilities are not currently available with every online journal. The technology to provide them exists, but online journals with some of these advanced technologies cover their costs by charging subscription fees.

Books

Research findings may be disseminated in printed reports and books. Foundations and federal agencies that sponsor a research project may provide paper-based reports of studies that have been conducted or are in progress. Due to the costs of printing, many of these organizations are publishing their reports online. Some qualitative studies and large, complex quantitative studies are published as chapters within books, as monographs, or as free-standing books. Publishing a book requires extensive commitment on the part of the researcher. In addition, the researcher must select a publisher and convince the publisher to support the book project. A prospectus must be developed that identifies the proposed content of the book, describes the market readership for the book, and includes a rationale for publishing the book. The publisher and researcher must negotiate a contract that is mutually acceptable regarding (1) the content and length of the book, (2) the time required to complete the book, (3) the percentage of royalties/fees the author will receive, (4) any financial coverage to be offered in advance, and (5) how the book will be marketed. The researcher must fulfill the obligations of the contract by producing the proposed book within the agreed time frame. Publishing a book is a significant accomplishment and an effective, but sometimes slow, means of communicating research findings.

Errors to Avoid

Plagiarism is a type of research misconduct that involves the appropriation of another person's ideas, processes, results, or words without giving appropriate credit. In a manuscript, this can include intentionally or inadvertently failing to cite a reference or properly attribute a quotation from another author. When this occurs, the author is implying that the words and ideas are his or her own (Shamoo & Resnik, 2015). Many journal editors screen a manuscript for plagiarism using software programs. Plagiarism is unethical (Gennaro, 2012). If portions of a manuscript have been presented at a scientific meeting in the form of an oral podium or poster presentation, this should be acknowledged along with funding sources and any potential conflict of interest.

Journals require the submission of an original manuscript, not previously published. Submitting a manuscript that has been previously published without referencing the duplicate work or notifying the editor of the previous publication is unethical and a form of scientific misconduct (Shamoo & Resnick, 2015). Duplicate publication is the practice of publishing the same article or major portions of an article in two or more print or electronic locations without notifying the editors and copyright holders or referencing the other publication in the reference list. It is not uncommon, however, to publish more than one article from a single study. However previous publications related to the study must be disclosed and cited in the text of the manuscript and the reference list (Shamoo & Resnick, 2015). Editors have the responsibility of developing a policy on duplicate

publications and informing all authors, reviewers, and readers of this policy (Committee on Publication Ethics [COPE], n.d.). In addition, editors must ensure that readers are informed of duplicate materials by adequate citation of the materials in the article's text and reference list. A duplicate publication can result in retractions and refusal to accept other manuscripts for review from the author (ICMJE, 2019). In keeping with the standards of nursing as a profession, dissemination of research findings must occur according to the highest standards of ethical behavior.

KEY POINTS

- Communicating research findings, the final step in the research process, involves developing a research report and disseminating it. Disseminating study findings is part of your obligation to your research participants, to the nursing profession, and to yourself.
- The greatest impact on nursing practice can be achieved by communicating nursing research findings to nurses, other health professionals, policymakers, and healthcare consumers.
- Both quantitative and qualitative research reports include four basic sections: (1) Introduction, (2) Methods, (3) Results, and (4) Discussion.
- The Introduction section provides background for the research topic and the significance of the study.
- The Methods section describes how the study was conducted, including any instruments, equipment, and other means of data collection such as interviews and observation.
- The Results sections of quantitative and qualitative research reports are similar in that each begins with a description of the sample, but they vary greatly for the rest of the report because of the type of data and methods of analysis.
- Quantitative research reports contain the presentation of statistical results in text, tables, or figures.
- Qualitative research reports contain the presentation of themes, sometimes supported by quotes from the participants, within context.
- The Discussion section includes validity-based limitations, conclusions that support or refute other published work, implications for nursing practice, and recommendations for further research.

- Research findings are presented at conferences and meetings through oral podium and poster presentations of selected portions of the study; the content of the report depends on the focus of the conference, the audience, and the time designated for each presentation.
- A poster presentation is a visual display of a study, presented at the "poster session" of a conference. Conference sponsors provide information concerning (1) size limitations or format restrictions for the poster and (2) the size of the poster display area. The home institution should provide (1) the institution's logo to place with your title and affiliations and (2) any requirements for the poster's color scheme. Your university or employer may have a template you are required to use.
- Developing a manuscript for publication includes the following steps: (1) selecting a journal, (2) writing a query letter, (3) preparing an original manuscript, (4) submitting the manuscript for review, and (5) responding to requests for revision of the manuscript.
- Selecting a journal for publication of a study requires knowledge of the basic requirements of the journal, the journal's refereed status, its impact factor, and recent articles published in the journal.
- Researchers must exercise care to avoid plagiarism, self-plagiarism, and duplicate publications by using plagiarism detection systems, receiving permission to use content previously published, and referencing their own and others' publications in the reference list.

REFERENCES

Adebiyi, M., Mosaku, S., Irinoye, O., & Oyelade, O. (2018). Socio-demographic and clinical factors associated with relapse in mental illness. *International Journal of Africa Nursing Sciences, 8*, 149–153. doi:10.1016/j.ijans.2018.05.007

Al-Ghareeb, A., McKenna, L., & Cooper, S. (2019). The influence of anxiety on student nurse performance in a simulated clinical setting: A mixed methods design. *International Journal of Nursing Studies, 98*, 57–66. doi:10.1016/j.ijnurstu.2019.06.006

American Psychological Association (APA). (2020). *Publication manual of the American Psychological Association* (7th ed.). Washington, DC: Author.

American Society of Agronomy, Crop Science Society of America, & Soil Science Society of America (ASA-CSSA-SSSA). (Updated 2019). *Publications handbook & style manual.* Retrieved from https://dl.sciencesocieties.org/files/publications/style/style-manual.pdf

Anderson, J. E., Ross, A. J., Lim, R., Kodate, N., Thompson, K., Jensen, H., & Cooney, K. (2019). Nursing teamwork in the care of older people: A mixed methods study. *Applied Ergonomics, 80*, 119–129. doi:10.1016/j.apergo.2019.05.012

Booth, W. C., Colomb, G. G., Williams, J. M., Bizup, J., FitzGerald, W. T., & The University of Chicago Press Editorial Staff (Eds.). (2018). *Kate L. Turabian: A manual for writers of research papers, theses, and dissertations: Chicago style for students and researchers* (9th ed.). Chicago, IL: University of Chicago Press.

Chan, H., Ng, J., Chan, K-S., Ko, P-S., Leung, D., Chan, C., ... Lee, D. (2018). Effects of a nurse-led post-discharge advance care planning programme for community-dwelling patients nearing the end of life and their family members: A randomised controlled trial. *International Journal of Nursing Studies, 87*, 26–33. doi:10.1016/j.ijnurstu.2018.07.008

Chapman, S. A., & Blash, L. K. (2017). New roles for medical assistants in innovative primary care practices. *Health Services Research, 52*(1), 383–406. doi:10.1111/1475-6773.12602

Chapman, S., Phoenix, B., Hahn, T., & Strod, D. (2018). Utilization and economic contribution of psychiatric mental health nurse practitioners in public behavioral health services. *American Journal of Preventive Medicine, 54*(6), S243–S249. doi:10.1016/j.amepre.2018.01.045

Chapman, S. A., Wides, C. D., & Spetz, J. (2010). Payment regulations for advanced practice nurses: Implications for primary care. *Policy, Politics, & Nursing Practice, 11*(2), 89–98. doi:10.1177/1527154410382458

Cleeland, C. (2009). *The brief pain inventory user guide.* Houston, TX: M. D. Anderson Cancer Center.

Colbert-Lewis, D. (2018). The Chicago manual of style (17th ed.). *Reference Reviews, 32*(4), 19–20. doi:10.1108/RR-02-2018-0024

Committee on Publication Ethics (COPE). (n.d.). *A short guide to ethical editing.* Retrieved from https://publicationethics.org/news/revised-and-updated-short-guide-ethical-editing-new-editors.

Consolidated Standards of Reporting (CONSORT). (2010). *CONSORT statement.* Retrieved from http://www.consort-statement.org/consort-2010

Craig, J. V., & Dowding, D. (2020). *Evidence-based practice in nursing* (4th ed.). Edinburgh, Scotland: Elsevier.

Creswell, J. W., & Creswell, J. D. (2018). *Qualitative inquiry and research design: Choosing among five approaches* (4th ed.). Thousand Oaks, CA: Sage.

Garfield, E. (2006). The history and meaning of the journal impact factor. *Journal of the American Medical Association, 295*(1), 90–93. doi:10.1001/jama.295.1.90

Gennaro, S. (2012). Ideas and words: The ethics of scholarship [Editorial]. *Journal of Nursing Scholarship, 44*(2), 109–110. doi:10.1111/j.1547-5069.2012.01450.x

Gennaro, S. (2018). Publishing success: Rules to live by [Editorial]. *Journal of Nursing Scholarship, 50*(3), 239–240. doi:10.1111/jnu.12382

Graves, J. M., Postma, J., Katz, J. R., Kehoe, L., Swalling, E., & Barbosa-Leiker, C. (2018). A national survey examining manuscript dissertation formats among nursing PhD programs in the United States. *Journal of Nursing Scholarship, 50*(3), 314–323. doi:10.1111/jnu.12374

Grove, S. K., & Cipher, D. J. (2020). *Statistics for nursing research: A workbook for evidence-based practice* (3rd ed.). St. Louis, MO: Saunders.

Hanneke, R., & Link, J. M. (2019). The complex nature of research dissemination practices among public health faculty researchers. *Journal of the Medical Library Association, 107*(3), 341–351. doi:10.5195/jmla.2019.524

Henderson, A., Ossenberg, C., & Tyler, S. (2015). "What matters to graduates": An evaluation of a structured clinical support program for newly graduated nurses. *Nurse Education in Practice, 15*(3), 225–231. doi:10.1016/j.nepr.2015.01.009

Inflexxion. (2010). *Current opioid misuse measure (COMM).* Retrieved from http://nationalpaincentre.mcmaster.ca/documents/comm_sample_watermarked.pdf

International Business Machines (IBM). (n.d.) *Statistical Package for Social Sciences.* https://www.ibm.com/products/spss-statistics

International Committee of Medical Journal Editors (ICMJE). (2019). *Uniform requirements for manuscripts submitted to biomedical journals: Writing and editing for biomedical publication.* Retrieved from http://www.icmje.org/recommendations/browse/roles-and-responsibilities/

International DOI Foundation. (2018). *DOI ® handbook*. Retrieved from https://www.doi.org/hb.html

International Journal of Nursing Studies (IJNS). (2019). *Guide for authors*. Retrieved from https://www.elsevier.com/journals/international-journal-of-nursing-studies/0020-7489/guide-for-authors#5021

Kroenke, K., Spitzer, R., Williams, J., & Löwe, B. (2010). The patient health questionnaire somatic, anxiety, and social depressive symptoms scales: A systematic review. *General Hospital Psychiatry*, *32*(4), 345–359. doi:10.1016/j.genhosppsych.2010.03.006

Lentz, M. (2011). *Writing a WINning abstract*. Retrieved from https://www.youtube.com/watch?v=d_Dmr4z17is

Mallah, Z., Nassar, N., & Kurdahi Badr, L. (2015). The effectiveness of a pressure ulcer intervention program on the prevalence of hospital acquired pressure ulcers: Controlled before and after study. *Applied Nursing Research*, *28*(2), 106–113. doi:10.1016/j.apnr.2014.07.001

Marshall, C., & Rossman, G. B. (2016). *Designing qualitative research* (6th ed.). Thousand Oaks, CA: Sage.

MedSurg Nursing. (2019). *Author guidelines*. Retrieved from http://www.medsurgnursing.net/cgibin/WebObjects/MSNJournal.woa/wa/viewSection?s_id=1073744511

Melnyk, B. M., & Fineout-Overholt, E. (2019). *Evidence-based practice in nursing & healthcare: A guide to best practice* (4th ed.). Philadelphia, PA: Lippincott Williams & Wilkins.

Miles, M., Huberman, A., & Saldaña, J. (2020). *Qualitative data analysis: A methods sourcebook* (4th ed.). Thousand Oaks, CA: Sage.

Mlinarić, A., Horvat, M., & Šupak Smolčić , V. (2017). Dealing with the positive publication bias: Why you should really publish your negative results. *Biochemia Medica*, *27*(3), 030201. doi:10.11613/BM.2017.030201

Morse, J. (2005). Feigning independence: The article dissertation [Editorial]. *Qualitative Health Research*, *15*(9), 1147–1148. doi:10.1177/1049732305281328

Munhall, P. (2012). *Nursing research: A qualitative perspective* (5th ed.). Sudbury, MA: Jones & Bartlett Learning.

Newnam, K., McGrath, J., Salyer, J., Estes, J., Jallo, N., & Bass, W. (2015). A comparative effectiveness study of continuous positive airway pressure-related skin breakdown when using different nasal interfaces in the extremely low birth weight neonate. *Applied Nursing Research*, *28*(1), 36–41. doi:10.1016/j.apnr.2014.05.005

New York University (NYU) Libraries. (2019). *How to create a research poster: Poster basics*. Retrieved from https://guides.nyu.edu/posters

Nursing and Allied Health Resources Section (NAHRS). (2016). *Selected list of nursing journals*. Retrieved from https://docs.google.com/viewer?a=v&pid=sites&srcid=ZGVmYXVsdGRvbWFpbnxuYWhyc251cnNpbmmdyZXNvdXJjZXN8Z3g6MmU4MTU4MDgwN2I4YjhkOA

Oermann, M. H., Nicoll, L. H, Chinn, P. L., Conklin, J. L., McCarty, M., & Amarasekara, S. (2018). Quality of author guidelines in nursing journals. *Journal of Nursing Scholarship*, *50*(3), 333–340. doi:10.1111/jnu.12383

Ot'Alora, G. M., Grigsby, J., Poulter, B., Van Derveer, J., Giron, S., Jerome, L., ... Doblin, R. (2018). 3,4-Methylenedioxymethamphetamine-assisted psychotherapy for treatment of chronic posttraumatic stress disorder: A randomized phase 2 controlled trial. *Journal of Psychopharmacology (Oxford, England)*, *32*(12), 1295–1307. doi:10.1177/0269881118806297

Public Library of Science (PLOS). (2019). *Submission guidelines*. Retrieved from https://journals.plos.org/plosone/s/submission-guidelines

Pyrczak, F., & Bruce, R. R. (2017). *Writing empirical research reports: A basic guide for students of the social and behavioral sciences* (8th ed.). New York, NY: Routledge.

Ruwaard, S., & Douven, R. (2018). Hospital choice for cataract treatments: The winner takes most. *International Journal of Health Policy and Management*, *7*(12), 1120–1129. doi:10.15171/ijhpm.2018.77

Sandelowski, M., & Barroso, J. (2002). Finding the findings in qualitative studies. *Journal of Nursing Scholarship*, *34*(3), 213–219. doi:10.1111/j.1547-5069.2002.00213.x

Sandelowski, M., & Leeman, J. (2012). Writing usable qualitative research findings. *Qualitative Health Research*, *22*(10), 1404–1413. doi: 10.1177/1049732312450368

Saver, C. (2006). Tables and figures: Adding vitality to your article. *AORN Journal*, *84*(6), 945–950. doi:10.1016/S0001-2092(06)63991-4

Schulz, K. F., Altman, D. G., & Moher, D. for the CONSORT Group. (2010). CONSORT 2010 statement: Updated guidelines for reporting parallel group randomised trials. *BMJ (Clinical Research Ed.)*, *340*(7748), C332. Retrieved from https://www.bmj.com/content/340/bmj.c332

Seth, U. (2019). How to read a forest plot. *Journal of the Practice of Cardiovascular Sciences*, *5*(2), 108–110. doi:10.4103/jpcs.jpcs_39_19

Shamoo, A., & Resnik, D. (2015). *Responsible conduct of research* (3rd ed.). Oxford, England: Oxford University Press.

Smith, M. (2018). Psychedelic drugs to treat depression, PTSD? *WebMD Health News*. Retrieved from https://www.webmd.com/mental-health/news/20180918/psychedlic-drugs-to-treat-depression-ptsd

Suhonen, R. (2016). Thoughts from an editor's desk [Editorial]. *Nursing Ethics*, *23*(8), 823–824. doi:10.1177/0969733016681679

Tong, A., Sainsbury, P., & Craig, J. (2007). Consolidated criteria for reporting qualitative research (COREQ): A 32-item checklist for interviews and focus groups. *International Journal for Quality in Health Care*, *19*(6), 349–357. doi:10.1093/intqhc/mzm042

Tonkin, L. (2008). The pain self-efficacy questionnaire. *The Australian Journal of Physiotherapy*, *54*(1), 77.

Web of Science Group. (2019). *2019 journal citation reports: Full journal list*. Retrieved from https://clarivate.com/webofsciencegroup/wp-content/uploads/sites/2/2019/10/WS407569850_JCR_Full_Journal_list-2.pdf

Wilson, M., Roll, J., Corbett, C., & Barbosa-Leiker, C. (2015). Empowering patients with persistent pain using an internet-based self-management program. *Pain Management Nursing*, *16*(4), 503–514. doi:10.1016/j.pmn.2014.09.009

Young, J., Bridgeman, M. B., & Hermes-De Santis, E. R. (2018). Presentation of scientific poster information: Lessons learned from evaluating the impact of content arrangement and use of infographics. *Currents in Pharmacy Teaching and Learning*, *11*, 204–210. doi:10.1016/j.cptl.2018.11.011

28

Writing Research Proposals

Suzanne Sutherland

http://evolve.elsevier.com/Gray/practice/

A **research proposal** is a formal written plan that identifies the major elements of a proposed study, such as the research problem, purpose, literature review, and framework, and communicates the methods and procedures for conducting a study. The purpose of writing a research proposal may be one or more of the following: (1) to seek approval from an educational institution to conduct research within the educational facility itself or elsewhere, under its auspices; (2) to seek approval from a healthcare institution for conduct of research that will obtain data from patients or institutional records; (3) to apply for research funding; (4) to fulfill a course requirement; and (5) to compete for a prize or honor. Researchers who seek approval to conduct a study submit a proposal to a select group for review and, in many situations, verbally defend the proposal. Receiving approval to conduct research has become more complicated because of the increasing intricacies of nursing studies, the difficulty involved in recruiting study participants, and escalating concerns over legal and ethical issues. In many large hospitals and healthcare corporations, both the institution's legal representatives and the institutional review boards (IRBs) evaluate research proposals. The expanded number of healthcare studies being conducted has led to competition for potential subjects in some settings, as well as increased competition for funding. A researcher must develop a quality study proposal to facilitate university and clinical agency IRB approval, obtain funding, and conduct a study successfully. This chapter provides students with guidelines for writing a research proposal and seeking approval to conduct a study. Chapter 29 presents the process of seeking funding for research.

WRITING A RESEARCH PROPOSAL

A well-written proposal communicates plans for a significant and carefully planned research project, displays the qualifications of the researcher, and generates support for the project. Conducting research requires precision and rigorous attention to detail. Reviewers judge a researcher's ability to conduct a study by the quality of the proposal, including the clarity of the writing. You are encouraged to access writing resources that present the rules of basic English usage and punctuation, such as *The Elements of Style* (Strunk & White, 2018). Writing resources often are available online from writing labs within your home institution or through your university library. A quality study proposal must be clear, concise, and complete. Writing such a proposal involves (1) developing ideas logically, (2) determining the depth or detail of the content of the proposal, (3) identifying critical points in the proposal, and (4) developing an

Acknowledgment: Drs. Gray, Grove, and Sutherland want to thank Kathy Daniels, RN, PhD, FAAN, for providing the example of a proposal.

aesthetically appealing copy (Merrill, 2011; Offredy & Vickers, 2010). But most of all, it involves reading instructions and following them, to the letter. Your thesis or dissertation advisor has experience navigating these instructions and can clarify details that seem contradictory or ambiguous.

Developing Ideas Logically

The ideas in a research proposal must build logically upon one another to justify or defend a study, just as a lawyer would construct a logical argument in defense of a client. The researcher builds a case to justify the reason a problem should be studied and proposes the appropriate means for doing so. Each step in the research proposal builds on problem and purpose statements to provide a clear picture of the study and its merit (Holtzclaw, Kenner, & Walden, 2018; Merrill, 2011).

Universities, medical centers, federal funding agencies, and grant-writing consultants have developed websites to help researchers write successful proposals. For example, the University of Michigan Department of Research and Sponsored Projects (2019) provides an online guide for proposal development with links to other resources. The National Institute of Nursing Research (NINR, 2019) provides online training on their website for developing nurse scientists. You can use a search engine of your choice, such as Google, and search for research proposal development training, proposal-writing tips, courses on proposal development, and proposal guidelines. In addition, several key publications have been developed to help individuals improve their scientific writing skills and adhere precisely to specific citation styles and formats (American Psychological Association [APA], 2020; Booth et al., 2018; The University of Chicago Press Staff, 2010). Various university writing labs provide online information that applies to different required citation styles: APA, MLA (Modern Language Association), Chicago, and others. For instance, the Purdue University Online Writing Lab (2019) maintains a search page from which you can obtain clear information and examples of correct APA formatting and style.

Determining the Depth of a Proposal

The depth or detail of content required for a proposal is determined by guidelines developed by colleges or schools of nursing, funding agencies, and institutions in which research is conducted. The website of the National Council of State Boards of Nursing (NCSBN) presents guidelines for proposal submission for research regarding the National Council Licensure Examination (NCLEX) (NCSBN, 2019). University of Oklahoma College of Nursing PhD program displays guidelines for dissertation proposals on its website (2019). National Institutes of Health (NIH, 2019) has a web page devoted to how to apply for a grant, including information about specific content that is highly valued in current proposals, such discussions of rigor and reproducibility (Holtzclaw et al., 2018). Guidelines provide specific directions for the development of a proposal and should be followed explicitly. Omission or misinterpretation of a guideline is frequently the basis for proposal rejection, or request for resubmission with revisions. In addition to following the guidelines, you should determine the amount of information necessary to describe each step of your study clearly. The reviewers of the proposal will have varied expertise in your area of study. The content in a proposal should be detailed and clear enough to inform different types of readers, yet concise enough to be interesting and easy to review. The guidelines often stipulate a page limit, which determines the depth of the proposal.

Identifying Critical Points

The key or critical points in a proposal must be evident, even to a hasty reader. Unless the guidelines prohibit it, highlighting critical points with bold or italicized type emphasizes essential points. Sometimes researchers create headings for emphasis of critical material, or they organize the content into tables or graphs. A research proposal should include the background and significance of the research problem and purpose, the study methodology, and the research implementation plans (data collection, data analysis, personnel, schedule, and budget) (APA, 2020; Booth et al., 2018; Holtzclaw et al., 2018).

Developing an Aesthetically Appealing Copy

An aesthetically appealing copy is typed without errors of spelling, punctuation, or grammar. A proposal with excellent content that is poorly typed or inaccurately formatted is not likely to receive the full attention or respect of reviewers. The format used in typing the proposal should follow exactly the guidelines developed by the reviewers or organization, with attention to correct font size, line spacing, and reference style. If no particular format is requested, nursing students and researchers tend to follow APA (2020) format. An appealing copy is legible and uses appropriate tables and figures to communicate essential information. You must submit the proposal by the means requested: mailed hard copy, e-mail attachment, or uploaded file.

TYPES OF RESEARCH PROPOSALS

This section introduces the most common proposals developed in nursing: (1) student proposals, (2) condensed research proposals, and (3) letters of intent or preproposals. The content of a proposal is written with the interest and expertise of prospective reviewers in mind. Proposals are typically reviewed by faculty, clinical agency IRB members, and representatives of funding institutions. The content and type of a proposal varies in accordance with the expected reviewers, the guidelines developed for the review, and the methodology of the proposed study (quantitative or qualitative).

This variation poses a problem. Because healthcare institutions, universities, and funding sources require differing formats and inclusions, nursing journal articles describing how to write a proposal are likely to contain helpful overall tips but no specific information. Several current articles address writing a proposal for funding in a specialty area (Knafl & Van Riper, 2017), or considerations for research that might impact another concern, such as policy (Bradbury-Jones & Taylor, 2014), but they are seldom of direct applicability to the nursing student planning a thesis or dissertation proposal. In addition, supporting material required by an educational institution, such as a form completed by your dissertation advisor, would not be applicable for other types of proposals. The proposal required by your educational institution is more detailed and complete than is the abbreviated proposal required by a healthcare human subjects committee. The proposal expected by a funding source demands other supporting materials not required by your university but may request less detail about published literature in your problem area.

The result is that a doctoral student who hopes to conduct research in a healthcare agency and who wishes to apply for a funding grant will generate three proposals, similar in some respects but all slightly different from one another. However, you must begin somewhere. Because the proposal for an educational institution is likely to have more detail and depth than any other proposal, we advise you to use the proposal development materials furnished by your university

and write the academic proposal first. Your thesis/dissertation advisor and the faculty who teach courses about academic proposal writing and crafting the proposal can provide insight into the university's requirements. After this is completed, you will edit down the large academic proposal into a shorter version, adding different foci, as needed, for healthcare agencies and funding sources.

Student Proposals

Student researchers develop proposals to communicate their research projects both to the faculty of their thesis or dissertation committee and to members of university and agency IRBs (see Chapter 9 for details on IRB membership and the approval process). Student proposals are written to satisfy requirements for a degree and are developed according to guidelines outlined by the university, the graduate division, and/or the faculty of the school or college. The faculty member who will be assisting with the research project (the chair of the student's thesis or dissertation committee) reviews these guidelines with the student. Each faculty member has a unique way of interpreting and emphasizing aspects of the guidelines.

As noted previously, the content of a student proposal submitted to the university usually requires greater detail than a proposal developed for an agency or funding organization. This proposal often consists of the introduction, literature review, theory review, and methodology chapters of the student's thesis or dissertation. The proposed study is discussed in the future tense—that is, what knowledge is identified by the student as being essential to investigate, and which the student will investigate in conducting the research. The initial page of a student research proposal is the title page, and it shows the full title of the proposal, the name and credentials of the investigator, the university name, and the date. You should devote time to developing the title so that it accurately reflects the scope and content of the proposed study (Martin & Fleming, 2010). The major content areas of quantitative and qualitative student research proposals are discussed later in this chapter.

Condensed Proposals

Condensed proposals may be requested for review by clinical agencies and funding institutions. Even though such proposals are condensed, the logical links among components of the study should be clearly articulated. A typical condensed proposal includes the problem and purpose; a short summary of previous research that has been conducted in an area (usually limited to three to five studies); the framework; the variables or factors of interest; the design and proposed sample; pertinent ethical considerations; and plans for data collection, data analysis, and dissemination of the findings.

A condensed proposal submitted to a clinical agency should identify the setting clearly, such as the intensive care unit or primary care clinic, and the projected time span for the study. Members of clinical agencies are particularly interested in the data collection process, especially if the data include protected health information or if institutional personnel are involved in data collection. The researcher must identify any likely disruptions in institutional functioning, presenting plans for preventing or minimizing the effects of this intrusion, when possible. Anything that impacts employee functioning negatively costs the agency money and can interfere with the quality of patient care. Showing that you are aware of these concerns and proposing ways to minimize their effects increases the probability of obtaining approval to conduct your study.

Various companies, corporations, and organizations provide funding for research projects. A condensed proposal developed for a funding source includes a brief description of the study, the significance of the study to the goals of the funding institution, a timetable, and a budget. Most of these proposals are brief. Some contain a single-page summary sheet or abstract at the beginning of the proposal that summarizes the steps of the study, worded in easy-to-read, nontechnical terminology. Some proposal reviewers for funding institutions are laypersons with no background in research or nursing, so you must write the proposal as if the reviewer knows nothing about the topic. Inability to understand the terminology might put the reviewer on the defensive or create a negative reaction, which could lead to disapproval of the study. When an institution is evaluating multiple studies for possible funding, the summary sheet can be the sole basis for final decisions. Consequently, the summary should be concise, informative, and designed to facilitate funding of the study.

In proposals for both clinical and funding agencies, the investigator documents his or her research background by supplying a resumé, known in academic circles as a **curriculum vitae**. The research review committee for approval of funding will be interested in the investigator's previous research, research publications, and clinical expertise, especially if a clinical study is proposed. If you are a graduate student, the committee may request the name of the chair or faculty sponsor for your study, and verification that your proposal has been approved by your school or college committee and by the university IRB.

Letters of Intent or Preproposals

Sometimes a researcher sends an initial **letter of intent**, also called a "pre-proposal" (Holtzclaw et al., 2018), rather than a full proposal, to a foundation or organization that accepts grant applications. The purpose of the letter of intent is to explore the match between your research plan and the goals of one or more funding agencies (Malasanos, 1976). If you choose to compose a letter of intent, you should include (1) a letter of transmittal, identifying who you are and why you are contacting the funding source; (2) the brief proposal of your study; (3) a listing of members of your research team and personnel, and the role of each in the proposed study; (4) an identification of the facility or facilities you will use as research sites; and (5) the budget for your study. The brief proposal provides an overview of the proposed project, including the research problem, purpose, and methodology (brief description), and, most important, a statement of the significance of the work for enhanced nursing knowledge in general and any potential benefit to the funding institution, in particular, such as meeting one of the institution's stated goals. By sending out a letter of intent or a preproposal to many potential sources, a researcher is able to determine the agencies interested in funding the study and limit submission of the full proposals to institutions that indicate an interest.

Sometimes a funding entity announces a call for research and requires potential researchers to submit letters of intent as the first step toward funding. The committee reviewing the letters will identify those studies that are the most rigorous and aligned with the intent of the call for research. The funding entity will then request full proposals from the researchers submitting the strongest letters of intent. For example, a funding institution announces a call for research related to community-based programs for substance abuse prevention and indicates that a letter of intent is due by a specific date. The funding institution may receive 75 letters of intent by the deadline, choose 25 letters representing the strongest studies, and invite the researchers for the 25 selected letters to submit full proposals. Then, based on the full proposals submitted, funding may be awarded for the researchers to conduct five studies.

CONTENT OF A QUANTITATIVE RESEARCH PROPOSAL

A **quantitative research proposal** usually includes a table of contents that reflects the following chapters or sections: (1) introduction, (2) review of relevant literature, (3) framework, and (4) methods and procedures. When the quantitative research proposed is for a thesis or dissertation, some graduate schools require in-depth development of these sections, which will become the first few chapters of the thesis or dissertation. Other institutions require only a condensed version of the same content. Another approach is that proposals for theses and dissertations may be required to be written in a format that can be transformed readily into one or more publications. Table 28.1 outlines the content often covered in the chapters of a student quantitative research proposal.

Chapter 1: Introduction

In the introductory chapter of a proposal, the researcher identifies the topic of the study and the research problem, discussing the significance and background of both. The discussion of the significance of the problem focuses on its importance for nursing practice, the socioeconomic impact of the research, and the expected usefulness of the findings (Bradbury-Jones & Taylor, 2014; Melnyk & Fineout-Overholt, 2019). The importance of a problem is partly determined by the interest of nurses, other healthcare professionals, policymakers, and healthcare consumers at the local, state, national, or international level, as reflected in the extent and depth of the professional literature, and you would document this interest with appropriate citations. The socioeconomic impact of a study addressing a clinical problem may be supported by the number of people affected, the expected morbidity and mortality of the health problem, and the cost of the problem in money and in human suffering. Your documentation would include statistics supporting prevalence, severity, cost of treatment, and outcomes. The background describes how the problem was identified and explains why the problem is within the purview of nursing practice. Your

background information might include one or two major studies conducted to resolve the problem, including some key theoretical ideas related to it as well as possible solutions. The background and significance form the basis for your problem statement, which identifies what is not known and establishes the need for further research. Follow your problem statement with a succinct statement of the research purpose or the goal of the study (see Chapter 5).

Chapter 2: Review of Relevant Literature

The review of relevant literature provides an overview of essential information that will guide you as you develop your study. It includes empirical literature that will allow you to write a cogent summary and critical appraisal of previous studies pertinent to your study. It usually includes theoretical literature with which you will present a background for defining and interrelating study concepts (see Table 28.1). In the summary of the current state of the empirical literature in your interest area, you will discuss recommendations made by other researchers, such as replicating, changing, or expanding a study, in relation to the approach you have chosen for your proposed study. This establishes your research as extending both the findings and the insights of previous researchers.

The depth of the literature review varies; it might include only recent studies and theorists' works, or it might be extensive and include a description and critical appraisal of many past and current studies and an in-depth discussion of theorists' works. The literature review is presented in a narrative format or in a table that summarizes relevant studies, or both (see Chapter 7). This review demonstrates to the reader that you have a command of current empirical and theoretical knowledge regarding the proposed problem (Offredy & Vickers, 2010). In the case of a dissertation, you are now an expert in the particular area of your research. This second chapter concludes with a summary. The summary includes a synthesis of the theoretical literature and the findings from previous empirical studies that describe the current knowledge of a problem. Gaps in the knowledge base are then identified, with a description of how the proposed study will address a research gap, thereby contributing to the body of nursing knowledge.

Some colleges and universities require an exhaustive review of the literature for dissertation research, meaning

TABLE 28.1	**Components of the Quantitative Research Proposal for Students**
Chapter 1	**Introduction** A. Background and significance of the problem B. Statement of the problem C. Statement of the purpose
Chapter 2	**Review of Relevant Literature** A. Review of theoretical literature B. Review of relevant research C. Summary

Chapter 3	**Framework**
	A. Identification of an appropriate framework
	  1. Presentation of a diagram or map of the study framework, definition of concepts in the diagram, description of relationships, or propositions in the diagram
	  2. Identify the focus of the study, and link framework concepts to study variables
	B. Formulation of objectives, questions, or hypotheses
	C. Definitions (conceptual and operational) of study variables
	D. Definition of relevant terms

Chapter 4	**Methods and Procedures**
	A. Description of the research design
	  1. Model of the design, strengths, and limitations of the design, in terms of threats to validity
	  2. If a pilot study is to be conducted, describe details and indicate how pilot findings will be incorporated
	B. Identification of the population and sample
	  1. Sampling methods, including strengths and weaknesses
	  2. Use of power analysis, sample size
	C. Selection of a setting
	  1. Approval to use site
	  2. Strengths and limitations of the setting
	D. Presentation of ethical considerations
	  Protection of subjects' rights and university and healthcare agency review processes
	E. Description of the intervention if one will be performed
	  1. Provide a protocol for the intervention, including who will implement
	  2. Describe how intervention fidelity is ensured
	F. Selection of measurement methods
	  1. Reliability, validity, scoring, and level of measurement of the instruments
	  2. Plans to examine rigor of measurement (reliability and validity or precision and accuracy)
	G. Plan for data collection
	  1. Data collection process, training of data collectors if appropriate, schedule
	  2. Management of data after collection
	H. Plan for data analysis
	  1. Sample and instrument descriptions
	  2. Analysis of objectives, questions, and hypothesis; level of significance
	I. Identification of limitations
	J. Discussion of communication of findings

References	References cited in the proposal, according to APA (2020) format
Appendices	Study budget, timetable, and tables or figures for projected results

that all available empirical literature pertaining to the problem is read and reviewed by the candidate. If the proposal in that educational institution is required to be equivalent to the first few chapters of the dissertation, the review of the literature that appears in the formal proposal might also be exhaustive. Because of the extent of an exhaustive literature review, several tables will be included that distill and synopsize the significance of each study for the dissertation. The results also may be synthesized within definable knowledge clusters and presented as group summaries and group critiques that represent the current state of the research in the dissertation problem area.

Chapter 3: Framework

A framework provides the basis for generating and refining the research problem and purpose and linking them to relevant theoretical knowledge in nursing or related fields. The framework includes concepts and relationships among concepts, or propositions, the latter of which are sometimes represented as models or maps (see Chapter 8). A middle-range theory from nursing or another discipline frequently is used as the framework for a quantitative study, and the proposition(s) to be tested that emanate from the theory are identified (Smith & Liehr, 2018). The framework needs to include concepts that will be examined in the study, their definitions, and their links to the study variables (see Table 28.1). If you use a theorist's or researcher's model from a journal article or book, letters documenting permission to use this model must be obtained from both the publisher and the theorist or researcher, and the letters will be included in your proposal appendices.

Sometimes a researcher develops objectives, questions, or hypotheses that will direct the study (see Chapter 6). All of these evolve from the research purpose and should reflect pertinent concepts within the study framework. Variables used in the objectives, questions, and hypotheses are first conceptually defined to establish their meaning in relationship to the framework, and then are operationally defined to determine how you plan to count or measure them. You also will define any relevant terms and identify assumptions that provide a basis for your study.

Chapter 4: Methods and Procedures

The researcher describes the design or general strategy for conducting the study, sometimes including a diagram of the design (see Chapters 10 and 11). Designs for descriptive and correlational studies are flexible and can be made unique for the study being conducted (see Chapter 10) (Creswell & Creswell, 2018; Kerlinger & Lee, 2000). Because of this uniqueness, the descriptions should specify the strengths and limitations posed by this study design, in particular, and not merely for the type of design, in general (see Chapter 10).

Presenting designs for quasi-experimental and experimental studies (see Chapter 11) involves (1) describing how the research situation will be structured; (2) detailing the treatment to be implemented (Cook & Campbell, 1986; Holtzclaw et al., 2018; Shadish, Cook, & Campbell, 2002); (3) explaining how the effect of the treatment will be measured; (4) specifying the extraneous variables for which the researcher will control and the methods for doing so; (5) identifying uncontrolled extraneous variables and determining their impact on the findings; (6) describing the methods for assigning subjects to the treatment, comparison, or control group, and/or usual care group; and (7) exploring strengths and limitations of the general type of design (see Chapters 10 and 11) (Campbell & Stanley, 1963). The design must be consistent with all the objectives, questions, and hypotheses identified in the proposal. If a pilot study is planned, the design should include the procedure for conducting this preliminary work and including the information obtained, and sometimes the raw data, into the proposed study (see Table 28.1). Your proposal should identify the target population to which study findings will be generalized and the accessible population from which the sample will be selected. Consequently, you must outline the inclusion and exclusion criteria you will use to select study participants and present the rationale for these sampling criteria (see Chapter 15). For example, a participant might be selected according to the following criteria: female, 18 to 60 years of age, hospitalized for abdominal surgery, and expected to remain in the hospital for at least 3 days postoperatively. The rationale for these criteria might be that the researcher will examine the effects of a selected in-hospital pain management intervention for women who have recently undergone abdominal surgery and will track pain for up to 3 days after surgery. Your proposal should include a discussion of the sampling method and the approximate sample size, in terms of their adequacy and limitations for investigating the research purpose. A power analysis should be conducted to determine an adequate sample size, with respect to the proposed statistical tests, level of significance, and expected effect size (see Chapter 15) (Aberson, 2019). Expected effect size is estimated, based on prior pilot work, as well as on other published studies in the literature.

A proposal includes a description of the proposed study setting, which frequently includes the name of the agency and the structure of the units or sites in which the study is to be conducted. Although it may be identified in the proposal, the name of the agency does not appear in the final research report. The agency you select should have the potential to generate the type and size of sample required for the study within a reasonable period of time. Your proposal would support this by including the number of individuals who would have met the sample criteria and been cared for by the agency during a recent time period. In addition, the structure and activities in the agency must be able to accommodate the proposed design of the study. If you are not affiliated with this agency, it is important for you to have a letter of support for your study from key agency personnel, such as the unit manager and medical director.

Ethical considerations in a proposal include the rights of the subjects and the rights of the agency, as well. Describe how you plan to protect subjects' rights and list the risks and potential benefits of your study. Also address the steps you will take to reduce any risks that the study might present. Healthcare agencies require a written consent form, and that form often is included in the appendices of the proposal (see Chapter 9). With the implementation of the Health Insurance Portability and Accountability Act (HIPAA), healthcare agencies and providers must have a signed authorization form from patients to release their health information for research. You must also address the risks and potential benefits of the study for the institution. If your study might place the agency at risk, outline the steps you will take to reduce or eliminate this type of risk. You must state that the proposal will be reviewed by the university IRB, as well as the IRB of the healthcare agency.

Some quantitative studies test the effectiveness of an intervention. If your study is interventional, you must describe the elements or stages of the intervention, as well as the way in which you will implement each step (Butcher, Bulecheck, Dochterman, & Wagner, 2018) (see Chapter 11 and see the example quasi-experimental study proposal at the end of this chapter). Consistent implementation, over time, represents intervention

fidelity, which must be present for the researcher to draw accurate conclusions about the effects of the intervention (Shadish et al., 2002).

When proposing a quantitative study, describe the methods you will use to measure study variables, including each instrument's reliability, validity, methods of scoring, and level of measurement (see Chapter 16). A plan for examining the reliability and validity of the instruments in the present study must be addressed. If an instrument has no reported reliability and validity, conducting a pilot study to examine these qualities is indicated. If the intent of the proposed study is to develop an instrument, describe the process of instrument development (Waltz, Strickland, & Lenz, 2017). If physiological measures are used, address the accuracy, precision, and error rate of the measures (Ryan-Wenger, 2017) (also see Chapter 16). A copy of the interview questions, questionnaires, scales, physiological measures, or other tools to be used in the study usually is included in the proposal appendices (see Chapter 17). You must obtain permission from the authors to use copyrighted instruments. Letters documenting that you have obtained that permission must be included in the proposal appendices.

The data collection plan clarifies what data are to be collected and the process for collecting the data. In this plan you will identify the data collectors, describe the data collection procedures, and present a schedule for data collection activities. If more than one person will be involved in data collection, it is important to describe methods used to train your data collectors and to document the interrater reliability achieved (see Chapter 16). The method of recording data often is described, and sample data recording sheets are placed in the proposal appendices. You also will discuss any special equipment to be used or developed to collect data for the study, and address data security, including methods of data storage (see Chapter 20).

The plan for data analysis identifies the statistical analysis techniques that will be used to summarize demographic data and to address the research objectives, questions, and hypotheses. The analysis section is best organized by the study objectives, questions, or hypotheses. The analysis techniques identified must be appropriate for the type of data collected (Grove & Cipher, 2020; Plichta & Kelvin, 2013). For example, if an associative hypothesis is developed, correlational analysis is planned. If a researcher plans to determine differences among groups, the analysis techniques might include a *t*-test or analysis of variance (ANOVA). A level of significance or alpha ($\alpha = 0.05, 0.01,$ or 0.001) also is identified, and it is usually set at $\alpha = 0.05$ in nursing studies (see Chapter 22). Often a researcher projects the type of results that will be generated from data analysis (see Chapters 22 through 25). Dummy tables, graphs, and charts can be developed to present these results and are included in the proposal appendices, if required by the guidelines. The researcher might project possible findings for a study and indicate what the implications for practice might be if a proposed hypothesis were supported, in light of the study framework and previous research findings.

The methods and procedures chapter of a proposal usually concludes with a discussion of the study's limitations and a plan for communication of the findings. Limitations discussed are those that are expected to be present, due to the chosen methodology. These might include an identification of what can and cannot be expected from the selected design, sampling method, sample size, measurement tools, data collection procedures, or data analysis techniques. For example, a descriptive design cannot be expected to establish causation. Similarly, a very large randomly selected sample is likely to provide evidence that can be generalized back to the study population. The accuracy with which the conceptual definitions and relational statements in a theory reflect reality also has a direct impact on the generalization of study findings. Theory that has withstood frequent testing through research provides a strong framework for the interpretation and generalization of findings. The plan for communicating research results should mention the researcher's intention to present the findings to audiences of nurses, other health professionals, policymakers, and healthcare consumers, as well as to submit the research report for publication (see Chapter 27).

Frequently, a budget and timetable are included in the proposal appendices. The budget projects expenses for the study, which might include costs for data collection tools and procedures, special equipment, consultants for data analysis, computer time, travel related to data collection and analysis, typing, copying, as well as developing, presenting, and publishing the final report. Study budgets requesting external funding for researchers' time include investigators' salaries and prorated benefit costs, as well as secretarial expenses. You should include a well-considered timetable that directs the

steps of your research project to assure the reviewer that you will complete the project on schedule. A timetable identifies tasks to be completed, the person responsible for each task, and when each one will be completed. An example proposal for a quasi-experimental study is presented at the end of this chapter to guide you in developing your proposal.

CONTENT OF A QUALITATIVE RESEARCH PROPOSAL

Qualitative research proposals are unique because the methods for the planned study are described, with the caveat that the methods may be revised as data are analyzed and new questions emerge. For example, during a phenomenological study, the researcher may learn that the lived experience of adaptation following a myocardial infarction is perceived by some participants to be overwhelming, due to the number of lifestyle changes that they are encouraged to make. The researcher, in subsequent interviews, may ask participants about lifestyle changes they have made, including one or more questions that were not listed in the initial interview schedule. A qualitative proposal usually includes the following sections: (1) introduction and background, (2) review of the literature, (3) philosophical foundation for the selected method, and (4) method of inquiry (Marshall & Rossman, 2016; Munhall, 2012; Munhall & Chenail, 2008). Guidelines are presented in Table 28.2 to assist you in developing a qualitative research proposal.

Chapter 1: Introduction and Background

The introduction usually provides a general background for the proposed study by identifying the phenomenon of interest (clinical problem, issue, or situation to be investigated) and linking it to the current state of nursing knowledge. The general aim or purpose of the study is identified and provides the focus for the qualitative study to be conducted. The study purpose might be followed by research questions that direct the investigation (Creswell and Poth, 2018; Munhall, 2012; Munhall & Chenail, 2008; Offredy & Vickers, 2010). For example, a possible aim or purpose for a phenomenological study might be to "describe the experience of losing an adult child to suicide." The corresponding research question may be a rephrasing of the purpose as a question: What is the lived experience of losing an adult child to suicide?" In phenomenological studies, the researcher may

TABLE 28.2 Qualitative Research Proposal Guidelines for Students

Chapter 1	**Introduction and Background**
	A. Identification of the phenomenon to be studied
	B. Description of the knowledge gap that the study will address
	C. The study purpose or aim and description of the qualitative approach to be used
	D. Study questions or objectives
	E. Background of the study
	    1. Rationale for conducting the study
	    2. Significance of the study to nursing

Chapter 2	**Review of Relevant Literature (the Depth and Breadth of the Initial Literature Review Will Vary, Depending on the Qualitative Method)** A. Review of theoretical literature pertinent to the topic B. Review of relevant research C. Summary
Chapter 3	**Philosophical Foundation for the Selected Method** A. Type of qualitative research to be conducted (phenomenological research, grounded theory research, ethnographical research, and exploratory-descriptive qualitative research) B. Philosophical basis of the research method C. Guiding theory, if one is being used D. Preliminary definitions of concepts or terms

Chapter 4	**Method of Inquiry**
	A. Overview of the qualitative approach
	B. Population and site
	C. The plan for each of the following:
	    1. Site access and approval to collect data
	    2. Selection of study participants
	    3. Addressing ethical concerns
	D. Data collection process:
	    1. What data will be collected
	    2. How raw data will be obtained (interview, focus groups, observation, etc.)
	    3. How raw data will be collected (audio recording, field notes, photography, etc.)
	    4. How raw data will be prepared for analysis
	E. Data analysis
	    1. Timing, who will be performing coding or other analyses
	    2. Use of specific data analysis procedures consistent with the specific research method, including computer analysis programs
	    3. Field notes and audit trail, how these will be collected, recorded, and reported
	    4. Steps to be taken to increase rigor and credibility (member checking, independent coding, etc.)
	    5. Limitations of the study
	    6. Plans for communication of findings

References	References cited in the proposal, according to the method that is required by chair or university
Appendices	Study budget and timetable

identify specific aspects of the experience to address, such as the following: "What life events preceded the suicide?" "Would you tell me about learning of the suicide?" and "How has your life changed since the suicide?"

The background is incorporated into the introduction and includes the study's potential significance for nursing practice, patients, the healthcare system, and health policy (Bradbury-Jones & Taylor, 2014; Liamputtong, 2013). Pertinent to this discussion are the researcher's personal and professional motivations for conducting the study, also called positioning. Depending on the topic, the way the problem developed over time may be described with reference to the literature (Munhall, 2012). The significance of a study could include the number of people affected, how this phenomenon affects health and quality of life, and the consequences of not understanding the phenomenon. Marshall and Rossman (2016) identified the following four questions to assess the significance of a qualitative study: (1) Who has an interest in this domain of inquiry? (2) What do we already know about the topic? (3) What has not been answered adequately in previous research and practice? and (4) How will this research add to knowledge, practice, and policy in this area? The introduction and background section concludes with an overview of the remaining sections that are covered in the proposal.

Chapter 2: Review of Relevant Literature

The role of the review of relevant literature depends on the qualitative approach being proposed (see Chapters 4 and 12). As a result, the breadth and depth of the initial literature review will vary among methods. A very limited review of literature will be performed prior to the study when conducting phenomenological and grounded theory studies. With both approaches, the researcher may conduct a preliminary review of the literature to document the need for the study but will otherwise defer the review until after data analysis is complete. At that point, the researcher compares the emerging themes and theory to published theories and research. In grounded theory research, the literature is used to explain, support, and extend the theory generated in the study (Glaser & Strauss, 1965). In ethnography and exploratory-descriptive qualitative studies, the review of the literature may be organized and presented very similarly to the review performed

for quantitative studies. The reports of completed qualitative studies, regardless of the qualitative approach, will include an examination of the findings in light of the existing literature.

Chapter 3: Philosophical Foundation for the Selected Method

This section introduces the philosophical and conceptual foundation for the qualitative research methodology (phenomenological research, ethnographical research, grounded theory research, or exploratory-descriptive qualitative research) selected for the proposed study. The researcher introduces the philosophy, the essential elements of the philosophy, and the assumptions for the specific type of qualitative research to be conducted (see Table 28.2).

The philosophy varies for the different types of qualitative research and guides the conduct of the study. For example, a proposal for a grounded theory study might indicate that the purpose of the study is to "to generate a theory explaining the process by which people with diabetes learn about their disease in Indonesia" (Ligita, Wicking, Francis, Harvey, & Nurjannah, 2019, p. 1). The researchers indicated that understanding the complexity in decision making for persons with diabetes would "assist healthcare professionals to engage effectively with people living with diabetes" (Ligita et al., 2019, p. 1). Consistent with the grounded theory approach to research, symbolic interactionism was the underlying philosophy (Ligita et al., 2019). Assumptions about the nature of the knowledge and the reality that underlie the type of qualitative research to be conducted also are identified. The assumptions and philosophy provide a theoretical perspective for the study that influences the focus of the study, data collection and analysis, and articulation of the findings. For exploratory-descriptive qualitative studies, and even some grounded theory and phenomenological studies, the researcher may approach the study from an additional specific theoretical perspective. The theoretical perspective may have no relationship to the type of qualitative research chosen. If such a theoretical perspective is identified, it is evident in the research questions being asked. As a doctoral student, you might propose a phenomenological study that explores the coping strategies of Hispanic first-time mothers. The theoretical perspective may be a theory of stress, appraisal, and coping (Lazarus & Folkman, 1984) or Roy's adaptation model (Roy & Andrews, 2008). Having a theoretical framework may help graduate students propose relevant interview questions or identify an appropriate sample.

Chapter 4: Method of Inquiry

Developing and implementing the methodology of qualitative research both require an expertise that some believe can be obtained only through a mentorship relationship with an experienced qualitative researcher. Through a one-to-one relationship, an experienced researcher can provide insights into the intricacies of data collection and be available for debriefing and exploring alternative meanings of the data. Planning the methods of a qualitative study requires knowledge of relevant sources that describe the different qualitative research techniques and procedures (Creswell & Creswell, 2018; Creswell & Poth, 2018; Marshall & Rossman, 2016). Chapter 12 provides details on qualitative research methods.

Identifying the methods for conducting a qualitative study is challenging because specifics of the design tend to emerge during the conduct of the study. Although the design for a quantitative study is decided before the study begins, the design for a qualitative study is expected to evolve during the study. The design will evolve in relation to the flow of data, the richness of various data sources, the explanations the participants provide, the insights the researcher experiences, and unexpected changes in the participants, setting, and researcher as the study is conducted (Denzin, 1970).

You, as a qualitative researcher, must document the logic and appropriateness of the qualitative method and develop a tentative plan for conducting your study. Because this plan is flexible, researchers include in formal proposals their intention to modify or change the data collection plan as needed during the conduct of the study. You will respond to the emerging narrative, theoretical insights, and intuitions that blossom during qualitative data collection and analysis (Miles, Huberman, & Saldaña, 2020). For instance, the number of participants in qualitative studies may be predetermined in some types of inquiry but often is driven by the quality and depth of the emerging data, especially in grounded theory and ethnography. However, the well-conceived design or plan must be consistent with the philosophical approach, study purpose, and specific research aims

or questions (Fawcett & Garity, 2009; Munhall, 2012). The tentative plan describes the process for selecting a site and population and the initial steps taken to gain access to the site. Having access to the site includes establishing relationships that facilitate recruitment of the participants necessary to address the research purpose and answer the research questions. For Ligita et al.'s (2019) study of people living with diabetes, participants were recruited in person from settings within the community, including a wound care clinic and two other public health venues. Data collection was completed in person through one-to-one interviews.

You, as a qualitative researcher, must achieve entry into the setting, developing a rapport with participants that will facilitate the detailed data collection process, but protecting their rights throughout the process (Jessiman, 2013; Marshall & Rossman, 2016). In planning entry, you should address the following questions in describing the researcher's role: (1) What is the best setting for the study? (2) What will facilitate entry into the research site? (3) How will I gain access to potential participants? (4) What actions will I take to encourage prospective participants to agree to be part of the study? and (5) What precautions will I take to protect the rights of the participants and to prevent the setting and the participants from being harmed? You will describe the process you will follow to obtain informed consent and the actions you will take to decrease study risks (see Chapter 9). The sensitive nature of some qualitative studies increases risk for participants, which makes ethical concerns and decisions a major focus of the proposal (Munhall, 2012). For studies on sensitive topics, the researcher makes a formal plan for participants to receive follow-up care with a counselor if they become distressed in telling their story. The researcher might choose to be debriefed with an experienced researcher when studying sensitive topics, or to obtain mental health support during the data collection and analysis phases of the study.

In qualitative research, the primary data collection techniques are observation, in-depth interviewing, focus groups, and document analysis. Observations can range from highly detailed, structured notations of behaviors to amorphous general descriptions of behaviors or events. An interview can range from a list of structured questions to one or two unstructured, open-ended questions (Marshall & Rossman, 2016; Munhall, 2012). Focus groups may be conducted with several different groups for one study, including persons with different perspectives, centering on a topic such as nurse burnout. In this case, one focus group might consist of administrators, another might be comprised of nurses who have worked for 10 years or more, and still a third could consist of nurses who have worked fewer than 10 years.

You will address several questions when describing the proposed data collection process. What data will be collected? For example, will the data consist of field notes from memory, audio recordings of interviews, transcripts of conversations, video recordings of events, or examination of existing documents? What techniques or procedures will the research team use to collect data? For example, if interviews are to be conducted, a list of the proposed questions would be included in the appendices. Another key point is deciding who will collect data and who will provide training to data collectors. As data collection transpires, how will data be recorded and stored?

The methods section must address how you will document the decision process that occurs regarding events that drive your intuitive judgments during data collection and analysis (see Chapter 12). This running account represents the audit trail that supports the logic and unbiased nature of your decisions. For example, you might keep a research journal or diary during the course of the study. These notes can document day-to-day activities, methodological decisions, data analysis processes, and personal notes about the informants. This information becomes part of the audit trail that you will provide to ensure the quality of the study (Creswell & Poth, 2018; Denizen & Lincoln, 2018; Marshall & Rossman, 2016).

The methods section of the proposal also includes the analysis techniques and the steps for conducting these techniques. In some types of qualitative research, data collection and analysis occur simultaneously. Usually, the data are in the form of notes, digital files, audio recordings, video recordings, and other material obtained from observation, interviews, and questionnaires. Through qualitative analysis, these data are organized to allow the researcher to examine the data in different ways, with the goal of promoting insight and revealing meaning (see Chapter 12). Researchers who plan to use data analysis software to assist in the coding and its documentation should provide the name of the software and describe the way in which it will be used.

Rigor, transferability, and credibility do not happen by accident. Specific actions that will be taken to demonstrate the quality of the study methods are specified in the proposal, such as decreasing bias by including a second person who will participate in data analysis (see Chapters 12) (Marshall & Rossman, 2016). Conclude your proposal by describing how you plan to communicate your findings to various audiences through presentations and publications. Often, a realistic budget and timetable are provided in the appendices. A qualitative study budget is similar to a quantitative study budget and includes costs for data collection tools, software, and recording devices; consultants for data analysis; travel related to data collection and analysis; transcription of recordings; copying related to data collection and analysis; and developing, presenting, and publishing the final report. However, one of the greatest expenditures in qualitative research is the researcher's time. Develop a timetable to project how long the study will take; often a period of several months is designated for data collection and analysis (Creswell & Poth, 2018; Marshall & Rossman, 2016). You can use your budget and timetable to make decisions regarding the need for funding.

Excellent websites have been developed to assist novice researchers in identifying an idea and developing a proposal for qualitative study. You can use these websites and other publications, such as those cited in this chapter, to promote the quality of your research proposal. The quality of a proposal will be evaluated according to the potential scientific contribution of the research to nursing knowledge; the congruence of the philosophical foundation and the research methods; and the knowledge, skills, and resources available to the investigators (Creswell & Creswell, 2018; Creswell & Poth, 2018; Marshall & Rossman, 2016; Miles et al., 2020).

SEEKING APPROVAL FOR A STUDY

Seeking approval to conduct a study is an action that should be based on knowledge and guided by purpose. Obtaining approval for a study from a research review committee or IRB requires understanding the approval process, writing a research proposal for review that addresses critical ethical concerns, and, in many cases, verbally defending the proposal. Little has been written to guide the researcher who is navigating approval mechanisms for the first time. This section provides a background for researchers seeking to obtain approval to collect data at the reviewing institution and obtain support for a proposed study.

Clinical agencies and healthcare corporations review studies to evaluate the quality of proposed studies and to ensure that adequate measures are being taken to protect human subjects. The administrators of an institution in which a study is planned also evaluate the impact of the activities of recruitment and data collection, as well as ensuing effects on the reviewing institution (Offredy & Vickers, 2010). IRB reviews sometimes identify potential risks or problems related to proposed research that must be resolved before studies are approved.

Approval Process

An initial step in seeking approval is to determine exactly what committees in which agencies must grant approval before the study can be conducted. You should take the initiative to determine the formal approval process rather than assume that you will be told whether a formal review system exists. Information about the formal research review system might be obtained from administrative personnel, an online website, special projects or grant officers, chairs of IRBs in clinical agencies, clinicians who have previously conducted research, university IRB chairs, and university faculty who are involved in research.

Graduate students require approval from their thesis or dissertation committee, the university IRB, and the agency IRB in which data are to be collected. University faculty members conducting research seek approval for their studies from the university IRB and the agency IRB. Nurses conducting research in an agency in which they are employed must obtain approval only from that agency. If researchers seek outside funding, or if they conduct research in several healthcare agencies, additional review committees may be involved. Not all studies require full review by the IRB (see Chapter 9 for the types of studies that qualify for exempt or expedited review). However, the chair and other members of the IRB, not the researcher, determine the type of review that the study requires for conduct in that agency.

When several committees must review a study, sometimes they agree mutually that one of them shall initiate the review for the protection of human subjects, with those findings receiving general acceptance by the other committees. For example, if the university IRB

examines and approves a proposal for the protection of human subjects, funding agencies usually recognize that review as sufficient. Reviews of other committees then focus on approval to conduct the study within the institution or decisions to provide study funding.

As part of the approval process, the researcher must determine the agency's policy regarding (1) the use of the name of the clinical facility in reporting findings, (2) the presentation and publication of the research report, and (3) the authorship of publications. The facility's name is used only with prior written administrative approval when presenting or publishing a study. The researcher may feel freer to report findings that could be interpreted negatively in terms of the institution when the name of the agency is not identified. Some institutions have rules that limit what is presented or published in a study, where it is presented or published, and who is the presenter or author. Before conducting a study, researchers, especially employees of healthcare agencies, must clarify the rules and regulations of the agency regarding authorship, presentations, and publications. In some cases, recognition of these rules must be included in the proposal if it is to be approved.

Preparing Proposals for Review Committees

The initial proposals for theses and dissertations may be developed as part of a formal class. In this case, the faculty members teaching the class provide students with specific proposal guidelines approved by the graduate faculty and assist them in developing their initial proposals. If students elect to conduct a thesis or dissertation, they ask an appropriate faculty member to serve as chair of their thesis or dissertation committee. With the assistance of the chair, the student identifies committee members with expertise in the focus of the proposed study or in conducting research who can work effectively together to refine the final proposal. The number of committee members varies across universities, but usually will include at least the chair and two additional faculty members. The thesis or dissertation committee members must approve the proposal before the student can seek IRB approval from the university. The student's chairperson usually provides direction and support in obtaining university IRB approval. The IRB review within universities usually requires the completion of a form related to the protection of study participants. These forms are similar but are particularized to meet university requirements. Once university IRB approval is obtained, students can submit required documents, including the letter indicating approval by the university IRB, and seek approval for their studies from agency IRBs.

Conducting research in a clinical agency requires approval by the agency IRB. The department that supports the IRB committee of the agency can provide researchers with copies of institutional policies and requirements, and they may assist the researcher with the IRB process. The staff in these departments can provide essential insight into studies that will be acceptable to the committee. Frequently, staff persons screen proposals for conducting research in the agency. The approval process policy and proposal guidelines are available from the designee of the chair of the IRB, usually a permanent staff person. Guidelines should be followed carefully, particularly those governing page limitations. Some committees refuse to review proposals that exceed page limitations. Reviewers on IRB committees evaluate proposals in addition to other full-time responsibilities, and their time is limited.

Investigators also should familiarize themselves with the IRB's process for screening proposals. In addition to scientific merit and human subjects' protection (Merrill, 2011), most agency IRBs evaluate proposals for the congruence of the study with the agency's research agenda and the impact of the study on patient care. This is why a support statement by a nurse manager or medical director is required by many institutional IRBs for research that involves the physical presence of the research team in patient care areas. Researchers should develop their proposals with these ideas in mind. They also must determine whether the committee requires specific forms to be completed and submitted with the research proposal. Other important information can be gathered by addressing the following questions: (1) How often does the committee meet? (2) When are the committee's regularly scheduled meetings? (3) What materials should be submitted before the meeting? (4) How far in advance of the scheduled meeting should these materials be submitted? (5) How many copies of the proposal are required? and (6) What is the turnaround time for committee review?

Social and Political Factors

Social and political factors play an important role in obtaining approval to conduct a study. The dynamics of the relationships among committee members are important to assess. Seek guidance from your chair when selecting committee members for your thesis or dissertation (Bradbury-Jones & Taylor, 2014).

Clinical agency IRBs may include nurse clinicians who have never conducted research, nurse researchers, and researchers in other disciplines. The reactions of each of these groups to a study could be very different. Sometimes IRB committees are made up primarily of physicians, which is frequently the case in health science centers. Physicians often are not oriented to nursing research methods, especially qualitative methods, and might need additional explanations related to the research methodology. However, most physicians are strong supporters of nursing research. They may be helpful in suggesting changes to strengthen the study and eager to facilitate access to study participants.

The researcher needs to anticipate potential responses of committee members and to prepare the proposal to elicit a favorable response. It is wise to meet with the chair of the agency IRB or a designee early in the development of a proposal. This meeting could facilitate proposal development, rapport between the researcher and agency personnel, and approval of the research proposal.

In addition to the formal committee approval mechanisms, you will need the tacit approval of the administrative personnel and staff who are affected by the conduct of your study. Obtaining informal approval and support often depends on the way in which a person is approached. Demonstrate interest in the institution and the personnel as well as interest in the research project. The relationships formed with agency personnel should be equal, sharing ones, because these key persons often can provide ideas and strategies for conducting the study that you may not have considered. The support of agency personnel during data collection also can determine the difference between a successful and an unsuccessful study.

Conducting nursing research can benefit the institution as well as the researcher. Clinicians have an opportunity to see nursing research in action, which can influence their thinking and clinical practice if the relationship with the researcher is positive. Conceivably, this is the first close contact some of these clinicians may have had with a researcher, and interpretation of the researcher's role and the aspects of the study may be necessary. In addition, clinicians tend to be more oriented in the present than researchers are, and they need to see the immediate impact that the study findings can have on nursing practice in their institution. Interactions with researchers might help clinicians see the importance of research in providing evidence-based practice and encourage them to become involved in study activities in the future (Offredy & Vickers, 2010). Conducting research and providing evidence-based practice are essential if a hospital is to achieve and maintain Magnet™ designation. The award of Magnet status from the American Nurses Credentialing Center (ANCC, 2018) is prestigious to an institution and validates the excellence in evidence-based care that nurses provide in that facility.

Be mindful of this, however. If you are to be a successful researcher, you must interact diplomatically with persons in positions of authority. In addition to the people who are in authority or are overtly involved in approving and implementing the study, there are other less obvious people, such as administrative assistants, nursing assistants, and housekeepers, with whom you may interact. Being consistently kind and respectful in all interactions often determines your success in implementing the study. The unit secretary you have treated with kindness may become committed to notifying you when potential study participants are admitted. The secretary in the Office of Research, whom you may have complimented for her extensive knowledge of the review process, may take time to peruse your paperwork before forwarding it and notify you that one required form lacks the signature page. The housekeeper whose contributions you have acknowledged may alert you to the pending discharge of a study participant from whom you hope to collect additional data. How you treat those who have no authority or power over you is a strong indicator of your authenticity as a nurse and a person.

Verbal Presentation of a Proposal

It is usually the case that graduate students writing theses or dissertations are required to present their proposals verbally to university committee members in meetings that are called thesis or dissertation proposal defenses. Many clinical agencies require researchers to meet with the IRB to discuss their proposals. In a verbal presentation of a proposal, reviewers can evaluate the researcher as a person, the researcher's knowledge and understanding of the content of the proposal, and his or her ability to reason and provide logical explanations related to the study. These face-to-face meetings give the researcher the opportunity to encourage committee members to approve the proposed study.

Appearance is important in a personal presentation because it can give an impression of competence or incompetence. Consider these presentations to be professional, with logical and rational interactions. Dress for the presentation should be dark toned, conservative, and businesslike. The committee might perceive individuals who are casually dressed as not valuing the review process or being careless about research procedures.

Nonverbal behaviors are important during the meeting as well; appearing calm, in control, and confident projects a positive image. Plan and rehearse your presentation to reduce anxiety. Try to obtain general information about the personalities of committee members, their relationships with one another, the vested interests of each member, and their areas of expertise, because this can increase your confidence and provide a sense of control.

It is important to arrive at the meeting early to see the room where the meeting will take place. If your presentation includes a slide presentation, you will want to familiarize yourself with the room's equipment and the location of electrical outlets. Bring your presentation with you. The presentation will, of course, be saved on your laptop. However, in case your computer is damaged or misplaced, making the presentation accessible in at least one additional way, such as a USB drive, a file on cloud-based storage, or an e-mail attachment to yourself, will allow you to retrieve it. As you assess the environment for the meeting, you can consider where you might prefer to sit so that all members of the committee will be able to see you. However, selecting a seat on one side of a table with all of the committee members on the other side could simulate an interrogation rather than a scholarly interaction. Sitting at the side of a table rather than at the head might be a strategic move to elicit support. As a guest, you may be invited into the meeting after the committee members are seated. In this case, the chair of the IRB will probably identify where you are to sit.

The verbal presentation of the proposal usually begins with a brief overview of the study. Your presentation should be carefully planned, timed, and rehearsed. Salient points should be highlighted, which you can accomplish with the use of audiovisuals. Anticipate questions from the committee members. Be prepared to defend or justify the methods and procedures used in your study. With your committee chair or mentor, practice answers to questions that you are likely to receive. This rehearsal will help you determine the best way to defend your ideas without appearing defensive. When the meeting ends, thank the members of the committee for their time and their input. If the committee does not come to a decision regarding the study during the meeting, ask when the decision will be made and how you will be notified.

Revising a Proposal

Reviewers sometimes suggest changes in a proposal that improve the study methodology; however, some of the changes requested may benefit the institution but not the study. Remain receptive to suggestions, explore with the committee the impact of changes on the proposed study, and try to resolve any conflicts. Usually reviewers make valuable suggestions that might improve the quality of a study or facilitate the data collection process. Revision of the proposal often is based on these suggestions.

Sometimes a study requires revision while it is being conducted because of problems with data collection tools or subjects' participation. However, if clinical agency personnel or representatives of funding institutions have approved a proposal, the researcher must consult with those who have approved and/or funded the study before making major changes. Before revising a proposal, address three questions: (1) What needs to be changed? (2) Why is the change necessary? and (3) How will the change affect implementation of the study and the study findings? Students must seek advice from the faculty committee members before revising their studies. Sometimes it is beneficial for seasoned researchers to discuss their proposed study changes with other researchers or agency personnel to elicit suggestions and additional viewpoints.

If a revision is necessary, revise your proposal and discuss the change with members of the IRB in the agency in which the study is to be conducted. Most IRB committees have a form you will complete when requesting a study modification. The IRB members might indicate that the investigators may proceed with the amended study or that the revised proposal requires another review. If a study is funded, the study changes must be discussed with the representatives of the funding agency. The funding agency has the power to approve or disapprove the changes. However, realistic changes that are clearly described and backed with rationale will probably be approved.

EXAMPLE QUANTITATIVE RESEARCH PROPOSAL

An example proposal of a quasi-experimental study is included to guide you in developing a research proposal for a thesis, dissertation, or research project in your clinical agency. The content of this proposal is brief and does not include the detail normally presented in a thesis or dissertation proposal. However, the example provides you with ideas regarding the content areas that would be covered in developing a proposal for a quantitative study. Dr. Kathryn Daniel (2015), an associate professor at the University of Texas at Arlington College of Nursing and Health Innovation, developed the proposal that is provided as the example.

"The Effect of Nurse Practitioner–Directed Transitional Care on Medication Adherence and Readmission Outcomes of Elderly Congestive Heart Failure Patients"

Kathryn Daniel, PhD, RN, ANP-BC, GNP-BC

Chapter 1

Introduction

Hospitalized patients with chronic health diagnoses such as congestive heart failure (CHF), pneumonia, and stroke are often readmitted to acute care hospitals within a 30-day interval for potentially preventable etiologies. These unnecessary readmissions carry a significant cost to Medicare and have been targeted for nonreimbursement. Hospitals and healthcare systems are eager to implement programs that can safely and effectively reduce unnecessary readmissions. Their interests are also tempered by the realization that either way, whether by administrative nonreimbursement policy or actual prevention of unnecessary readmissions, such admissions will no longer be

"The Effect of Nurse Practitioner–Directed Transitional Care on Medication Adherence and Readmission Outcomes of Elderly Congestive Heart Failure Patients"—cont'd

the source of revenue, but rather a cost to the organization. Even though some readmissions will not be preventable, the burden will likely be on the hospital organization to justify payment (Stauffer et al., 2011).

Estimates of the prevalence of heart failure vary. However, older adults, defined as those 65 years of age and older, have documented higher rates of CHF, 6%–10%. The trends over the past decade are an older age at first hospital admission for adults with CHF and an older age at death. This is probably secondary to technological advances and evidence-based guidelines for the care of individuals with heart failure. Despite these trends, the cost for management of CHF in the United States accounts for nearly 2% of the total cost of health care in the country (Mosterd & Hoes, 2007; Solomon et al., 2005).

CHF patients have one of the highest readmission rates to the hospital within 30 days of any diagnosis. Nationally 25% of patients discharged from the hospital after an acute care stay for heart failure are readmitted to the hospital within 30 days (Jencks, Williams, & Coleman, 2009). Reports are as high as 50% of those readmitted from the community had no follow-up with their primary care provider prior to readmission. When patients are readmitted to the hospital within the 30-day period, hospitals may not be reimbursed for subsequent hospitalizations. In 2004, premature CHF readmissions cost the Medicare system an estimated $17.4 billion (Jencks et al., 2009).

Prognosis remains poor once CHF is diagnosed. From the date of index hospitalization, the 30-day mortality rate is between 10% and 20%. Mortality at 1 year (and 5 years) is estimated between 30% and 40% (and 60% and 70%), respectively. Most individuals will die with progressively worsening symptoms while others will succumb to fatal arrhythmias (Mosterd & Hoes, 2007; Solomon et al., 2005). With these high morbidity and mortality rates, individuals with CHF need additional health care in the community to manage their disease and decrease their rates of premature hospital readmission.

Chapter 2
Review of Relevant Literature
Care for this population is fragmented and uncoordinated. Systems of care today often are connected to sites of care, so when patients are discharged from acute care settings to home or to other settings and back again, there are many opportunities for gaps in care. Vulnerable complex frail patients with new problems or questions about management of existing problems have few knowledgeable resources to help them navigate the new landscape of their health. More and more hospital care is rendered by hospitalist providers who do not follow patients after discharge from the acute care setting, but refer patients back to their outpatient providers for care after discharge. Communication between inpatient and outpatient silos of care may be absent and is frequently delayed. Studies designed to use predictive modeling to identify patients at risk for readmission have had low predictive sensitivity (Billings et al., 2012).

Medically complex patients who have multiple chronic diseases and few socioeconomic resources are the most vulnerable within this group and most likely to be readmitted. Silverstein, Qin, Mercer, Fong, and Haydar (2008) found that male African American patients over age 75 with multiple medical comorbidities, admitted to a medicine service (not surgical), and who had Medicare only as a payer source have the highest risk of readmission. CHF was the highest single predictor of readmission, but other comorbidities such as cancer, chronic obstructive pulmonary disease (COPD), or chronic renal failure were also contributing factors. The period of greatest vulnerability for readmission is the first month after hospitalization, before patients have been seen by their primary care provider (PCP).

Adverse drug events are a leading cause of readmission (Morrissey, McElnay, Scott, & McConnell, 2003). Medication reconciliation and adherence are important in the postdischarge situation. Patients and families do their best to relay their drug information to inpatient providers, but they may forget things or assume the provider knows what they are taking. Because patients have had an acute change in their health, their medication regimens are often modified during their hospital stay. In addition, inpatient medication choices are influenced by hospital formularies. Even when diligent providers discharge patients with prescriptions for their new or modified medications, these choices may not be available on the patients' drug formulary plan. So, when they present these prescriptions to their local pharmacy after discharge from the hospital, the new medication may not be available to them or is too costly for them to afford. Inpatient providers may also be unaware of all the medications that the patient already has at home and duplicate drugs or drug classes that the patient has on hand (Corbett, Setter, Daratha, Neumiller, & Wood, 2010).

Continued

"The Effect of Nurse Practitioner–Directed Transitional Care on Medication Adherence and Readmission Outcomes of Elderly Congestive Heart Failure Patients"—cont'd

Early physician follow-up (within 7 days) has been identified as a possible target for reducing readmissions (Hernandez et al., 2010), but in most cases requires that the patient be capable of navigating and transferring within an ambulatory care practice rapidly after hospital discharge. Home visits by nurse practitioners (NPs) are an efficient and logical method of delivering a similar quality service.

NPs are educated to manage chronic diseases and understand systems of care. Thus they are in a unique position within the healthcare system to have significant positive effects on patient outcomes, thereby decreasing readmissions, improving patient physical and mental health outcomes, and decreasing the costs of care (Naylor, 2004). Trials using the transitional care model have been very favorable, both in controlled research settings and in real-world settings. Patients followed by a transitional care NP have had substantial reduction in 30-day readmissions (Naylor, 2004; Neff, Madigan, & Narsavage, 2003; Stauffer et al., 2011; Zhao & Wong, 2009). Yet, in spite of success in prevention of unnecessary readmissions, balancing the cost of such programs must be weighed against decreasing revenue streams before hospitals will support them (Stauffer et al., 2011).

Within the past 10 years, multiple interventions regarding medication reconciliation (Young, Barnason, Hays, & Do, 2015), discrepancies (Kostas et al., 2013), and management (Crotty, Rowett, Spurling, Giles, & Phillips, 2004; Davis, 2015) have been implemented to address management of medications across care transitions. Although NPs were among the treating providers within these study samples, they were not identified or controlled for in the studies. Medication discrepancies, reconciliation, and adherence all continue to be targets in the quest to reduce readmissions (Coleman, Smith, Raha, & Min, 2005).

We know that transitional care programs utilizing advanced practice nurses have consistently reduced readmissions of vulnerable patients. Medication management is an important part of the transitional care NP role. What is not known is the effect of a transitional care NP program focused on medication management on readmission rates and medication adherence of elderly individuals with CHF. Thus the purpose of this study is to examine the effects of an NP-directed transitional care program on the hospital readmission rate and medication adherence of elderly CHF patients.

Chapter 3
Framework
The transitional care model provides comprehensive in-hospital planning and home follow-up for chronically ill, high-risk older adults hospitalized for common medical and surgical conditions (Fig. 28.1). This model was initially developed by Dorothy Brooten in the 1980s with a population of high-risk pregnant women and low-birthweight infants (Brooten et al., 1987, 1994). Later, Naylor and colleagues developed it further in high-risk elderly populations focusing on patients with CHF (Brooten et al., 2002; Naylor, 2004). Multiple randomized controlled trials (RCTs) support its effectiveness in reducing unnecessary readmissions (Naylor, 2004; Neff et al., 2003; Ornstein, Smith, Foer, Lopez-Cantor, & Soriano, 2011; Williams, Akroyd, & Burke, 2010; Zhao & Wong, 2009).

The goals of care provided by the transitional care model focus on empowering the patient and family through coordination of care and medical management of disease and comorbidities as needed with the ability to make changes immediately based on set protocols, health literacy, self-care management, and collaboration with other providers and families to prevent unnecessary hospital readmissions. Fig. 28.1 illustrates the interrelationship of concepts in this model (transitional care model—when you or a loved one requires care). Patients who are more vulnerable, either socially or physically, or complex, would utilize more aspects of the transitional care model, whereas patients with more resources (social and physical) need less support during transitions of care. According to this model's conceptual relationships, when advanced practice nurses educate patients about self-management skills, they are more adherent to the overall plan of care. Thus these chronically ill individuals have fewer unnecessary readmissions and greater medication adherence (Brooten, Youngblut, Kutcher, & Bobo, 2004).

The purpose of this study is to determine the effect of an NP-directed transitional care program on medication adherence and hospital readmission rate of discharged elderly adults with CHF. The independent variable (IV) is the NP-directed transitional care program and the dependent variables (DVs) are medication adherence and hospital readmission rates. This study will compare the medication adherence and readmission rate of medically complex elderly CHF patients who receive NP-directed transitional

"The Effect of Nurse Practitioner–Directed Transitional Care on Medication Adherence and Readmission Outcomes of Elderly Congestive Heart Failure Patients"—cont'd

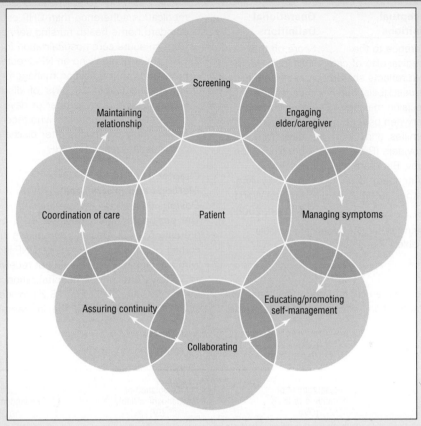

Fig. 28.1 Transitional care model. (Naylor, M. D. [2012] Advancing high value transitional care: the central role of nursing and its leadership. *Nursing Administration Quarterly, 36*[2], 115–126. doi:10.1097/NAQ.0b013e31824a040b.)

care with medication management, and those who receive standard home health nursing services. The following table summarizes the conceptual and operational definitions for the IV and DVs in this study.

Variables	Conceptual Definitions	Operational Definitions	Variables	Conceptual Definitions	Operational Definitions
IV: Nurse practitioner (NP)–directed transitional care program	Time-limited services delivered by specially trained NPs to at-risk populations designed to ensure continuity and avoid preventable poor outcomes as they move across sites of care and among multiple providers (Brooten et al., 1987; Coleman & Boult, 2003).	Enrollment and participation in a NP-directed transitional care program, including medication management after an acute care hospital stay for CHF (see protocol in Appendix A).	DV: Hospital readmission rate	Outcome that reflects inadequate training and preparation of patients/family to manage new/chronic health conditions or breakdown in communication between patient/family and provider (Coleman & Boult, 2003).	Any unplanned readmission to an acute care hospital reported to study investigators within 30 days of hospital discharge. Number of days from hospital discharge to readmission will be measured.

Continued

"The Effect of Nurse Practitioner–Directed Transitional Care on Medication Adherence and Readmission Outcomes of Elderly Congestive Heart Failure Patients"—cont'd

Variables	Conceptual Definitions	Operational Definitions
DV: Medication adherence	Adherence to the medical plan of care that reflects shared values, goals, and decision making between patients, families, and providers (Rich, Gray, Beckham, Wittenberg, & Luther, 1996).	Score on the Morisky Medication Adherence Scale measured on intake and 30 days from index hospitalization discharge (Morisky, Ang, Krousel-Wood, & Ward, 2008).

CHF, Congestive heart failure; *DV*, dependent variable; *IV*, independent variable.

Hypotheses

1. CHF patients receiving an NP-directed transitional care program with medication management have greater medication adherence than CHF patients who receive standard home health nursing services after discharge from an acute care hospitalization for CHF.

2. CHF patients receiving an NP-directed transitional care program with medication management have fewer readmissions within 30 days of discharge from index hospitalization, and number of days to readmission is greater than CHF patients who receive standard home health nursing services after discharge from an acute care hospitalization for CHF.

Chapter 4
Methods and Procedures
Design

The design for this study will be a quasi-experimental pretest-posttest design comparing readmission outcomes of patients who received NP-led transitional care with similar patients who did not receive transitional care at 30 days after index hospitalization discharge (Grove, Burns, & Gray, 2013). Fig. 28.2 provides a model of the study design identifying the implementation of the IV

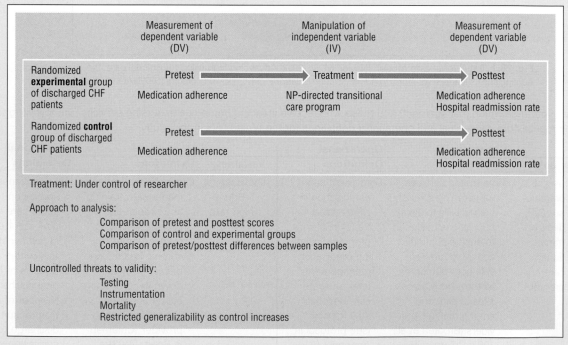

Fig. 28.2 Classic experimental design. *CHF*, Congestive heart failure.

"The Effect of Nurse Practitioner–Directed Transitional Care on Medication Adherence and Readmission Outcomes of Elderly Congestive Heart Failure Patients"—cont'd

(see Appendix A) and measurement of the DVs. The study will also compare pretest-posttest medication adherence scores between the experimental and standard care groups at 30 days. The protocol for conducting the study is presented in Appendix B. The proposal will be submitted to the institutional review boards (IRBs) of The University of Texas at Arlington (UTA) and a selected healthcare system for approval. After approvals are obtained, patients admitted to one of the participating hospitals in the system who have an admitting diagnosis of CHF will be screened for eligibility. Eligible patients will be approached by study personnel who will explain the opportunity to participate in the study after discharge from the hospital. Patients who consent to participate will be randomized into either the experimental (intervention) group or the comparison (standard care) group. Demographic information, medical status, and pretest medication adherence will be collected from all patients who consent to be in the study before discharge from the hospital. Outcome measures (hospital readmission rate and posttest medication adherence) will be recorded at 30 days after discharge using the data collection form in Appendix C. The pretest and posttest design with a comparison group has uncontrolled threats to validity due to selection, maturation, instrumentation, and the possible interaction between selection and history (Grove et al., 2013; Shadish, Cook, & Campbell, 2002). Randomization of subjects to the treatment, controlled implementation of the study treatment, and quality measurement methods strengthen the study design.

Ethical Considerations
University and clinical agency IRB approvals will be obtained. All study personnel who have access to the data or to participants will complete human subject protection training before beginning to participate in study delivery. All participants will have the study explained to them in detail and have all of their questions answered before signing consent forms to participate in the study. The consent form for this study is presented in Appendix D. The participants will receive a copy of their signed consent form

Time frame: This entire study is projected to take 1 year. Subject recruitment will begin after IRB approval and informational in-services are presented to the nursing and social work staff in the participating hospitals. Data collection and analysis of readmission outcomes and mortality will begin with the recruitment of participants and will end 30 days after the last participant is recruited (see the Study Protocol in Appendix B).

Intervention and Procedures
Patients who consent to participate in the study will be visited by the transitional care NP who will be following them after discharge for an intake visit before they are discharged from the hospital. The same NP will visit the patient in his or her home within 24 hours of discharge from the hospital to monitor the patient's condition, review the goals and plans for care, provide patient education as needed, and manage any new issues as they emerge. The NP will also manage all aspects of the patients' medications. The NP will make at least weekly home visits for the entire study period, carefully inquiring about any interval emergency department visits or hospital admissions. Patients who are readmitted to the hospital may be retained in the study for the full study period (30 days) even though they have already reached the end point of readmission so that medication adherence can be measured. At the end of the 30 days, all patients in the study will be contacted and/or visited at home by study staff to capture outcome measures. The intervention and study protocols were developed to ensure intervention fidelity (see Appendices A and B) (Dumas, Lynch, Laughlin, Smith, & Prinz, 2001; Erlen & Sereika, 2006; Moncher & Prinz, 1991).

NPs who will be delivering transitional care to study patients will receive study-related training that explicitly reviews the 2009 Focused Update incorporated into the American College of Cardiology Foundation/American Heart Associated (ACCF/AHA) 2005 Guidelines for the Diagnosis and Management of Heart Failure in Adults (Jessup et al., 2009) as well as training in study protocols (weekly visits) and study-related measures. Because only 40 patients will be in the intervention group, one NP is expected to be able to manage 40 patients over a 1-year period. To ensure study continuity and coverage for holidays and scheduled absences, a second NP employed in the agency will also be trained. Study recruitment and outcome measures will be accomplished via a study registered nurse (RN) who will be trained on study information and procedures (see Appendix B and the patient consent process).

Subjects and Setting
Sample criteria: An electronic search of the inpatient database each night at midnight will reveal all patients in

Continued

"The Effect of Nurse Practitioner–Directed Transitional Care on Medication Adherence and Readmission Outcomes of Elderly Congestive Heart Failure Patients"—cont'd

the participating hospitals with qualifying diagnosis of CHF who are age 75 or older. Other inclusion criteria are as follows: The patient must have a minimum of three chronic disease states, be of male gender, and have Medicare, Medicaid, and or charity status as a payer source. These criteria are selected based on information from Billings and Silverstein (Billings et al., 2012; Silverstein et al., 2008), which revealed these characteristics specifically increased risk of readmission in a similar population. Study personnel will eliminate any patients who have already been offered participation. Patients who are on ventilator support or vasoactive drips will be deferred until they are stable enough to begin discharge planning. Patients who are being discharged on hospice or who have already participated are not eligible to participate. Patients who are on dialysis will be excluded due to their unique needs and resources.

A power analysis was conducted to determine the desired sample size. Because this intervention is known to be effective in preventing readmission with a moderate effect size, the effect size of 0.45 was chosen with $\alpha = 0.05$ and power of 0.80, indicating a sample size of 70 was required for the study with 35 participants in both the intervention and comparison groups (Aberson, 2019). Ten percent will be added to each group to accommodate for attrition. This leaves a final required sample size of 40 for each group. When the required sample size of 80 has been secured, recruitment will stop. Due to the large population of elderly CHF patients in these hospitals, the sample is hoped to be obtained in 4 to 6 months.

Demographic variables of interest will be collected to describe the study sample and compare the sample with the population for representativeness. Race, gender, age, chronic illnesses, marital status, educational level, and healthcare insurance will be collected using the data collection form in Appendix C. Socioeconomic status and literacy are known predictors of health status and utilization (Silverstein et al., 2008). Describing relationships between these factors and patient outcomes may be important in explaining study outcomes. The study participants' addresses will be obtained also for contact by NPs following hospital discharge.

Instruments
The Morisky Medication Adherence Scale will be administered to all subjects who agree to participate in the study during intake and at 30 days post initial hospital discharge (Morisky et al., 2008). This tool has established

sensitivity of 93% and specificity of 53% when used with a similar population of older adults taking antihypertensive medications. It consists of eight questions, seven asking for yes/no answers about the patient's self-reported adherence over the preceding 2 weeks and a final question with a 5-point Likert-style question. High adherence is associated with a score greater than 6 points on the scale (see Appendix E). Low/medium adherence was significantly associated with poor blood pressure control, while high-adhering patients (80.3%) were more likely to have blood pressure controlled (Morisky et al., 2008). Test-retest procedures were utilized to produce consistency of performance measures from one group of subjects on two separate occasions, which were then correlated with the norm reference of actual blood pressure measurements (Waltz, Strickland, & Lenz, 2017). Item-total correlations were > 0.30 for each of the eight items in the scale with Cronbach alpha of 0.83. Confirmatory factor analysis revealed a unidimensional scale with all items loading to a single factor.

The Morisky Medication Adherence Scale is appropriate for the proposed study because it was validated on a similar population of older outpatients who were mostly minority (76.5% black). The questions specifically ask about "blood pressure medicines," which are the primary medications used in CHF management. This eight-question instrument is derived from a previously validated four-question version (Morisky, Green, & Levine, 1986).

Procedure
Eligible participants will have the study explained to them by the study recruiter who will obtain consent from those who are willing to participate. The recruiter, a RN who is part of the study team, will also capture demographic and medical data, and administer the Morisky Medication Adherence Scale to all participants (see Appendix E). Patients assigned to the transitional care intervention will be visited by a transitional care NP before being discharged home (see Appendix B for Study Protocol).

On the day after discharge, the transitional care NP will visit the patients in their home to evaluate their home situation and resources as well as review the plan of care. For the next 30 days, the transitional care NP will visit the patient on at least a weekly basis. The visit will conform to the transitional care visit guideline in Appendix A so that intervention fidelity will be maintained. At all times a transitional care NP will be available by telephone. Outcome measures (hospital readmissions and medication

"The Effect of Nurse Practitioner–Directed Transitional Care on Medication Adherence and Readmission Outcomes of Elderly Congestive Heart Failure Patients"—cont'd

adherence) will be measured at 30 days after discharge using the data collection form in Appendix C and the Morisky Medication Adherence Scale in Appendix E. The study recruiter will also do these measures to decrease potential for bias.

Plan for Data Management and Analysis

Demographic data will be analyzed and NP actions and their frequency of use will be examined using descriptive statistics. All encounter content with patients will be recorded in the electronic health record, which all transitional care staff will have access to at all times. The documentation of weekly scheduled visits from the transitional care NP will follow a template so that all areas are consistently addressed with all study participants, and intervention fidelity is assured (Erlen & Sereika, 2006). Differences in the interval-level data produced by the Morisky Medication Adherence Scale will be examined with a t-test at pretest between the intervention and comparison groups to ensure the groups were similar at the start of the study. Differences will also be examined between pretest and posttest, and at posttest between the intervention and comparison groups. Differences in readmission rates will be examined at 30 days between the intervention and comparison groups. IBM Statistical Package for Social Sciences Statistics 21 will be used to analyze the data. Alpha will be set at 0.05 to conclude statistical difference. The statistical tests will be an independent t-test between two groups and a dependent t-test comparing pretest and posttest. Bonferroni correction for multiple t-tests will be done to reduce the risk of a Type I error (Grove & Cipher, 2020; Plitchta & Kelvin, 2013).

References

Aberson, C. L. (2019). *Applied power analysis for the behavioral sciences*. (2nd ed.) New York, NY: Routledge.

Billings, J., Blunt, I., Steventon, A., Georghiou, T., Lewis, G., & Bardsley, M. (2012). Development of a predictive model to identify inpatients at risk of re-admission within 30 days of discharge (PARR-30). *BMJ Open, 2*(4), 2012. doi:10.1136/bmjopen-2012-001667

Brooten, D., Kumar, S., Brown, L. P., Butts, P., Finkler, S. A., Bakewell-Sachs, S., et al. (1987). A randomized clinical trial of early hospital discharge and home follow-up of very-low-birth-weight infants. In L. T. Rinke (Ed.), *Outcome measures in home care: Research* (pp. 95–106). New York, NY: National League for Nursing.

Brooten, D., Naylor, M. D., York, R., Brown, L. P., Munro, B. H., Hollingsworth, A. O., et al. (2002). Lessons learned from testing the quality cost model of advanced practice nursing (APN) transitional care. *Journal of Nursing Scholarship, 34*(4), 369–375.

Brooten, D., Roncoli, M., Finkler, S., Arnold, L., Cohen, A., & Mennuti, M. (1994). A randomized trial of early hospital discharge and home follow-up of women having cesarean birth. *Obstetrics and Gynecology, 84*(5), 832–838.

Brooten, D., Youngblut, J. M., Kutcher, J., & Bobo, C. (2004). Quality and the nursing workforce: APNs, patient outcomes and health care costs. *Nursing Outlook, 52*(1), 45–52.

Coleman, E. A., & Boult, C. (2003). Improving the quality of transitional care for persons with complex care needs. *Journal of the American Geriatrics Society, 51*(4), 556–557.

Coleman, E. A., Smith, J. D., Raha, D., & Min, S. (2005). Posthospital medication discrepancies: Prevalence and contributing factors. *Archives of Internal Medicine, 165*(16), 1842–1847.

Corbett, C. F., Setter, S. M., Daratha, K. B., Neumiller, J. J., & Wood, L. D. (2010). Nurse identified hospital to home medication discrepancies: Implications for improving transitional care. *Geriatric Nursing, 31*(3), 188–196.

Crotty, M., Rowett, D., Spurling, L., Giles, L. C., & Phillips, P. A. (2004). Does the addition of a pharmacist transition coordinator improve evidence-based medication management and health outcomes in older adults moving from the hospital to a long-term care facility? Results of a randomized, controlled trial. *The American Journal of Geriatric Pharmacotherapy, 2*(4), 257–264.

Davis, D. (2015). *A medication management intervention across care transitions*. University of Massachusetts Amherst, Amherst, MA: Capstone DNP Project.

Dumas, J. E., Lynch, A. M., Laughlin, J. E., Smith, E. P., & Prinz, R. J. (2001). Promoting intervention fidelity: Conceptual issues, methods, and preliminary results from the EARLY ALLIANCE prevention trial. *American Journal of Preventive Medicine, 20*(1), 38–47.

Erlen, J. A., & Sereika, S. M. (2006). Fidelity to a 12-week structured medication adherence intervention in patients with HIV. *Nursing Research, 55*(2), S17–S22.

Grove, S. K., Burns, N., & Gray, J. (2013). *The practice of nursing research: Appraisal, synthesis, and generation of evidence* (7th ed.). St. Louis, MO: Elsevier/Saunders.

Grove, S. K., & Cipher, D. (2020). *Statistics for nursing research: A workbook for evidence-based practice* (3rd ed.). St. Louis, MO: Saunders.

Hernandez, A. F., Greiner, M. A., Fonarow, G. C., Hammill, B. G., Heidenreich, P. A., Yancy, C. W., et al. (2010). Relationship between early physician follow-up and 30-day readmission among Medicare beneficiaries hospitalized for heart failure. *Journal of the American Medical Association, 303*(17), 1716–1722.

Jencks, S. F., Williams, M. V., & Coleman, E. A. (2009). Rehospitalizations among patients in the Medicare fee-for-service program. *The New England Journal of Medicine, 360*(14), 1418–1428.

Jessup, M., Abraham, W. T., Casey, D. E., Feldman, A. M., Francis, G. S., Ganiats, T. G., et al. (2009). 2009 focused update: ACCF/AHA guidelines for the diagnosis and management of heart

Continued

"The Effect of Nurse Practitioner–Directed Transitional Care on Medication Adherence and Readmission Outcomes of Elderly Congestive Heart Failure Patients"—cont'd

failure in adults: A report of the American College of Cardiology Foundation/American Heart Association task force on practice guidelines: Developed in collaboration with the International Society for Heart and Lung Transplantation. *Circulation, 119*(4), 1977–2016.

Kostas, T., Paquin, A. M., Zimmerman, K., Simone, M., Skarf, L. M., & Rudolph, J. L. (2013). Characterizing medication discrepancies among older adults during transitions of care: A systematic review focusing on discrepancy synonyms, data sources and classification terms. *Aging Health, 9,* 497–508.

Moncher, F. J., & Prinz, R. J. (1991). Treatment fidelity in outcome studies. *Clinical Psychology Review, 11*(3), 247–266.

Morisky, D. E., Ang, A., Krousel-Wood, M., & Ward, H. J. (2008). Predictive validity of a medication adherence measure in an outpatient setting. *Journal of Clinical Hypertension, 10*(5), 348–354.

Morisky, D. E., Green, L. W., & Levine, D. M. (1986). Concurrent and predictive validity of a self-reported measure of medication adherence. *Medical Care, 24*(1), 67–74.

Morrissey, E. F. R., McElnay, J. C., Scott, M., & McConnell, B. J. (2003). Influence of drugs, demographics and medical history on hospital readmission of elderly patients: A predictive model. *Clinical Drug Investigation, 23*(2), 119–128.

Mosterd, A., & Hoes, A. W. (2007). Clinical epidemiology of heart failure. *Heart (British Cardiac Society), 93*(9), 1137–1146.

Naylor, M. (2004). Transitional care for older adults: A cost-effective model. *LDI Issue Brief, 9*(6), 1–4.

Neff, D. F., Madigan, E., & Narsavage, G. (2003). APN-directed transitional home care model: Achieving positive outcomes for patients with COPD. *Home Healthcare Nurse, 21*(8), 543–550.

Ornstein, K., Smith, K. L., Foer, D. H., Lopez-Cantor, M., & Soriano, T. (2011). To the hospital and back home again: A nurse practitioner-based transitional care program for hospitalized homebound people. *Journal of the American Geriatrics Society, 59*(3), 544–551.

Plichta, S. B., & Kelvin, E. (2013). *Munro's statistical methods for health care research* (6th ed.). Philadelphia, PA: Lippincott Williams & Wilkins.

Rich, M. W., Gray, D. B., Beckham, V., Wittenberg, C., & Luther, P. (1996). Effect of a multidisciplinary intervention on medication compliance in elderly patients with congestive heart failure. *The American Journal of Medicine, 101*(3), 270–276.

Shadish, W. R., Cook, T. D., & Campbell, D. T. (2002). *Experimental and quasi-experimental designs for generalized causal inference.* Boston, MA: Houghton Mifflin.

Silverstein, M. D., Qin, H., Mercer, S. Q., Fong, J., & Haydar, Z. (2008). Risk factors for 30-day hospital readmission in patients <GT> or = 65 years of age. *Baylor University Medical Center Proceedings, 21*(4), 363–372.

Solomon, S. D., Zelenkofske, S., McMurray, J. J. V., Finn, P. V., Velazquez, E., Ertl, G., et al. (2005). Sudden death in patients with myocardial infarction and left ventricular dysfunction, heart failure, or both. *The New England Journal of Medicine, 352*(25), 2581–2588.

Stauffer, B., Fullerton, C., Fleming, N., Ogola, G., Herrin, J., Stafford, P., et al. (2011). Effectiveness and cost of a transitional care program for heart failure: A prospective study with concurrent controls. *Archives of Internal Medicine, 14*(14), 1238–1243.

Waltz, C. F., Strickland, O. L., & Lenz, E. R. (2017). *Measurement in nursing and health research* (5th ed.). New York, NY: Springer.

Williams, G., Akroyd, K., & Burke, L. (2010). Evaluation of the transitional care model in chronic heart failure. *British Journal of Nursing, 19*(22), 1402–1407.

Young, L., Barnason, S., Hays, K., & Do, V. (2015). Nurse practitioner-led medication reconciliation in critical access hospitals. *The Journal for Nurse Practitioners, 11*(5), 511–518.

Zhao, Y., & Wong, F. K. Y. (2009). Effects of a postdischarge transitional care programme for patients with coronary heart disease in China: A randomised controlled trial. *Journal of Clinical Nursing, 18*(17), 2444–2455.

APPENDIX A   Intervention Protocol for Transitional Care Nurse Practitioner (TCNP) Visit Protocol

1. Patients are initially visited within 24 to 48 hours of discharge from the hospital.
2. Only NPs who have been trained on CHF protocols and transitional care protocols and are included on the study IRB protocol may visit/interact with study patients.
3. On the first visit the TCNP will review the hospital discharge plan of care with the patient. A family caregiver is identified on the hospital visit or first home visit. This person should be present and included in all visits and supervise the patient's needs in the home. On every visit the following will be addressed by the TCNP.

a. Review the plan of care given to the patient on discharge from the hospital.
b. On all visits after the initial visit, inquire about any unplanned visits to any hospital.
c. Ask about any new problems, issues, or symptoms that have arisen since hospital discharge.
d. Conduct a brief review of systems, looking specifically for any changes since discharge from the hospital.
e. Review log of daily weights/teach if needed to do daily weights before breakfast and after voiding each morning.

APPENDIX A Intervention Protocol for Transitional Care Nurse Practitioner (TCNP) Visit Protocol—cont'd

f. Conduct a focused physical exam with careful attention to cardiovascular and respiratory exam on every visit, and other systems as indicated by any patient complaints.

g. Review all recommended medications with the patient and caregiver by physically viewing the supply. On the first visit to the home, if the patient does not have a "medminder," the TCNP will provide one to the patient/family at no cost and set up the medications for the first week. The available quantities and dosages on hand will be monitored on all medications, not just CHF medications. (Anticipate unexpected problems to arise here with possible duplication of drug classes, unavailable meds, etc.)

h. Review indication, rationale, schedule, and possible side effects of every medication.

i. Provide patient/family education as needed on dietary choices, exercise, as-needed medications, and so forth.

j. When possible and needed the TCNP will adjust medications as required to accommodate individual patient plan formulary.

k. Adjust/titrate meds as indicated to achieve goals of care.

l. Order lab tests necessary to monitor patient response to medication changes.

m. Order any other medications/tests/referrals indicated by patient exam and complaints.

n. Consult immediately with primary care provider (PCP)/cardiologist for any unexpected deterioration in patient condition.

o. Communicate any changes in medication regimen in writing for patient/caregiver.

p. Record visit in electronic health record (EHR); forward copy to patient's PCP for review. Visit template in EHR will include fields to capture items (c) through (p).

q. On final home visit at the end of the fourth week, collect Morisky Medication Adherence Scale for study.

r. After final visit at the end of the fourth week, compose discharge summary and send to PCP.

Study RN Protocol for Comparison Group

a. The study RN will recruit, consent, and randomize patients. After consent is obtained, the RN will also obtain demographic information and the pretest Morisky Medication Adherence Scale on all participants.

b. The study RN will contact all usual care patients by telephone at the end of each week during the study period of 4 weeks to inquire about any interval hospital admissions.

c. On the final telephone call to the usual care participant at the end of week 4, the study RN will also collect the posttest Morisky Medication Adherence Scale.

d. The study RN will also contact all transitional care participants at the end of week 4 to collect posttest Morisky Medication Adherence Scale.

APPENDIX B Study Protocol

Recruiting/Intake—Study RN

1. Generate CHF list from hospital IT.
2. Compare list to track daily discharges of patients already recruited.
3. Screening for eligibility: Inclusion sample criteria
   a. Service area is 30 miles from the hospital: Use GPS if you are unsure about how far the patient lives from the facility.
   b. Must have heart failure diagnosis
   c. Age 75+
   d. African American
   e. Male gender
   f. Medicare, nonfunded or Medicaid
   g. Patient resides in a private residence, assisted living facility, or residential care home.

4. Exclusion sample criteria:
   a. Patients discharged home on hospice
   b. Patients on dialysis
   c. Patients on ventilators or vasoactive drips should not be approached until they are in the discharge planning stage.
5. If patient meets all of the previous inclusion and exclusion sample criteria, they will be approached for study participation.
6. Introduce yourself to the patient and family.
7. Explain the opportunity to participate in the study after discharge from the hospital and what is involved. If patients agree to participate, give them consent to read or read to them if desired.
8. Ask them to sign consent if they wish to participate.

Continued

APPENDIX B   Study Protocol—cont'd

9. If they decline to participate, thank them for giving of their time. Make a note in the chart that they were offered study participation and have refused, that they are not in the study.

10. For those patients who consent to participate in the study:
    a. Collect patients' demographic, medical, and educational information.
    b. Administer the Morisky Medication Adherence Scale.
    c. Confirm their address and phone number.
    d. Give them your card and phone number.
    e. Randomize participant to either the intervention or comparison group. Let them know which group they will be in and when to expect contact again.
    f. Intervention group will be visited by NP in hospital and within 24 hours of discharge from hospital in their residence, then weekly throughout study period. Place a transitional care "sticker" on the chart to alert inpatient staff that we are following the patient who was assigned to the intervention group.
    g. Usual care group will receive weekly phone call from study RN to determine any hospital readmissions, plus one end-of-study data collection of Morisky Medication Adherence Scale.

Intervention Group

A transitional care nurse practitioner is preferably certified as an adult/gerontology primary care NP, although other NPs with significant geriatric expertise will be considered. Other types of advanced practice nurses will not be included in this trial although they were included in much of the original studies by Brooten et al. (2004) and Naylor (2004). All transitional care NPs will complete a standardized orientation and training program focusing on a review of national heart failure guidelines as well as principles of geriatric care, patient and caregiver goal setting, and educational and behavioral strategies focused on patient and caregiver needs.

Scripting for Transitional Care Program Introduction During Inpatient Visit

1. Introduce yourself to the patient/family.
2. You were randomly chosen to be in the transitional care group. The goal of the program is to help people (and their families) with heart problems learn how to best manage their illness at home.
    a. Heart failure has more hospital readmissions than any other problem in the United States.
    b. Of all people discharged with this problem, 20% return to the hospital within 30 days.
    c. Patients followed in transitional care programs have had lower readmission rates.
3. This is how the program works:
    a. I meet you here in the hospital (probably one time only).
    b. I come to see you very soon after you go home; I will be there within 24 to 48 hours.
    c. I will see you every week for 1 month at a minimum; we can add more visits to this if needed for you and your family.
4. I work with your doctors and keep them informed of how things are going at home. I am an NP; I am not a home healthcare nurse, although I will work with your home healthcare nurse as needed. Go into more explanation regarding differences, etc. as needed, give them brochure on "What is an NP?"
    a. Why NPs can do more.
    b. NP can prescribe and make medication changes if necessary and keep your physician informed.
    c. NPs can address new problems that might come up.
    d. Your Medicare benefit and supplemental insurance will pay for my visits; you will not be billed for any uncovered copays.
5. The goal of the program is not to slow you down; we do not want to interfere with your other activities, and we want you to continue to be able to do as much as you can do.
    a. We will review your medications at every visit.
    b. I will ask you each week about any readmissions to any hospital since the previous visit.
    c. Each week we will review your plan of care, how you are doing, and about any new problems or issues that arise.
    d. The study RN who recruited you to the study will contact you at the end of the study and ask you the same questions that she asked after you initially consented to participate (Morisky Medication Adherence Scale).
6. There will be different levels of coordination involved with each patient.
    a. I may discuss your case with your hospital nurse and hospitalist/cardiologist if needed.
    b. I may discuss your case with your primary care provider if needed during intervention period; he or she will receive a copy of the record for every visit.
    c. I will provide a comprehensive discharge summary to your PCP when discharged from transitional care service after 1 month.

APPENDIX B   Study Protocol—cont'd

Study RN—Data Collection on Comparison Group Patients

1. Call all usual care patients at day 7, 14, 21, and 30 after discharge. On each occasion, he or she will update the database on any hospitalizations that have occurred since the last interval data collection (specifically how many days since discharge to readmission). On the final call, the Morisky Medication Adherence Scale will also be collected.

APPENDIX C   Data Collection Form

Data Collection Form					Pretest Morisky Medication Adherence Score	Heart Failure Diagnosis (ICD-9 Code)	All Other Diagnoses (One Line/ ICD-9 Code)	Days Since Discharge without Readmission				Posttest Morisky Medication Adherence Score
Study ID	Age	Gender	Race	Years of Education				End of Week 1	End of Week 2	End of Week 3	End of Week 4	

ICD-9, International Classification of Diseases, Ninth Revision.

APPENDIX D   Informed Consent

Principal Investigator Name
Kathryn Daniel, PhD, RN, ANP-BC, GNP-BC

Title of Project
The Effect of Nurse Practitioner–Directed Transitional Care on Medication Adherence and Readmission Outcomes of Elderly Congestive Heart Failure Patients

Introduction
You are being asked to participate in a research study. Your participation is voluntary. Please ask questions if there is anything you do not understand.

Purpose
This study is designed to examine the effects of nurse practitioner–directed transitional care program on medication adherence and hospital readmission of elderly patients who have congestive heart failure. Nationally, 20% or more of patients who are hospitalized with congestive heart failure are readmitted to the hospital within 30 days, often for reasons that are preventable. Transitional care using nurse practitioners has been shown to have positive benefits for many

Continued

people like you after they are discharged from the hospital. This study is designed to determine whether medication adherence is also related to decreased hospital readmissions.

Duration
This study will last for 4 weeks after you are discharged from the hospital.

Procedures
After you have read this form and agreed to participate, the intake nurse will gather some basic information from you. Then you will be randomly assigned to receive usual care or transitional care after you are discharged from the hospital.

If you are assigned to the **usual care group**, you will be given the care your physician orders for you to receive upon discharge from the hospital. In addition, you will be telephoned at your home once per week for 4 weeks by a study nurse who will ask you whether you have been back to the hospital. On the fourth and final week's call, the nurse will ask you some additional questions about how you take your medications.

If you are assigned to the **transitional care nurse practitioner group**, your assigned transitional care nurse practitioner will come to your room and introduce herself or himself to you before you are discharged from the hospital. You will also receive the care ordered by your doctor after you are discharged from the hospital, including at least weekly visits and telephone support from the transitional care nurse practitioner. The transitional care nurse practitioner will work with you and your doctors to bridge the gap between hospital discharge and your return to your usual PCP as you learn to manage the changes in your health.

Possible Benefits
There are no direct benefits to you for participating in this research; however, your participation will help us determine whether nurse practitioner–led transitional care can decrease unnecessary hospital readmissions and improve medication adherence. It is possible that having direct access to the transitional care nurse practitioner may provide you with more timely evaluation and management of problems that occur during the 4 weeks after discharge from the hospital.

Compensation
You will not receive any compensation for your participation in this study.

Possible Risks/Discomforts
You may return to your usual state of health and activities rapidly and thus not feel the need for a visit from the nurse practitioner or a phone call from the study nurse every week for 4 weeks.

Alternative Procedures/Treatments
There are no alternatives to participation, except not participating. You will always receive the care ordered by your physician.

Withdrawal From the Study
You may discontinue your participation in this study at any time without any penalty or loss of benefits.

Number of Participants
We expect 80 participants to enroll in this study.

Confidentiality
If in the unlikely event it becomes necessary for the institutional review board (IRB) to review your research records, then the University of Texas at Arlington (UTA) will protect the confidentiality of those records to the extent permitted by law. Your research records will not be released without your consent unless required by law or a court order. The data resulting from your participation may be made available to other researchers in the future for research purposes not detailed within this consent form. In these cases, the data will contain no identifying information that could associate you with it or with your participation in any study.

If the results of this research are published or presented at scientific meetings, your identity will not be disclosed.

APPENDIX D   Informed Consent—cont'd

Contact for Questions

Questions about this research or your rights as a research subject may be directed to Kathryn Daniel at (xxx)-xxx-xxxx. You may contact the chairperson of the UTA IRB at (xxx)-xxx-xxxx in the event of a research-related injury to the subject.

Consent Signatures

As a representative of this study, I have explained the purpose, the procedures, the benefits, and the risks that are involved in this research study:

_____   _____
Signature   Date

(Signature and printed name of principal investigator or person obtaining consent / Date)

   By signing below, you confirm that you have read or had this document read to you.

   You have been informed about this study's purpose, procedures, possible benefits and risks, and you have received a copy of this form. You have been given the opportunity to ask questions before you sign, and you have been told that you can ask other questions at any time. You voluntarily agree to participate in this study. By signing this form, you are not waiving any of your legal rights. Refusal to participate will involve no penalty or loss of benefits to which you are otherwise entitled, and you may discontinue participation at any time without penalty or loss of benefits, to which you are otherwise entitled.

_____   _____
Signature   Date

(Signature of volunteer / Date)

APPENDIX E   Morisky Medication Adherence Scale

Please complete the following scale by circling the best response that fits you.

1. Do you sometimes forget to take your medications? Yes/No
2. Over the past 2 weeks, were there any days when you did not take your medication? Yes/No
3. Have you ever cut back or stopped taking your medication without telling your doctor because you felt worse when you took it? Yes/No
4. When you travel or leave home, do you sometimes forget to bring along your medications? Yes/No
5. Did you take your medicine yesterday? Yes/No
6. When you feel like your blood pressure is under control, do you sometimes stop taking your medication? Yes/No

7. Taking medication every day is a real inconvenience for some people. Do you ever feel hassled about sticking to your blood pressure treatment plan? Yes/No
8. How often do you have difficulty remembering to take all of your medications? (Select one.)
Never
Occasionally, but less than half of the time
About half of the time
More than half of the time
Almost all of the time

Morisky, D. E., Ang, A., Krousel-Wood, M., & Ward, H. J. (2008). Predictive validity of a medication adherence measure in an outpatient setting. *Journal of Clinical Hypertension, 10*(5), 348–354.

KEY POINTS

- This chapter focuses on writing a research proposal and seeking approval to conduct a study.
- A research proposal is a written plan that identifies the major elements of a study, such as the problem, purpose, review of literature, and framework, and outlines the methods and procedures that will be used to conduct the study.
- Writing a quality proposal involves (1) developing ideas logically, (2) determining the depth or detail of the proposal content, (3) identifying critical points

in the proposal, and (4) developing an aesthetically appealing copy.

- Most clinical agencies and funding institutions require a condensed proposal, which usually includes a problem and purpose, an overview of previous research conducted in the area, a framework, variables, design, sample, ethical considerations, a plan for data collection and analysis, and a plan for dissemination of findings.
- Sometimes a researcher will send a preproposal or letter of intent to funding organizations, rather than a proposal. The parts of the preproposal are logically ordered as follows: (1) a letter of transmittal, (2) proposal for a study, (3) personnel, (4) facilities, and (5) budget.
- A quantitative research proposal usually has four chapters or sections: (1) introduction and background, (2) review of relevant literature, (3) framework, and (4) methods and procedures.
- A qualitative research proposal generally includes the following chapters or sections: (1) introduction and background, (2) review of relevant literature, (3) philosophical foundation of the selected method, and (4) identification and description of the method of inquiry.
- Seeking approval for the conduct or funding of a study is a process that involves submission of a proposal to a selected group for review and, in many situations, verbal defense of that proposal.
- Research proposals are reviewed to (1) evaluate the quality of the study, (2) ensure that adequate measures are being taken to protect human subjects, and (3) evaluate the impact of conducting the study on the reviewing institution.
- Proposals sometimes require revision before or during the implementation of a study; if a change is necessary, the researcher should discuss the change with the members of the university and clinical agency IRBs and the funding institution.
- An example of a brief quantitative research proposal of a quasi-experimental study is provided.

REFERENCES

Aberson, C. L. (2019). *Applied power analysis for the behavioral sciences* (2nd ed.). New York, NY: Routledge.

American Nurses Credentialing Center (ANCC) (2018). *Magnet Recognition Program® overview*. Retrieved from https://www.nursingworld.org/ancc/

American Psychological Association (APA). (2020). *Publication manual of the American Psychological Association* (7th ed.). Washington, DC: Author.

Booth, W. C., Colomb, G. G., Williams, J. M., Bizup, J., FitzGerald, W.T., & The University of Chicago Press Editorial Staff (Eds.). (2018). *Kate L. Turabian: A manual for writers of research papers, theses, and dissertations: Chicago style for students and researchers* (9th ed.). Chicago, IL: University of Chicago Press.

Bradbury-Jones, C., & Taylor, J. (2014). Applying social impact assessment in nursing research. *Nursing Standard, 28*(48), 45–49. doi:10.7748/ns.28.48.45.e8262

Brown, S. J. (2018). *Evidence-based nursing: The research-practice connection* (4th ed.). Sudbury, MA: Jones & Bartlett.

Butcher, H. K., Bulecheck, G. M., Dochterman, J. M., & Wagner, C. M. (Eds.). (2018). *Nursing interventions classification* (NIC) (7th ed.). St. Louis, MO: Elsevier.

Campbell, D. T., & Stanley, J. C. (1963). Experimental and quasi-experimental designs for research on teaching. In N. L. Gage (Ed.), *Handbook of research on teaching* (pp. 171–246). Chicago, IL: Rand McNally.

Cook, T. D., & Campbell, D. (1986). The causal assumptions of quasi-experimental practice. *Synthese, 68*(1), 141–180.

Creswell, J., & Creswell, D. (2018). *Research design: Qualitative, quantitative and mixed methods approaches* (5th ed.). Thousand Oaks, CA: Sage.

Creswell, J., & Poth, C. (2018). *Qualitative inquiry & research design: Choosing among five approaches* (4th ed.). Thousand Oaks, CA: Sage.

Daniel, K. (2015). *The effect of nurse practitioner directed transitional care on medication adherence and readmission outcomes of elderly congestive heart failure patients*. Unpublished proposal.

Denizen, N., & Lincoln, Y. (Eds.). (2018). *The Sage handbook of qualitative research* (5th ed.). Thousand Oaks, CA: Sage.

Denzin, N. (1970). *The research act*. Chicago, IL: Aldine.

Fawcett, J., & Garity, J. (2009). *Evaluating research for evidence-based nursing practice*. Philadelphia, PA: F. A. Davis.

Glaser, B., & Strauss, A. L. (1965). Discovery of substantive theory: A basic strategy underlying qualitative research. *American Behavioral Scientist, 8*(1), 5–12.

Grove, S. K., & Cipher, D. J. (2020). *Statistics for nursing research: A workbook for evidence-based practice* (3rd ed.). St. Louis, MO: Saunders.

Holtzclaw, B. J., Kenner, C., & Walden, M. (2018). *Grant writing handbook for nurses and health professionals*. New York, NY: Springer Publishing Company.

Jessiman, W. (2013). 'To be honest, I haven't even thought about it'—recruitment in small-scale, qualitative research in primary care. *Nurse Researcher*, *21*(2), 18–23. doi:10.7748/nr2013.11.21.2.18.e226

Kerlinger, F. N., & Lee, H. B. (2000). *Foundations of behavioral research* (4th ed.). Fort Worth, TX: Harcourt College.

Knafl, K., & Van Riper, M. (2017). Tips for developing a successful family research proposal. *Journal of Family Nursing*, *23*(4), 450–460. doi:10.1177/1074840717743248

Lazarus, R., & Folkman, S. (1984). *Stress, appraisal, and coping*. New York, NY: Springer.

Liamputtong, P. (2013). *Qualitative research methods* (4th ed.). South Melbourne, AU: Oxford University Press.

Ligita, T., Wicking, K., Francis, K., Harvey, N., & Nurjannah, I. (2019). How people living with diabetes in Indonesia learn about their disease: A grounded theory study. *PLoS ONE*, *14*(2), E0212019. doi:10.1371/journal.pone.0212019

Malasanos, L. J. (1976). What is the preproposal? What are its component parts? Is it an effective instrument in assessing funding potential of research ideas? *Nursing Research*, *25*(3), 223–224.

Marshall, C., & Rossman, G. B. (2016). *Designing qualitative research* (6th ed.). Los Angeles, CA: Sage.

Martin, C. J. H., & Fleming, V. (2010). A 15-step model for writing a research proposal. *British Journal of Midwifery*, *18*(12), 791–798.

Melnyk, B. M., & Fineout-Overholt, E. (2019). *Evidence-based practice in nursing & healthcare: A guide to best practice* (4th ed.). Philadelphia, PA: Lippincott Williams & Wilkins.

Merrill, K. C. (2011). Developing an effective quantitative research proposal. *Journal of Infusion Nursing: The Official Publication of the Infusion Nurses Society*, *34*(3), 181–186. doi:10.1097/NAN.0b013e3182117204

Miles, M. B., Huberman, A. M., & Saldaña, J. (2020). *Qualitative data analysis: A methods sourcebook* (4th ed.). Beverly Hills, CA: Sage.

Munhall, P. L. (2012). *Nursing research: A qualitative perspective* (5th ed.). Sudbury, MA: Jones & Bartlett.

Munhall, P. L., & Chenail, R. (2008). *Qualitative research proposals and reports: A guide* (3rd ed.). Boston, MA: Jones and Bartlett.

National Council of State Boards of Nursing (NCSBN). (2019). *Request for proposals for research related to the NCLEX: Guidelines for proposal submission to the Joint Research Committee (JRC)*. Retrieved from https://www.ncsbn.org/Guidelines_for_Proposals.pdf

National Institute of Nursing Research (NINR). (2019). *Developing nurse scientists*. Retrieved from http://www.ninr.nih.gov/training/online-developing-nurse-scientists#.Vav4aPlVhBc

National Institutes of Health (NIH). (2019). *Office of Extramural Research. Grants and funding: How to apply*. Retrieved from https://grants.nih.gov/grants/how-to-apply-application-guide.html

Offredy, M., & Vickers, P. (2010). *Developing a healthcare research proposal: An interactive student guide*. Oxford, UK: Wiley-Blackwell.

Plichta, S.B., & Kelvin, E. (2013). *Munro's statistical methods for health care research* (6th ed.). Philadelphia, PA: Lippincott Williams & Wilkins.

Purdue University Online Writing Lab. (2019). *APA formatting and style guide*. Retrieved from https://owl.purdue.edu/owl/research_and_citation/apa_style/apa_formatting_and_style_guide/general_format.html

Roller, M., & Lavrakas, P. (2015). *Applied qualitative research design: A total quality framework approach*. New York, NY: Guilford Press.

Roy, C., & Andrews, H. A. (2008). *Roy's adaptation model for nursing* (3rd ed.). Stamford, CT: Appleton & Lange.

Ryan-Wenger, N. A. (2017). Precision, accuracy, and uncertainty of biophysical measurements for research and practice. In C. F. Waltz, O. L. Strickland, & E. R. Lenz (Eds.), *Measurement in nursing and health research* (5th ed., pp. 427–446). New York, NY: Springer.

Shadish, W. R., Cook, T. D., & Campbell, D. T. (2002). *Experimental and quasi-experimental designs for generalized causal inference*. Chicago, IL: Rand McNally.

Smith, M. J., & Liehr, P. R. (2018). *Middle range theory for nursing* (4th ed.). New York, NY: Springer.

Strunk Jr., W., & White, E. B. (2018). *The elements of style* (4th ed.). Retrieved from http://www.jlakes.org/ch/web/The-elements-of-style.pdf

The University of Chicago Press Staff. (2010). *The Chicago manual of style* (16th ed.). Chicago, IL: University of Chicago Press.

University of Michigan. (2019). *University of Michigan research and sponsored projects: The proposal writer's guide*. Retrieved from https://orsp.umich.edu/proposal-writers-guide-overview

University of Oklahoma College of Nursing. (2019). *Oklahoma University College of Nursing: Dissertation guidelines*. Retrieved from https://nursing.ouhsc.edu/Portals/1303/Assets/documents/New%202016%20Dissertation%20Proposal%20Guidelines.pdf?ver=2016-06-28-105026-460

Waltz, C. F., Strickland, O. L., & Lenz, E. R. (2017). *Measurement in nursing and health research* (5th ed.). New York, NY: Springer.

Seeking Funding for Research

Suzanne Sutherland

http://evolve.elsevier.com/Gray/practice/

Research funding is necessary for implementation of complex, well-designed studies. Simpler studies may be completed with fewer resources, but associated costs, such as mailing a survey to an adequate-sized sample, can be expensive. As the rigor and complexity of a study's design increase, cost tends to increase proportionately. In addition to paying for expenses, funding adds credibility to a study because it indicates that others have reviewed the proposal and recognized its scientific and social merit. The scientific credibility of the profession is related to the quality of studies conducted by its researchers. Thus scientific credibility and funding for research are interrelated.

The nursing profession has invested a great deal of energy toward increasing both the funding sources and the size of grants awarded annually for nursing research. Receiving funding not only enhances the professional status of the recipient, but also increases the likelihood of funding for subsequent studies. In an academic setting, funding is advantageous for faculty members because a grant may reimburse part or all of their salary and release them from other institutional responsibilities, allowing the research team to devote time to conducting the study. Funding also may be utilized to hire assistants and coordinators who assist with conducting various parts of the study, thereby enhancing the team's productivity. Skills in seeking funding for research are essential for developing an ongoing research program that will generate knowledge in your area of specialization.

This chapter describes building a program of research, different sources of funding, and strategies to increase your success in obtaining a grant.

BUILDING A PROGRAM OF RESEARCH

As a novice researcher, you may have the goal of writing a grant proposal to the federal government or a national foundation for your first study and receiving a large grant that covers your salary, equipment, computers, payments to participants for their time and effort, and salaries of research assistants and secretarial support. In reality, this scenario rarely occurs for an inexperienced researcher. Even experienced researchers with previous federal funding are not always successful when they submit grant proposals. A new researcher is caught in the difficult position of needing to demonstrate prior experience to receive funding but needing funding to be able to have time away from normal duties to conduct research and disseminate the findings. One way of resolving this dilemma is to design initial studies that can realistically be completed without release time and with little or no funding. This approach requires a commitment to put in extra hours of work, which is often unrewarded monetarily or socially. However, when they are well conducted and the findings are published, small unfunded studies provide the credibility one needs to begin the process toward receiving major grant funding. Guidelines for proposals for federal funding usually include a section of the proposal in which applicants are expected to describe their own prior research, either completed or in progress, especially studies that are precursors to the one proposed. Grant reviewers want evidence of the researcher's ability to conceptualize and implement a study and to disseminate findings. Funders seek assurance that if they fund a proposal, their money will not be wasted and that the findings of the study will be published.

An aspiring career researcher should plan to initiate a program of research in a specific area of study and seek funding in that area. A program of research consists of the studies a researcher conducts, starting with small, simple ones and moving to larger, complex endeavors, usually focusing on closely related problem areas. It sounds simplistic, but if your research interest is promotion of health in rural areas, you need to plan a series of studies that focus on promoting rural health. Early studies may be small, with each successive effort building on the findings of the previous one. Successive findings can suggest new solutions or provide evidence that a hoped-for solution is ineffective or that a learning program is promising. Trend analyses can reveal unforeseen patterns in health and illness or demonstrate that an old strategy has a new application.

Jean McSweeney is a nurse and educator who has sustained a valuable program of research over more than two decades. She is a professor at the College of Nursing, University of Arkansas for Medical Sciences, where she serves as director of the PhD nursing program. In her first nursing position, McSweeney's area of clinical practice was critical care. Early in her practice, she became interested in cardiac patients (American Nurses Association [ANA], 2008). Her doctoral dissertation was a qualitative study exploring behavior changes after myocardial infarction (MI). She received an American Nurses Foundation grant for a second qualitative study focusing on women's motivations to change their behavior after an MI. She based subsequent research, a series of quantitative studies, on her own qualitative findings. She was the first researcher to document the ways in which women's symptoms of an MI, such as severe fatigue without chest pain, were different from men's typical symptoms, which often include crushing chest pain. Her research findings provided the impetus for recognition of these differences as diagnostic symptoms as they apply to the assessment of women experiencing emergent cardiac events. While pursuing publication in peer-reviewed journals, McSweeney also capitalized on opportunities to share her findings in the mass media by agreeing to be interviewed by reporters for newspapers and national news programs. Box 29.1 provides examples of McSweeney's publications focusing upon cardiovascular disease and health. Her approximately six dozen publications include several

in different areas, as well, reflecting collaboration with clinical partners and doctoral students, but perusal of the titles of the articles reveals the common thread of cardiac disease in women. Publication of funded studies increased her credibility and provided the foundation for future funding.

After a researcher has received a major grant, subsequent funding tends to be substantial. Munro et al. (2019) reported survey results of the Nursing Research Initiative (NRI) of the Veterans Affairs grant recipients and the amounts of their subsequent grant awards. Of the 61 major grant recipients, the 52 who could be contacted were sent the survey, with 28 surveys returned. All of the 28 returning the survey were PhD-prepared recipients. Collectively, the 28 reported that, after the NRI grant, they had received subsequent grants totaling $167,535,623, for a mean of $7,777,136 per person (Munro et al., 2019, p. 9). Even if the other 33 researchers who received NRI grants had received no subsequent funding, the average received by all 61 of the recipients after the initial grant would be $2,746,485.

However, there is a downside. The process of applying for a major grant, such as a National Institutes of Health (NIH) grant, requires substantial time. Kulage et al. (2015) examined the time and cost of preparing NIH grants at Columbia School of Nursing. Three principal investigators (PIs) within the department agreed to document the time and cost of preparing NIH applications. PIs' time expended ranged from 69.8 to 162.3 hours, and administrators' time expenditures ranged from 33.9 to 56.4 hours. This was found to be equivalent in costs for personnel salaries to $4784 to $13,512 per grant.

Deciding on the Research Focus

How do you decide on the focus of your program of research? The ideal focus of a program of research is the intersection of a potential contribution to science, your capacity, and the capital that you can assemble. Fig. 29.1 highlights areas of McSweeney's program of research, reflecting overlapping circles of contribution, capacity, and capital—the three Cs.

Contribution

Contribution refers to the gap in knowledge that your research will address. Is there a contribution to be made in this area? Reviewing the literature and finding a

BOX 29.1   A Program of Research: Exemplars Excerpted From McSweeney's More Than 70 Publications

Citations From Oldest to Most Recent

McSweeney, J. (1993). Making behavior changes after a myocardial infarction. *Western Journal of Nursing Research*, 15(4), 441–455.

McSweeney, J. (1998). Women's narratives: Evolving symptoms of myocardial infarction. *Journal of Women & Aging*, 10(2), 67–83.

McSweeney, J., & Crane, P. (2000). Challenging the rules: Women's prodromal and acute symptoms of myocardial infarction. *Research in Nursing & Health*, 23(2), 135–146.

McSweeney, J. C., Cody, M., O'Sullivan, P., Elberson, D., Moser, D. K., & Gavin, B. J. (2003). Women's early warning symptoms of acute myocardial infarction. *Circulation*, 108(21), 2619–2623.

McSweeney, J. C., O'Sullivan, P., Cody, M., & Crane, P. B. (2004). Development of the McSweeney Acute and Prodromal Myocardial Infarction Symptom Survey. *Journal of Cardiovascular Nursing*, 19(1), 58–67.

McSweeney, J. C., & Coon, S. (2004). Women's inhibitors and facilitators associated with making behavioral changes after myocardial infarction. *Medsurg Nursing*, 13(1), 49–56.

McSweeney, J. C., Lefler, L. L., & Crowder, B. F. (2005). What's wrong with me? Women's coronary heart disease diagnostic experiences. *Progress in Cardiovascular Nursing*, 20(2), 48–57.

McSweeney, J. C., Lefler, L. L., Fischer, E. P., Naylor, A. J., & Evans, L. K. (2007). Women's prehospital delay associated with myocardial infarction: Does race really matter? *The Journal of Cardiovascular Nursing*, 22(4), 279–285.

McSweeney, J. C., Pettey, C. M., Fischer, E. P., & Spellman (2009). Going the distance: Overcoming challenges in recruitment and retention of Black and White women in multisite, longitudinal study of predictors of coronary heart disease. *Research in Gerontological Nursing*, 2(4), 256–264.

McSweeney, J. C., Cleves, J. A., Zhao, W., Lefler, L. L., & Yang, S. (2010). Cluster analysis of women's prodromal and acute myocardial infarction symptoms by race and other characteristics. *The Journal of Cardiovascular Nursing*, 25(4), 104–110.

McSweeney, J. C., Pettey, C. M., Souder, E., & Rhoads, S. (2011). Disparities in women's cardiovascular health. *Journal of Obstetric, Gynecologic, and Neonatal Nursing*, 40(3), 362–371.

Cole, C., McSweeney, J., Cleves, M., Armbya, N., Bliwise, D., & Pettey, C. (2012). Sleep disturbance in women before myocardial infarction. *Heart & Lung: The Journal of Critical Care*, 41(5), 438–445.

McSweeney, J., Cleves, M., Fischer, E., Rojo, M., Armbya, N., & Moser, D. (2013). Reliability of the McSweeney Acute and Prodromal Myocardial Infarction Symptom Survey among black and white women. *European Journal of Cardiovascular Nursing: Journal of the Working Group on Cardiovascular Nursing of the European Society of Cardiology*, 12(4), 360–367.

McSweeney, J., Cleves, M., Fischer, E., Moser, D., Wei, J., Pettey, C., . . . Armbya, N. (2014). Predicting coronary heart disease events in women: A longitudinal cohort study. *The Journal of Cardiovascular Nursing*, 29(6), 482–492.

Pettey, C., McSweeney, J., Stewart, K., Price, E., Cleves, M., Heo, S., & Souder, E. (2015). Perceptions of family history and genetic testing and feasibility of pedigree development among African Americans with hypertension. *European Journal of Cardiovascular Nursing: Journal of the Working Group on Cardiovascular Nursing of the European Society of Cardiology*, 14(1), 8–15.

Heo, S., McSweeney, J., Tsai, P., & Ounpraseuth, S. (2016). Differing effects of fatigue and depression on hospitalizations in men and women with heart failure. *American Journal of Critical Care*, 25(6), 526–534.

McSweeney, J., Cleves, M., Fischer, E., Pettey, C., & Beasley, B. (2017). Using the McSweeney Acute and Prodromal Myocardial Infarction Symptom Survey to predict the occurrence of short-term coronary heart disease events in women. *Women's Health Issues: Official Publication of the Jacobs Institute of Women's Health*, 27(6), 660–665.

Heo, S., McSweeney, J., Ounpraseuth, S., Shaw-Devine, A., Fier, A., & Moser, D. (2018). Testing a holistic meditation intervention to address psychosocial distress in patients with heart failure: A pilot study. *The Journal of Cardiovascular Nursing*, 33(2), 126–134.

Heo, S., McSweeney, J., Tsai, P., Ounpraseuth, S., Moser, D., & Kim, J. (2019). The associations of diagnoses of fatigue and depression with use of medical services in patients with heart failure. *The Journal of Cardiovascular Nursing*, 34(4), 289–296.

significant gap in knowledge is where you start. McSweeney identified that little was known about patients' adherence patterns related to behavioral changes after an MI nor about interindividual difference in symptoms during an acute cardiac event. The research focus is broader than a single study and implies the potential for a continuing research program. There is no need to develop a program of research in an area that has been extensively studied unless you identify a major gap or perspective that is missing.

Capacity

Once you identify an area in which there is a research gap, assess your capacity (the second C) to address the gap. Capacity may be divided into two parts: your connection to the topic and your relevant expertise. Which areas of nursing and health stimulate your curiosity and sustain your interest? Think about the topics or areas of nursing practice in which you are the most interested. Which patients or clinical areas stimulate your curiosity? Maybe you have a personal connection

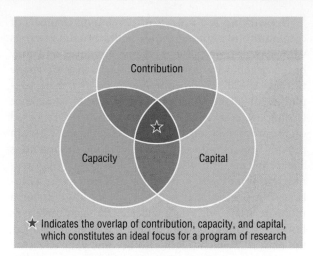

Fig. 29.1 Ideal focus for a program of research: The intersection of contribution, capital, and capacity.

(Within figure)

Contribution

Capacity   Capital

★ Indicates the overlap of contribution, capacity, and capital, which constitutes an ideal focus for a program of research

to a particular area, such as a nurse researcher who is interested in autism because of being the parent of a child with autism. Maybe you work in the newborn nursery and notice the challenges of helping mothers with a history of substance abuse bond with their babies. Your research focus may evolve over time and, ideally, your passion for a specific topic or group of patients would provide the basis for a long research career. Research is hard work, and a personal connection can lend perseverance for sustained work in an area.

Capacity includes internal resources you possess, such as experience, emotional maturity, intellect, knowledge, skills, and tenacity. Your expertise may arise from educational programs, personal study, and clinical experience. If you are interested in genomics research, what is your knowledge of genes and the interactions between them and the environment? Have you completed a course in genetics or mastered the laboratory skills to gather and analyze cellular-level data? If you are interested in the effects of positioning on the hemodynamics of unstable, acutely ill patients, have you ever worked in a critical care unit? One aspect of building a research career is to continue to expand your capacity in a focus area but, in the beginning, it is helpful to select an area in which you have firsthand practice or personal knowledge.

Capital

Capital refers to resources and, specifically, to available funding, institutional support, and people. The primary purpose of this chapter is to describe how to increase your monetary capital. Review the websites of organizations, foundations, and agencies, including NIH, to learn their research priorities and the types of grants they fund. Although you may have a passion for understanding nurses' experiences in caring for terminally ill patients, you may be unable to find a funder with that priority. If your goal is a lifelong career as a full-time researcher, you must select a topic that is fundable.

Evaluate the institution in which you work. Is the environment supportive of research? Administrators of a non-Magnet hospital may be less supportive of research than those of a hospital designated by the American Nurses Credentialing Center as a Magnet hospital through the Magnet Recognition Program®. A teaching hospital or a clinic in a health sciences center may be more supportive of research than a community hospital or private physician's office would be. If you are a nurse faculty member, a research-intensive university with graduate programs is more likely to demonstrate support of research than is a liberal arts university focused on undergraduate education. In an institution with a research focus, you are more likely to find a group of like-minded individuals who can lend social support and critique.

Peers who share common values, ways of thinking, and activities can be a **reference group** for a novice researcher. Generally speaking, a reference group is the cluster of associates with whom a person identifies and from whom a person assimilates standards and attitudes. You tend to evaluate your own values and behavior in relation to those of the group. A new researcher may choose to gravitate toward a reference group that values research and grant writing, rather than perceiving it as too difficult or irrelevant. From this new group, you are likely to receive the support and feedback necessary to encourage you, as you develop grant-writing skills and enact a program of research. In addition, you will have the opportunity to provide similar support and feedback to your peers. There are additional people who can support your program of research, including mentors and experienced researchers with whom you can interact in an apprentice role. These support persons will be discussed later in the chapter.

When a potential contribution to science, your capacity, and available capital overlap, you have found an ideal focus for your research career (see Fig. 29.1). Over time, your focus may shift based on findings of your early studies, new developments in scientific publications, changes in the healthcare environment, and the availability of funding. However, an initial focus that considers possible contribution, capital, and capacity is a secure place to begin.

BUILDING CAPITAL

Your personal capital may need to be enhanced. How can you build your capital? What type and level of commitment do you have? Who are your support persons and mentors? Do you have a reference group that will provide feedback and encouragement?

Level of Commitment

Writing proposals for funding is hard work. Before beginning, reflect on whether your motivation is external or internal. If your motivation is external, you are committed to seeking funding because of the potential to receive rewards from your employer, to earn the high regard of your peers, or to be eligible for a promotion or for a different position. If your motivation is internal, you are convinced that more knowledge is needed to benefit your patients. Both external and internal motivation are valid reasons to be committed to a program of research; however, an internally motivated researcher may be more likely to conduct studies with limited funding and continue to seek additional support, even in the absence of external funding. As an element of capacity, your level of commitment will determine your ability to persevere and develop a program of research.

Support of Other People

Even the most internally motivated person may experience times of discouragement and need the support of peers. Rarely, if ever, is an investigator funded to conduct a major study alone. Funded research projects usually require a team of people with varied skills. As a novice researcher, it is important to work with others who have more experience in seeking and receiving funding (Holtzclaw, Kenner, & Walden, 2018).

Networking is a process of developing channels of communication among people with common interests who may not work for the same employer and may be geographically scattered. Contacts may be made through social media, computer networks, mail, telephone, or arrangements to meet at a conference (Holtzclaw et al., 2018). Strong networks are based on reciprocal relationships. A professional network can provide opportunities for brainstorming, sharing ideas and problems, and discussing grant-writing opportunities. In some cases, networking may lead to the members of a professional network writing a grant for a multisite study with data collected in each member's home institution. When a proposal is being developed, the network, which might also become your reference group, can provide feedback at various stages of proposal development. Adegbola (2011) suggested that an effective way to begin to develop a professional network is to send a follow-up e-mail to researchers with whom you interact at a conference when their areas of interest overlap with yours.

Through networking, nurses interested in a particular area of study can find peers, content experts, and mentors. A **content expert** may be a clinician or researcher who is known for his or her work in the area in which you are interested. Through your review of the literature, you might identify a researcher who has developed an instrument to measure a variable that you have decided to include in your proposed study. For example, you want to measure a biological marker of stress and you have read several studies in which an experienced researcher measured the variable using a specific piece of equipment. Contact the researcher through e-mail and make a telephone appointment to discuss the strengths and weaknesses of this particular measurement. If you are more comfortable with face-to-face interactions, request a web-facilitated meeting. You might also arrange to meet at an upcoming conference.

A **mentor** is a person who is rich in professional experience and willing to work with someone with less experience in order to advance his or her professional goals. Even among nursing faculty members, there is perceived to be a need for increased faculty-to-faculty support in academic pursuits such as research (Hershberger et al., 2019). Because the process of mentoring is very time intensive, finding a mentor may require significant effort. Grant-writing activities are best learned in a mentor relationship that includes actual participation, because mastery evolves from hands-on activities such as developing a convincing narrative, writing to a grant's specifications, and conducting ongoing revisions. This type of relationship requires a willingness by both professionals to invest time and energy. A mentor relationship at this level has characteristics of both a teacher-learner relationship and a close friendship. Each individual must have an affinity for the other from which a close working relationship can be developed. The relationship usually continues for a long period of time.

Grantsmanship

Grantsmanship, the ability to write proposals that are funded, is not an innate skill; it must be learned. Learning grant-related skills requires a commitment of both time and energy. However, the rewards can be great. Strategies used to learn grantsmanship are described in the following sections and are listed in order of increasing time commitment, involvement, and level of expertise needed. These strategies are attending grantsmanship courses, working with experienced researchers, joining research organizations, and participating on research committees or review panels.

Attending Courses and Workshops

Some universities offer elective courses on grantsmanship. Continuing education programs or professional conferences sometimes offer topics related to grantsmanship. The content of these sessions may include the process of grant writing, techniques for obtaining grant funds, and sources of grant funds. In some cases, representatives of funding agencies are invited to explain funding procedures. This information is useful for understanding agency priorities and developing skill in writing proposals. Not all courses or educational opportunities for learning grantsmanship require attendance at a conference because some seminars are offered as webinars or online courses.

Experienced Researchers

Volunteering to assist with the activities of an experienced researcher is an excellent way to learn research and grantsmanship. As a graduate student, you can be paid while you gain this experience by becoming a graduate research assistant. Through working directly with a funded researcher, you can gain experience in writing grants and reading proposals that have been funded. Examining proposals that have been rejected and the comments of the review committee can be useful as well.

The criticisms of the review committee point out the weaknesses of the study and clarify the reasons the proposal was rejected. Examining these comments on the proposal can increase your insight as a new grant writer and prepare you for similar experiences. Some researchers are sensitive about these criticisms and may be reluctant to share them. If an experienced researcher is willing, however, it is enlightening to hear his or her perceptions and opinions about the criticisms. Ideally, by working closely with an experienced researcher, you will have the opportunity to demonstrate your commitment, and the researcher may invite you to become a permanent member of the research team.

Regional Nursing Research Organizations

In the United States, nurse researchers in each region have formed regional research organizations. Table 29.1 lists these organizations and their websites. Each regional organization holds an annual conference and provides opportunities for nursing students to display posters or present findings of pilot studies or initial phases of a study in progress. These conferences are excellent opportunities to network and meet more experienced researchers. Regional research organizations may also fund small grants for which members can apply.

Serving on Research Committees

Research committees and institutional review boards exist in many healthcare and professional organizations. Hospitals, healthcare systems, foundations, and professional nursing organizations have research committees. Through membership on these committees, contacts with researchers can be made. Also, many research committees are involved in reviewing proposals for the

TABLE 29.1 **Regional Nursing Research Organizations**	
US Region	**Website**
Eastern Nursing Research Society	http://www.enrs-go.org
Southern Nursing Research Society	http://www.snrs.org
Midwest Nursing Research Society	http://www.mnrs.org
Western Institute of Nursing	http://www.winursing.org

funding of small grants or granting approval to collect data in an institution. Often reading proposals for approval for research involving human subjects or for funding can give the novice researcher insight into the importance of clarity and organization in the research proposal. Reviewing proposals and making decisions about funding are experiences that may help researchers become better able to critique and revise their own proposals before submitting them for review.

IDENTIFYING FUNDING SOURCES

Each funding source seeks proposals for research to advance the source goals, mission, and agenda. Consequently, the types of studies funded vary. For instance, the American Heart Association may decline to fund a study of social factors that are associated with successes in obsessive-compulsive disorder (OCD) desensitization, whereas a mental health funding source may be quite willing to do so. The next section provides an overview of a few types of grants and donors.

Types of Grants

Two main types of grants are sought in nursing: project grants and research grants. **Project grant proposals** are written to obtain funding for the development of new educational programs in nursing, such as an accelerated baccalaureate plus master's program or a project to buy out salaries for two hospital shifts a week for staff nurses seeking advanced degrees. These grants also may fund a project manager to achieve the goals of the grant. Although these funded programs may involve evaluation, they seldom involve research. For example, the effectiveness of shift buyouts for education may be evaluated, but the findings can seldom be generalized beyond the unit or institution in which funded release time for education was provided. The emphasis is on implementing the project, not on conducting research.

Research grants provide funding to conduct a study. Although the two types of grant proposals have similarities, they have important differences in writing techniques, flow of ideas, and content. This chapter focuses on seeking funding for research. Research grant proposals vary in both scope and style, depending on the source of funding. Proposals for federal funding are the most complex and include a significant amount of information about your institution's resources and capacity to support the study. The section "Government Funding" provides additional information on types of federal proposals.

Private or Local Funding

The first step for obtaining funding is to determine potential sources for small amounts of research money. In some cases, management in your work institution can supply limited funding for research activities when a logical, compelling argument is presented for the usefulness of the study to the institution. Healthcare institutions, for example, are already invested in saving money and decreasing patient risk. A funding proposal is stronger when it enumerates anticipated benefits to the institution. In many universities, funds are available for intramural grants, which you can obtain competitively by submitting a brief proposal to a university committee.

Local chapters of nursing organizations have money available for research activities. Sigma, the honor society for nurses, provides small grants for nursing research that can be obtained through submission to local, regional, national, or international review committees. Many nursing organizations are sources of funding. For instance, the Emergency Nurses Association (ENA) Foundation offers several small seed grants annually (ENA, 2019). Generally, applications for these small grants include a less sophisticated grant application process than would applying for substantial funding.

Private individuals who are locally active in philanthropy may be willing to provide financial assistance for a small study in an area appealing to them. You need to know of the person whom you might approach and how and when to make that approach to increase the probability of successful funding. Sometimes this approach requires knowing someone who knows someone who might be willing to provide financial support. Acquiring funds from private individuals requires more assertiveness than do other approaches to funding.

Requests for funding need not be limited to a single source. If you anticipate requiring a larger amount of money than one source can supply, seek funds from one source for a specific research need and from another source for another research need, within that line of inquiry. For example, one funder may support the preliminary phase of the research while another funder supports the next phase of the study. Another strategy is to approach different funders about different budget items, such as asking one for mailing costs and another for the salary of a research assistant.

Seeking funding from local sources is less demanding in terms of formality and length of the proposal than is the case with other types of grants. Often the process is informal and may require only a short description (two or three pages) of the study. Provide a clear, straightforward description of the study and the way in which the findings will contribute to practice or to subsequent research. The important thing is to know what funds are available and how to apply for them. Some funding earmarked for research goes unused each year because nurses are unaware of its existence or believe that they are unlikely to be successful in obtaining the money. This unused money leads granting agencies or potential donors to conclude that nurses do not need more money for research and to decrease or cease budgeting for nursing research.

Small grants do more than merely provide the funds necessary to conduct the research. They are the first step you take toward being recognized as a credible researcher and in being considered for more substantial grants for later studies. When you receive a grant, no matter how small, include this information on your curriculum vitae or resumé. Also, list your participation in funded studies, even if you were not the primary investigator (PI). These entries are evidence of first-level recognition as a researcher.

National Nursing Organizations

Many nursing specialty organizations provide support for studies relevant to that specialty, such as the American Association of Nurse Practitioners (AANP, 2019). These organizations often provide guidance to new researchers or those with less experience who need assistance in beginning the process of planning and seeking funding. To determine the resources provided by a particular nursing organization, search the organization's website or contact the organization by e-mail, letter, or telephone. Table 29.2 provides information about a select group of large nursing specialty organizations that provide grant funding.

Two national nursing organizations that provide small grants not linked to a specialty are the American Nurses Foundation and Sigma. These grants are usually for less than $7500 each year, are very competitive, and are awarded to new investigators with promising ideas. Receiving funding from these organizations is held in high regard. Information about these grants is available from the American Nurses Foundation (2019) and Sigma Theta Tau International (2019).

TABLE 29.2 US National Specialty Nursing Organizations That Fund Research	
Organization or Association	**Website**
Academy of Medical-Surgical Nurses	http://www.amsn.org
American Association of Critical-Care Nurses	http://www.aacn.org
Association of Nurses in AIDS Care	http://www.nursesinaidscare.org
Association of Women's Health, Obstetric and Neonatal Nurses	http://www.awhonn.org
Emergency Nurses Association	http://www.ena.org
Hospice and Palliative Nurses Association	https://advancingexpert-care.org
National Association of Orthopaedic Nurses	http://www.orthonurse.org
National Gerontological Advanced Practice Nurses	https://www.gapna.org/welcome-former-ngna-members
Oncology Nursing Society	http://www.ons.org
Society of Pediatric Nurses	http://www.pedsnurses.org
Wound Ostomy and Continence Nurses Society	http://www.wocn.org

AIDS: Acquired immune deficiency syndrome.

Industry

Industry may be a good source of funding for nursing studies, particularly if one of the company's products is involved in the study. For example, if a particular type of equipment is being used during an experimental treatment, the company that developed the equipment may be willing to provide equipment for the study without charge or may be willing to fund the study. Similarly, if a comparison study examining outcomes of one type of dressing versus another is to be conducted, the company that produces one of the products might provide the product or fund the study. Industry-supported research has been heavily scrutinized because of publicized incidents in which possible conflicts of interest resulted in harm to a subject or may have prevented the publication of unfavorable findings

(Iyioke, 2016). Iyioke emphasized the point that society should be able to hold biomedical business concerns to the same general expectations of ethical behavior and social responsibility that nations expect from individuals, groups, and non-healthcare business entities. The ethics of seeking such funding should be carefully considered because there is a risk that the researcher might find it difficult to be unbiased in interpreting study results. Consequently, when an independent researcher accepts funding from industry, a written statement must be agreed upon by the researcher, employing institution, and company prior to the conduct of the study, describing in detail what will be provided and the rights of the researcher to publish all findings, regardless of the nature of the results.

Foundations

Many foundations in the United States provide funding for research, but the challenge is to determine which foundations have current interest in a particular field of study. The board of a foundation may evaluate priorities annually, resulting in different general areas of research interest each year. You must learn the characteristics of the foundation, including what it will fund in the coming cycle. A foundation may fund studies only by female researchers, or it may be interested only in studies of low-income groups or in research that addresses prevention of a small cluster of diagnoses or societal problems. A foundation may fund only studies being conducted in a specific geographical region.

The average amount of money awarded for a single grant and the range of awards are determined by each foundation. If the average award of a particular foundation is $2500 but the researcher needs $30,000, that source of funding is not the most desirable. Identify foundations that match your research topic, geographical location, and funding needs. Review carefully the foundation's guidelines for submitting funding requests. Making a personal visit to the foundation or contacting the staff person responsible for funding is desirable in some cases. You can increase the likelihood of funding by revising your proposal to align with the foundation's priorities.

There are several sources that list foundations and their agendas. If you work in a hospital or university, the development department or other department responsible for institutional fundraising can be very helpful because it has access to information about foundations. That department is likely to have access to a computerized information system, the Sponsored Programs Information Network. This system allows searches for information on specific foundations or about specific health conditions that are funded. You can then locate the most appropriate funding sources to support your research interests. The database contains approximately 2000 programs that provide information on federal agencies, private foundations, and corporate foundations. Check with your development office or administrators to find out whether you have access to this resource, without cost to yourself. If so, they can arrange for you to receive periodic computer listings of current research opportunities and contact information for each.

Other sources are available but at a price. The largest comprehensive resource is Candid, which requires a paid subscription. Candid is a reputable resource for information on foundations; it is an outgrowth of a combination of two previous foundation sources, Foundation Center and GuideStar. Candid (2019) provides information about 2.7 million nonprofit foundations worldwide and lists current calls for proposals.

Other Funders

Despite federal agencies distributing billions of dollars for health research, gaps continue to exist regarding understanding the benefits and risks inherent in different treatments of health disorders. Today's **comparative effectiveness research** (CER) focuses on "evaluating and comparing the implications and outcomes of two or more health care strategies to address a particular medical condition" (Johns Hopkins Medicine, 2019). Studies that are classified as being CER are those in which different treatments are evaluated for their outcomes within a select group of people, such as adults with hypertension and hypercholesteremia. These comparisons may be performed in real time using randomized clinical trials, or they may be reviews and statistical analyses of earlier similar method studies. While it is heartening to hear a patient's subjective account of the efficacy of a newly trialed intervention, CER addresses only objective measures and provides detailed statistical analyses of the effectiveness of two or more strategies. An example of this is a current treatment for posttraumatic stress disorder (PTSD) with psychedelics, namely 3,4-methylenedioxymethamphetamine (MDMA, also called Ecstasy). A phase III trial is in progress (Smith, 2018), measuring the frequency, duration, and severity of acute PTSD symptoms, comparing MDMA plus psychotherapy with the usual treatment of conventional medications plus therapy. A patient's account of MDMA's efficacy cannot present objective measures but merely provides a powerful story: When one patient discussed his traumatic wartime incidents in a therapy session with MDMA, "the adrenaline kick didn't happen. The hair didn't stand up on my neck. It's like doing therapy while being hugged by everyone who loves you in a bathtub full of puppies licking your face" (Smith, 2018). You can't measure the sensory glow of warm puppies, but in CER you can certainly quantify the reported symptoms, establishing evidence for best practice recommendations.

In 2006, the Institute of Medicine (IOM) convened a committee of distinguished researchers, healthcare professionals, and policymakers to set priorities for CER and patient-focused research (Frank et al., 2015). Their report, *Knowing What Works in Health Care*, was published by the IOM (2008).

Based on the IOM report, the Patient Protection and Affordable Care Act of Recovery and Revitalization (US Congress, 2010) contained a section (6301) that authorized the Patient-Centered Outcomes Research Institute (PCORI) to fund CER. PCORI is a nongovernmental, nonprofit corporation run by a board of governors. Patients, healthcare professionals, and insurance companies are involved in studies from conceptualization to dissemination of the findings to the end users (PCORI, 2019).

Other sources of funding may be condition-specific organizations in which patients and families are involved, such as the Multiple Sclerosis Association or the National Organization for Rare Disorders. These organizations are similar to foundations in that they have specific funding priorities. A proposal seeking funding must target one of the organization's priorities and the patients with this condition to be successful.

Government Funding

The largest source of grant monies in the United States (US) is the federal government—so much so that the federal government influences what is studied and what is not. Information on funding agencies will soon be available from the government's Catalog of Federal Domestic Assistance (2019), which allows persons seeking

a grant to search for all types of government funding, including funding for healthcare research. This will be available through the new general governmental website, SAM.gov, now in beta testing. For now, however, the grants website of the US Department of Health and Human Services (HHS, 2019) is a practical stepping-off site from which to search for government-sponsored funding. The NIH, particularly the National Institute of Nursing Research (NINR) and the Agency for Healthcare Research and Quality (AHRQ), solicit nursing proposals. Each agency has areas of focus and priorities for funding that change over time.

Federal agencies seek researchers through two paths (Fig. 29.2). As the researcher, you can identify a significant problem, develop a study to examine it, and submit a proposal for the study to the appropriate federal funding agency. This type of proposal is called an **investigator-initiated research proposal**. Periodically, an agency or group of agencies releases a **program announcement** (PA) to remind researchers of priority areas and generate interest in these areas. Proposals submitted in response to a PA are considered investigator-initiated proposals. Alternatively, an agency within the federal government identifies a significant problem, develops a plan by which the problem can be studied, and publishes a **request for proposals** (RFP) or a **request for applications** (RFA) from researchers.

When preparing an investigator-initiated proposal, refine your ideas and contact an official within the government agency early in the planning process to inform the agency of your intent to submit a proposal. Each

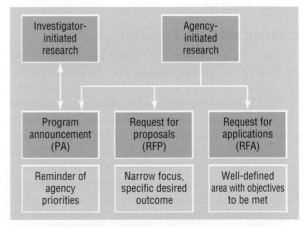

Fig. 29.2 Types of federal research proposals.

agency has established dates, usually three times a year, when proposals are reviewed. You will need to start preparing your proposal months ahead of this deadline, and some agencies are willing to provide assistance and feedback to researchers during proposal development. This assistance may occur through e-mail or telephone conversations. NIH program officers and NIH staff members responsible for specific areas of research frequently attend regional and national research conferences and make themselves available for appointments to discuss research ideas.

The NIH issues an RFP when scientists advising the institutes identify a specific gap in the professional literature that represents a focus for research within a partially researched area of knowledge. An RFA may be broader than an RFP but still may have a focus and a list of objectives that an institute or center within the NIH has identified. An RFA has a single application deadline. The amount that has been budgeted for the successful applications is indicated, and the RFA remains open for several funding cycles.

SUBMITTING A PROPOSAL FOR A FEDERAL GRANT

Federal funding for research is very competitive. To be successful in obtaining funding, you need strong institutional support and must propose an innovative study. The review process has multiple layers at the federal level. You need to allocate extensive time for writing the study plan and for completing all the required application components. If a proposal is not funded, be prepared to revise and resubmit by the next funding deadline.

Ensuring a Unique Proposal

During your review of the literature, you may have read the findings of funded studies, but the literature does not include recently completed or ongoing funded studies. Early in the process of planning a study for which you intend to seek federal funding, it is wise to determine the studies on your topic of interest that have been funded previously and the funded studies currently in process. This information is available at the website, NIH Research Portfolio Online Reporting Tools—Expenditures and Results (RePORTER), which is maintained by the NIH Office of Extramural Research (NIH, 2019a). The institutes and agencies that fund studies and projects, and are included in the

RePORTER, are listed in Table 29.3. You can search the database by state, subject, type of grant, funding agency, or investigator.

Reviewing proposals that are funded by a particular agency can be helpful. Although the agency cannot provide access to these proposals, researchers can sometimes obtain copies of them by contacting the PI of the study personally. In some cases, a researcher writing a proposal may choose to travel to Washington to meet with an agency representative. Project officers, the agency personnel who manage studies on a specified topic, may also travel to regional and national research conferences to be available to meet with potential researchers. This type of contact allows the

TABLE 29.3 Federal Agencies That Fund Grants and Are Included in the National Institutes of Health Research Portfolio Online Reporting Tools—Expenditures and Results (RePORTER)

Agency	Types of Projects Funded
Agency for Health Care Research and Quality (AHRQ)	Projects to produce evidence to improve the quality, safety, and accessibility of health care
Centers for Disease Control and Prevention (CDC)	Research studies and projects to improve public health
Food and Drug Administration (FDA)	Grants and cooperative agreements to protect food and drug safety
Health Resources and Services Administration (HRSA)	Program grants to prepare and develop health professionals to care for diverse populations and improve access to care
National Institutes of Health (NIH)	Studies and research training programs on wide range of topics, through its centers and institutes
Substance Abuse and Mental Health Services Administration (SAMHSA)	Research studies and projects to prevent and treat substance abuse and mental illness
US Department of Veterans Affairs	Projects and studies to benefit military veterans

individual researcher to modify a proposal to fit more closely within agency guidelines, increasing the probability of funding. In many cases, proposals will fit within the interests of more than one government agency at the time of submission. It is permissible and perhaps desirable to request that the proposal be assigned to two agencies for review and potential funding.

Verifying Institutional Support

Grant awards are most commonly made to institutions rather than to individuals. It is important to determine the willingness of the institution to receive the grant and support the study. This willingness needs to be documented in the proposal. Supporting the study involves agreeing with the appropriateness of the study topic, ensuring the adequacy of facilities and services, providing space needed for the study, contributing to the study in nonmonetary ways (e.g., staff time, equipment, data processing), and overseeing the rights of human subjects. The study's budget will include a category called **indirect costs** to pay the institution's expenses, as compared to **direct costs**, which are the funds necessary to conduct the study. Direct costs are used to pay a portion of the researcher's salary and the salaries of data collectors or other research assistants, obtain equipment for the study, and provide a small payment to study participants to acknowledge their time and effort. For federal grants, indirect costs may be equal to direct costs, meaning that 50% of the requested amount would cover direct costs and the other half the indirect costs.

Making Time to Write

Recognize that writing a proposal requires a significant amount of time (see Chapter 28 for how to write a proposal). Kulage et al.'s (2015) study of the time required to submit a proposal for an NIH grant required 69.8 to 162.3 hours for the PI alone. The required time will be shorter for less complex grants. However, even for a rather simple grant, budgeting at least an entire workweek of 40 or more hours is wise because of the many tasks to address. Allow sufficient time to write the proposal. Read the funding agency's guidelines carefully and completely before starting to write. Keep the guidelines nearby as you write for easy reference. Strictly adhere to the page limitations and required font sizes. Check, check, and double-check your work, using spellcheck, grammar-check, and point-by-point confirmation that each requisite component has been completed perfectly and that all details such as formatting, variable names and spellings, inclusion criteria, titles of tools and measurement strategies, planned statistical tests, and references, agree across the several sections of the proposal. The sections of the proposal are uploaded separately into an online system. All details must match.

Writing your first proposal on a tight timeline is unwise. Proposal writing for a novice researcher demands refining the idea and method as you develop and articulate your plans for all steps of the process, as well as rewriting the text several times. Before any writing occurs, allow 6 to 12 months for proposal development, beginning from the point of early development of your research ideas. Jot down your thoughts and questions early in the process. Read available current literature on your topic. Confirm the availability of data collection sites. Discuss the topic with peers. Review potential research methodologies. As soon as you have a first draft, ask a peer or mentor to read the proposal to check for errors in logic. As people review your proposal informally, recognize that their questions are indications that an idea was not clearly presented and may need to be rewritten. Remember, their questions and comments are valuable. Before submission, it is highly recommended that you have a content expert or other researcher who is not at your institution critique the proposal.

Understanding the Review Process

The Center for Scientific Review has the administrative responsibility for ensuring a fair, equitable review of all proposals submitted to the NIH and to other Public Health Services agencies. After submission, the staff person assigned to your grant will determine which integrated review group will review your proposal for its technical and scientific merit. Within the integrated review group, each grant is assigned to a study section for scientific evaluation. The study section is comprised of active funded researchers.

Peer review of research funding proposals is what gives research its scientific credibility because of the expressed intent to evaluate submission "on the basis of a process that strives to be fair, equitable, timely, and free of bias" (NIH, 2019b). The study sections have no alignment with the funding agency. Thus staff persons in the agencies have no influence on the committee's work of judging the scientific merit of the proposal. The proposal is given to two or more reviewers who are

BOX 29.2   Review Criteria for NIH Research Grant Proposals

- Overall impact
- Significance
- Investigator(s)
- Innovation
- Approach
- Environment

Extracted from https://grants.nih.gov/grants/peer/guidelines_general/Review_Criteria_at_a_glance.pdf
NIH: National Institutes of Health.

considered qualified to evaluate the proposal and have no conflicts of interest. The reviewers rate the proposal on the core criteria and overall impact and then submit a written critique of the study. Box 29.2 lists the core criteria on which proposals are evaluated. Each member may have 50 to 100 proposals to read in a period of 1 to 2 months. A meeting of the full study section is then held. The persons who critiqued the proposal discuss each application, and other members comment or ask questions before recording their scores.

Proposals are assigned a numerical score used to develop a priority rating for ranking. A study that is scored is not necessarily funded. The PI may review the progress of the proposal through the stages of review by accessing an online system, the Electronic Research Administration (eRA) Commons. Funding begins with the proposal that has the highest rank order and continues until available funds are depleted. This process can take 6 months or longer. Because of this process, researchers may not receive grant money for up to a year after submitting the proposal.

Many proposals are rejected (or scored but not funded) with the first submission. The critique of the scientific committee, called a **summary statement**, is available to the researcher via his or her eRA Commons account. Frequently the agency staff encourages the researcher to rewrite the proposal with guidance from the comments and resubmit it to the same agency. The probability of funding is greater the second time if the researcher has followed the suggestions.

Responding to Rejected Grant Proposals

If your proposal is unfunded, you are not alone. In 2018, only 20.2% of all proposals submitted to NIH were funded (NIH, 2019c). For NINR, the overall rate in 2018

was only 17.1% (NIH, 2019d). The researcher's reaction to a rejected proposal is usually anger and then depression. The frustrated researcher may want to abandon the proposal. There seems to be no way to avoid the subjective reaction to a rejection because of the significant emotion and time invested in the processes of writing and submission. However, after a few weeks, it is advisable to examine the rejection letter and summary statement again. The comments can be useful in revising the proposal for resubmission. The learning experience of rewriting the proposal and evaluating the comments will provide a background for seeking funding for another study. Considering the low rate of acceptance, the researcher must be committed to submitting proposals a number of times to achieve grant funding.

GRANT MANAGEMENT

Receiving notice that a grant proposal is funded is one of the highlights in a researcher's career and warrants a celebration. However, work on the study must begin as soon as possible. You included a detailed plan of activities in the proposal that is ready to be implemented. To avoid problems, you need to consider the practicalities of managing the budget, hiring and training research personnel, maintaining the promised timetable, and coordinating activities of the study.

Managing the Budget

Although the supporting institution is ultimately responsible for dispensing and controlling grant monies, the PI is responsible for monitoring budget expenditures and making decisions about how the money is to be spent (Holtzclaw et al., 2018). If this grant is the first one received, a PI who has no previous administrative experience may need guidance in how to keep records and make reasonable budget decisions. If funding is through a federal agency, the PI will be required to provide interim reports and updates on the progress of the study.

Training Research Personnel

When a new grant is initiated, set aside time to interview, hire, and train grant personnel (Holtzclaw et al., 2018). The personnel who will be involved in data collection must learn the process. Then data collection needs to be refined to ensure that all data collectors are consistent with one another. This process helps evaluate interrater reliability. The PI needs to set aside time to oversee the work of personnel hired for the grant.

Maintaining the Study Schedule

The PI must adhere to the timetable submitted with the proposal, whenever possible. This requires careful planning and frequent monitoring for assessment of progress and delays. Otherwise, work activities and other responsibilities are likely to take precedence and delay the grant work. Unexpected events do happen. However, establishment of tight monitoring oversight early in the process can minimize the impact of unforeseen happenings. If the project falls behind schedule, action must be taken to return to the original schedule or to readjust the timetable.

Coordinating Activities

During a large study with several investigators and other grant personnel, coordinating activities can be a problem. Arrange meetings of all grant workers at predetermined intervals to share ideas and solve problems. These meetings should be either face time or electronically mediated real time, in nature. Keep records of the discussions at these meetings. These actions can lead to a more smoothly functioning team. In all the flurry of activity, it is tempting to think of the research site as a stable factor. In truth, the PI must maintain contact with site personnel, as well, to maintain good relations and resolve conflicts as early as possible.

Submitting Reports

As mentioned, federal grants require the submission of interim reports according to preset deadlines. The notice of a grant award sent as a Portable Document Format (PDF) document via e-mail will include guidelines for the content of the reports, which will consist of a description of grant activities. Set aside time to prepare the report, which usually requires uploading data and other information about the study into the federal electronic record system. In addition to electronic reports, it is often useful to maintain contact with the appropriate staff at the federal agency.

PLANNING YOUR NEXT GRANT

The researcher should not wait until funding from the first grant has ended to begin seeking funds for a second study, because of the length of time required to obtain funding. It may be wise to have several ongoing studies in various stages of implementation. For example, you could be planning one study, collecting data on a second study, analyzing data on a third, and writing papers for publication on a fourth. A full-time researcher could have completed one funded study, be in the last year of funding for a second, be in the first year of funding for a third study, and be seeking funding for a fourth. This scenario may sound unrealistic, but with planning it is not. This strategy not only provides continuous funding for research activities but also facilitates a rhythm of research that prevents time pressures and makes use of lulls in activity in a particular study. To increase the ease of obtaining funding, all studies should be within the same area of research, each building on the last.

KEY POINTS

- Building a program of research requires conducting a series of studies on a topic, with each study building on the findings of the previous one.
- The ideal topic around which to build a research program can be identified by considering topics for which the researcher has or can gain the expertise to conduct studies (capacity), funding is available (capital), and the potential exists for the researcher to make a difference (contribution). Capacity can be expanded by working with others with different types of skills and knowledge.

- Writing a grant proposal for funding requires a commitment to working extra hours.
- To receive funding, researchers need to learn grantsmanship skills.
- The first studies a researcher completes usually are conducted with personal funding or small grants.
- Nongovernmental sources of funding include private donors, local organizations, nursing organizations, and foundations.
- Before submitting a proposal to seek federal funding, the researcher should successfully complete

two or more small studies and disseminate the findings.

- The researcher identifies a significant problem, develops a study to examine it, and submits a proposal for the study to an appropriate funding source.
- The PI is responsible for keeping within the budget, training research personnel, maintaining the schedule, and coordinating activities.

- Grants require the submission of interim and final reports of expenditures, activities, and achievements.
- A researcher should not wait until funding from one grant ends before seeking funds for the next grant.

REFERENCES

Adegbola, M. (2011). Soar like geese: Building developmental network relationships for scholarship. *Nursing Education Perspectives*, *32*(1), 51–53.

American Association of Nurse Practitioners. (2019). *AANP grants*. Retrieved from https://www.aanp.org/education/professional-funding-support/aanp-grants

American Nurses Association. (2008). Leading the way in research on women and heart disease. *The American Nurse*, *40*(1), 12.

American Nurses Foundation. (2019). *Nursing research grants*. Retrieved from https://www.nursingworld.org/~49eb64/globalassets/get-involved/2019-nrg-grants-list-pdf

Candid. (2019). *Candid gets you the information you need to do good*. Retrieved from https://candid.org/

Catalog of Federal Domestic Assistance (CFDA). (2019). *[to be renamed SAM.gov]* Retrieved from https://beta.sam.gov/?s=generalinfo&mode=list&tab=list&tabmode=list

Emergency Nurses Association (ENA). *Foundation*. (2019). Retrieved from https://www.ena.org/foundation#research

Frank, L., Forsythe, L., Ellis, L., Schrandt, S., Sheridan, S., Gerson, J., ... Daugherty, S. (2015). Conceptual and practical foundations of patient engagement in research at the Patient Centered Outcomes Research Institute. *Quality of Life Research*, *24*(5), 1033–1041. doi:10.1007/s11136-014-0893-3

Hershberger, P., Minton, M., Voss, J., McCarthy, A., Murrock, C., Topp, R., & Talsma, A. (2019). Midcareer faculty needs identified by the Midwest Nursing Research Society Midcareer Scholars Task Force. *Western Journal of Nursing Research*, *41*(5), 762–783. doi:10.1177/0193945918798634

Holtzclaw, B. J., Kenner, C., & Walden, M. (2018). *Grant writing handbook for nurses and health professionals*. New York, NY: Springer Publishing Company.

Institute of Medicine (IOM). (2008). *Knowing what works in health care: A roadmap for the nation*. Washington, DC: National Academies Press.

Iyioke, I. (2016). *Re-conceptualizing responsibility in clinical trials (an insight with the African notion of self)*. Unpublished doctoral dissertation. ProQuest Dissertations and Theses.

Johns Hopkins Medicine. (2019). *Comparative effectiveness research*. Retrieved from https://www.hopkinsmedicine.org/gim/research/method/comp_eff.html

Kulage, K. M., Schnall, R., Hickey, K. T., Travers, J., Zezulinski, K., Torres, F., ... Janine, L. E. (2015). Time and costs of preparing and submitting an NIH grant application at a school of nursing. *Nursing Outlook*, *63*(6), 639–649. doi:10.1016/j.outlook.2015.09.003

Munro, S., Hendrix, C. C., Cowan, L. J., Battaglia, C., Wilder, V. D., Bormann, J. E., ... Sullivan, S. C. (2019). Research productivity following nursing research initiative grants. *Nursing Outlook*, *67*(1), 6–12. doi:10.1016/j.outlook.2018.06.011

National Institutes of Health (NIH). (2019a). *Research portfolio online reporting tools (RePORT)* [Excel file]. Retrieved from https://projectreporter.nih.gov/reporter.cfm

National Institutes of Health (NIH). (2019b). *Peer review*. Retrieved from https://grants.nih.gov/grants/peer-review.htm

National Institutes of Health (NIH). (2019c). *Research project grants and other mechanisms: Funding: Fiscal year 2018*. Retrieved from http://report.nih.gov/success_rates/index.aspx

National Institutes of Health (NIH). (2019d). *Research portfolio online reporting tools (RePORT)* [Excel file]. Retrieved from https://report.nih.gov/success_rates/

Patient-Centered Outcomes Research Institute (PCORI). (2019). *About us*. Retrieved from http://www.pcori.org/about-us

Sigma. (2019). *Nursing research grants*. Retrieved from https://www.sigmanursing.org/advance-elevate/research/research-grants

Smith, M. (2018). *Psychedelic drugs to treat depression, PTSD? WebMD Health News*. Retrieved from https://www.webmd.com/mental-health/news/20180918/psychedelic-drugs-to-treat-depression-ptsd

US Congress. (2010). *Patient Protection and Affordable Care Act, Subtitle D of Title VI, §§ 6301 Patient-Centered Outcomes Research*. Retrieved from http://www.pcori.org/sites/default/files/PCORI_Authorizing_Legislation.pdf

US Department of Health and Human Services (HHS). (2019). *Grants*. Retrieved from https://www.grants.gov/learn-grants/grant-making-agencies/department-of-health-and-human-services.html

z Values Table

z Score	From Mean to z (%)	z Score	From Mean to z (%)	z Score	From Mean to z (%)
.00	.00	.36	14.06	.72	26.42
.01	.40	.37	14.43	.73	26.73
.02	.80	.38	14.80	.74	27.04
.03	1.20	.39	15.17	.75	27.34
.04	1.60	.40	15.54	.76	27.64
.05	1.99	.41	15.91	.77	27.94
.06	2.39	.42	16.28	.78	28.23
.07	2.79	.43	16.64	.79	28.52
.08	3.19	.44	17.00	.80	28.81
.09	3.59	.45	17.36	.81	29.10
.10	3.98	.46	17.72	.82	29.39
.11	4.38	.47	18.08	.83	29.67
.12	4.78	.48	18.44	.84	29.95
.13	5.17	.49	18.79	.85	30.23
.14	5.57	.50	19.15	.86	30.51
.15	5.96	.51	19.50	.87	30.78
.16	6.36	.52	19.85	.88	31.06
.17	6.75	.53	20.19	.89	31.33
.18	7.14	.54	20.54	.90	31.59
.19	7.53	.55	20.88	.91	31.86
.20	7.93	.56	21.23	.92	32.12
.21	8.32	.57	21.57	.93	32.38
.22	8.71	.58	21.90	.94	32.64
.23	9.10	.59	22.24	.95	32.89
.24	9.48	.60	22.57	.96	33.15
.25	9.87	.61	22.91	.97	33.40
.26	10.26	.62	23.24	.98	33.65
.27	10.64	.63	23.57	.99	33.89
.28	11.03	.64	23.89	1.00	34.13
.29	11.41	.65	24.22	1.01	34.38
.30	11.79	.66	24.54	1.02	34.61
.31	12.17	.67	24.86	1.03	34.85
.32	12.55	.68	25.17	1.04	35.08
.33	12.93	.69	25.49	1.05	35.31
.34	13.31	.70	25.80	1.06	35.54
.35	13.68	.71	26.11	1.07	35.77

Continued

z Score	From Mean to z (%)	z Score	From Mean to z (%)	z Score	From Mean to z (%)
1.08	35.99	1.57	44.18	2.06	48.03
1.09	36.21	1.58	44.29	2.07	48.08
1.10	36.43	1.59	44.41	2.08	48.12
1.11	36.65	1.60	44.52	2.09	48.17
1.12	36.86	1.61	44.63	2.10	48.21
1.13	37.08	1.62	44.74	2.11	48.26
1.14	37.29	1.63	44.84	2.12	48.30
1.15	37.49	1.64	44.95	2.13	48.34
1.16	37.70	1.65	45.05	2.14	48.38
1.17	37.90	1.66	45.15	2.15	48.42
1.18	38.10	1.67	45.25	2.16	48.46
1.19	38.30	1.68	45.35	2.17	48.50
1.20	38.49	1.69	45.45	2.18	48.54
1.21	38.69	1.70	45.54	2.19	48.57
1.22	38.88	1.71	45.64	2.20	48.61
1.23	39.07	1.72	45.73	2.21	48.64
1.24	39.25	1.73	45.82	2.22	48.68
1.25	39.44	1.74	45.91	2.23	48.71
1.26	39.62	1.75	45.99	2.24	48.75
1.27	39.80	1.76	46.08	2.25	48.78
1.28	39.97	1.77	46.16	2.26	48.81
1.29	40.15	1.78	46.25	2.27	48.84
1.30	40.32	1.79	46.33	2.28	48.87
1.31	40.49	1.80	46.41	2.29	48.90
1.32	40.66	1.81	46.49	2.30	48.93
1.33	40.82	1.82	46.56	2.31	48.96
1.34	40.99	1.83	46.64	2.32	48.98
1.35	41.15	1.84	46.71	2.33	49.01
1.36	41.31	1.85	46.78	2.34	49.04
1.37	41.47	1.86	46.86	2.35	49.06
1.38	41.62	1.87	46.93	2.36	49.09
1.39	41.77	1.88	46.99	2.37	49.11
1.40	41.92	1.89	47.06	2.38	49.13
1.41	42.07	1.90	47.13	2.39	49.16
1.42	42.22	1.91	47.19	2.40	49.18
1.43	42.36	1.92	47.26	2.41	49.20
1.44	42.51	1.93	47.32	2.42	49.22
1.45	42.65	1.94	47.38	2.43	49.25
1.46	42.79	1.95	47.44	2.44	49.27
1.47	42.92	1.96	47.50	2.45	49.29
1.48	43.06	1.97	47.56	2.46	49.31
1.49	43.19	1.98	47.61	2.47	49.32
1.50	43.32	1.99	47.67	2.48	49.34
1.51	43.45	2.00	47.72	2.49	49.36
1.52	43.57	2.01	47.78	2.50	49.38
1.53	43.70	2.02	47.83	2.51	49.40
1.54	43.82	2.03	47.88	2.52	49.41
1.55	43.94	2.04	47.93	2.53	49.43
1.56	44.06	2.05	47.98	2.54	49.45

z Score	From Mean to *z* (%)	*z* Score	From Mean to *z* (%)	*z* Score	From Mean to *z* (%)
2.55	49.46	2.71	49.66	2.87	49.795
2.56	49.48	2.72	49.67	2.88	49.801
2.57	49.49	2.73	49.68	2.89	49.807
2.58	49.51	2.74	49.69	2.90	49.813
2.59	49.52	2.75	49.702	2.91	49.819
2.60	49.53	2.76	49.711	2.92	49.825
2.61	49.55	2.77	49.720	2.93	49.831
2.62	49.56	2.78	49.728	2.94	49.836
2.63	49.57	2.79	49.736	2.95	49.841
2.64	49.59	2.80	49.744	2.96	49.846
2.65	49.60	2.81	49.752	2.97	49.851
2.66	49.61	2.82	49.760	2.98	49.856
2.67	49.62	2.83	49.767	2.99	49.861
2.68	49.63	2.84	49.774	3.00	49.865
2.69	49.64	2.85	49.781		
2.70	49.65	2.86	49.788		

B APPENDIX

Critical Values for Student's *t* Distribution

Level of Significance (α), One-Tailed Test						
	0.001	0.005	0.01	0.025	0.05	0.10

Level of Significance (α), Two-Tailed Test						
df	0.002	0.01	0.02	0.05	0.10	0.20
2	22.327	9.925	6.965	4.303	2.920	1.886
3	10.215	5.841	4.541	3.182	2.353	1.638
4	7.173	4.604	3.747	2.776	2.132	1.533
5	5.893	4.032	3.365	2.571	2.015	1.476
6	5.208	3.707	3.143	2.447	1.943	1.440
7	4.785	3.499	2.998	2.365	1.895	1.415
8	4.501	3.355	2.896	2.306	1.860	1.397
9	4.297	3.250	2.821	2.262	1.833	1.383
10	4.144	3.169	2.764	2.228	1.812	1.372
11	4.025	3.106	2.718	2.201	1.796	1.363
12	3.930	3.055	2.681	2.179	1.782	1.356
13	3.852	3.012	2.650	2.160	1.771	1.350
14	3.787	2.977	2.624	2.145	1.761	1.345
15	3.733	2.947	2.602	2.131	1.753	1.341
16	3.686	2.921	2.583	2.120	1.746	1.337
17	3.646	2.898	2.567	2.110	1.740	1.333
18	3.610	2.878	2.552	2.101	1.734	1.330
19	3.579	2.861	2.539	2.093	1.729	1.328
20	3.552	2.845	2.528	2.086	1.725	1.325
21	3.527	2.831	2.518	2.080	1.721	1.323
22	3.505	2.819	2.508	2.074	1.717	1.321
23	3.485	2.807	2.500	2.069	1.714	1.319
24	3.467	2.797	2.492	2.064	1.711	1.318
25	3.450	2.787	2.485	2.060	1.708	1.316
26	3.435	2.779	2.479	2.056	1.706	1.315
27	3.421	2.771	2.473	2.052	1.703	1.314
28	3.408	2.763	2.467	2.048	1.701	1.313
29	3.396	2.756	2.462	2.045	1.699	1.311
30	3.385	2.750	2.457	2.042	1.697	1.310

Level of Significance (α), One-Tailed Test—cont'd					
0.001	0.005	0.01	0.025	0.05	0.10

Level of Significance (α), Two-Tailed Test—cont'd						
df	0.002	0.01	0.02	0.05	0.10	0.20
31	3.375	2.744	2.453	2.040	1.696	1.309
32	3.365	2.738	2.449	2.037	1.694	1.309
33	3.356	2.733	2.445	2.035	1.692	1.308
34	3.348	2.728	2.441	2.032	1.691	1.307
35	3.340	2.724	2.438	2.030	1.690	1.306
36	3.333	2.719	2.434	2.028	1.688	1.306
37	3.326	2.715	2.431	2.026	1.687	1.305
38	3.319	2.712	2.429	2.024	1.686	1.304
39	3.313	2.708	2.426	2.023	1.685	1.304
40	3.307	2.704	2.423	2.021	1.684	1.303
45	3.281	2.690	2.412	2.014	1.679	1.301
50	3.261	2.678	2.403	2.009	1.676	1.299
55	3.245	2.668	2.396	2.004	1.673	1.297
60	3.232	2.660	2.390	2.000	1.671	1.296
65	3.220	2.654	2.385	1.997	1.669	1.295
70	3.211	2.648	2.381	1.994	1.667	1.294
75	3.202	2.643	2.377	1.992	1.665	1.293
80	3.195	2.639	2.374	1.990	1.664	1.292
85	3.189	2.635	2.371	1.988	1.663	1.292
90	3.183	2.632	2.368	1.987	1.662	1.291
95	3.178	2.629	2.366	1.985	1.661	1.291
100	3.174	2.626	2.364	1.984	1.660	1.290
200	3.131	2.601	2.345	1.972	1.653	1.286
300	3.118	2.592	2.339	1.968	1.650	1.284
∞	3.1	2.58	2.33	1.96	1.65	1.28

df, Degrees of Freedom.

Critical Values of *r* for Pearson Product Moment Correlation Coefficient

Level of Significance (α), One-Tailed Test								
0.05	0.025	0.01	0.005		0.05	0.025	0.01	0.005

Level of Significance (α), Two-Tailed Test								
df = N − 2	0.10	0.05	0.02	0.01	*df* = N − 2	0.10	0.05	0.02	0.01

df = N − 2	0.10	0.05	0.02	0.01	*df* = N − 2	0.10	0.05	0.02	0.01
1	0.9877	0.9969	0.9995	0.9999	39	0.2605	0.3081	0.3621	0.3978
2	0.9000	0.9500	0.9800	0.9900	40	0.2573	0.3044	0.3578	0.3932
3	0.8054	0.8783	0.9343	0.9587	41	0.2542	0.3008	0.3536	0.3887
4	0.7293	0.8114	0.8822	0.9172	42	0.2512	0.2973	0.3496	0.3843
5	0.6694	0.7545	0.8329	0.8745	43	0.2483	0.2940	0.3458	0.3801
6	0.6215	0.7067	0.7887	0.8343	44	0.2455	0.2907	0.3420	0.3761
7	0.5822	0.6664	0.7498	0.7977	45	0.2429	0.2876	0.3384	0.3721
8	0.5493	0.6319	0.7155	0.7646	46	0.2403	0.2845	0.3348	0.3683
9	0.5214	0.6021	0.6851	0.7348	47	0.2377	0.2816	0.3314	0.3646
10	0.4973	0.5760	0.6581	0.7079	48	0.2353	0.2787	0.3281	0.3610
11	0.4762	0.5529	0.6339	0.6835	49	0.2329	0.2759	0.3249	0.3575
12	0.4575	0.5324	0.6120	0.6614	50	0.2306	0.2732	0.3218	0.3542
13	0.4409	0.5140	0.5923	0.6411	55	0.2201	0.2609	0.3074	0.3385
14	0.4259	0.4973	0.5742	0.6226	60	0.2108	0.2500	0.2948	0.3248
15	0.4124	0.4821	0.5577	0.6055	65	0.2027	0.2404	0.2837	0.3126
16	0.4000	0.4683	0.5426	0.5897	70	0.1954	0.2319	0.2737	0.3017
17	0.3887	0.4555	0.5285	0.5751	75	0.1888	0.2242	0.2647	0.2919
18	0.3783	0.4438	0.5155	0.5614	80	0.1829	0.2172	0.2565	0.2830
19	0.3687	0.4329	0.5034	0.5487	85	0.1775	0.2108	0.2491	0.2748
20	0.3598	0.4227	0.4921	0.5368	90	0.1726	0.2050	0.2422	0.2673
21	0.3515	0.4132	0.4815	0.5256	95	0.1680	0.1996	0.2359	0.2604
22	0.3438	0.4044	0.4716	0.5151	100	0.1638	0.1946	0.2301	0.2540
23	0.3365	0.3961	0.4622	0.5052	120	0.1496	0.1779	0.2104	0.2324
24	0.3297	0.3882	0.4534	0.4958	140	0.1386	0.1648	0.1951	0.2155
25	0.3233	0.3809	0.4451	0.4869	160	0.1297	0.1543	0.1827	0.2019
26	0.3172	0.3739	0.4372	0.4785	180	0.1223	0.1455	0.1723	0.1905
27	0.3115	0.3673	0.4297	0.4705	200	0.1161	0.1381	0.1636	0.1809
28	0.3061	0.3610	0.4226	0.4629	250	0.1039	0.1236	0.1465	0.1620
29	0.3009	0.3550	0.4158	0.4556	300	0.0948	0.1129	0.1338	0.1480
30	0.2960	0.3494	0.4093	0.4487	350	0.0878	0.1046	0.1240	0.1371
31	0.2913	0.3440	0.4031	0.4421	400	0.0822	0.0978	0.1160	0.1283
32	0.2869	0.3388	0.3973	0.4357	450	0.0775	0.0922	0.1094	0.1210
33	0.2826	0.3338	0.3916	0.4297	500	0.0735	0.0875	0.1038	0.1149
34	0.2785	0.3291	0.3862	0.4238	600	0.0671	0.0799	0.0948	0.1049
35	0.2746	0.3246	0.3810	0.4182	700	0.0621	0.0740	0.0878	0.0972
36	0.2709	0.3202	0.3760	0.4128	800	0.0581	0.0692	0.0821	0.0909
37	0.2673	0.3160	0.3712	0.4076	900	0.0548	0.0653	0.0774	0.0857
38	0.2638	0.3120	0.3665	0.4026	1000	0.0520	0.0619	0.0735	0.0813

df, Degrees of Freedom.

Critical Values of *F* for α = 0.05 and α = 0.01

Critical Values of *F* For α = 0.05

df Denominator	DEGREES OF FREEDOM (df) NUMERATOR

df Denominator	1	2	3	4	5	6	7	8	9	10	12	15	20	24	30	40	60	120	∞
1	161.4	199.5	215.7	224.6	230.2	234.0	236.8	238.9	240.5	241.9	243.9	245.9	248.0	249.1	250.1	251.1	252.2	253.3	254.3
2	18.51	19.00	19.16	19.25	19.30	19.33	19.35	19.37	19.38	19.40	19.41	19.43	19.45	19.45	19.46	19.47	19.48	19.49	19.50
3	10.13	9.55	9.28	9.12	9.01	8.94	8.89	8.85	8.81	8.79	8.74	8.70	8.66	8.64	8.62	8.59	8.57	8.55	8.53
4	7.71	6.94	6.59	6.39	6.26	6.16	6.09	6.04	6.00	5.96	5.91	5.86	5.80	5.77	5.75	5.72	5.69	5.66	5.63
5	6.61	5.79	5.41	5.19	5.05	4.95	4.88	4.82	4.77	4.74	4.68	4.62	4.56	4.53	4.50	4.46	4.43	4.40	4.36
6	5.99	5.14	4.76	4.53	4.39	4.28	4.21	4.15	4.10	4.06	4.00	3.94	3.87	3.84	3.81	3.77	3.74	3.70	3.67
7	5.59	4.74	4.35	4.12	3.97	3.87	3.79	3.73	3.68	3.64	3.57	3.51	3.44	3.41	3.38	3.34	3.30	3.27	3.23
8	5.32	4.46	4.07	3.84	3.69	3.58	3.50	3.44	3.39	3.35	3.28	3.22	3.15	3.12	3.08	3.04	3.01	2.97	2.93
9	5.12	4.26	3.86	3.63	3.48	3.37	3.29	3.23	3.18	3.14	3.07	3.01	2.94	2.90	2.86	2.83	2.79	2.75	2.71
10	4.96	4.10	3.71	3.48	3.33	3.22	3.14	3.07	3.02	2.98	2.91	2.85	2.77	2.74	2.70	2.66	2.62	2.58	2.54
11	4.84	3.98	3.59	3.36	3.20	3.09	3.01	2.95	2.90	2.85	2.79	2.72	2.65	2.61	2.57	2.53	2.49	2.45	2.40
12	4.75	3.89	3.49	3.26	3.11	3.00	2.91	2.85	2.80	2.75	2.69	2.62	2.54	2.51	2.47	2.43	2.38	2.34	2.30
13	4.67	3.81	3.41	3.18	3.03	2.92	2.83	2.77	2.71	2.67	2.60	2.53	2.46	2.42	2.38	2.34	2.30	2.25	2.21
14	4.60	3.74	3.34	3.11	2.96	2.85	2.76	2.70	2.65	2.60	2.53	2.46	2.39	2.35	2.31	2.27	2.22	2.10	2.13
15	4.54	3.68	3.29	3.06	2.90	2.79	2.71	2.64	2.59	2.54	2.48	2.40	2.33	2.29	2.25	2.20	2.16	2.11	2.07
16	4.49	3.63	3.24	3.01	2.85	2.74	2.66	2.59	2.54	2.49	2.42	2.35	2.28	2.24	2.19	2.15	2.11	2.06	2.01
17	4.45	3.59	3.20	2.96	2.81	2.70	2.61	2.55	2.49	2.45	2.38	2.31	2.23	2.19	2.15	2.10	2.06	2.01	1.96
18	4.41	3.55	3.16	2.93	2.77	2.66	2.58	2.51	2.46	2.41	2.34	2.27	2.19	2.15	2.11	2.06	2.02	1.97	1.92
19	4.38	3.52	3.13	2.90	2.74	2.63	2.54	2.48	2.42	2.38	2.31	2.23	2.16	2.11	2.07	2.03	1.98	1.93	1.88
20	4.35	3.49	3.10	2.87	2.71	2.60	2.51	2.45	2.39	2.35	2.28	2.20	2.12	2.08	2.04	1.99	1.95	1.90	1.84
21	4.32	3.47	3.07	2.84	2.68	2.57	2.49	2.42	2.37	2.32	2.25	2.18	2.10	2.05	2.01	1.96	1.92	1.87	1.81
22	4.30	3.44	3.05	2.82	2.66	2.55	2.46	2.40	2.34	2.30	2.23	2.15	2.07	2.03	1.98	1.94	1.89	1.84	1.78
23	4.28	3.42	3.03	2.80	2.64	2.53	2.44	2.37	2.32	2.27	2.20	2.13	2.05	2.01	1.96	1.91	1.86	1.81	1.76
24	4.26	3.40	3.01	2.78	2.62	2.51	2.42	2.36	2.30	2.25	2.18	2.11	2.03	1.98	1.94	1.89	1.84	1.79	1.73
25	4.24	3.39	2.99	2.76	2.60	2.49	2.40	2.34	2.28	2.24	2.16	2.09	2.01	1.96	1.92	1.87	1.82	1.77	1.71
26	4.23	3.37	2.98	2.74	2.59	2.47	2.39	2.32	2.27	2.22	2.15	2.07	1.99	1.95	1.90	1.85	1.80	1.75	1.69
27	4.21	3.35	2.96	2.73	2.57	2.46	2.37	2.31	2.25	2.20	2.13	2.06	1.97	1.93	1.88	1.84	1.79	1.73	1.67
28	4.20	3.34	2.95	2.71	2.56	2.45	2.36	2.29	2.24	2.19	2.12	2.04	1.96	1.91	1.87	1.82	1.77	1.71	1.65
29	4.18	3.33	2.93	2.70	2.55	2.43	2.35	2.28	2.22	2.18	2.10	2.03	1.94	1.90	1.85	1.81	1.75	1.70	1.64
30	4.17	3.32	2.92	2.69	2.53	2.42	2.33	2.27	2.21	2.16	2.09	2.01	1.93	1.89	1.84	1.79	1.74	1.68	1.62
40	4.08	3.23	2.84	2.61	2.45	2.34	2.25	2.18	2.12	2.08	2.00	1.92	1.84	1.79	1.74	1.69	1.64	1.58	1.51
60	4.00	3.15	2.76	2.53	2.37	2.25	2.17	2.10	2.04	1.99	1.92	1.84	1.75	1.70	1.65	1.59	1.53	1.47	1.39
120	3.92	3.07	2.68	2.45	2.29	2.17	2.09	2.02	1.96	1.91	1.83	1.75	1.66	1.61	1.55	1.50	1.43	1.35	1.25
∞	3.84	3.00	2.60	2.37	2.21	2.10	2.01	1.94	1.88	1.83	1.75	1.67	1.57	1.52	1.46	1.39	1.32	1.22	1.00

From Merrington, M., & Thompson, C.M. (1943). Tables of percentage points of the inverted beta (F) distribution. *Biometrika, 33*(1), 80-81.

Critical Values of F For $\alpha = 0.01$

df Denominator	\multicolumn{19}{c}{df NUMERATOR}																		
	1	2	3	4	5	6	7	8	9	10	12	15	20	24	30	40	60	120	∞
1	4052	4999.5	5403	5625	5764	5859	5928	5982	6022	6056	6106	6157	6209	6235	6261	6287	6313	6339	6366
2	98.50	99.00	99.17	99.25	99.30	99.33	99.36	99.37	99.39	99.40	99.42	99.43	99.45	99.46	99.47	99.47	99.48	99.49	99.50
3	34.12	30.82	29.46	28.71	28.24	27.91	27.67	27.49	27.35	27.23	27.05	26.87	26.69	26.60	26.50	26.41	26.32	26.22	26.13
4	21.20	18.00	16.69	15.98	15.52	15.21	14.98	14.80	14.66	14.55	14.37	14.20	14.02	13.93	13.84	13.75	13.65	13.56	13.46
5	16.26	13.27	12.06	11.39	10.97	10.67	10.46	10.29	10.16	10.05	9.89	9.72	9.55	9.47	9.38	9.29	9.20	9.11	9.02
6	13.75	10.92	9.78	9.15	8.75	8.47	8.26	8.10	7.98	7.87	7.72	7.56	7.40	7.31	7.23	7.14	7.06	6.97	6.88
7	12.25	9.55	8.45	7.85	7.46	7.19	6.99	6.84	6.72	6.62	6.47	6.31	6.16	6.07	5.99	5.91	5.82	5.74	5.65
8	11.26	8.65	7.59	7.01	6.63	6.37	6.18	6.03	5.91	5.81	5.67	5.52	5.36	5.28	5.20	5.12	5.03	4.95	4.86
9	10.56	8.02	6.99	6.42	6.06	5.80	5.61	5.47	5.35	5.26	5.11	4.96	4.81	4.73	4.65	4.57	4.48	4.40	4.31
10	10.04	7.56	6.55	5.99	5.64	5.39	5.20	5.06	4.94	4.85	4.71	4.56	4.41	4.33	4.25	4.17	4.08	4.00	3.91
11	9.65	7.21	6.22	5.67	5.32	5.07	4.89	4.74	4.63	4.54	4.40	4.25	4.10	4.02	3.94	3.86	3.78	3.69	3.60
12	9.33	6.93	5.95	5.41	5.06	4.82	4.64	4.50	4.39	4.30	4.16	4.01	3.86	3.78	3.70	3.62	3.54	3.45	3.36
13	9.07	6.70	5.74	5.21	4.86	4.62	4.44	4.30	4.19	4.10	3.96	3.82	3.66	3.59	3.51	3.43	3.34	3.25	3.17
14	8.86	6.51	5.56	5.04	4.69	4.46	4.28	4.14	4.03	3.94	3.80	3.66	3.51	3.43	3.35	3.27	3.18	3.09	3.00
15	8.68	6.36	5.42	4.89	4.56	4.32	4.14	4.00	3.89	3.80	3.67	3.52	3.37	3.29	3.21	3.13	3.05	2.96	2.87
16	8.53	6.23	5.29	4.77	4.44	4.20	4.03	3.89	3.78	3.69	3.55	3.41	3.26	3.18	3.10	3.02	2.93	2.84	2.75
17	8.40	6.11	5.18	4.67	4.34	4.10	3.93	3.79	3.68	3.59	3.46	3.31	3.16	3.08	3.00	2.92	2.83	2.75	2.65
18	8.29	6.01	5.09	4.58	4.25	4.01	3.84	3.71	3.60	3.51	3.37	3.23	3.08	3.00	2.92	2.84	2.75	2.66	2.57
19	8.18	5.93	5.01	4.50	4.17	3.94	3.77	3.63	3.52	3.43	3.30	3.15	3.00	2.92	2.84	2.76	2.67	2.58	2.49
20	8.10	5.85	4.94	4.43	4.10	3.87	3.70	3.56	3.46	3.37	3.23	3.09	2.94	2.86	2.78	2.69	2.61	2.52	2.42
21	8.02	5.78	4.87	4.37	4.04	3.81	3.64	3.51	3.40	3.31	3.17	3.03	2.88	2.80	2.72	2.64	2.55	2.46	2.36
22	7.95	5.72	4.82	4.31	3.99	3.76	3.59	3.45	3.35	3.26	3.12	2.98	2.83	2.75	2.67	2.58	2.50	2.40	2.31
23	7.88	5.66	4.76	4.26	3.94	3.71	3.54	3.41	3.30	3.21	3.07	2.93	2.78	2.70	2.62	2.54	2.45	2.35	2.26
24	7.82	5.61	4.72	4.22	3.90	3.67	3.50	3.36	3.26	3.17	3.03	2.89	2.74	2.66	2.58	2.49	2.40	2.31	2.21
25	7.77	5.57	4.68	4.18	3.85	3.63	3.46	3.32	3.22	3.13	2.99	2.85	2.70	2.62	2.54	2.45	2.36	2.27	2.17
26	7.72	5.53	4.64	4.14	3.82	3.59	3.42	3.29	3.18	3.09	2.96	2.81	2.66	2.58	2.50	2.42	2.33	2.23	2.13
27	7.68	5.49	4.60	4.11	3.78	3.56	3.39	3.26	3.15	3.06	2.93	2.78	2.63	2.55	2.47	2.38	2.29	2.20	2.10
28	7.64	5.45	4.57	4.07	3.75	3.53	3.36	3.23	3.12	3.03	2.90	2.75	2.60	2.52	2.44	2.35	2.26	2.17	2.06
29	7.60	5.42	4.54	4.04	3.73	3.50	3.33	3.20	3.09	3.00	2.87	2.73	2.57	2.49	2.41	2.33	2.23	2.14	2.03
30	7.56	5.39	4.51	4.02	3.70	3.47	3.30	3.17	3.07	2.98	2.84	2.70	2.55	2.47	2.39	2.30	2.21	2.11	2.01
40	7.31	5.18	4.31	3.83	3.51	3.29	3.12	2.99	2.89	2.80	2.66	2.52	2.37	2.29	2.20	2.11	2.02	1.92	1.80
60	7.08	4.98	4.13	3.65	3.34	3.12	2.95	2.82	2.72	2.63	2.50	2.35	2.20	2.12	2.03	1.94	1.84	1.73	1.60
120	6.85	4.79	3.95	3.48	3.17	2.96	2.79	2.66	2.56	2.47	2.34	2.19	2.03	1.95	1.86	1.76	1.66	1.53	1.38
∞	6.63	4.61	3.78	3.32	3.02	2.80	2.64	2.51	2.41	2.32	2.18	2.04	1.88	1.79	1.70	1.59	1.47	1.32	1.00

From Merrington, M., & Thompson, C.M. (1943). Tables of percentage points of the inverted beta (F) distribution. *Biometrika, 33*(1), 84–85.
df, Degrees of Freedom.

Critical Values of the χ^2 Distribution

Degrees of Freedom (df)	ALPHA (α) LEVEL			Degrees of Freedom (df)	ALPHA (α) LEVEL		
	0.05	0.01	0.001		0.05	0.01	0.001
1	3.842	6.635	10.828	24	36.415	42.980	51.179
2	5.992	9.210	13.816	25	37.653	44.314	52.620
3	7.815	11.345	16.266	26	38.885	45.642	54.052
4	9.488	13.277	18.467	27	40.113	46.963	55.476
5	11.071	15.086	20.515	28	41.337	48.278	56.892
6	12.592	16.812	22.458	29	42.557	49.588	58.301
7	14.067	18.475	24.322	30	43.773	50.892	59.703
8	15.507	20.090	26.125	31	44.985	52.191	61.098
9	16.919	21.666	27.877	32	46.194	53.486	62.487
10	18.307	23.209	29.588	33	47.400	54.776	63.870
11	19.675	24.725	31.264	34	48.602	56.061	65.247
12	21.026	26.217	32.910	35	49.802	57.342	66.619
13	22.362	27.688	34.528	36	50.999	58.619	67.985
14	23.685	29.141	36.123	37	52.192	59.893	69.347
15	24.996	30.578	37.697	38	53.384	61.162	70.703
16	26.296	32.000	39.252	39	54.672	62.428	72.055
17	27.587	33.409	40.790	40	55.759	63.691	73.402
18	28.869	34.805	42.312	41	56.942	64.950	74.745
19	30.144	36.191	43.820	42	58.124	66.206	76.084
20	31.410	37.566	45.315	43	59.304	67.459	77.419
21	32.671	38.932	46.797	44	60.481	68.710	78.750
22	33.924	40.289	48.268	45	61.656	69.957	80.077
23	35.173	41.638	49.728				

GLOSSARY

absolute zero point Point at which a value of zero indicates the absence of the property being measured. Ratio-level measurements, such as weight scales, vital signs, and laboratory values, all have an absolute zero point.

abstract Clear, concise summary of a study, usually limited to 100 to 250 words.

abstract thinking Thinking that is oriented toward the development of an idea without application to or association with a particular instance and is independent of time and space. Abstract thinkers tend to look for meaning, patterns, relationships, and philosophical implications.

acceptance rate Number or percentage of the subjects who agree to participate in a study. The percentage is calculated by dividing the number of subjects agreeing to participate by the number of subjects approached. For example, if 100 subjects are approached and 90 agree to participate, the acceptance rate is 90% ($[90 \div 100] \times 100\% = 90\%$).

accessible population Portion of a target population to which the researcher has reasonable access.

accidental or convenience sampling Nonprobability sampling technique in which subjects are included in the study because they happen to be in the right place at the right time. Available subjects who meet inclusion criteria are entered into the study until the desired sample size is reached.

accuracy The closeness of agreement between the measured value and the true value of the quantity being measured.

accuracy in physiological measures Comparable to validity, the extent to which the instrument measures the concept that is defined in the study.

accuracy of a screening test The ability of a screening test to assess correctly the true presence or absence of a disease or condition.

administrative databases Databases with standardized sets of data for enormous numbers of patients and providers that are created by insurance companies, government agencies, and others not directly involved in providing patient care.

Agency for Healthcare Research and Quality (AHRQ) Federal government agency originally created in 1989 as Agency for Health Care Policy and Research. The mission of the AHRQ is to carry out research; establish policy; and develop evidence-based guidelines, training, and research dissemination activities with respect to healthcare services and systems. The focus of this agency is to promote evidence-based health care.

allocative efficiency The degree to which resources go to the area in which they will do the most good in terms of delivery of services: effectiveness, usefulness to persons served, number of persons actually reached, and adherence rates.

alpha (α) Level of significance or cut-off point used to determine whether the samples being tested are members of the same population (nonsignificant) or different populations (significant); alpha is commonly set at 0.05, 0.01, or 0.001. Alpha is also the probability of making a Type I error.

alternate-forms reliability Also referred to as *parallel forms reliability* and involves comparing the scores for two versions of the same paper-and-pencil instrument, as a test of equivalence.

analysis of variance (ANOVA) A statistical test that enables the researcher to determine whether there is a difference between or among groups with regard to a continuous dependent or outcome variable.

ancestry search Examination of the references of relevant studies in order to identify previous studies that are pertinent to the search; used when conducting research syntheses or an exhaustive literature search for a study.

anonymity Meaning literally "without a name"; in research, the removal of all names and identifiers from data.

applied research Scientific investigation conducted to generate knowledge, the results of which have potential for direct application to practice.

assent The affirmative agreement to participate in research provided by a person not legally able to provide consent, usually a child or a person with permanently or temporarily diminished capacity.

associative hypothesis Statement of a proposed noncausative relationship between or among variables. None of the variables in the hypothesis are posited to cause any of the other variables: two or more of them merely may vary in unison.

associative relationship A noncausative relationship between or among concepts or variables.

assumption A belief that is accepted as true, without proof. In statistical testing, a belief related to a data set that, if untrue, may invalidate the test's results for that particular set.

attrition A threat to internal validity that results from subjects withdrawing from a study before its completion. Attrition makes the originally-assigned groups less similar to one another.

attrition rate The number or percentage of subjects or study participants who withdraw from a study before its completion. For example, if the sample size is 100 subjects and 20 subjects drop out of the study, the attrition rate is 20% ($[20 \div 100] \times 100\% = 20\%$).

authority Person with expertise and power who is able to influence opinion and behavior.

background for a research problem Part of the research problem that summarizes what is known about the phenomenon of interest.

bar graph Figure or illustration that uses a series of rectangular bars to provide a representation of the results of statistical analysis of a data set. These graphs consist of horizontal or vertical bars that represent the size or amount of the group or variable studied.

basic research Scientific investigation directed toward better understanding of physical or psychological processes, without any emphasis on application.

being A term in phenomenological research indicating a person's subjective awareness of experiencing life in relation to self and others.

beneficence, principle of The ethical position that compels the researcher to actively strive to do good and confer benefit, in respect to the study subjects or participants. Its ethical counterpart is nonmaleficence, which compels the researcher to actively strive to do no harm to research participants.

benefit-risk ratio Means by which researchers and reviewers of research judge the potential gains posed to a subject as a result of research participation in comparison with the potential harm posed. The benefit-risk ratio is one determinant of the ethics of a study.

best research evidence The strongest empirical knowledge available that is generated from the synthesis of quality study findings to address a practice problem.

between-groups variance A measurement used in analysis of variance (ANOVA) and similar tests in order to determine whether a difference exists between groups.

bias Any influence or action in a study that distorts the findings or slants them away from the true or expected, a distortion. Also used to refer to a point of view that differs from the objective truth.

bibliographical database Database that either consists of citations relevant to a specific discipline or is a broad collection of citations from a variety of disciplines.

bimodal Distribution of scores that has two modes (most frequently occurring scores).

bivariate analysis Any of a number of statistical procedures that involve comparison of the same variable measured in two different groups or measurement of two distinct variables within a single group.

bivariate correlation analysis Any of a number of analysis techniques that measure the extent of the linear relationship between two variables within a single sample.

Bland and Altman chart or plot A graphical method of displaying agreement between measurement techniques, which may be used to compare repeated measurements of a single method of measurement or to compare a new technique with an established one. Accompanied by a Bland and Altman analysis, which determines extent of agreement.

blinding Strategy in interventional research by which the patient's status as an experimental subject versus a control subject is hidden from the patient, data collectors, and/or those providing care to the patient.

blocking In research design, the strategy of assigning subjects to groups in two or more stages so as to assure equal distribution of a potentially extraneous variable between or among groups.

body of knowledge The total of all information, principles, theories, and empirical evidence that is organized by the beliefs accepted within a discipline at a given time.

Bonferroni procedure Post hoc analysis that determines differences among three or more groups without inflating Type I error. When a design involves multiple comparisons, the procedure may be done during the planning phase of a study to adjust the significance level so as not to inflate the Type I error.

borrowing Appropriation and use of knowledge from other disciplines to guide nursing practice.

bracketing Practice used in some forms of Husserlian phenomenology in which the researcher identifies personal preconceptions and beliefs and consciously sets them aside for the duration of the study.

breach of confidentiality Accidental or direct action that allows an unauthorized person to have access to a subject's identity information and study data.

C

calculated variable A variable used in data analysis that is not collected but is calculated from other variables.

care maps Flow diagrams that display usual care for treatment of an injury or illness, depicting anticipated patient progress. Synonymous with care pathways, clinical pathways, and critical pathways.

carryover effect Effects from a previous intervention that may continue to affect the dependent variable in subsequent interventions. A type of carryover effect is the order effect in which two interventions are applied and the order in which they are enacted determines the magnitude of the dependent variable.

case study design A design that guides the intensive exploration of a single unit of study, such as a person, family, group, community, or institution. It is similar to a life history, in that it tells the story of the unit of study. Can be quantitative, qualitative, or mixed methods research.

case-control design An epidemiological design in which subjects or "cases" are members of a certain group and "controls" are not members of that group. The case group is most commonly comprised of individuals with a certain condition or disease that the control group lacks. Selection of controls is made on the basis of demographic similarity, yielding a control group that is demographically almost identical to that of the "cases."

causal connection The link between the independent variable (cause) and the dependent variable (outcome or effect) that is examined in quasi-experimental and experimental research.

causal hypothesis or relationship A relationship between two variables in which one variable (independent variable) is thought to cause the presence of the other variable (dependent variable). Some causal hypotheses include more than one independent or dependent variable.

causality A relationship in which one variable causes a change in another. Causality has three conditions: (1) there must be a strong relationship between the proposed cause and effect, (2) the proposed cause must precede the effect in time, and (3) the cause must be present whenever the effect occurs.

cell Intersection between the row and column in a table or matrix into which a specific value is inserted.

censored data A data point that is known to exceed the limits of measurement parameters but whose exact value is unknown. Examples of this are "relapsed before three months," "beyond retirement age," "survived more than five years," and "too young to attend kindergarten."

chain sampling See *network sampling*.

chi-square test Compares differences in proportions of nominal-level (categorical) variables.

citation The act of quoting a source, using it as an example, or presenting it as support for a position taken. A citation should be accompanied by the appropriate reference to the source.

classical hypothesis testing Refers to the process of testing a hypothesis so that the researcher can infer that a relationship exists.

cleaning data   Checking raw data to determine errors in data recording, coding, or entry and to eliminate impossible data points.

clinical databases   Databases of patient, provider, and healthcare agency information that are developed by healthcare agencies and sometimes providers to document care delivery and outcomes.

clinical expertise   In health care, the cumulative effect of a practitioner's knowledge, skills, and past experience in accurately assessing, diagnosing, and managing an individual's health needs. Presumably, expertise increases with experience and may not be translatable from one practice area to another.

clinical guidelines   Standardized, current guidelines for the assessment, diagnosis, and management of patient conditions developed by clinical guideline panels or professional groups to improve the outcomes of care and promote evidence-based health care.

clinical importance   The impact a positive statistical finding would have if applied to clinical practice. The sensible question associated with this is, "Will this make a meaningful difference to the patient experience or outcomes?"

clinical judgment   The quality of reasoned decision-making in healthcare practice.

clinical trial   Any study that prospectively assigns human participants or groups of humans to one or more health-related interventions to evaluate the safety of the intervention and/or the effects on health outcomes as defined in 2014 by the National Institutes of Health.

cloud storage   Multiple-server storage of electronic data for the purpose of convenient retrieval and assurance against loss.

cluster sampling   A sampling method in which locations, institutions, or organizations are chosen from among all possible options, instead of individual subjects, because individual subjects' identities are not yet known. It is used most often when the accessible population is widespread, and the research is multisite in nature.

code   In qualitative research, a symbol or abbreviation used to label words or phrases in data sets during the data-analysis phase.

codebook   In quantitative research, the listing of each variable in a study, including

the full name, definition, an abbreviated variable name, a descriptive variable label, and the range of possible numerical values for each. This "book" may exist in either physical or virtual form.

coding   In qualitative studies, the process of naming or labeling phrases, quotations, and other raw data and later of sorting them so as to identify themes and patterns. In quantitative research, the process of transforming raw quantitative or qualitative data into numerical symbols that can be analyzed statistically.

coefficient of determination *(r²)*   The square of the correlation value, which represents the percentage of variance two variables share.

coefficient of multiple determination *(R²)*   The percentage of the total variation that can be explained by all the variables the researcher includes in the final predictive equation.

coefficient of stability   Result of a correlational analysis of the values of a measurement, educational test, or scale administered at two different measurement times (test-retest reliability).

coercion   Overt threat of harm or excessive reward intentionally presented by one person to another to obtain compliance.

cohort   Usually synonymous with group. Used in medical and epidemiological studies to refer to a group that shares at least one characteristic that is the focus of the research.

communicating research findings   Sharing the findings of a study, either verbally or in print and informally or formally.

comparative analysis   Examination of methodology and findings across studies for similarities and differences.

comparative descriptive design   A design used to describe differences in a variable's value in two or more different groups.

comparative effectiveness research   Descriptive or correlational research that compares different treatment options for their risks, outcomes, and costs.

comparative evaluation   The part of the Stetler Model in which research findings are assessed for accuracy, fit in a given healthcare setting, feasibility, and the likelihood that the intervention will produce change in current practice.

comparison group   A group of subjects that is not selected through random sampling and, because of design structure,

does not control for the effects of extraneous variables.

compensatory equalization of treatment   Extra attention or advantages provided to control group subjects by staff or family members in compensation for what experimental subjects receive.

complete observation   Data collection strategy in which the researcher maintains only the role of observer during data collection and refrains from all direct social interaction in the setting.

complete participation   Qualitative data collection strategy in which the researcher becomes a member of the social or work group and does not reveal the role of researcher.

concept   An abstract idea. A concept is a term that abstractly describes and names an object, a phenomenon, or an idea, thus providing it with a distinct identity or meaning.

concept analysis   Strategy through which the set of characteristics essential to the connotative meaning or conceptual definition of a concept is identified.

concept derivation   Process of extracting and defining concepts from theories in other disciplines. The derived concepts describe or define an aspect of nursing in an innovative way that is meaningful.

concept synthesis   Process of describing and naming a previously unidentified concept, using sources in which the concept is used in order to establish common elements.

conceptual definition   A definition that provides a variable or concept with connotative (abstract, comprehensive, theoretical) meaning and is established through concept analysis, concept derivation, or concept synthesis. Often, the conceptual definition of a variable in a study is developed from the study framework and is the link between the study framework and the operational definition of the variable.

conceptual map   The visual representation of a research framework. It depicts the study's concepts and relational statements by use of a diagram.

conceptual model   Set of highly abstract, related constructs that broadly explains phenomena of interest, expresses assumptions, and usually reflects a philosophical stance.

conclusions Syntheses and clarifications of the meanings of study findings. They provide a basis for identifying nursing implications and suggesting further studies.

concrete thinking Thinking that is oriented toward and limited by tangible things or events observed and experienced in reality.

concurrent validity The extent to which a subject's individual score on an instrument or scale can be used to estimate concurrent performance for a different instrument, scale, quality, criterion, or other variable.

condensed proposal A brief or shortened proposal developed for review by clinical agencies and funding institutions.

confidence interval The probability of including the value of a parameter within an interval estimate.

confidentiality Management of data that has been provided by a subject so that the information will not be shared with others without that subject's authorization. This implies that access to data will be guarded carefully to prevent breaches of confidentiality.

confirmatory studies Research conducted only after a large body of knowledge has been generated with exploratory studies. Confirmatory studies are expected to have large samples and to use random sampling techniques. The results are intended for wide generalization.

confounding variables A special subtype of extraneous variable, unique in that it is embedded in the study design because it is intertwined with the independent variable. It is the result of poor initial operationalization of the independent variable.

connotative Something suggested by a word external to its literal meaning. A connotative definition captures the conceptual definition of an idea and may include emotional as well as objective meaning.

consent form Printed form containing the requisite information about a study to ensure that a potential subject has been adequately informed and can decide whether to participate. The subjects sign consent forms to indicate agreement and willingness to participate.

construct validity The degree to which a study measures all aspects of the concept it purports to measure. This depends on the skill with which the researcher has conceptually defined and then operationally defined a study variable.

constructs Concepts at very high levels of abstraction that have general meanings.

content analysis Qualitative analysis technique whereby the words in a text are classified into categories according to repeated ideas or patterns of thought.

content expert A clinician or researcher who is known for broad and deep knowledge in a specific content area.

content validity The extent to which a measurement method includes all the major elements relevant to the construct being measured. Evidence for this type of validity is obtained from the literature, representatives of the relevant populations, and relevant experts.

content validity index A calculation by researchers of each item on a scale, made by rating each item a 0 (not necessary), 1 (useful), or 3 (essential).

content validity ratio A ratio score of the proportion of the number of experts who agree that the items of an instrument measure the desired concept to the total number of experts performing the review. The score is calculated for a complete instrument.

contingent relationship A statistical relationship between two variables that exists only if a third variable or concept is present. The third variable is called either an *intervening* or a *mediating* variable.

continuous variable Variable with an unlimited number of potential values, including decimals and fractions. Values in the "gaps" between whole numbers are possible. If a variable is not continuous, it is termed a *discrete variable*.

control Design decisions made by the researcher to decrease the intrusion of the effects of extraneous variables that could alter research findings and consequently force an incorrect conclusion.

control group Group of elements or subjects not exposed to the experimental treatment. The term *control group* is always used in studies with random assignment to group and sometimes used for research without random assignment if the presence of the group allows control of the effects of extraneous variables.

convenience sampling See *accidental sampling.*

convergent concurrent strategy A mixed methods strategy selected when a researcher wishes to use quantitative and qualitative methods in an attempt to confirm, cross-validate, or corroborate findings within a single study. Quantitative and qualitative data collection processes are conducted at the same time.

convergent validity Type of measurement validity obtained by using two instruments to measure the same variable, such as depression, and correlating the results from these instruments. Evidence of validity from examining convergence is achieved if the data from the two instruments have a moderate to strong positive correlation.

correlation coefficient Numerical value that indicates the magnitude or strength of relationship between two variables; coefficients range in value from $+1.00$ (perfect positive relationship) to 0.00 (no relationship) to -1.00 (perfect negative or inverse relationship).

correlation matrix A table of the bivariate correlations of every pair of variables in a data set. Along the diagonal through the matrix the variables are correlated with themselves, with the left and right sides of the table being mirror images of each other.

correlational analysis Statistical procedure conducted to determine the direction (positive or negative) and magnitude (or strength) of the relationship between two variables.

correlational designs A variety of study designs (descriptive correlational, predictive correlational, model-testing) that are used to examine relationships among variables.

correlational research Systematic investigation of relationships between two or more variables to explain the direction (positive or negative) and strength of the relationship but never cause and effect.

costs of care In outcomes research, costs to the patient or family. Costs of care can be direct or indirect.

counterbalancing A strategy used in research that consists of administration of various treatments in random order rather than consistently in the same sequence. This is used when the researcher suspects that one or more of the treatments administered may produce a carryover effect.

covert data collection Data collection that occurs when subjects are unaware that research data are being collected.

criterion sampling Recruiting participants for a qualitative study who do or do not have specific characteristics relevant to the phenomenon. Criterion sampling may be used to create homogenous samples or focus groups.

criterion-referenced testing Comparison of a subject's score with a criterion of achievement that includes the definition of target behaviors. When the subject has mastered the behaviors, he or she is considered proficient in these behaviors, such as being proficient in the behaviors of a nurse practitioner.

critical appraisal of research Systematic, unbiased, careful examination of all aspects of a study to judge the merits, weaknesses, meaning, and significance, based on previous research experience and knowledge of the topic. The following three steps are used in the process: (1) identifying the steps of the research process, (2) determining the study's strengths and weaknesses, and (3) evaluating the credibility, trustworthiness, and meaning of a study to nursing knowledge and practice.

critical appraisal process for qualitative research Evaluating the quality of a qualitative study using standards appropriate for qualitative research, such as congruence of the methods to the philosophical basis of the research approach and transferability of the findings.

critical appraisal process for quantitative research Examination of the quality of a quantitative study using standards appropriate for quantitative research, such as threats to design validity (construct, internal, external, and statistical conclusion validity).

critical pathways Flow diagrams that display usual care for treatment of an injury or illness, depicting anticipated patient progress. Synonymous with care maps, care pathways, and clinical pathways.

critical value In quantitative data analysis, the value at which statistical significance is achieved in a study.

crossover or counterbalanced design Two-phase design in which half of the sample is administered an intervention, with the other half acting as the control group; then, in a second phase, assignments are reversed so that the initial control group receives the intervention while the initial experimental group does not. This type of research sometimes is conducted using more than two groups or more than two phases.

cross-sectional designs Research strategies used to simultaneously examine groups of subjects in various stages of a process, with the intent of inferring trends over time.

cultural immersion The spending of extended periods of time in the culture one is studying using ethnographical methods to gain increased familiarity with elements of that culture, such as language, sociocultural norms, and traditions.

curvilinear relationship A relationship between two variables in which the strength of the relationship varies over the range of values so that the graph of the relationship is a curved line rather than a straight line.

D

data (plural) Pieces of information that are collected during a study (singular: datum).

data analysis In quantitative studies, organization and statistical testing of data to determine prevalence, relationship, and cause. In qualitative research, reduction and organization of data and revelation of meaning.

data collection Precise, systematic gathering of information relevant to the research purpose and the specific objectives, questions, or hypotheses of a study.

data collection forms Hardcopy or virtual forms that researchers develop or adapt and use for collecting or recording demographic data, information excerpted from patient records, observations, and values from physiological measures.

data collection plan A detailed flowchart of the chronology of interactions with subjects and investigator responses at different points during data collection.

data saturation The point in the qualitative research process at which new data begin to be redundant with what already has been found and no new themes can be identified.

data use agreement Preexistent document that limits how the data set for a study may be used and how it will be protected to meet Health Insurance Portability and Accountability Act (HIPAA) requirements. This usually stipulates that data accessed must not contain names or personal identifiers.

datum (singular) One piece of information collected for research (plural: data).

debriefing Meeting at the end of a process, intended for exchange of factual information. In research, may refer to conferences among the researchers or between a researcher and a subject. When data collection has been clandestine or deception of subjects has occurred, debriefing is used to disclose hidden information to subjects, including the true purpose of the study and its results.

deception Deliberate deceit. In research, refers to misinforming subjects for research purposes.

decision making Cognitive process of assessing a situation and deciding on a course of action, which is important for conducting research and providing health care. Phase III in the Stetler Model of Research Utilization to Facilitate Evidence-Based Practice.

Declaration of Helsinki Ethical code based on the Nuremberg Code (1964) that described necessary components of subject consent, such as knowledge of the risks and benefits of a study, and differentiated therapeutic from nontherapeutic research, among other points.

deductive reasoning Reasoning from the general to the specific or from a general premise to a particular situation.

degrees of freedom (df) Freedom of a score's value to vary, given the other existing scores' values and the established sum of these scores. The numerical value for degrees of freedom counts the number of values that are truly independent (formula for degrees of freedom varies according to statistical test).

de-identification of health data Removal of the 18 elements that could be used to identify an individual, including relatives, employer, or household members. This term is part of the Health Insurance Portability and Accountability Act (HIPAA).

Delphi technique Method of measuring the judgments of a group of experts for assessing priorities or making forecasts.

demographic variables Specific variables such as age, gender, and ethnicity that are collected in a study to describe the sample.

denotative definition The literal meaning of a word.

dependent groups Groups in which the subjects or observations selected for data collection are in some way related to the selection of other subjects or observations. For example, if subjects serve as their own controls by using the pretest as a control, the observations (and therefore the groups) are dependent. Use of twins in a study or matching subjects on a selected variable, such as medical diagnosis or age, results in dependent groups.

dependent variable Response, behavior, or outcome that is predicted and measured in research. In interventional research, changes in the dependent variable are presumed to be caused by the independent variable.

description Involves identifying and understanding the nature and attributes of nursing phenomena and sometimes the relationships among these phenomena. Description is one possible outcome of research.

descriptive correlational design A research design used when the primary research goal is to describe relationships between or among variables.

descriptive design A design used to provide information about the prevalence of a variable or its characteristics in a data set, in quantitative research.

descriptive research Provides an accurate portrayal of what exists, determines the frequency with which something occurs, and categorizes information. Quantitative descriptive research generates statistics describing the prevalence of its variables, such as percentages, ratios, raw numbers, ranges, means, and standard deviations. In qualitative research, *descriptive* refers to studies of various designs that investigate new areas of inquiry.

descriptive statistics Summary statistics that describe a sample's average and uniformity.

descriptive study designs Quantitative research designs that produce a statistical description of the phenomenon of interest.

design, research The researcher's choice of the best way in which to answer a research question with respect to several considerations, including number of subject groups, timing of data collection, and researcher intervention, if any.

design validity Design-dependent truthfulness of a study: the degree to which an entity that the researcher believes is being performed, evaluated, measured, or represented is actually what is being performed, evaluated, measured, or represented. Its four components are construct validity, internal validity, external validity, and statistical conclusion validity.

deterministic relationship Causal statement of what always occurs in a particular situation, such as a scientific law.

deviation score See *difference score.*

dialectic reasoning A type of reasoning that involves the holistic perspective, in which the whole is greater than the sum of the parts, and examining factors that are opposites and making sense of them by merging them into a single unit or idea that is greater than either alone.

diary A written record of personal experiences and reflections, maintained over time. In research, this refers to a research participant's record of experiences and reflections that may be used as data by a researcher. Use of diaries as data sources is more common in qualitative or mixed methods research than in quantitative research.

difference score A measure of dispersion that is obtained by subtracting the mean from an individual variable value, indicating the magnitude of its difference from the mean. The mean deviation is the average of all difference scores and represents average spread around the mean. Also known as the deviation score.

diffusion of an intervention or treatment Threat to internal validity in which experimental and control subjects interact and become aware of their group membership, leading to the intervention or treatment "leaking" or diffusing into the control group.

diminished autonomy Describes subjects with decreased ability to voluntarily give informed consent to participate in research, because of temporary or permanent inability to fully deliberate all aspects of the research consent process or because of legal or mental incompetence.

direct costs The researcher's costs for materials and equipment to conduct a study that are identified in a proposal and included in the study's budget. Also, in outcomes research, refers to specific costs the patient incurs for insurance payments and copayments associated with health care.

direct measurement Used for quantification of a simple, concrete variable, such as a strategy that measures height, weight, or temperature.

direction of a relationship Refers to whether two variables are positively or negatively related. In a positive relationship, the two variables change in the same

direction (increase or decrease together). In a negative relationship, the variables change in opposite directions (as one variable increases, the other decreases).

directional hypothesis A hypothesis that predicts the direction of the relationship between or among variables (e.g., A causes an increase in the value of B, H eliminates D).

disproportionate sampling Selection of the sample for a study so that the number of subjects within identifiable strata are equal and do not reflect actual population proportions. Disproportionate sampling is used to eliminate bias introduced by stratum membership, such as gender, race, or area of residence.

dissemination of research findings Communication of research findings by means of presentation or publication.

dissertation An exhaustive and usually original research work, completed by a doctoral student under the supervision of faculty in the discipline. A dissertation is the final requirement for a doctoral degree.

distribution In statistics, the relative frequency with which a variable assumes certain values.

distribution-free Term used to refer to statistical analyses that do not assume that data are normally distributed. Distribution-free analyses usually are nonparametric statistical techniques.

divergent validity Type of measurement validity established by correlation of an instrument that measures a certain concept with another instrument that measures its opposite. Negative correlation supports the divergent validity of both instruments.

double-blinding A strategy in which neither subjects nor data collectors are aware of subject assignment to group. Double-blinding avoids several threats to construct validity.

dummy variables Assignment of one or more numbers to categorical or dichotomous variables so that they can be included in a regression analysis.

duplicate publication bias Appearance of more research support for a finding than is accurate, because a study's findings have been published by the authors in more than one journal without cross-referencing the other journal.

dwelling with the data Taking time to reflect on qualitative data before initiating analysis.

E

effect size Degree to which the phenomenon is present in the population or to which the null hypothesis is false. In examining relationships, it is the magnitude or size of the association between variables. Also refers to the effectiveness of an intervention in quasi-experimental and experimental research.

effectiveness The extent to which something produces a projected effect.

element Person (subject or participant), event, behavior, or any other single unit of a study.

eligibility criteria See *sampling criteria*.

embodied Heideggerian phenomenologist's belief that the person is a self within a body and that events, perceptions, and feelings are experienced through the body and accompanied by physical sensations; thus, the person is referred to as *embodied*.

emergent concepts The ideas related to the phenomenon of interest that the researcher discovers during the processes of data collection and data analysis. Also referred to as *themes*, *essences*, *truths*, *factors*, and *factors of interest*, among other terms.

emic view In ethnographical research, a point of view that consists of studying the natives or insiders in a culture and reporting the results from their point of view.

empirical generalizations Inferences based on accumulated research evidence.

empirical literature Relevant studies published in journals, in books, and online, as well as unpublished studies, such as master's theses and doctoral dissertations.

empirical world The sum of reality experienced through our senses; the concrete portion of our existence.

endogenous variables Variables in a path analysis, or structured equation model whose values are influenced and possibly caused by exogenous variables and other endogenous variables.

environmental variable A variable that emanates from the research setting.

epistemology A point of view related to knowing and knowledge generation. Epistemology is the study of knowledge and of what distinguishes belief from evidenced knowing.

equivalence reliability A type of reliability that compares two versions of the same instrument (alternate forms reliability) or two observers measuring the same event (interrater reliability).

error in physiological measures Inaccuracy of data obtained from physiological instruments related to environment, user, subject, equipment, and interpretation errors.

error score Amount of random error in the measurement process, which is equal to the observed score minus the true score.

ethical principles Principles of respect for persons, beneficence, and justice.

ethnographical research Qualitative research methodology developed within the discipline of anthropology for investigating cultures. Ethnographical research is one of the principal qualitative strategies used in nursing research.

ethnographies The written reports of a culture from the perspective of insiders. These reports were initially the products of anthropologists who studied primitive, foreign, or remote cultures.

ethnography A word derived by combining the Greek roots of *ethno* (folk or people) and *graphos* (picture or portrait). An ethnography presents the portrait or word picture of a people.

ethnonursing research A type of nursing research that focuses on nursing and health care within a culture. Ethnonursing research emerged from Leininger's theory of transcultural nursing.

etic approach Anthropological research approach of studying behavior from outside the culture and examining similarities and differences across cultures. It yields the outsider's point of view.

evaluation step of critical appraisal Determining the validity, credibility, significance, and meaning of the study by examining the links among the study process, study findings, and previous studies.

evidence-based practice (EBP) Conscientious integration of best research evidence with clinical expertise and patient values and needs in the delivery of quality, cost-effective health care.

evidence-based practice centers Universities and healthcare agencies identified by the Agency for Healthcare Research and Quality (AHRQ) as centers for the conduct, communication, and synthesis of research knowledge in selected areas to promote evidence-based health care.

evidence-based practice guidelines Rigorous, explicit clinical guidelines developed on the basis of the best research evidence available (such as findings from systematic reviews, meta-analyses, mixed methods research syntheses, meta-syntheses, and extensive clinical trials); supported by consensus from recognized national experts and affirmed by outcomes obtained by clinicians.

exclusion sampling criteria Descriptive criteria that must be absent for the prospective subject to be included in the research sample. Exclusion criteria eliminate some elements or subjects from inclusion for the purpose of eliminating or minimizing the effects of known extraneous variables.

exempt from review One of the three types of designations related to the extent of review required for a study. Exempt from review status is reserved for studies that meet federally established criteria for exemption because they pose no discernible risk to participating subjects.

exogenous variables Variables in a path analysis, or structured equation model, whose values influence the values of the other variables in the model but whose own causes are not explained within the model.

expedited IRB review One of the three types of institutional review board reviews that may be required for a study. In expedited review, risks posed to research subjects are determined to be no greater than those ordinarily encountered in daily life or during performance of routine physical or psychological examinations.

experimental group Subjects who are exposed to the experimental treatment or intervention.

experimental research Objective, systematic investigation that examines causality and is characterized by (1) researcher-controlled intervention (manipulation of the independent variable), (2) the presence of a distinct control group, (3) random assignment of subjects to either the experimental or the control group, and (4) attenuation of threats of design validity, as much as is possible.

experimenter expectancies A threat to construct validity, characterized by a belief of the person collecting the data that may encourage certain responses from subjects, either in support of those beliefs or opposing them.

explanatory sequential design A mixed methods approach in which the researcher collects and analyzes quantitative data and then collects and analyzes qualitative data to explain the quantitative findings.

exploratory factor analysis A subtype of factor analysis in which the researcher explores different solutions in choosing factors and their corresponding items. It is performed when the researcher has few prior expectations about the factor structure.

exploratory-descriptive qualitative research Qualitative research that lacks a clearly identified qualitative methodology (neither phenomenology, grounded theory, nor ethnography). In this text, a default term used for studies that the researchers have identified as being qualitative without indicating a specific approach or underlying philosophical basis.

exploratory sequential design A mixed methods approach in which the collection and analysis of qualitative data precede the collection of quantitative data.

exploratory studies Research designed to increase the knowledge of a field of study and not intended for generalization to large populations. Exploratory studies provide the basis for confirmatory studies.

external validity Extent to which study findings can be generalized beyond the sample included in the study.

extraneous variables Variables that are neither the independent nor the dependent variable but that intrude upon the analysis and affect the strength of statistical results. Extraneous variables exist in all studies and can affect the measurement of study variables and the relationships among these variables.

F

F **statistic** Value or result obtained from conducting an analysis of variance.

fabrication in research Type of scientific misconduct that involves creating data or study results and recording or reporting them as true.

face validity A subjective assessment, usually by an expert, that verifies that a measurement instrument appears to measure the content it is purported to measure.

factor Hypothetical construct created by factor analysis that represents several separate measured variables and whose name reflects the focus of the variables with which it is associated.

factor analysis Statistical strategy in which variables or items in an instrument are evaluated for interrelationships, identifying those that are closely related. In explanatory factor analysis, the clusters or factors are then named, representing constructs or concepts of importance. The two types of factor analysis are exploratory and confirmatory.

factor loading In factor analysis, the magnitude of the correlation of a variable or item with the principal factors, ultimately the central concepts of the data set.

factor scores The sum of the factor loadings for each variable for each study participant that is associated with one of the factors in a factor analysis. Thus, each subject will have a score for each factor in the instrument.

factorial design In its original form, an experimental design in which two independent variables are tested for their effects upon one or more dependent variables, using four study groups. Its advantage is that it also provides results of the combined effect of both variables.

fair treatment Ethical principle that promotes selection and treatment of subjects in a way that does not exclude some individuals or groups because of personal characteristics unrelated to the study.

false negative Result of a diagnostic or screening test that indicates a disease is not present when it is.

false positive Result of a diagnostic or screening test that indicates a disease is present when it is not

falsification of research Type of research misconduct that involves either manipulating research materials, equipment, or processes or changing or omitting data or results in such a manner that the study results are not accurately represented in the research record.

feasibility of a study Whether or not resources are sufficient for study completion.

field notes Notes that a qualitative researcher makes during data collection.

field work Qualitative data collection that occurs in a naturalistic setting.

findings The researcher's explanation of the study results.

fishing and the error rate problem A threat to statistical conclusion validity that exists when a researcher conducts multiple statistical analyses of relationships or differences, "fishing" for statistically

significant findings, when the analyses are not required by the study questions or hypotheses. Error is additive, so if hundreds of tests are performed, it is likely that one or more will produce positive results, resulting in a Type I error.

fixed-effect model A model in which the working assumption is that the effect size of an intervention or change is constant across studies and that observed differences are due to error.

focus groups Groups constituted with the purpose of collecting data about a specific topic from more than one research participant at the same time.

forced choice item A questionnaire item with an even number of choices indicating opinion, at various levels of emphasis (agree strongly, agree somewhat, agree slightly, disagree slightly, etc.): there is no neutral position.

forest plots A graphical display of results of the individual studies examined in a quantitative meta-analysis or systematic review.

framework The abstract, logical structure of meaning that guides development of the study and enables the researcher to link the findings to the body of knowledge for nursing. A framework is a combination of concepts, and the connections between them are used to explain relationships.

frequency distribution Statistical procedure that involves listing all possible values of a variable and tallying the number for each value in the data set. Frequency distributions may be either ungrouped or grouped.

frequency table A visual display of the results of a frequency distribution in which possible values appear in one column of a table and the frequency of each value in the other column.

funnel plot Used in a meta-analysis in several studies, a graphical display of effect sizes or odds ratios for a given intervention.

G

gap In a research problem statement, an area that is unresearched or underresearched and that consequently represents incomplete knowledge for theory or practice.

general proposition Highly abstract statement of the relationship between or among concepts that is found in a conceptual model.

generalization The act of applying the findings from a study to identical or similar people or situations.

geographical analyses Analysis of a variable, with respect to the co-variable of geography. Geographical analysis is a focus of spatial analysis in epidemiology and is used in health care to examine variations in health status, health services, patterns of care, or patterns of resource use. Sometimes referred to as *small area analyses*.

gold standard The accepted benchmark for commodities, assessments, or analyses that serves as a basis of comparison with other commodities, assessments, or analyses. In medicine, the most accurate means of diagnosing a particular disease.

government report Document generated by a governmental agency, often quantitative and descriptive in nature. Government reports may be useful for providing information about incidence and status of a condition, disease, or social process to be cited in the significance and background section of the problem of a research proposal or report.

grant Research funding from a private or public institution that supports the conduct of a study.

grantsmanship Expertise and skill in successfully developing proposals to obtain funding for selected studies.

grey literature Studies that have limited distribution, such as theses and dissertations, unpublished research reports, articles in obscure journals, some online journals, conference papers and abstracts, conference proceedings, research reports to funding agencies, and technical reports.

grounded theory research Qualitative, inductive research technique based on symbolic interaction theory that is conducted to investigate a human process within a sociological focus. Its result is the generation of conceptual categories, and sometimes theory.

grouped frequency distribution Visual presentation of a count of variable values divided into subsets. For example, instead of providing numbers of subjects for all ages, the grouped frequency distribution provides numbers of subjects from ages 20 to 29, 30 to 39, and so forth.

Grove Model for Implementing Evidence-Based Guidelines in Practice Model developed by one of the textbook authors (Grove) to promote the use of national, standardized evidence-based guidelines in clinical practice.

H

Hawthorne effect A threat to construct validity in which subjects alter their normal behaviors because they are being scrutinized. This is also referred to as *reactivity*. The Hawthorne effect can exist in both noninterventional and interventional studies.

hazard ratio (HR) The ratio of the likelihood of an event occurring, in the presence of a predictor variable, as compared with its likelihood in the absence of a predictor variable. Interpreted almost identically to an odds ratio (*OR*).

hazard risk In research, the risk or possibility of event occurrence.

heterogeneity Variety. In research, a heterogeneous sample is a varied sample, with respect to at least one characteristic. Use of a heterogeneous sample tends to reduce bias but in interventional research may introduce potentially extraneous variables.

hierarchical statement set A set of three statements representing decreasing levels of abstraction, composed of a general proposition, a specific proposition, and a hypothesis or research question.

highly controlled setting A structured environment, artificially developed for the sole purpose of conducting research, such as a laboratory, experimental center, or medical research unit. Highly controlled settings are used for basic research studies and occasionally for applied research.

HIPAA Privacy Rule A United States set of standards federally implemented in 2003 to define protected health information, limiting its use or disclosure by covered entities, such as healthcare providers and health plans, in order to protect an individual's health information. The HIPAA Privacy Rule pertains not only to the healthcare environment but also to the research conducted in that environment.

history threat A threat to internal validity that exists when an event external to a study occurs and affects the value of the dependent variable.

homogeneity Sameness. In research, a homogeneous sample includes participants who are similar with respect to one or more characteristics. Use of a homogeneous sample eliminates potential extraneous variables but may produce results with limited generalizability, because the sample may be poorly representative of the target population.

homoscedastic Even dispersion of data on a scatter diagram, both above and below the regression line, which indicates that variance is similar throughout the range of values.

horizontal axis The *x*-axis of a graph. The horizontal axis is oriented in a left-right plane across the graph.

human rights Claims and demands related to legitimate expectations of safety, fairness, entitlement, and freedom that have been justified in the eyes of an individual or by the consensus of a group of individuals. Human rights are protected in research.

hypothesis Formal statement of a proposed relationship(s) between two or more variables. In research, a hypothesis is situated within a specified population.

hypothesis guessing within experimental conditions A threat to construct validity that occurs when subjects within a study guess the hypothesis of the researcher and modify their behavior so as to support or undermine that hypothesis.

hypothetical population A population that is inferred because the members of the actual population are unknown. According to sampling theory rules, a list of all members of a known population must be generated before sampling occurs.

I

immersion in the data Initial phase of qualitative data analysis in which researchers become very familiar with the data by spending extensive time reading and rereading notes and transcripts, recalling observations and experiences, listening to audio tapes, and viewing videos.

implications of research findings for nursing Meaning of research conclusions for the body of knowledge, theory, and practice in nursing, a term analogous to "usefulness."

inclusion sampling criteria Sampling requirements identified by the researcher that must be present for the element or subject to be included in the sample.

incomplete disclosure Failure to disclose to subjects the exact purpose of a study, based on the belief that subjects might alter their actions if they were made aware of the true purpose. After study completion, subjects must be debriefed about the complete purpose and the findings of the study.

independent groups Groups of subjects assigned to one or another condition so that the assignment of one is totally unrelated to the assignment of others. An example is the random assignment of subjects to treatment versus control groups.

independent samples *t*-test Common parametric analysis technique used in nursing studies to test for significant differences between two groups unrelated to each other. Scores of one group are not linked to scores of the other group. See *paired or dependent samples* t-*test.*

independent variable In interventional research, the treatment, intervention, or experimental activity that is manipulated or varied by the researcher to create an effect on the dependent variable. In correlational research, a variable that predicts the occurrence of the dependent variable. In the latter case, the predictive variable may or may not be found to be causative in subsequent research.

indirect costs The researcher's costs that are not specified in a grant proposal, such as use of space and some administrative costs. The amount of a grant may be increased to provide support to the institution to cover these costs. In outcomes research, the "hidden" costs the patient and family incur during hospitalization or treatment, such as loss of employment, lodging and meals away from home, and parking fees.

indirect measurement The strategy of quantification used with variables that cannot be measured directly but whose attributes can be quantified. Most measurement tools are examples of indirect measurement, such as the State-Trait Anxiety Inventory (STAI).

individually identifiable health information (IIHI) Any information collected from a person, including demographic information, that is created or received by healthcare providers, a health plan, or a healthcare clearinghouse, that is related to the past, present, or future physical or mental health or condition of an individual, and that identifies the person.

inductive reasoning Reasoning from the specific to the general in which particular instances are observed and then combined into a larger whole or general statement. It involves observing a connection or pattern and then attempting to derive a general explanation of that pattern.

inference Use of inductive reasoning to move from a specific case to a general truth. Inference is one basis of the qualitative analysis process. It is also the basis of inferential statistics used in quantitative research.

inferential statistics Statistics designed to allow inference from a sample statistic to a population parameter; commonly used to test hypotheses of similarities and differences in subsets of the sample under study.

informed consent Prospective subject's agreement to participate voluntarily in a study, which is reached after the subject assimilates essential information about the study.

institutional review Process of examining the design and methods of a proposed study for ethical considerations and also for overseeing studies in progress. Institutional review is undertaken by an independent committee of peers at an institution to determine the extent to which the proposed study protects the rights of subjects.

institutional review board (IRB) The committee of peers that reviews research to ensure that the investigator conducts the research ethically. Universities, hospital corporations, and many managed care centers maintain IRBs for the purpose of promoting the conduct of ethical research and protecting the rights of prospective subjects at their institutions.

instrumentation A component of measurement that involves the application of specific rules to develop a measurement device or instrument. Also, a threat to internal validity that exists when changes to an instrument, to its calibration, or to the way in which it is used occur while a study is in progress.

integration Making connections among ideas, theories, and experience.

intention to treat An analysis based on the principle that participant data are analyzed according to the groups into which they were randomly assigned regardless of whether or not they complete the study.

interaction of different treatments A threat to construct validity in which two independent variables are tested and the interaction between them is measured inadequately.

interaction effects Threats to internal or external validity composed by the interaction of two separate threats. Examples are selection of subjects and treatment, setting and treatment, or history and treatment.

intercept In regression analysis, the point at which the regression line crosses (or intercepts) the *y*-axis. The intercept is represented by the letter *a.*

internal consistency reliability Type of reliability testing used with multiple-item scales that addresses the correlation of the items within an instrument to determine the consistency of the scale in measuring a study variable. Also referred to as *homogeneity reliability.*

internal validity The degree to which measured relationships among variables are truly due to their interaction and the degree to which other intrusive variables might have accounted for the measured value.

interpretation of research outcomes In quantitative research, the formal process by which a researcher considers the results of data analysis within contexts of previous research in the area, representativeness of the sample, usefulness within nursing, and state of the body of knowledge. In qualitative research, the researcher's understanding of the meaning of the results of research and the research's usefulness in the context of existing knowledge.

interrater reliability Degree of consistency between two or more raters who independently assign ratings or interpretations to a variable, factor of interest, attribute, behavior, or other phenomenon being investigated.

interval data Numerical information that has equal distances between value points. Interval data are mutually exclusive and exhaustive, and they are artificial in that they are obtained through artificial measurement instruments, such as scales, or devices with arbitrary values, such as a thermometer. Interval data are analyzed with parametric statistics.

interval estimate The researcher's approximation of the range of probable values of a population parameter.

interval level of measurement A measurement that exists at the interval level. See *interval data.*

intervening variable A variable that occurs between the independent variable and the dependent variable and whose existence explains the relationship between them. An intervening variable, unlike a mediating variable, is often a psychological construct.

intervention fidelity Reliable and competent implementation of an experimental treatment that includes two core components: (1) adherence to the delivery of the prescribed treatment behaviors, session, or course and (2) competence in the researcher's or interventionalist's skill in the administration of the intervention.

interventional research Research that examines causation by means of an intervention administered to the subjects and a subsequent measure of its effects. Interventional research may be experimental or quasi-experimental.

interventions In research, treatments, therapies, procedures, or actions that are implemented to determine their outcomes. In healthcare practice, interventions are actions implemented by professionals to and with patients, in a particular situation, to promote beneficial health outcomes.

interview Structured or unstructured verbal communication between the researcher and subject during which information is obtained for a study.

introspection Process of turning one's attention inward, toward thoughts and feelings, to provide increased awareness and understanding of their flow and interplay.

intuition Insight or understanding of a situation or event as a whole that usually cannot be logically explained. It is reasoning-free knowledge, claimed to lack support from data.

invasion of privacy Ethical violation of an individual's right to privacy that occurs when private information is shared without that individual's knowledge or against his or her will.

inverse linear relationship See *negative linear relationship.*

investigator-initiated research proposal Research proposal in which the principal investigator identifies a significant problem, develops a study to examine it, and submits a proposal for the study to the appropriate federal funding agency.

Iowa Model of Evidence-Based Practice Model developed in 1994 and revised in 2001 by Titler and colleagues to promote evidence-based practice in clinical agencies. The most current revision and validation of the Iowa Model was published in 2017 by the Iowa Model Collaborative.

iteration A term used in mathematics and statistics that refers to repeating sequential operations, using early solutions in subsequent calculations. In research, iteration refers to the ongoing process of revision of both design and methods while research is still in the planning stages and to revision of interpretation during the latter phases of a study.

J

justice, principle of Ethical principle that states that human subjects should be treated fairly, as groups and as individuals.

K

key informants Participants in ethnographical studies whom the researcher purposely chooses for in-depth data collection because they are both knowledgeable about the culture and articulate.

keywords Major concepts or variables that may be used in literature searches to find relevant references. Keywords or terms can be identified by determining the concepts, the populations of particular interest, interventions, measurement methods, and possible outcomes for the study.

knowledge Essential content or body of information for a discipline that is acquired through traditions, authority, borrowing, trial and error, personal experience, role-modeling and mentorship, intuition, reasoning, and research. It is expected to be an accurate representation of reality.

Kolmogorov-Smirnov two-sample test Nonparametric test used to determine whether two independent samples have been drawn from the same population.

kurtosis Degree of peakedness (platykurtic, mesokurtic, or leptokurtic) of the curve shape that is related to the spread or variance of scores.

L

landmark studies Published research that led to an important development or a turning point in a certain field of study.

Landmark studies are well known by individuals in a specialty area, representing a change in conceptualization.

language bias Bias that may affect meta-analyses and reviews when the search includes articles written in only one language, such as English, when important studies are written in other languages, as well.

legally authorized representative In research, an individual or group authorized under applicable law to consent on behalf of a prospective participant to the procedures involved in the research.

leptokurtic Term used to describe an extremely peaked-shape distribution of a curve, which means that the scores in the distribution are similar and have limited variance.

level of significance See *alpha* (α).

levels of measurement Scheme of hierarchical differentiation denoting the type of information inherent, and degree of precision, in a given measurement. The four levels, from low to high, are nominal (differentiation by names, not amounts), ordinal (differentiation by general magnitude), interval (differentiation by total number assigned by scale or by artificial numbering that uses whole numbers), and ratio (differentiation by the real number scale).

Likert scale Instrument designed to determine the opinion or attitude of a subject; it contains a number of declarative statements with a scale after each statement.

limitations Aspects of a study that decrease the generalizability of the findings and conclusions or restrict the population to which findings can be generalized. Limitations are based on the design's validity. Construct validity-based limitations, sometimes called *theoretical limitations*, relate to faulty operationalization of variables or faulty execution of the study. Other limitations are embedded in the study's methods or design and are termed *methodological limitations*.

line of best fit The regression line drawn schematically that best fits all paired variable values. The line of best fit is represented by the regression equation.

line graphs Graphical representations of point variable values joined by lines. A line graph may represent two different variables, or one variable over time, or one variable value and its frequency.

linear relationship Numerical relationship between two variables in which the values are proportional to one another, in which the formula $y = ax + b$ remains true for all variable values, and which is represented graphically by a straight line.

literature review See *review of relevant literature.*

location bias Bias that may affect meta-analyses and systematic reviews in which the search retrieves studies only in high-impact journals and commonly-searched databases.

logic A branch of philosophy based on the study of valid reasoning. Also used to refer to valid reasoning and is inclusive of both abstract and concrete thinking.

logical positivism The branch of philosophy on which the scientific method is based. Logical positivists consider empirical discovery the only dependable source of knowledge. Quantitative research emerged from logical positivism.

longitudinal designs Noninterventional research in which data are collected on several occasions in order to examine change in a variable over time within a defined group.

low statistical power Power to detect relationships or differences that is below the acceptable standard power (0.8) needed to conduct a study. Low statistical power increases the likelihood of a Type II error.

M

manipulation The quantitative researcher's action of changing the value of the independent variable in order to measure its effect on the dependent variable.

Mann-Whitney *U* test A statistical test conducted to determine whether two samples with nonparametric data are from the same population.

matching Technique by which subjects for a control or comparison group are purposively selected from a larger pool on the basis of their demographic similarity to the experimental group. This process results in dependent or related groups.

maturation The threat to internal validity in which normal changes that occur because of the passage of time affect the value of the dependent variable. An example of this might be improvement in gross motor task performance over a seven-hour testing period.

mean Statistical measure of central tendency used with ratio-level and interval-level data. The mean is the arithmetic average of all of the values of a variable, calculated by dividing the sum of all the values by the total number of data points.

mean deviation Statistical measure of dispersion used with ratio-level and interval-level data. The mean deviation is the average magnitude of the difference between the mean and each individual score, using the absolute values.

mean difference A standard statistic that is calculated to determine the absolute difference between the means of two groups.

measurement Process of assigning values to objects, events, or situations in accord with some rule. The measurement method in quantitative research is determined by a concept's operational definition.

measurement error Difference between what exists in reality and what is measured by a research instrument.

measures of central tendency Statistical procedures (mode, median, and mean) calculated to determine the center of a distribution of scores.

measures of dispersion Statistical procedures (range, difference scores, sum of squares, variance, and standard deviation) conducted to determine the degree of distance between values in a set and their mean or median.

median Score at the exact center of an ungrouped frequency distribution. The median is the middle value; if the number of data points is even, the median value is the average of the two middle values.

mediating variables Variables that occur as intermediate links between independent and dependent variables. Often, they provide insight into the proposed relationship between cause and effect.

memo A reminder written by a qualitative researcher that contains insights or ideas related to data and pertinent to data analysis.

mentor Someone who serves as a teacher, sponsor, guide, exemplar, or counsellor for a novice or protégé. For example, an expert nurse serves as a guide or role model for a novice nurse or mentee.

mentorship Intense form of role-modeling in which a more experienced person works with a less experienced person to impart information about a new skill or way of being.

mesokurtic Term that describes a normal curve with an intermediate degree of kurtosis and intermediate variance of scores.

meta-analysis A technique that statistically pools data and results from several studies into a single quantitative analysis that provides one of the highest levels of evidence for practice. The studies in the pool all must share a similar design.

metasummary, qualitative Description of findings across qualitative reports performed in order to determine the current knowledge in an area.

metasynthesis, qualitative Integration of qualitative study findings that provides a novel description or explanation of a target event or experience versus a summary view of that event or experience. Metasynthesis requires more complex, integrative thought than does metasummary in developing a new perspective or theory based on the findings of previous qualitative studies.

method of least squares Procedure in regression analysis for developing the line of best fit.

methodological congruence The extent to which the methods of a qualitative study are consistent with the philosophical tradition and qualitative approach identified by the researchers.

methodology, research The general type of the research selected to answer the research question: quantitative research, qualitative research, outcomes research, or mixed methods research.

methods, research The specific ways in which the researcher chooses to conduct the study, within the chosen design. Methods include subject selection, choice of setting, attempts to limit factors that might introduce error, the manner in which a research intervention is strategized, ways in which data are collected, and choice of statistical tests.

metric ordinal scale Scale that has unequal intervals; its use in data collection yields ordinal-level data.

middle-range theory A theory that is less abstract than and addresses more specific phenomena than does a grand theory; that is directly applicable to practice; and that focuses on explanation and implementation. Often, a middle-range theory provides the conceptual framework for a quantitative research study. Also known as *practice theory.*

minimal risk Studies in which the potential for harm is not greater than what a person might encounter in everyday life or in routine health care.

mixed methods approach A research methodology in which two types of data are collected to better represent truth. The vast majority of mixed methods studies combine a quantitative design with a qualitative design.

mixed methods research synthesis A synthesis of studies, having more than one methodology, conducted in order to determine the current knowledge in a problem area.

mixed results When more than one relationship or difference is examined, study results that are contradictory, such as opposite results of the effect of an independent variable.

mode Numerical value or score that occurs with the greatest frequency in a distribution. The mode does not necessarily indicate the center of the data set.

model-testing design Correlational research, such as structural equation modeling and path analysis, that measures proposed relationships within a theoretical model.

moderator A facilitator for a focus group, preferably one who reflects the age, gender, and race/ethnicity of the group members. The moderator, if not a member of the research team, must understand the purpose of the study and be trained to promote interaction.

modifying variable Variable that alters the strength and occasionally the direction of the relationship between other variables.

monographs Books, booklets of conference proceedings, or pamphlets, which are written and published for a specific purpose and may be updated with a new edition, as needed.

monomethod bias A threat to construct validity in which the dependent variable is measured in several similar ways, for instance by use of three self-assessment instruments to measure life stress.

mono-operation bias A threat to construct validity in which a given variable, especially a complex one like pain, is measured in only one way.

multicollinearity The case in which independent variables in a regression equation are strongly correlated with one another, making generalizability difficult.

multidimensional scaling A measurement method that was developed to examine many aspects or elements of a concept or variable and that results in a spatial representation with three or more dimensions.

multimethod-multitrait technique A method for assessing construct validity in which the concepts in a study are measured in multiple ways to assess both the convergent and divergent validity of the testing methods.

multimodal A distribution of two or more scores selected equally by the highest number of participants.

multiple regression analysis A regression analysis of three of more variables and their interactions. Extension of simple linear regression with more than one independent variable entered into the analysis.

N

narrative analysis Qualitative approach that uses stories as its data. The narratives that comprise the data may originate from interviews, informal conversations, and field notes, as well as from tangible sources, such as journals and letters.

natural settings Settings in which data are collected without any attempts by the researcher to control for the effects of extraneous variables.

necessary relationship One variable or concept must occur in order for a second variable or concept to occur.

negative likelihood ratio Ratio of true-negative results to false-negative results; is calculated as follows: Negative likelihood ratio = (100% − Sensitivity) ÷ Specificity.

negative linear relationship A statistical finding in which as one variable or concept changes, the other variable or concept changes in the opposite direction, and both occur according to the standard regression formula of $y = ax + b$. It is also referred to as an inverse *linear relationship*.

negative results See *nonsignificant results*.

negatively skewed An asymmetry in a data set in which, instead of a bell curve shape, the resultant shape is more elongated on the left side. This means that the smaller values are further from the mean than the larger values, but the majority of data points are larger than the mean.

network sampling Nonprobability sampling method in which the first subjects are obtained through convenience or purposive sampling and the remainder of the subjects are recruited through assistance or suggestions made by the initial subjects. Network sampling is synonymous with *chain sampling* and *snowball sampling*.

networking Process of developing channels of communication among people with common interests.

nominal data Lowest level of data that can be organized into exclusive and exhaustive categories but the categories cannot be compared or rank-ordered. These data are analyzed using nonparametric statistical techniques. Also called *categorical data*.

nominal level of measurement Lowest level of measurement that is used when data can be organized into categories that are exclusive and exhaustive, but the categories cannot be compared or rank-ordered, such as gender, race, marital status, and diagnosis. See *nominal data*.

nondirectional hypothesis States that a relationship exists but does not predict the exact direction of the relationship, positive versus negative.

noninterventional research Studies in which researchers observe, measure, or test subjects, but do not enact experimental interventions. Within quantitative research, correlational studies and descriptive studies are noninterventional types of designs.

nonparametric statistical analyses Statistical techniques used when one or both of the first two assumptions of parametric statistics cannot be met: normal distribution and data that are at least at the interval level of measurement.

nonprobability sampling Nonrandom sampling technique in which not every element of the population has an opportunity for selection in the sample, such as convenience (accidental) sampling, quota sampling, purposive sampling, and network sampling.

nonsignificant results Study results not strong enough to reach statistical significance: the null hypothesis cannot be rejected. Nonsignificant results are synonymous with negative results.

nontherapeutic research Research conducted to generate knowledge for a discipline and in which the results from the study might benefit future patients but will probably not benefit those acting as research subjects.

normal curve A symmetrical, unimodal bell-shaped curve that is a theoretical distribution of all possible scores but is rarely seen in real data sets. The normal curve is also called a *bell curve* because of its shape.

normally distributed Distribution of data points that follows the spread or distribution of a normal curve.

norm-referenced testing A type of evaluation that yields an estimate of the performance of the tested individual in comparison to the performance of a large set of other individuals on whom the test was "normed."

null hypothesis A hypothesis that is the opposite of the research hypothesis, stating there is no significant difference between study groups or no significant relationship among the variables. The null hypothesis is tested during data analysis and is used for interpreting statistical outcomes.

Nuremberg Code Ethical code of conduct developed in 1949 after the trial for Nazi researchers. The code's purpose is to guide investigators conducting research.

Nursing Care Report Card A set of nurse-sensitive quality indicators that were developed in 1994 to evaluate hospital nursing care. Its purpose is to facilitate benchmarking and comparison of nursing care among hospitals.

nursing interventions Deliberative cognitive, physical, or verbal actions performed with or on behalf of individuals and their families to accomplish particular therapeutic objectives relative to health and well-being. Nursing interventions are tested in quasi-experimental and experimental nursing studies.

nursing research Formal inquiry through quantitative, qualitative, outcomes, or mixed methods research that validates and refines existing knowledge and generates new knowledge that directly and indirectly influences the delivery of evidence-based nursing practice.

nursing-sensitive patient outcomes Patient outcomes that are influenced by or associated with nursing care.

O

observation Collection of data through listening, smelling, touching, and seeing, with an emphasis on what is seen.

observational checklist A form used to collect observational data on which a tally mark is used to count each occurrence of a listed behavior.

observational measurement Use of structured and unstructured observations to quantify study variables.

observed score Actual score or value obtained for a subject on a measurement tool. Observed score = true score + random error.

odds ratio (*OR*) The ratio of the odds of an event occurring in one group, such as the treatment group, to the odds of it occurring in another group, such as the standard care or control group.

one-group pretest-posttest design A quasi-experimental design in which subjects act as their own controls, with data collected before and after the intervention. Because it exerts almost no control over the effects of extraneous variables, interpretation of results is difficult.

one-tailed test of significance Analysis used with directional hypotheses in which extreme statistical values of interest are hypothesized to occur in a single tail of the distribution curve.

one-way chi-square A statistic that compares the distribution of a nominal-level variable with expected probability statistics for random occurrence.

operational definition Description of how concepts will be measured in a study, essentially converting them to variables.

operational reasoning Involves identification and discrimination among many alternatives or viewpoints and focuses on the process of debating alternatives.

operationalizing a variable or concept Establishing a description of how a variable or concept will be measured.

operator In a computer search, a set of directions that permits grouping of ideas, selection of places to search in a database record, and ways to show relationships within a database record, sentence, or paragraph. The most common operators are Boolean, locational, and positional.

operator, Boolean The three words AND, OR, and NOT are used with the researcher's identified concepts in conducting searches of databases.

operator, locational Search operator that identifies terms in specific areas or fields of a record, such as article title, author, and journal name.

operator, positional Search operator used to look for requested terms within certain distance of one another. Common positional operators are NEAR, WITH, and ADJ.

ordinal data Data that can be ranked, with intervals between the ranks that are not necessarily equal. Ordinal data are analyzed using nonparametric statistical techniques.

ordinal level measurement Measurement that yields ordinal or ranked data, such as levels of coping. See *ordinal data.*

outcome reporting bias Type of bias that occurs when study results are not reported clearly and with complete accuracy.

outcomes of care The dependent variables or clinical results of health care that are measured to determine quality. The outcomes from the Medical Outcomes Study Framework include clinical end points, functional status, general well-being, and satisfaction with care.

outcomes research Research that examines quality of care, as quantified by selected outcomes. It utilizes predominantly noninterventional quantitative designs from epidemiology, as well as other disciplines.

outliers Extreme scores or values in a set of data that are exceptions to the overall findings.

out-of-pocket costs Those expenses incurred by the patient, family, or both that are not reimbursed by the insurance company and might include noncovered expenses, copayments, cost of travel to and from care, and the costs of buying supplies, dressings, selected medications, or special foods.

P

paired or dependent samples Samples that are related or matched in some way. See *dependent groups.*

paired or dependent samples *t*-test Parametric statistical test conducted to examine differences between dependent groups. The groups are dependent in repeated measures and case-control designs and when participants in two groups are matched for relevant characteristics or variables. See *independent samples* t-test.

paradigm A set of philosophical or theoretical concepts that characterizes a particular way of viewing the world.

parallel-forms reliability See *alternate-forms reliability.*

parameter The measure or numerical value of a characteristic of a population.

parametric statistical analyses Statistical techniques used when three assumptions are met: (1) the sample was drawn from a population for which the variance can be calculated, and the distribution is expected to be normal or approximately normal, (2) the level of measurement is interval or ratio, with an approximately normal distribution, and (3) the data can be treated as though they were obtained from random samples.

paraphrasing Restating an author's ideas in other words that capture the meaning. Paraphrasing implies understanding and, consequently, is preferred to direct quotation for theoretical content that is part of a scholarly paper.

partially controlled setting A naturalistic environment that the researcher modifies temporarily in order to control for the effects of extraneous variables. Partially controlled settings are the most prevalent settings of experimental and quasi-experimental nursing research.

participant observation A form of observation used in qualitative research in which researchers either are already participants in a society or culture or they become participants in order to provide the insider view.

participants Individuals who participate in qualitative and quantitative research; also referred to as *subjects* in quantitative research. In ethnographical research, participants may also be called *informants*.

partitioning Strategy in which a researcher analyzes subjects according to a variable that can be regarded as dichotomous (smoking versus nonsmoking) but actually has a number of different values (number of years smoked x packs per day). Partitioning provides more nuanced results than would be obtained from a dichotomously defined variable.

path analysis In a proposed model, the diagrammed relationships among pairs of variables, in which each is tested for its strength and direction, yielding a correlational value.

patient Someone who has gained access to care in a given healthcare setting.

pattern A repeated word, phrase, or occurrence. In qualitative data, a pattern may indicate similarities across participants and may be identified as an emergent concept or theme.

Pearson's product-moment correlation coefficient (r) Parametric statistical test conducted to determine the linear relationship between two variables, both of which must be at the ratio or interval level.

percentage distribution Indicates the percentage of the sample with scores falling within a specific group or range.

percentage of variance Amount of variability explained by a linear relationship; the value is obtained by squaring Pearson's product-moment correlation coefficient (r). For example, if $r = 0.5$ in a study, the percentage of variance explained is $r^2 = 0.25$, or 25%.

periodicals Subset of serials with predictable publication dates, such as journals that are published over time and are numbered sequentially for the years published.

permission to participate in a study Agreement of parents or guardians that their child or ward of the state can be a subject in a study.

personal experience Gaining knowledge by being individually or personally involved in an event, situation, or circumstance.

phenomenological research Inductive, descriptive qualitative methodology developed from phenomenological philosophy. Conducted for the purpose of describing experiences as they are lived by the study participants and, often, the meaning of such experiences to the participants.

phenomenon (singular) Literally, a happening. In research, often means an idea or concept of interest (plural: phenomena).

phenomenon of interest The central topic of a quantitative, qualitative, outcomes, or mixed methods study. Also known as the *phenomenon*, the *study focus*, the *concept of interest*, and the *central issue*, among other terms.

philosophy Broad, global explanation of the world that provides a framework within which thinking, knowing, and doing occur. In nursing research, the overriding philosophical perspective that determines how reality is viewed, what is knowable, and how research is conducted.

photovoice A qualitative research method that uses images taken by participants as data for analysis.

physiological measures Techniques and equipment used to measure physiological variables either directly or indirectly, such as techniques to measure heart rate or mean arterial pressure.

PICOS or PICO Format An acronym for Population or participants of interest; Intervention needed for practice; Comparisons of the intervention with control, placebo, standard care, variations of the same intervention, or different therapies; Outcomes needed for practice; and Study design. PICOS is one of the most common formats used to delimit a relevant clinical question.

pilot study Smaller-sample version of a proposed study conducted with the same research population, setting, intervention, and plans for data collection and analysis. The purpose of a pilot study is to determine whether the proposed methods are effective in locating and consenting subjects, in collecting useful data, and in providing adequate data for analysis.

placebo In pharmacology, a substance without discernible effect, administered in research studies to the control group. Broadly, an intervention intended to have no effect.

plagiarism Type of research misconduct that involves the appropriation of another person's ideas, processes, results, or words without giving appropriate credit, including those obtained through confidential review of others' research proposals and manuscripts.

platykurtic Term that indicates a relatively flat curve and a large variance for the set of scores.

population The particular group of elements (individuals, objects, events, or substances) that is the focus of a study.

population-based studies Cohort studies conducted so as to discover information about an entire population. In epidemiology and health fields, such studies often are conducted after the occurrence of an event that affects health, such as a treatment, an outbreak, or an exposure. Also referred to as *population studies*.

population parameter A true but unknown numerical characteristic of a population. Parameters of the population are estimated with statistics.

position paper A formal essay authored by an individual or group and disseminated in order to present an opinion or viewpoint regarding an issue of debate or disagreement. Position papers often are disseminated by professional organizations and government agencies to represent that agency's position on an issue.

positive likelihood ratio Ratio calculated to determine the likelihood that a positive test result is a true positive. Positive Likelihood Ratio = Sensitivity ÷ (100% − Specificity).

positive linear relationship A numerical relationship between two variables such that as one variable changes (value of the variable increases or decreases), the other variable will change in the same direction.

post hoc tests (Latin for *after this one*). Statistical tests developed specifically to determine the location of differences in studies with more than two groups. They are performed after an initial test demonstrates a difference. When performed after an ANOVA to pinpoint location of differences, frequently-used post hoc tests are Bonferroni's procedure, the Newman-Keuls test, the Tukey Honestly Significant Difference (HSD) test, the Scheffé test, and Dunnett's test. Also called *post hoc analyses.*

poster session A time during a professional conference when the results of selected studies are visually presented, usually on a two-dimensional surface, and include text, pictures, and illustrations. Other topics of general interest to conference attendees may also be presented in this way.

posttest-only control group design An experimental design in which there is no preintervention measurement of the value of the dependent variable in either the experimental group or the control group.

posttest-only design with comparison group Quasi-experimental study, conducted to examine the difference between the experimental group that receives a treatment and the comparison group that does not. The design provides very poor control for threats to internal validity; however, with a very strong comparison group and concurrent data collection, the design can generate useful information about causation.

posttest-only design with comparison to norms A quasi-experimental design in which the results of an intervention in a single group are compared with average population values.

power Probability that a statistical test will detect a significant difference or relationship if one exists, which is the capacity to correctly reject a null hypothesis.

power analysis Statistical test conducted before a study to determine the risk of Type II error so that the study can be modified to decrease the risk, if necessary. Conducting a power analysis uses alpha (level of significance), effect size, and standard power of 0.8 to determine the sample size for a study. Because effect size of an intervention varies from study to study, a power analysis often is conducted after a study when nonsignificant results are obtained to determine the actual power of the analysis.

practice pattern The pattern of *what* care is provided by a certain healthcare professional. Practice pattern is a term usually applied to physicians' practices, but it can refer to usual nursing care that is provided on a hospital unit or in a clinic setting.

practice pattern profiling Epidemiological technique used in outcomes research that focuses on patterns of care rather than individual occurrences of care. Practice pattern profiling was originally used to compare outcomes of physicians' practice patterns with one another, usually in the same type of practice and in the same region or specialty, and it may include patterns of referrals and resource utilization, as well. Practice pattern profiling now also includes comparisons among types of healthcare providers, such as advanced practice nurses and physician assistants.

practice style The pattern of *how* care is provided. This includes the skill of a practitioner in interpersonal relationships in such aptitudes as communication skills. Practice style is part of the construct *processes of care* from Donabedian's theory of health care.

precision In general, a high degree of exactness with a small amount of variability. In statistics, accuracy with which the population parameters have been estimated within a study. Also used to describe the degree of consistency or reproducibility of data collected using physiological instruments.

prediction The offering of an opinion or guess about an unknown or future event, amount, outcome, or result. In statistics, a part of the process of inference.

predictive design Correlational design used to establish strength and direction of relationships between or among variables. Predictive correlational research is often the prelude to construction of a theoretical model.

predictive validity A type of criterion-related instrument validity reflecting the extent to which an individual's score on a scale or instrument can be used to predict future performance or behavior on a criterion.

premise In research, a statement that identifies the proposed relationship between two or more variables or concepts. In a logical argument, a proposition from which a conclusion is drawn.

preproposal Short document (usually four to five pages plus appendices) written to explore the funding possibilities for a research project.

presentation A formal report of research findings made at a professional meeting or conference either orally as a podium presentation or visually as a poster presentation.

pretest-posttest control group design A experimental design in which, after random assignment to group, the intervention is applied to the experimental group, and both experimental and control groups are measured (tested) before and after the intervention so that the effect of the intervention can be measured. It is often called the *classic experimental design.*

pretest-posttest design with nonrandom control group A quasi-experimental design in which the intervention is applied to the experimental group, and both experimental and control groups are measured (tested) before and after the intervention so that the effect of the intervention can be measured. This design is essentially the pretest-posttest control group design without random assignment to experimental/control group.

primary source Source that is written by the person who originated or is responsible for generating the ideas published.

principal investigator (PI) The researcher who takes the major responsibility for developing the research proposal, the execution of the study, and the writing of the research report. When multiple authors' names appear in a published report, the first author is usually the PI. In a research grant, the PI is the individual who will have primary responsibility for administering the grant and interacting with the funding agency. Also *primary investigator*.

privacy In research, the freedom of an individual to determine the time, extent, and general circumstances under which personal information will be shared with or withheld from others.

probability Likelihood. In statistics, probability refers to the percentage of chance that the result of a certain statistical test performed with a sample actually represents the population from which the sample was drawn.

probability distributions Distributions of values for different statistical analysis techniques, such as tables of r values for Pearson product-moment correlation, t values for t-test, or F values for analysis of variance. Some common probability distribution tables are found in the appendices of this text.

probability sampling method Any random sampling technique in which each member (element) in the population has a greater than zero opportunity to be selected for the sample. The four types of probability sampling described in this text are simple random sampling, stratified random sampling, cluster sampling, and systematic sampling.

probability theory The branch of mathematics and statistics that addresses likelihood of occurrence and, in research, the likelihood that the findings or statistics of a sample are the same as the population parameters.

probing The act of posing secondary questions or questions during a qualitative interview so that the researcher can elicit contextual detail, clarification, and additional information.

problem statement The statement that briefly synopsizes the state of the research and identifies the gap in research knowledge. Therefore the problem statement identifies the main concepts upon which the study will focus.

problematic reasoning Involves identifying a problem, selecting solutions to the problem, and resolving the problem.

process of care Construct that includes the actual care delivered by healthcare persons, both in a technical sense and in relation to patient–practitioner interactions with patients. Process of care is one of the three components (structure, process, and outcomes of care) of Donabedian's theory of quality of health care.

project grant proposal An application for a nonresearch grant to develop a new education program or implement an idea in clinical practice.

proportionate sampling A sampling strategy wherein subjects are selected from various strata so that their proportions are identical to those of the population.

proposal, research Written plan identifying the major elements of a study, such as the problem, purpose, and framework, and outlining the methods to conduct the study. The research proposal is written to request approval to conduct a study; also, a request for funding must be accompanied by a research proposal.

proposition Abstract, formal statement of the relationship between or among concepts.

prospective Looking forward in time. In data collection, refers to measurements made during the course of a study. Prospective is the opposite of retrospective.

prospective cohort study A study that uses a longitudinal design, either descriptive or correlational, in which a researcher identifies a group of persons at risk for a certain event, with data collection occurring at intervals. The prospective cohort study originated in the field of epidemiology.

protection from discomfort and harm A right of research participants based on the ethical principle of beneficence, which holds that one should do good and, above all, do no harm. The levels of discomfort and harm are (1) no anticipated effects, (2) temporary discomfort, (3) unusual levels of temporary discomfort, (4) risk of permanent damage, and (5) certainty of permanent damage.

providers of care Individuals responsible for delivering care, such as nurse practitioners and physicians, who are part of the structures of care of Donabedian's theory of health care.

publication bias Bias that occurs when studies with positive results are more likely to be published than studies with negative or inconclusive results.

published research Studies that are permanently recorded in hard copies of journals, monographs, conference proceedings, or books, or are posted online for readers to access.

purposive sampling Judgmental or selective sampling method that involves conscious selection by the researcher of certain subjects or elements to include in a study. Purposive sampling is a type of nonprobability or nonrandom sampling.

Q

Q-sort methodology Technique of comparative ratings in which a subject sorts cards with statements on them into designated piles (usually 7–10 piles in the distribution of a normal curve) that might range from best to worst. Q-sort methodology might be conducted to identify important items when developing a scale or for determining research priorities in specialty nursing areas.

qualitative research A scholarly and rigorous approach used to describe life experiences, cultures, and social processes from the perspectives of the persons involved.

qualitative research proposal A document developed by the researcher of a proposed qualitative study that often includes an introduction, a review of the literature, the philosophical foundation for the selected approach, and identification of the method of inquiry.

qualitative research reports The written report of the results of qualitative inquiry intended to describe the dynamic implementation of the research project and the unique, creative findings obtained. The report usually includes introduction, review of the literature, methods, results, and discussion sections.

qualitative research synthesis Process and product of systematically reviewing and formally integrating the findings from qualitative studies. Qualitative research synthesis produces either metasummary or metasynthesis.

quantitative research Formal, objective, systematic study process that counts or measures in order to answer a research question. Its data are analyzed numerically.

quantitative research proposal A document developed by the researcher of a proposed quantitative study that often includes the introduction, review of the literature, framework, and methodology proposed for the study.

quantitative research report A written report that includes an introduction, review of the literature, methods, results, and a discussion of findings for a quantitative study.

quasi-experimental research Type of quantitative research conducted to test a cause-and-effect relationship but which lacks one or more of the four essential elements of experimental research: (1) rigorously implemented intervention, (2) a control group, (3) random assignment of subjects to groups, and (4) attenuation of threats to design validity.

query letter Letter sent to an editor of a journal to ask about the editor's interest in reviewing a manuscript.

questionnaire Self-report form designed to elicit information that can be obtained through the subject's selection from a list of predetermined options or through textual responses of the subject.

quota sampling Nonprobability convenience sampling technique in which the proportion of identified groups is predetermined by the researcher. Quota sampling may be used to ensure the inclusion of subject types likely to be underrepresented in the convenience sample, such as women, minority groups, and the undereducated, or to constitute the sample in order to achieve some sort of representativeness.

R

random assignment to groups Procedure used to assign subjects to the treatment or control group in which each subject has an equal opportunity to be assigned to either group.

random error Error that causes individuals' observed scores to vary haphazardly around the true score without a pattern.

random heterogeneity of participants The threat to design validity that exists when subjects in a treatment or intervention group differ in ways that correlate with the dependent variable.

random sampling methods See *probability sampling method.*

random variation Normally-occurring and expected difference in values that occurs when one examines different subjects from the same sample.

randomization Term used in medical and biological research that is equivalent to random assignment.

randomized controlled trial (RCT) A study of an intervention using the pretest-posttest control group design, or another experimental design closely related to it,

in order to produce definitive evidence for an intervention. It is considered the gold standard for interventional testing in health care. An RCT may be single-site or multisite.

range Simplest measure of dispersion, obtained by subtracting the lowest score from the highest score ("range of 63") or by identifying the lowest and highest scores in a distribution of scores ("range from 118 to 181").

rating scales A method of measurement in which the rater or the research subject assigns a value, sometimes numeric and sometimes not, from among an ordered set of predefined categories. A rating scale can be used to measure quantitative information, such as frequency, size, and level of activity, or perceptive/emotional information, such as feelings and preferences. FACES Pain Rating Scale is a commonly used rating scale to measure pain in pediatric patients.

ratio data Numerical information based on the real number scale. Ratio data are mutually exclusive and mutually exhaustive, and they are real in that they represent actual quanta and are capable of representing values between the numerals such as fractions and decimals. Ratio data are analyzed with parametric statistics.

ratio level of measurement The highest level of measurement. As such, it meets all the rules of other levels of measurement: mutually exclusive categories, exhaustive categories, rank ordering, equal spacing between intervals, and a continuum of values; also it has an absolute zero, such as measurement of weight. See *ratio data.*

readability The degree of difficulty with which a text may be read and comprehended, often applied to a scale or survey instrument. Most available readability tools are based on the length of phrases or sentences and the number of syllables in the words of the scale. The readability of a scale can influence its reliability and validity when used in a study.

reasoning Processing and organizing ideas to reach conclusions. Some types of reasoning described in this text are problematic, operational, dialectic, and logistical.

recommendations for further research An objective assessment of the state of the current research-generated body of knowledge in a discipline based on the findings of the current study and a review of the literature

and the logical steps subsequent researchers might take in the future in order to expand that knowledge. Based on the limitations of the research, recommendations may also include suggestions for subsequent refinements to the research design and methods.

recruiting research participants The process of obtaining subjects or participants for a study that includes identifying potential subjects, approaching them to participate in the study, and gaining their agreement to participate.

refereed journal Publication that is peer-reviewed, using expert reviewers (referees) to determine whether a manuscript is suitable for publication in that particular journal.

reference group In research, the group of individuals or other elements that constitutes the standard against which individual subjects' scores are compared. In sociology, the group of people with whom one makes self-comparison, whether or not one considers oneself to be part of that group.

referencing Comparing a subject's score against a standard, which is used in norm-referenced and criterion-referenced testing.

reflexivity A qualitative researcher's introspective self-awareness and critical examination of the interaction between self and the data during data collection and analysis. Reflexivity may lead the researcher to explore personal feelings and experiences that could introduce bias into the data analysis process.

refusal rate Percentage of potential subjects who decide not to participate in a study. The refusal rate is calculated by dividing the number refusing to participate by the number of potential subjects approached. For example, if 100 subjects are approached and 15 refuse to participate, the refusal rate is $(15 \div 100) \times 100\% = 0.15 \times 100\% = 15\%$.

regression analysis Analysis by which the statistical relationship between or among variables is measured and characterized. The independent (predictor) variable or variables are analyzed to determine the influence upon variation or change in the value of the dependent variable.

regression equation Outcome of regression analysis, whereby a formula or equation is developed to predict a dependent variable.

regression line Line that best represents the linear relationship between two variables and may be depicted amidst the values of the raw scores plotted on a scatter diagram.

relational statement Explanation of the connection between or among concepts. Within theories, relational statements also are called *propositions* and become the focus of testing in quantitative research.

relative risk A quantification of an occurrence, comparing two groups, sometimes comparing subjects in an experimental group and subjects in a control group. Relative risk is used most frequently to describe the risk associated with treated versus untreated conditions, with screening versus nonscreening, or with exposure versus nonexposure. Also referred to as *risk ratio*.

reliability The consistency of an obtained measurement. Also see *reliability testing*.

reliability testing Measure of the amount of random error in the instrument, or measurement technique, as it is used in a study. Reliability testing of measurement methods focuses on the following three aspects of reliability: stability, equivalence, and internal consistency or homogeneity.

repeated measures design A research design that repeatedly assesses or measures study variables, alternating intervention with lack of intervention, in the same group of subjects. Also referred to as a within-subjects design or a repeated reversal design.

replication The act of reproducing or repeating a study in order to determine whether similar findings will be obtained, thus assessing the possibility of Type I or Type II error in the original study and sometimes allowing extension of findings to a larger population.

replication, approximate Operational replication that involves repeating the original study under similar conditions and following the methods as closely as possible.

replication, exact A type of replication that involves precise or exact duplication of the initial researcher's study to confirm the original findings. Exact replication is an ideal, not a reality.

replication, systematic Constructive replication that is done under distinctly new conditions in which the researchers conducting the replication follow the design but not the methods of the original researchers. The goal of such replication is to extend the findings of the original study to different settings or to clients with different disease processes.

representativeness of the sample The degree to which the sample is like the population it purportedly represents.

request for applications (RFA) An opportunity for funding similar to the request for proposals (RFP), except that the government agency not only identifies the problem of concern but also describes what the goal of the research is. For example, an RFA may be released to discover the psychological characteristics of patients seeking bariatric surgery. Researchers design their own research and compete for this type of contract.

request for proposals (RFP) An opportunity for funding in which an agency within the federal government seeks proposals from researchers dealing with a specific clinical or system problem. The goal of the research is unspecified.

research Diligent, systematic inquiry or investigation, the goal of which is to validate and refine existing knowledge and generate new knowledge.

research benefit Something of health-related, psychosocial, or other value to an individual research subject or something that will contribute to the acquisition of generalizable knowledge. Assessing research benefits is part of the ethical process of balancing benefits and risks for a study.

research design See *design, research*.

research grant Funding awarded specifically for conducting a study.

research hypothesis Alternative hypothesis to the null hypothesis stating that there is a relationship or a difference between two or more variables.

research methodology See *methodology, research*.

research methods See *methods, research*.

research misconduct Deliberate fabrication, falsification, or plagiarism in processing, performing, or reviewing research or in reporting research results. Falsification does not include honest error or differences in opinion.

research objectives (or aims) The researcher's formal stated goal or goals of the study: its desired outcomes. If quantitative research has several articulated objectives or aims, each addresses the outcome of a specific statistical test or comparison.

research problem An area in which there is a gap in the knowledge base.

research proposal See *proposal, research*.

research purpose Concise, clear statement of the researcher's specific over-riding focus or aim: the reason for conducting the study.

research questions Concise, interrogative statements developed to direct research studies.

research report The written description of a completed study designed to communicate study findings efficiently and effectively to nurses and other healthcare professionals.

research topics Concepts or broad problem areas that indicate the foci of essential research knowledge needed to provide evidence-based nursing practice. Research topics include numerous potential research problems.

research utilization Process of synthesizing, disseminating, and using research-generated knowledge to make an impact on or a change in a practice discipline.

research variable or concept A default term used to refer to a variable that is the focus of a quantitative study but that is not identified as an independent or a dependent variable.

researcher–participant relationships In qualitative research, the specific interactions between the researcher and the study participants that are initiated by the researcher to establish rapport, encouraging both information exchange and communication of the participants' perceptions, feelings, and opinions.

respect for persons, principle of Ethical principle that indicates that persons have the right to self-determination and the freedom to participate or not participate in research.

response set Parameters or possible answers within which a question or item is to be answered in a questionnaire. For example, a response set for a questionnaire might include a range of options between "strongly agree" and "strongly disagree."

results Outcomes from data analysis that are generated for each research objective, question, or hypothesis.

retaining research participants Keeping subjects participating in a study and preventing their attrition. A high retention rate provides a more representative sample and decreases the threats to design validity.

retention rate The number and percentage of subjects completing a study.

retrospective Looking backward in time. In data collection, refers to measurements made in the past that are retrieved by the research team from existent records in the course of a study. Retrospective is the opposite of prospective.

retrospective study Literally a study that looks back. Retrospective research retrieves existent data and analyzes them.

review of relevant literature Synthesis of sources that are pertinent or highly important in providing the in-depth knowledge needed to synthesize the state of the body of knowledge within a problem area.

right to self-determination See *self-determination, right to.*

rigor Literally, hardness or difficulty. In research, rigor is associated with paying attention to detail and exerting unflagging effort to adhere to scientific standards. In quantitative research, rigor implies a high degree of accuracy, consistency, attention to all measurable aspects of the research, and strictly logical deductive reasoning. In qualitative research, rigor implies ensuring congruence between the philosophical foundation, qualitative approach, and methods, with the goal of using openness and flexibility to produce trustworthy and unbiased findings.

risk ratio See *relative risk.*

rival hypothesis A second hypothesis that serves as an alternate explanation for the study findings. Although the researcher may state a rival hypothesis in a research design, in nursing research the rival hypothesis usually represents a dichotomy in interpretation introduced by an extraneous variable.

role-modeling Learning by imitating the behavior of a person who is admired.

S

sample Subset of the population that is selected for a study.

sample attrition See *attrition rate.*

sample characteristics Description of the research subjects who actually participate in a study, obtained by analyzing data acquired from the measurement of their demographic variables (e.g., age, gender, ethnicity, annual income) and health information (e.g., previous history, functional status, current medical diagnosis).

sample size Number of subjects or participants who actually participate in at least the first phase of a study.

sampling Selecting groups of people, events, behaviors, or other elements with which to conduct a study.

sampling criteria List of the characteristics essential for membership in the target population (inclusion criteria), and those undesirable for membership (exclusion criteria). Sampling criteria are *not* the same as sample characteristics.

sampling error Difference between a sample statistic used to estimate a population parameter and the actual but unknown value of the parameter.

sampling frame A listing of every member of the accessible population with membership defined by the sampling criteria.

sampling method The process of selecting a group of people, events, behaviors, or other elements that meet sampling criteria. Sampling methods may be random or nonrandom.

sampling plan A description of the strategies that will be used to obtain a sample for a study. The sampling plan may include either probability or nonprobability sampling methods.

scale Form of measurement composed of several related items that are thought to measure the construct being studied. A scale may be observational or self-report. The rater or subject responds to each item on the continuum or scale provided, such as a pain perception scale, behavioral scale, or state anxiety scale.

scatter diagrams or scatterplots Graphs that provide a visual array of data points. Scatter diagrams provide a useful preliminary impression about the nature of the relationship between variables and the distribution of the data.

science Coherent body of knowledge composed of research findings, tested theories, scientific principles, and laws for a discipline.

scientific method All procedures that scientists have used, currently use, or may use in the future to pursue knowledge. "The scientific method," however, is a means of testing hypotheses, using deduction and hypothetical reasoning. It rests on the process of stating a hypothesis, testing it, and then either disproving it or testing it more fully.

scientific theory Theory with valid and reliable methods of measuring each concept and relational statements that has been tested repeatedly through research and demonstrated to be valid.

secondary analysis A strategy in which a researcher performs an analysis of data collected and originally analyzed by another researcher or agency or collected by the researcher during a prior study. It may involve the use of administrative or research databases.

secondary source Source that summarizes or quotes content from a primary source.

seeking approval to conduct a study Process that involves submission of a research proposal to an authority or group for review.

selection The process by which subjects are chosen to take part in a study.

selection threat A threat to internal validity in which subject assignment to a group occurs in a nonrandom way. Selection threat occurs most frequently because of subject self-assignment to a group or because experimental and control groups represent distinctly different populations.

selection-maturation interaction A threat to internal design validity. In a study with nonrandom group assignment, selection-maturation interaction occurs when the naturally occurring attributes change due to the passage of time but at different rates in the study groups, independent of the study treatment.

self-determination, right to A right that is based on the ethical principle of respect for persons, which states that because humans are capable of making their own decisions, they should be treated as autonomous agents who have the freedom to conduct their lives as they choose, without external controls.

seminal study Study that prompted the initiation of a field of research.

sensitivity, physiological measure The extent to which a physiological measure can detect a small change. Higher sensitivity means more precision.

sensitivity of screening or diagnostic test The ability of a screening or diagnostic test to correctly detect the presence of a disease; the proportion of patients with the disease who have a true-positive test result.

sequential relationship Relationship in which one concept occurs later than the other.

serendipitous results Research results that were not the primary focus of a study but that reveal new information that may prove useful.

serials Literature published over time or in multiple volumes at one time. Serials do not necessarily have a predictable publication date.

setting, research Location for conducting research. A research setting may be natural, partially controlled, or highly controlled.

sham Something that appears to be something it is not: a deceit. A sham intervention may be used with a control group so that the subjects perceive that they have received an intervention, such as an intravenous medication. Use of a sham intervention prevents subjects from knowing their group assignment, avoiding potential threats to construct validity.

Shapiro-Wilk *W* test A statistical test of normality that assesses whether a variable's distribution is skewed, kurtotic, or both.

significance of a problem Part of the research problem. In nursing, the significance statement expresses the importance of the problem to nursing and to the health of individuals, families, or communities.

significant and not predicted results Significant results that are the opposite of those predicted by the researcher. These also are referred to as *unexpected results*.

significant results Results of statistical analyses that are highly unlikely to have occurred by chance. Statistically significant results are those that are in keeping with the researcher's predictions, if predictions were made.

simple hypothesis A statement of the posited relationship (associative or causal) between only two variables.

simple linear regression Parametric analysis technique that provides a means to estimate the value of an outcome (dependent) variable based on the value of a predictor (independent) variable.

simple random sampling Selection of elements at random from a sampling

frame for inclusion in a study. Each study element has a probability greater than zero of being selected for inclusion in the study.

situated The time and place in which a person lives that shape one's life experiences. Cultural, societal, relationship, and environmental factors create the unique context in which a person lives.

situated freedom The amount of flexibility a person has to make certain choices based on one's placement in history, the societal hierarchy, and the physical world in addition to demographic variables such as race, ethnicity, gender, age, income, and education.

skewed A curve that is asymmetrical (positively or negatively) because of an asymmetrical (non-normal) distribution of scores from a study.

slope The amount by which a line deviates from the horizontal. In statistics, the direction and angle of the regression line on a graph, represented by the letter *b*.

small area analyses See *geographical analyses*.

snowball sampling See *network sampling*.

Spearman rank-order correlation coefficient Nonparametric analysis technique for ordinal data that is an adaptation of the Pearson's product-moment correlation used to examine relationships among variables in a study.

specific propositions Statements found in theories that are at a moderate level of abstraction and provide the basis for the generation of hypotheses to guide a study.

specificity of a screening or diagnostic test Proportion of patients without a disease who are actually identified as disease-free, as shown by negative test results (true negative).

split-half reliability Process used to determine the homogeneity of an instrument's items. The instrument items are split in half, and a correlational procedure is performed, comparing the two halves for degree of similarity.

spurious correlations Correlational tests found to be statistically significant when, in fact, the relationships they affirm as existing are not present. These represent a Type I error. Replication of the research usually results in statistically nonsignificant findings.

stability reliability The degree to which a measurement instrument produces the same score on repeated administration.

standard of care The norm on which quality of care is judged. Standards of care are based on research findings in conjunction with current practice patterns. According to Donabedian, a standard of care is considered one of the processes of care.

standard deviation (*SD*) A measure of the amount of dispersion from the mean that characterizes a data set.

standardized mean difference Calculated in a meta-analysis when the same outcome, such as depression, is measured by different scales or methods.

statement synthesis Combining information across theories and research findings about relationships among concepts to propose specific new or restated relationships among the concepts being studied. This step is a part of developing a framework for a study.

statistic Numerical value obtained from a sample that is used to estimate a population parameter.

statistical conclusion validity The degree to which the researcher makes decisions about proper use of statistics so that the conclusions about relationships and differences drawn from the analyses are accurate reflections of reality.

statistical hypothesis See *null hypothesis*.

statistical regression toward the mean A threat to internal validity that is present when subjects display extreme scores of a variable. On remeasurement, the value tends to be closer to the population mean, so attribution of true cause is complicated.

statistical significance The condition in which the value of the calculated statistic for a certain test exceeds the predetermined cut-off point. Statistical significance means that the null hypothesis is rejected.

Stetler Model of Research Utilization to Facilitate Evidence-Based Practice Model developed by Stetler that provides a comprehensive framework to enhance the use of research findings by nurses to facilitate evidence-based practice.

stratification A strategy used in one type of random sampling in which the researcher predetermines the desired subject proportion of various levels (strata) of a characteristic of interest in the study population. Stratification may be used to create a sample proportionate to the population or one that is intentionally disproportionate, depending on the study purpose and research question.

stratified random sampling Method of random sampling used to predetermine the desired proportion to be selected for several values of a variable (often demographic). It is used when the researcher knows some of the variables in the population that are critical to achieving representativeness.

strength of a relationship Amount of variation explained by a relationship. A value of the statistic r that is close to 1 or to -1 represents a very strong relationship; a value of r close to 0 represents a very weak relationship.

structural equation modeling (SEM) A complex analysis of theoretical interrelationships among variables displayed in a diagrammed model. Using multiple regression analysis, its complex calculations allow the researcher to identify the best model that explains interactions among variables, yielding the greatest explained variance.

structured interview A set of interview questions in which questions are asked in the same order with all subjects. The answer options in a quantitative structured interview are predefined and limited, while the answer options in qualitative structured interviews are flexible. Interviews in qualitative studies are more commonly semistructured interviews.

structured observation Observations that are clearly identified regarding what is to be observed and precisely defining how the observations are to be made, recorded, and coded. Structured observations are used in quantitative research.

structures of care Set entities that affect quality of care in a healthcare environment, according to Donabedian. Some structures of care are the overall organization and administration of the healthcare agency, the essential equipment of care, educational preparation of qualified health personnel, staffing, and workforce size, as well as patient characteristics and the physical plant of the agency within its neighborhood.

study protocol A step-by-step, detailed plan for implementing a study, beginning with recruitment and concluding with final data collection.

study validity Measure of the truth or accuracy of research. It includes the degree to which measured variables represent what they are thought to represent.

study variables Concepts at various levels of abstraction that are defined and measured or manipulated during the course of a study.

subject attrition See *attrition rate*.

subject term Frequently searched term included in a database thesaurus.

subjects Individuals participating in a study. See *participants*.

substantive theory A theory that is contextual and that applies directly to practice. Synonymous with *middle-range theory*.

substitutable relationship Relationship in which a similar concept can be substituted for the first concept and the second concept will occur.

substruction, theoretical The technique of diagramming a research study's constructs, concepts, variables, relationships, and measurement methods for easy review of logical consistency among levels.

sufficient relationship States that when the first variable or concept occurs, the second will occur, regardless of the presence or absence of other factors.

sum of squares Mathematical manipulation involving summing the squares of the difference scores that is used as part of the analysis process for calculating the standard deviation.

summary statistics See *descriptive statistics*.

summated scales Scales in which various items are summed to obtain a single score.

survey Data collection technique in which questionnaires are used to gather data about an identified population.

symbolic meaning In symbolic interaction, the meaning attached to particular ideas or clusters of data. A shared symbol is one for which the meaning is the same for a group of persons or a society.

symmetrical curve A curve in which the left side is a mirror image of the right side.

synthesis of sources Clustering and interrelating ideas from several sources to promote a new understanding or provide a description of what is known and not known in an area.

systematic bias or variation Bias or variation obtained when subjects in a study share various characteristics, making the sample less representative than desired. Their resemblance to one another makes it more likely that demographics and measurements of effects of interventions will be quite similar for most of them.

systematic error Measurement error that is not random but occurs consistently with the same magnitude and in the same direction each time the measurement is applied.

systematic review Structured, comprehensive synthesis of quantitative studies in a particular healthcare area to determine the best research evidence available for expert clinicians to use to promote an evidence-based practice.

systematic sampling Conducted when an ordered list of all members of the population is available and involves selecting every kth individual on the list, starting from a point that is selected randomly.

T

table Presentation of data, study results, or other information in columns and rows for easy review by the reader.

tails Extremes of the normal curve where significant statistical values can be found.

target population All elements (individuals, objects, events, behaviors, or substances) that meet the sampling criteria for inclusion in a study and to which the study findings might be generalized.

technical efficiency The degree to which there is waste-minimum utilization of precious resources, which are usually inadequate for serving an entire population and can be scarce.

tentative theory Theory that is newly proposed, has had minimal exposure to critical appraisal by the discipline, and has had little testing.

testable Study that contains variables that are measurable or can be manipulated in the real world.

test-retest reliability Determination of the stability or consistency of a measurement technique by correlating the scores obtained from repeated measures.

textbooks Monographs written to be used in formal educational programs.

themes See *emergent concepts*.

theoretical limitations Inability to conceptually define and operationalize study variables adequately or inadequate connections among construct, concept, variable, and measurement. Theoretical limitations imply illogical or incomplete reasoning and substantially restrict abstract generalization of the findings.

theoretical literature Published concept analyses, conceptual maps, theories, and conceptual frameworks.

theoretical sampling A method of sampling often used in grounded theory research to advance the development of a theory throughout the research process. The researcher recruits eligible subjects on the basis of their ability to advance the emergent theory.

theory An integrated set of defined concepts, existence statements, and relational statements that are defined and interrelated to present a systematic view of a phenomenon.

therapeutic research Research that provides the patient an opportunity to receive an experimental treatment that might have beneficial results.

thesis Research project completed by a master's student as part of the requirements for a master's degree. A thesis usually is a culminating or capstone accomplishment.

threat to construct design validity Design flaw in which the measurement of a variable is not suitable for the concept it represents. In most cases, this threat occurs because of the researcher's imprecise operational definition of the variable.

threat to validity A factor or condition that decreases the validity of research results. The four threats to design validity are threats to construct validity, internal validity, external validity, and statistical conclusion validity.

threat to external design validity A limit to generalization based on differences between the conditions or participants of the study and the conditions or characteristics of persons or settings to which generalization is considered.

threat to internal design validity In interventional research, a factor that causes changes in the dependent variable that are not a result of the independent variable's influence. Two common reasons for these threats are that experimental and control groups are fundamentally dissimilar at the onset of the study or as the study progresses and that groups are exposed in a dissimilar way to outside influences during the course of the study.

threat to statistical conclusion design validity A factor that produces a false data analysis conclusion. Usually these threats occur because of inadequate sample size or inappropriate use of a statistical test.

time-dimensional designs Designs used extensively within the discipline of epidemiology to examine change over time in relation to disease occurrence. In nursing, that change over time is often development, learning, personal growth, disease progression, exposure, aging, or deterioration.

time series design with comparison group Quasi-experimental design in which simultaneous data are collected repeatedly for two groups. One of the groups reflects an intervention; the other does not.

time series design with repeated reversal Quasi-experimental design in which data are collected repeatedly for a single group. An intervention is introduced and a measurement made; then the intervention is removed and another measurement made. This process of reapplying the intervention with a measurement and removing it, followed by another measurement, is repeated for at least two complete cycles. The design is also called the repeated-reversal design and sometimes the single subject research.

time series designs One of a related set of quantitative quasi-experimental designs in which data are collected repeatedly for a single group both before and following an intervention.

total variance The sum of the within-group variance and the between-group variance determined by conducting analysis of variance (ANOVA).

traditions Truths or beliefs that are based on customs and past trends that provide a way of acquiring knowledge.

translational research An evolving concept that is defined by the National Institutes of Health as the translation of basic scientific discoveries into practical applications.

treatment Independent variable or intervention that is enacted in a study by the researcher to produce an effect on the dependent variable.

trend design A design used to examine changes over time in the value of a variable in an identified population.

trial and error An approach with unknown outcomes that is used in a situation of uncertainty when other sources of knowledge are unavailable.

triangulation The integration of data from two sources or sets of data. A metaphor taken from ship navigation and land surveying in which measurements are taken from two perspectives and the point of intersection is the location of a distant object.

true negative Result of a diagnostic or screening test that indicates accurately the absence of a disease/condition.

true positive Result of a diagnostic or screening test that accurately indicates the presence of a disease/condition.

true score Score that would be obtained if there were no error in measurement. Theoretically, some measurement error always occurs when a sample is used to estimate a population parameter.

t-test A parametric analysis technique used to determine significant differences between measures of two samples. See *independent samples* t-*test* and *paired samples* t-*test*.

two-tailed test Type of analysis used for a nondirectional hypothesis in which the researcher assumes that an extreme score can occur in either tail of the distribution curve.

two-way chi-square A nonparametric statistic that tests the association between two categorical variables.

Type I error Error that occurs when the researcher concludes that the samples tested are from different populations (the difference between groups is significant) when, in fact, the samples are from the same population (the difference between groups is not significant). The null hypothesis is rejected when it is, in fact, true.

Type II error Error that occurs when the researcher concludes that there is no significant difference between the samples examined when, in fact, a difference exists. The null hypothesis is regarded as true when it is, in fact, false. Type II error often occurs when a sample is of insufficient size to demonstrate a difference.

U

ungrouped frequency distribution A table or display listing all values of a variable and next to them the number of times in the set that the value was recorded.

unimodal Distribution of scores in a sample that displays one mode (most frequently occurring score).

unstructured interview Interview initiated with a broad question, after which subjects are encouraged to elaborate by telling their stories. The unstructured interview is a common data collection method used in some types of qualitative research.

unstructured observations Spontaneously observing and recording what is seen with a minimum of planning. Unstructured observation is a common data collection method used in qualitative research.

V

validation phase Second phase of the Stetler Model in which the research reports are critically appraised to determine their scientific soundness.

validity, instrument The extent to which an instrument actually reflects or is able to measure the construct being examined.

variables Concrete or abstract ideas that have been made measurable. In quantitative research, variables are studied in order to establish their incidence, the connections that may exist among them, or cause-and-effect relationships.

variance Measure of dispersion that is the mean or average of the sum of squares. Also, in a prediction model, the total amount of the dependent variable that is explained by the predictor variables.

variance analysis Outcomes research strategy that defines expected outcomes and the approximate points at which they are expected to occur and then tracks delay or nonachievement of these outcomes.

vary Assume more than one value. Numerical values associated with variables may vary or change from one measurement to the next, or they may remain unchanged.

verbal presentation The communication of a research report at a professional conference or meeting.

vertical axis The y-axis in a graph of a regression line or scatterplot. The vertical axis is oriented in a top-to-bottom direction across the graph.

visual analog scale A line 100 mm in length with right-angle stops at each end on which subjects are asked to record their response to a study variable. Also referred to as *magnitude scale*.

voluntary consent Indication that prospective participant has decided to take part in a study of his or her own volition without coercion or any undue influence.

volunteer sample Those willing to participate in the study. All human participants must be volunteers.

W

wait-listed In experimental research, refers to a control group guaranteed to receive the treatment at the completion of the study. The strategy of wait-listing is sometimes used in the first tests of a new therapeutic medical intervention.

washout period The amount of time that is required for the effects of an intervention to dissipate and the subject to return to baseline.

Wilcoxon matched-pairs test Nonparametric analysis technique conducted to examine changes that occur in pretest-posttest measures or matched-pairs measures.

within-group variance Variance that results when individual scores in a group vary from the group mean.

Y

y-intercept Point at which the regression line crosses (or intercepts) the y-axis. At this point on the regression line, $x = 0$.

Z

z scores Standardized scores developed from the normal curve.

INDEX

Note: Page numbers followed by "*b*," "*f*," and "*t*" indicate boxes, figures, and tables, respectively.

Designs for Quantitative Nursing Research in This Text: Quick Access Chart

Noninterventional Study Designs

Descriptive Study Designs
- Longitudinal designs, 245
- Trend analysis design, 246
- Cross-sectional designs, 247
- Simple descriptive study design, 249
- Comparative descriptive design, 250

Correlational Study Designs
- Descriptive correlational design, 252
- Predictive correlational design, 253
- Model-testing design, 255

Interventional Study Designs

Quasi-experimental Study Designs
- One-group posttest-only design, 287
- Posttest-only design with comparison group, 287
- One-group pretest-posttest design, 287
- Pretest and posttest design with a comparison group, 288
- Pretest and posttest design with two comparison treatments, 289
- Pretest and posttest design with a removed treatment, 290
- Simple interrupted time-series designs, 292
- Interrupted time-series design with a no-treatment comparison group, 293
- Interrupted time-series design with multiple treatment replications, 293

Experimental Study Designs
- Pretest/posttest control group design, 295
- Solomon four-group design, 296
- Experimental posttest-only control group design, 297
- Within subjects design, 298
- Factorial design, 300
- Clinical trials, 302
- Randomized controlled trials, 303
- Pragmatic clinical trials, 304

Other Designs
- Comparative effectiveness research, 307
- Methodological designs, 308